Tourette Syndrome

TOURETTE SYNDROME

Edited by

DAVIDE MARTINO, MD, PHD
NEUROSCIENCE TRAUMA CENTER
BARTS AND THE LONDON SCHOOL OF MEDICINE AND DENTISTRY
DEPARTMENT OF NEUROLOGY
QUEEN ELIZABETH HOSPITAL
SOUTH LONDON HNS TRUST
LONDON, UK

JAMES F. LECKMAN, MD
CHILD STUDY CENTER
DEPARTMENTS OF PSYCHIATRY,
PEDIATRICS AND PSYCHOLOGY
YALE UNIVERSITY SCHOOL OF MEDICINE
NEW HAVEN, CT

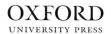

OXFORD
UNIVERSITY PRESS

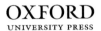

OXFORD
UNIVERSITY PRESS

Oxford University Press is a department of the University of Oxford.
It furthers the University's objective of excellence in research, scholarship,
and education by publishing worldwide.

Oxford   New York
Auckland   Cape Town   Dar es Salaam   Hong Kong   Karachi
Kuala Lumpur   Madrid   Melbourne   Mexico City   Nairobi
New Delhi   Shanghai   Taipei   Toronto

With offices in
Argentina   Austria   Brazil   Chile   Czech Republic   France   Greece
Guatemala   Hungary   Italy   Japan   Poland   Portugal   Singapore
South Korea   Switzerland   Thailand   Turkey   Ukraine   Vietnam

Oxford is a registered trademark of Oxford University Press
in the UK and certain other countries.

Published in the United States of America by
Oxford University Press
198 Madison Avenue, New York, NY 10016

Library of Congress Cataloging-in-Publication Data
Tourette syndrome / [edited by] Davide Martino, James F. Leckman.
p. ; cm.
Includes bibliographical references and index.
ISBN 978–0–19–979626–7 (hardcover : alk. paper)
I. Martino, Davide.   II. Leckman, James F.
[DNLM: 1. Tourette Syndrome. WM 197]
616.8'3—dc23
2012040644

The science of medicine is a rapidly changing field. As new research and clinical experience broaden our
knowledge, changes in treatment and drug therapy occur. The author and publisher of this work have
checked with sources believed to be reliable in their efforts to provide information that is accurate and
complete, and in accordance with the standards accepted at the time of publication. However, in light
of the possibility of human error or changes in the practice of medicine, neither the author, nor the
publisher, nor any other party who has been involved in the preparation or publication of this work
warrants that the information contained herein is in every respect accurate or complete. Readers
are encouraged to confirm the information contained herein with other reliable sources, and are
strongly advised to check the product information sheet provided by the pharmaceutical
company for each drug they plan to administer.

1 3 5 7 9 8 6 4 2
Printed in the United States of America
on acid-free paper

We dedicate this book:

To the real experts on Tourette—the individuals with this disorder and their families;

To all of our mentors and teachers and to Donald J. Cohen, in particular, for his vision and encouragement over the decades;

To our dedicated colleagues across the globe in the advocacy organizations and academic centers who continue to seek ways to improve the wellbeing of individuals with Tourette by reducing stigma, advancing our scientific understanding of this enigmatic disorder, and helping us prepare this volume; and

To our families

Table of Contents

Foreword

IT IS critical that we understand and develop better treatments for diseases that can be labeled as "early onset." Tourette syndrome (TS) is one of those "early onset diseases," typically beginning in childhood or in adolescence. TS is very common in the population at large, and it has the potential to influence a person over an entire lifetime. In 1885 George Albert Edouard Brutus Gilles de la Tourette described nine patients with a mixture of motor and behavioral manifestations. The original descriptions were vivid and personal, and these descriptions underscored the tremendous variety of challenges that a patient with TS may experience over a lifetime.

We now understand that Tourette syndrome is much more than a disease of simple motor or vocal tics. We understand that not all patients have coprolalia, or vulgar utterances. We now recognize a variety of disabling comorbidities. This recognition has led to improvements in educating society on what is and what is not TS.

It has also allowed a new generation of sufferers to live happy and hopeful lives.

What became known as TS in 1885 had in fact been present in society for hundreds and maybe thousands of years. The origins of TS can be traced back to at least the fifteenth century, and there are many documented cases of religious persecution associated with TS. Those with this syndrome have, over many generations, been misunderstood, persecuted, and victimized by both organized religion and society. Many have also been incredibly successful and amazingly productive. Some notables include Mozart and the author of the modern dictionary, Samuel Johnson.

Over the past three decades there has been an explosion of basic knowledge about TS, and there have been critical improvements, especially in terms of earlier diagnosis and in the approach to treatment. This book, by Martino and Leckman, is the most comprehensive and up-to-date volume on TS available anywhere. It summarizes the relevant science and the important behavior associated with this syndrome.

Martino and Leckman have assembled the best physicians and the highest-quality scientists from around the world to contribute chapters. Together, this expert group addresses the most important contemporary topics related to TS. In the first section of the book, the experts answer critical questions about tic phenomenology, the premonitory urge, related comorbidities, the clinical course, and the epidemiology of the illness. In the second section, they explore the genetics, the environment, and the overlap between them. The authors do not shy away from tackling the issues of perinatal risk and the highly controversial issues surrounding infection and PANDAS. Next, an entire section is devoted to pathology, physiology, neurobiology, immunity, and animal models. Finally, the editors have asked some of the best TS clinicians in the world to summarize the issues related to diagnosis, outcome measures, and various treatment approaches (including cognitive-behavioral therapy and deep brain stimulation).

TS patients, family members, and medical providers are all aware that addressing the science behind this disease without addressing the social issues would be a huge mistake.

The disability caused by TS is not just medical; indeed, in many cases, the more devastating consequences are social. The issues facing each patient and each family member often begin at a very early age, and these issues can quickly accumulate and become complex and difficult to manage. Martino and Leckman, as two of the leading experts in the field, have addressed these social issues by adding three final chapters containing many pearls and tips for patients, families, and teachers, and also for those interested in TS support groups.

Those familiar with this disease will immediately recognize that Martino and Leckman have assembled a comprehensive volume that will be practical and useful for scientists, health care workers, residents, students, patients and families touched by TS. Many of the contributors to this book will, over the next decade, undoubtedly make important discoveries. We hope that together these leaders will move us closer to better addressing this highly prevalent and important "early onset disease."

Michael S. Okun, M.D.
Adelaide Lackner Professor of Neurology
University of Florida Center for Movement
Disorders and Neurorestoration
Gainesville, FL

Introduction

The first and best victory is to conquer one's self.
—Plato

THIS BOOK is intended to provide an unbiased summary of the current knowledge on Tourette syndrome (TS). We hope that patients, parents, and policymakers as well as clinicians, professionals, and scientists across a broad range of disciplines will find the content to be readily accessible. This was our primary goal.

Scientific and public interest in TS is not new. With the formation of advocacy organizations, notably the Tourette Syndrome Association in the United States (http://www.tsa-usa.org/), a rapid expansion of interest started more than two decades ago and accelerated throughout the "decade of the brain" and the first decade of the new millennium. As stated by Donald J. Cohen, Joseph Jankovic, and Christopher G. Goetz in the preface to their seminal monograph on this condition from 2001, TS continues to be considered and explored by clinicians and neuroscientists as "a model developmental neuropsychiatric disorder." The primary goal of increasing knowledge of TS remains the improvement of the quality of life and well-being of the individuals and families affected by this condition.

As stated by Donald J. Cohen, Joseph Jankovic, and Christopher G. Goetz in the preface to their seminal monograph on this condition from 2001, TS continues to be considered and explored by clinicians and neuroscientists as "a model developmental neuropsychiatric disorder." Increasing knowledge of the underlying neural mechanisms and psychological processes of TS has prompted fascinating spin-offs for the understanding of complex processes like inhibition, sensory gating, self-awareness, self-regulation, motor regulation, and emotional processing, as well as of the intricate relationship between genetic background and environmental influences over the course of neural development. Several aspects related to the etiology and pathophysiology of TS are objects of controversy and are increasingly attracting the attention of researchers.

TS is a complex disorder and a common one as well. Only recently, the increasing application of meta-analyses to the ocean of clinical studies dedicated to neurodevelopmental disorders has yielded estimates of the prevalence of TS to a figure very close to 1% of the general population of children and adolescents in Europe, Asia, as well as North and South America. At the same time, the improvement in the understanding of this multifaceted phenomenology has clearly taught us that TS encompasses a heterogeneous and multidimensional spectrum of clinical presentations. Early on there was the hope, indeed the expectation, that a single gene would be discovered that would provide a clear path to understanding the pathogenesis of TS. While this may be true in some rare families, it is now clear that a multiplicity of genetic and environmental factors contribute to its pathogenesis and broad range of clinical expression. Efforts to define clinically homogenous subtypes are now under way. Time will tell how beneficial this approach will be.

More work needs to be done. Although the absolute number of peer-reviewed articles dedicated to TS and tic disorders has increased every year by at least 30% over the past decade, the prevalence and social burden of the disorder call for the substantial deployment of resources into this field by investigators from around the world. Knowledge gaps still exist in crucial areas that directly affect the delivery of care to individuals and families affected by TS and related disorders. TS remains an orphan disorder. Large-scale, methodologically robust treatment trials are rare. Consequently, well-validated therapeutic algorithms, guidelines, and pathways of care are limited and depend on the expertise of experienced clinicians.

A major aim of this book was to identify crucial questions that remain unanswered. We invited leading scientists, clinicians, and educators active in the field to summarize their understanding of TS and to identify gaps in our knowledge base and pose innovative ways of filling these gaps. Consequently, a brief summary of "Questions for Future Research" concludes each chapter, emphasizing that this is one of the core messages our book intends to convey. In the decades to come we hope that many of these questions will be answered. Part of our optimism comes from the formation of the European Society for the Study of Tourette Syndrome (http://tourette-eu.org) and more recently its Asian counterpart. This has led to the formation of new networks of researchers within Europe and Asia and to the initiation of major European and Asian research projects.

From its conception, this book has been thought of as an opportunity to combine expertise from around the globe. This is represented both by the editors and by the list of distinguished contributors. The first section of the volume, "Clinical Phenomenology and Epidemiology," outlines some of the fundamental issues upon which research will likely focus in the next years. Some clinical and epidemiological features of TS provide direct hints toward disease mechanisms. The male predominance within TS patients clearly suggests a role for a complex interrelation between endocrine, molecular, and neural mechanisms during development, the details of which remain unexplained. The neurobiological origin of premonitory urges and their role in tic expression needs to be explored more deeply to better capture the real essence of tics. Particularly, we need to understand whether these urges and the tics are two phases of the same behavioral pattern or whether urges are "simply" positive reinforcers for tics. Just as much as the onset of tics, patients and health professionals need to know more about their course over time. How can we prevent the waxing phase of the course of tic severity? Neurobiological researchers should delve deeper to discover whether the peculiar dynamics of tics are subdued by the temporal pattern of neural activity present in specific neuronal types, and how this is genetically determined and/or environmentally modified. Another crucial question raised almost inevitably in the physician's office is whether tics will get better over time, or whether the patient is destined to "tic" lifelong, and how badly. Novel, truly longitudinal studies performed during crucial temporal windows throughout the developmental period are necessary to understand which clinical features are important predictors of future outcome, and whether the course of illness of parents or older siblings is informative in this respect in familial cases. Also, we have very limited knowledge of the effect of treatment upon the clinical course of illness, and whether disease modification will become soon a reachable therapeutic goal in TS. Most importantly, longitudinal studies are essential to identify new "endophenotypes," state and trait markers of the condition, that could help in this prediction by tapping into the central mechanisms of the disorder with greater accuracy than clinical phenomenology. Structural and functional MRI, the measurement of cortical excitability, prepulse inhibition, and behavioral and cognitive performance should all be explored to identify the most suitable "intermediate phenotypes" of TS. Psychiatric comorbidities are not a collateral issue in TS: it is well recognized that conditions like attention-deficit/hyperactivity disorder, obsessive-compulsive disorder, anxiety, depression, and important behavioral symptoms such as rage attacks or self-injurious behaviors represent in many cases the major source of disability. Moreover, in the wake of dividing the TS spectrum into different subtypes, the comorbidity pattern is likely to be crucial to inform the clinical and neurobiological substrate of each of these subtypes.

Sections 2 and 3, "Etiology" and "Pathophysiology," are meant to expand the most relevant issues highlighted in the first section. It is quite intuitive that in the *splitting* process of TS the relative contributions of genes and environment, and their interaction, will provide enormous insight. Studying large cohorts and having access to larger populations of twins or siblings from families manifesting TS, although highly demanding in terms of time and resources, seems the best way forward. The tremendous advances in genetics during the past decade, with the advent of new-generation sequencing techniques, offer the rare opportunity to investigate both common and rare variation in large populations. With such a high-throughput technology, we guess the challenge will be to pursue successful biobanking programs, and this will inevitably change the mentality behind collaborative research in the field of TS, as is already

happening for other complex diseases, fostering the establishment of larger, worldwide consortia. This will allow us also to better understand the role of variants in the "non-coding" genome, epistatic effects, and epigenetics in the etiology of TS. Likewise, large-scale populations will be the best setting to explore the effect of environmental factors, such as perinatal adversities and group A streptococcal infections or other types of infections. These continue to be an object of intense debate, giving rise to many review articles and viewpoints but fewer valuable original research contributions. Neuropathology and animal model researchers should work in an integrated fashion to generate new knowledge on the molecular pathways affected in tic disorders and explore *in vivo* the effect of their dysfunction on behavior. Brain banking is definitely more cumbersome to develop in a neurodevelopmental, nonfatal condition like TS, but even small databases can provide highly valuable information, thanks to the application of microarray transcriptome approaches. This will potentially inspire the creation of new animal models with greater face and concept validity to this perplexing human disorder.

Sections 4 and 5, "Diagnosis and Assessment" and "Treatment," take us back into the physician's office, but this time as a full immersion on how best to approach patients to improve their functioning and quality of life. TS is a multidisciplinary condition requiring, ideally, a multidisciplinary team for its management. This is undoubtedly one of the reasons why, unlike in other neurological and psychiatric illnesses, the number of qualified tertiary referral centers for TS is limited around the world. Advances in clinimetric research are of great importance to provide clinicians and clinical researchers with the best tools to measure in the office the heterogeneous constellation of symptoms and clinical features presented by people with TS. Big steps ahead in this direction have been made in the way we measure nonmotor symptoms, such as premonitory urges, or quality of life, but surely more work is needed to homogenize protocols. Deciding how much importance should be given to cognitive neuropsychological assessments in the routine evaluation of TS patients is another challenge. We expect that the improvement of clinimetric rating and the greater attention given by clinical researchers to the impact of comorbidities will accelerate the undertaking of novel, breakthrough research in the field of clinical neuropsychology of TS.

What treatment, and when? Is this still a question without a clear answer, or are existing data helpful in providing a solution to this issue, albeit preliminary? *Primum non nocere* (first, do not harm): the basic proverbial teaching from classical medicine is more pertinent to TS today than it has ever been before. Given its potentially self-limiting course, it is essential to identify as early as possible which patients should be managed with less-invasive approaches and which should, instead, be treated more aggressively. Psychoeducation is clearly a key ingredient and an important starting point for clinicians. Likewise, building on the strengths and interests of the affected individual is another fundamental goal if we are to ensure the lifelong success of our patients. It is also crucial to establish continuity of care, given the chronic nature of this disorder and its fluctuating character. Although behavioral interventions are increasingly being accepted as a front-line approach, many aspects of the management of TS are still bitterly debated. Sadly, there is very limited experimental evidence in favor of this or that specific intervention. The methodology of clinical trials in TS is a little-discussed aspect, but we believe it is of fundamental strategic importance to advance research in the field. This is why meta-analyses and systematic reviews of clinical trials are so important, and relatively new, in TS, provided they are able to not only convey the obvious limitations of existing studies, but also guide progress in methodology of clinical trials in the disorder.

We thought it was useful to dedicate the final section of the volume to social support and psychoeducation. Although the stigmatization of TS sufferers has declined in many cultures, largely due to the tireless efforts of patient advocacy organizations around the world, social support to patients with severe life-long TS is more often than not a theoretical concept rather than a practical reality. Up-to-date peer education programs on TS for schoolchildren across the globe (as well as parents and teachers) and techniques to increase productivity in students with tics or TS (e.g., based on assistive technology) are needed and should be tested experimentally. Finally, the value of patient advocacy groups and patients' associations throughout the world cannot be stressed enough. The Tourette Syndrome Association USA continues to be a beacon for all patient advocacy groups on TS around the world, with its outstanding educational support and the invaluable program funding research on the condition from everywhere in the world. We hope that they will continue to translate new knowledge into increasing public awareness and scientific interest in this "model developmental neuropsychiatric disorder."

Davide Martino
James F. Leckman

Contributors

Pedro G. de Alvarenga
Department of Psychiatry
University of São Paulo Medical School
São Paulo, Brazil

Kevin J. Black
Department of Psychiatry
Washington University School of Medicine
St. Louis, MO

Michael H. Bloch
Child Study Center and Department of
    Psychiatry
Yale University
New Haven, CT

Kathryn Bradbury
Department of Psychology
University of Connecticut
Storrs, CT

Matthew R. Capriotti
Department of Psychology
University of Wisconsin-Milwaukee
Milwaukee, WI

Francesco Cardona
Department of Pediatrics and Child
    Neuropsychiatry
University La Sapienza of Rome
Rome, Italy

Danielle C. Cath
Department of Clinical & Health Psychology
Utrecht University
Utrecht, The Netherlands

Andrea E. Cavanna
Department of Neuropsychiatry
Birmingham and Solihull
    Mental Health National Health Service
    Foundation Trust
School of Clinical and Experimental Medicine
University of Birmingham
Birmingham, UK

Barbara J. Coffey
Department of Psychiatry
Icahn School of Medicine at Mount Sinai
New York, NY

Soren Dalsgaard
Department for Child and Adolescent
    Psychiatry
University of Southern Denmark
Odense, Denmark

Valsamma Eapen
Department of Infant, Child and Adolescent
    Psychiatry
University of New South Wales
South West Sydney, Australia

Clare M. Eddy
Department of Neuropsychiatry
Birmingham and Solihull
    Mental Health National Health Service
    Foundation Trust
School of Clinical and Experimental Medicine
University of Birmingham
Birmingham, UK

Virginia W. Eicher
Child Study Center
Yale University
New Haven, CT

Thomas V. Fernandez
Child Study Center
Yale University
New Haven, CT

Ygor A. Ferrao
Department of Psychiatry
Federal University School of Health Sciences
Porto Alegre, Brazil

Deanna J. Greene
Department of Neurology
Washington University School of Medicine
St. Louis, MO

Pieter J. Hoekstra
Department of Child and Adolescent
    Psychiatry
University Medical Center Groningen
Groningen, The Netherlands

Peter J. Hollenbeck
Department of Biological Sciences
Purdue University
West Lafayette, IN

Ana G. Hounie
Department of Psychiatry
University of São Paulo Medical School
São Paulo, Brazil

Yukio Imamura
Unit on Neural Systems and Behavior
Okinawa Institute of Science and Technology
Onna Son, Okinawa, Japan

Masaki Isoda
Unit on Neural Systems and Behavior
Okinawa Institute of Science and Technology
Onna Son, Okinawa, Japan

Yuko Kataoka-Sasaki
Department of Neural Regenerative Medicine
Sapporo Medical University School of
    Medicine
Sapporo, Hokkaido, Japan

Robert A. King
Child Study Center
Yale University
New Haven, CT

Roger Kurlan
Atlantic Neuroscience Institute
Overlook Medical Center
Summit, NJ

Angeli Landeros-Weisenberger
Child Study Center
Yale University
New Haven, CT

Eli R. Lebowitz
Child Study Center
Yale University
New Haven, CT

James F. Leckman
Child Study Center and Departments of
    Psychiatry, Pediatrics and Psychology
Yale University
New Haven, CT

Jessica B. Lennington
Child Study Center
Yale University
New Haven, CT

Andrea G. Ludolph
Department of Child and Adolescent
    Psychiatry
University of Ulm
Ulm, Germany

Davide Martino
Barts and The London School Medicine and
    Dentistry
Queen Mary University of London
London, UK

Maria A. de Mathis
Department of Psychiatry
University of São Paulo Medical School
São Paulo, Brazil

Kevin W. McCairn
Unit on Neural Systems and Behavior
Okinawa Institute of Science and Technology
Onna Son, Okinawa, Japan

Euripedes C. Miguel
Department of Psychiatry
University of São Paulo Medical School
São Paulo, Brazil

Kirsten R.Müller-Vahl
Department of Social Psychiatry and
    Psychotherapy
Hannover Medical School
Hannover, Germany

Tanya K. Murphy
Departments of Pediatrics and Psychiatry
University of South Florida
Gainesville, FL

Tara Murphy
Great Ormond Street Hospital
National Health Service Trust
London, UK

Michael Orth
Department of Neurology
University of Ulm
Ulm, Germany

Leslie E. Packer
Independent Practice
North Bellmore, NY

John C. Pansaon Piedad
Department of Neuropsychiatry
Birmingham and Solihull Mental Health
    National Health Service Foundation Trust
School of Clinical and Experimental Medicine
University of Birmingham
Birmingham, UK

Mauro Porta
Tourette Clinic and Functional
    Neurosurgery Unit
Istituto Di Ricovero e Cura a Carattere
    Scientifico Galeazzi
Milan, Italy

Sheryl K. Pruitt
Parkaire Consultants, Inc.
Marietta, GA

Hugh E. Rickards
Department of Neuropsychiatry
Birmingham and Solihull Mental Health
    National Health Service Foundation Trust
School of Clinical and Experimental Medicine
University of Birmingham
Birmingham, UK

Renata Rizzo
Department of Medical and Pediatric Sciences
University of Catania
Catania, Italy

Mary M. Robertson
Department of Neurology
St. George's Hospital and Medical School
London, UK

Veit Roessner
Clinic and Policlinic of Child and Adolescent
    Psychiatry and Psychotherapy
Dresden University of Technology
Dresden, Germany

Louise Roper
University of Birmingham
Birmingham, UK

Maria C. do Rosário
Department of Psychiatry
Federal University of São Paulo
São Paulo, Brazil

Aribert Rothenberger
Department of Child and Adolescent
    Psychiatry
University Medical Center
Goettingen, Germany

Marco Sassi
Tourette Clinic and Functional
    Neurosurgery Unit
Istituto Di Ricovero e Cura a Carattere
    Scientifico Galeazzi
Milan, Italy

Lawrence Scahill
Marcus Autism Center
School of Medicine, Emory University
Atlanta, GA

Bradley L. Schlaggar
Department of Neurology
Washington University School of Medicine
St. Louis, MO

Domenico Servello
Tourette Clinic and Functional
    Neurosurgery Unit
Istituto Di Ricovero e Cura a Carattere
    Scientifico Galeazzi
Milan, Italy

Harvey S. Singer
Departments of Neurology and Pediatrics
Johns Hopkins Hospital
Johns Hopkins University School of Medicine
Baltimore, MD

Matthew W. State
Department of Psychiatry
University of California San Francisco
San Francisco, CA

Denis G. Sukhodolsky
Child Study Center
Yale University
New Haven, CT

Flora M. Vaccarino
Child Study Center and the Department of
    Neurobiology
Yale University
New Haven, CT

Douglas W. Woods
Department of Psychology
University of Wisconsin-Milwaukee
Milwaukee, WI

Beata Zolovska
Department of Child and Adolescent
    Psychiatry
New York University School of Medicine
NYU Child Study Center
New York, NY

SECTION 1

CLINICAL PHENOMENOLOGY AND EPIDEMIOLOGY

1

Phenomenology of Tics and Sensory Urges: The Self Under Siege

JAMES F. LECKMAN, MICHAEL H. BLOCH, DENIS G. SUKHODOLSKY,
LAWRENCE SCAHILL AND ROBERT A. KING

Abstract

The origin of tics may be related to a heightened and selective sensitivity to cues from within the body or from the outside world, possibly as a result of reduced ability to suppress irrelevant information in sensory, motor, and cognitive domains. The temporal pattern of tics, which are known to occur in bouts and wax and wane in severity, and their long-term outcome might represent important clues to the neurobiology of tics. Moreover, the role played by the environmental context in modulating tic expression may be key to refining and developing novel behavioral interventions. The association of tics with comorbid behavioral problems has a very strong impact on social, emotional, and academic outcomes in adulthood. This chapter will introduce the reader to the wide phenomenological spectrum of Tourette syndrome and other tic disorders. The key phenomenological features of Tourette syndrome and related disorders represent crucial educational objectives for clinicians, teachers, parents, and peers and may lead to better clinical, social, and academic outcomes.

There is really no adequate description of the sensations that signal the onset of the actions. The first one seems irresistible, calling for an almost inevitable response ... Intense concentration on the site can itself precipitate the action ... Tourette's syndrome movements are intentional body movements ... The end of the Tourette's syndrome action is the "feel" that is frequently accompanied by a fleeting and incomplete sense of relief.
—Joseph Bliss (1980)

I finally apprehend the magnitude of the background noise that I have been experiencing for decades ... the people around me do not share my tics because they do not hear the drumbeat. They do not feel the sensations without sources, do not have irresistible urges to pause in

mid-sentence ... and so on in endless, bewildering variety ... Finally and most important, I feel convinced that this complex challenging enigmatic internal world is the obvious core of Tourette.
—Peter Hollenbeck (2001)

The human body is the best picture of the human soul.
—Ludwig Wittengenstein (1958)

WORKING IN close collaboration with patients and their families, we and other clinical investigators have endeavored to characterize both the overt features of tics and the associated sensory and mental states. Insights gained in these areas have deepened our understanding of tics and their impact on an individual's development. In this chapter we initially focus on the phenomenology of tics, premonitory urges, and the fleeting and incomplete sense of relief that frequently follows the completion of a tic. We then turn to the other sensory phenomena and "disinhibition"—the urge to do exactly what should not be done that is present in many individuals with Tourette syndrome (TS). Next, we consider the context and timing of tics and their quasi-volitional character as well as the important role of psychosocial stress and its impact on future tic severity. We then discuss how this complex interface of acts, urges, and sensations can influence the individual's internal sense of himself or herself over the course of a lifetime. Many mysteries and unanswered questions await future research. We close the chapter by highlighting key points and unanswered questions.

WHAT ARE TICS?

When Gilles de la Tourette (1885) first described the syndrome that bears his name, he used the designation *maladie des tics*. So what are tics? **Tics** are a bewildering collection of abrupt movements and sounds. Often more easily recognized than precisely defined, tics are sudden, rapid, motor movements or sounds that recur for unpredictable durations. Virtually any movement or sound that the human body is capable of making can become a tic. Indeed, we think of tics as simply fragments of normal behavior that appear without any logical reason. Usually, tics can be easily mimicked, and they can be confused with normal movements or sounds. However, they have a "stereotyped" quality, which simply means that the tic looks or sounds more or less the same each time it occurs. Their sudden unexpected nature can excite surprise. If the observer (a parent, teacher, or a peer) does not know better, he or she may think that tics are being done "on purpose."

With few exceptions, including Janet (1903) and Freud (1913), clinical descriptions from the nineteenth century onward, including those of J. M. G. Itard (1825) and Georges Gilles de la Tourette (1885), have largely focused on cataloguing and classifying tics as viewed from the outside. We first discuss these overt phenomena before considering the internal sensory states

that surround them. Tics are characterized based on their anatomical location, number, frequency, and duration. Another useful descriptor is the intensity or "forcefulness" of the tic, as some tics call attention to themselves simply by virtue of their exaggerated, forceful character. The variation in intensity ranges from behaviors that are not noticeable (a slight shrug or a hushed guttural noise) to strenuous displays (arm thrusts or loud barking) that are frightening and exhausting. Tics can also be described in terms of their "complexity." Complexity refers to how simple or involved a movement or sound is, ranging from brief, meaningless, abrupt fragments (simple tics) to ones that are longer, more involved, and seemingly more purposive in character (complex tics).

As described in Chapter 19, although several scales are available for the rating of tic severity, the Yale Global Tic Severity Scale (YGTSS) is the most widely used instrument in clinical trials (Leckman, Riddle, Hardin et al., 1989). The YGTSS includes separate ratings of the number, frequency, intensity, complexity, and interference associated with motor and vocal tics as well as an overall impairment rating. However, distinctions between motor and vocal tics have been questioned, as vocal tics are due to muscle contractions of the oropharynx or diaphragm. Another useful tool to characterize the tic phenotype of an individual is the Tourette Syndrome Diagnostic Confidence Index, which documents many relevant characteristics mentioned in this review, including the range and complexity of tics, their changeable nature, the temporal features of tic expression, and the fact they are usually associated with specific subjective and cognitive experiences (Robertson et al., 1999).

Motor Tics

Motor tics usually begin with brief bouts of transient tics involving the face or head. A typical report involves bouts of eye blinking of variable intensity beginning in kindergarten or in the early school years. For example, Shapiro and colleagues (1988) reported that among the 666 TS cases seen in their specialty clinic from 1965 to 1981, 538 (83%) of the cases had a motor tic at onset, and in 297 (44.6%) cases, the initial tic was a simple motor tic involving the eyes or the face. These initial symptoms often disappear after a few weeks, only to reappear at a later point in time. As depicted in Figure 1.1, there is often a rostral–caudal progression of motor tics, with tics of the face, head, and shoulders appearing earlier and in a higher proportion of patients than motor tics involving the extremities or the torso (Jagger et al., 1982; Leckman, King, & Cohen, 1998; Shapiro et al., 1988). The observed range of motor tics is extraordinary, so that virtually any voluntary motor movement can emerge as a motor tic. Table 1.1 presents a brief compendium of some of the more common motor tics.

Motor tics are frequently described as "simple" or "complex." **Simple motor tics** are sudden, brief (usually less than 1 second in duration), meaningless movements. Common examples include eye blinking, facial grimacing, mouth movements, head jerks, shoulder shrugs, and arm and leg jerks. Younger patients often are totally unaware of their simple motor tics.

Over time, many individuals develop **complex motor tics**, which are sudden, more purposive-appearing, stereotyped movements of longer duration. Examples are myriad and include facial gestures and movements such as brushing hair back, possibly in combination with head jerk, and body shrugs. Gyrating, bending, and twisting movements of the head or torso are also seen. These slow twisting movements are usually referred to as **dystonic tics**, while isometric contractions such as tensing of the abdominal muscles are considered **tonic tics**. Complex motor tics rarely are seen in the absence of simple motor tics. Paroxysms, or continuous orchestrated displays of simple and complex motor tics, can occur in more severe cases. Lewd and obscene gestures with the hands or tongue (**copropraxia**) and self-injurious acts (hitting the face, biting a hand or wrist) are observed in a small number of patients. At times, it may be difficult to distinguish complex tics from motor dyskinesias, choreas, and other hyperkinetic movement disorders. See Chapter 17 for a full discussion of the differential diagnosis of tic disorders.

The degree of impairment and disruption associated with particular motor tics is variable and is a salient clinical feature. Partly dependent on the frequency, intensity, complexity, and duration of specific tics, estimates of impairment

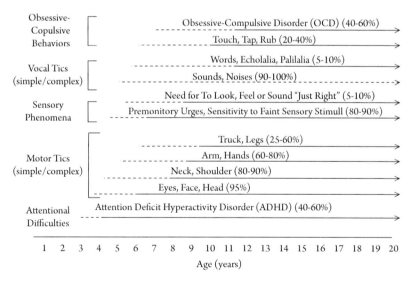

FIGURE 1.1   Natural history of tics and associated behaviors.   The occurrence of motor and vocal tics and related behaviors progressing at different ages from transient episodes (*broken lines*) to sustained periods (*solid lines*).

(Adapted from Jagger et al., 1982.)

Table 1.1 Simple and Complex Motor and Vocal Tics

Tic Symptoms	Examples
Simple motor tics: Sudden, brief, meaningless movements	Eye blinking, eye movements, grimacing, nose twitching, mouth movements, jaw snaps, lip pouting, head jerks and turns, shoulder shrugging, arm jerks, abdominal tensing, kicks, finger movements, rapid jerking of any part of the body
Complex motor tics: Slower, longer, more "purposeful" movements	Sustained "looks," facial gestures, biting, touching objects or self, throwing, banging, thrusting arms, gestures with hands, gyrating and bending, twisting dystonic postures, copropraxia (obscene gestures)
Simple phonic tics: Sudden, meaningless sounds or noises	Throat clearing, coughing, sniffling, spitting, screeching, barking, grunting, gurgling, clacking, hissing, sucking, and innumerable other sounds
Complex phonic tics: Sudden, more "meaningful" utterances	Syllables, words, phrases, statements such as "oh, okay," "I've got to," "stop that," "shut up," "what makes me do this?," "how about it," or "now you've seen it," speech atypicalities (usually rhythms, speed, tone, accents, intensity of speech); echo phenomenon (echolalia [i.e., the immediate repetition of one's own or another's words or phrases]); and coprolalia (obscene, inappropriate, and aggressive words and statements)

also need to include the impact on the individual's self-esteem, family life, social acceptance, school or job functioning, and physical well-being. For example, a very frequent simple motor wrist tic may be less impairing than an infrequently occurring, forceful copropraxic gesture. Patients are often aware of their complex motor tics and their impact on other people, setting the stage for detrimental intrapsychic consequences. The mental elaborations associated with the behaviors may also have a detrimental effect on self-esteem and limit socialization. Physical injuries, including blindness from retinal detachment, also can occur in a small minority of adolescent and adult cases secondary to severe self-injurious tics.

VOCAL TICS

On average, vocal or phonic tics begin 1 to 2 years after the onset of motor symptoms and are usually simple in character (e.g., throat clearing, grunting, squeaks) (see Fig. 1.1). Vocal tics often show a progression similar to that seen in motor tics from transient episodes to more sustained periods of phonic symptoms (Jagger et al., 1982; Shapiro et al., 1988). Again, the range of possible phonic or vocal symptoms is extraordinary, with any noise or sound having the potential to be enlisted as a tic (see Table 1.1). As with motor tics, phonic symptoms are characterized by their number, frequency, duration, intensity (volume), and complexity (noises vs. syllables or words).

Simple vocal tics are fast, meaningless sounds or noises that can be characterized by their frequency, duration, volume intensity, and potential for disrupting speech. Sniffing, throat clearing, grunting, barks, and high-pitched squeaks are common simple phonic symptoms. **Complex vocal tics** are quite diverse and can include syllables, words, or phrases, as well as odd patterns of speech in which there are sudden changes in the rate, volume, and/or rhythm. Cavanna and colleagues (2010) recently reported the occurrence of episodic and contextually inappropriate outbursts of laughter in eight adults with TS. Not surprisingly, this rare complex vocal tic was invariably described as distressing and socially disabling. Immediate echo phenomena such as repeating words and phrases are common in some patients (*echolalia* and *palilalia*). In a minority of patients *coprolalia* is present, in which socially inappropriate syllables, words, or phrases are expressed, at times in a loud explosive manner. Shapiro and colleagues (1988) reported that among the 666 TS cases evaluated in their specialty clinic, 30% endorsed the presence of one or more of these vocal echophenomena. Current prevalence estimates of coprophenomena in TS cases treated in specialty clinics are in the range of 15% to 20% (Freeman et al., 2009).

Complex vocal tics are rarely if ever present in the absence of simple vocal tics and motor tics of one sort or another. Provocative and insulting phonic tics and motor tics of one sort or another have a high potential for stigmatizing the patient and his or her family, and can indirectly lead to emotional and/or physical injury and at times posttraumatic stress disorder and retreat from life. As reviewed in Chapter 16, there is preliminary evidence that there may be distinctive subtypes of tic disorders, such as one characterized by predominantly simple tics versus those with multiple complex tics. For example, Mathews and colleagues (2007) analyzed the lifetime tic and related symptom data in 121 TS subjects from the Central Valley of Costa Rica and 133 TS subjects from the Ashkenazi Jewish population in the United States. Remarkably, in both of these genetically distinct populations, the presence of multiple complex tics was associated with increased tic severity, global impairment, medication treatment, and presence of a family history of tics.

The study by Mathews and colleagues (2007) is just one of several studies that have subjected individual tic symptoms to cluster and factor analyses in an effort to identify possible tic symptom dimensions (Alsobrook & Pauls, 2002; Kircanski et al., 2010; Robertson & Cavanna, 2007; Robertson et al., 2008). Typically the tic symptoms separated along dimensions of simple versus complex tics. Most recently, Kircanski and colleagues (2010) reported the results of an investigation of tic symptom clusters using a sample of 99 youth diagnosed with a primary tic disorder (TS or chronic tic disorder) across two university-based outpatient clinics. Their cluster analysis of the inventory of more than 40 tics included in the YGTSS identified four symptom dimensions: predominantly complex tics; simple head/face tics; simple body tics; and simple vocal/facial tics (Fig. 1.2). Similar to the results of the study by Mathews and colleagues, these clusters were shown to be differentially associated with demographic and clinical characteristics. For example, their Cluster 1, comprising predominantly complex tics, was large and diverse and included motor and vocal tics that were generally characterized by movements or vocalizations of relative intricacy and/or duration (see Fig. 1.2). These results may suggest that the multiple complex tics and several simple tics within this cluster tend to co-occur. Of note, their Cluster 1 scores were also positively associated with number of concurrent diagnoses and demonstrated a trend toward a positive association with duration of illness. The continued study of symptom dimensions in tic disorders is needed. Prospective within-person longitudinal analyses will be particularly valuable and may lead to the identification of tic clusters differentially associated with long-term outcomes.

In summary, tics present as fragments of innate behavioral routines that are expressed inappropriately. This viewpoint leads naturally to questions about the neurobiological substrates of TS and related conditions. Although this topic is addressed in greater depth in Section 3 (Pathophysiology), it is worth pointing out that many of our behavioral programs are selected and integrated within the circuitry of the basal ganglia and its connections with the thalamus and cortex, and that the circuits contained in these structures are somatotopically organized (Hampson et al., 2009; Leckman et al., 2010).

Next, we turn to the sensory and mental phenomena that are commonly associated with tics. Some of these symptoms differentially aggregate with particular types of motor and vocal tics. For example, a study by Kircanski and colleagues

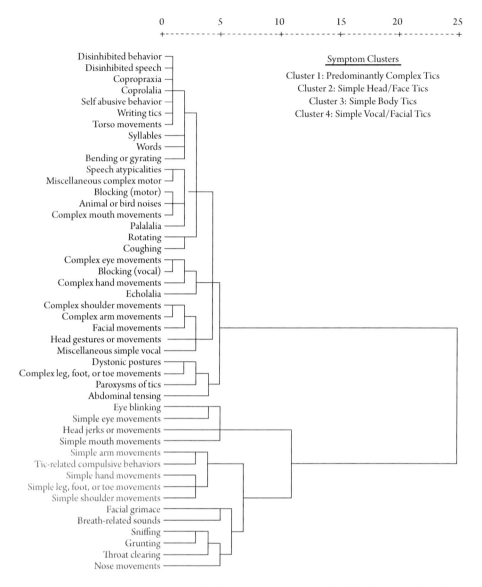

FIGURE 1.2 **Tic symptom dimensions.** This figure presents the rescaled dendrogram of agglomerative hierarchical cluster analysis using Ward's method of 46 YGTSS symptom checklist items. Text colors indicate clustered symptoms. (See color insert.)

(From Kircanski K, Woods DW, Chang SW, Ricketts EJ, Piacentini JC. Cluster analysis of the Yale Global Tic Severity Scale (YGTSS): Symptom dimensions and clinical correlates in an outpatient youth sample. *J Abnorm Child Psychol* 2010; 38:777–788.)

(2010) found that their Cluster 1 was associated with premonitory urges.

PREMONITORY URGES

Although overt tics are the defining feature of TS, many individuals report experiencing "urges," which are usually difficult to describe. Most frequently, individuals with TS will refer to unpleasant somatic phenomena that build up prior to the tic (or upon attempts to resist ticcing) and are momentarily alleviated by performance of the tic (Leckman, Walker, & Cohen, 1993). In some instances, individuals report that these ***premonitory urges*** are more bothersome than the tics themselves (Kane, 1994). The initial research on this topic stemmed primarily from detailed anecdotal accounts provided by individuals with TS. Bliss (1980) described sensory signals that preceded his tics along with "a very rapidly escalating desire to satisfy the sensations with movements intended to free oneself from the insistent feeling" (p. 37). Kane (1994) echoed this description and added, "these sensations are not mere precursors to tics … they precipitate tics more than providing a signal of imminence, the pre-tic sensation acts as the aversive stimulus toward which tics are directed" (p. 806). Some individuals perceive these urges and other sensory phenomena as being the "core" of TS (Hollenbeck, 2001). Although these urges are often difficult to describe in words, some precocious young children spontaneously assign names to specific urges (e.g., "tight feelings," "cramps," "my 'cocky' feeling") that reflect their presence in the child's internal subjective world. Other individuals with TS describe their urges as a type of discomfort or a feeling of pressure or tingling localized in the muscles involved in the performance of the tics. As with tics, the occurrences of urges vary in their frequency, intensity, and duration. The intensity of the urge can vary from fleeting and easily ignored to irresistible and inevitably leading to a tic (Woods et al., 2005).

In the first of two formal investigations of the premonitory urge phenomena, we conducted a cross-sectional study with 28 individuals (aged 9–60 years) with TS (Cohen & Leckman, 1992). Twenty-two (82%) of the 28 subjects experienced premonitory urges prior to motor and vocal tics. Of these 22, 13 (57%) found the premonitory urges more bothersome than the tics themselves, and 12 (55%) thought the premonitory urges enhanced their ability to suppress tics.

In the second study, a larger group of 135 individuals with TS (aged 8–71 years) were asked to describe and characterize their premonitory urges (Leckman, Walker, & Cohen, 1993). A substantial majority (92%) of the individuals indicated that their tics were either fully or partially a voluntary response to their premonitory urges. Consistent with Joseph Bliss' account of his tics, 84% of these subjects also reported that tics were associated with a momentary feeling of relief.

In addition, we found that premonitory urges often are focal in character and limited to a specific anatomical location. Figure 1.3 presents a body map depicting the body location and density of the premonitory urges. Tics involving the head, neck, shoulders, or the midline abdomen were most frequently preceded by urges, whereas simple tics such as eye blinking and mouth movements were less likely to be preceded by urges. More rarely, the urges were exclusively on the right side (5%) or the left side (5%). For others, these urges are more generalized and are best captured by a sense of inner tension. These sensory urges have also been described as *sensory tics* (Chee & Sachev, 1997; Kurlan et al., 1989). Many individuals reported having both focal and more generalized antecedent urges and sensations.

Developmentally, these individuals reported that they first became aware of their premonitory urges at an average of 3.1 years after tic onset, suggesting that premonitory urges may be absent during early stages of the disorder and emerge only at a later point in time. This suggests tics may begin as nonfunctional responses that, with the development of premonitory urges, become strengthened and maintained by automatic negative (the urges themselves) and positive (the momentary relief) reinforcement (Evers & van de Wetering, 1994; Woods et al., 2005). Alternatively, it is possible that younger children with tics (7- to 8-year-olds) may be less able to recognize and describe the experience sensation of premonitory urge. This suggestion is supported by clinical observations during the Habit Reversal Training (HRT) for tics with younger children. When asked to suppress or "hold their tics in" during the awareness training portion of HRT, many children are indeed able to report sensory discomfort that builds up during tic suppression.

Subsequent investigations have largely confirmed these initial observations. Kwak and colleagues (2003) administered a questionnaire to 50 individuals (mean age 24 years) with TS and found that 92% reported the presence of premonitory urges. Sixty-eight percent

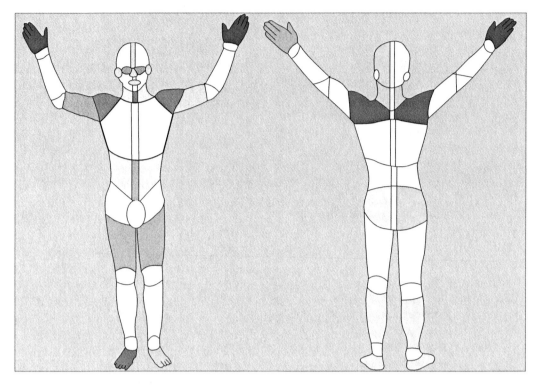

FIGURE 1.3 **Density of premonitory urges.** The densities of premonitory urges for each of 89 anatomical regions are depicted, indicating the proportion of cases that identify that body region as a site of premonitory urges. The highest density (intensity of the red color) on the scale represents the total premonitory urges per region per person, the lowest represents 0 urges per region per person, and the midpoint represents 20 urges per region per person. These data are based on current premonitory urges ever experienced as assessed in a self-report questionnaire (N = 135). (See color insert.)

(From Leckman JF, Walker DE, Cohen DJ. Premonitory urges in Tourette syndrome. *Am J Psychiatry* 1993; 150:98–102.)

of these subjects also reported that their urges disappeared with the performance of the tic. Banaschewski and colleagues (2003) administered a comparable questionnaire to 254 children with TS and documented more exactly the developmental progression of the premonitory urges; 24% of those aged 8 to 10 years, 34% of those aged 11 to 14, and 57% of those aged 15 to 19 endorsed the presence of premonitory urges.

Advances in this field include the development of the Premonitory Urge for Tics Scale (PUTS) (Woods et al., 2005). In the initial description of the PUTS, Woods and colleagues (2005) assessed premonitory urge phenomena in 42 children and adolescents with TS or a chronic tic disorder (aged 8–16 years)

and found that 98% of surveyed youth reported the presence of premonitory urges. The PUTS was found to have excellent psychometric properties for children above the age of 10 years. PUTS scores were correlated with overall tic severity as measured by the YGTSS ($r = 0.31$, $p < .05$). Among the subscales of the YGTSS, the number, complexity, and interference domains were significantly correlated with premonitory urge severity, but frequency and intensity domains were not.

The development of the PUTS has made it possible to better characterize and monitor changes in the intensity of premonitory urges. For example, the severity of premonitory urges has been shown to improve as the tics improve with some medications, including topiramate and Botulinum toxin (Jankovic et al., 2010; Rath et al., 2010).

As reviewed in Chapter 23, an increased awareness of premonitory urges has also enhanced various cognitive-behavioral interventions for tics. Comprehensive Behavioral Intervention for Tics (C-BIT) differs from the standard HRT by enhancing the patient's awareness of premonitory urges and teaching the patient how to perform a competing behavior just when he or she senses the tic symptoms are about to occur (Piacentini et al., 2010). Preliminary data also suggest that Exposure to Premonitory Sensations and Response Prevention of Tics (ERP) is another promising treatment for TS (Verdellen et al., 2007, 2008).

TOO EASILY CAPTURED BY EXTERNAL PERCEPTIONS

In addition to premonitory urges, many individuals with TS are remarkably sensitive to perceptions arising from the external world. As first noted by Gilles de la Tourette and described above, individuals may unconsciously mirror the behavior (echopraxia) and speech (echolalia) of others as well as of themselves (palilalia): they do and say what they have just seen or heard. Other examples include *site sensitization*; the need for things to be *"just right"* based on visual, tactile, and/or auditory perceptions; and *disinhibited behavior*.

Site Sensitization

In the case of site sensitization, the individual with TS is acutely aware of, distracted, and distressed by faint sensory stimuli. A classic example involves the sensations associated with tags in new clothing. Unless they are removed, some children with TS find it difficult to attend to more salient stimuli. In the study by Cohen and Leckman (1992), 70% of the TS subjects questioned reported that they had heightened sensitivity to tactile, auditory, and/or visual stimuli. More recently, Belluscio and colleagues (2011) administered questionnaires and performed in-depth interviews with 19 adult TS subjects and 19 age-matched healthy controls. Eighty percent of their subjects described a heightened sensitivity to external stimuli in at least one sensory modality: smell (70%) > tactile (65%) > light (60%) > sound (55%) > taste (50%). They reported that the most bothersome stimuli were those that were faint, repetitive or constant, and nonsalient. Intense stimuli were less problematic. These investigators then empirically evaluated this phenomenon using actual olfactory and tactile stimuli. Two alternative hypotheses were tested: Is this heightened sensitivity due to an increased ability to detect faint stimuli, or is it due to some alteration in sensory processing? The results indicated that there were no differences between TS cases and controls with regard to their ability to detect specific olfactory and tactile stimuli. However, they did find differences in sensory processing: TS subjects were more likely than the healthy controls to rate these stimuli as being at the lowest end of the intensity scale.

In addition to the PUTS scale, investigators have sought to advance our understanding of the processing of sensory stimuli through the use of behavioral and neurophysiological tests. Specifically, the presence of premonitory urges and hypothesized abnormalities in cortical-subcortical circuits in TS have led to studies using behavioral paradigms to detect inhibitory deficits, such as prepulse inhibition (PPI; Swerdlow et al., 2001). PPI is a simple behavioral measure of inhibition of the startle blink reflex, referring to reduction in startle blink magnitude when a stimulus (prepulse) occurs 30 to 500 ms before a startle stimulus. The prepulse is believed to activate automatic brain mechanisms that protect or "gate" the processing of that stimulus for a brief window of time. Several studies have shown reduced PPI in TS subjects compared to healthy controls (Castellanos et al., 1996; Smith & Lees, 1989; Swerdlow et al., 2001; Zebardast et al., in press). PPI may also emerge as an endophenotype of TS that can be utilized both in human and animal studies. These topics are further explored in Sections 2 (Etiology) and 3 (Pathophysiology).

It may also be possible to use self-report instruments to assess deficits in sensory motor gating. The Sensory Gating Inventory (SGI) is a self-report instrument that includes many items relevant to the sensory phenomena associated with TS (Hetrick et al., 2012). Recently, Sutherland Owens and colleagues (2011) found that 18 TS subjects (aged 10–41 years) had significantly elevated mean scores on the SGI relative to the healthy controls. However, the SGI scores were not correlated with either the YGTSS tic severity ratings or the PUTS scores.

"Just Right" Phenomena

Another set of sensory phenomena frequently encountered in TS subjects involves a need for things to feel, look, or sound *"just right"* (Leckman, Walker, Goodman et al., 1994). In our second study of more than 130 subjects with tic disorders (aged 9–71 years), 59 (44%) reported the presence of "just right" phenomena. Most individuals could readily distinguish these "just right" sensations from the premonitory urges associated with tic behavior. Frequently, this took the form of pointing out that the "just right" perception was more of a mental phenomenon than a bodily sensation. The "just right" awareness most commonly referred to was for visual (31%) or tactile (25%) as opposed to auditory (10%) perceptions. These symptoms were far more common in individuals with comorbid obsessive-compulsive disorder (OCD; 81%) compared to those individuals with subclinical OCD (61%). More recently, Worbe and colleagues (2010), using a semistructured interview, also found that 30% of 166 consecutive patients with TS (aged 15–68 years) endorsed the presence of "just right" perceptions. When the TS cases were stratified according to whether or not they had repetitive behaviors and thoughts that were "tic-like" versus "OCD-like," the tic-like group had significantly higher rates of the "just right" perceptions.

As discussed in Chapter 3, the University of São Paulo Sensory Phenomena Scale (UPS-SPS) (Miguel et al. 2000; Rosario et al., 2009) was developed to characterize the sensory abnormalities frequently encountered in individuals with OCD and tic disorders. In the initial study, Miguel and colleagues (2000) performed in-depth interviews with 61 adults (aged >17

years), including 21 adult TS subjects without OCD, 20 TS cases with comorbid OCD, and 20 with OCD alone. They found that 90% of the TS-plus-OCD cases versus 48% of the TS-alone cases reported the presence of one or more "just right" (visual > tactile > auditory) perceptions. The rate in the OCD-alone cases was just 35%.

Although "just right" sensations appear to be distinct from premonitory urges, one study did report a correlation between PUTS and UPS-SPS scores (Sutherland Owens et al., 2011). However, this association may well be due to the presence of the other sensory domains included in the UPS-SPS.

CONTEXT AND TIMING OF TICS

Waxing and Waning of Tics

Virtually all descriptions of TS mention the **waxing and waning** course of this disorder. This simply means that over a period of weeks to months, a person's tics get better or worse. We still do not understand why this happens. Is it due to changes in stress levels or the season of the year? Or perhaps it is due to some intrinsic properties of the neurons and neural circuits that underlie tics (Leckman, Vaccarino, Kalanithi, & Rothenberger, 2006).

One of the few studies that have been performed suggested the presence of a fractal process in the tic time series (Peterson & Leckman, 1998). If true, this simply means that for any temporal dimension (minutes, hours, days, weeks, months, or years), the same pattern of tics is evident. Hence, during the course of minutes, individual tics occur in discrete bursts or **bouts** with very brief inter-tic intervals (measured in seconds or fractions of seconds). Similarly, for the time scale measured in hours, these bouts of tics occur in bouts so that on any given day there are both tic-free periods as well as periods of intense ticcing. For long time scales measured in months, a waxing and waning pattern emerges as well (Fig. 1.4).

In that project, we videotaped 22 medication-free TS subjects (aged 8–49 years) (Chappell et al., 1994). The intervals between temporally adjacent tics were measured, and

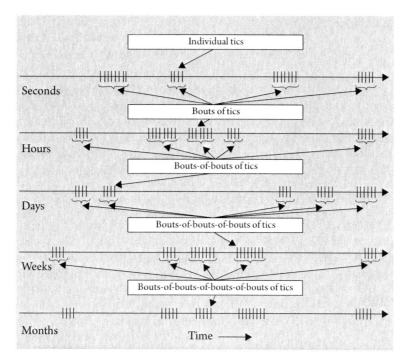

FIGURE 1.4 **Fractal character of the temporal occurrence of tics.** Progressively longer time dimensions (seconds to months) are depicted in this figure. Tics occur in bouts, and bouts of tics occur in bouts. We predict that regardless of the temporal dimension, the bout-like appearance of tics (or higher-order combinations of bouts and bouts of bouts of tics) will be observed. This fractal quality may well underlie the waxing and waning of tics observed over weeks to months as well as other features of the natural history of TS.

(From Leckman JF. Tourette syndrome. *Lancet* 2002; 360:1577–1586.)

the statistical properties of these intervals were assessed through graphical representation of frequency distributions, autoregressive integrated moving average (ARIMA) modeling, spectral analysis, and construction of first return maps. The frequency distribution of tic interval durations followed an inverse power law of temporal scaling, which is typical of fractal processes (Fig. 1.5). Spectral analyses similarly demonstrated that the spectral power density of tic interval duration is related inversely to frequency. The first return maps revealed the "burst-like" behavior and short-term periodicity in tics (Peterson & Leckman, 1998). Given the time-intensive nature of this research, the development of automated tic-counting devices will be of value (Bernabei et al., 2010).

If this study is replicated, tics then might best understood as being the product of nested processes that unfold over many time scales, from milliseconds to years or even decades. As

such, they may be exemplars of a dynamic system at work in the development of the central nervous system (Smith & Thelen, 2003). At the other end of the time scale, it is possible that an examination of the neural mechanisms underlying this fractal phenomenon may identify related events that can be measured in milliseconds or even shorter intervals that are associated with the generation of tic phenomena. The timing of the firing of brain cells may also provide some important clues to identifying, in very rare severe cases where an individual has treatment-resistant, self-injurious tics, where to place the electrodes that are used in deep brain stimulation (see Chapter 26).

Tic Exacerbations

Although there are compelling preliminary data to support the inherent nature of the waxing and waning of tics, the description of tics as simply

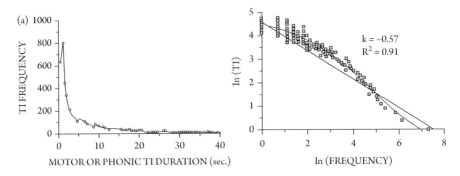

FIGURE 1.5 Tics in time, evidence for the inverse power law. A. Group composite inverse power law frequency distributions. Tic interval (TI) frequency count plotted as a function of TI duration (in seconds) for time series in which both motor and phonic tics were regarded as "events." **B.** The log-log transforms of the frequency distributions produce a straight-line relationship between TI duration and TI frequency. The slope (k) of this descending line segment was estimated using simple linear regression; R2 is the amount of variance in the distribution explained by the regression equation.

(From Peterson BS, Leckman JF. Temporal characterization of tics in Gilles de la Tourette syndrome. *Biol Psychiatry* 1998; 44:1337–1348.)

intermittent trains of involuntary motor discharge is incomplete. The severity of tic symptoms varies over time. In some instances there appears to be a sudden exacerbation of symptoms. Is this simply due to the waxing and waning of tic symptoms, or is it due to some other factors that cause the symptoms to be outside the normal range of fluctuation? In an effort to establish an objective, prospective, and quantitative method for identifying symptom exacerbations in individuals with TS, Lin and colleagues (2002) modeled monthly consecutive YGTSS scores, prospectively obtained, in 64 youth (aged 7–16 years) diagnosed with TS for periods ranging from 3 to 39 months (Luo et al., 2004). Exacerbation thresholds were estimated by using state-of-the-art bootstrap methods. These thresholds were then independently evaluated by asking two expert clinicians to identify clinically significant exacerbations based on a review of all available clinical and research records. The severity of tic symptoms displayed a high degree of intrasubject variability. Exacerbation thresholds, which incorporated the change score from the previous month and the current symptom score, provided the best agreement with those of expert clinicians. Interestingly, when both tic and obsessive-compulsive symptoms were present, there was a significant degree of covariation. Thus far, this approach has been used in

three articles describing the results of two prospective longitudinal studies to study the effects of antecedent group A beta-hemolytic streptococcal infections (Leckman, King, Gilbert et al., 2011; Lin et al., 2010; Luo et al., 2004). The results of these and related studies are reviewed in Chapters 9 and 14.

Antecedent and Contextual Factors

Tic expression (choice of tics as well as their severity) can be influenced (both exacerbated and attenuated) by environmental contingencies involving both internal and external stimuli. A large number of antecedent environmental and emotional factors have been implicated; a partial list of some of the factors that have thus far been implicated is presented in Table 1.2. Data supporting each of these factors have come from clinical experience and anecdotal self-reports (Bornstein et al., 1990; Eapen et al., 2004; Robertson et al., 2002; Silva et al., 1995) and daily diaries (O'Connor et al., 1994, 2003) and from small-N functional behavioral analyses and experimental studies (Conelea, Woods, & Brandt, 2011; Meidinger et al., 2005; Piacentini et al., 2006; Scahill et al., 2001; Watson et al., 2005; Wood et al., 2003; Woods et al., 2001) as well as from prospective longitudinal studies (Hoekstra et al., 2004; Lin et al., 2007). Conelea

Table 1.2 What Makes Tics Better or Worse?

Better	Sleep (almost always the tics will disappear)
	Doing something that requires focused attention and motor control, like riding a bicycle or playing ping-pong or playing a musical instrument (almost always)
	Relaxation (variable)
	Verbal instructions to suppress tics, especially with incentives
	During and after physical exercise (usually the tics will diminish or be less forceful)
Worse	Stressful life events (50–90%)
	Returning to school (60–70%)
	Being anxious or upset or noticing stress in a loved one (80–90%)
	Excitement, like going to Disney World for the first time, birthdays, holidays, especially with presents (60–70%)
	Watching exciting movies (in the theater) or television shows (almost always)
	Fatigued, being tired but not quite ready to fall asleep (almost always) (50–75%)
	Being alone (40–50%)
	Quiet reading tasks
	Talking about tics, tics are "suggestible" (almost always)
	Menstruation (only for some women)
	Eating (only for some individuals)
	Drinking coffee (only for some individuals)
	Being too hot, hot weather (only for some individuals)

Based in part on the review of this field by Conelea & Woods (2008a). The self-report and anecdotal data are drawn from descriptive studies (Bornstein et al., 1990; Eapen et al., 2004; Robertson et al., 2002; Silva et al., 1995; Zinner et al., 2011), self-report diaries (O'Connor et al., 1994, 2003), experimental studies (Conelea, Woods, & Brandt, 2011; Kobets et al., submitted; Meidinger et al., 2005; Piacentini et al., 2006; Scahill et al., 2001; Watson et al., 2005; Woods et al., 2001; Wood et al., 2003), and prospective longitudinal studies (Hoekstra et al., 2004; Lin et al., 2007).

and Woods (2008a) have thus far provided the most comprehensive review of this field. Although self-reports do not always agree with objective ratings, a compelling case can be made that current levels of psychosocial stress are associated with future levels of tic severity (Bornstein et al., 1990; Cohen & Leckman, 1992; Eapen et al., 2004; Hoekstra et al., 2004; Lin et al., 2007, 2010; Robertson et al., 2002; Silva et al., 1995). It is also clear that emotional factors, including excitement, such as at birthday parties or visits to Disneyland, as well as returning to school, are frequently associated with transient increases in tic severity (Bornstein et al., 1990).

Tics are *suggestible*. A classic example regularly occurs in the consulting room when we inquire about a broad range of tic phenomena. In this context it is not unusual for a patient or even a family member with a lifetime history of tics to display tics just after a particular type of

tic is mentioned. Remarkably, some of these tics may not be part of the individual's current tic repertoire, but had been present in the distant past.

Another potentially related phenomenon is senseless, inappropriate, and at times even dangerous responses to sensory cues in the environment. In children and adolescents with TS this may take the form of having a prominent tic just when the teacher is trying to get the attention of her class. Not surprisingly, these behaviors can contribute to a teacher's negative appraisal of some children with TS. In the study by Cohen and Leckman (1992), 10 (36%) of the 28 TS subjects reported examples of *reflexive tics* in response to specific sensory cues. Other examples include the urge to make a loud vocal tic in a quiet library immediately upon seeing the sign "Quiet Please." We have also heard individuals describe the "need" to touch a hot iron or to put the car in reverse gear while driving down a highway, or to touch the foot of an adjacent person. Another extreme example was related by a physicist who during World War II had to give up a job in a high-energy physics laboratory because whenever he saw the sign "Danger High Voltage" he had the strong urge to touch the apparatus. Cavanna and colleagues (2010) reported that two of the eight individuals with laughing tics reported that their tic was cued by hearing certain words or phrases. In one instance this tic occurred only when an adolescent subject heard the word "tree." When his classmates realized this, he was subjected to unrelenting teasing in the school environment that subsided only through the active intervention of another student and school personnel.

Experimental studies have also documented that tic-related conversations can prompt transient tic worsening in some individuals. For example, Woods and colleagues (2001) performed a functional analysis of the effects of "tic-related" talk on the frequency of vocal and motor tics in two boys (aged 6 and 16 years) with TS. Using A-B-A-B withdrawal designs, these two boys were alternately exposed to conditions with and without talk of their tics. They found that vocal tics markedly increased when talk pertained to tics and decreased when talk did not pertain to tics, but motor tic covariance was less consistent. Contextual distractions do not appear to affect tic frequency (Conelea & Woods, 2008b).

Interestingly, Wood and colleagues (2003) found that, while monitoring four children (aged 8–14 years) as they watched a movie known to elicit emotional responses, their tics were more frequent during periods associated with anticipation and resolution of emotional changes and lowest during periods of overt anger and happiness. This finding is perhaps consistent with the observation by Belluscio and colleagues (2011) that individuals with TS show a greater sensitivity to faint versus more intense sensory stimuli.

Tic Suppression

For many individuals tics are under partial voluntary control, evidenced by their capacity to suppress them for brief periods of time. There is also increasing recognition that individuals with TS vary in terms of their ability to suppress tics. Some describe the process of tic suppression to be relatively effortless and requiring minimal amount of self-monitoring. Others report that they can suppress their tics, but that this process requires tremendous mental effort, associated with the discomfort of premonitory urges, and takes away from the ability to perform tasks at hand. We also acknowledge a possible connection of tic severity with the *need to suppress tics* and the *success of tic suppression*. For example, individuals with mild tics might not feel the need to suppress their tics because the tics are not bothersome. In contrast, individuals with severe tics might try to suppress their tics but fail in their efforts.

In one of the few experimental studies to examine this phenomenon, Meidinger and colleagues (2005) recruited seven TS subjects (aged 7–20 years) to test their ability to suppress their tics using an A-B-A design consisting of baseline, suppression, and postsuppression conditions. Following baseline observation, participants were instructed to refrain from exhibiting tics while watching videotapes, while engaging in conversation, or while alone in a room with no activity. Each of the three experimental conditions (baseline, alone suppression or social suppression, and postsuppression) was approximately 30 minutes in length and was repeated across two, three, or four sessions over the course of several weeks. The results of this experiment showed suppression of tics in almost half of all sessions, with the older individuals being more effective at suppressing their tics. The results of this experiment also failed to support a commonly held belief that following a period of voluntary suppression tics will rebound in frequency and severity.

Subsequently, Himle and colleagues (2007) investigated the effects of tic suppression on premonitory urge ratings and found that some children reported higher urge ratings during periods of tic suppression. Himle and colleagues (2008) also documented that differential reinforcement of effective tic suppression (with coin-like tokens) resulted in lower tic frequencies in three of the four children (aged 8–10 years) compared to the tic rates recorded when tokens were delivered noncontingently.

Experiments are continuing to explore the factors that influence tic suppression, and whether or not reinforcement could be used to create some degree of stimulus control over tic expression. For example, Woods and colleagues (2009) studied ten youth with TS or a chronic tic disorder (aged 9–15 years) who completed four training sessions. Each session consisted of three exposures to each of three 5-minute conditions presented in a random order. In one condition, participants were reinforced for tic absence on a 10-second fixed-interval schedule in the presence of a purple light. Confirming findings from other studies, results showed that reinforcing tic suppression reduced tic frequency to a greater extent than only providing instructions to suppress. Of interest, this suppression effect (conditioned on the presence of a purple light, but not lights of any other color) persisted during a fifth session even though no instructions to suppress (or not suppress) tics and no reinforcers were delivered. Results indicated that in the presence of the purple light, tics were significantly lower than when neither light was illuminated. These findings provide preliminary support for the idea that a history of differential reinforcement in various contexts may play a role explaining variability in tic symptom expression.

As discussed in Chapter 23, perhaps the most promising preliminary finding related to tic suppression is that a behavioral intervention consisting of exposure to premonitory sensory experiences during prolonged tic suppression may be beneficial in the treatment of tics (Verdellen et al., 2007, 2008).

Tic Disappearance During Periods of Focused Attention and Motor Control

Oliver Sacks, in his 1995 book *An Anthropologist on Mars*, describes his interactions with Carl Bennett, a surgeon and amateur pilot with TS. The surgeon is often beset by tics, but they vanish when he is operating. Tim Howard, the goalkeeper for the U.S. soccer team, describes

a similar phenomenon when a member of the opposing team approaches the goal he is guarding. Clinically, similar accounts are common, ranging from musicians to athletes to surgeons. Although few studies in the medical literature have focused on this aspect of TS, it appears that when someone with TS engages in an activity that requires focused attention and motor control, his or her tics often disappear. Kobets and colleagues (submitted), in a recent case report, describe the "Wii effect" where an individual with serious TS shows a marked reduction of his tics while playing the tennis Wii game. We can only surmise that when the neural circuitry of individuals with TS is fully engaged in a familiar activity, the events that prompt tics are markedly diminished. If these preliminary findings are confirmed, they may point the way to novel therapeutic interventions.

NATURAL HISTORY OF TICS AND TIC DISORDERS

Tics usually have their onset in the first decade of life. Boys are more commonly affected, as documented in both clinically referred and population-based studies (Centers for Disease Control, 2009; Freeman et al., 2000; Khalifa & von Knorring, 2003). Most investigators report a median onset of simple motor tics between 5 and 7 years of age (Freeman et al., 2000; Khalifa & von Knorring, 2003). Figure 1.6 presents age-of-onset data for 221 patients with TS evaluated at Yale.

Subsequently, as discussed above, the classic history includes a waxing and waning course and a changing repertoire of tics. Typically, in cases of TS, the symptoms multiply and worsen, so that even during the waning phases the tics are troublesome. In our experience, for a majority of patients, the period of worst tic severity usually falls between the ages of 7 and 15 years of age, after which tic severity gradually declines (Leckman et al. 1998). This falloff in tic symptoms is consistent with available epidemiological data that indicate a much lower prevalence of TS among adults than children (Peterson et al., 2001). As discussed in Chapter 5, this decline

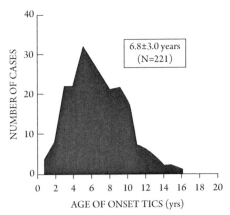

FIGURE 1.6 **Age-of-onset distribution.** This figure presents the age of onset of tics in a series of 221 individuals with TS evaluated at the Yale Child Study Clinic.

(From Leckman JF, Cohen DJ. *Tourette syndrome: Tics, obsessions, compulsions—Developmental psychopathology and clinical care.* New York: John Wiley and Sons, 1998.)

in tic severity is also present in follow-up studies of clinically referred TS patients (Bloch et al., 2006; Gorman et al., 2010). In many instances, the phonic symptoms become increasingly rare or may disappear altogether, and the motor tics may be reduced in number and frequency.

Complete remission of both motor and phonic symptoms has also been reported, but estimates vary considerably, with some studies reporting rates of remission as high as 30% to 50% (Bloch et al., 2006; Torup, 1962). In such cases, the legacy of TS in adult life is most closely associated with what it "meant" to have severe tics as a child. For example, individuals who were misunderstood and punished at home and at school for their tics or who were teased mercilessly by peers and stigmatized by their communities will fare worse than children whose interpersonal environment was more understanding and supportive (Chao et al., 2010; Conelea, Woods, Zinner et al., 2011; Zinner et al., 2012).

In contrast, adulthood is also the period when the most severe and debilitating forms of tic disorder can be seen. In this small minority of adult patients, severe tics can persist or re-emerge with frightening intensity. At their worst, these tics can be self-injurious and disabling, placing in serious jeopardy an individual's accomplishments and aspirations. In our clinical experience, adults with persistent severe tics often feel socially excluded and have symptoms of a posttraumatic stress disorder.

THE SELF UNDER SIEGE

In 1999, Donald Cohen, who founded the Tic Disorder Clinic at the Yale Child Study Center in the 1970s, first used the phrase "the self under siege" to describe the internal experience of individuals suffering with a chronic tic disorder and all of the accompanying sensory and mental states (Cohen & Leckman, 1998). He pointed out that often children with TS become expert observers of their own experiences and how these mental representations can shape and mold their sense of self. As reviewed in Chapters 18, 22, and 30, he championed the need for clinicians, parents, and teachers to build on children's strengths and to keep their development on track despite the challenges posed by their tics and the complexities of their internal sensory world.

Cohen also remarked on the increased self-awareness of one's own feelings and the feelings of others that we often encounter in our clinical practice. In a majority of cases, when parents are asked to describe the strengths of their child, they point to how "sensitive" their child is to the emotional states of others. This can be a burden as well as a strength. Some adolescents and adults with TS also describe a phenomenon we have termed "somatic empathy" in which they seem to be able to "sense" what someone in their immediate physical presence is about to do, whether it be in the context of jazz ensemble, a soccer match, or a martial arts competition (Sides, 2010).

It is also clear that for many children and adults, their tics are just part of the story. Indeed, the remaining chapters in this initial section focus on the range of other difficulties frequently encountered by individuals with chronic tic disorders, including OCD, attention-deficit/ hyperactivity disorder (ADHD), mood disorders, anger control problems, and in a minority autism spectrum disorders and learning disabilities (see Fig. 1.1). These comorbid conditions occur more frequently in individuals with a full case of TS compared to those with a chronic tic disorder (Khalifa & von Knorring, 2006) and often are of greater emotional and prognostic significance than are the tics themselves, given their impact on self-esteem, family and peer relationships, academic performance, and peer acceptance (Gorman et al., 2010; Sukhodolsky et al., 2003).

As reviewed in Chapters 2 and 3, the presence of comorbid ADHD and OCD may be differentially associated with specific tic symptoms. Thus far at least eight studies have examined symptom factors/clusters in cohorts of well-characterized TS cases. For example, Cavanna and colleagues (2011) analyzed symptom data from a sample of 639 TS patients and identified three factors that in total accounted for ~45% of the phenotypic variance: (1) complex motor tics and echophenomena (echolalia, echopraxia, and palilalia) and obsessive-compulsive behaviors; (2) complex vocal tics and coprolalia and copropraxia; and (3) attention-deficit and hyperactivity symptoms plus aggressive behaviors and obsessive-compulsive behaviors. A better characterization of the TS phenotypes may help to identify the molecular and neural pathways underlying this etiologically heterogeneous condition.

CONCLUSIONS AND QUESTIONS FOR FUTURE RESEARCH

As briefly summarized in Box 1.1, for over 150 years, a growing literature has focused on the phenomenology of tics and tic disorders. The past

---

Box 1.1. Key Points

- Tics often arise from a *heightened and selective sensitivity* to cues from within the body or from the outside world. This may be due in part to a loss in the normal "automatic" ability to suppress or "gate" irrelevant information in sensory, motor, and cognitive domains.
- Motor and phonic tics occur in bouts over the course of a day and wax and wane in severity over the course of weeks to months. Less well known is the "self-similarity" of these temporal patterns across different time scales. Understanding the dynamic patterns of tics may be useful to families, clinicians, and teachers. If confirmed, it may also provide deeper insights into the neurobiology of tics.
- Tic expression, the choice of tics as well as their severity, can be influenced (both exacerbated and attenuated) by environmental contingencies involving both internal and external stimuli. Understanding the cues and contextual factors that influence tic expression is key to refining and developing novel behavioral interventions.
- Tics are worse during periods of fatigue, stress, and excitement and better during periods of goal-directed behavior that requires motor control, such as playing a musical instrument.
- In most cases, motor and vocal tic severity peaks early in the second decade, with many patients showing a marked reduction in tic severity by the age of 19 or 20 years.
- Tics, in some form, persist in the majority of cases well into adulthood.
- The presence of chronic motor and vocal tics *alone* in the absence of other difficulties often heralds a positive outcome—especially in the presence of other strengths; *however, tics alone are the exception rather than the rule.*
- Social, emotional, and academic outcomes in adulthood are *not* synonymous with tic outcomes.
- Clinicians, teachers, parents, and peers need to be educated about the key phenomenological features of TS and related disorders to ensure the best outcomes.
- Future progress in this field depends on close interdisciplinary collaboration among *teams* of scientists, parents, teachers, and advocacy groups working together.

two decades has seen an increased attention to the sensory, subjective, and contextual experiences associated with TS, which in turn has led to refinements of existing cognitive-behavioral interventions. We have also found that when clinicians, parents, teachers, and peers understand the sensory aspects of TS, they "understand" at some level why the child is doing what he or she is doing.

Experimental approaches have also done much to focus on the contextual factors that influence tic suppression. Preliminary data suggest the potentially important role that tic suppression may play in behavioral techniques that depend on exposure to premonitory urges and response prevention. Other major advances concern the timing of tics and their inherent waxing and waning character. It has also become clear that motor and vocal tic severity typically peaks early in the second decade, with many patients showing a marked reduction in tic severity by 19 or 20 years of age. Clusters of tic symptoms and co-occurring OCD and ADHD may also be of value in sorting out vulnerability genes and neural pathways (Cavanna et al., 2011; Matthews et al., 2007). As discussed in more detail in Chapter 5, tics, in some form, persist in the majority of cases well

---

Box 1.2. Questions for Future Research

1. Why are males more commonly affected with TS than females? What endocrine, molecular, and neural mechanisms play a role, and at what point in development do these events unfold?

2. What determines tic onset? What are the underlying processes that lead tics to appear during a specific phase of neural development?

3. What is the neurobiological origin of premonitory urges, and what functional role do they play in tic expression? Are they causally related, or are they simply nonfunctional responses that become strengthened and maintained by automatic negative (the urges themselves) and positive (the momentary relief) reinforcement? How can we diminish the intensity of tic urges?

4. How can we better understand the nonlinear dynamics of the waxing and waning of tics, particularly with regard to its neural origins and its potential prognostic value? Is a similar temporal pattern of neural activity present in certain classes of neurons? If it were possible to monitor in real time patient-specific variables, would that provide us with more accurate tools to assess tic severity?

5. What genetic, environmental, and neurobiological factors influence the natural history of tic disorders, leading in some cases to a marked attenuation or remission of tics in early adulthood? Is there an endophenotype of TS, such as diminished prepulse inhibition, that remains even if the tics largely remit? Is remission a return to a "normal" state of neural function, or does it reflect a progressive adaptation to the anomalous motor and sensory states associated with tics and associated behaviors? Prospective longitudinal studies are needed to clarify the patterns of neural interconnectivity seen in TS.

6. How can we best understand the range of comorbid conditions associated with TS? Why is the rate of these disorders higher in TS cases compared to individuals with a chronic tic disorder?

7. Are there unique etiological subtypes of TS that can be identified based on their clinical presentation? Why are certain clusters of tic symptoms differentially associated with premonitory urges and co-occurring ADHD and OCD symptoms? Will these phenotypes be useful in clarifying the vulnerability genes and other aspects of the developmental pathobiology of TS?

into adulthood. The presence of chronic motor and vocal tics *alone* in the absence of other difficulties often heralds a positive outcome—especially in the presence of other strengths; *however, tics alone are the exception rather than the rule.*

Close collaborations between clinicians and the designers of model intervention programs have been longstanding. These collaborations are now beginning to include scientists from a broad range of disciplines: neuroimagers, developmental and behavioral neuroscientists, geneticists, and immunologists as well as representatives of advocacy organizations. Indeed, many of the scientific advances of the past two decades began with initiatives funded by organizations such as the Tourette Syndrome Association and affiliated organizations across the globe. Box 1.2 points to some of the unanswered questions regarding the "enigmatic world" of TS.

REFERENCES

Alsobrook, JP Pauls DL. A factor analysis of tic symptoms in Gilles de la Tourette's syndrome. *Am J Psychiatry*, 2002; *159*:291–296.

Banaschewski T, Woerner W, Rothenberger A. Premonitory sensory phenomena and suppressibility of tics in Tourette syndrome: Developmental aspects in children and adolescents. *Dev Med Child Neurol* 2003;*45*:700–703.

Belluscio BA, Jin L, Watters V et al. Sensory sensitivity to external stimuli in Tourette syndrome patients. *Mov Disord* 2011; *26*: 2538–2543.
This is the first study to document that individuals with TS show the greatest sensitivity to faint sensory stimuli.

Bernabei M, Andreoni G, Mendez Garcia MO et al. Automatic detection of tic activity in the Tourette Syndrome. *Conf Proc IEEE Eng Med Biol Soc* 2010; 2010:422–425.

Bliss, J. Sensory experiences of Gilles de la Tourette syndrome. *Arch Gen Psychiatry* 1980; 37:1343–1347.
A graphic first-person account of what it is like to live with TS.

Bloch MH, Peterson BS, Scahill L et al. Clinical predictors of future tic and OCD severity in children with Tourette syndrome. *Arch Pediatr Adolesc Med* 2006; *160*:65–69.

Bornstein RA, Stefl ME, Hammond L. A survey of Tourette syndrome patients and their families: the 1987 Ohio Tourette survey. *J Neuropsychiatry Clin Neurosci* 1990; *2*:275–281.

Castellanos FX, Fine EJ, Kaysen D et al. Sensorigating in boys with Tourette syndrome and ADHD: Preliminary results. *Biol Psychiatry* 1996; *39*:33–41.

Cavanna AE, Ali F, Leckman JF, Robertson MM. Pathological laughter in Gilles de la Tourette syndrome: an unusual phonic tic. *Mov Disord* 2010; 25:2233–2239.

Cavanna AE, Critchley HD, Orth M et al. Dissecting the Gilles de la Tourette spectrum: a factor analytic study on 639 patients. *J Neurol Neurosurg Psychiatry* 2011; *82*:1320–1323.

Centers for Disease Control and Prevention. Prevalence of diagnosed Tourette syndrome in persons aged 6–17 years—United States, 2007. *MMWR Morb Mortal Wkly Rep*. 2009; 58:581–585.

Chao KY, Wang HS, Chang HL et al. Establishment of the reliability and validity of the Stress Index for Children or Adolescents with Tourette Syndrome (SICATS). *J Clin Nurs* 2010; *19*:332–340.

Chappell PB, McSwiggan-Hardin MT, Scahill L et al. Videotape tic counts in the assessment of Tourette's syndrome: Stability, reliability, and validity. *J Am Acad Child Adolesc Psychiatry* 1994; 33:386–393.

Chee KY, Sachdev P. A controlled study of sensory tics in Gilles de la Tourette syndrome and obsessive-compulsive disorder using a structured interview. *J Neurol Neurosurg Psychiatry* 1997; 62:188–192.

Cohen AJ, Leckman JF. Sensory phenomena associated with Gilles de la Tourette's syndrome. *J Clin Psychiatry* 1992; 53:319–323.

Cohen DJ, Leckman JF. Introduction: The self under siege. In: Leckman JF, Cohen DJ (eds.), *Tourette's Syndrome: Tics, Obsessions, Compulsions—Developmental Psychopathology and Clinical Care*. New York: John Wiley and Sons, 1998, pp.1–20.

Conelea CA, Woods DW. The influence of contextual factors on tic expression in Tourette's syndrome: a review. *J Psychosom Res* 2008a; 65:487–496.
The best review to date on contextual factors that can influence tic expression.

Conelea CA, Woods DW. Examining the impact of distraction on tic suppression in children and adolescents with Tourette syndrome. *Behav Res Ther* 2008b; 46:1193–1200.

Conelea CA, Woods DW, Brandt BC. The impact of a stress induction task on tic frequencies in youth with Tourette Syndrome. *Behav Res Ther* 2011; 49:492–497.

Conelea CA, Woods DW, Zinner SH et al. Exploring the impact of chronic tic disorders on youth: results from the Tourette Syndrome Impact Survey. *Child Psychiatry Hum Dev* 2011; 42:219–242.

Eapen V, Fox-Hiley P, Banerjee S, Robertson M. Clinical features and associated psychopathology in a Tourette syndrome cohort. *Acta Neurol Scand* 2004; 109:255–260.

Evers RAF, van de Wetering BJM. A treatment model for motor tics based on specific tension-reduction technique. *J Behav Ther Exp Psychiatry* 1994; 25:255–260.

Freeman RD, Fast DK, Burd L et al. An international perspective on Tourette syndrome: selected findings from 3,500 individuals in 22 countries. *Dev Med Child Neurol* 2000; 42:436–447.

Freeman RD, Zinner SH, Müller-Vahl KR et al. Coprophenomena in Tourette syndrome. *Dev Med Child Neurol* 2009; 51:218–227.

Freud S. The disposition to obsessional neurosis. *In* Strachey J, Freud A, Strachey A, Tyson A (Eds.), *The Complete Psychological Works of Sigmund Freud, Vol. XII.* 1913. London: Hogarth Press.

Gilles de la Tourette G. Etude sur une affection nerveuse caracterisee par de l'incoordination motrice accompagnee de l'echolalie et de la coprolalie. *Arch Neurol* (Paris) 1885; 9:19–42, 158–200.

Gorman DA, Thompson N, Plessen KJ et al. Psychosocial outcome and psychiatric comorbidity in older adolescents with Tourette syndrome: controlled study. *Br J Psychiatry* 2010; 197:36–44.

Hampson M, Tokoglu F, King RA et al. Brain areas coactivating with motor cortex during chronic motor tics and intentional movements. *Biol Psychiatry* 2009; 65:594–599.

Hetrick WP, Erickson MA, Smith DA. Phenomenological dimensions of sensory gating. *Schizophr Bull* 2012; 38:178–191.

Himle MB, Woods DW, Bunaciu L. Evaluating the role of contingency in differentially reinforced tic suppression. *J Appl Behav Anal* 2008; 41:285–289.

Himle MB, Woods DW, Conelea CA et al. Investigating the effects of tic suppression on premonitory urge ratings in children and adolescents with Tourette's syndrome. *Behav Res Ther* 2007; 45:2964–2976.

Hoekstra PJ, Steenhuis MP, Kallenberg CG, Minderaa RB. Association of the small life events with self reports of tic severity in pediatric and adult tic disorder patients: a prospective longitudinal study. *J Clin Psychiatry* 2004; 65:426–431.

Hollenbeck PJ. Insight and hindsight into Tourette syndrome. *Adv Neurol* 2001; 85:363–367.
Another excellent first-person account that highlights the importance of sensory urges in TS.

Itard JMG. Mémoire sur quelques fonctions involontaires des appareils de la locomotion, de la préhension et de la voix. *Archives Générales de Médecins* 1825; 8:385–407.

Jagger J, Prusoff BA, Cohen DJ et al. The epidemiology of Tourette's syndrome: a pilot study. *Schizophr Bull* 1982; 8:267–278.

Janet P. *Les Obsessions et la Psychiasthenie, Vol. 1.* Paris, Alcan, 1903 (reprinted in New York, Arno, 1976).
Janet, a colleague of Freud and student of Charcot, argued that both obsessions and tics shared common origin in a sense of "incompleteness."

Jankovic J, Jimenez-Shahed J, Brown LW. A randomised, double-blind, placebo-controlled study of topiramate in the treatment of Tourette syndrome. *J Neurol Neurosurg Psychiatry* 2010; 81:70–73.

Kane MJ. Premonitory urges as "attentional tics" in Tourette's syndrome. *J Am Acad Child Adolesc Psychiatry* 1994; 33:805–808.

Khalifa N, von Knorring AL. Prevalence of tic disorders and Tourette syndrome in a Swedish school population. *Dev Med Child Neurol* 2003; 45:315–319.

Khalifa N, von Knorring AL. Psychopathology in a Swedish population of school children with tic disorders. *J Am Acad Child Adolesc Psychiatry* 2006; 45:1346–1353.

Kircanski K, Woods DW, Chang SW et al. Cluster analysis of the Yale Global Tic Severity Scale (YGTSS): Symptom dimensions and clinical correlates in an outpatient youth sample. *J Abnorm Child Psychol* 2010; 38:777–788.
A recent study suggesting the existence of clusters of tic symptoms that may be differentially associated with various clinical features of tic disorders.

Kobets AJ, Pittenger C, Leckman JF. Focused, goal-oriented movement and tics in Tourette syndrome: Evidence for a "Wii effect" (submitted).

Kurlan R, Lichter D, Hewitt D. Sensory tics in Tourette's syndrome. *Neurology* 1989; 39:731–734.

Kwak C, Dat Vuong K, Jankovic J. Premonitory sensory phenomenon in Tourette's syndrome. *Mov Disord* 2003; 18:1530–1533.

Leckman JF. Tourette's syndrome. *Lancet* 2002; 360:1577–1586.

Leckman JF, Bloch MH, Smith ME et al. Neurobiological substrates of Tourette's disorder. *J Child Adolesc Psychopharmacol* 2010; 20:237–247.

Leckman JF, Cohen DJ. *Tourette's Syndrome: Tics, Obsessions, Compulsions—Developmental Psychopathology and Clinical Care*. New York, John Wiley and Sons, 1998.

Leckman JF, King RA, Cohen DJ. Tics and tic disorders. In: Leckman JF, Cohen DJ (eds.), *Tourette's Syndrome Tics, Obsessions, Compulsions—Developmental Psychopathology and Clinical Care*. New York: John Wiley and Sons, 1998, pp. 23–42.

Leckman JF, King RA, Gilbert DL et al. Streptococcal upper respiratory tract infections and exacerbations of tic and obsessive-compulsive symptoms: a prospective longitudinal study. *J Am Acad Child Adolesc Psychiatry* 2011; *50*:108–118.

Leckman JF, Riddle MA, Hardin MT et al. The Yale Global Tic Severity Scale (YGTSS): Initial testing of a clinician-rated scale of tic severity. *J Am Acad Child Adolesc Psychiatry* 1989; *28*:566–573.

The first study reporting the psychometric properties of the most widely used tic severity scale.

Leckman JF, Vaccarino FM, Kalanithi PS, Rothenberger A. Tourette syndrome: a relentless drumbeat—driven by misguided brain oscillations. *J Child Psychol Psychiatry* 2006; *47*:537–550.

Leckman JF, Walker DE, Cohen DJ. Premonitory urges in Tourette's syndrome. *Am J Psychiatry* 1993; *150*:98–102.

One of the initial descriptive cross-sectional studies of premonitory urges.

Leckman JF, Walker DE, Goodman WK et al. "Just right" perceptions associated with compulsive behavior in Tourette's syndrome. *Am J Psychiatry* 1994; *151*:675–680.

Leckman JF, Zhang H, Vitale A et al. Course of tic severity in Tourette syndrome: The first two decades. *Pediatrics* 1998; *102*:14–19.

The first study to use growth curve analyses and other statistical technique to model the course of tic severity over the first two decades of life.

Lin H, Katsovich L, Ghebremichael M et al. Psychosocial stress predicts future symptom severities in children and adolescents with Tourette syndrome and/or obsessive-compulsive disorder. *J Child Psychol Psychiatry* 2007; *48*:157–166.

Lin H, Williams KA, Katsovich L et al. Streptococcal upper respiratory tract infections and psychosocial stress predict future tic and obsessive-compulsive symptom severity in children and adolescents with Tourette syndrome and obsessive-compulsive disorder. *Biol Psychiatry* 2010; *67*:684–691.

Lin H, Yeh CB, Peterson BS et al. Assessment of symptom exacerbations in a longitudinal study of children with Tourette's syndrome or obsessive-compulsive disorder. *J Am Acad Child Adolesc Psychiatry* 2002; *41*:1070–1077.

Luo F, Leckman JF, Katsovich L et al. Prospective longitudinal study of children with tic disorders and/or obsessive-compulsive disorder: relationship of symptom exacerbations to newly acquired streptococcal infections. *Pediatrics* 2004; *113*:e578–585.

Mathews CA, Jang KL, Herrera LD et al. Tic symptom profiles in subjects with Tourette Syndrome from two genetically isolated populations. *Biol Psychiatry* 2007; *61*:292–300.

Meidinger AL, Miltenberger RG, Himle M et al. An investigation of tic suppression and the rebound effect in Tourette's disorder. *Behav Modif* 2005; *29*:716–745.

A seminal experimental study documenting the potential for enhancing tic suppression as a therapeutic avenue.

Miguel EC, do Rosário-Campos MC, Prado HS et al. Sensory phenomena in obsessive-compulsive disorder and Tourette's disorder. *J Clin Psychiatry* 2000; *61*:150–156.

O'Connor K, Brisebois H, Brault M et al. Behavioral activity associated with onset in chronic tic and habit disorder. *Behav Res Ther* 2003; *41*:241–249.

O'Connor KP, Gareau D, Blowers GH. Personal constructs associated with tics. *Br J Clin Psychol* 1994; *33*:151–158.

Peterson BS, Leckman JF. The temporal dynamics of tics in Gilles de la Tourette syndrome. *Biol Psychiatry* 1998; *44*:1337–1348.

An underappreciated report that likely points to a core aspect of what determines the timing of tics.

Peterson BS, Pine DS, Cohen P, Brook JS. Prospective, longitudinal study of tic, obsessive-compulsive, and attention-deficit/hyperactivity disorders in an epidemiological sample. *J Am Acad Child Adolesc Psychiatry* 2001; *40*:685–695.

Piacentini J, Himle MB, Chang S et al. Reactivity of observation procedures to situation and setting. *J Abnorm Child Psychol* 2006; *34*:647–656.

Piacentini J, Woods DW, Scahill L et al. Behavior therapy for children with Tourette disorder: a randomized controlled trial. *JAMA* 2010; *303*:1929–1937.

A multisite randomized controlled clinical trial documenting the benefits of Comprehensive

Behavioral Treatment for Tics for children with TS.

Rath JJ, Tavy DL, Wertenbroek AA et al. Botulinum toxin type A in simple motor tics: short-term and long-term treatment-effects. *Parkinsonism Relat Disord* 2010; 16:478–481.

Robertson MM, Althoff RR, Hafez A, Pauls DL. Principal components analysis of a large cohort with Tourette syndrome. *Br J Psychiatry* 2008; 193:31–36.

Robertson MM, Banerjee S, Eapen V, Fox-Hiley P. Obsessive compulsive behaviour and depressive symptoms in young people with Tourette syndrome: a controlled study. *Eur Child Adolesc Psychiatry* 2002; 11:261–265.

Robertson MM, Banerjee S, Kurlan R et al. The Tourette syndrome diagnostic confidence index: development and clinical associations. *Neurology* 1999; 53:2108–2112.

Robertson MM, Cavanna AE. The Gilles de la Tourette syndrome: a principal component factor analytic study of a large pedigree. *Psych Genet* 2007; 17:143–152.

Rosario MC, Prado HS, Borcato S. Validation of the University of São Paulo Sensory Phenomena Scale: initial psychometric properties. *CNS Spectr* 2009; 14:315–323.

Sacks O. *A surgeon's life. In: An Anthropologist on Mars: Seven Paradoxical Tales.* New York, Alfred A. Knopf, 1995.

Scahill L, Lombroso PJ, Mack G et al. Thermal sensitivity in Tourette syndrome: preliminary report. *Percept Motor Skills* 2001; 92:419–443.

Shapiro AK, Shapiro ES, Young JG, Feinberg TE. *Gilles de la Tourette Syndrome*, 2nd ed. New York, Raven Press, 1988.

Sides H. The sporting scene, "National Defense," *The New Yorker*, June 7, 2010, p. 54.

Silva RR, Munoz DM, Barickman J, Friedhoff AJ. Environmental factors and related fluctuation of symptoms in children and adolescents with Tourette's disorder. *J Child Psychol Psychiatry* 1995; 36:305–312.

Smith LB, Thelen E. Development as a dynamic system. *Trends Cogn Sci* 2003; 7:343–348.

Smith SJ, Lees AJ. Abnormalities in the blink reflex in Gilles de la Tourette syndrome. *J Neurol Neurosurg Psychiatry* 1989; 52:895–898.

Sukhodolsky DG, Scahill L, Zhang H et al. Disruptive behavior in children with Tourette's syndrome: Association with ADHD comorbidity, tic severity, and functional impairment. *J Am Acad Child Adolesc Psychiatry* 2003; 42: 98–105.

Sutherland Owens AN, Miguel EC, Swerdlow NR. Sensory gating scales and premonitory urges in Tourette syndrome. *Sci World Journal* 2011; 22:736–741.

Swerdlow NR, Karban B, Ploum Y et al. Tactile prepuff inhibition of startle in children with Tourette's syndrome: in search of an "fMRI-friendly" startle paradigm. *Biol Psychiatry* 2001; 50:578–585.

Torup E. A follow-up study of children with tics. *Acta Paediatr* 1962; 51:261–268.

Verdellen CW, Hoogduin CA, Kato BS et al. Habituation of premonitory sensations during exposure and response prevention treatment in Tourette's syndrome. *Behav Modif* 2008; 32:215–227.

A preliminary study pointing to the potential therapeutic value of Exposure and Response Prevention in TS.

Verdellen CW, Hoogduin CA, Keijsers GP. Tic suppression in the treatment of Tourette's syndrome with exposure therapy: the rebound phenomenon reconsidered. *Mov Disord* 2007; 22:1601–1606.

Watson TS, Dufrene B, Weaver A et al. Brief antecedent assessment and treatment of tics in the general education classroom: a preliminary investigation. *Behav Modif* 2005; 29:839–857.

Wittgenstein, L. *Philosophical Investigations.* Oxford, Blackwell, 1958.

Wood BL, Klebba K, Gbadebo O et al. Pilot study of effect of emotional stimuli on tic severity in children with Tourette's syndrome. *Mov Disord* 2003; 18:1392–1395.

Woods DW, Piacentini J, Himle MB, Chang S. Premonitory Urge for Tics Scale (PUTS): initial psychometric results and examination of the premonitory urge phenomenon in youths with tic disorders. *J Dev Behav Pediatr* 2005; 26:397–403.

The first published study reporting the psychometric properties of a scale specifically developed to rate the intensity of premonitory urges.

Woods DW, Walther MR, Bauer CC et al. The development of stimulus control over tics: a potential explanation for contextually-based variability in the symptoms of Tourette syndrome. *Behav Res Ther* 2009; 47:41–47.

Woods DW, Watson TS, Wolfe E et al. Analyzing the influence of tic-related talk on vocal and motor tics in children with Tourette's syndrome. *J Appl Behav Anal* 2001; 34:353–356.

Worbe Y, Mallet L, Golmard JL et al. Repetitive behaviours in patients with Gilles de la Tourette syndrome: tics, compulsions, or both? *PLoS One* 2010; 5:e12959.

Zebardast N, Crowley MJ, Bloch MH et al. Brain mechanisms for prepulse inhibition in adults with Tourette syndrome. *(submitted)*.

Zinner SH, Conelea CA, Glew GM et al. Peer victimization in youth with Tourette syndrome and other chronic tic disorders. *Child Psychiatry Hum Dev* 2012; 43: 124–136.

2

The Phenomenology of Attention-Deficit/ Hyperactivity Disorder in Tourette Syndrome

ARIBERT ROTHENBERGER AND VEIT ROESSNER

Abstract

This chapter focuses on the complex epidemiological and phenomenological aspects of attention-deficit/hyperactivity disorder (ADHD) in Tourette syndrome (TS). Research on this topic is relatively recent and has elucidated the importance of comorbidity in TS and the need for an early assessment for ADHD in TS. Several observational studies confirmed that ADHD is the most common comorbidity in TS (present in about 60% of cases), possibly anticipating TS onset and influencing the male gender predominance of TS. ADHD exerts a negative impact on externalizing and internalizing symptoms as well as on psychosocial functioning and quality of life in TS. The impact of comorbid ADHD upon sleep disturbances in TS remains a neglected issue. Approaches to model the coexistence of TS and ADHD are ongoing. Whereas basic neurobiological aspects fit with an additive model, complex cognitive functioning supports an interactive model. Specific pathophysiological features for TS plus ADHD have not yet been identified, but common heritability between TS and ADHD might be explained, at least in part, by the comorbidity of ADHD and OCD. Future studies on the phenomenology of TS plus ADHD should consider not only the core symptoms of TS and ADHD, but also obsessive-compulsive traits, emotional aspects, neuropsychological aspects, quality of life, early risk factors, resilience, and other possible mediators and moderators.

INTRODUCTION

The presentation of Tourette syndrome (TS) in the absence of other childhood-onset neuropsychiatric disorders is the exception rather than the rule. In TS as well as in attention-deficit/hyperactivity disorder (ADHD), about 80% of individuals show at least one additional behavioral problem. In tic disorders, ADHD coexists in about 50% of patients, while in ADHD cases, chronic tic disorders are seen in about 20%; both of these percentages are well above what would be expected by chance alone. The background of overlap and relationship, especially long term, between these two neuropsychiatric disturbances has been recognized as critical. Both TS and ADHD are common pediatric psychiatric disorders (with approximate frequency rates of 1% and 5%, respectively), which change in their symptom profile and prevalence rate during development.

In this chapter, we explore the co-occurrence of TS and ADHD. Initially, we provide some background information concerning ADHD before exploring the available epidemiological data. We then move on to focus on the diverse clinical consequences of the co-occurrence of TS and ADHD by initially taking a historical perspective. Subsequently, we review the complex, and at times contradictory, empirical data from cross-sectional and a few longitudinal studies with respect to clinical consequences and mutual modification associated with the co-occurrence of these two conditions. Relevant domains include the co-occurrence of other neuropsychiatric and behavioral disorders, as well as its adverse impact on cognitive performance, psychosocial functioning, and quality of life. We also highlight its negative impact on other crucially important biobehavioral domains, including the sleep–wake cycle.

In closing, we note that many important questions remain for future research, including how best to understand the diversity of the clinical presentation of TS and ADHD, and how that maps onto the etiological factors that contribute to these potentially disabling disorders.

CORE FEATURES OF ADHD

ADHD is characterized by the core symptoms of developmentally inappropriate levels of inattention, hyperactivity, and impulsivity. As Preuss and colleagues (2006) point out, the diagnosis is best made on the basis of observational data, parent and teacher reports, and a detailed clinical history. There are different approaches to the diagnosis of ADHD, with both the DSM-IV criteria of the American Psychiatric Association (1994) and the ICD-10 criteria for hyperkinetic disorder (HD) of the World Health Organisation (1992) being used. According to the DSM-IV criteria, symptoms of inattention and/or hyperactivity/impulsivity must persist for at least 6 months, be present before the age of 7 years, and cause impairment in two or more settings (e.g., at school and at home), and there must be clear evidence of clinically important impairment in social, academic, or occupational functioning. The ICD-10 criteria for HD are similar to DSM-IV criteria for ADHD-combined type, requiring all symptoms of inattention, hyperactivity, and impulsiveness to be present and pervasive and to result in functional impairment. Thus, the ICD-10 criteria select a smaller subgroup of children with more severe symptoms than those identified by the DSM-IV criteria (Taylor et al., 2004). Estimates of the prevalence of ADHD vary depending on the diagnostic criteria used within a study. However, there is general agreement that the prevalence of DSM-IV-defined ADHD is between 5% and 8%, and that of ICD-10-defined HD is around 1.5% (Taylor et al., 2004). Although ADHD is diagnosed in many European countries, the rates of diagnosis are much lower than those reported in the United States, and it is recognized that, in general, ADHD is underdiagnosed and undertreated by clinicians across Europe and in other parts of the world. Data from the United Kingdom and the Netherlands suggest low rates of referral and diagnosis and skepticism of medical professionals regarding the disorder (Ralston & Lorenzo, 2004). Both the DSM and ICD classification systems are currently under revision, with DSM-V expected to be released in 2013. Major changes in the diagnostic criteria for TS and ADHD are not expected (Coghill & Seth, 2011). The main suggestions for change are focused on improving the criteria for use in adults and making relatively minor adjustments to the content and number of criteria for the various subtypes (combined type vs. predominantly inattentive vs. predominantly hyperactive-impulsive), as well as changes to the inclusion and exclusion criteria.

CO-OCCURRENCE OF ADHD WITH OTHER EARLY-ONSET NEUROPSYCHIATRIC DISORDERS

ADHD rarely presents as an isolated disorder, frequently coexisting with other conditions, such as oppositional defiant disorder (ODD), conduct disorder (CD), learning disorders, anxiety, depression, epilepsy, and chronic tic disorders, including TS (Biederman et al., 1991; Pliszka, 2000). The presence of these coexisting conditions can complicate the diagnosis of ADHD, as well as contribute to the severity of the hyperactive/inattentive/impulsive symptoms (Taylor, 1998). ADHD also often results in significant academic, social, and emotional problems both at home and school. Children with severe ADHD often have low self-esteem, develop emotional and social problems due to difficulties with their peers, and frequently underachieve at school. Moreover, ADHD is a chronic disorder that often persists into adolescence and adulthood and is associated with continued impairment (Faraone & Tsuang, 2001). ADHD affects the daily lives not only of the affected child, but also of his or her family, and has a relevant impact on society in general. These difficulties can be compounded by the economic stress associated with parental work disruptions and medical care costs (Anastopoulos et al., 1992). For example, a European naturalistic observational trial (ADORE-Study, Ralston & Lorenzo,

2004) studied in 1,478 patients the impact of coexisting psychiatric problems with ADHD on a number of important outcomes, including psychosocial functioning and quality of life. Not surprisingly, having multiple coexisting neuropsychiatric disorders (including ODD/CD, anxiety/depression, chronic tic disorders, and developmental coordination disorder) increased the severity of ADHD in all domains. Hence, the ADORE-Study provided impressive evidence for the far-reaching consequences of coexisting psychiatric problems in children with ADHD that warrant intensive consideration in clinical assessment and treatment. However, these findings do not support the hypothesis that ADHD in combination only with TS forms a valid nosological subtype (Steinhausen et al., 2006).

EPIDEMIOLOGICAL AND HISTORICAL PERSPECTIVES ON TS/ADHD COMORBIDITY

Systematic research on the TS/ADHD comorbidity is relatively recent. Lucas and colleagues (1967) reported that 10 of 15 patients with tics had signs of minimal brain dysfunction (MBD), which during that period represented a proxy of what we call today ADHD. Only about 10 years later, Shapiro and colleagues (1978) tried to evaluate their sample of 145 TS patients by analyzing systematically the coexistence of MBD. Quoting from this publication, these "children were described as irritable, impulsive, never at rest, into everything, and having short attention spans and other symptoms of MBD" (Shapiro et al., 1978; pp. 114–118). Their TS sample yielded a surprisingly high frequency of 57.9% of patients with coexisting MBD, many of whom showed both tics and choreiform movements. The relationship between MBD and TS remained unclear.

A decade later, Shapiro and colleagues (1988) had gathered a much larger clinical sample of 666 TS patients, and diagnosed "attention deficit disorder plus hyperactivity" [ADD(+H)] along DSM-III criteria. Their retrospective analysis revealed the following main behavioral results: higher male/female ratio among TS+ADD(+H) patients; decreased ability to inhibit tics among TS+ADD(+H) patients; anticipation

of pleasant stimuli increased tics more among TS+ADD(+H) patients; listening to a lecture or sermon decreased symptoms only among TS-only and TS+ADD(-H) patients, but not among TS+ADD(+H) patients. Shapiro and colleagues (1988) concluded that, so far, studies of TS were confounded by the presence of TS+ADD(+H) patients, and that there was a need to control for this comorbidity to obtain clearer and more specific information on the phenomenology of TS. It became obvious that in clinical samples of children with tics, about 40% to 60% also had ADHD (Comings & Comings, 1988).

The frequency of co-occurrence of TS and ADHD from community samples was estimated to be around 10% to 20% (Rothenberger, 1991; Schlander et al., 2011). In particular, Schlander and colleagues (2011) provided information on the 12-month "administrative prevalence" of TS and other tic disorders. The highest rate of ADHD co-occurring with tic disorders was observed among adolescents, within an age range of 13 to 18 years (15.1%). Tic disorders were observed in 2.3% of patients with ADHD. Compared to other previous community-based epidemiological studies (e.g., Khalifa & von Knorring, 2006), these rates were rather low, suggesting that a large number of cases may remain undetected under the present conditions of routine outpatient care.

The Swedish study by Khalifa and von Knorring (2006) was conducted retrospectively over 1 year in a population of 4,479 children aged 7 to 15 years: 25 children had a diagnosis of TS, 34 had a chronic motor tic disorder (CMTD), 24 had a chronic vocal tic disorder (CVTD), and 214 had transient tics. In 92%, a comorbid disorder was found, consistent with other large clinical samples (Freeman, 2007; Freeman et al., 2000). Khalifa and von Knorring (2006) reported comorbid ADHD in 68% of TS patients (60% ADHD combined type), 33% of CVTD patients, 12% of CMTD patients, and 4% of patients with transient tics.

Olfson and colleagues (2011) reviewed U.S. health insurance company databases focusing on claims of TS diagnosis in a 4- to 18-year-old population over a 12-month period. Compared with privately insured youth, children under Medicaid diagnosed with TS had higher rates of ADHD

(50.2% vs. 25.9%). These rates of ADHD are somewhat lower than rates in samples drawn from specialty clinics (range 54–77%; Roessner et al., 2007a). The latter may be more liable to a referral bias, leading to the ascertainment of cases with higher rates of co-occurring conditions. It is also possible that community clinicians do not diagnose ADHD when tics dominate the clinical picture, and vice versa (Olfson et al., 2011). Consistent with this, in a naturalistic-observational study with a design similar to the one used by Schlander and colleagues (2011), Steinhausen and colleagues (2006) reported a prevalence of tic disorders of only about 9% in approximately 1,500 children with ADHD. The authors of these studies also underline that important differences exist in service use for different socioeconomic groups with TS plus ADHD. Overall, these findings suggest that our knowledge of ADHD phenomenology within TS might be, to a certain degree, biased by sample characteristics and related medical advice-seeking behavior. A challenge to this statement comes from another study (Coffey et al., 1997) that showed how previously undiagnosed patients with TS from the community shared essentially the same phenotypic, sociodemographic, and clinical correlates, including patterns of Axis I comorbidity, with TS patients who had been referred to and directly evaluated at a specialized TS clinic.

Overall, the similarity in the rates of co-occurrence of TS and ADHD in community and service-based populations, combined with the progressively increasing frequency of comorbid ADHD along a spectrum ranging from patients with transient tics to those with chronic tic disorder and then to TS, raises important issues concerning the role of genetic and environmental factors over the course of brain development (Shaw et al., 2007, 2011).

THE INFLUENCE OF ADHD/TS COMORBIDITY ON THE CLINICAL PRESENTATION OF THE TWO DISORDERS

The issue of ADHD modification with coexisting TS was addressed by Walkup and colleagues (1999) in a book chapter entitled "Phenomenology and natural history of

tic-related ADHD and learning disabilities." These authors noted the lack of studies rigorously comparing subjects with TS plus ADHD to those with ADHD only in order to identify differences in ADHD symptoms. On the other hand, the same authors stated that "compared to children with TS only, children with TS plus ADHD and those with only ADHD share a similar profile of co-morbid conditions—depression, anxiety, and disruptive behaviour—suggesting that the presence of multiple co-morbidities in TS is perhaps a function of the presence of ADHD and not specific to TS."

In a subsequent work, Spencer and colleagues (2001a) evaluated primarily differences in the course and neuropsychiatric features between five different subgroups of children (TS only, TS plus ADHD, ADHD only, psychiatric controls, normal controls). Although ADHD severity was rated as minimally more severe in children with TS plus ADHD compared to those with ADHD only, age of onset and duration of ADHD symptoms did not differ between these two groups. The frequencies of mood, disruptive, psychotic, and most of the anxiety disorders were identical in children with TS plus ADHD and children with ADHD only. In addition, the frequency of other psychiatric comorbidities was higher in children with ADHD and/or TS than in other psychiatric patients without ADHD or TS. The frequency of OCD was higher in children with TS (with or without comorbid ADHD) than in children with ADHD only. Of note, children with TS plus ADHD and children with ADHD only had greater psychosocial impairment (measured by Global Assessment of Functioning) than other psychiatric patients without ADHD or TS. In another work, children with TS plus ADHD were found to be more psychosocially impaired than children with ADHD only (Erenberg et al., 1987).

Other authors have identified subtle differences between patients with TS plus ADHD and TS only in some cognitive aspects, which are reviewed in greater detail in Chapter 20. Most of these differences can be attributed primarily to the diagnosis of ADHD (Greimel et al., 2011; Roessner et al., 2007b). In particular, given the well-established abnormality of executive functioning in ADHD, Denckla (2006) compared children with TS only,

TS plus ADHD, and ADHD only on the Behavior Rating Inventory of Executive Function (BRIEF). Both ADHD-only and TS-plus-ADHD groups were impaired on the five primary indices of the BRIEF. The BRIEF indices in the TS-only group were almost identical to those of the healthy control group, consistent with previous findings (Mahone et al., 2002). This direction of results was confirmed in several neuropsychological experiments from our group (Greimel et al., 2011; Roessner et al., 2006a, 2007b). A similar change was found also in motor coordination. Denckla (2006) points out:

> in many previous studies using the physical and neurological examination for soft signs (PANESS) for developmental neuromotor integrity, children with ADHD and TS plus ADHD showed slow-for-age timed movements, whereas most children with TS only performed all movements with normal speed and half of all movements faster than average [see also Schuerholz et al., 1997]. It can be stated that 76% of children who have TS only are faster than average on timed motor coordination.

INFLUENCE OF ADHD/TS COMORBIDITY ON CLINICAL ASSESSMENT OF TS

In the context of TS, the clinical recognition and assessment of comorbid ADHD, as well as the influence of ADHD comorbidity on the general assessment of TS patients, may represent challenges even for the well-trained and experienced clinician. For children, it is crucially important to secure data from multiple informants, including parents and school personnel. Direct observation in the classroom setting, when possible, is also highly desirable. Personalized treatment strategies are often necessary and may be aided by consulting experts' viewpoints and guidelines (Cath et al., 2011, Roessner et al., 2011). In addition, the core features of each of these two disorders may in some instances make the recognition of the core features of the other disorder difficult. Indeed, the phenomenology of the ADHD triad—hyperactivity, inattention, impulsivity—may in some cases be hardly differentiated from core elements of TS (e.g., bouts/series of tics, distraction by tics, rage tantrums related to urges associated with tics). If both these phenomenological triads are present, the complexity of the clinical picture may be difficult to disentangle, and the overall severity of this combination of symptoms quite high. Tables 2.1 and 2.2 summarize clinical features useful for a correct interpretation of TS and ADHD core phenomenology.

Moreover, choreiform movements and motor coordination problems belong to the spectrum of ADHD and are highly associated with the coexistence of a developmental coordination disorder (Fliers et al., 2012). An accurate neurological examination is warranted to

Table 2.1 Main Distinctive Features of Motor Abnormalities in Tic Disorders and ADHD

Tic Disorders	ADHD
Fragments of normal movements	Generally increased motor activity
Circumscribed functional muscle groups	Whole motor system involved
Suddenly occurring(independent of waiting situation)	Slowly increasing (intensified by waiting situation)
Fixed pattern of quick actions	Disorganized, tempo change
Badly modulated	Badly modulated
Uniformly repeated (often in timed bouts)	Irregular-intermittent, variable in timing(changing intensity)

Adapted from Cath et al., 2011.

Table 2.2 Distinctive Features of Tics and Stereotypies

Feature	Tics	Stereotypies
Age at onset (years)	6–7	<2
Pattern	Variable	Fixed, identical, foreseeable
Movement	Blinking, grimacing, warping, jerking	Arm-hands, wavelike, fluttering, jiggling
Rhythm	Quick, sudden, aimless, but not rhythmic	Rhythmic
Duration	Intermittent, short, abrupt	Intermittent, repeated, prolonged
Pre-movement sensorimotor phenomena	Yes1	No
Trigger	Excitement, stress	Excitement, stress, also in case of demands
Suppressibility	Self-directed, short (associated with increased inner pressure)	By external distraction, seldom conscious effort
Family history	Often positive	May be positive
Treatment	Primarily neuroleptics	Rarely responsive to medication

[1] Not always; increase in reported frequency with age
Stereotypies may constitute one of the behavioral abnormalities observed in TS plus ADHD.
Adapted from Cath et al., 2011.

differentiate tics from these other motor deficits and to assess their respective contribution to the overall impairment of patients (Kompoliti & Goetz, 1998).

Neuropsychological test batteries are generally recommended to assess overall cognitive functioning in both disorders (Cath et al., 2011; see Chapter 20). In this setting, the most psychometrically robust and easily applicable rating scale for this purpose is probably the BRIEF. Using this tool, Mahone and colleagues (2002) showed abnormalities of executive functions in ADHD patients, whereas executive functions seemed preserved in patients with TS only; in addition, both patients with ADHD only and patients with TS plus ADHD were rated as more impaired compared to patients with TS without ADHD and healthy controls. There was no significant correlation between data obtained from the inventory and performance-based executive functions or measures of psychoeducational competence; however, the BRIEF showed a strong relationship with interviews and other parent-based behavioral measures relevant to

ADHD. Hence, the BRIEF may aid the practitioner in screening for executive functions, which are important to predict the outcome of behavioral therapy (Döpfner & Rothenberger, 2007).

Finally, in addition to motor phenomena and executive functions, the co-occurrence of TS and ADHD presents with a complexity of psychopathological phenomena, which usually play a major role in long-term clinical care. This relevant aspect will be discussed in greater detail below.

ADHD/TS COMORBIDITY AND PSYCHOPATHOLOGICAL SPECTRUM OF TS PATIENTS

Reports from clinicians in 27 countries confirm that ADHD is the most common comorbidity in TS, estimated to affect approximately 60% of TS cases. The strength of the relationship between TS and ADHD is supported by a prospective study of at-risk young children with TS parents (McMahon et al., 2003). In this cohort,

29% of the children developed a tic disorder, whereas 41% received a diagnosis of ADHD at follow-up. In a subsequent worldwide clinical dataset of TS (Freeman, 2007), the prevalence of comorbid ADHD in TS, the relative proportions of the three ADHD subtypes, and the male predominance of comorbid ADHD were in line with other studies (Kurlan et al., 2002; Millstein et al., 1997; Murphy et al., 2002; Palumbo et al., 2005). Highly TS-specific features, such as coprophenomena, did not appear to be significantly associated with comorbid ADHD on logistic regression analyses. On the other hand, the presence of ADHD was associated with anticipation of the diagnosis of TS by 3.5 years, similar to previous works (Spencer et al., 2001b); this was more related to comorbidity for the ADHD combined subtype than for the ADHD inattentive subtype.

The effect of comorbid ADHD over the complex phenomenology of the TS spectrum has been analyzed in the context of factor analytic studies. For example, Robertson and colleagues (2008) included 410 TS patients in a factor analysis, observing the existence of five factors: (1) socially inappropriate behaviors and other complex vocal tics, (2) complex motor tics, (3) simple tics, (4) compulsive behaviors, and (5) touching self. Of note, individuals with co-occurring ADHD had significantly higher factor scores on factors (1) and (3). Another interesting input from factor analysis came from Grados and colleagues (2008) and from Mathews and Grados (2011), who observed that the subgroup of patients with the triple comorbidity TS plus OCD plus ADHD may represent a highly heritable phenotype. These authors suggest that the high degree of heritability of this triple comorbidity "may be due to a genetic association between OCD and ADHD and in part to shared environmental factors." Support for this finding came from O'Rourke and colleagues (2011), who concluded that the presence of OCD or subclinical OCD in a proband is associated with a significantly increased risk of comorbid tic disorder plus ADHD in his or her relatives. Additional research exploring in detail obsessive-compulsive behavior (OCB; i.e., the dimensional obsessive-compulsive symptoms

profile in the absence of a categorical diagnosis of OCD; see Chapter 3) could add further insight to this aspect, since patients with anxiety-related OCB might be more prone to OCD plus ADHD comorbidity. In contrast, non–anxiety-related OCB (e.g., a need for things to be "just right," and compulsions about symmetry, ordering, doing and redoing, as well as sensory phenomena) might be closer to TS only or TS plus ADHD. Interestingly, a recent study on children with chronic tic disorder aged 7 to 15 years suggested that the premonitory urge did not correlate with ADHD or anxiety but with OCB and depression (Steinberg et al., 2012).

The complex spectrum of psychiatric disorders that may occur in comorbidity with TS will be analyzed in greater detail in Chapter 4. In respect to the influence of ADHD comorbidity upon the full spectrum of psychopathology in TS patients, several works showed the most severe psychopathology and psychosocial impairment in patients with TS plus ADHD (Carter et al., 2000; Gadow et al., 2002; Kurlan et al., 2002; Pierre et al., 1999; Spencer et al., 1998; Sukhodolsky et al., 2003). Roessner and colleagues (2007c) showed that all comorbid disorders, with the exception of anxiety disorders, are significantly associated with ADHD comorbidity. Moreover, these authors reported that emotional problems are present in both chronic tic disorders and ADHD, while externalizing behavior is more closely related to ADHD. In particular, anger control problems, sometimes referred to as "rage," were shown to be related to comorbid ADHD, but neither to tic disorders without ADHD nor to other comorbidities (Budman et al., 2003; Freeman et al., 2000).

The relationship between the psychopathology spectrum and ADHD comorbidity in TS is still, however, an object of debate (Carter et al., 2000; Hoekstra et al., 2004, 2006; Lebowitz et al., 2012; Pierre et al., 1999; Spencer et al., 1998; Stephens & Sandor, 1999; Sukhodolsky et al., 2003). To gain further insight into the relationship between the psychopathology spectrum in children with chronic tic disorders (CTD, including CMTD, CVTD, and TS) and coexisting ADHD, Roessner and colleagues

(2007c) used the optimal 2 × 2 design analyzing the broad psychopathological profile of four large age- and gender-matched groups of patients (CTD only, n = 112; CTD plus ADHD, n = 82; ADHD only, n = 129; controls, n = 144). The eight subscales of the Child Behavior Checklist (CBCL; Achenbach, 1991) were used to evaluate similarities and differences in dimensional psychopathology in children with CTD and/or ADHD. This revealed the highest levels of psychopathology in patients with CTD plus ADHD, except on the Somatic Complaints subscale; no interaction was observed between CTD and ADHD on any subscales except on the Somatic Complaints subscale, strongly supporting the existence of an additive effect of CTD and ADHD on comorbid psychopathological profile. The contrasted analysis also revealed a greater weight of ADHD, compared to CTD, in determining the psychopathology of the comorbid group. The higher scores of psychopathology in the comorbid group (CTD plus ADHD) compared to both "pure" groups (CTD only, ADHD only) are consistent with other studies on children (Gadow et al., 2002; Kurlan et al., 2002; Pierre et al., 1999; Shin et al., 2001; Spencer et al., 1998), children and adults combined (Comings & Comings, 1987), and adolescents/adults (Comings 1985a, 1985b) with CTD. The main effect of ADHD on the subscales Aggressive Behavior and Delinquent Behavior is also in agreement with previous literature (Pierre et al., 1999; Sukhodolsky et al., 2003) and underlines the strong relationship of ADHD to externalizing psychopathology measured by the CBCL. Also, this finding is in line with prior observation that disruptive behavior and impairment of psychosocial functioning is associated with ADHD and not with the existence or severity of tics *per se* (Carter et al., 2000; Hoekstra et al., 2004; Shin et al., 2001; Spencer et al., 2001b; Stephens & Sandor, 1999; Sukhodolsky et al., 2003). For internalizing behaviors, the highest scores in both groups with CTD (CTD plus ADHD and CTD only) on the subscale Somatic Complaints is also consistent with other results (Carter et al., 2000; Hoekstra et al., 2004; Shin et al., 2001; Termine et al., 2006). In conclusion, Roessner and colleagues (2007c) showed that ADHD was strongly related to externalizing as well as internalizing psychopathology, whereas CTD was related to internalizing psychopathology in patients with coexisting CTD plus ADHD. There was only some overlap in a few scales reflecting internalizing behavior, supporting an additive model at this level of investigation.

This evidence supports the recommendation that treatment of ADHD should be the main focus of intervention in patients with TS plus ADHD, as suggested already by different authors (Banaschewski et al., 2006; Peterson & Cohen, 1998). This is also in accordance with the fact that ADHD symptoms generally impair cognitive, emotional, and social skills more severely than tics (Como, 2005; Roessner et al., 2007a; Sukhodolsky et al., 2003). In addition, TS follows a largely remitting course and has a limited impact on the course and outcome of individuals with ADHD across the life cycle (Spencer et al., 2001b). Furthermore, the mental effort required to suppress tics may accentuate inattention in ADHD (Brown & Dure, 2005), and attentional problems are negatively correlated with the ability to suppress tics (Himle & Woods, 2005) and positively with the severity of TS (Cardona et al., 2004). On the other hand, it has been shown that the TS diagnosis contributes to internalizing psychopathology in a similar way as ADHD. This should be considered for treatment planning when internalizing psychopathology contributes substantially to individual impairment, and implies that both tics and ADHD symptoms should be the target of therapy for such cases (Allen et al., 2005; Van Brunt et al., 2005).

Although several studies have been performed to disentangle the overlap between TS and ADHD (Spencer et al., 1998) using psychopathological (Roessner et al., 2007c), neurophysiological (Kirov et al., 2007a, 2007b, 2007c; Moll et al., 2001; Yordanova et al., 1996, 1997), neuropsychological (Mahone et al., 2002; Roessner et al., 2006a, 2006b, 2007b; Sherman et al., 1998; Shin et al., 2001), and other approaches, a definitive picture cannot be drawn yet. Family studies (Pauls et al., 1994) led to divergent hypotheses concerning the nature of the TS plus ADHD comorbidity (Banaschewski et al., 2007). Also, tics usually follow a remitting course after childhood, with improvement in late adolescence or early adulthood (Pappert et al., 2003). Further, comorbid ADHD commonly antedates tic onset, while OCB or OCD typically follows tic onset (Leckman, 2002). These observations on the natural history of these disorders strongly suggest that cross-sectional studies analyzing patients with TS plus ADHD are able to offer only a snapshot of a dynamic condition that changes rapidly and substantially over the years.

IMPACT OF ADHD/TS COMORBIDITY UPON DEVELOPMENTAL ASPECTS OF OTHER PSYCHIATRIC COMORBIDITIES IN CHRONIC TIC DISORDERS

Psychopathological studies of patients with TS have neglected to some extent the issue of multiple psychopathological comorbidity during the developmental period (Bruun & Budman, 2005), although the few prospective studies have provided data of great value (Peterson et al., 2001). Roessner and colleagues (2007a) conducted a study aimed at documenting the developmental aspects of other comorbidities in children and adolescents with TS without ADHD compared to TS plus ADHD using cross-sectional data from a large, worldwide clinical dataset (TIC database) of 5,060 individuals. The impact of ADHD upon characteristics related to developmental aspects of other psychiatric comorbidities was examined year-wise by logistic regression analysis. The evaluation yielded a complex picture of comorbid developmental psychopathology in TS that can be summarized by five main results:

1. There was a higher rate of comorbid conditions in the TS-plus-ADHD group compared to the TS-without-ADHD group in both children (5–10 years) and adolescents (11–17 years), although the increased rate of general comorbidity over time was more pronounced in the group without ADHD (Fig. 2.1A).

2. In the presence of ADHD there was a higher rate of OCD in children (5–10 years) but not in adolescents (11–17 years), congruent with the more pronounced, year-wise increase of comorbid OCD in the latter group (Fig. 2.1B).

3. Mood disorders were more frequent in children and adolescents with TS if ADHD was coexisting, but the increasing rate with age was independent of comorbidity with ADHD (Fig. 2.1C).

4. Although in children (5–10 years) there were slightly more anxiety disorders in TS plus ADHD compared to TS without ADHD, this difference was no longer detectable in adolescents (11–17 years). This is congruent with the higher year-wise increase of anxiety problems in TS without ADHD (Fig. 2.1D).

5. The rate of comorbid conduct disorder (CD) and oppositional defiant disorder (ODD) was much higher in children and adolescents with TS plus ADHD: in both groups (TS without ADHD and TS plus ADHD), there was a similar year-wise increase of comorbid CD/ODD (Fig. 2.1E).

Two aspects of these findings deserve a more detailed consideration. First, with respect to tics, comorbid ADHD was associated with an earlier onset of tics, while the presence or absence of further comorbid conditions did not seem to play a major role. This is in line with the findings by Shapiro and colleagues (1988) and Spencer and colleagues (2001a) that younger age of onset predicted comorbid ADHD. This was not found for lifetime peak tic severity: children with TS plus ADHD showed the same lifetime peak tic severity of those without ADHD. Consistent with the earlier reports, a more recent study of 158 youth with TS found that individuals with TS plus ADHD did not differ from those with TD only on measures of tic severity (Lebowitz et al., 2012). In contrast, several earlier studies reported an association of severity of tic symptoms with behavioral disturbances (Comings & Comings, 1987; de Groot et al., 1995; Randolph et al., 1993; Rosenberg et al., 1995), although with some exceptions (Edell-Fischer & Motta 1990; Singer & Rosenberg, 1989; Stokes et al., 1991). Hence, tic severity might be partly related to comorbid conditions but not to ADHD *per se*. The same could be stated in terms of the

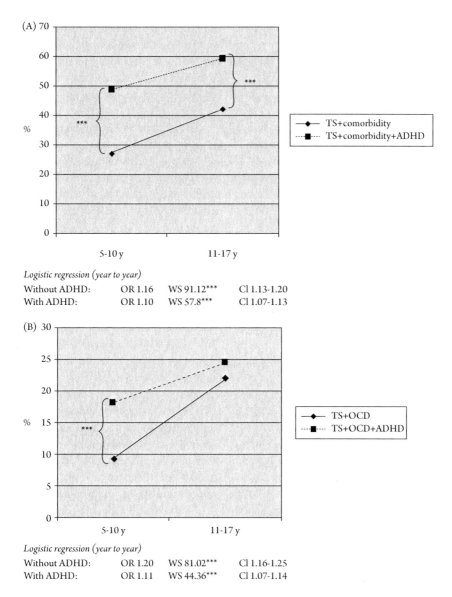

Logistic regression (year to year)
Without ADHD: OR 1.16 WS 91.12*** CI 1.13-1.20
With ADHD: OR 1.10 WS 57.8*** CI 1.07-1.13

Logistic regression (year to year)
Without ADHD: OR 1.20 WS 81.02*** CI 1.16-1.25
With ADHD: OR 1.11 WS 44.36*** CI 1.07-1.14

FIGURE 2.1 Year-wise changes in comorbidity rates in children and adolescents with TS without ADHD versus TS plus ADHD in (**A**) proportion of children with comorbid conditions, (**B**) obsessive-compulsive disorders (OCD), (**C**) anxiety disorders, (**D**) conduct disorder (CD)/oppositional defiant disorder (ODD), and (**E**) mood disorders. The asterisks at brackets give level of significance of group comparison (TS without ADHD vs. TS plus ADHD) for both age groups (5–10 years, 11–17 years). OR, odds ratio; WS, Wald statistic, CI, confidence interval. OR indicates year-wise change in the rate of comorbidities, WS gives level of significance; if CI of TS without ADHD and TS plus ADHD are not overlapping, there is a group difference in the year-wise change of rate of comorbidities; $p < .05$, *** $p < .001$. (See color insert.)

(From Roessner et al., 2007a.)

duration between onset of first tics and diagnosis of TS—that is, in the "comorbidity groups" the diagnosis of TS might have been given later than in TS-only patients. Similarly, further comorbidities are much more strongly associated with later referral to one of the tertiary centers after the onset of first tics than the presence of ADHD *per se*.

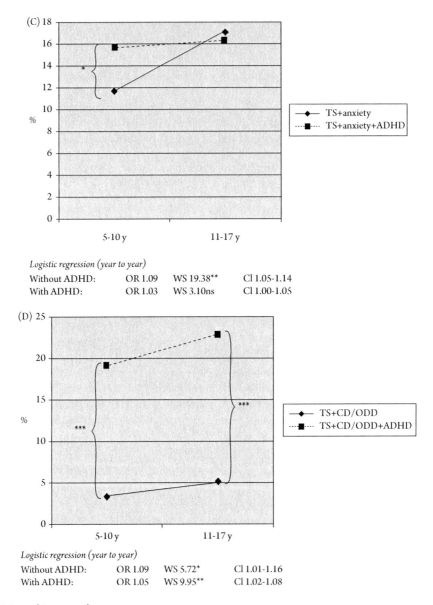

(C)

Logistic regression (year to year)
Without ADHD: OR 1.09   WS 19.38**   CI 1.05-1.14
With ADHD: OR 1.03   WS 3.10ns   CI 1.00-1.05

(D)

Logistic regression (year to year)
Without ADHD: OR 1.09   WS 5.72*   CI 1.01-1.16
With ADHD: OR 1.05   WS 9.95**   CI 1.02-1.08

FIGURE 2.1   (*Continued*)

A second aspect to consider is that data on the influence of age on the rate of comorbidity in TS are limited. In a study of 21 children with TS, where the parent-completed Behavior Problem Checklists was applied, the authors failed to reveal a relationship to age (Wodrich et al., 1997), while the incidence of behavioral and social problems, measured with the CBCL, in a group of children and adolescents with TS aged 6 to 11 years (n = 48) was higher than in a group aged 12 to 16 years (n = 30)

(Singer & Rosenberg, 1989). Excluding CD/ODD and OCD, Gadow and colleagues (2002) found in a sample of preschool children that the TS-without-ADHD group had more comorbidities than the TS-plus-ADHD group, whereas in schoolchildren the opposite was observed, and in adolescents the two groups were indistinguishable. Nevertheless, longitudinal data (Burd et al., 2001) on intraindividual comorbid psychopathology throughout development revealed a decrease of the number of comorbidities at a

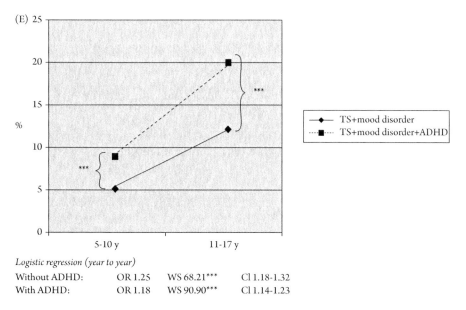

Logistic regression (year to year)

Without ADHD:	OR 1.25	WS 68.21***	Cl 1.18-1.32
With ADHD:	OR 1.18	WS 90.90***	Cl 1.14-1.23

FIGURE 2.1   (*Continued*)

follow-up of 13 years, which was less pronounced than the decrease of tic severity. The presented rates of OCD (including its increase with older age) are in accordance with previous studies in children with TS from clinic-based (Bloch et al., 2006; Cardona et al., 2004; Coffey et al., 2000; Freeman et al., 2000; Peterson et al., 2001) as well as community-based samples (Burd et al., 2001; Kadesjö & Gillberg 2000; Khalifa & von Knorring, 2006). The similar rate of comorbid OCD between the TS-without-ADHD and the TS-plus-ADHD groups of adolescents is in line with the findings of Spencer and colleagues (1998) but in contrast to the statement by Budman and colleagues (1998) that OCD is closely associated with ADHD in this age group. Gadow and colleagues (2002) reported in preschool children of their community-based sample a lack of difference between the TS-without-ADHD and the TS-plus-ADHD groups on OCD symptom scores. This is in contrast with the higher rate in younger children with TS plus ADHD observed by Roessner and colleagues (2007a). However, Gadow and colleagues (2002) found a strong co-occurrence of OCD and ADHD among younger schoolchildren (6–12 years), which reversed among older schoolchildren (13–18 years): this may

reflect the well-known decrease of ADHD and increase of OCD in the older schoolchildren (Bloch et al., 2006; Leckman et al., 2003). The higher rate of comorbid anxiety disorders in the presence of ADHD in younger patients was no longer detectable in older patients, because only in the TS-without-ADHD group did the rate of comorbid anxiety disorders increase with age. These findings are in line with previous reports. Generally, elevated rates (8–51%) of trait anxiety, phobias, generalized anxiety disorder, and separation anxiety have been described in people with TS (Coffey et al., 1992, 2000; Comings & Comings, 1987; Erenberg et al., 1987; Freeman et al., 2000; Pauls et al., 1994) and seem to change in profile along child development. Whereas the frequency of multiple anxiety disorders in TS children was estimated by Spencer and colleagues (2001b) to be approximately 40% independently from comorbid ADHD, the percentage of categorically defined social phobia was greater in children with TS plus ADHD compared to children with TS without ADHD (18% vs. 6%). This conflicts with the dimensional finding of more specific phobias (adolescents only) and social phobias (children only) in the TS-without-ADHD than in the TS-plus-ADHD group in a large, community-based sample of children and adolescents (Gadow et al., 2002). In contrast, higher generalized anxiety symptom scores were found in the TS-plus-ADHD group than in the TS-without-ADHD group independently of age. This seems to reflect that both TS and ADHD might independently be related to anxiety problems in children with TS plus ADHD.

The higher rate of comorbid CD/ODD independently of age in the present TS-plus-ADHD group compared to the TS-without-ADHD group is in line with several other studies that have found a higher incidence of CD/ODD behavior in the TS-plus-ADHD group compared to TS-only groups and healthy controls, but was at the same level as seen in ADHD-only groups (Carter et al., 2000; Stephens & Sandor, 1999; Sukhodolsky et al., 2003). This view is also supported by studies reporting that ODD is present in 71% of children with TS plus ADHD (Biederman et al., 1992, Randolph et al., 1993) but in only 39% of children with TS without ADHD (Spencer et al., 1998). Furthermore, CD was present more rarely: in 20% of children with TS plus ADHD (Milberger et al., 1997; Randolph et al., 1993) and in 11% of children with TS without ADHD (Erenberg et al., 1987). Accordingly, Comings and Comings (1987) also found higher rates of CD symptoms in the TS-plus-ADHD group than in the TS-without-ADHD group. In the sample studied by Roessner and colleagues (2007a), the rate of comorbid CD/ODD increased with age in TS independently of comorbid ADHD. In the epidemiological study by Gadow and colleagues (2002), the symptom scores of CD/ODD remained stable throughout development only in the TS-plus-ADHD group. In sum, the data indicate heterogeneous developments for CD/ODD in relation to TS and ADHD, with a stronger impact of ADHD. This assumption might be supported by the impression from Roessner and colleagues (2007a) that the rate of comorbid CD/ODD was higher in the TS-plus-ADHD group regardless of age, which might reflect a reduction of behavioral inhibition in patients with TS plus ADHD, contributing to their externalizing problems. Roessner and colleagues (2007a) also found that the presence of ADHD was associated with a higher

rate of comorbid mood disorders in younger as well as in older children. The rate of comorbid mood disorders, however, increased with age in TS, independently of co-occurring ADHD. Comings and Comings (1987) found no differences in the frequency of depression between children with TS with (n = 246) and without ADHD (n = 15). Accordingly, there was no difference in 16 children with TS without ADHD and 33 children with TS plus ADHD on the Kovacs Child Depression Inventory (Carter et al., 2000). In contrast, the symptom scores in all age groups (3–18 years) of a community-based sample of children and adolescents were higher in the TS-plus-ADHD group than in the TS-without-ADHD group (Gadow et al., 2002). In another study, slightly more children in the TS-plus-ADHD group (10 of 52) had depression, compared to 6 of 42 children with TS without ADHD (Sukhodolsky et al., 2003). In terms of mania, finally, no categorical data on the impact of ADHD have been published. It has been reported that there was a higher percentage of patients with TS plus ADHD with elevated mania scores (24.3%) compared to patients with TS without ADHD (10.7%) (Kerbeshian et al., 1995). Given the difference in assessment protocols, inventories, age groups, sample size, and the definition of mania used in children and adolescents, further research on mood disorders is needed to clarify this issue (Gaze et al., 2006).

Children and adolescents with tics need a comprehensive assessment of comorbid symptoms, given the implications on psychosocial impairment (Casey et al., 2000) and clinical management (Robertson, 2006; Robertson & Stern, 2000). In particular, comorbid ADHD has a negative impact on several psychopathological (Roessner et al., 2007a, 2007c), cognitive (Roessner et al., 2006a), and psychosocial (Carter et al., 2000) domains. It seems unlikely that the behavioral problems intervening during childhood in TS patients are predominantly transient phenomena (Carter et al., 1994); on the contrary, the rate of behavioral problems tends to increase over time in many children, even in the face of seemingly improved tics (Bruun et al., 2005).

IMPACT OF ADHD ON SLEEP DISTURBANCES IN TS

Sleep disturbances represent a relevant and peculiar aspect of ADHD psychopathology (Taylor, 2009), to the extent that sleep problems—including REM sleep (Kirov et al., 2007a, 2007b) abnormalities and increased nocturnal motor activity (Konofal et al., 2001) or restlessness (restless legs-like symptoms)—may be related to the appearance of ADHD symptoms and cognition during the day (Brown & McMullen, 2001; Corkum et al., 2001; Kirov et al., 2011; Lewin & DiPinto, 2004, Rothenberger & Kirov, 2005). Also, patients with TS plus ADHD present as many sleep problems as TS patients with a burden of five other comorbidities (TIC consortium, unpublished observation). Further, parents of ADHD patients report in their children resistance to going to bed, difficulty falling asleep, night awakenings, breathing problems such as snoring, and excessive daytime sleepiness (Taylor, 2009). Similarly, sleep disturbances (e.g., tics during the night, parasomnias) in patients with TS are frequent and may worsen daytime tic severity (Cohrs et al., 2001; Kostanecka-Endress et al., 2003; Rothenberger et al., 2001). Along with the high rate of coexistence of TS and ADHD, these observations point to the great clinical importance of sleep research in patients with this comorbidity. Research should address the issue as to whether these sleep problems appear additively as expected from polysomnographic parameters (Kirov et al., 2007a, 2007b, 2007c) or, alternatively, children with TS plus ADHD exhibit sleep patterns that are qualitatively different from each of the two isolated conditions.

To the best of our knowledge, only two studies used sleep questionnaires in patients with TS plus ADD/H (Comings & Comings, 1987) and TS plus ADHD (Allen et al., 1992), both cited and critically evaluated by Rothenberger and colleagues (2001). A higher frequency of sleep difficulties was related to comorbidity with ADD/H and ADHD, respectively, as well as to the severity of TS, but Allen and colleagues (1992) found similar percentages in ADHD-only patients (48%) and TS-plus-ADHD patients (41%), while sleep problems were present in only 26% of TS-only patients and in 10% of normal control subjects. Freeman (2007) also suggested that TS plus ADHD carries a higher risk for sleep difficulties in children. It would appear that new studies with updated methodology and sufficiently large and well-characterized samples are needed to gain further insight into behavioral sleep disorders in children with TS plus ADHD.

IMPACT OF ADHD ON PSYCHOSOCIAL IMPAIRMENT AND QUALITY OF LIFE

When parents bring their child with tics for a specialist consultation, the final and probably most important question for them is if there is a chance that their child will be able to function as well as other children in school, with peers, and in the community—that is, psychosocial functioning is a primary objective of consultation. Thus, after the assessment, the physician should consider carefully the profile of psychopathology (e.g., co-occurring ADHD) and symptom severity (e.g., frequent and severe coprolalia).

From cross-sectional as well as longitudinal research on TS samples, we know that mainly ADHD and OCB/OCD are associated with psychosocial impairment, while tic severity seems less important. For example, Spencer (1998) showed that 49% of children with TS and severe ADHD were enrolled in special classes, compared to only 18% of children with TS and no, mild, or moderate ADHD. In these patients, the average level of psychosocial functioning was unaffected by tic severity. In contrast, the severity of ADHD symptoms was associated with a significantly lower Global Activity Scale (GAS) score; functional characteristics of the Global Assessment Functioning (GAF) revealed a similar direction (TS plus ADHD 47.3; ADHD-only 50.0; TS without ADHD 52.5; psychiatric controls 56.3; normal controls 68.7). These results further support that psychosocial impairment of TS seems secondary to comorbidity with ADHD.

Disruptive behavior in children with TS and its relationship to ADHD is still a topic of investigation (Gorman et al., 2010; Rothenberger et al., 2007a, 2007b). Sukhodolsky and colleagues (2003) focused on this point, studying four large groups of children (42 TS only, 52 ADHD only, 52 TS plus ADHD, 61 unaffected controls). All three groups with psychiatric diagnoses scored significantly below controls on the Social Competence scale of the CBCL, not differing from each other. The TS-only group did not differ from unaffected controls in the Vineland Communication and Socialization domains and was significantly better than the TS-plus-ADHD and ADHD-only groups in the Socialization domain. The TS-plus-ADHD and ADHD-only groups did not differ from each other and were significantly below unaffected controls in all three domains. With respect to family functioning, significant main effects of diagnostic status were also observed on the Family Environment Scale (FES) Conflict and Cohesion scales, but not on the Control scale. The TS-plus-ADHD children lived in families with significantly greater levels of family dysfunction than unaffected controls, reflected by the higher mean scores on the Conflict and Cohesion scales. There was no significant mean score difference between the TS-plus-ADHD and ADHD-only groups in any area of family functioning. The TS-only group did not differ from unaffected controls on any of the Family Environment scales. There was an additional impact of disruptive behavior on Functional Outcome. A diagnosis of TS significantly predicted impairment only on the CBCL Social Competence scale. ADHD, on the other hand, significantly predicted all measures of functional outcome included in the regression analysis. A smaller study (Carter et al., 2000) reached similar results, namely that "much of the social and behavioural dysfunction in children with TS is ADHD-specific and children with TS alone have a very different social-emotional profile than do those with TS plus ADHD. Finally, social-emotional adjustment in children with TS is best understood within the family context." This study also stressed that the psychosocial resources of TS families depend on the coping capabilities of their members. For example, if a child has TS plus ADHD and another member (sibling, parent) suffers from ADHD

(even subclinical), an adequate regulation of interactive stress might be difficult, with the risk of increasing symptomatology and psychological family burden. Hence, psychoeducation related to the greater social and emotional risk of children with TS plus ADHD is important, as well as long-term monitoring and guidance of the family in order to minimize family stress (for a more detailed review of social functioning and psychoeducational interventions in TS, see Chapters 21 and 22).

A second highly important question of parents is if the child will grow out of the disorder or what psychosocial outcome might be expected in the future, given the variability of long-term course in TS (reviewed in greater detail in Chapter 5). Previous longitudinal studies found that patients with TS functioned quite well when followed up into early adulthood. This was supported by a study by Gorman and colleagues (2010), who compared psychosocial outcomes and lifetime comorbidity rates in 65 adolescents with TS followed up to around 18 years of age to age-matched healthy controls. Although adolescents with TS had lower GAS scores (56.4 vs. 70.4) and Vineland Socialization domain standard scores (84.5 vs. 101.1) at the end of the follow-up period, their poorer psychosocial outcome was associated mainly with their ADHD symptomatology, and to a lesser extent with OCD and tic severity.

The negative influence of ADHD on psychosocial outcome was also underlined by the follow-up study by Spencer and colleagues (2001b) on 132 adults with TS plus ADHD and 252 with TS without ADHD. Comparing ADHD patients with (n = 36) and without (n = 27) tics yielded differences that were accounted for by ADHD only in most outcome measures related to school performances (e.g., number of repeated grades, placement in special classes, in-school tutoring, GAF score). Also, the presence of tic disorder in children with ADHD had no discernible impact on ADHD outcome assessed in multiple noncompeting domains of functioning.

Finally, studies using quality-of-life (QoL) measurements came to the conclusion that also tics in their own right, especially when severe, may reduce QoL (Eddy et al., 2011). The degree of QoL impairment is highly dependent on the subjective view and family context, and coexisting psychopathological conditions like OCD and ADHD make an important contribution in determining which aspects of QoL are most affected in the individual.

RECENT ADVANCES IN MODELING THE COEXISTENCE OF TS AND ADHD AND CONCLUDING REMARKS

The overlap and relationship between CTD (including TS) and ADHD have been recognized as critical with respect to clinical as well as pathophysiological aspects (Doepfner & Rothenberger 2007; Poncin et al., 2007; Rothenberger & Banaschewski 2006). Accordingly, the question as to whether the co-occurrence of CTD and ADHD in children represents a combination of two independent pathologies (additive model), a separate nosological entity manifested by both tics and ADHD symptoms (interactive model), or a phenotypical subgroup of one of the two major clinical forms (phenotype model) has received increased attention (Banaschewski et al., 2006; Kirov et al., 2007a, 2007b; Moll et al., 2001; Rothenberger et al., 2000; Sukhodolsky et al., 2007; Yordanova et al., 2006). So far, a stepwise model is proposed (Banaschewski et al., 2006; Yordanova et al., 2006) according to which CTD/ADHD comorbidity can be classified at different levels, from basic neurobiological aspects to complex cognitive functions, showing that basic features like motor inhibition and sleep-profile impairment are merely additive, while data from higher mental functions, like cognitive stimulus evaluation, support the interactive model for CTD plus ADHD—that is, the higher the cognitive impact for task performance or behavior, the more the interaction of neuronal networks comes into play and displays the special characteristics of CTD/ADHD comorbidity, including neurobiological markers that can be found only in the comorbid condition. Also, the neurodynamics of brain oscillations have to be taken into account in this respect (Leckman et al., 2006; Rothenberger, 2009; Sukhodolsky

et al., 2007; Yordanova et al., 2006). Fortunately, research interest in the comorbidity of CTD plus ADHD has increased. For example, the specific PubMed search "Tourette and ADHD" rose from 340 titles up to June 2005 to 616 titles up to July 2011. Using a combination of these two words with the third word "comorbidity," we found 90 titles up to June 2005 and 160 titles up to July 2011, reflecting both increasing clinical impact and future needs.

The main conclusions from recent empirical studies on CTD/ADHD comorbidity are summarized below, giving some indications on possible main objectives for future research (see Rothenberger et al., 2007b):

- CTD and ADHD do not seem to be alternate phenotypes of a single underlying genetic cause. The increasing risk of comorbid CTD and ADHD in affected families might, however, reflect etiological commonalities between CTD and ADHD (Banaschewski et al., 2007; Stewart et al., 2006; Yordanova et al., 2006).
- In CTD plus ADHD, the ADHD component does not seem to be associated with tic severity but rather with learning disabilities, cognitive dysfunction, disruptive behavior, emotional problems, and social dysfunction. The direct influence of tic severity and persistence on these aspects is less clear and needs further investigation (Burd et al., 2005, 2006; Carter et al., 2000; Denckla, 2006; Erenberg, 2005; Khalifa & von Knorring 2006; Lebowitz et al., 2012; Roessner et al., 2006a, 2007a, 2007b; Scahill et al., 2005, 2006; Spencer et al., 1998; Sukhodolsky et al., 2003; Zhu et al., 2006).
- In CTD plus ADHD, the CTD component does not seem to increase significantly ADHD and other psychopathological symptoms, nor the clinical severity of ADHD or psychosocial functioning or QoL (Steinhausen et al., 2006).
- CTD plus ADHD has many neurophysiological and neuropsychological similarities to ADHD only (Banaschewski et al., 2006; Denckla, 2006; Kirov et al., 2007a, 2007b, Roessner et al., 2007a; Sukhodolsky et al., 2003).

- Children with CTD only appear to have a unique pattern of deficits in procedural learning that are distinct from the pattern of motor or executive control deficits seen in children with ADHD (Denckla, 2006; Roessner et al., 2007b; Marsh et al., 2004).

At the level of broadband psychopathology, an additive model of CTD plus ADHD is suggested by the available data. However, it should be noted that children with comorbidity are often more impaired than children with the isolated disorders. Suppression of tics may accentuate inattention in ADHD (Brown & Dure, 2005); correspondingly, attentional problems are correlated with the severity of TS (Cardona et al., 2004) but inversely associated with the ability to suppress tics (Himle & Wood, 2005). In children with comorbidity, ADHD has been identified as more disruptive than TS, but anxiety and depressive symptoms were equally or more strongly influenced by TS (Peterson et al., 2001; Roessner et al., 2007c; Spencer et al., 2001a). Thus, ADHD-related symptomatology is the primary treatment target in most comorbid patients (Peterson & Cohen, 1998).

Within this framework it seems important to control precisely for *confounders* like gender, since the frequency of CTD plus ADHD may be different between boys and girls. For example, Freeman (2007) found TS plus ADHD in 55% of boys but only 36% of girls from a population of 1,703 pediatric patients. Also, this study showed that the ratio of boys versus girls was higher for CTD plus ADHD (7:1; n = 47) and ADHD only (8:1; n = 289) compared to CTD only (3:1, n = 119), suggesting that ADHD but not CTD increased the rates of boys in CTD plus ADHD.

In conclusion, the characterization of the comorbidity of TS and ADHD has been significantly refined during the past decade (Box 2.1). Early screening and assessment of TS patients for ADHD is recommended (see also Chapter 18). Even subclinical (below diagnostic threshold) ADHD symptoms deserve close monitoring and, in some cases, multimodal treatment, given the associated risk for psychosocial impairment. Box 2.2 summarizes the main aspects that should be addressed by future studies exploring phenomenological aspects of TS plus ADHD.

Box 2.1. Key Points

- Research on the phenomenology of TS plus ADHD is relatively recent and has elucidated the importance of comorbidity in TS and the need for an early assessment of ADHD in TS.
- Several observational studies have confirmed that ADHD is the most common comorbidity in TS (present in about 60% of cases), possibly anticipating TS onset and influencing the male gender predominance of TS. ADHD exerts a negative impact on externalizing and internalizing symptoms, as well as on psychosocial functioning and QoL in TS.
- The impact of comorbid ADHD upon sleep disturbances in TS remains a neglected issue.
- Approaches to model the coexistence of TS and ADHD are ongoing. Whereas basic neurobiological aspects fit with an additive model, complex cognitive functioning supports an interactive model.
- Specific pathophysiological features for TS plus ADHD have not yet been identified, but common heritability between TS and ADHD might be explained, at least in part, by the comorbidity of ADHD and OCD.
- Future studies on the phenomenology of TS plus ADHD should consider not only the core symptoms of TS and ADHD, but also OCB traits, emotional aspects, neuropsychological aspects, QoL, early risk factors, resilience, and other possible mediators and moderators.

REFERENCES

Achenbach TM. *Manual for the Child Behavior Checklist/4–18 and 1991 Profile*. Burlington, VT: University of Vermont, Department of Psychiatry, 1991.

Allen AJ, Kurlan RM, Coffey BJ et al. Atomoxetine treatment in children with ADHD and comorbid tic disorders. *Neurology* 2005; 65:1941–1949.

Allen RP, Singer HS, Brown JE, Salam MM. Sleep disorder in Tourette syndrome: a primary or unrelated problem? *Pediatr Neurol* 1992; 8:275–280.

American Psychiatric Association. Diagnostic and Statistical Manual of Mental Disorders (4th ed.). American Psychiatric Association, Washington, DC., 1994.

Anastopoulos AD, Guevremont DC, Shelton TL, DuPaul GJ. Parenting stress among families of children with attention deficit hyperactivity disorder. *J Abn Child Psychol* 1992; 20:503–520.

Banaschewski T, Coghill D, Santosh P et al. Long-acting medications for the hyperkinetic disorders: a systematic review and European treatment guideline. *Eur Child Adolesc Psychiatry* 2006; 15:476–495.

Banaschewski T, Hollis C, Oosterlaan J et al. Towards an understanding of unique and shared pathways in the psychopathophysiology of ADHD. *Dev Sci* 2005; 8:132–140.

Banaschewski T, Neale BM, Rothenberger A, Roessner V. Comorbidity of tic disorders and ADHD—conceptual and methodological considerations. *Eur Child Adolesc Psychiatry* 2007; 16 (Suppl 1):I/5–I/14. **A comprehensive commentary on TS-plus-ADHD modeling.**

Biederman J, Faraone SV, Keenan K et al. Further evidence for family-genetic risk factors in attention deficit hyperactivity disorder. Patterns of comorbidity in probands and relatives psychiatrically and pediatrically referred samples. *Arch Gen Psychiatry* 1992; 49:728–738.

Biederman J, Newcorn J, Sprich S. Comorbidity of attention deficit hyperactivity disorder with conduct, depressive, anxiety, and other disorders. *Am J Psychiatry* 1991; 148:564–577.

Bloch MH, Peterson BS, Scahill L et al. Adulthood outcome of tic and obsessive-compulsive symptom severity in children with Tourette syndrome. *Arch Pediatr Adolesc Med* 2006; 160:65–69.

Brown L, Dure LS. The treatment of comorbid attention-deficit disorder and Tourette's syndrome. In: Kurlan R (Ed.), *Handbook of Tourette's syndrome and related tic and behavioural disorders*. Marcel Dekker, New York, 2005, pp. 455–465.

Brown TE, McMullen WJ. Attention deficit disorders and sleep/arousal disturbance. *Ann NY Acad Sciences* 2001; 931:271–286.

Bruun RD, Budman CL. The natural history of Gilles de la Tourette Syndrome. In: Kurlan R (Ed.), *Handbook of Tourette's syndrome and related tic and behavioral disorders*. Marcel Decker, New York, 2005, pp. 23–38.

Budman CL, Bruun RD, Park KS, Olson ME. Rage attacks in children and adolescents with Tourette's disorder: a pilot study. *J Clin Psychiatry* 1998; 59:576–580.

Budman CL, Rockmore L, Stokes J, Sossin M. Clinical phenomenology of episodic rage in children with Tourette syndrome. *J Psychosom Res* 2003; 55:59–65.

Burd L, Freeman RD, Klug MG, Kerbeshian J. Tourette syndrome and learning disabilities. *BMC Pediatr* 2005; 5:34–40.

Burd L, Freeman RD, Klug MG, Kerbeshian J. Variables associated with increased tic severity in

5,500 patients with Tourette syndrome. *J Dev Phys Disabil* 2006; *18*:13–24.

Burd L, Kerbeshian PJ, Barth A et al. Long-term follow-up of an epidemiologically defined cohort of patients with Tourette syndrome. *J Child Neurol* 2001; *16*:431–437.

Cardona F, Romano A, Bollea L, Chiarotti F. Psychopathological problems in children affected by tic disorders—study on a large Italian population. *Eur Child Adolesc Psychiatry* 2004; *13*:166–171.

Carter AS, O'Donnell DA, Schultz RT et al. Social and emotional adjustment in children affected with Gilles de la Tourette's syndrome: associations with ADHD and family functioning. *J Child Psychol Psychiatry* 2000; *41*:215–223.

Carter AS, Pauls DL, Leckman JF, Cohen DJ. A prospective longitudinal study of Gilles de la Tourette's syndrome. *J Am Acad Child Adolesc Psychiatry* 1994; *33*:377–385.

Casey MB, Cohen M, Schuerholz LJ et al. Language-based cognitive functioning in parents of offspring with ADHD comorbid for Tourette syndrome or learning disabilities. *Dev Neuropsychol* 2000; *17*:85–110.

Cath DC, Hedderly T, Ludolph AG et al. European clinical guidelines for Tourette syndrome and other tic disorders. Part I: assessment. *European Child and Adolescent Psychiatry* 2011; *20*:155–171.

The first European guidelines on the assessment of TS.

Coffey B, Frazier J, Chen S. Comorbidity, Tourette syndrome, and anxiety disorders. In: Chase TN, Friedhoff AJ, Cohen DJ (Eds.), *Advances in Neurology, Tourette syndrome: Genetics, neurobiology, and treatment*. Raven, New York, 1992, pp. 95–104.

Coffey BJ, Biederman J, Geller DA et al. Distinguishing illness severity from tic severity in children and adolescents with Tourette's disorder. *J Am Acad Child Adolesc Psychiatry* 2000; *39*:556–561.

Coghill D, Seth S. Do the diagnostic criteria for ADHD need to change? Comments on the preliminary proposals of the DSM-5 ADHD and Disruptive Behavior Disorders Committee. *Eur Child Adolesc Psychiatry* 2011; *20*:75–81.

Cohrs S, Rasch T, Altmeyer S et al. Decreased sleep quality and increased sleep related movements in patients with Tourette's syndrome. *J Neurol Neurosurg Psychiatry* 2001; *70*:192–197.

One of the rare polysomnographic reports in ADHD.

Comings DE. The role of genetic factors in conduct disorder based on studies of Tourette syndrome and attention-deficit hyperactivity disorder probands and their relatives. *J Dev Behav Pediat* 1985a; *16*:142–157.

Comings DE. Role of genetic factors in depression based on studies of Tourette syndrome and ADHD probands and their relatives. *Am J Med Genet* 1985b; *60*:111–121.

Comings DE, Comings BG. A controlled study of Tourette syndrome, I-VII. *Am J Hum Genet* 1987; *41*:701–866.

Comings DE, Comings BG. Tourette's syndrome and attention deficit disorder. In: Cohen DJ, Bruun RD, Leckman JF (Eds.), *Tourette's syndrome and tic disorders*. Wiley, New York, 1988, pp. 119–135.

Comings DE, Wu S, Chiu C et al. Polygenic inheritance of Tourette syndrome, stuttering, attention deficit hyperactivity, conduct, and oppositional defiant disorder: The additive and subtractive effect of the three dopaminergic genes—DRD2, D beta H, and DAT1. *Am J Med Gen* 1996; *67*:264–288.

Como PG. Neuropsychological function in Tourette's syndrome. In: Kurlan R (Ed.), *Handbook of Tourette's syndrome and related tic and behavioral disorders*. New York, Marcel Dekker, 2005, pp. 237–252.

Corkum P, Tannock R, Moldofsky H et al. Actigraphy and parental ratings of sleep in children with attention deficit/hyperactivity disorder (ADHD). *Sleep* 2001; *24*:303–312.

de Groot CM, Janus MD, Bornstein RA. Clinical predictors of psychopathology in children and adolescents with Tourette syndrome. *J Psychiatr Res* 1995; *29*:59–70.

Denckla MB. Attention deficit hyperactivity disorder. The childhood comorbidity that most influences the disability burden in Tourette syndrome. In: Walkup JT, Mink JW, Hollenbeck PT (Eds.), *Advances in Neurology, vol. 99: Tourette syndrome*. Lippincott Williams and Wilkins, New York, 2006, pp. 17–21.

Doepfner M, Rothenberger A. Behavior therapy in tic disorders with co-existing ADHD. *Eur Child Adolesc Psychiatry* 2007; *16* (Suppl 1):I/89–I/9.

A commentary on the impact of ADHD comorbidity upon response to cognitive-behavioral interventions.

Dooley JM , Brna PM, Gordon KE. Parent percep- tions of symptom severity in Tourette's syndrome. *Arch Dis Child* 1999; 81:440–441.

Eddy CM, Rizzo R, Gulisano M et al. Quality of life in young people with Tourette syndrome: a control- led study. *J Neurol* 2011; 258:291–301.

Edell-Fisher BH, Motta RW. Tourette syndrome: relation to children's and parents' self-concepts. *Psychol Rep* 1990; 66:539–545.

Erenberg G. The relationship between Tourette syndrome, attention deficit hyperactivity disorder, and stimulant medication: a critical review. *Semin Pediatr Neurol* 2005; 12:217–221.

Erenberg G, Cruse RP, Rothner AD. The natural his- tory of Tourette syndrome: A follow-up study. *Ann Neurol* 1987; 22:383–385.

Faraone SV, Tsuang MT. Adult attention deficit hyperactivity disorder. *Curr Psychiatry Rep* 2001; 3:129–130.

Fliers EA, Vasquez AA, Poelmans G et al. Genome-wide association study of motor coor- dination problems in ADHD identifies genes for brain and muscle function. *World J Biol Psychiatry* 2012; 13:211–222.

Freeman RD, Fast DK, Burd L et al. An international perspective on Tourette syndrome: selected find- ings from 3,500 individuals in 22 countries. *Dev Med Child Neurol* 2000; 42:436–447.
The first worldwide clinical database on TS.

Freeman RD and the Tourette Syndrome International Database Consortium. Tic disorders and ADHD: answers from a World-wide Clinical Dataset on Tourette Syndrome. *Eur Child Adolesc Psychiatry* 2007; 16 (Suppl 1):I/15–I/23.
A work that expands the population sample and the qualitative data provided in the previous work.

Gadow KD, Nolan EE, Sprafkin J, Schwartz J. Tics and psychiatric comorbidity in children and adoles- cents. *Dev Med Child Neurol* 2002; 44:330–338.

Gaze C, Kepley HO, Walkup JT. Co-occurring psychiatric disorders in children and adolescents with Tourette syndrome. *J Child Neurol* 2006; 21:657–664.

Gorman DA, Thompson N, Plessen KJ et al. Psychosocial outcome and psychiatric comorbid- ity in older adolescents with Tourette syndrome: a controlled study. *Br J Psychiatry* 2010; 197:36–44.

Grados MA, Mathews CA and Tourette Syndrome Association International Consortium for Genetics. Latent class analysis of Gilles de la Tourette syndrome using comorbidities: clinical and genetic implications. *Biol Psychiatry* 2008; 64:219–225.

Greimel E, Wanderer S, Rothenberger A et al. Attentional performance in children and ado- lescents with tic disorder and co-occurring attention-deficit/hyperactivity disorder: New insights from a 2×2 factorial design study. *J Abnorm Child Psychol* 2011; 39:819–828.
A recent work exploring attention abilities in patients with tic disorders plus ADHD.

Himle, MB, Woods DW. An experimental evaluation of tic suppression and the tic rebound effect. *Behav Res Ther* 2005; 43:1443–1451.

Hoekstra PJ, Steenhuis MP, Kallenberg CG, Minderaa RB. Association of small life events with self-reports of tic severity in pediatric and adult tic disorder patients: a prospective longitudinal study. *J Clin Psychiatry* 2004; 65:426–431.

Kadesjö B, Gillberg C. Tourette's disorder: epidemiol- ogy and comorbidity in primary school chil- dren. *J Am Acad Child Adolesc Psychiatry* 2000; 39:548–555.

Kerbeshian J, Burd L, Klug MG. Comorbid Tourette's disorder and bipolar disorder: an etiologic per- spective. *Am J Psychiatry* 1995; 152:1646–1651.

Khalifa N, von Knorring AL. Psychopathology in a Swedish population of school children with tic dis- orders. *J Am Acad Child Adolesc Psychiatry* 2006; 45:1346–1353.

Kirov R, Banaschewski T, Uebel H et al. REM-sleep alterations in children with tic disorder and ADHD comorbidity—impact of hypermotor symptoms. *Eur Child Adolesc Psychiatry* 2007b; 16 (Suppl 1):I/45–I/50.

Kirov R, Kinkelbur J, Banascheski T, Rothenberger A. Sleep patterns in children with attention-deficit/ hyperactivity disorder, tic disorder, and comorbid- ity. *J Child Psychol Psychiatry* 2007a; 48: 561–570.

Kirov R, Uebel H, Albrecht B et al. Two faces of REM sleep in normal and psychopathological development. *Eur Psychiatry* 2011; 26 (Suppl. 1) P01–419;422–423.
The first 2×2 factor analysis showing additive effects of tic disorders and ADHD upon sleep patterns.

Kirov R, Roessner V, Uebel H et al. Schlafverhalten bei Kindern mit Tic-Störungen—eine polysom- nographische Studie. *Zeitschrift für Kinder- und Jugendpsychiatrie und Psychotherapie* 2007c; 35:119–126.

Kompoliti K, Goetz CG. Hyperkinetic move- ment disorders misdiagnosed as tics in Gilles de la Tourette syndrome. *Mov Disord* 1998; 13:477–480.

Konofal E, Lecendreux M, Bouvard MP, Mouren-Simeoni MC. High levels of nocturnal activity in children with attention-deficit hyperactivity disorder: a video analysis. *Psychiatry Clin Neurosci* 2001; 55:97–103.

Kostanecka-Endress T, Banaschewski T, Kinkelbur J et al. Disturbed sleep in children with Tourette syndrome: A polysomnographic study. *J Psychosom Research* 2003; 55:23–29.

Kurlan R, Como PG, Miller B et al. The behavioural spectrum of tic disorders: a community-based study. *Neurology* 2002; 59:414–420.

Lebowitz ER, Motlagh MG, Katsovich L et al. Tourette syndrome in youth with and without obsessive-compulsive disorder and attention deficit hyperactivity disorder. *European Child and Adolescent Psychiatry* 2012 Apr 28 [E-pub ahead of print].

Leckman JF. Tourette's syndrome. *Lancet* 2002; 360:1577–1586.

Leckman JF. Phenomenology of tics and natural history of tic disorders. *Brain Dev* 2003; 25 Suppl 1:S24–S28.

Leckman JF, Vaccarino FM, Kalanithi PS, Rothenberger A. Annotation: Tourette syndrome: a relentless drumbeat—driven by misguided brain oscillations. *J Child Psychol Psychiatry* 2006; 47:537–550.

Lewin DS, Di Pinto M. Sleep disorders and ADHD: Shared and common phenotypes. *Sleep* 2004; 27:188–189.

Lucas AR, Kauffman PE, Morris EM. Gilles de la Tourette's disease: a clinical study of fifteen cases. *J Am Acad Child Psychiatry* 1967; 6:700–722.

Mahone EM, Cirino PT, Cutting LE et al. Validity of the behavior rating inventory of executive function in children with ADHD and/or Tourette syndrome. *Arch Clin Neuropsychol* 2002; 17:643–662.

Marsh R, Alexander GM, Packard MG et al. Habit learning in Tourette syndrome: a translational neuroscience approach to a developmental psychopathology. *Arch Gen Psychiatry* 2004; 61:1259–1268.

Mathews CA, Grados MA. Familiality of Tourette syndrome, obsessive-compulsive disorder, and attention-deficit/hyperactivity disorder: heritability analysis in a large sib-pair sample. *J Am Acad Child Adolesc Psychiatry* 2011; 50:46–54.

An influential work exploring the complex genetic relationship between TS and ADHD, and the related impact of concurrent OCB and OCD.

McMahon WM, Carter AS, Fredine N, Pauls DL. Children at familial risk for Tourette's disorder: child and parent diagnoses. *Am J Med Gen B (Neuropsychiatric Genetics)* 2003; 121B:105–111.

Millstein RB, Wilens T, Biederman J, Spencer TJ. Presenting ADHD symptoms and subtypes in clinically referred adults with ADHD. *J Atten Disord* 1997; 2:159–166.

Moll GH, Heinrich H, Trott GE et al. Children with comorbid attention-deficit-hyperactivity disorder and tic disorder: evidence for additive inhibitory deficits within the motor system. *Ann Neurol* 2001; 49:393–396.

A work that supports an additive effect of tic disorders and ADHD upon inhibitory circuits.

Murphy KR, Barkley RA, Bush T. Young adults with attention deficit hyperactivity disorder: subtype differences in comorbidity, educational, and clinical history. *J Nerv Ment Dis* 2002; 190:147–157.

Olfson M, Crystal S, Gerhard T et al. Patterns and correlates of tic disorder diagnoses in privately and publicly insured youth. *J Am Acad Child Adolesc Psychiatry* 2011; 50:119–131.

O'Rourke JA, Scharf JM, Platko J et al. The familial association of Tourette's disorder and ADHD: the impact of OCD symptoms. *Am J Med Genet B Neuropsychiatr Genet* 2011; 156B:553–560.

Palumbo D. New directions in the treatment of comorbid attention deficit hyperactivity disorder and Tourette's syndrome. In: Kurlan R (Ed.), *Handbook of Tourette's syndrome and related tic and behavioral disorders* (2nd ed.). Marcel Dekker, New York, 2005, pp. 89–108.

Pappert EJ, Goetz CG, Louis ED et al. Objective assessments of longitudinal outcome in Gilles de la Tourette's syndrome. *Neurology* 2003; 61:936–940.

Pauls DL, Leckman JF, Cohen DJ. Evidence against a genetic relationship between Tourette's syndrome and anxiety, depression, panic and phobic disorders. *Br J Psychiatry* 1994; 164:215–221.

Pauls DL, Leckman JF, Cohen DJ. Familial relationship between Gilles de la Tourette's syndrome, attention deficit disorder, learning disabilities, speech disorders, and stuttering. *J Am Acad Child Adolesc Psychiatry* 2003; 32:1044–1050.

Peterson BS, Cohen DJ. The treatment of Tourette's syndrome: multimodal, developmental intervention. *J Clin Psychiatry* 1998; 59 (Suppl 1):62–72.

Peterson BS, Pine DS, Cohen P, Brook JS. Prospective, longitudinal study of tic, obsessive-compulsive, and attention-deficit/hyperactivity disorders in an epidemiological sample. *J Am Acad Child Adolesc Psychiatry* 2001; 40:685–695.

A highly influential work exploring the course of TS plus ADHD.

Pierre CB, Nolan EE, Gadow KD et al. Comparison of internalizing and externalizing symptoms in children with attention-deficit hyperactivity disorder with and without comorbid tic disorder. *J Dev Behav Pediatr* 1999; 20:170–176.

Pliszka SR. Patterns of psychiatric comorbidity with attention deficit/hyperactivity disorder. *Child Adolesc Psychiatr Clin North Am* 2000; 9:525–540.

Poncin Y, Sukhodolsky D, McGuire J, Scahill L. The drug and non-drug treatment of children with ADHD and tic disorders. *Eur Child Adolesc Psychiatry* 2007; 16 (Suppl 1):I/78–I/88.

Preuss U, Ralston SJ, Baldursson G et al. Study design, baseline patient characteristics and intervention in a cross-cultural framework: results from the ADORE study. *Eur Child Adolesc Psychiatry* 2006; 15 (Suppl 1):I5–14.

Ralston SJ, Lorenzo MJ. ADORE—Attention-Deficit Hyperactivity Disorder Observational Research in Europe. *Eur Child Adolesc Psychiatry* 2004; 13 (Suppl 1):36–42.

Randolph C, Hyde TM, Gold JM et al. Tourette's syndrome in monozygotic twins. Relationship of tic severity to neuropsychological function. *Arch Neurol* 1993; 50:725–728.

Robertson MM. Attention deficit hyperactivity disorder, tics and Tourette's syndrome: the relationship and treatment implications. A commentary. *Eur Child Adolesc Psychiatry* 2006; 15:1–11.

Robertson MM. The prevalence and epidemiology of Gilles de la Tourette syndrome. Part 2: tentative explanations for differing prevalence figures in GTS, including the possible effects of psychopathology, aetiology, cultural differences, and differing phenotypes. *J Psychosom Res* 2008; 65:473–486.

Robertson MM, Althoff RR, Hafez A, Pauls DL. Principal components analysis of a large cohort with Tourette syndrome. *Br J Psychiatry* 2008; 193:31–36.

Robertson MM, Stern JS. Gilles de la Tourette syndrome: symptomatic treatment based on evidence. *Eur Child Adolesc Psychiatry* 2000; 9 Suppl 1:I60–75.

Roessner V, Banaschewski T, Rothenberger A. Neuropsychologie bei ADHS und Tic-Störungen—eine Follow-up-Untersuchung [Neuropsychology in ADHD and tic disorders—a follow-up investigation]. *Praxis der Kinderpsychologie und Kinderpsychiatrie* 2006a; 55:314–327.

Roessner V, Becker A, Banaschewski T et al. Developmental psychopathology of children and adolescents with Tourette syndrome—impact of ADHD. *Eur Child Adolesc Psychiatry* 2007a; 16 (Suppl 1):24–35.

A work that characterizes the impact of ADHD upon the course of TS, including its impact on the psychopathological comorbid profile.

Roessner V, Becker A, Banaschewksi T, Rothenberger A. Executive functions in children with chronic tic disorders with/without ADHD—new insights. *Eur Child Adolesc Psychiatry* 2007b; 16 (Suppl 1):I/36–I/44.

Roessner V, Becker A, Banaschewski T, Rothenberger A. Psychopathological profile in children with chronic tic disorder and co-existing ADHD: additive effects. *J Abnorm Child Psychol* 2007c; 35:79–88.

The impact of ADHD comorbidity in TS upon the behavioral profile of the condition is analyzed in detail in this paper.

Roessner V, Robatzek M, Knapp G et al. First-onset tics in patients with attention-deficit-hyperactivity disorder: impact of stimulants. *Dev Med Child Neurol* 2006b; 48:616–621.

Roessner V, Rothenberger A, Rickards H, Hoekstra PJ. European clinical guidelines for Tourette syndrome and other tic disorders. *Eur Child Adolesc Psychiatry* 2011; 20:153–154.

Rosenberg LA, Brown J, Singer HS. Behavioral problems and severity of tics. *J Clin Psychol* 1995; 51:760–767.

Rothenberger A. *Wenn Kinder Tics entwickeln: Beginn einer komplexen kinderpsychiatrischen Störung.* G. Fischer, Stuttgart, 1991.

Rothenberger A. Brain oscillations forever—neurophysiology in future research of child psychiatric problems. *J Child Psychol Psychiatry* 2009; 50:79–86.

Rothenberger A, Banaschewski T. Tic disorders. In: Gillberg C, Harrington R, Steinhausen HC (Eds.), *A clinician's handbook of child and adolescent psychiatry.* Cambridge Univ. Press, 2006, pp. 598–624.

Rothenberger A, Banaschewski T, Heinrich H et al. Comorbidity in ADHD children: coexisting conduct disorder but not tic disorder accompanied by brain electrical deficit in an auditory selective attention task. *Eur Arch Psychiat Clin Neurosci* 2000; 250:101–110.

Rothenberger A, Banaschewski T, Roessner V. Tic-Störungen [Tic disorders]. In: Herpertz-Dahlmann B, Resch F, Schulte-Markwort M, Warnke A (Eds.), *Entwicklungspsychiatrie [Developmental psychiatry]* (2nd ed.). Schattauer, Stuttgart, 2007a, pp. 694–718.

Rothenberger A, Kirov R. Changes in sleep-wake behaviour may be more than just an epiphenomenon of ADHD (open peer commentary). *Behav Brain Sci* 2005; *28*:439.

Rothenberger A, Kostanecka T, Kinkelbur J et al. Sleep and Tourette's syndrome. In: Cohen DJ, Jankovic J, Goetz C (Eds.), *Tourette syndrome. Advances in Neurology, Vol. 85.* Lippincott Williams and Wilkins, Philadelphia, 2001, pp. 245–259.

One of the few review articles on sleep pattern in TS and the role played by ADHD comorbidity upon sleep abnormalities in this condition.

Rothenberger A, Roessner V, Banaschewski T, Leckman J. Co-existence of tic disorders (TIC) and ADHD—recent advances in understanding and treatment. *Eur Child Adolesc Psychiatry* 2007b; *16* (Suppl 1): i1–i99.

The first complete issue of a journal devoted to tic disorder plus ADHD.

Scahill L, Sukhodolsky DG, Williams SK, Leckman JF. Public health significance of tic disorders in children and adolescents. *Adv Neurol* 2005; *96*:240–248.

Scahill L, Williams S, Schwab-Stone M et al. Disruptive behavior problems in a community sample of children with tic disorders. In: Walkup JT, Mink JW, Hollenbeck PT (Eds.), *Advances in Neurology, vol. 99: Tourette syndrome.* Lippincott Williams and Wilkins, New York, 2006, pp. 184–190.

Schlander M, Schwarz O, Rothenberger A, Roessner V. Tic disorders: Administrative prevalence and co-occurrence with attention-deficit/hyperactivity disorder in a German community sample. *Eur Psychiatry* 2011; *26*:370–374.

Many children with tics seem not to be referred.

Schuerholz LJ, Cutting L, Mazzocco MM et al. Neuromotor functioning in children with Tourette syndrome with and without attention deficit hyperactivity disorder. *J Child Neurol* 1997; *12*:438–442.

Shapiro AK, Shapiro ES, Bruun RD, Sweet RD. Gilles de la Tourette syndrome. Raven Press, New York, 1978.

Shapiro AK, Shapiro ES, Young JG, Feinberg TE. Gilles de la Tourette syndrome. New York, Raven Press, 1988.

Shaw P, Eckstrand K, Sharp W et al. Attention-deficit/hyperactivity disorder is characterized by a delay in cortical maturation. *Proc Natl Acad Sci USA* 2007; *104*:19649–19654.

Shaw P, Gilliam M, Liverpool M et al. Cortical development in typically developing children with symptoms of hyperactivity and impulsivity: support for a dimensional view of attention deficit hyperactivity disorder. *Am J Psychiatry* 2011;*168*:143–151.

Sherman EM, Shepard L, Joschko M, Freeman RD. Sustained attention and impulsivity in children with Tourette syndrome: comorbidity and confounds. *J Clin Exp Neuropsychol* 1998; *20*:644–657.

Shin MS, Chung SJ, Hong KE. Comparative study of the behavioural and neuropsychologic characteristics of tic disorder with or without attention-deficit hyperactivity disorder (ADHD). *J Child Neurol* 2001; *16*:719–726.

Singer HS, Rosenberg LA. Development of behavioral and emotional problems in Tourette syndrome. *Pediatr Neurol* 1989; *5*:41–44.

Spencer T, Biederman J, Coffey B et al. Tourette disorder and ADHD. *Adv Neurol* 2001a; *85*:57–77.

Spencer TJ, Biederman J, Faraone S. Impact of tic disorders on ADHD outcome across the life cycle: findings from a large group of adults with and without ADHD. *Am J Psychiatry* 2001b; *158*:611–617.

Spencer T, Biederman J, Harding M et al. Disentangling the overlap between Tourette's disorder and ADHD. *J Child Psychol Psychiatry* 1998; *39*:1037–1044.

One of the landmark articles highlighting the importance of ADHD comorbidity in TS.

Steinberg T, Baruch SS, Harush A et al. Tic disorders and the premonitory urge. *J Neural Transm* 2012; *117*:277–284.

Steinhausen HC, Novik TS, Baldursson G et al. Co-existing psychiatric problems in ADHD in the ADORE cohort. *Eur Child Adolesc Psychiatry* 2006; *15* (Suppl 1):i25–i29.

Stephens RJ, Sandor P. Aggressive behaviour in children with Tourette and comorbid attention-deficit hyperactivity disorder and obsessive–compulsive disorder. *Can J Psychiatry* 1999; *44*:1036–1042.

Stewart SE, Illmann C, Geller DA et al. A controlled family study of attention-deficit/hyperactivity disorder and Tourette's disorder. *J Am Acad Child Adolesc Psychiatry* 2006; *45*:1354–1362.

Stokes A, Bawden HN, Camfield PR et al. Peer problems in Tourette's disorder. *Pediatrics* 1991; *87*:936–942.

Sukhodolsky DG, Scahill L, Zhang H et al. Disruptive behavior in children with Tourette's syndrome: association with ADHD comorbidity, tic severity, and functional impairment. *J Am Acad Child Adolesc Psychiatry* 2003; *42*:98–105.

Sukhodolsky D, Leckman JF, Rothenberger A, Scahill L. The role of abnormal neural oscillations in the pathophysiology of co-occurring Tourette syndrome and ADHD. *Eur Child Adolesc Psychiatry* 2007; *16* (Suppl 1):I/51–I/59.

Taylor E. Clinical foundations of hyperactivity research. *Behav Brain Res* 1998; *94*:11–24.

Taylor E. Sleep and tics problems associated with ADHD. *J Am Acad Child Adolesc Psychiatry* 2009; *48*:877–878.

Taylor E, Dopfner M, Sergeant J et al. European clinical guidelines for hyperkinetic disorder—first upgrade. *Eur Child Adolesc Psychiatry* 2004; *13* (Suppl 1):7–30.

Termine C, Balottin U, Rossi G et al. Psychopathology in children and adolescents with Tourette's syndrome: A controlled study. *Brain Dev* 2006; *28*:69–75.

Van Brunt DL, Johnston JA, Ye W et al. Predictors of selecting atomoxetine therapy for children with attention-deficit/hyperactivity disorder. *Pharmacotherapy* 2005; *25*:1541–1549.

Walkup JT, Khan S, Schuerholz L et al. Phenomenology and natural history of tic-related ADHD and learning disabilities. In: Leckman JF, Cohen DJ (Eds.), *Tourette's syndrome: Developmental psychopathology and clinical care.* Wiley, New York, 1999, pp. 63–79.

Wodrich DL, Benjamin E, Lachar D. Tourette's syndrome and psychopathology in a child psychiatry setting. *J Am Acad Child Adolesc Psychiatry* 1997; 36:1618–1624.

World Health Organization. *The ICD-10 classification of mental and behavioural disorders: clinical descriptions and diagnostic guidelines.* WHO, Geneva, Switzerland, 1992.

Yordanova J, Dumais-Huber C, Rothenberger A. Coexistence of tics and hyperactivity in children: no additive effect at the psychophysiological level. *Int J Psychophysiology* 1996; *21*:121–133.

Yordanova J, Dumais-Huber C, Rothenberger A, Woerner W. Frontocortical activity in children with comorbidity of tic disorder and attention-deficit hyperactivity disorder. *Biol Psychiatry* 1997; 41:585–594.

Yordanova J, Heinrich H, Kolev V, Rothenberger A. Increased event-related theta activity as a psychophysiological marker of comorbidity in children with tics and attention-deficit/hyperactivity disorders. *NeuroImage* 2006; 32:940–955.

Zhu Y, Leung KM, Liu P et al. Comorbid behavioural problems in Tourette's syndrome are positively correlated with the severity of symptoms. *Aust N Z J Psychiatry* 2006; 40:67–73.

3

The Phenomenology of Obsessive-Compulsive Symptoms in Tourette Syndrome

YGOR A. FERRÃO, PEDRO G. DE ALVARENGA, ANA G. HOUNIE, MARIA A. DE MATHIS, MARIA C. DE ROSÁRIO AND EURÍPEDES C. MIGUEL

Abstract

In clinical practice, the boundary between symptoms arising from obsessive-compulsive disorder (OCD) and Tourette syndrome (TS) is not easily determined, with important areas of overlap between tics and compulsions. The frequency of this behavioral comorbidity varies across studies, and rates differ between those of obsessive-compulsive symptoms and those of obsessive-compulsive disorder. Psychiatric comorbid diagnoses are more frequent in TS with comorbid OCD and include separation anxiety disorder, attention-deficit/hyperactivity disorder, grooming behaviors, posttraumatic stress disorder, and social and simple phobias. This chapter describes the complex phenomenology of obsessive-compulsive symptoms in TS and highlights the impact of this comorbidity on the occurrence of other behavioral problems and the burden of other psychiatric comorbidities.

We fear things in proportion to our ignorance of them.

—Titus Livius

An unwanted thought is like an unwanted guest. Pay no attention to the guest, don't feed the guest, don't talk to the guest. The guest will leave eventually.

—Unknown

You cannot prevent the birds of sorrow from flying over your head, but you can prevent them from building a nest in your hair.

—Chinese proverb

INTRODUCTION

Obsessions (i.e., unwanted thoughts, ideas, or images), and compulsions (i.e., repetitive behaviors performed in response to or to relieve an obsession or abnormal feelings), the hallmark of the clinical picture of obsessive-compulsive disorder (OCD), have been described in Tourette syndrome (TS) since its earliet reports. Since then, the relationship between OCD and TS has been extensively studied.

Comorbidity in psychiatric disorders is a common phenomenon. Therefore, the association between OCD and TS could be a coincidence. However, as will be discussed in the next pages, there are several sources of evidence suggesting that at least for some forms of OCD and TS, this association is not by chance.

This topic has been investigated from different perspectives. Some authors focused on the manifestations of obsessive-compulsive symptoms (OCS) in TS, while others explored the phenotypic impact of tics in OCD. In this chapter we will explore both perspectives.

Thus, in the following pages, we will first give a historical overview of the association between

OCD and TS. Then we will explore the current epidemiological and common environmental and genetic factors that support this association. Further, we will present the clinical features of OCS in TS and OCD with tics as well as the basis of the phenomenological continuum between the two disorders. Finally, we will describe the current data on treatment response of patients who present with both OCD and tics or TS. We will conclude by discussing the limitations of the current knowledge in this field and possible future developments.

HISTORICAL OVERVIEW

Obsessions and compulsions were first described by John Climacus in the sixth century. Until the Renaissance, however, there were very few scholarly works on the subject. OCS were identified, as they are currently defined, in the seventeenth century. At that time, obsessions and repetitive behaviors were often described as symptoms of religious melancholy, and sufferers were considered to be possessed by outside forces (Salzman & Thaler, 1981). Influenced by intellectual currents and the advent of the biological sciences, the modern concepts of OCD and TS began to evolve in the nineteenth century (Alvarenga et al., 2008). A psychiatric condition quite similar to the contemporary concept of OCD was first described in a case report ("Mademoiselle F") by Jean-Etienne Dominique Esquirol, who classified it as a form of monomania, a kind of partial insanity (Esquirol, 1838). The overlap between OCS and tics was noted as early as 1825, in the first clinical report of TS, in which Jean-Marc Gaspard Itard described a noblewoman who presented with motor and vocal tics, together with obsessive thoughts (cited in Como, 1995). Itard described the case of Marquise de Dampierre, an important noblewoman of her time, whose episodes, later understood to be coprolalia, "were obviously in stark contrast to the lady's background, intellect, and refined manners." Sixty years later, Jean-Martin Charcot and his student Gilles de la Tourette described a series of nine clinical cases of what they called *maladie des tics* ("tic disease") and reported OCS in several cases, including the

case originally described by Itard (Kushner, 2000). In fact, Charcot considered OCS to be part of the clinical profile of tic disorders (Shapiro et al., 1978). Together with Georges Guinon and Bernard Grasset, de la Tourette illustrated the psychopathology of patients with "compulsive tic disorder," within which the authors included checking rituals, arithmomania, *délire de toucher* ("delusion of touch"), *folie du doute* ("madness of doubt"), and "mania for order" (Robertson, 1991). Likewise, when discussing the case of "Frau Emmy Von N," diagnosed with hysteria, Sigmund Freud noted that *tic convulsif* (his term for TS) was characterized by involuntary movements such as grimaces, coprolalia, echolalia, and obsessions, thus falling within the "madness of doubt" spectrum (Freud, 1916–17).

At the beginning of the twentieth century, Pierre Janet published various works related to a total of 325 patients with obsessions, compulsions, tics, and body dysmorphic features. Janet proposed that obsessions and compulsions arise in the final (third) stage of psychasthenic neurosis (which encompasses OCS, tics, and body dysmorphic features). He described symptoms referred to as "forced agitations," which he categorized as either mental (obsessions) or motor (tics), stating that these symptoms play an important role in the psychasthenic mental state (Janet, 1903; Pitman, 1987). Janet also described the successful treatment of compulsions and rituals with techniques we now know to be consistent with concepts of cognitive-behavioral therapy, which was developed much later (Pitman, 1987; Rachman & Hodgson, 1967).

During the first half of the twentieth century, the prevailing etiological theories suggested that OCS and tics were both treatable through psychoanalysis (Alvarenga et al., 2008). In 1968, a 24-year-old woman with various motor and vocal tics was successfully treated with haloperidol (Shapiro & Shapiro, 1968). After many years of being conceptualized as psychogenic, tics began to be understood as a neurochemical malfunction potentially responsive to antipsychotic treatment (Hounie et al., 2006a). The first neurobiological models of TS were particularly important for the development of an evidence-based approach to OCD, previously considered an emotional disorder. In the past three decades, a variety of epidemiological and family studies have demonstrated that OCD and TS aggregate in families (Nestadt et al., 2000; Rosário-Campos et al., 2005), and new methods that emerged with the advance of neurosciences were applied to the study of OCD and TS.

As we will see further in this chapter, due to the high rates of comorbidity and high familial loading, as well as similarities in terms of the underlying mechanisms and clinical presentation, TS and OCD are currently viewed as part of the same neuropsychiatric spectrum (Hollander et al., 2009; Phillips et al., 2010).

EPIDEMIOLOGY OF OCS IN TS AND TICS IN OCD

Prevalence

TS has been described worldwide, presenting with virtually the same symptoms across cultures. The same is true for OCD. However, there is evidence to suggest that TS varies in its presentation, especially with regard to associated features such as OCS. For example, in a cohort of TS patients in Korea (Min & Lee, 1986), the number of OCS and behavioral problems was found to be lower than that reported for Western populations, whereas a greater predominance of males and lower rates of coprolalia were noted among TS patients in Japan (Kano et al., 1998).

It has been reported that TS affects 0.3% to 1.0% of the population, depending on the age of the subjects, as well as on the diagnostic criteria and sampling method used. The lifetime prevalence of OCD in the general population is higher, between 1.9% and 3.2% (Heyman et al., 2003; Ruscio et al., 2010). Although OCS may be present in up to 60% to 90% of TS subjects (Cath et al., 2001; Comings & Comings, 1987; Robertson et al., 2002), the rates of OCD in TS subjects vary from 10% to 35% (Cavanna et al., 2009). Similarly, the rates range from 7% of TS in OCD patients (Miguel et al., 2008) to 37.5% of tics in OCD patients (de Mathis et al., 2009). The discrepancy in the results may reflect the variance of methodologies and the recruited sample (i.e., if the sample was recruited from the community or from clinical services).

A large cross-sectional study comprising 813 consecutive OCD outpatients from the Brazilian OCD Research Consortium reported a general prevalence of tic disorders (TD) (including TS and other chronic TD) of 29.0%, with 8.9% presenting TS, 17.3% chronic motor tic disorder, and 2.8% chronic vocal tic disorder (Alvarenga et al., 2012).

Gender and Age Distribution

Gender also plays a role in OCD and TS. Studies examining the clinical features of TS in North America and Europe have consistently shown that the disorder is more common in males, with a male-to-female ratio ranging from 3:1 to 4:1 (Tanner et al., 1997). Although OCD also affects both genders, it has a bimodal distribution, early-onset OCD being more common among males. Obsessive-compulsive phenomena are present in TS patients of both genders, especially if there is a family history of OCD. Among children with OCD, tic disorders are more common in boys. Santangelo and colleagues (1994) examined TS patients by gender, evaluating several variables. Although the overall experience of TS appeared to be similar for both genders, males more often presented rage symptom at onset and more often had a history of any form of simple tics. Females more often presented compulsive tics at onset than did males. TS patients with comorbid OCD were more likely than were those without OCD to present with complex tics at onset. Females were typically older at diagnosis of TS than were males (Pauls & Leckman, 1986).

Age at onset of OCS in OCD patients also influences the relationship with gender and tics. Early-onset OCD is associated with a greater likelihood that the males in the family will develop tics. Since puberty changes the clinical expression of both disorders, the importance of the age at onset of OCS was investigated in studies using child and adolescent OCD probands (de Mathis et al., 2009; Leonard et al., 1992). For instance, in one cohort study, 20% of carefully screened male preschoolers presenting with OCD eventually developed tics (Cath et al., 1992).

PHENOMENOLOGY OF OCS IN TS AND OCD WITH TICS

As mentioned above, since the earliest descriptions, obsessions and compulsions, typical OCD phenomena, have also been present in patients with TS. The differences between these symptoms are probably consequences of the diverse brain structures involved in the TS and OCD neurocircuitry (Singer, 2003; Stein, 2000) and may help in differentiating diagnoses and making therapeutic decisions. The general psychopathological aspects of obsessions and compulsions and how they occur in patients with TS are presented below. The "continuum" between OCD and TS will also be briefly discussed. Finally, the sensory phenomena, a key psychopathological manifestation of both OCD and TS, are presented.

Obsessions and Compulsions

An **obsession** may be defined as thoughts, images, sounds, fears, memories, and doubts that are intrusive and repetitive and that result in distress and/or any kind of discomfort (anxiety, fear, sadness, anguish). The patient realizes, in most cases, that the content of the obsessions is egodystonic but is not able to avoid them; if he or she is able to avoid them, it is only for short periods of time. Any theme may become an obsession, but the most frequent contents are contamination, sex, religion and moral aspects, aggression, symmetry, and hoarding. Obsessions may lead patients to perform repetitive behaviors (compulsions) or mental rituals (e.g., counting, praying, remembering), which are attempts to relieve the suffering caused by obsessions. The length of a single obsession may be seconds to hours. The severity of an obsession varies from individual to individual, and in the same individual it may vary according to the moment and to the content, tending to present in a "waxing-and-waning" course.

Compulsions may be defined as repetitive behaviors and/or mental acts performed to reduce the anxiety, discomfort, or distress caused by an obsession or without any specific reason. The compulsion may provide temporary relief of the discomfort. The most frequent compulsions are counting specific things (such as footsteps) or in specific ways (for instance, by intervals of two), washing hands or cleaning objects, arranging, ordering, organizing symmetrically, checking, repeating (e.g., turning lights on and off, closing and opening doors, touching objects a certain number of times). Whether or not behaviors are compulsions or mere habits depends on the context in which they are performed. For example, arranging and ordering books for 8 hours a day would be expected of one who works in a bookstore but would seem abnormal in other situations. In other words, habits tend to bring efficiency to one's life while compulsions tend to disrupt it, and when severe enough may lead patients to familial and social isolation and academic or professional disabilities, resulting in social or familial burdening in more severe cases. Figure 3.1 presents the most common OCS in a large sample of OCD patients according to the Dimensional Yale-Brown Obsessive-Compulsive Scale (DY-BOCS, see below) checklist (Miguel et al., 2008).

Specific Features of OCS or OCD in TS: Categorical Approach

Several studies were performed looking for specific clinical features to differentiate OCS in TS and a possible "OCD with tics" subtype. Pauls and Leckman began the important work of distinguishing these OCD subgroups on the basis of family genetic data and referred to these subgroups as tic-related OCD and non–tic-related OCD (Leckman et al., 1994-1995; Pauls et al., 1986b). The most frequent obsessions in TS patients are sexual/religious, aggressive, symmetry/ordering/arrangement, and hoarding (Baer et al., 1994; Diniz et al., 2006; George et al., 1993; Kono et al., 2010; Leckman et al., 2003; Torres et al., 2012; Zohar et al., 1997). Other authors also described somatic obsessions as being frequent in TS patients (de Groot et al., 1994, 1995). Diniz and colleagues (2006) compared patients with OCD plus TS and OCD alone and found that subjects with OCD alone were characterized by a higher frequency of contamination obsessions and cleaning compulsions. They also found that OCD patients with chronic motor or vocal tics were similar to OCD patients with TS in terms of the frequency of intrusive sounds, but these symptoms were more frequent in those groups than in OCD patients without tics. The severity and content of the obsessions do not seem to be associated with tic severity (de Groot et al., 1994, 1995). Tic-related OCD, in contrast to non–tic-related OCD, is characterized by higher frequencies of touching, tapping, and rubbing (also called "tic-like" compulsions); a higher percentage of violent and aggressive intrusive thoughts and images; and concerns about symmetry and exactness (Leckman et al., 1997). TS patients with "compulsions" or OCD patients with tics often report a relative absence of elaborated obsessions and beliefs in catastrophic consequences associated with their compulsions. Instead they may report explicit discomforts or subjective feelings and concerns that these feelings will be intolerable and possibly unending if their intentional repetitive behaviors are not performed. These compulsions typically involve just-right or just-so requirements with an emphasis on symmetry, arrangement, positioning, hoarding, ordering, touching, and counting (Diniz et al., 2006; Rosario-Campos et al., 2001; Summerfeldt, 2004). Therefore, in these patients the repetitive behaviors are less frequently associated with cognitions, but rather with different forms of subjective feelings that we call sensory phenomena, as described in detail below (Coffey et al., 1998; Mansueto et al., 2005; Rosário et al., 2009; Sutherland et al., 2011).

Specific Features of OCS or OCD in TS: Dimensional Approach

As described above, OCD is a heterogeneous disorder, and its complex phenotypes have variable clinical expressions across and within subjects. In the search for more homogeneous subgroups of patients, a dimensional approach has proven to be of extreme value. Recent factor analytic studies have reduced the OCS to a few fairly consistent and clinically meaningful symptom

dimensions (Bloch et al., 2008; Mataix-Cols et al., 2005). Both in adult (Leckman et al., 2003) and pediatric samples (Stewart et al., 2005), many factor and cluster analytical studies, involving more than 6,000 patients, have consistently identified at least four OCS dimensions, often named contamination/cleaning, obsessions/checking, symmetry/ordering, and hoarding. These studies have demonstrated that these dimensions are temporally stable and correlate meaningfully with various clinical, genetic, neuroimaging, and treatment-response variables (Bloch et al., 2008; Mataix-Cols et al., 2005).

The first longitudinal twin study of OCS stability in children aged 7 to 12 years was performed by van Grootheest and colleagues (2007). They found that the obsessive-compulsive behavior in childhood was moderately stable. When categorical approaches were used, the symptom stability was lower than when quantitative and dimensional approaches were used. They also found that stability was influenced by genetic factors, by environmental factors shared by children growing up in the same family, and by nonshared environmental factors.

More recently, the Dimensional Yale-Brown Obsessive-Compulsive Scale (DYBOCS) was developed to evaluate OCS according to specific dimensions, which include obsessions and related compulsions. The DYBOCS can assess the presence and severity of each dimension independently but also provides a global severity of all OCS. Other advantages of the DYBOCS are the investigation of avoidant behaviors and mental and repetitive rituals within each dimension. It also investigates the time spent with OCS and the level of anxiety and interference, with scores ranging from 0 to 5 (maximum of 15 for each dimension). The negative impact of the OCS on the person's life is also measured (maximum score of 30). The DYBOCS has demonstrated excellent psychometric properties (Rosario-Campos et al., 2006).

Figure 3.1 highlights the differences of DYBOCS dimensions rates between patients with pure OCD and patients with OCD plus tics in a large Brazilian sample (n = 1,001) collected by the Brazilian Research Consortium on Obsessive-Compulsive Spectrum Disorders

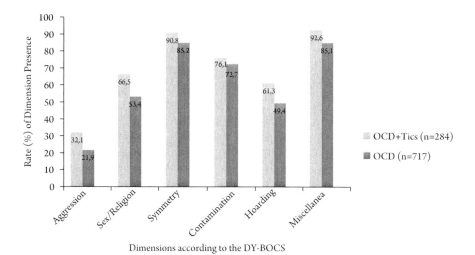

FIGURE 3.1   OCS, obsessive-compulsive symptoms; OCD, obsessive-compulsive disorder; DY-BOCS, Dimensional Yale-Brown Obsessive-Compulsive Scale; n, absolute values; percent, relative values.

(CTOC). The sample presented significant differences in the severity of specific dimensions ("aggression," "sexual/religion," and "hoarding"), which were more severe in the OCD plus tic disorders group (Alvarenga et al., 2012), giving support to previous findings (de Mathis et al., 2008). These same dimensions have been reported as more frequent in the early-onset OCD group (de Mathis et al., 2006, 2008; Leckman et al., 2009).

A recent study (Kono et al., 2010) assessed 40 Japanese TS outpatients (29 males, 11 females) with the DYBOCS (Rosário-Campos et al., 2006). OCS were present in 80% of the total sample. The miscellaneous and the symmetry dimensions were the most frequent in the "current" and "lifetime" surveys, respectively. The aggression dimension had the smallest difference between "worst ever" and current ratings among all the OCS dimensions. TS patients with the aggression dimension (n = 7) had significantly lower scores in the Global Assessment Function Scale (GAF) and higher frequencies of coprolalia. In another interesting study of the same group, 88 young Japanese TS patients (67 males and 21 females; mean age 15.2 years) were assessed; OCS were present in 42.% of the subjects, while attention-deficit/hyperactivity disorder (ADHD) was present in 28.4%. In the group with TS plus OCS and/or ADHD, coprophenomena,

impulsiveness/aggression, school refusal, and self-injurious behaviors were significantly more frequent than in the TS-only group, even correcting by age (Kono et al., 2010).

One clear example of OCD with tics can be seen at the movie "Matchstick Men," based on Eric Garcia's novel "Matchstick Men: A Novel about Grifters with Issues" (2002). Roy Waller (Nicolas Cage) is a con artist residing in Los Angeles. Alongside his partner and protégé Frank Mercer (Sam Rockwell), Roy operates a fake lottery, selling overpriced water filtration systems to unsuspecting customers. Roy suffers from several mental disorders, including OCD and tic disorders (eye blinking, yelling "pygmies" whenever something surprises or upsets him, head movements, other vocal tics). Other suggested movies or pictures exploring OCD are "The Aviator" (2004), the TV series "Monk" (2002–09), and the motion picture "As Good as It Gets" (1997), whereas TS is represented in films such as "Dodes'ka-den" (1970) and "The Big White" (2005).

The Continuum Between Descriptive Phenomenology of OCD and TS

In clinical practice, the boundaries between symptoms arising from OCD and TS are not easily determined. The TS Classification Study Group (1993) described tics as an "involuntary" (i.e., completely unintentional) response to either an urge or an unpleasant sensation (i.e., sensory phenomena) perceived as "voluntary." Nevertheless, there are areas of phenomenological overlap between tics and compulsions. For instance, repetitive behaviors such as touching or eye blinking may result from a need to relieve an urge or an unpleasant sensation (as defined above) but also to neutralize an obsession. Thus, depending on the nature of the subjective experience, the same repetitive behavior may be labeled differently (Miguel et al., 1995) as tics or compulsions.

To study the phenomenological continuum along these disorders, we proposed the term "intentional repetitive behavior," which has the advantage of encompassing various presentations of stereotyped repetitive behaviors reported in TS and OCD patients while at the same time allowing a clear differentiation from unintentional or involuntary tic phenomena, such as simple tics (Miguel et al., 1995).

Therefore, patients with TS can present with intentional repetitive behaviors exactly as they occur in OCD (e.g., touching). The nature of these behaviors, however, may differ in tic-related OCD compared to pure OCD. For instance, repetitive behavior (compulsions) in classic pure OCD is usually performed to relieve an unwanted thought, idea, or image (obsessions). Most patients with TS do not report obsessions preceding their repetitive behavior, but they describe uncomfortable sensations named sensory phenomena, as described in more detail below (Miguel et al., 1995). In addition, pure OCD patients more often report symptoms of autonomic anxiety (e.g., tachycardia, shortness of breath, sweating, pallor) preceding their repetitive behavior, while TS patients usually do not (Miguel et al., 1995).

Other authors suggested the name "Tourettic OCD" for tic-like compulsions (Mansueto et al., 2005). For these authors, TS patients with "compulsions," or "Tourettic OCD" patients, often report a relative absence of elaborate obsessions and of the belief in catastrophic consequences, although some report vague notions that something bad might happen if they do not perform their compulsions. They also frequently report explicit concerns that their discomfort will be intolerable and possibly unending if their intentional repetitive behaviors are not performed. "Compulsions" themselves typically involve just-right or just-so requirements with an emphasis on symmetry, arranging, positioning, hoarding, ordering, touching, and numbers (Diniz et al., 2006). The repetitive behaviors reportedly are not associated with anxiety but with sensory phenomena such as localized physical tension, generalized somatic discomfort, and diffuse psychological distress, such as feelings of incompleteness (Mansueto et al., 2005; Rosário et al., 2009; Sutherland et al., 2011). The performance of the intentional repetitive behavior tends to serve the express purpose of reducing the focal, localized, or general discomfort as opposed to playing a more central role in the modulation of anxiety and prevention of catastrophic consequences (Cath et al., 2001; Coffey & Rapoport, 2010; Mansueto et al., 2005; Summerfeldt et al., 2004). Box 3.1 summarizes the differences and similarities between TS and OCD in terms of obsessions and compulsions (adapted from Ferrão et al., 2009).

SENSORY PHENOMENA

As mentioned above, often in addition to obsessions, many OCD patients (especially those with OCD plus TS) report that other kinds of subjective experiences may precede or accompany their compulsions. Initially described in the literature on TS patients, these subjective experiences may be reported by almost 70% of OCD subjects (Ferrão et al., 2006; Rosario-Campos et al., 2001; Shavitt et al., 2006) and by up to 81% of OCD patients with comorbid TS (Cohen & Leckman, 1992; Leckman et al., 1993, 1997).

Besides the high frequencies in TS and OCD patients, other reasons reinforce the relevance of investigating sensory phenomena in these patients. For instance, some patients report that they may cause even more distress than the obsessions and/or compulsions (Cohen & Leckman, 1992; Prado et al., 2008). It has also been noted that a better recognition of the presence of these sensory phenomena may increase the patients' ability to redirect their attention or suppress their symptoms (Cohen & Leckman, 1992) and that they may be a predictive factor of treatment response (Leckman et al., 1993; Shavitt, 2006).

Box 3.1. Key Points

- In clinical practice, the boundary between symptoms arising from OCD and TD is not easily determined. Nevertheless, there are areas of phenomenological overlap between tics and compulsions.
- OCS may be present in up to 90% of TS subjects. The rates of OCD in TS subjects vary from 10% to 35%. Otherwise, the rates range from 7% of TS in OCD patients to 37.5% of tics in OCD patients. Most common obsessions are symmetry and exactness, aggressive, hoarding, and sounds.
- Other repetitive behaviors in TS include compulsions (exactly like they occur in OCD) and tic-like compulsions. Tics and tic-like compulsions are usually not preceded by obsessions but by sensory phenomena, and are frequently less rigid.
- Sensory phenomena are present in OCD with or without TS. Sensory phenomena are more prevalent in TS and in OCD+TS than in pure OCD. These include just-right phenomena, localized physical tension, generalized somatic discomfort, and diffuse psychological distress (such as feelings of incompleteness) (see Chapter 1).
- OCS and OCD in TS are more prevalent in males. Males more often present at onset with rage and have ever experienced any form of simple tics. Females usually present at onset with tic-like compulsions.

OCS and OCD in TS have earlier onset than pure OCD.
- Patients with TS+OCD present more frequently with separation anxiety disorder, ADHD, grooming behaviors, PTSD, and social and simple phobia.
- There are higher rates of OCD and OCS in the TS first-degree relatives. Female relatives of TS probands more often express OCS, while male relatives more often express TS or chronic tics.
  - Cortico–striatum–thalamocortical circuits (caudate nucleus for cognitive and putamen for motor aspects) are involved in OCD in TS.

More recently, a new scale was developed to assess the presence and severity of different types of SP occurring before or during the performance of repetitive behaviors, the University of São Paulo Sensory Phenomena Scale (USP-SPS) (Rosário et al., 2009). This is a semi-structured scale divided in two parts, a checklist and a severity scale. The checklist comprises items assessing past and current examples of the different types of sensory phenomena described above. If symptoms were endorsed, patients were also asked to provide their age of onset. The USP-SPS severity scale assesses the severity of sensory phenomena by using three ordinal scales with six anchor points that focus on the frequency of the sensory phenomena (0–5), the

amount of distress they cause (0–5), and the degree to which they interfere with the patient's functioning (0–5). The total score is obtained by combining the three scores (0–15). Scores are obtained both for current severity and the time when the sensory phenomena were at their worst. The USP-SPS has shown excellent initial psychometric properties (Rosário et al., 2009).

Other studies have reported that these sensory phenomena may be useful to identify more homogeneous subgroups of OCD and TS patients. Miguel and colleagues (1995, 1997, 2000) and Leckman and colleagues (1994) reported that the need to perform a behavior until feeling "just right" was reported in 90% of the OCD+TS group compared to 48%

of the TS group and 35% of the OCD group. Feelings of incompleteness were even more distinctive in the OCD+TS group. Diniz and colleagues (2006) investigated possible differences in the expression of sensory phenomena in OCD patients without tics, OCD patients with chronic motor or vocal tics, and OCD patients with TS. Interestingly, patients with OCD with chronic motor or vocal tics were intermediate between OCD+TS and OCD patients without tics in terms of the frequency and severity of sensory phenomena, providing further evidence that sensory phenomena may prove to be useful in subtyping OCD not only as a categorical but also as a dimensional measure.

An early onset of OCD (<10 years) has also been associated with significantly higher frequencies of sensory phenomena compared to the late-onset group (>18 years) (Rosário-Campos et al., 2001).

The presence and severity of sensory phenomena has also shown high convergent validity with the "symmetry/ordering" dimension, frequently described as a component of the tic-related OCD phenotype (Miguel et al., 2005; Rosário et al., 2009). Lee and colleagues (2009), investigating the association of sensory phenomena and perfectionism, found that all sensory phenomena subtypes were significantly more frequent and more severe in OCD than in control subjects, suggesting that the presence and severity of sensory phenomena and specific elements of perfectionism clearly distinguish OCD patients from healthy control subjects.

The Brazilian Consortium on OCD Research assessed the clinical correlates of the presence and severity of sensory phenomena in 1,001 consecutive OCD patients. Six hundred fifty-one (65.0%) subjects reported at least one type of sensory phenomena preceding their repetitive behaviors. Interestingly, sensory phenomena were described as being more severe than were obsessions by 102 patients. Logistic regression analysis showed that the presence of sensory phenomena was associated with a higher frequency and a greater severity of the symmetry/ordering/arranging and contamination/washing symptom dimensions; comorbidity with TS; and a family history of tic disorders (Ferrão et al., 2011).

In summary, sensory phenomena are not restricted to TS patients and can be an important phenotypic variable in the characterization of the tic-related OCD subtype and can help to understand the phenomenological continuum between OCD and TS. In addition, they are also more frequently associated with some clinical features in OCD patients, such as an early age at obsessive-compulsive symptom onset; higher frequency and severity of the symmetry/ordering dimension; certain perfectionism characteristics; comorbidity with chronic tics and/or TS; and a family history of tics. Future studies are warranted to better determine whether these sensory phenomena have specific neuroimaging, genetic, and treatment-response correlates. In addition, future studies should investigate whether sensory phenomena are prevalent in other psychiatric disorders, particularly anxiety and impulse-control disorders.

NATURAL COURSE AND PSYCHIATRIC COMORBIDITIES

The natural history of tics and TS is described in Chapters 1 and 5. Briefly, tics typically have an onset between the ages of 4 and 6 years (i.e., before the OCS or OCD onset) and reach their worst-ever severity between the ages of 10 and 12 years (Bloch & Leckman, 2009; Neuner & Ludolph, 2009). Symptoms usually begin with transient bouts of simple motor tics. By age 10 years, most children are aware of nearly irresistible somatosensory urges that precede the tics. A momentary sense of relief typically follows the completion of a tic. Over the course of hours, tics occur in bouts, with a regular inter-tic interval (Leckman et al., 2006). On average, tic severity declines during adolescence. By early adulthood, roughly three quarters of children with TS will have greatly diminished tic symptoms and over one third of these will be tic-free.

In contrast with tic disorders, OCS can start in different phases of development. Half of OCD patients start their OCS before age 10, 25% between 10 and 18, and 25% after 18 (deMathis et al., 2012; Miguel et al., 2008). As mentioned before, the OCD associated with tics or TS starts early, before age 10 (de Mathis et al., 2012;

Miguel et al., 2008). Typically, like OCS, TS shows a waxing-and-waning course (Leckman et al., 2006; Muller, 2007). Like OCS, tics increase during periods of emotional excitement and fatigue. Worst-ever OCD symptoms occur approximately 2 years later than worst-ever tic symptoms (Bloch et al., 2006). Thus, OCS associated with TS appears similar to the spectrum of the tic disorder with regard to onset, severity, and course (Como et al., 2005).

Regarding comorbidities (Fig. 3.2), the Brazilian OCD Consortium study reported that the tic-related OCD group, compared to pure OCD patients, showed increased rates of anxiety disorders, especially specific and social phobia, generalized anxiety disorder, and posttraumatic stress disorder (PTSD). Separation anxiety disorder, ADHD, skin picking, and impulse-control disorders in general were also more frequent in the group with tic disorders-related OCD compared to the pure OCD group (Coffey et al., 1998; Petter et al., 1998).

The association between tic-related OCD and PTSD is an interesting finding, since psychological trauma may play an etiological role not only in PTSD and tic disorders, but also in OCD (Grabe et al., 2008). Moreover, the high prevalence of impulsivity and ADHD in this population might also have increased the chance of exposure to traumatic situations. Higher rates of ADHD and impulse-control disorders, which have been frequently described in both TD and early-onset OCD, might be related to a continuum of impulsivity and motor disinhibition observed in TS patients (Ferrão, 2009).

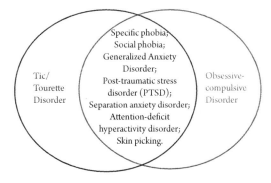

FIGURE 3.2   Common psychiatric comorbidities in patients with tics/Tourette disorder and OCD.

The comorbidity of ADHD and TS is more thoroughly discussed in Chapter 2.

Using data from the Brazilian Research Consortium on Obsessive-Compulsive Spectrum Disorders, de Mathis and colleagues (personal communication) developed a study with the goal of understanding the trajectory of comorbid disorders according to the first manifested psychiatric diagnosis and their impact on the clinical development of OCD and subsequent psychiatric comorbidities. Briefly, the authors first investigated the mean age at onset and frequency of Axis I comorbidity distribution in the 1,001 OCD patients. In the whole sample the first comorbidity to appear was separation anxiety disorder, followed by ADHD, and tic disorders. Afterwards, they chose to describe how each one of these disorders would influence the course of clinical and comorbidity patterns along the lifespan if they were the first diagnosis manifested.

The findings are reported in Figure 3.3 (courtesy of Maria Alice de Mathis, 2011). It shows the mean age at onset of psychiatric comorbidities in OCD patients throughout the lifespan (Fig. 3.3A) and the comorbidities distribution when tics (Fig. 3.3B), ADHD (Fig. 3.3C), and separation anxiety (Fig. 3.3D) precede OCD.

Interestingly, OCD patients who presented with separation anxiety disorder as their first diagnosis tended to have higher frequencies of anxiety disorders, somatoform disorders, and posttraumatic stress disorders afterwards. OCD patients who presented with ADHD as their first diagnosis had higher frequencies of substance abuse and dependence. Finally, OCD patients who presented with tic disorders as their first diagnosis had higher frequencies of OC spectrum disorders (i.e., trichotillomania, body dysmorphic disorder, and skin picking and grooming behaviors) (de Mathis, personal communication).

We observed the density curves of the average age at onset for each one of the different comorbidities. These posterior distributions are the normalized likelihood functions. In other words, for a specific comorbidity, the respective curve represents the density function of the age average for the comorbidity. The curve indicates that the true population average (parameter) is more likely to be at some point under the curve,

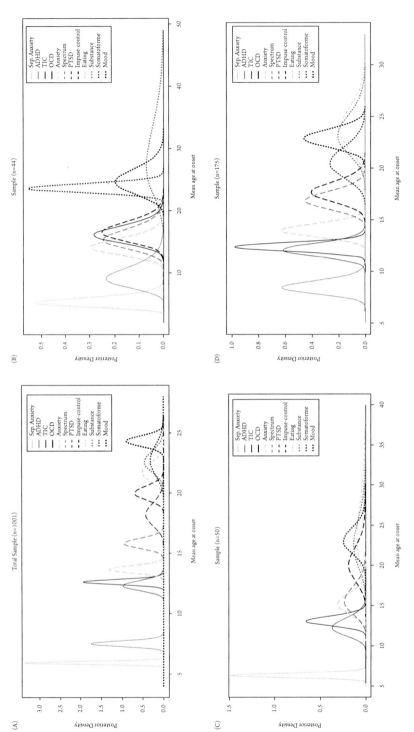

FIGURE 3.3   Psychiatric comorbidities distribution throughout the lifespan and when OCD is preceded by specific psychiatric comorbidities. Sep Anxiety, separation Anxiety; ADHD, attention-deficit/hyperactivity disorder; TIC, tic disorders; OCD, obsessive-compulsive disorder; Anxiety, generalized anxiety disorder; Spectrum, other obsessive-compulsive spectrum disorders; PTSD, posttraumatic stress disorder; impulse-control, impulse-control disorders; eating, eating disorders; Substance, substance dependence; somatoform, somatoform disorders; Mood, mood disorders; n, absolute values. (See color insert.)

with the highest probability near the peak. For instance, the average age at onset of separation anxiety disorder (close to 6 years old) happens most likely before the onset of eating disorders (close to 22 years old). The first is highly probable at 6 years, with little chance of being far from this age. The second can occur at any point between 20 and 24 years old, with the highest probability being near 22 years old. It is worth mentioning that when the distribution of the probabilities is applied, the area under the curve is always one. In Figure 3.4 we tried to reconcile the findings of Mathis and colleagues (personal communication) with previous models (Miguel et al., 2005) proposed by our group to subtype OCD, each one related to specific psychiatric comorbidities, according to its onset and

familial load: one group related to anxiety disorders, another to impulse-control disorders, and another related to tic disorder (Fig. 3.4). Further aspects on the differential diagnosis of tic disorders are discussed in Chapter 17.

ETIOLOGY AND PATHOGENESIS

Current theories about the etiology of TS and OCD, as for most psychiatric disorders, suggest that these disorders are the result of an abnormal interaction of environmental and genetic factors during critical periods of development. This may influence the formation of specific neuronal circuits of neural networks that form the neurobiological substrates associated with the expression of the phenotype. Therefore in this section we

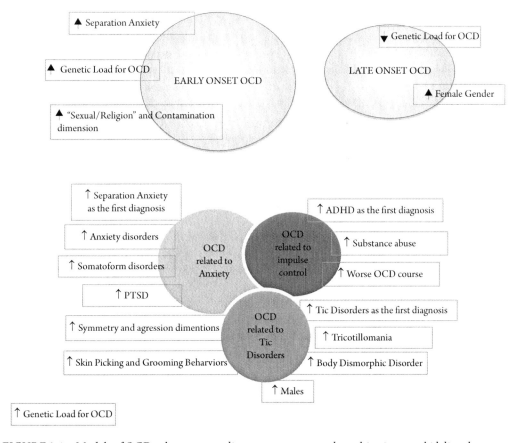

FIGURE 3.4   Models of OCD subtypes according to age at onset and psychiatric comorbid disorders. ADHD, attention-deficit/hyperactivity disorder; OCD, obsessive-compulsive disorder; PTSD, posttraumatic stress disorder. (See color insert.)

(Adapted from de Mathis et al., personal communication).

will briefly discuss the environmental and genetic risk factors associated with OCS in TS and tics in OCD, followed by findings that support the role of specific neurobiological substrates associated with this complex phenotypic expression. A comprehensive understanding about genetic susceptibility for TS is given in Chapter 7, and a more detailed discussion of the neurobiology of TS is given in Chapters 12 and 13.

RISK FACTORS ASSOCIATED WITH OCS IN TS AND TICS IN OCD

General Environmental Risk Factors

In predisposed subjects, environmental factors (Fig. 3.5), emotional stress, traumatic brain injury, and exposure to certain substances (cocaine, stimulants in general, and hormones) early in development can act as triggers for OCD and tics (Motlagh et al., 2010). In the study by Santangelo and colleagues (1994) a history of birth complications during delivery, especially forceps deliveries, was found to be associated with male gender and co-morbid OCD in TS

patients. Fetal exposure to relatively high levels of caffeine, nicotine, or alcohol was also found to be predictive of OCD in TS probands. Vasconcelos and colleagues (2006) found that edema of the hands, feet, or face and excessive weight gain during gestation; hyperemesis gravidarum; prolonged labor; preterm birth; and jaundice could be prenatal, perinatal, and postnatal risk factors associated with the expression of OCD later in life (see also Chapter 8 for more details on this aspect).

In the past two decades an elegant field of research has investigated the association between group A β-hemolytic streptococcal (GABHS) infection as well as rheumatic fever (systemic autoimmune disease triggered by GABHS) and the arousal of neuropsychiatric disorders, especially tics and/or OCD (Alvarenga et al., 2006; Mercadante et al., 2005). The model for pathophysiology suggests that GABHS infection in a susceptible host initiates the production of autoantibodies that cross-react with the cellular components of the basal ganglia, particularly in the caudate nucleus and putamen (Arnold & Richter, 2001; Mercadante et al., 2005). This

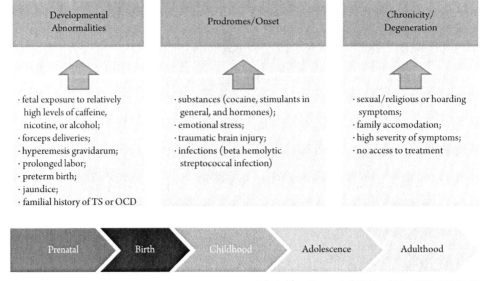

Environmental Risk Factors Associated with OCS and OCD in TS

Developmental Abnormalities	Prodromes/Onset	Chronicity/ Degeneration
· fetal exposure to relatively high levels of caffeine, nicotine, or alcohol; · forceps deliveries; · hyperemesis gravidarum; · prolonged labor; · preterm birth; · jaundice; · familial history of TS or OCD	· substances (cocaine, stimulants in general, and hormones); · emotional stress; · traumatic brain injury; · infections (beta hemolytic streptococcal infection)	· sexual/religious or hoarding symptoms; · family accomodation; · high severity of symptoms; · no access to treatment

Prenatal ▷ Birth ▷ Childhood ▷ Adolescence ▷ Adulthood

Adapted from Tsuang et al. Br J Psychiatry 1990; 156:17-26

FIGURE 3.5   Environmental risk factors associated with OCS in TS and tics in OCD. OCS, obsessive-compulsive symptoms; OCD, obsessive-compulsive disorder; TS, Tourette syndrome.

hypothesis was supported by neuroimaging (Giedd et al., 1996) and immunological assays (Hoekstra et al., 2004). In 1998 Swedo and colleagues characterized 50 prepubertal children with acute onset of OCD, TS, and other neuropsychiatric disorders after streptococcal infection and proposed the acronym PANDAS (pediatric autoimmune neuropsychiatric disorders associated with streptococcal infection) as a novel diagnosis (Swedo et al., 1998). PANDAS were postulated to represent a more homogeneous subgroup of children with tics and/or OCD who may experience symptom exacerbation after GABHS infection. PANDAS children are significantly more likely to present with separation anxiety, urinary urgency, hyperactivity, impulsivity, and decline in school performance during their initial episode of neuropsychiatric disorder compared to non-PANDAS children (Bernstein et al., 2010). Although the PANDAS concept has been widely accepted, many controversies remain. More recently, the new concept "pediatric acute onset neuropsychiatry syndrome" (PANS) has been proposed, emphasizing the acute "overnight" onset of OCD in these cases. The PANS criteria also deemphasize tic symptoms compared to their more prominent place in the PANDAS criteria (Swedo et al., 2012). More detailed information about streptococcal infection, PANDAS, and PANS will be presented in Chapters 9 and 14.

Genetic Risk Factors Associated with OCD in TS and Tics in OCD

The genetics of TS is thoroughly discussed elsewhere in this book (Chapter 7). We will summarize here the main findings regarding the genetics of TS and OCD comorbidity. Although genetic research in OCD and TS has evolved substantially in the past 30 years, the precise genetic abnormalities underlying the pathophysiology of both disorders remain unknown.

Briefly, family studies have demonstrated that the frequency of OCD without tics among first-degree relatives is significantly elevated in the families of patients with TS or OCD, as well as in those of TS-without-OCD probands, and that these rates are higher than in the general population (Grados et al., 2001; Pauls et al., 1995; Rosario-Campos et al., 2005).

Studies have also found that childhood-onset OCD is a highly familial disorder, and that these early-onset cases might represent a valid subgroup, with higher genetic loading and shared vulnerability with chronic tic disorders (O'Rourke et al., 2009; Rosario-Campos et al., 2005). In addition, specific OCS are likely to be integral to the TS clinical profile (Leckman et al., 2003). Alsobrook and colleagues (1999) were the first to use OCS dimensions in a genetic study. They found that the relatives of OCD probands who had high scores on the obsessions/checking and symmetry/ordering factors (factors that are also associated with tic-related OCD) were at greater risk for OCD than were relatives of probands who had low scores on those factors.

A few segregation analyses have been performed on TS datasets. Using data collected by the Tourette Syndrome Association International Consortium for Genetics (TSAICG) Affected Sibling Pair Study, Leckman and colleagues (2003) selected all available affected TS pairs and their parents for whom these obsessive-compulsive symptom dimensions (factor scores) could be generated using the four-factor algorithm first presented by Leckman and colleagues (1997). Remarkably, over 50% of the TS siblings were found to have comorbid OCD and more than 30% of mothers and 10% of fathers also had a diagnosis of OCD. The factor scores for aggressive, sexual, and religious obsessions; checking compulsions; and symmetry and ordering obsessions and compulsions were significantly correlated in sibling pairs concordant for TS. In addition, the mother–child correlations, but not father–child correlations, were significant for these two factors. On the basis of the results of the complex segregation analyses, significant evidence for genetic transmission was obtained for all factors.

PATHOPHYSIOLOGICAL MODEL OF OCS IN TS OR TICS IN OCD

The prefrontal cortices and striatum (caudate + putamen) are interlinked by a web of pathways that form the cortical–striatum–thalamocortical circuits (Bolam et al., 2000; Mink, 1996). This same circuit is involved in tics and in OCS (Mink, 2001; Saxena & Rauch, 2000), but for each patient, other structures and/or pathways (involving, for example, amygdala, hippocampus, and nucleus accumbens) may contribute to the different symptom presentations. There seem to be two distinct pathways of functioning in the cortical–striatum–thalamocortical circuits: the direct and the indirect ones (Mercadante et al., 2004). While there is a balance between these two pathways in healthy individuals, some authors speculate that TS and OCD sufferers show a preference for the direct pathway, thereby increasing activity in the orbitofrontal cortex, ventromedial caudate, and medial dorsal thalamus, which results in tics, obsessions, or compulsions (Govindan et al., 2010; Jang et al., 2010; Lewis & Kim, 2009; Saxena et al., 2000; Mink, 2001; Muller-Vahl et al., 2009; Stern et al., 2011), depending on what structure is more or less involved in the specific pathway.

In the prefrontal cortex, dopaminergic and serotonergic terminals mutually contact both pyramidal neurons and nonpyramidal interneurons (Lambe et al., 2000). From clinical and anatomical considerations, it has been inferred that TS and OCD are disorders associated primarily with alterations in the basal ganglia and, based on the dense dopaminergic and serotonergic innervations of the striatum, these are specifically disorders of striatal organization and/or function (Wong et al., 2008). For example, the dorsal striatum is crucial for some appropriate sequencing of repetitive movements, such as grooming (Aldridge & Berridge, 1998; Cromwell & Berridge, 1996). Berridge and colleagues (2005) suggested that stereotypies are analogous to complex tics or obsessive-compulsive behaviors. Another important concept is that the basal ganglia participate in brain circuits responsible for habit formation and maintenance. Tics (and tic-like compulsions) could represent a form of inappropriate habit formation in which inappropriate stimulus–response associations are formed. This interpretation might correlate with the fluctuating nature and "sensory" component of tics (Marsh et al., 2004).

Worbe and colleagues (2010) compared patients with simple tics, with complex tics, and with tics associated with OCS and found that the pattern of cortical thinning differed among the clinical subgroups of patients. In patients with simple tics, cortical thinning was mostly found in primary motor regions. In patients with simple and complex tics, thinning extended into larger premotor, prefrontal, and parietal regions. In patients with associated obsessive-compulsive disorders, there was a trend for reduced cortical thickness in the anterior cingulate cortex, and hippocampal morphology was altered.

The cortico–striatal–thalamocortical neurocircuitry model considers the tonically active inhibitory output of the basal ganglia as a "brake" on motor pattern generators (MPGs) in the cerebral cortex and brainstem (Mink, 1996). For a desired movement controlled by a particular MPG, a specific set of striatal neurons is activated; these neurons inhibit basal ganglia output neurons in the globus pallidus pars interna (GPi) and substantia nigra pars reticulata (SNr) that project back, via the thalamus, to the cortical MPGs. The removal of tonic inhibition from the GPi and SNr (the "brake") enables the desired motor pattern to proceed. In parallel, neurons in the subthalamic nucleus (STN) excite the surrounding majority of GPi and SNr output neurons. These surrounding neurons project via the thalamus to competing MPGs, increasing their inhibitory output and applying the "brake" to competing MPGs. The net result is facilitation of intended movement with inhibition of competing movements. In the generation of tics, it is hypothesized that an aberrant focus (with or without repetitive overactivity) of striatal neurons becomes inappropriately active, causing unwanted inhibition of a group of basal ganglia output neurons, which in turn disinhibit an MPG leading to an involuntary movement (tics) or intentional repetitive behaviors (tic-like compulsion and/or compulsions) (Albin & Mink, 2006). According to this hypothesis, each repetitive movement or behavior corresponds to the activity of a discrete set of striatal neurons (Mink, 2001), possibly within striatal matrisomes (Graybiel et al., 1994). Matrisomes are thought to be zones of functional homogeneity defined to a large extent by the pattern of corticostriate inputs.

Graybiel (1997) proposed that some basal ganglia neuronal loops that are involved in motor aspects (tics, compulsions, and tic-like compulsions) may also be involved in cognitive processes (obsessions), since the ventral striatum is connected to the hippocampal system, where the cognitive maps and declarative memories are grounded. The striosomes, especially in the caudate nucleus, receive inputs from the limbic system (especially from the orbitofrontal cortex, anterior cingulate, and amygdala). Because the striosomes are surrounded by the tissue matrix (matrisomes), which itself has clear sensorimotor connections, the striosomes may also have local connections that interfere with the occurrence of cognitive, emotional, and motor aspects simultaneously, justifying the intersection of psychopathological phenomena in patients with TS and OCD (tics, obsessions, compulsions, tic-like compulsions, anxiety, and sensory phenomena).

The model of deficient frontostriatal circuits (especially those including the dorsomedial striatum) in OCD and in TS is supported by studies of impaired sensorimotor gating, as assessed with the prepulse inhibition (PPI) paradigm (Baldan et al., 2011; Hoenig et al., 2005; Swerdlow et al., 2001). Hoenig and colleagues (2005) found that PPI was reduced in OCD patients, and this deficit was most pronounced for most intense (16 dB(A)) prepulses, where mean PPI was 39.6% in unmedicated patients (n = 4), 45.8% in medicated patients, and 58.9% in controls. De Leeuw and colleagues (2010) measured PPI of the startle reflex and P50 suppression paradigms and found that sensorimotor and sensory gating were not impaired in drug-free OCD patients. Thus, PPI deficits (related or not related to pharmacological and behavioral treatment and to possible subtypes of OCD [i.e., tic-related OCD]) merit further studies in TS and OCD patients.

In summary, the cortico–striatum–thalamo-cortical circuits are involved in tics and in OCS. The different symptom presentations for each patient may be the result of other involved structures connected to the direct and the indirect pathways. The dense dopaminergic and serotonergic innervations imbalance, especially in orbitofrontal cortex, ventromedial caudate, and medial dorsal thalamus, may result in tics or compulsions, as corroborated by neuroimaging and neurophysiological studies. More detailed aspects of neurobiology of TS are discussed in Chapters 12 and 13.

TREATMENT RESPONSE OF OCS IN TS AND TICS IN OCD

Chapter 25 covers the most relevant aspects related to the treatment of OCD comorbid with TS. Initial studies looking for treatment response in OCD found that the presence of tics in OCD patients was associated with a worse response to monotherapy with a selective serotonin reuptake inhibitor (SSRI; McDougle et al., 1993), and that adding haloperidol to an SSRI was especially effective for OCD patients with comorbid tic disorders (McDougle et al., 1994a). However, subsequent studies did not confirm these findings (Bloch et al., 2009; Husted et al., 2007; Shavitt et al., 2006). Therefore, more studies are necessary to determine the role of tics in the OCD treatment response. Basically, the treatment of OCD in TS should start with the first-line therapies for OCD (March et al., 1997), plus a first-line treatment for tics or TS when necessary (Cath et al., 2011; McDougle et al., 1990, 1994b).

COMMENTARY

The findings reported above support the notion that OCD and TS are commonly associated. Moreover, there are some specific features that differentiate OCD in TS from other forms of OCD. Some of these clinical features are male predominance, early onset of symptoms, the presence of sensory phenomena (e.g., somatic urges and "just-right" perceptions), the OCS dimensions "aggression" and "symmetry" (Diniz et al., 2006; Miguel et al., 2005), and a higher genetic load for OCD and TS. Comorbid disorders such as trichotillomania, body dysmorphic disorder, and skin picking and grooming behaviors are also more frequent in these patients.

Interestingly, patients with OCS and TS, or OCD with tics, share some common environmental and genetic factors, which interact with one other, enhancing the chance of this specific phenotype. For instance, in genetically susceptible families, streptococcal strains might provide the environmental triggers for a variety of psychiatric conditions, particularly OCD and TS (Alvarenga et al., 2008; Hounie et al., 2007).

Recent studies designed to identify valid endophenotypes have suggested that OCD and TS also share certain neurobiological substrates. Structural and functional neuroimaging studies have provided extensive evidence of deregulation of frontostriatal control systems (Marsh et al., 2009), as well as of specific neuropsychological abnormalities, such as fine motor deficits, visual-motor impairment, and cognitive inflexibility (Chang et al., 2007).

Clinical trials in OCD patients and TS patients have shown that cognitive-behavioral treatments (either exposure or response prevention for OCD or habit reversal for TS) have higher effect sizes and provoke fewer side effects than do any pharmacological agents (Mancuso et al., 2010; Piacentini et al., 2010). For patients with OCD who do not respond to cognitive-behavioral treatment or have moderate to severe symptoms, SSRIs are still the pharmacological agents of choice (Mancuso et al., 2010). More studies are necessary to understand and predict the effect of the presence of tics in OCD treatment response. As most clinical trials for OCD exclude patients with TS, the data are scarce. However, instead of being a predictor of worse response as first thought, the presence of tics may, in fact, be associated with a better OCD course (Bloch et al., 2009).

Treatment approaches could be improved, though, if the phenomenological continuum between OCD and TS could be better understood. For instance, specific behavioral approaches could improve tic-related OCD patients who report absence of obsessions, and alternatively present with sensory phenomena preceding their repetitive behaviors. Instead of looking for obsessions on these cases, clinicians should focus on helping the patient to recognize these subjective experiences. To recognize these behaviors in clinical practice, more descriptive terms, such as repetitive behaviors, in the place of compulsions or complex motor tics may be helpful. Although great strides in refining phenotypic knowledge about OCD and TS has allowed us to find more homogeneous phenotypes of the disorders,

---

Box 3.2. Questions for Future Research

- How can the differences between OCD in TS versus other forms of OCD be explained? What environmental, genetic, neurobiological, and neurophysiological mechanisms contribute to those differences?
- Which environmental risk factors for OCD or TS can be identified—and hence prevented or corrected? Are there other external risk factors (other than streptococcal infections)?
- How can we predict the role of the presence of tics in OCD treatment response? Does the presence of tics worsen or improve OCD treatment response to medication, psychotherapies, and neurobiological approaches?
- How can we predict the role of the presence of OCD or other common comorbidities in Tourette syndrome treatment response? Do OCD or other common comorbidities worsen or improve TS treatment response?
  - How can we best understand the range of comorbid conditions associated with OCS and OCD in TS? What makes one patient present with "x" or "y" psychiatric condition associated with OCD and/or TS? Understanding those mechanisms would help us to better treat and rehabilitate patients.

as shown above, this approach has not yet brought what was expected in terms of genetic discovery (i.e., replicable results) or specific treatments.

Therefore, a possible new endeavor for the progress of the field may include the characterization of subjects by using a variety of concurrent neurobiological measures (e.g., different genes, response to neurophysiological paradigms—startle, PPI, EEG findings, findings from neuroimaging techniques, and neuropsychological measures with endophenotypic value), which combined with clinical features could help to identify more specific profiles of subjects with OCD and/or TS for whom adequate and effective personalized treatments could be designed.

An additional strategy to be explored is the investment in longitudinal studies in which individuals at risk (e.g., children of parents with TS or tic-related OCD), during the premorbid phase, can be followed, controlling for the environmental factors during development. In these children, proper therapeutic interventions designed to prevent the beginning of the disorder could be then tested in the prodromal phase.

In conclusion, while we wait for future developments in this intriguing field, the identification of a specific tic-related OCD group can not only increase the knowledge of this specific phenotypic expression and help patients to understand their symptoms, but can also foster the development of specific behavioral and pharmacological treatments (Miguel et al., 2005).

REFERENCES

Albin RL, Mink JW. Recent advances in Tourette syndrome research. *Trends in Neurosciences* 2006; 29(3):175–82.

Aldridge J, Berridge K. Coding of serial order by neostriatal neurons: a 'natural action' approach to movement sequences. *J Neurosci* 1998; 18: 2777–2787.

Alsobrook II JP, Leckman JF, Goodman WK et al. Segregation analysis of obsessive-compulsive disorder using symptom-based factor scores. *Am J Med Genet* 1999; 88: 669–675.

Alvarenga PG, Hounie AG, Mercadante MT et al. Obsessive-compulsive symptoms in heart disease patients with and without history of rheumatic fever. *J Neuropsychiatry Clin Neurosci* 2006; 18:405–408.

Alvarenga PG, Hounie AG, Miguel EC. The role of group A beta-hemolytic streptococcal infection in neuropsychiatric disorders. *Pediatrics* 2008; 122(5):1157.

Alvarenga PG, Mathis MA, Dominguez A et al. Clinical features of tic-related obsessive-compulsive disorder: results from a large multicenter study. *CNS Spectrums* 2012; 17:87–93.

Arnold PD, Richter MA. Is obsessive-compulsive disorder an autoimmune disease? *CMAJ* 2001; 165:1353–1358.

Baer L. Factor analysis of symptom subtypes of obsessive compulsive disorder and their relation to personality and tic disorders. *Journal of Clinical Psychiatry* 1994; 55 Suppl:18–23.

Baldan Ramsey LC, Xu M, Wood N, Pittenger C. Lesions of the dorsomedial striatum disrupt prepulse inhibition. *Neuroscience* 2011; 180:222–228.

Bernstein GA, Victor AM, Pipal AJ, Williams KA. Comparison of clinical characteristics of pediatric autoimmune neuropsychiatric disorders associated with streptococcal infections and childhood obsessive-compulsive disorder. *J Child Adolesc Psychopharmacol* 2010; 20:333–340.

Berridge KC, Aldridge JW, Houchard KR, Zhuang X. Sequential super-stereotypy of an instinctual fixed action pattern in hyper-dopaminergic mutant mice: a model of obsessive compulsive disorder and Tourette's. *BMC Biol* 2005; 3:4.

Bloch MH, Craiglow BG, Landeros-Weisenberger A et al. Predictors of early adult outcomes in pediatric-onset obsessive-compulsive disorder. *Pediatrics*. 2009; 124:1085–1093.

Bloch MH, Landeros-Weisenberger A, Kelmendi B et al. A systematic review: antipsychotic augmentation with treatment refractory obsessive-compulsive disorder. *Mol Psychiatry* 2006; 11:622–632.

An excellent review about therapeutic options for refractory OCD.

Bloch MH, Landeros-Weisenberger A, Rosario MC et al. Meta-analysis of the symptom structure of obsessive-compulsive disorder. *Am J Psychiatry* 2008; 165:1532–1542.

Bloch MH, Leckman JF. Clinical course of Tourette syndrome. *J Psychosom Res* 2009; 67:497–501.

Bolam JP, Hanley JJ, Booth PA, Bevan MD. Synaptic organisation of the basal ganglia. *J Anat* 2000; 196:527–542.

Cath DC, Hoogduin CA, van de Wetering BJ et al. Tourette syndrome and obsessive-compulsive disorder. *An analysis of associated phenomena.* Adv Neurol 1992; 58:33–41.

Cath DC, Hedderly T, Ludolph AG et al. ESSTS Guidelines Group. European clinical guidelines for Tourette syndrome and other tic disorders. Part I: assessment. *Eur Child Adolesc Psychiatry* 2011; 20(4):155–171.

Cath DC, Spinhoven P, Hoogduin CA et al. Repetitive behaviors in Tourette's syndrome and OCD with and without tics: what are the differences? *Psychiatry Res* 2001; 101(2):171–85.

An interesting paper that shows the distinction between obsessions, compulsions and impulsions in Tourette-related repetitive behaviors.

Cavanna AE, Servo S, Monaco F, Robertson MM. The behavioral spectrum of Gilles de la Tourette syndrome. *J Neuropsychiatry Clin Neurosci* 2009; 21(1):13–23.

Chang SW, McCracken JT, Piacentini JC. Neurocognitive correlates of child obsessive compulsive disorder and Tourette syndrome. *J Clin Exp Neuropsychol* 2007; 29(7): 724–33.

Coffey BJ, Miguel EC, Biederman J et al. Tourette's disorder with and without obsessive-compulsive disorder in adults: are they different? *J Nerv Ment Dis* 1998; 86(4):201–206.

This paper highlights the importance of assessing the full spectrum of psychiatric comorbidity in patients with TD and OCD.

Coffey BJ, Rapoport J. Obsessive-compulsive disorder and Tourette's disorder: where are we now? *J Child Adolesc Psychopharmacol* 2010; 20(4): 235–6.

Cohen AJ, Leckman JF. Sensory phenomena associated with Gilles de la Tourette's syndrome. *J Clin Psychiatry* 1992; 53(9):319–323.

Comings DE, Comings BG. A controlled study of Tourette syndrome. IV. Obsessions, compulsions, and schizoid behaviors. *Am J Human Genetics* 1987; 41(5):782–803.

Como PG. Obsessive-compulsive disorder in Tourette's syndrome. In: Weiner WJ, Lang AE (Eds.), *Advances in Neurology.* Raven Press, New York, 1995.

Como PG, LaMarsh J, O'Brien KA. Obsessive-compulsive disorder in Tourette's syndrome. *Adv Neurol* 2005; 96:249–261.

A comprehensive review about OCD in TS, including neurobiological aspects.

Cromwell HC, Berridge KC. Implementation of action sequences by a neostriatal site: a lesion mapping study of grooming syntax. *J Neurosci* 1996;16: 3444–3458.

de Groot CM, Bornstein RA. Obsessive characteristics in subjects with Tourette's syndrome are related to symptoms in their parents. *Comp Psychiatry* 1994; 35(4):248–51.

de Groot CM, Bornstein RA, Janus MD, Mavissakalian MR. Patterns of obsessive compulsive symptoms in Tourette subjects are independent of severity. *Anxiety* 1994–1995; 1(6):268–74.

de Leeuw AS, Oranje B, van Megen HJ et al. Sensory gating and sensorimotor gating in medication-free obsessive-compulsive disorder patients. *Int Clin Psychopharmacol* 2010; 25(4):232–240.

de Mathis MA, Diniz JB, do Rosário MC et al. What is the optimal way to subdivide obsessive-compulsive disorder? *CNS Spectr* 2006 ; 11(10):762–768, 771–774, 776–779.

de Mathis MA, Diniz JB, Shavitt RG et al. Early onset obsessive-compulsive disorder with and without tics. *CNS Spectr* 2009; 14(7):362–370.

This paper highlights the differences between OCD with and without tics according to the age at onset of OCS.

de Mathis MA, do Rosario MC, Diniz JB et al. Obsessive-compulsive disorder: influence of age at onset on comorbidity patterns. *Eur Psychiatry* 2008; 23(3):187–194.

de Mathis MA, Diniz JB, Hounie AG et al. Trajectory in obsessive-compulsive disorder comorbidities. *Eur Neuropsychopharmacol* 2012. (accepted)

Diniz JB, Rosario-Campos MC, Hounie AG et al. Chronic tics and Tourette syndrome in patients with obsessive-compulsive disorder. *J Psychiatric Res* 2006; 40(6):487–493.

This paper compared OCD not only versus OCD+TS, but also versus OCD+chronic tics, showing differences in OCS according to different tic features exhibited by patients.

Esquirol JED. *Des maladies mentales considérées sous les rapports médical, hygiénique et médico-légal.*

[Mental illnesses considered by medical, hygienic and medico-legal aspects] Ed. Balliere, Librairie de l'Académie de Médecine, Paris, 1838.

A classic on OCD that should not be missed in your library.

Ferrão YA, Miguel E, Stein DJ. Tourette's syndrome, trichotillomania, and obsessive-compulsive disorder: how closely are they related? *Psychiatry Res* 2009; *170*(1):32–42.

Ferrão YA, Shavitt RG, Bedin NR et al. Clinical features associated to refractory obsessive-compulsive disorder. *J Affect Disord* 2006; *94*(1-3):199–209.

Ferrão YA, Shavitt RG, Prado H et al. Sensory phenomena associated with repetitive behaviors in obsessive-compulsive disorder: an exploratory study of 1,001 patients. *Psychiatry Research* 2011 (ahead of print). Available online (http://dx.doi.org/10.1016/j.psychres.2011.09.017)

The study on the largest sample to date in which sensory phenomena in OCD were explored.

Freud S. *Introductory lectures on psycho-analysis. Parts I & II, SE*, 1916-17: 15–16.

George MS, Trimble MR, Ring HA et al. Obsessions in obsessive-compulsive disorder with and without Gilles de la Tourette's syndrome. *Am J Psychiatry* 1993; *150*(1):93–97.

Giedd JN, Rapoport JL, Leonard HL et al. Case study: acute basal ganglia enlargement and obsessive-compulsive symptoms in an adolescent boy. *J Am Acad Child Adolesc* 1996; *35*: 913–915.

Graybiel AM et al. The basal ganglia and adaptive motor control. *Science* 1994; *265*, 1826–1831.

Govindan RM, Makki MI, Wilson BJ et al. Abnormal water diffusivity in corticostriatal projections in children with Tourette syndrome. *Hum Brain Mapp* 2010; *31*(11):1665–1674.

Grabe HJ, Ruhrmann S, Spitzer C et al. Obsessive-compulsive disorder and posttraumatic stress disorder. *Psychopathology* 2008; *41*(2):129–134.

Grados MA, Riddle MA, Samuels JF et al. The familial phenotype of obsessive-compulsive disorder in relation to tic disorders: the Hopkins OCD family study. *Biol Psychiatry* 2001; *50*(8):559–565.

This paper "links" genetically OCD to TS.

Graybiel AM. The basal ganglia and cognitive pattern generators. *Schizophrenia Bull* 1997; *23*(3): 459–469.

Heyman I, Fombonne E, Simmons H et al. Prevalence of obsessive-compulsive disorder in the British nationwide survey of child mental health. *Int Rev Psychiatry* 2003;*15* (1-2):178–184.

Hoekstra PJ, Minderaa RB, Kallemberg CG. Lack of effect of intravenous immunoglobulins on tics: a double-blind placebo-controlled study. *J Clin Psychiatry* 2004; *65*(4): 537–42.

Hoenig K, Hochrein A, Quednow BB et al. Impaired prepulse inhibition of acoustic startle in obsessive-compulsive disorder. *Biol Psychiatry* 2005; *57*(10):1153–1158.

Hollander E, Kim S, Braun A et al. Cross-cutting issues and future directions for the OCD spectrum. *Psychiatry Res* 2009; *30;170*(1):3–6.

Houeto JL, Giré P. Tics and Tourette syndrome: diagnosis, course and treatment principles. *Presse Med* 2008; *37*(2 Pt 2):263–270.

Hounie AG, do Rosario-Campos MC, Diniz JB et al. Obsessive-compulsive disorder in Tourette syndrome. *Advances in Neurology* 2006b; *99*:22–38.

Hounie AG, Rosario-Campos, Sampaio AS et al. Tourette Syndrome: treatment. In: Marazziti D, Vitiello B, Masi G. *Handbook of Child and Adolescent Psychopharmacology* (1st ed.). Informa *Healthcare New York*, 2006a. Vol. 1, pp. 145–194.

Hounie AG, Pauls DL, do Rosario-Campos MC et al. Obsessive-compulsive spectrum disorders and rheumatic fever: a family study. *Biol Psychiatry* 2007; *61*:266–272.

Husted DS, Shapira NA, Murphy TK et al. Effect of comorbid tics on a clinically meaningful response to 8-week open-label trial of fluoxetine in obsessive compulsive disorder. *J Psychiatr Res* 2007; *41*(3-4):332–337.

Janet P. *Les Obsessions et La Psychasthenie [Obsessions and the Psychasthenie]* (Vol. 1). Alcan, Paris, 1903.

Another classic that should not be missed in your library.

Jang JH, Kim JH, Jung WH et al. Functional connectivity in fronto-subcortical circuitry during the resting state in obsessive-compulsive disorder. *Neurosci Lett* 2010; *474*(3):158–162.

Kano Y, Ohta M, Nagai Y. Tourette syndrome in Japan: a nationwide questionnaire survey of psychiatrists and pediatricians. *Psychiatry Clin Neurosci* 1998;*52* (4):407–411.

Kono T, Shishikura K, Konno C et al. Obsessive-compulsive symptom dimensions in Japanese Tourette syndrome subjects. *CNS Spectrum* 2010; *15*(5):296–303.

Kushner HI. A brief history of Tourette syndrome. *Rev Bras Psiquiatria* 2000; *22*(2):76–79.

Lambe EK, Krimer LS, Goldman-Rakic PS. Differential postnatal development of catecholamine and serotonin inputs to identified neurons in prefrontal cortex of rhesus monkey. *J Neurosci* 2000; *20*: 8780–8787.

Leckman JF, Bloch MH, King RA. Symptom dimensions and subtypes of obsessive-compulsive disorder: a developmental perspective. *Dialogues Clin Neurosci* 2009; *11*(1):21–33.

Leckman JF, Bloch MH, Scahill L, King RA. Tourette syndrome: the self under siege. *J Child Neurol* 2006; *21*(8):642–649.

Leckman JF, Grice DE, Barr LC et al. Tic-related vs. non-tic-related obsessive compulsive disorder. *Anxiety* 1994-1995; *1*(5):208–215.

This work identifies the specific OCS exhibited by patients with both OCD and tics.

Leckman JF, Grice DE, Boardman J et al. Symptoms of obsessive-compulsive disorder. *Am J Psychiatry* 1997; *154*(7):911–917.

Leckman JF, Pauls DL, Zhang H et al. Obsessive-compulsive symptom dimensions in affected sibling pairs diagnosed with Gilles de la Tourette syndrome. *Am J Med Genetics B Neuropsychiatric Genetics* 2003; *116B*(1):60–68.

Leckman JF, Walker DE, Cohen DJ. Premonitory urges in Tourette's syndrome. *Am J Psychiatry* 1993; *150*(1):98–102.

Leckman JF, Walker DE, Goodman WK et al. "Just right" perceptions associated with compulsive behavior in Tourette's syndrome. *Am J Psychiatry* 1994;*151*(5):675–680.

Lee JC, Prado HS, Diniz JB et al. Perfectionism and sensory phenomena: phenotypic components of obsessive-compulsive disorder. *Compr Psychiatry* 2009; *50*(5):431–436.

Leonard HL, Lenane MC, Swedo SE et al. Tics and Tourette's disorder: a 2- to 7-year follow-up of 54 obsessive-compulsive children. *Am J Psychiatry* 1992;*149*(9):1244–1251.

Lewis M, Kim SJ. The pathophysiology of restricted repetitive behavior. *J Neurodev Disord* 2009; *1*(2):114–132.

Mancuso E, Faro A, Joshi G, Geller DA. Treatment of pediatric obsessive-compulsive disorder: a review. *J Child Adolesc Psychopharmacol* 2010; *20*(4):299–308.

Mansueto CS, Keuler DJ. Tic or compulsion? It's Tourettic OCD. *Behavior Modification* 2005; *29*(5):784–799.

An interesting and comprehensive review about OCD associated with TS, focusing also on treatment options.

March JS, Frances A, Carpenter D, Kahn DA. The expert consensus guideline series— treatment of obsessive-compulsive disorder. *J Clin Psychiatry* 1997;*58* (suppl. 4).

Marsh R, Alexander GM, Packard MG et al. Habit learning in Tourette syndrome: a translational neuroscience approach to a developmental psychopathology. *Arch Gen Psychiatry* 2004; *61*:1259–1268.

Marsh R, Maia TV, Peterson BS. Functional disturbances within frontostriatal circuits across multiple childhood psychopathologies. *Am J Psychiatry* 2009; *166*(6): 664–674.

Mataix-Cols D, Rosario-Campos MC, Leckman JF. A multidimensional model of obsessive-compulsive disorder. *Am J Psychiatry* 2005; *162*(2):228–238.

McDougle CJ, Goodman WK, Leckman JF et al. The efficacy of fluvoxamine in obsessive-compulsive disorder: effects of comorbid chronic tic disorder. *J Clin Psychopharmacol* 1993; *13*:354–358.

McDougle CJ, Goodman WK, Leckman JF et al. Haloperidol addition in fluvoxamine-refractory obsessive-compulsive disorder: a double-blind, placebo-controlled study in patients with and without tics. *Arch Gen Psychiatry* 1994a; *51*:303–308.

McDougle CJ, Goodman WK, Price LH et al. Neuroleptic addition in fluvoxamine-refractory obsessive-compulsive disorder. *Am J Psychiatry* 1990; *147*(5):652–654.

McDougle CJ, Goodman WK, Price LH. Dopamine antagonists in tic-related and psychotic spectrum obsessive-compulsive disorder. *J Clin Psychiatry* 1994b; *55*(Suppl. 3):24–31.

Mercadante MT, Diniz JB, Hounie AG et al. Obsessive-compulsive spectrum disorders in rheumatic fever patients. *J Neuropsych Clin Neurosci* 2005; *17*(4):544–547.

Mercadante MT, Rosario-Campos MC, Quarantini LC, Sato FP. The neurobiological bases of obsessive-compulsive disorder and Tourette syndrome. *Jornal de Pediatria* 2004; *80*(2 Suppl):S35–44.

The next three references explore comprehensively the phenomenology of OCD and TS and their possible overlap.

Miguel EC, Baer L, Coffey BJ et al. Phenomenological differences appearing with repetitive behaviours in obsessive-compulsive disorder and Gilles de la Tourette's syndrome. *Br J Psychiatry* 1997; *170*:140–145.

Miguel EC, Coffey BJ, Baer L et al. Phenomenology of intentional repetitive behaviors in obsessive-compulsive disorder and Tourette's disorder. *J Clin Psychiatry* 1995; *56*(6):246–255.

Miguel EC, do Rosário-Campos MC, Prado HS et al. Sensory phenomena in obsessive-compulsive disorder and Tourette's disorder. *J Clin Psychiatry* 2000; *61*(2):150–156.

Miguel EC, Leckman JF, Rauch S et al. Obsessive-compulsive disorder phenotypes: implications for genetic studies. *Mol Psychiatry* 2005; *10*(3):258–275.

Miguel EC, Ferrão YA, Rosário MC et al. The Brazilian Research Consortium on Obsessive-Compulsive Spectrum Disorders: recruitment, assessment instruments, methods for the development of multicenter collaborative studies and preliminary results. *Rev Bras Psiquiatr* 2008; *30*(3):185–196.

Mink JW. The basal ganglia: focused selection and inhibition of competing motor programs. *Prog Neurobiol* 1996; *50*:381–425.

Mink JW. Basal ganglia dysfunction in Tourette's syndrome: a new hypothesis. *Pediatr Neurol* 2001; *25*:190–198.

Min SK, Lee H. A clinical study of Gilles de la Tourette's syndrome in Korea. *Br J Psychiatry* 1986; *149*:644–647.

Motlagh MG, Katsovich L, Thompson N et al. Severe psychosocial stress and heavy cigarette smoking during pregnancy: an examination of the pre- and perinatal risk factors associated with ADHD and Tourette syndrome. *Eur Child Adolesc Psychiatry* 2010; *19*(10):755–764.

Müller N. Tourette's syndrome: clinical features, pathophysiology, and therapeutic approaches. *Dialogues Clin Neurosci* 2007; *9*(2):161–171.

Müller-Vahl KR, Kaufmann J, Grosskreutz J et al. Prefrontal and anterior cingulate cortex abnormalities in Tourette Syndrome: evidence from voxel-based morphometry and magnetization transfer imaging. *BMC Neurosci* 2009; *10*:47.

Nestadt G, Samuels J, Riddle M et al. A family study of obsessive-compulsive disorder. *Arch General Psychiatry* 2000; *57*(4):358–363.

Neuner I, Ludolph A. Tics and Tourette's syndrome throughout the life span. *Nervenarzt* 2009; *80*(11):1377–1387.

O'Rourke JA, Scharf JM, Yu D, Pauls DL. The genetics of Tourette syndrome: a review. *J Psychosom Res* 2009; *67*(6):533–545.

Pauls DL, Alsobrook JP 2nd, Goodman W et al. A family study of obsessive-compulsive disorder. *Am J Psych* 1995; *152*(1):76–84.

Pauls DL, Leckman J. The inheritance of Gilles de la Tourette's syndrome and associated behaviors. Evidence for autosomal dominant transmission. *N Engl J Med* 1986a; *315*(16):993–997.

Pauls DL, Towbin KE, Leckman JF et al. Gilles de la Tourette's syndrome and obsessive-compulsive disorder. Evidence supporting a genetic relationship. *Arch Gen Psychiatry* 1986b; *43*(12):1180–1182.

One of the first (and most valuable) papers that associate OCD and TS genetically.

Petter T, Richter MA, Sandor P. Clinical features distinguishing patients with Tourette's syndrome and obsessive-compulsive disorder from patients with obsessive-compulsive disorder without tics. *J Clin Psychiatry* 1998; *59*(9):456–459.

Similar to the Miguel et al. papers above, this work explores the overlap of phenomenology of OCD and TS.

Phillips KA, Stein DJ, Rauch SL et al. Should an obsessive-compulsive spectrum grouping of disorders be included in DSM-V? *Depression Anxiety* 2010; *27*(6):528–555.

Piacentini J, Woods DW, Scahill L et al. Behavior therapy for children with Tourette disorder: a randomized controlled trial. *JAMA* 2010; *303*(19):1929–1937.

Pitman RK. Pierre Janet on obsessive-compulsive disorder: review and commentary. *Arch Gen Psychiatry* 1987; *44*:226–232.

Prado HS, Rosário MC, Lee J et al. Sensory phenomena in obsessive-compulsive disorder and tic disorders: a review of the literature. *CNS Spectrums* 2008; *13*(5):425–432.

Rachman S, Hodgson RJ. Studies in desensitization. IV. Optimum degree of anxiety-reduction. *Behavioral Research Therapy* 1967; *5*(3):249–250.

Robertson MM. The Gilles de la Tourette syndrome and obsessional disorder. *Int*

Clin Psychopharmacol 1991; 6 (Suppl 3): 69–82.

Robertson MM, Banerjee S, Eapen V, Fox-Hiley P. Obsessive-compulsive behaviour and depressive symptoms in young people with Tourette syndrome. *A controlled study. Eur Child Adolesc Psychiatry* 2002; 11(6):261–265.

Rosario-Campos MC, Leckman JF, Curi M et al. A family study of early-onset obsessive-compulsive disorder. *Am J Medical Genetics B Neuropsychiatric Genetics* 2005; 136(1): 92–97.

Rosario-Campos MC, Leckman JF, Mercadante MT et al. Adults with early-onset obsessive-compulsive disorder. *Am J Psych* 2001; 158(11):1899–1903.

Rosario-Campos MC, Miguel EC, Quatrano S et al. The Dimensional Yale-Brown Obsessive-Compulsive Scale (DY-BOCS): an instrument for assessing obsessive-compulsive symptom dimensions. *Mol Psychiatry* 2006; 11(5):495–504.

A paper demonstrating the importance of the dimensional approach in OCD.

Rosario MC, Prado HS, Borcato S et al. Validation of the University of São Paulo Sensory Phenomena Scale: initial psychometric properties. *CNS Spectrums* 2009; 14(6):315–323.

Ruscio AM, Stein DJ, Chiu WT, Kessler RC. The epidemiology of obsessive-compulsive disorder in the National Comorbidity Survey Replication. *Mol Psychiatry* 2010; 15(1):53–63.

Salzman L, Thaler F. Obsessive-compulsive disorder: A review of the literature. *Am J Psychiatry* 1981; 138, 286–296.

Santangelo SL, Pauls DL, Goldstein JM et al. Tourette's syndrome: what are the influences of gender and comorbid obsessive-compulsive disorder? *J Am Acad Child Adolesc Psychiatry* 1994; 33(6):795–804.

This work explores the influence of a specific aspect (gender) in the phenomenological overlap between OCD and TS.

Saxena S, Rauch SL. Functional neuroimaging and the neuroanatomy of obsessive–compulsive disorder. *Psychiatric Clin North Am* 2000; 23:563–586.

Shapiro AK, Shapiro E. Treatment of Gilles de la Tourette's syndrome with haloperidol. *Br J Psychiatry* 1968; 114(508):345–350.

Shapiro AK, Shapiro ES, Bruun RD, Sweet RD. Gilles de la Tourette syndrome. Raven Press, New York, 1978.

Shavitt RG, Belotto C, Curi M et al. Clinical features associated with treatment response in obsessive-compulsive disorder. *Compr Psychiatry* 2006; 47(4):276–281.

Singer H. Neurobiology of Tourette's syndrome: concepts of neuroanatomic localization and neurochemical abnormalities. *Brain and Development* 2003; 25:S70–S84.

Stein DJ. Neurobiology of the obsessive-compulsive spectrum disorders. *Biol Psychiatry* 2000; 47(4):296–304.

Stern ER, Welsh RC, Fitzgerald KD et al. Hyperactive error responses and altered connectivity in ventromedial and frontoinsular cortices in obsessive-compulsive disorder. *Biol Psychiatry* 2011; 69(6):583–591.

Stewart SE, Ceranoglu TA, O'Hanley T, Geller DA. Performance of clinician versus self-report measures to identify obsessive-compulsive disorder in children and adolescents. *J Child Adolesc Psychopharmacol* 2005; 15(6):956–963.

Summerfeldt LJ. Understanding and treating incompleteness in obsessive-compulsive disorder. *J Clin Psychol* 2004; 60(11):1155–1168.

Sutherland Owens AN, Miguel EC, Swerdlow NR. Sensory gating scales and premonitory urges in Tourette syndrome. *Scientific World Journal* 2011; 11:736–741.

Swedo SE, Leonard HL, Garvey M et al. Pediatric autoimmune neuropsychiatric disorders associated with streptococcal infections (PANDAS): a clinical description of the first fifty cases. *Am J Psychiatry* 1998; 155:264–271.

Swedo SE, Leckman JF, Rose NR. From research subgroup to clinical syndrome: Modifying the PANDAS criteria to describe PANS (pediatric acute-onset neuropsychiatric syndrome). *Pediatr Therapeut* 2012; 2:113–120.

Swerdlow NR, Karban B, Ploum Y et al. Tactile prepuff inhibition of startle in children with Tourette's syndrome: in search of an "fMRI-friendly" startle paradigm. *Biol Psychiatry* 2001; 50(8):578–585.

Tanner CM, Goldman SM. Epidemiology of Tourette syndrome. *Neurolologic Clinics* 1997; 15(2):395–402.

The Tourette Syndrome Classification Study Group. Definitions and classification of tic disorders. *Arch Neurol* 1993; *50*(10):1013–1016.

Torres AR, Fontenelle LF, Ferrão YA et al. Clinical features of obsessive-compulsive disorder with hoarding symptoms: a multicenter study. *J Psychiatr Res* 2012; *46*(6):724–732.

van Grootheest DS, Bartels M, Cath DC et al. Genetic and environmental contributions underlying stability in childhood obsessive-compulsive behavior. *Biol Psychiatry* 2007; *61*(3):308–315.

Vasconcelos MS, Sampaio AS, Hounie AG et al. Prenatal, perinatal, and postnatal risk factors in obsessive-compulsive disorder. *Biol Psychiatry* 2006; *61*(3):301–307.

Wong DF, Brasic JR, Singer HS et al. Mechanisms of dopaminergic and serotonergic neurotransmission in Tourette syndrome: clues from an in vivo neurochemistry study with PET. *Neuropsychopharmacology* 2008; *33*(6):1239–1251.

Worbe Y, Gerardin E, Hartmann A et al. Distinct structural changes underpin clinical phenotypes in patients with Gilles de la Tourette syndrome. *Brain* 2010; *133*(Pt 12):3649–3660.

Zohar AH, Pauls DL, Ratzoni G et al. Obsessive-compulsive disorder with and without tics in an epidemiological sample of adolescents. *Am J Psychiatry* 1997; *154*(2):274–276.

This work explores the overlap between OCD and TS in a significant sample of adolescents.

4

Other Psychiatric Comorbidities in Tourette Syndrome

DANIELLE C. CATH AND ANDREA G. LUDOLPH

Abstract

This chapter will examine in detail the phenomenology, comorbidity profile, and impact on outcome of all the major psychiatric comorbidities observed in Tourette syndrome (TS) patients in addition to attention-deficit/hyperactivity disorder (ADHD) and obsessive-compulsive disorder. Symptoms of anxiety and depression are frequent in patients with TS and in their family members, but the relationship is complex and still incompletely defined. Whereas obsessive-compulsive symptoms, more than tics, may be associated with later development of anxiety and depressive symptoms, anxiety symptoms in childhood and adolescence may influence the risk of tic persistence into adulthood. The role of environmental adversities also needs to be underscored as a contributing factor to comorbidity with anxiety and depression in this condition. Specific personality disorders are more common than others in TS, although this remains an underinvestigated aspect. There seem to be similarities between executive function problems typical of autistic spectrum disorders and those typical of TS, and this may in part be accounted for by the comorbidity profile in TS, with cognitive flexibility and planning more impaired in patients with comorbid obsessive-compulsive disorder and autistic traits and inhibition problems more often linked to comorbid ADHD. Likewise, the association with learning disabilities seems related to comorbidity with ADHD particularly. Finally, the impact of rage attacks in TS patients and their association with comorbidities will be discussed.

INTRODUCTION

Since the 1970s there has been increasing awareness of the wide range of psychiatric comorbidities of Tourette syndrome (TS). Up to 79% of cases have comorbid psychopathology, comprising, in addition to attention-deficit/hyperactivity disorder (ADHD) and obsessive-compulsive disorder (OCD) (the subject of Chapters 2 and 3), mood and anxiety disorders, autism spectrum disorders, learning disorders, anger-control problems, conduct and oppositional defiant disorders (CD/ODD), and impulsive, self-injurious, and aggressive behavior (Freeman et al., 2000; Robertson, 2000). In this overview of psychiatric comorbidities of TS, we will address the relevant issue of whether these comorbidities are intrinsic to the TS phenotype, or, alternatively, whether they are consequential to the tic disorder.

ANXIETY AND DEPRESSION IN TS

Clinical Vignette: Robert, a 25-year-old single man with a well-documented history of moderate Tourette disorder (multiple facial tics, throat clearing, and shoulder shrugs) and mild OCD (aggressive obsessions and checking), is referred to the outpatient clinic because of worrying and depressed mood. Lately, his OCD complaints have increased, with more persistent checking of the door, gas, and staring at light switches before leaving his house, and extra checking of his work as an administrator. Checking rituals have taken 2 hours per day for the past 3 months and are highly distressing for him. For 2 months now, he has had difficulties falling asleep due to worrying and wakes up early, with the result that he sleeps less than 5 hours per night. He has lost 4 kg of weight and is unable to concentrate at work. He is very worried that he will not be able to carry on working, will be fired, and will get into financial trouble. Finally, he is worrying that he will be unable to find a partner.

Lifetime prevalence rates for anxiety disorders and depressive symptoms in the general adult population are 19% to 25% and 15%, respectively, are twofold higher in women (Bijl et al., 2002), and are among the top five disorders in terms of health-related costs (Beekman et al., 1997). Depressive and anxiety disorders can, however, already be apparent at age 6 (Bolton et al., 2007). In adults, depressive symptoms appear to be the most important predictor of impaired quality of life in TS (Muller-Vahl et al., 2010), leading to considerably increased health costs, both directly (due to treatment) and indirectly (secondary to loss of productivity) (Dodel et al., 2010; Eddy et al., 2011a). In children, comorbid anxiety or depression is often referred to as "internalizing" behavior; therefore, when logical, we will also use this term in this chapter. Internalizing behavior refers to behavior directed toward the self (e.g., somatic complaints and anxiety/depression). Internalizing behavior is usually measured by the Child Behavior Checklist (CBCL; Achenbach & Ruffle, 2000).

Epidemiology of Anxiety and Depression in TS: Clinic-Based Studies

In an early report (1969) of 34 cases with TS, increased rates of "inhibition of hostility" have been described in patients, but no specific mention was made of comorbid anxiety or depression (Corbett et al., 1969). One of the earliest large-scale studies on comorbidity in TS was a survey of 431 members of the Ohio chapter of the Tourette Syndrome Association, in which 33% of the TS patients reported extreme anxiety and 32% reported mood swings (Stefl et al., 1984). Comings and Comings (1987) reported that simple phobias occurred in 26% of their TS population (n = 246), compared to 8.5% of a control population (n = 47), with a female preponderance (55%) for simple phobias (Comings & Comings, 1987a, 1987b). Panic attacks were recorded in 33% of the patients

(with up to 16% of patients reporting more than two panic attacks per week) compared to 8% of the controls. Elevated depression scores were found in 22.9% of the patients compared to 2% of the controls. Other studies confirmed elevated rates of anxiety and depression, with rates of major depressive disorder or depressive symptoms up to 41%, phobias up to 37%, and generalized anxiety disorder up to 16% in TS groups across different ages (Pauls et al., 1994; Rosenberg et al., 1995; Spencer et al., 1995). More recent clinical studies confirmed elevated rates of depression in TS children as well as in adults compared to controls, with approximately 45% of patients labeled as depressed and 12% who fulfilled ICD-10 criteria for major depressive disorder (Eapen et al., 2004; Robertson, 2006). Estimates appear to be influenced by the type of referral: higher rates have been reported in series from specialized TS clinics (Coffey et al., 2000), whereas studies from very large clinical databases, such as the Tourette Syndrome International Consortium (TIC) database, provided lower rates (Freeman, 2007; Freeman et al., 2000). Finally, when directly compared to patients with major depressive disorder (MDD) and isolated OCD, TS patients score between MDD or OCD patients and controls on quantitative measures of depression (e.g., Beck Depression Inventory) (George et al., 1993; Robertson et al., 1993).

Epidemiology of Anxiety and Depression in TS: Community-Based Studies

Patients with multiple comorbidities are more likely to be referred to specialty clinics than patients with isolated tic disorder. Community-based studies can therefore provide more realistic estimates of the comorbidity of tics, anxiety, and depression, since population-based studies on tics are likely to include more cases with TS who are only mildly affected and not in treatment. Few population-based studies have been conducted on this issue (Table 4.1). In a study of 166 school children age 13 or 14 years, 30 (18%) were diagnosed with possible tics, and 5 with definite TS; rates of self-reported depression were not elevated in the possible tics or TS cases of this cohort (Mason et al., 1998). In a subsequent study by Hornsey and colleagues (2001), tics were identified in 189 (18.7%) of 918 schoolchildren aged 13 or 14, and 7 (0.8%) fulfilled diagnostic criteria for TS: individuals with mild tics (n = 42; 4.5%) did not differ from the unaffected group on quantitative depression scores using the Birleson Depression self-rating scale (Hornsey et al., 2001).

Kurlan and colleagues (2002) conducted a community-based study with direct interviews in 1596 schoolchildren between 9 and 17 years of age (Kurlan et al., 2002). When compared to children without tics (n = 1,257; 78%), children with tics (n = 339; 22%) had significantly more over-anxious disorder (21% vs. 15%), separation anxiety disorder (15% vs. 7%), simple phobias (29% vs. 19%), social phobia (28% vs. 18%), and agoraphobia (9.4% vs. 6.3%). Rates of panic disorder (4.7% vs. 4.1%), major depressive disorder, and dysthymia were similar across children with and without tics (9.7% vs. 7.5% and 5% vs. 4%, respectively). A drawback of the study was that only 11% of the selected subjects agreed to participate in the study; therefore, the representativeness of the sample is unclear. One recent study reviewed insurance claims from private and public insurances across a 1-year period focusing on tic diagnoses. Interestingly, the children under Medicaid insurance (representing public insurance) had significantly higher comorbidities, including higher rates of depression (14% vs. 9.8%), than the privately insured children (Olfson et al., 2011).

In conclusion, there seems to be some divergence between the information gathered from clinical studies and population-based studies. Clinical studies in TS indicate elevated rates of both anxiety and depression, whereas population-based studies seem to confirm the elevated rates of anxiety disorders (particularly separation anxiety and social and specific phobias) in TS, but not of depression. An age factor might be involved, since most epidemiological studies were conducted in children and adolescents. Thus, as expected, the occurrence of depression seems to be more prominent in clinically referred cases and in adults, suggesting that depression develops with age and as a consequence of disease burden. In contrast, tics and phobias co-occurring in community-based samples of children might share underlying genetic mechanisms. However, due to the cross-sectional nature of the studies and the paucity of community-based studies, plus the lack of studies across different age windows, no definite conclusions can be inferred from these data with respect to etiology. Longitudinal studies, as well as family and twin studies, are more suitable to investigate the nature of the relationship between TS and comorbidity.

Table 4.1 Overview of Epidemiological Studies on Mood and Anxiety Disorders in Tourette Syndrome

Reference	Population	Age (yrs)	N	Outcome
Mason et al., 1998	Schoolchildren	13–14	166	N = 30 tic possible, n = 5 TS No elevated depression rates
Hornsey et al, 2001	Schoolchildren	13–14	918	N = 42 tic possible, n = 7 TS No elevated depression rates
Kurlan et al., 2002	Schoolchildren	10–15	1,596	N = 339 tic disorder Elevated anxiety disorder rates No elevated depression rates
Olfson et al., 2011	Insurance registry of publicly & privately insured children		>26 million	Elevated depression rates (9.8–14.6%) depending on type of insurance

Course of Anxiety and Depression Comorbidity in Relation to Tic Persistence Across the Lifespan

A number of clinical studies have examined the time course between onset of tics and onset of anxiety or depressive symptoms in TS. Coffey and colleagues (2004) re-examined a group of 50 children with TS between 6 and 17 years who had been thoroughly examined 2 years earlier, in order to assess the relationship between tic persistence and tic-associated impairment (including anxiety and depression). At baseline, 88% of subjects met threshold criteria for at least mild tics, and 30% of them showed tic-associated impairment. At the 2-year follow-up, tics persisted in 82% of them, but tic-associated impairment was still present in only 14%, suggesting that future overall impairment is not necessarily predicted by the persistence of tics in TS. This aspect has been explored in the literature with contrasting results, with some authors reporting slightly higher rates of internalizing behavior in children and adults with isolated tic disorder compared to the general population (Carter et al., 1994; Rizzo et al., 2011) and others failing to report any difference (Sukhodolsky et al., 2003).

What about the relationship the other way around? Are there studies available on the predictive value of comorbid anxiety and depression on later tic persistence? Peterson and colleagues (2001) performed an epidemiological longitudinal study in 976 schoolchildren, with three measurement points, studying the relationships between tics and comorbidities and the persistence/occurrence of tics and comorbidities over time. Interestingly, the authors found that tic persistence into adulthood was predicted by simple phobias and by comorbid OCD in early adolescence, suggesting that these comorbidities—rather than tic occurrence at adolescence—determine tic persistence into adulthood.

Anxiety and Depression Comorbidity in Relation to Tic Severity Across the Lifespan

Several cross-sectional studies have found positive relationships between tic severity (as measured with the Yale Global Tic Severity Scale) and rates of depression and anxiety (Cath et al., 2001; Coffey et al., 2000; Comings & Comings, 1987a, 1987b; Gorman et al., 2010). However, as noted by Rosenberg and colleagues (1995), the relationship between depressive symptoms and tic severity is not strictly linear: some children with severe tics are remarkably resilient with respect to possible consequences and social reactions to the tics, and others with only mild tics report severe depressive symptoms as a result of their mild tic disorder. Although the literature is somewhat contradictory, recent studies have found that tic severity either does not affect or only slightly affects quality of life (Eddy et al., 2011a). In contrast, comorbid anxiety and depression do have a substantial impact on quality of life in TS (Eddy et al., 2011b). Further, in a clinical study in 190 children and adolescents with various degrees of TS symptom severity, Coffey and colleagues (2000b) found that anxiety disorders were overrepresented among subjects with severe TS in comparison to patients with mild TS; separation anxiety disorder most robustly and independently predicted tic severity, irrespective of the presence of OCD or other anxiety disorders. In a related study, Coffey and colleagues (2000a) examined 156 TS patients between 5 and 20 years of age. Of the 19 (12%) TS patients who required psychiatric hospitalization, major depression, bipolar disorder, panic disorder, and overanxious disorder were significant predictors of hospitalization, whereas tic severity only marginally predicted whether hospitalization was needed. Another more recent study (Cohen et al., 2008) found that in 65 TS children between 9 and 16 years, tic severity—as reported by the mothers—correlated with comorbid depression, but not with comorbid anxiety symptoms.

To summarize, both anxiety disorders and depression are associated with tic severity. However, the direction of the relationships—whether more severe tics lead to more severe anxiety or depressive symptoms or vice versa—cannot be inferred from these cross-sectional studies. Prospective longitudinal studies can shed more light on the direction of the relationship between tic severity, anxiety, and depression (Lin et al., 2007; Peterson et al., 2001). One 2-year prospective study with between 4 and 24 measurements in the 2 years has specifically addressed this issue, using structural equation modeling (Lin et al., 2007). This study was performed in 45 patients (age 7–17 years) with TS alone, TS+OCD, or OCD alone, and in 41 matched controls, to study the temporal relationship between psychosocial stress and the severity of tics, obsessive-compulsive symptoms, and depressive symptoms. Current obsessive-compulsive symptom severity (and worsening of obsessive-compulsive symptoms), as well as psychosocial adversity, mostly predicted future depressive symptoms. Further, and importantly, current depression was an independent predictor of future tic symptom severity, independent of antecedent psychosocial stress. In contrast, tic severity only very modestly predicted future depression. Thus, depressive symptoms in children and adolescents seem to be markers of later tic severity, rather than tic severity predisposing to later depressive symptoms. The temporal relationship between tic severity and anxiety symptoms was not directly addressed in this study.

et al., 2002), these findings support the hypothesis that, in adult women more so than in adult men, tic persistence and severity have a direct impact on quality of life, and—as a result—might lead to depressive and (non-OCD) anxiety symptoms. The authors suggest that the reason is that women are generally more sensitive to negative social feedback (as a result of their tics) than men.

In sum, the overall rather complex picture that emerges from these studies on the relation of tics with anxiety and depression diverges between children and adults. Children (as well as adolescents and adults) with "tics only" only very modestly differ from healthy controls in terms of anxiety and depression. Neither the persistence of tics into adolescence and adulthood nor tic severity at a young age sufficiently explain the development of anxiety or depressive disorders later in life. In adults, the picture is slightly different, especially in women with TS. Adult women seem to be more sensitive to social signals from the environment and therefore, with increasing tic severity, seem to be more at risk to develop comorbid anxiety and depressive symptoms due to tic disease burden.

Gender Issues in the Relation Between Tics and Comorbid Anxiety and Depression

A recent Internet-based survey in a nonclinical sample of 460 adults, comparing 185 women with 275 men with self-reported TS, found that women in the survey reported twice as many comorbid conditions as the men, despite similar tic frequencies and severity rates (Lewin et al., 2011). The comorbid disorders reported by the women encompassed 1.75 times more non-OCD anxiety disorders, 1.8 times more mood disorders, and 11 times more eating problems than men. Further, in women, tic severity was found to be associated with anxiety, depression, and functional impairment. Despite several limitations of this study, including Web-based data collection and therefore no verification of tic diagnoses by independent observers, and considering the fact that internalizing behaviors overall occur more frequently in women (Bijl

Relation Between Anxiety and Depression in TS with Comorbid ADHD and OCD

Comorbidity between TS and OCD and between TS and ADHD has been addressed in Chapters 2 and 3. Generally, in TS comorbid ADHD and OCD significantly contribute to lower psychosocial functioning (Gorman et al., 2010) and to lower quality of life (Eddy et al., 2010a, 2010b). To what extent do these comorbidities drive the elevated rates of anxiety and depression in both children and adults with TS? In a recent study in 65 TS children between 9 and 16 years of age (predominantly boys; Cohen et al., 2008), comorbid ADHD was found to correlate with comorbid depression as well as with comorbid anxiety symptoms. In another study, using the TIC database in 5,060 patients, the impact of comorbid ADHD on comorbid psychopathology has been investigated across two age groups—children (5–10 years) and adolescents (11–17 years)—and TS patients with and without comorbid ADHD were compared (Roessner et al., 2007). In the children with TS+ADHD, higher rates of OCD, anxiety disorders, CD/ODD, and mood disorders were found than in TS children without ADHD. In the adolescents with TS+ADHD, higher rates of CD and ODD were found. However, as rates of anxiety disorders, mood disorders, and OCD increased in adolescence in both the TS group without ADHD and in the TS+ADHD group, no between-group differences persisted with respect to internalizing behaviors. Although this was a cross-sectional study, and therefore no definite conclusions can be drawn on the development of internalizing and externalizing behavior from childhood to adolescence, these findings indicate that in children comorbid ADHD is associated with a broad spectrum of internalizing as well as externalizing problems, whereas in adolescence comorbid ADHD seems to be associated predominantly with externalizing behavior. Partly in line with this, a comparative study in children with TS+ADHD (n = 52), children with TS only (n=42), children with ADHD only (n = 52), and control children (n = 61) (Sukhodolsky et al., 2003) found that the group with TS+ADHD and with ADHD only showed considerably more disruptive behavior than the TS-only group, suggesting that externalizing but not internalizing behavior is mostly associated with comorbid ADHD.

With respect to the relationship with OCD, in the 2-year longitudinal study performed by Lin and colleagues (2007), current obsessive-compulsive symptom severity (and worsening of obsessive-compulsive symptoms) predicted future depressive symptoms in children and adolescents in the TS-alone, TS+OCD, or OCD-alone diagnostic groups. A parallel study, using the TIC database, investigated the impact of comorbid OCD on anxiety and depressive symptoms across two different age groups: children (5–10 years) and adolescents (11–17 years) (Wanderer et al., 2012). As expected, both children and adolescents with TS+OCD showed higher rates of internalizing (i.e., anxiety and mood) disorders than individuals with TS without OCD. A year-wise increase

of coexisting mood disorders but not of anxiety disorders was found both for subjects with TS with and without OCD, suggesting that specifically mood disorders develop in the course of the illness, and are associated with cognitive development and illness awareness.

From a somewhat different angle, a recent comparative study investigated the impact of tics, OCD, and ADHD on internalizing and externalizing behaviors, using CBCL data of 180 referred children and adolescents with TS only (n = 38), TS+ADHD (n = 142), or ADHD only (n = 121) and unaffected controls (n = 48) (Pollak et al., 2009). In the TS group, externalizing behaviors were predicted by tic severity, inattention, and hyperactivity/impulsivity, whereas internalizing behaviors were predicted by inattention and OCD symptoms. The authors conclude that tics, ADHD, and OCD symptoms differentially explain the variance in externalizing and internalizing behavioral problems in individuals with TS.

Finally, another prospective study (Peterson et al., 2001) followed 976 schoolchildren from childhood (age range between 1 and 10 years) into early adulthood, with reassessments after 8, 10, and 15 years. Emphasis was placed on the associations between tics, OCD, and ADHD over time, but the development and predictive value of other comorbidities were taken into account as well. A complex picture emerged. Young children with tics were more likely to develop anxiety disorders at adolescence. Adolescents with tics were more likely to develop depression at late adolescence. In young adolescents, childhood tics and early adolescent separation anxiety (measured at time point 2) predicted the development of OCD symptoms in late adolescence. Depression, anxiety, and disruptive behaviors broadly predicted future ADHD symptoms at time points 2 and 3. Finally, comorbid OCD and simple phobias at time point 2 predicted persistence of tics into early adulthood.

In conclusion, the predictive value of OCD and ADHD symptoms in TS patients for the development of symptoms of anxiety disorder and depression in adulthood seems—to a certain extent—to depend on the age of the child at which comorbid OCD and ADHD have occurred.

There seem to be differential age windows at which tics and OCD and ADHD symptoms are more disruptive, with greater impact on functioning later in life. Especially comorbid OCD seems to put persons at risk for developing subsequent anxiety and depression, and has a large impact on disease burden, to a larger extent than tic occurrence or persistence or the occurrence of ADHD.

Family Studies Exploring Anxiety and Depression Comorbidity in TS

Family studies or twin studies specifically targeting comorbidity with anxiety and depression in families of TS patients present an opportunity for exploring underlying relationships among these conditions (Wickramaratne & Weissman, 1993). However, twin studies on the comorbidity between tics, anxiety, and depression have not been done. As in all complex disorders, both environmental and genetic factors seem to contribute to the development and clinical expression of TS and its most prominent comorbidities. Family studies of TS to date have mainly focused on the relation between tic disorders, OCD, and ADHD (Grados & Mathews, 2008). These studies have strongly indicated a fully shared genetic basis between TS and (tic-related) OCD (Pauls et al., 1991; Pauls & Leckman, 1986), and—in a more complex way—shared etiologies between TS and ADHD (Stewart et al., 2006). What about a shared genetic relationship between TS and anxiety and depression? Two early papers by Comings and Comings (1987, 1990) have proposed that anxiety and depressive disorders represent variant expressions of a shared genetic background for TS (Comings, 1990; Comings & Comings, 1987a, 1990). Comings and Comings suggested that, in addition to chronic tics, ADHD and OCD, conduct disorder, learning and speech problems, phobic disorder, and major depressive disorder were all variant manifestations of the TS genotype. Subsequently, one large-scale family study has been performed to study the genetic relationship between mood, anxiety disorders, and TS in 338 biological first-degree relatives of 85 TS probands, 92 biological first-degree relatives of 27 unaffected control probands, and 21 nonbiological first-degree relatives of 6 adopted TS probands. Increased rates of major depressive disorder, panic disorder, simple phobia, and generalized anxiety disorder (GAD) were found in the biological relatives of the probands with TS (Pauls et al., 1994). If a comorbid disorder represents a variant expression of the TS +/- OCD phenotype, then the rate of the comorbid disorder should be elevated in the relatives, independent of whether they have TS, and also independent of whether the proband has the comorbidity. In this study, this was not the case; therefore, the authors concluded that neither anxiety disorders nor comorbid depression are part of the TS phenotype and argued against a genetic relationship between TS and comorbid anxiety and depression. The elevated rates of anxiety and depression symptoms in relatives of TS probands were predominantly found in those relatives who also had comorbid OCD, and symptoms of anxiety and depression were most often preceded by OCD symptoms in these relatives. Apparently, as confirmed by Lin and colleagues (2007), comorbid OCD puts persons at risk for the subsequent development of anxiety and depressive symptoms. However, although the study clearly pointed out that full genetic overlap between TS and phobic and depressive disorders is unlikely, this one study does not rule out partly shared and more complex genetic relationships between TS, TS-related OCD, and anxiety and depressive comorbidity.

Environmental Influences on the Relationship Between TS, Anxiety, and Depression

Environmental adversity such as negative psychosocial influences in childhood, traumatic life events, a negative family environment (Carter et al., 2000; Cohen et al., 2008), or maternal smoking during pregnancy (Mathews et al., 2006) all seem to contribute to the development of anxiety and depression in TS (for further details, see Chapter 8). An important study on environmental adversity in TS has been conducted by Carter and colleagues (1994), examining family functioning and adaptation in 22 families including one person (a parent or child) affected with TS and unaffected high-risk siblings (Carter et al., 1994). Children were followed between 1 and 4 years. No family variables were identified that predicted tic occurrence/severity. However, low family cohesion, low recreational activities, and low independence predicted affective and attentive problems among the children. A more recent study investigated the contribution of family locus of control and perceived parenting style on the presence of internalizing behaviors (anxiety and depression) in 65 TS children (Cohen et al., 2008). External locus of control was an important predictor of anxiety and depression levels in the children. These findings suggest that symptoms of anxiety and depression in children with TS are influenced by family-environment factors that extend beyond the influence of comorbid ADHD and OCD. An internal locus of control, associated with an accepting and autonomy-granting parenting style, appears to protect against anxiety and depression in TS children. The extent to which this finding is specific for TS is debatable. Finally, the 2-year prospective study by Lin and colleagues (2007), described above, found that "current" psychosocial stressors were predictive of future depressive symptoms and of obsessive-compulsive and tic symptom severity, indicating that environmental adversity has an impact on the TS (plus obsessive-compulsive) phenotype as well as on comorbid depressive symptoms.

PERSONALITY DISORDERS AND TS

Very few studies have addressed the occurrence of personality disorders in TS. Personality disorders are defined, according to DSM-IV-TR criteria, as enduring patterns of inner experiences and pervasive and inflexible behaviors that deviate markedly from the expectations of the person's culture. Personality disorders have their onset in adolescence or early adulthood, are stable over time, and lead to distress and impairment (First & Pincus, 2002).

The earliest uncontrolled study conducted on DSM-IV–defined personality disorders in TS, using nonstandardized interviews, reported on 36 adult patients with TS, 75% of whom had a personality disorder (Shapiro et al., 1978).

A later study compared 39 adult TS patients to 34 controls and found that 64% of the patients had one or more DSM-III-R personality disorders, compared to 6% of the controls (Robertson et al., 1997). Taking into account that patients could present with more than one personality disorder, 78% of patients in this small sample showed a cluster B personality disorder, 44% a cluster C personality disorder, and 36% a cluster A personality disorder. Finally, elevated scores on aggression and hostility were found in the TS group. Cath and colleagues (2001) investigated 51 patients with OCD +/- TS in comparison with 26 controls, using dimensional measures of personality. The impulsivity subscale of the Emotionality Activity Sociability Impulsivity Scale Third Version (EASI-III) was used to measure impulsivity (Buss & Plomin, 1975), and the extraversion and neuroticism subscales of the Eysenck Personality Questionnaire (EPQ) were used (Eysenck & Eysenck, 1975). The presence of OCD resulted in lower extraversion scores (F = 11.6, p = .001) and in higher neuroticism scores (F = 11.2, p = .001) of the EPQ. Further, the presence of tics resulted in higher neuroticism scores (F = 6.4, p = .001). Neither EASI-III impulsivity nor EPQ extraversion scores—the latter reflecting impulsivity in a more indirect way—were elevated across or within the patient groups, and no effect of tics was found on EASI-III impulsivity scores or on EPQ extraversion ratings. These findings suggest that the presence of tics is not necessarily related to increased impulsivity, but might be related to increased neuroticism, especially when patients have OCD comorbidity.

Finally, based on previous reports of elevated rates of "schizophrenia-like" symptoms (especially ideas of persecution and of being controlled, and paranoid ideation) in 95 children with TS (Kerbeshian & Burd, 1987), Cavanna and colleagues (2007) evaluated schizotypical traits in 102 patients with TS who were referred to a tertiary clinic. The instrument used was the Structured Clinical Interview on DSM-IV Personality Disorders (SCID-II), supplemented by a self-report scale, the Schizotypal Personality Questionnaire (SPQ) (Raine, 1991). The SPQ has a cognitive-perceptual factor (reality distortion), a disorganized factor (odd behavior, odd speech), and an interpersonal factor (excessive social anxiety, constricted affect, suspiciousness). Fifteen percent of the patients met the criteria for schizotypal personality disorder. Further, in the TS patients, scores were higher on the disorganized factor and on the interpersonal factor, with anxiety, obsessionality, and comorbid OCD being most predictive of schizotypy. Investigations in OCD patients have revealed that patients with comorbid OCD plus schizotypy exhibit a more deteriorative course and poorer prognosis (Gelernter et al., 1995; Poyurovsky & Koran, 2005). In analogy with OCD patients, this might well be the case in TS as well. As the authors state, the TS subgroup with OCD plus schizotypy may share specific dopaminergic striatal dysfunctional similarities with OCD and with schizotypy, as reflected in smaller caudate nucleus volumes in patients with TS (Levitt et al., 2002).

In sum, very few studies have been performed on personality disorder in TS. The most important reason for this is that TS is predominantly a disorder of childhood, a period in which personality disorders might develop but are by definition not present yet. In general, most studies in TS have focused on children and adolescents, and adults have been relatively understudied. Considering the paucity of data available and the absence of epidemiological studies on TS and comorbid personality disorder, it is hard to draw any specific conclusions about comorbidity with personality disorders in TS from the studies carried out to date. In clinical populations rates of personality disorder are increased in general, and comorbid OCD appears to further increase the risk of a comorbid personality disorder and of neuroticism (but not impulsivity) in general.

AUTISM SPECTRUM DISORDERS AND TS

Clinical Vignette: Marc, age 24, has moderate to severe TS with multiple simple and complex motor and vocal tics. He presents at our outpatient clinic because of severe obsessions about contact with girls. He has always been a solitary boy, very attached to his home environment, reluctant to change in any daily routine, with very few friends,

and he has never had a romantic relationship. His worries and subsequent obsessions started 5 years ago at school, after his teacher had made jokes and suggestions about him being in love with a girl in his class. After that, he became increasingly avoidant of young women, producing checking behavior as to whether he had looked at them or spoken with them, avoiding looking at them, and trying to avoid thinking of girls. He has always had a particular interest in agricultural machines, frequently studying their manuals on the Internet, and knowing some of them by heart. Family history reveals that his father is extremely solitary and has set many rules for the family with respect to daily routines that the family has to obey.

Historical Overview

In 1943, Leo Kanner provided the first (and critically important) clinical description of 11 children with "autistic disturbances of affective contact" (Kanner & Eisenberg, 1957). He was the first to conceptualize the lack of autistic children's motivation to engage in social interaction, viewing the disorder as an inborn constitutional disorder. He introduced the term "autism" for these children, borrowing the term from Eugene Bleuler, who had used this term to describe self-centered thinking in schizophrenia patients. Kanner described the sometimes remarkable failure of autistic children to engage in communication, the difficulties they can have in using the first person to describe themselves, and the occasional overresponsiveness of children to sounds or to small changes in daily routine. With respect to the classification of autism spectrum disorders, in DSM-I and DSM-II, the term "childhood schizophrenia" was used to describe autistic children. In DSM-III, autism as a separate disorder was first incorporated into the classification system. In DSM-IV, autism spectrum disorders are positioned within the disorders usually first diagnosed in infancy, childhood, and adolescence. Autism spectrum disorders encompass autistic disorder, Rett's disorder, childhood disintegrative disorder, Asperger disorder, and pervasive developmental disorder not otherwise specified. Since Rett's disorder and childhood disintegrative disorder entail highly characteristic degenerative and specific disorders, further elaboration of their relationship with TS is outside the scope of this chapter. We will focus on the relationship between TS and autism spectrum disorders, including autism, Asperger disorder, and pervasive developmental disorder not otherwise specified. Population prevalence rates of autism spectrum disorders range—depending on the definition of autism (narrow vs. broad)—between 0.07 and 6 per 1,000 persons (Chakrabarti & Fombonne, 2005). The narrowly defined classification includes autistic disorder only, whereas in the broadly defined classification persons with Asperger syndrome and autism spectrum disorders not otherwise specified are included as well. Currently, the concept of a broad autism phenotype of autism spectrum disorders that is continuously distributed in the population, with a population prevalence of about 0.6%, has been adopted (Gillberg & Wing, 1999).

Phenomenology of Autism Coexisting with TS: Similarities and Differences

The comorbidity of autism spectrum disorders with TS has been relatively understudied. At first sight there are some demographic similarities between (some forms of) TS and autism spectrum disorders, with both disorders starting in childhood and having a male preponderance. The male-to-female ratio is about 3:1 in TS (Robertson, 2008) and between 1.5:1 and 6:1 in autism spectrum disorders, depending on the child's intelligence (Muhle et al., 2004). Further, some TS patients, like autism spectrum disorder patients, have academic problems (Rapin, 2001) that might be caused by similar language impairments and/or uneven cognitive profiles that are reported in autism spectrum disorders (Legg et al., 2005).

Tics in TS patients have been observed to also share some phenomenological overlap with the rigid and ritualistic behavior and motor stereotypies of autism spectrum disorders (Baron-Cohen et al., 1999; Rapin, 2001). For example, TS patients as well as autism spectrum disorder patients can display repetitive sniffing and smelling of objects (Comings et al., 1991).

Motor stereotypies are rather variably defined as repetitive simple movements that can easily be suppressed (Singer, 2011). Stereotypies include movements such as hand flapping, rocking, head nodding, and finger wriggling (Singer, 2009). Stereotypies are sometimes misdiagnosed as complex motor tics. However, tics and stereotypies differ in several aspects; whereas tics on average start by age 5 to 6, stereotypies mostly have a very early age of onset (before age 2). Further, tics are predominantly displayed in head, neck, and shoulders; are nonrhythmical, abrupt, and fluctuating; and vary in type and expression; in contrast stereotypies are rhythmical, often predictable, and fixed; are more prolonged in duration; and occur predominantly in the hands and arms or the whole body (Table 4.2; Singer, 2009). Although exact prevalence rates are unknown due to the large differences in definitions, stereotypies occur much more often in children with autism spectrum disorder and in children with developmental delay than in control children (Goldman et al., 2009). Little is known about the course of stereotypies. Although this has not been thoroughly investigated, stereotypies seem to run a rather chronic course. One follow-up study in typically developing children showed persistence of stereotypies in 94% between 6 and 12 years of age (Harris et al., 2008). In contrast, in more than 75% of TS patients, tics tend to decrease in frequency and intensity at adolescence (Leckman et al., 1998). Further, both stereotypies and tics are suppressible, although stereotypies seem to be more easily suppressible than tics (Singer, 2009).

Both in autism spectrum disorders and in TS patients, sensory phenomena sometimes occur. Thus, at first glance the sensory phenomena preceding tics in TS, especially in older children, adolescents, and adults (Leckman et al., 1993), might bear some resemblance to the sensory features in autism (Baranek et al., 2005). For example, patients with tics might experience distress (and tics) provoked by the feeling of cloth or tightness of clothes on the skin (Cath et al., 1992). The sensory phenomena in autistic children have been described to include underresponsiveness as well as overresponsiveness to all sensory modalities (including auditory, visual,

Table 4.2 Tics Versus Stereotypies: Clinical Features

Characteristics	Tics	Stereotypies
Age at onset	>5 yrs	<3 yrs
Course	Decrease in intensity, frequency in adolescence	? More chronic course
Movement characteristics	Brief, sudden, nonrhythmical, variable, brief duration	Rhythmic, predictable, fixed, prolonged duration
Suppressibility	Yes, but variable	Yes, instantaneously
Localization	Predominance for face, head, shoulders, variance in localization	Predominance for hands and arms, whole body, fixed localization
Premonitory urges	In most cases (after age 12)	No
Environmental mediators	Excitement, stress, fatigue	Excitement, stress, fatigue
Goal-directedness	Often in response to internal or external environmental cues	Mostly self-directed

olfactory, and tactile modalities) and occur in up to 88% of children with autism spectrum disorders (Volkmar & Cohen, 1986). Auditory sensitivities seem to be most common (Baranek et al., 2005) and are expressed as sensory fascinations (for instance, being fascinated by certain sounds or covering the ears against specific sounds). However, the sensitivities in autistic children seem to reflect direct defensive motor responses (or lack of responses) to external sensory stimuli, or conversely result in fascinated listening to a specific sound while excluding all other auditory input. On the contrary, the premonitory urges described in TS, which precede tics, are reported as unpleasant somatosensory sensations, either in muscles or in parts of the body or the head (Leckman et al., 1993). Premonitory urges can be bound to discrete corporeal regions, with "hot spots" in the shoulder girdle, hands, feet, and front of the thighs. They can also be more generalized and reported as a sense of "inner tension." These phenomena are very different from the hypersensitivities described in autistic patients.

With respect to motor coordination problems, both children with autism spectrum disorders and with TS may show some impairment. In one study in 109 children with a broad range of autism spectrum disorders, 79% showed marked impairments on the Movement Assessment Battery for Children, with children with low IQ being more impaired than the children with normal IQ (Green et al., 2009). Likewise, although differently assessed, TS children show motor coordination problems on the Purdue Pegboard Test (Bloch et al., 2006). The Purdue Pegboard Test tests gross movements of hands, fingers, and arms and "fingertip" dexterity in assembly tasks. Worse performance on the Purdue Pegboard Test in children with TS predicted poorer outcome with respect to tic severity and psychosocial functioning in early adulthood (Bloch et al., 2006). Whether these findings reflect similar fine-motor skills problems in autism spectrum disorders and TS children warrants further comparative research.

Finally, with respect to neuropsychological functioning, various studies have investigated executive functioning in TS (see Chapter 20) as well as in autism. Executive function refers to those neuropsychological processes that involve planning, strategic organization of complex processes, flexible adaptation to novel stimuli, and ability to shift mental sets, to inhibit irrelevant (motor) responses, and to engage in trial-and-error learning. Pennington and Ozonoff (1996) have defined executive functions: inhibition, visual working memory, planning, cognitive flexibility, and verbal fluency. Multiple studies have identified executive function deficits in older children and adults with autism (Geurts et al., 2004; Sergeant et al., 2002). Usually, few executive function problems are found in preschoolers, but autism-specific executive function deficits become clearer with age, possibly due to maturation of the frontal lobe. School-age children with autism have problems in planning, cognitive flexibility, working memory, and verbal fluency, but usually have no difficulty with motor inhibition (Ozonoff & Strayer, 1997). In TS, no specific executive function problems have been found in children with "pure" TS, but executive function deficits in TS have been linked to comorbid ADHD or OCD, in most studies regardless of comorbid tic number or severity (Cath et al., 2011; see also Chapter 20). Two research groups have directly compared executive function in TS and autism patients (Geurts et al., 2008; Ozonoff et al., 1994; Verte et al., 2005). The results of these studies are somewhat contradictory. As might have been expected, Ozonoff and colleagues (1994) found that TS patients showed deficits in motor inhibition, whereas autism subjects were impaired on measures of cognitive flexibility. In contrast, in later studies, children with high-functioning autism (HFA), with TS, and with HFA+TS, compared with a control group, showed that children with HFA scored lower than the control children on all the executive functions measured, and lower than the TS group on inhibition of a prepotent response and cognitive flexibility (Verte et al., 2005). Remarkably, children with "pure" HFA performed worse than children with comorbid HFA+TS on all functions, with the exception of inhibiting an ongoing response, interference control, and verbal fluency. Importantly, and in line with previous studies in pure TS children, children with TS only and children with TS+HFA were similar to controls on all measures of executive function. Thus, children with HFA+TS seem to resemble a TS group rather than an HFA group. There even seems to be a positive influence of comorbid TS on autism-related executive function, a finding that has been observed previously (Burd et al., 1987; Burd & Kerbeshian, 1988).

Burd and Kerbeshian suggested that the development of TS subsequent to the onset of autism may mark an improved developmental outcome with respect to IQ and receptive or expressive language. Possibly, "pure" HFA groups etiologically differ from HFA+TS patients. Interestingly, in this study, comorbid ADHD was the most significant predictor of inhibition failure across all study groups. Unexpectedly, the HFA group had difficulties with inhibiting a prepotent and ongoing response, as well as with interference control. Thus, inhibition problems in TS are likely to be driven by comorbidity (with ADHD or with autism) rather than by TS itself.

Epidemiology: Comorbidity Rates in TS and Autism

TS is estimated to occur in 0.95% of the population across large epidemiological cohorts (Robertson, 2008; see also Chapter 6 for further details), whereas autism spectrum disorders occur in 0.6% of the population. Therefore, if TS and autism spectrum disorders were truly independent disorders, the rate of co-occurrence expected by chance would be about 0.006%, or about 6 in 100,000. However, rates of tics and TS among individuals with autism spectrum disorders are well documented and are estimated across studies to be 6.5% to 50%, depending on the definition of autism (broad vs. narrow) and on characteristics of the study populations (clinical vs. outpatient populations; low vs. high cognitive abilities; absence or presence of brain damage, absence or presence of pre- or perinatal adversities) (Baron-Cohen et al., 1999; Burd et al., 1986; Simonoff et al., 2008). Thus, the co-occurrence of tics in autism spectrum disorders far exceeds the frequencies expected by chance alone.

To our knowledge very little research has been performed on the occurrence of autism spectrum disorder or autistic traits in TS. One large-scale study has been conducted in the TIC database, which largely depends on clinician-based diagnoses, currently comprising 7,288 patients with TS (Burd et al., 2009). A point prevalence rate of 4.6% (n = 334) of pervasive developmental disorder was found. Thus, TS patients seem to run a 13-fold increased risk of developing comorbid pervasive developmental disorder compared to the normal population. Predictive of the combination of TS and pervasive developmental disorder were male sex, absence of a family history of TS, and elevated number of comorbidities. Recently, in a first exploratory study on the occurrence of autism traits in TS patients with or without comorbid OCD and ADHD, we compared 121 adult TS patients (mean age 36.8 ± 14.1 years; 61% males) to 93 controls (mean age 37.7 ± 13.5 years; 46% males) on autism symptoms (Cath et al., personal communication). The Autism Spectrum Quotient (AQ) for adults was used to screen for autism symptoms (Baron-Cohen et al., 2001; Hoekstra et al., 2007). The AQ is a 50-item self-administered screening instrument specifically developed for adults with normal intelligence, a classic rating scale in a 4-point Likert format. Either dichotomous ratings (range 0–50, by dichotomizing the 4-point Likert scale with the most conservative cut-off of ≥32 indicative of an autism spectrum disorder) or continuous ratings are used to measure autistic traits. Five subscales are provided: social skills, attention switching, attention to detail, communication problems, and imagination. The association between autism symptoms, tics (YGTSS scores), obsessive-compulsive symptom severity (Yale-Brown Obsessive-Compulsive scale [YBOCS]), and ADHD behavior (Conners Adult ADHD Rating Scale [CAARS]) was investigated. The TS group as a whole was compared with controls, and subanalyses were performed after dividing the TS group into TS-only patients (n = 36), TS+OCD patients (n = 15), TS+ADHD patients (n = 28) and TS+OCD+ADHD patients (n = 34). Covariance analyses were performed, with education level as covariate, Spearman's rho correlations were calculated, and stepwise regression analyses were performed. Using the Baron-Cohen cut point, 12% of the TS patients scored above the AQ threshold suggestive for autism spectrum disorder, versus 1% in the control group. Further, scores on both AQ total and on all subscales were elevated in the TS group when compared to controls. Interestingly, there were significant positive correlations between AQ total and subscale scores, on the one hand, and CAARS total and subscale scores, YBOCS

severity scores, and YGTSS scores in the whole study group (Spearman's rho coefficients 0.4–0.6). Analyses of covariance (with education level as covariate) revealed higher AQ total scores in all subgroups of TS patients. The "pure" TS group had the lowest total AQ scores (but elevated compared to controls), followed by the TS+OCD group. Only the subscale attention to detail was elevated in the "pure" TS group compared to controls. The TS+OCD+ADHD group showed the highest scores on the AQ total and subscale scores, followed by the TS+ADHD group. When compared to the "pure" TS group, the TS+ADHD and TS+OCD+ADHD groups showed elevated scores on (lack of) social skills and attention switching. Finally, stepwise regression analyses to investigate which variables predicted AQ scores revealed that CAARS total scores, CAARS hyperactivity/impulsivity, and YBOCS severity explained 24% of the variance in AQ scores in the TS group.

In summary, considering that 12% of TS patients have a positive screen for autism, there is a relationship between TS and autism spectrum disorders, which is predominantly driven by comorbidity with ADHD and—to a lesser extent—with OCD. In other words, in TS patients, comorbid ADHD and OCD seem to be related to autistic symptoms. Further, in the TS+ADHD group, the association with autistic symptoms does not seem to be restricted to a dysfunction in attention switching—to direct alternating behaviors, but extends to social skill problems (as reflected in the social skill AQ subscale). These findings are in line with the general notion that "pure" TS patients are less affected with autism-related features than TS+ADHD patients, who can exhibit autism-related deficits in social interaction, communication, and play that characterize autism spectrum disorders individuals (Rapin, 2001).

Considerations on Etiology

Although no conclusions can be inferred from this descriptive phenomenological study, these data present evidence in favor of viewing TS (especially the type with comorbidity with OCD, ADHD, and autism spectrum disorders) as a spectrum disorder with partly overlapping etiologies with the "pure" forms of OCD, ADHD, and autism spectrum disorders. In line with this notion, a recent genetic study on rare copy number variations (CNVs) in 460 TS subjects revealed enrichment of genes within histamine receptor (subtypes 1 and 2) signaling pathways (Fernandez et al., 2012). Moreover, three *de novo* events were identified, including one disrupting multiple gamma-aminobutyric acid (GABA) receptor genes. These findings show significant overlap with genes identified in autism spectrum disorders (see Chapter 7 for further details).

Concluding Remarks

Strikingly little attention has been paid to date to studying the direct relationship between TS and autism symptoms or autism spectrum disorders. Although both disorders are neurodevelopmental and have a childhood onset, and in both disorders repetitive movements are frequently reported, the characteristics of these movements largely differ between the disorders. In both disorders an increased prevalence of comorbid ADHD and OCD has been reported. Further, elevated frequencies of autism spectrum disorders have been reported in TS with or without comorbidity. Conversely, elevated rates of tics have been reported in autism spectrum disorders populations, strongly suggesting a relationship between autism symptoms and (subgroups of) TS. Elevated frequencies of autism symptoms seem to be particularly associated with comorbidity with ADHD and—to a lesser extent—with comorbid OCD, although tic severity seems to be modestly associated as well. Neuropsychological studies, focusing on executive functions in TS compared to autism spectrum disorders children (Ozonoff et al., 1994; Verte et al., 2005), have revealed that executive function problems in TS (i.e., problems with motor inhibition, cognitive flexibility, and planning) are more convincingly explained by comorbid psychopathology than by tic number or severity. Dysfunctions of cognitive flexibility and planning are likely to be related to comorbid OCD and autism traits in TS, and inhibition problems are likely to be linked to comorbid

ADHD in TS. Interestingly, the development of tics in children with HFA seems to be a marker of improved outcome with respect to cognitive functioning and language development. As TS and autism (as well as OCD, ADHD, and learning disorders) are all frontostriatal neurodevelopmental disorders, both similarities and differences in etiology with respect to executive function between the disorders are likely to converge at the level of frontostriatal circuits (Palumbo & Maughan, 1997; State, 2010). Future studies should focus on the neurobiological mechanisms involved in TS and its comorbid conditions, classifying different types of repetitive behavior by their neuroanatomical correlates in corticostriatal circuits (Langen et al., 2011).

LEARNING DISABILITIES

Clinical Vignette: Mrs. M seeks advice about her 9-year-old son, Thomas. He has mild tics, including eye blinking and a discrete throat clearing once every few minutes. Thomas does not mind his tics and gets along with his classmates, who do not tease him, but he seems to be really unhappy and depressed. He detests going to school and needs hours and hours for his homework. A recent intelligence test revealed an average cognitive ability. His teacher noticed that he reads very slowly and does not seem to be interested in learning.

Historical Overview

Learning disabilities (or learning disorders, LD) were first recognized in the early 1800s, when a German physician, Franz Joseph Gall, conducted research on acquired brain pathology in adults and saw a relationship between brain injury and mental impairment (http://www.nrcld.org/resources/ldsummit/hallahan.pdf). Current research gives evidence that learning disabilities cannot be considered as a unitary entity but rather as a composition of disabilities in different academic domains as instantiated in U.S. federal regulations in 1977 (Fletcher et al., 2007)—that is, in listening comprehension (receptive language), oral expression (expressive language), basic reading skills (decoding and word recognition), reading comprehension, written expression, mathematical calculation, and mathematical reasoning.

What about the history of learning disabilities in TS? A study by Comings and Comings (1987) that included 3,034 students with learning disabilities in three schools in a single school district in California found a prevalence of definite TS for males of about 1% and for females of about 0.13%. Seventy percent of all students with TS were in special education classes, where the prevalence of TS was 12%. The 10 TS patients in this study who were additionally evaluated in a TS clinic also had definite ADHD. Kurlan (1994) found a 26% incidence of tics among special education students compared with only 6% in regular classroom students. Further studies reported that up to 50% of children with TS also have learning disabilities, as assessed by parent-derived questionnaires or by interviewing the parents (Burd et al., 1992). In one standardized study by Burd and colleagues (1992), 42 children with TS were examined and IQ level and achievement was examined using standardized testing; a discrepancy between IQ level and achievement had to be 1.5 standard deviations to consider a child to have a learning disorder. In this study 51% of the children met the criteria for a specific learning disability in at least one academic area (reading, math, or spelling). In all the studies mentioned above, if comorbidities were evaluated, there was a strong association between learning disabilities and ADHD. Subsequent studies revealed that the presence of comorbidities, notably ADHD and OCD, appears to significantly increase the incidence of learning disabilities (Como, 2005).

Definitions

The term "learning disability" was initially defined by Kirk (1962) as "a retardation, disorder, or delayed development in one or more of the processes of speech, language, reading, writing, arithmetic, or other school subject resulting from a psychological handicap caused by a possible cerebral dysfunction and/or emotional or behavioral disturbances. Learning disorders do not result from mental retardation, sensory deprivation, or cultural and instructional factors." Currently, learning disabilities are diagnosed on the basis of the discrepancy between students' IQ and achievement scores (Aaron et al., 2008). In contrast to other neuropsychiatric diagnoses there are no specific criteria given in DSM-IV-TR, but simply the hint that "reading achievement (or mathematical ability or writing skills) ... as measured by individually administered standardized tests ... is substantially below that expected given the person's chronological age, measured intelligence, and age-appropriate education."

The diagnostic process in learning disabilities takes place under varying circumstances. Teachers and school psychologists in public schools may use other testing methods because of a different theoretical background than psychologists and (child and adolescent) psychiatrists in private practice. The latter may preponderantly apply the DSM or International Classification of Diseases (ICD) clinical classification systems.

Different ways to diagnose and referral bias might contribute to the wide range in prevalence rates. In an epidemiological sample of 215 girls and 199 boys followed up from second to third grade, Shaywitz and colleagues (1990) pointed out the discrepancy in prevalence estimates of learning disabilities derived from research-identified versus school-identified reading-disabled children. In research populations, 8.7% of the boys and 6.9% of the girls were diagnosed with reading disorder in the second grade (9.0% of the boys and 6.0% of the girls in the third grade). School identification classified 13.6% of the boys and only 3.2% of the girls in the second grade and 10.0% of the boys and 4.2% of the girls in the third grade as reading-disabled. Depending on which IQ test and which reading or mathematics test is used, a student may qualify as having a learning disability or not. Thus, in public schools, standards and practices for the diagnoses of learning disabilities may differ from state to state.

The fact that to some extent a final definition is still missing on learning disabilities has caused a serious delay in recognition of learning disorders such as dyslexia. For instance, New

Zealand did not recognize dyslexia as a disorder until 2008 because "defining dyslexia is a complex and contested process in which there are no agreed definitions internationally" (Tunmer & Greaney, 2010).

Phenomenology

Learning difficulties can account for impairment in reading, writing, listening, speaking, reasoning, and doing mathematics. Reading disability is the most common type of learning disability: nearly 80% to 90% of all diagnosed learning disabilities cases involve reading disabilities (Pennington, 1991; St Sauver et al., 2001). Especially at a young age, learning disabilities often go unrecognized and children present with school refusal and social phobia and might develop somatic symptoms. Children with TS and learning disabilities are twice as impaired as children with only one of these disorders. The fear of humiliation—because of disturbing tics and because of possible school failure—can also lead to symptoms of oppositional defiant disorder, in the sense of "offense being the best defense." These children have to defend their self-esteem and need to avoid further humiliation at all cost. These problems might also lead to continuous tension in children with TS; learning disabilities may eventually contribute also to rage attacks (see below).

Epidemiology

Prevalence data of learning disabilities in the general population depend on the samples, diagnostic criteria, and assessment procedures; therefore, estimates range from 5% to 20% (AACAP, 1998; Rutter et al., 2004; St Sauver et al., 2001). The discrepant definitions of learning disabilities give rise to even higher prevalence rates in some studies (Aaron et al., 2008). An epidemiological sample of 9- to 10-year-old British schoolchildren (n = 1,206) revealed a prevalence of 1.3% specific arithmetic difficulties, 2.3% combined arithmetic and reading difficulties, and 3.9% specific reading difficulties. Only in reading difficulties was a preponderance of boys seen (Lewis et al., 1994). In 2004, Rutter

and colleagues presented data of four epidemiological studies: the Dunedin Multidisciplinary Health and Development Study, with 989 participants (52.1% male); the Christchurch Health and Development Study, with 895 participants (50% male); the Office for National Statistics (ONS) Study, with 5,752 children from the UK (50.1% male); and the Environmental Risk Longitudinal Twin Study (E-Risk), with 2,163 twin children from England and Wales (49.1% male). The main outcome measure, reading performance, was assessed in boys and girls separately (Rutter et al., 2004). In all four studies, the rates of reading disability were significantly higher in boys: in the Dunedin study, 21.6% in boys and 7.9% in girls; in the Christchurch study, 20.6% in boys and 9.8% in girls; in the ONS study, 17.6% in boys and 13.0% in girls; and in the E-Risk study, 18.0% in boys and 13.0% in girls. The authors concluded that reading disabilities are clearly more common in boys than in girls.

As can be seen from the above-mentioned epidemiological studies, male sex is a strong risk factor for learning disabilities. Boys have a 2.0- to 2.5-fold higher risk of learning disabilities than girls. In a case-control study (n = 5,701), St Sauver and colleagues (2001) examined whether boys and girls are differentially affected by risk factors. Also in this study, boys were more often impaired by reading disability than girls (49.0% males in the non-reading disability group vs. 71.0% males in the reading disability group). Girls of low birth weight and girls whose mothers had 12 or fewer years of education were twice as likely to be identified as having reading disorder. For boys, only 12 or fewer years of paternal education was associated with the diagnosis of reading disorder. The authors concluded that there was a differential susceptibility to risk factors in boys and girls with reading disorder, possibly based on a different gender-specific pathophysiology (St Sauver et al., 2001).

Subsequently, the effect of comorbid ADHD on the prevalence of learning disabilities was determined in boys and girls with learning disabilities in a population-based birth cohort (n = 5,718) (Yoshimasu et al., 2010). In children with ADHD the incidence of reading disability was significantly higher (51% in boys, 46.7% in girls) than in children without ADHD (14.5% in boys, 7.7% in girls). Whereas boys without ADHD were twice as likely as girls to be affected by reading disability, this preponderance for boys was not detectable among the children with ADHD.

Learning Disabilities in TS Patients

Burd and colleagues (2005) performed analyzes using the clinical TIC database mentioned above (Burd et al., 2005). The majority of the cases from this registry were from Canada (40.6%), the United States (22.6%), and Europe (25.1%); other cases were from the Middle East, South America, Asia, Australia, and Africa. The standardized data entry form is available online (http://www.biomedcentral.com/content/supplementary/1471-2431-5-34S1.doc). The diagnosis of learning disabilities was supposed to be given as defined in the DSM-IV, including specific learning disorders and also the less verifiable category of learning disorders not otherwise specified. The authors compared subjects with TS with and without learning disabilities. Among 5,450 subjects they found 1,235 subjects with TS + learning disabilities (22.7%). In all TS patients, ADHD was the most prevalent comorbid disorder (58%). Whereas only 51.3% of the subjects with TS without learning disabilities had ADHD, in the subjects with both TS and learning disabilities, 80.2% were affected by this comorbidity. Whereas 31% of children with TS and ADHD (58% of the whole population) also had learning disabilities, in the TS group without ADHD only 11% had learning disabilities, a prevalence that can also be found in the general population (AACAP, 1998). Importantly, these results indicate that co-occurring ADHD is responsible for the increased prevalence of learning disabilities in youth with TS, not the tic disorder itself. A major drawback that might have contributed to the high rates of learning disabilities in this study might have been the diagnostic criteria that were operant in the registry. For instance, the diagnosis "learning disabilities not otherwise specified" could be entered in the data form. Another drawback is that possible relations to other comorbidities (including OCD) were not explored in this study.

Most studies investigating the relationship between learning disabilities and other comorbidities in TS patients have been conducted in clinical samples with an oversampling of males (up to 90% in some studies). For instance, in a Swedish school population (n = 4,479), the male-to-female radio in the children with TS (n = 25) was 10:1 in the younger age groups (7–9 and 10–12 years old) (Khalifa & von Knorring, 2003, 2006). In the 13- to 15-year-old TS subjects the sex ratio was 2:2. Four (16%) of the 25 TS subjects also fulfilled the criteria for a learning disorder (dyslexia). Taking into account that 90% of the young TS subjects in this sample were male, the prevalence of learning disabilities in this sample was not significantly higher than in the general population.

In conclusion, the accumulated body of the literature suggests that the prevalence of learning disabilities in TS is quite similar to rates in the general population. However, the most common comorbidity in childhood, ADHD, is very often associated with learning disabilities, and thus in TS+ADHD subjects an increased prevalence of learning disabilities is found.

Natural History

Of all learning disabilities, the outcome of dyslexia has been the most extensively studied (AACAP, 1998). Adults who were diagnosed with reading disorder in childhood demonstrate a wide range of reading disabilities and reading problems (Hallahan et al., 1996). There are no long-term outcome studies of learning disabilities available in adult subjects with TS. The accumulated literature on learning disabilities in TS suggests that learning disability is highly associated with ADHD and to a lesser extent with other comorbidities such as OCD. Therefore, these comorbidities are the major contributors to the outcome. Most studies assessing the long-term outcome in adult TS patients do not consider learning disabilities (Eapen et al., 2004). Individuals, although leading a successful life as adults, might still suffer from self-esteem problems due to their early learning disorders (Walkup et al., 1999).

Interplay Between Learning Disabilities and Tics

As mentioned above, learning disabilities are strongly associated with the comorbidity ADHD in TS patients. Learning disabilities do not correlate with tic severity. However, combined with tics, learning disabilities—even in a mild form— might significantly aggravate school problems for the TS-affected child who already has to struggle for his or her position in the peer group. Thus, unrecognized learning disabilities might contribute to low self-esteem, school phobia, and mood disorders in a child with TS. We strongly agree with Como's recommendation to use specific neuropsychological testing to identify the cognitive deficits common in TS, in particular visuomotor integration, motor skill, and executive function (Como, 2005; see also Chapter 20).

Etiology

As mentioned in the Practice Parameters of the American Academy of Child and Adolescent Psychiatry (AACAP, 1998; Pennington, 1995), "evidence from family and twin studies suggests that reading disabilities are familial and heritable and that they are genetically heterogeneous" (Pennington, 1995). Across family studies, the familial risk in first-degree relatives has been found to be 35% to 45%, compared with the population risk of 3% to 10%. The precise mode of transmission is not known, but there is evidence for a single major locus (Pennington et al., 1991), a polygenic or a multifactorial mode of transmission (Pennington, 1995), or a quantitative trait locus (QTL) (Cardon et al., 1994). Pauls and colleagues (1993) conducted a study to investigate familial relationship between TS, attention-deficit disorder (ADD), learning disabilities, speech problems, and stuttering. The authors examined 338 first-degree relatives of 85 TS patients and 113 controls and found no evidence that ADD, learning disabilities, speech problems, or stuttering were variant forms of TS.

Rage Attacks

"If there was a single word that best characterized the behavioral problems in TS it would be 'anger'" (Comings & Comings, 1985). Even though "rage attacks" is not a diagnostic term in the classification systems DSM-IV or ICD-10, every clinician dealing with TS patients and all affected families can immediately relate to the phrase. A significant number of clinically referred subjects with TS, especially children and adolescents, seem to be affected by behavioral abnormalities characterized by rage attacks, meaning sudden and unpredictable anger, irritability, temper outbursts, and also aggression up to marked verbal and physical violence (Budman et al., 1998, 2000; Neuner & Ludolph, 2009). A comprehensive definition of a "rage attack" is given by Leslie E. Packer, PhD, on http://www.schoolbehavior.com/disorders/rage-attacks-or-storms: "a sudden, out-of-control explosive outburst that appears—to the observer and the individual experiencing it—to be without warning and totally out of proportion to any triggering event in the environment. It is also experienced as being a somewhat (but not completely) uncontrollable event that once started, just has to run its course." Similar symptom clusters have been described by the DSM-IV diagnosis of intermittent explosive disorder with the following criteria:

A. Several discrete episodes of failure to resist aggressive impulses that result in serious assaultive acts or destruction of property.

B. The degree of aggressiveness expressed during the episodes is grossly out of proportion to any precipitating psychosocial stressors.

C. The aggressive episodes are not better accounted for by another mental disorder (e.g., Antisocial Personality Disorder, Borderline Personality Disorder, a Psychotic Disorder, a Manic Episode, Conduct Disorder, or Attention-Deficit/Hyperactivity Disorder) and are not due to the direct physiological effects of a substance (e.g., a drug of abuse, a medication) or a general medical condition (e.g., head trauma, Alzheimer's disease).

Since recent studies showed that nearly all children, adolescents, and adults with TS and rage attacks have at least one other neuropsychiatric disorder, mostly ADHD, OCD, and/or conduct disorder, criterion C is not fulfilled in TS patients with rage attacks. Therefore, these explosive outbursts should not be considered as a discrete disorder but instead as one of the extreme ends of the broad spectrum of disinhibited behavior that TS patients are prone to.

Historical Background

In a book chapter entitled "Phenomenology and natural history of tic-related ADHD and learning disabilities," Walkup and colleagues (1999) wrote: "Georges Gilles de la Tourette stated in his initial article that his subjects' mental state was perfectly normal." Tourette mainly concentrated on the description of the motor and vocal abnormalities of his adult patients. However, a closer look at the original descriptions of the childhood histories of these first nine cases reveals that he did mention—among others— sudden explosive outbursts of behavior (Gilles de la Tourette, 1885). In Case 6, he describes an 11-year-old boy, J. L. The boy's father mentioned that "J. has always been nervous. In general, he is quite a likeable child, but very easily upset. By an unpleasant event, for example a just punishment, he is immediately thrown into turmoil." In Case 9, he tells the story of a 23-year-old man, "born in Havre, who lost his parents in early childhood and was raised by a wet nurse. He tended to have ferocious fits of rage. The disease he currently suffered from had begun at the age of 14 for no apparent reason. He was seized by "convulsions," in one leg, then in both legs, subsequently in one arm, and finally in both arms and legs. These rhythmic convulsions emerged in sudden attacks ... For four years now he has got the irresistible urge to repeat his own words." In sum, Gilles de la Tourette did not consider rage attacks as part of the disorder, but he mentioned them in two of his nine case reports.

Searching PubMed using the terms "tics and aggression," the first reference dates back to 1968. Bruch and Thum (1968) reported the case of 12-year-old Harry, who was referred to the clinic for the first time in October 1959 and suffered from severe vocal and motor tics. His behavior was described as follows: "During the preceding 2 or 3 years he had been an inactive,

oppositional and lonely boy who hated to be told what to do. His main interests were guns, knives, forts, and, at times, vigorous physical activity. It was very difficult to get him to do anything around the house, and his school record, too, suffered from his oppositional behavior. ... Getting his homework done was a recurrent 'battle royal'."

More than 40 years later, these lines read like a typical description of a boy with ADHD and ODD. Back then the authors emphasized the psychodynamic background and the intrafamilial interaction as reasons for the tic disorder and aggressive behavior and argued that "the early development of this patient was not incompatible with a later schizophrenic reaction." The old literature emphasized a close association between *maladie des tics* and schizophrenia. Bruch and Thum mentioned that "the literature on the tic syndrome has oscillated between organic and psychodynamic etiological considerations." They cited Mahler and her extensive psychoanalytic studies of the tic syndrome describing "the mother and child interdependence as having been quite extreme at all times" (Mahler, 1949). In conclusion, from the psychoanalytical point of view, parents with children with tic disorders might tend to display an overcontrolling attitude and an exaggerated inhibition of aggressive behavior, which in turn leads the child to demonstrate even more tics and disruptive behavior.

Modern parent training, one of the best-evaluated behavioral therapies for children with ADHD and disruptive behavior, starts right here (van den Hoofdakker et al., 2007). The influence of parenting styles and aggressive behavior in youth is well investigated (Dishion & Patterson, 2006). Today the "neglectful parenting style" is considered a major risk factor for aggression in offspring (Hoeve et al., 2009). Behavioral parent training (BPT) is an evidence-based treatment for disruptive behavior disorder in childhood. This treatment of choice for oppositional behaviors, although probably the best-studied and most efficacious psychosocial treatment, is not commonly used in patients with TS and has not been studied yet (Gaze et al., 2006). A recent study showed that generally mothers' parenting self-efficacy is a major moderator of the effectiveness of BPT (van den Hoofdakker et al., 2010). Moreover, the genetic background seems to play a moderating role in BPT: in children with ADHD and with no or one DAT1 10-repeat allele, BPT was highly effective, but that was not the case in children with two DAT1 10-repeat alleles (van den Hoofdakker et al., 2012).

Phenomenology

Signs and symptoms of rage attacks are best described in the definition above. Explosive outbursts seem to appear from nowhere. The abrupt onset is unpredictable for the surroundings. Some patients feel a kind of hyperarousal or increasing tension just before an attack similar to the premonitory urge prior to tics. As in the case of the tic, after a rage attack there is a short sensation of relief. However, the child may also have regrets, in particular if he or she has destroyed something or even hurt someone. Budman and colleagues (2000) suggested that the explosive outbursts—usually lacking antecedents—may be triggered by "situational predispositions, such as sleep deprivation, hunger, or a particular activity." With respect to specific activities related to rage attacks, a few parents in the Ulmer outpatient clinic, which specializes in tic disorders, reported an increased frequency and ferocity of the outbursts after the child had been playing computer games, whether a sports game or a shooting game. These attacks can last from minutes to less than an hour and sometimes occur several times per day; they happen more often at home than in school or outside the family.

Epidemiology

The phenomenology of rage attacks resembles that of intermittent explosive disorder. Intermittent explosive disorder is a much more common condition than previously recognized. Depending upon how broadly it is defined, it affects as many as 7.3% of adults—11.5 to 16 million Americans—in their lifetimes (Kessler et al., 2006). The study by Kessler and colleagues is based on data from the National Comorbidity Survey Replication, a nationally representative, face-to-face household survey of 9,282 U.S. adults, conducted between 2001 and 2003.

Among clinically referred patients with TS, rage attacks occur in 23% to 40% (Budman et al., 2000; Comings & Comings, 1985; Eapen et al., 2004). Considering anger-control problems, irritability, and recurrent behavioral outbursts, the prevalence increases to 70% of TS patients (Budman et al., 2005). Frank and colleagues (2011) found a prevalence of intermittent explosive disorder of 51.6% in the 31 adult TS patients participating in the exploratory study investigating impulse-control disorders as defined by DSM-IV: intermittent explosive disorder, kleptomania, pathological gambling, pyromania, trichotillomania, and impulse-control disorders not otherwise specified (including compulsive Internet usage disorder, compulsive sexual behavior, and compulsive shopping disorder). Seventy-two percent of the patients had at least one impulse-control disorder (Frank et al., 2011).

Many studies investigating aggressive behavior in TS patients did not distinguish between male and female patients. Since the study groups investigated are usually small, sex differences in the occurrence of rage attacks are not always mentioned (Cardona et al., 2004). The studies looking at gender differences have been inconclusive. Some studies have found a similar sex ratio in TS groups with and without rage attacks (Budman et al., 2000; Comings & Comings 1985). In another study by Budman and colleagues (2003), 83% of the participating 48 subjects were male and 17% were female, not allowing conclusions to be drawn with respect to the male-to-female ratio in the frequencies of rage attack. In the TIC database analyzed by Freeman and colleagues (2000), the gender difference in the history of anger-control problems was significant ($p < .0001$; 38% of males [n = 2,846] and 30% of females [n = 654]).

Natural History

Cardona and colleagues (2004), in a cross-sectional study, reported aggressive behavior in 10% of the 5- to 11-year-old children with TS (N = 100), and in 6% of the 12- to 17-year-old patients (N = 25). Since the studies mentioned above including adult TS patients revealed an even higher prevalence of rage attacks, this behavioral problem does not seem to alleviate with age. However, no longitudinal studies have been performed, so no adequate information is currently available on the course of rage attacks in TS.

Interplay Between Rage Attacks and Tics

The literature is ambiguous on whether rage attacks are associated with tic severity or not. The stigmatization by provocative phonic and/or motor tics can be extremely stressful for patients and their families, even leading to posttraumatic stress disorder and complete social withdrawal. Moreover, the extraordinary burden caused by extreme tics along with recurrent frustration might also trigger disruptive behavior, especially in children and adolescents, and thus might contribute to rage attacks. Most recent studies draw the conclusion that rage attacks are significantly related to comorbid psychiatric diagnoses, especially ADHD and OCD rather than tic severity (Budman et al., 1998, 2000; Rizzo et al., 2007).

In one of the first studies investigating rage attacks in children and adolescents with TS, Budman and colleagues (1998) presented 12 children with TS and rage attacks. All of them had comorbid ADHD or OCD, and two children were additionally diagnosed with oppositional defiant disorder. Surprisingly, no internalizing symptoms were described. In a larger group of 68 children and adolescents with TS (37 children with TS and rage attacks and 31 children with TS without rage attacks), every child in the subgroup of the TS patients with rage attacks had at least one comorbidity. Four subjects in the TS group without rage attacks had no comorbidity (13%), and 32% in the TS group without rage attacks had only one comorbidity (Budman et al., 2000). In contrast, in the TS group with rage attacks, only one TS patient had only one comorbidity (2.7%), and 12 patients (32%) had two, three, or even four comorbidities. Tic severity was mild in both patient groups, and tics did not differ in type or severity. However, the TS group with rage attacks scored significantly higher on the Tourette Syndrome Global Scale (TSGS) because of two elevated dimensions of social functioning: motor restlessness and behavioral problems.

Etiology

Rage attacks—like TS and its comorbidities—are probably caused by a number of environmental and biological factors. As Budman and colleagues (2003) concluded, "episodic rage in TS has stereotypic features, but diverse and complex etiologies." Research on these etiological determinants in TS patients is scarce. Rage attacks seem to be highly correlated with ADHD and OCD symptom severity. Little is known about internalizing disturbances and rage attacks in TS patients. In general, anger attacks are fairly common in depressed patients, as shown in several studies (Brody et al., 1999; Fava et al., 1991). However, no research has been performed on the association between rage attacks and depression or anxiety in TS.

Psychoanalytic theorists have historically proposed that feelings of guilt and depression are a result of anger directed toward oneself. Depressed people also report stronger subjective experiences of anger and greater efforts to suppress expression of anger (Riley et al., 1989). Further, a history of depression seems to be associated with anger attacks. In a small-scale study (n = 30 depressed patients vs. 25 controls), 36% (n = 9) of the patients who recovered from a major depression (N = 9) reported having experienced at least one anger attack, compared with just 4% (N = 1) of the healthy control group (Brody et al., 1999). Rosenbaum and colleagues (1993) tried to distinguish depressed patients with anger attacks from those without by the thyrotropin-releasing hormone (TRH) test and found a reduced prolactin response in depressed patients with anger attacks compared to the depressed patients without anger attacks. Fluoxetine treatment increased the prolactin response to TRH in the depressed patients with anger attacks. The authors concluded that central serotonergic dysregulation is increased

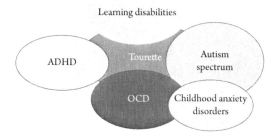

FIGURE 4.1 The spectrum of neurodevelopmental disorders.

in the depressed patients with anger attacks. Extrapolating these findings to TS patients with rage attacks, involvement of serotonin metabolism can also be hypothesized in the pathophysiology of rage attacks in TS patients, since serotonin regulates behavioral inhibition.

Concluding Remarks

Strikingly little research has been performed on rage attacks in TS. The range of prevalence estimates of rage attacks in TS has led to inconclusive results due to differences in sample ascertainment, assessment methods, and diagnostic thresholds (Scahill et al., 2006). Further, the association of rage attacks in TS with gender, environmental triggers, tic severity, and comorbid ADHD and OCD; the course in development; etiological aspects; and finally treatment aspects all need further research. Whereas the association between anxiety disorders and disruptive behavior disorders in children and adolescents, as well as the association between depressive disorders and disruptive behavior in adults, and some of their underlying mechanisms, are well recognized (Bubier & Drabick, 2009), this association has never been investigated within TS patients, to the best of our knowledge. Further, a possible relationship between (the intensity of) sensorimotor urges and rage attacks in TS has never been investigated. However, the frequent distraction by these annoying sensations in TS individuals, along with the anxiety of loss of control, might contribute to the outbursts.

CONCLUSIONS

In this chapter, we aimed at elucidating several aspects of the relationship between TS and "other" comorbidities, exploring the extent to which these comorbidities are etiologically (genetically) related to the TS phenotype or the consequence of disease burden. Although no definite answers can be given, and especially depression and anxiety symptoms can be exacerbated by various environmental adversities, at least in children and young adolescents most of the evidence leads to a genetic link between TS, OCD, and anxiety disorders. The relationship between TS and autism spectrum disorder, ADHD, and learning difficulties seems to be due to partly overlapping genes as well. TS and these comorbid disorders can to a certain extent be fitted into a cluster of neurodevelopmental disorders as formulated by Langen and colleagues (2011) and Palumbo (1997; Fig. 4.1). With respect to comorbid depression in TS, more evidence converges toward environmental stressors (such as family dysfunction, psychosocial adversities, being bullied at school as a result of an eye-catching disease, etc.) or disease burden (e.g., concurrent obsessive-compulsive symptoms), which may exacerbate depression in TS.

In reviewing the literature, one final question comes to mind. Across the various comorbid disorders reviewed in this chapter, strikingly, there seems to be a difference between the groups with "pure" TS without comorbidity, and TS with comorbid ADHD, OCD, autism, internalizing disorders, and learning difficulties. The "pure" TS group seems to show few differences with normal control groups in terms of course, cognitive functioning, development of comorbidities, and long-term outcome. On the other hand, the TS groups with comorbid psychopathology develop anxiety disorders, depression, and other comorbidities and seem to run a more deleterious course. One might ask to what extent these groups reflect distinct etiologies. Interestingly, one important study in TS has performed latent class analyses and heritability analyses in a large sample of 952 individuals from 222 TS families in order to identify TS sub-phenotypes and assess

Box 4.1. Key Points

Comorbidity with Anxiety and Depression

- Symptoms of anxiety and depression are more common in patients with TS and in their family members.
- There is hardly any relationship between tic persistence into adulthood and development of anxiety or depression comorbidity.
- In children and young adolescents anxiety symptoms put persons at risk for later tic persistence.
- OCD symptoms in childhood put persons at risk for later development of anxiety and depressive symptoms.
- In adults (specifically women), there is a relationship between tic severity and anxious and depressive symptoms. Anxious and depressive symptoms in this group seem to be the result of disease burden.
- Specifically, comorbid OCD in children and adolescents puts TS individuals at risk to develop (internalizing) anxiety and depressive symptoms, whereas comorbid ADHD mostly puts individuals at risk to develop disruptive and externalizing behaviors.
- The strikingly few longitudinal studies to explore relationships between the development of tics, OCD, ADHD, anxiety, and depressive symptoms from childhood into adulthood suggest that there are specific although not yet clarified age windows in development in which internalizing behaviors predict tic persistence and OCD occurrence in adulthood.
- One family study on the relationship between TS and comorbid anxiety and depression argues against a completely shared background between TS, anxiety, and depression.
- Environmental adversities (negative family environment factors, psychosocial stressors) strongly contribute to comorbidity with anxiety and depression in TS.

Comorbidity with Personality Disorders

- In adults with TS, personality disorders are prevalent, with cluster B personality disorder being most prevalent, cluster A personality disorder being least prevalent, and schizotypal personality disorder occurring in 15% of patients.
- Dimensional personality ratings indicate that neuroticism, but not impulsivity or extraversion, seems to be mostly associated with tics.

Comorbidity with Autism Spectrum Disorders

- Elevated rates of pervasive developmental disorder (autism spectrum disorders) symptoms occur in TS patients, and occur in all three domains of autism spectrum disorders symptomatology.
- Autism spectrum disorders symptoms are more common in TS subjects with comorbidities, especially with ADHD and to a lesser extent with OCD. In children with autism spectrum disorders, comorbid tics seem to have a protective effect on adult outcome with respect to cognitive and psychosocial functioning.
- Executive function problems in TS bear similarities to executive function problems in autism spectrum disorders (i.e., problems with motor inhibition and with cognitive flexibility and planning). Executive function problems in TS are more convincingly explained by comorbid pathology than by tic number or severity. Dysfunctions of cognitive flexibility and planning are more often related to comorbid OCD and autism traits in TS, and inhibition problems are more often linked to comorbid ADHD in TS.

Box 4.1. (*Continued*)

Comorbidity with Learning Disabilities
• Intellectual ability is normally distributed in TS.
• The prevalence of learning disabilities in TS is similar to the prevalence in the general population.
• There is a clear preponderance of the male sex for learning disabilities.
• Comorbidities with ADHD and to a lesser extent with OCD seem to increase the prevalence of learning disabilities.
• Besides the fact that dyslexia is by far the most common learning disability in general, children with TS tend to have problems with mathematics and written language.

Comorbidity with Rage Attacks
• Rage attacks are common in TS, causing severe impairment.
• Rage attacks are far more common in TS subjects with comorbidities, with a particular contribution of comorbid ADHD.
• The sex ratio of rage attacks in TS subjects is still unclarified.

Box 4.2. Questions for Future Research

Comorbidity with Anxiety and Depression
1. Which factors determine the onset and development of anxiety and depressive symptoms in subjects with TS and TS+OCD?
2. What is the exact relationship between anxiety and depressive symptoms and the onset, persistence, and reduction of tics and of OCD across the lifespan?
3. How exactly do tics influence the onset and course of anxiety and depressive symptoms across the lifespan in TS? What is the direction of the relationship between tics on the one hand and anxiety and depressive symptoms at various stages of development across the lifespan?
4. Which environmental factors at which age determine the onset and persistence of anxiety and depressive symptoms in children, adolescents, and adults with TS? Can we identify environmental factors that protect against the development of comorbid anxiety and depressive symptoms?
5. What is the genetic relationship between comorbid OCD and comorbid anxiety and depression in TS individuals and their family members?

Comorbidity with Personality Disorders
1. Which personality disorders are associated with TS? Are there differential patterns of personality disorder in pure TS patients versus those with TS+OCD or TS+ADHD?
2. What is the association between the onset and course of anxiety and depression in TS and personality disorders?
3. What is the nature of the etiological relationship between TS, comorbid OCD, ADHD, anxiety, depression, and TS-related personality disorders?

(Continued)

Box 4.2. (*Continued*)

4. What is the relationship between comorbid personality disorders in TS and the course of tics, OCD, ADHD, and quality of life?
5. Which environmental factors can be determined to predict later development of personality disorders in TS?

Comorbidity with Autism Spectrum Disorders

1. What is the exact relationship of autism spectrum disorders with TS? What is the nature of the relationship between autism spectrum disorders signs and symptoms in "pure TS" individuals and their family members, versus autism spectrum disorders signs and symptoms in those with TS plus a comorbidity and their family members?
2. What is the impact of autism spectrum disorders symptoms on the development and course of tics and of comorbid conditions such as OCD and ADHD and quality of life across the lifespan in TS subjects? How exactly do autism spectrum disorders symptoms influence quality of life at various ages? And, conversely, can we replicate the suggestion that tic symptoms are markers of more favorable cognitive development in later life in autism disorder subjects? If so, can we find neurobiological explanations for this effect?
3. To what extent can TS plus comorbid ADHD/OCD be regarded as neurobiologically and genetically related to autism spectrum disorders, in contrast to "pure" TS? Can we explore genetic and endophenotypic relationships between autism spectrum disorders and TS using large enough samples of "pure" TS patients and families, of TS+OCD/ADHD patients and families, and "pure" autism spectrum disorder patients and families?
4. When hypothesizing that tics and autism spectrum disorders symptoms are both part of a spectrum of neurodevelopmental disorders, what are the shared genetic and neurobiological underpinnings in comparative studies on TS and autism spectrum disorders when exploring cortico–striato–thalamocortical circuitry pathways in genetic and neuroimaging studies?

Comorbidity with Learning Disabilities

1. Why are learning disorders more common in boys than girls?
2. How does learning disorder affect the long-term prognosis in patients with TS? What is the influence of an early learning disorder on tics and on quality of life in later life?
3. What is the long-term outcome of learning disabilities in childhood?

Comorbidity with Rage Attacks

1. What is the long-term outcome of TS subjects who suffer from rage attacks in childhood with respect to later-life comorbidity and quality of life? Is their prognosis worse?
2. What exactly are the frequencies of rage attacks in boys/men and girls/women with TS, and to what extent is the phenotypic expression of rage attacks different for boys/men and girls/women across different ages?
3. What is the relationship between rage attacks and comorbidities with internalizing and externalizing behaviors across different ages in TS?

heritability of these classes (Grados & Mathews, 2008). Latent class analyses identified three TS-affected groups: TS+OCS/OCB, TS+OCD, and TS+OCD+ADHD, in addition to a minimally affected class and a small chronic tics + OCD class. A preponderance of males and younger age at onset were found in the more comorbidly affected classes. Only the TS+OCD+ADHD class was highly heritable. The authors conclude that these various TS classes may represent genetically distinct entities, with both shared and unique etiologies. The TS+OCD+ADHD class in particular seems to represent a specific heritable phenotype that can be used to further inform genetic studies. In light of the evidence reviewed here, we would recommend that future studies focus specifically on the groups of patients with TS plus comorbid disorders. Further, future research should study patients affected by TS, autism, ADHD, OCD, and learning disabilities in cohesion, looking for phenotypic and endophenotypic similarities across disorders, linking these similarities (repetitive or stereotyped behaviors) to genetic, neuroanatomical, cognitive, and longitudinal course findings, and to environmental stressors and protective factors.

ACKNOWLEDGMENTS

We are very grateful to Mathilde Huisman, MSc, and Rianne Boerstra, MSc, who have helped with providing relevant literature and organizing tables for this chapter.

REFERENCES

AACAP. Practice parameters for the assessment and treatment of children and adolescents with language and learning disorders. *J Am Acad Child Adolesc Psychiatry* 1998; 37:46S–62S.

Aaron PG, Joshi RM, Gooden R, Bentum KE. Diagnosis and treatment of reading disabilities based on the component model of reading: an alternative to the discrepancy model of learning disabilities. *J Learn Disabil* 2008; 41:67–84.

Achenbach TM, Ruffle TM. The Child Behavior Checklist and related forms for assessing behavioral/emotional problems and competencies. *Pediatr Rev* 2000; 21:265–271.

Baranek G, Parham D, Bodfish JW. Sensory and motor features in autism: assessment and intervention. In: Eds Vokmar FR, Paul R, Klin A, Cohen D (Eds.), *Handbook of autism and pervasive developmental disorders*, pp. 831–862. John Wiley & Sons, Hoboken, NJ, 2005.

Baron-Cohen S, Mortimore C, Moriarty J et al. The prevalence of Gilles de la Tourette's syndrome in children and adolescents with autism. *J Child Psychol Psychiatry* 1999; 40:213–218.

A large-scale clinical study showing prevalence rates of TS in a clinical group of autism children to be between 4.3% and 6.5%.

Baron-Cohen S, Wheelwright S, Skinner R et al. The autism-spectrum quotient (AQ): evidence from Asperger syndrome/high-functioning autism, males and females, scientists and mathematicians. *J Autism Dev Disord* 2001; 31:5–17.

Beekman AT, Deeg DJ, Braam AW et al. Consequences of major and minor depression in later life: a study of disability, well-being and service utilization. *Psychol Med* 1997; 27:1397–1409.

Bijl RV, de Graaf R, Ravelli A et al. Gender and age-specific first incidence of DSM-III-R psychiatric disorders in the general population. Results from the Netherlands Mental Health Survey and Incidence Study (NEMESIS). *Soc Psychiatry Psychiatr Epidemiol* 2002; 37:372–379.

Bloch MH, Sukhodolsky DG, Leckman JF, Schulz RT. Fine-motor skill deficits in childhood predict adulthood tic severity and global psychosocial functioning in Tourette's syndrome. *J Child Psychol Psychiatry* 2006; 47:551–559.

A small-scale prospective study indicating that fine-motor skill deficits may be a predictor of future tic severity and global psychosocial function in children with TS.

Bolton D, Rijsdijk F, O'Connor TG et al. Obsessive-compulsive disorder, tics and anxiety in 6-year-old twins. *Psychol Med* 2007; 37:39–48.

Brody CL, Haaga DA, Kirk L, Solomon A. Experiences of anger in people who have recovered from depression and never-depressed people. *J Nerv Ment Dis* 1999; 187:400–405.

Bruch H, Thum LC. Maladie des tics and maternal psychosis. *J Nerv Ment Dis* 1968; 146:446–456.

Bubier JL, Drabick DA. Co-occurring anxiety and disruptive behavior disorders: the roles of anxious symptoms, reactive aggression, and shared risk processes. *Clin Psychol Rev* 2009; 29:658–669.

Budman CL, Bruun RD, Park KS et al. Explosive outbursts in children with Tourette's disorder. *J Am Acad Child Adolesc Psychiatry* 2000; 39:1270–1276.

A study investigating TS and explosive outbursts in 68 children, pointing to the significant association of rage attacks and comorbidities.

Budman CL, Bruun RD, Park KS, Olson ME. Rage attacks in children and adolescents with Tourette's disorder: a pilot study. *J Clin Psychiatry* 1998; 59:576–580.

Budman CL, Rockmore L, Bruun RD. Aggressive symptoms and Tourette's syndrome. In: Kurlan R (Ed.), *Handbook of Tourette's syndrome and related tic and behavioral disorders*, pp. 127–154. Marcel Dekkers, New York, 2005.

Budman CL, Rockmore L, Stokes J, Sossin M. Clinical phenomenology of episodic rage in children with Tourette syndrome. *J Psychosom Res* 2003; 55:59–65.

Burd L, Fisher WW, Kerbeshian J, Arnold ME. Is development of Tourette disorder a marker for improvement in patients with autism and other pervasive developmental disorders? *J Am Acad Child Adolesc Psychiatry* 1987; 26:162–165.

Burd L, Freeman RD, Klug MG, Kerbeshian J. Tourette syndrome and learning disabilities. *BMC Pediatr* 2005; 5:34.

A study using the Tourette Syndrome International Consortium database reporting that the high prevalence of learning disabilities in TS is associated with ADHD.

Burd L, Kauffman DW, Kerbeshian J. Tourette syndrome and learning disabilities. *J Learn Disabil* 1992; 25:598–604.

Burd L, Kerbeshian J. Familial pervasive development disorder, Tourette disorder and hyperlexia. *Neurosci Biobehav Rev* 1988; 12:233–234.

Burd L, Kerbeshian J, Wikenheiser M, Fisher W. A prevalence study of Gilles de la Tourette's syndrome in North Dakota school-aged children. *J Am Acad Child Psychiatry* 1986; 25:552–553.

Burd L, Li Q, Kerbeshian J et al. Tourette syndrome and comorbid pervasive developmental disorders. *J Child Neurol* 2009; 24:170–175.

Buss AH, Plomin R. *A temperament theory of personality development*. New York, 1975.

Cardona F, Romano A, Bollea L, Chiarotti F. Psychopathological problems in children affected by tic disorders—study on a large Italian population. *Eur Child Adolesc Psychiatry* 2004; 13:166–171.

Cardon LR, Smith SD, Fulker DW et al. Quantitative trait locus for reading disability on chromosome 6. *Science* 1994; 266:276–279.

Carter AS, O'Donnell DA, Schultz RT et al. Social and emotional adjustment in children affected with Gilles de la Tourette's syndrome: associations with ADHD and family functioning. *J Child Psychol Psychiatry* 2000; 41:215–223.

Carter AS, Pauls DL, Leckman JF, Cohen DJ. A prospective longitudinal study of Gilles de la Tourette's syndrome. *J Am Acad Child Adolesc Psychiatry* 1994; 33:327–338.

This study examined social-emotional functioning and contribution of family functioning in children with TS only, TS+ADHD, and controls. Social and behavioral dysfunction in children with TS is ADHD-specific, and TS-only children differ largely on social-emotional profile compared to those with TS+ADHD.

Cath DC, Hedderly T, Ludolph AC et al. European Clinical guidelines for Tourette syndrome and other tic disorders. Part I: assessment and medical examination. *Eur Child Adolesc Psychiatry* 2011; 20:147–172.

Cath DC, Hoogduin CAL, van de Wetering BJM et al. Tourette syndrome and obsessive-compulsive disorder: An analysis of associated phenomena. In: Chase TN, Friedhoff AJ, & Cohen DJ (Eds.), *Advances in Neurology Series*, pp. 33–41. Raven Press, New York, 1992.

Cath DC, Spinhoven P, Landman AD et al. Psychopathology and personality ratings in relation to 5-HT blood measures in Tourette's syndrome and obsessive-compulsive disorder. *J Psychopharmacol* 2001; 15:111–119.

This cross-sectional controlled study investigated personality dimensions in TS-only and TS+OCD patients and found that the comorbid OCD was associated with lower extraversion and higher neuroticism, and that tics were associated with higher neuroticism but not with higher impulsivity or exraversion.

Cavanna AE, Robertson MM, Critchley HD. Schizotypal personality traits in Gilles de la Tourette syndrome. *Acta Neurol Scand* 2007; 116:385–391.

Chakrabarti S, Fombonne E. Pervasive developmental disorders in preschool children: confirmation of high prevalence. *Am J Psychiatry* 2005; 162:1133–1141.

Coffey BJ, Biederman J, Geller D et al. Reexamining tic persistence and tic-associated impairment in Tourette's disorder: findings from a naturalistic follow-up study. *J Nerv Ment Dis* 2004; 192:776–780.

Coffey BJ, Biederman J, Geller D et al. Distinguishing illness severity from tic severity in children and adolescents with Tourette's disorder. *J Am Acad Child Adolesc Psychiatry* 2000a; 39:556–561.

Coffey BJ, Biederman J, Smoller JW et al. Anxiety disorders and tic severity in juveniles with Tourette's disorder. *J Am Acad Child Adolesc Psychiatry* 2000; 39, 562–569.

This follow-up study investigated tic persistence and tic-associated impairment in 50 youth (ages 6–17 years) with TS. Results showed a dissociation between tic persistence and tic-associated dysfunction.

Coffey BJ, Biederman J, Smoller JW et al. Anxiety disorders and tic severity in juveniles with Tourette's disorder. *J Am Acad Child Adolesc Psychiatry* 2000b; 39:562–568.

Cohen E, Sade M, Benarroch F et al. Locus of control, perceived parenting style, and symptoms of anxiety and depression in children with Tourette's syndrome. *Eur Child Adolesc Psychiatry* 2008; 17:299–305.

Comings DE, Comings BG. Tourette syndrome: clinical and psychological aspects of 250 cases. *Am J Hum Genet* 1985; 37:435–450.

Comings DE, Comings BG. A controlled study of Tourette syndrome. I. Attention-deficit disorder, learning disorders, and school problems. *Am J Hum Genet* 1987; 41:701–741.

Comings DE, Comings BG. A controlled study of Tourette syndrome III: Phobias and panic attacks. *Am J Hum Genet* 1987a; 41:761–780.

Comings DE, Comings BG. A controlled study of Tourette syndrome V: Depression and mania. *Am J Hum Genet* 1987b; 41: 804–821.

Comings DE, Comings BG. A controlled family history study of Tourette's syndrome III: Affective and other disorders. *J Clin Psychiatry* 1990; 51:288–291.

Comings DE, Comings BG, Muhleman D et al. The dopamine D2 receptor locus as a modifying gene in neuropsychiatric disorders. *JAMA* 1991; 266:1793–1800.

Como PG. Neuropsychological function in Tourette's syndrome. In: Kurlan D (Ed.), *Handbook of Tourette's syndrome and related tic and behavioral disorders*, pp. 237–252. Marcel Dekker, New York, 2005.

Corbett JA, Mathews AM, Connell PH, Shapiro DA. Tics and Gilles de la Tourette's syndrome: a follow-up study and critical review. *Br J Psychiatry* 1969; 115:1229–1241.

Dishion TJ, Patterson GR. The development and ecology of antisocial behavior in children and adolescents. In: Cichetti D, Cohen DJ (Eds.), *Developmental psychopathology, vol. 3: Risk, disorder and adaptation*, pp. 503–541. Wiley, Hoboken, NJ, 2006.

Dodel I, Reese JP, Muller N et al. Cost of illness in patients with Gilles de la Tourette's syndrome. *J Neurol* 2010; 257:1055–1061.

Eapen V, Fox-Hiley P, Banerjee S. Clinical features and associated psychopathology in a Tourette syndrome cohort. *Acta Neurol Scand* 2004; 109:255–260.

Eddy CM, Cavanna AE, Gulisano M et al. Clinical correlates of quality of life in Tourette syndrome. *Mov Disord* 2011a; 26:735–738.

This study investigated quality of life in young people with TS and found that depression and behavioral difficulties, including symptoms of OCD, predicted poor quality of life best in TS.

Eddy CM, Rizzo R, Gulisano M et al. Quality of life in young people with Tourette syndrome: a controlled study. *J Neurol* 2011b; 258:291–301.

Eysenck J, Eysenck S. *Manual of the Eysenck Personality Questionnaire*. Hodder and Stroughton Educational, London, 1975.

Fava M, Rosenbaum JF, McCarthy M et al. Anger attacks in depressed outpatients and their response to fluoxetine. *Psychopharmacol Bull* 1991; 27:275–279.

Fernandez TV, Sanders SJ, Yurkiewicz IR et al. Rare copy number variants in Tourette syndrome disrupt genes in histaminergic pathways and overlap with autism. *Biol Psychiatry* 2012; 71: 392–402.

First MB, Pincus HA. The DSM-IV Text Revision: rationale and potential impact on clinical practice. *Psychiatr Serv* 2002; 53:288–292.

Fletcher JM, Lyon GR, Fuch LS, Barnes MA. *Learning disabilities: From identification to intervention*. 2007 New York: Guilford.

Frank MC, Piedad J, Rickards H, Cavanna AE. The role of impulse control disorders in Tourette syndrome: an exploratory study. *J Neurol Sci* 2011; *310*:276–278.

Freeman RD, Fast DK, Burd L et al. An international perspective on Tourette syndrome: selected findings from 3500 individuals in 22 countries. *Dev Med Child Neurol* 2000; *42*:436–447.

This paper describes a collaborative effort of a multisite, international database of 3,500 individuals diagnosed with TS. Specifically, behavioral problems are associated with comorbidity.

Freeman RD. Tic disorders and ADHD: answers from a world-wide clinical dataset on Tourette syndrome. *Eur Child Adolesc Psychiatry* 2007; *16* Suppl 1: 15–23.

Gaze C, Kepley HO, Walkup JT. Co-occurring psychiatric disorders in children and adolescents with Tourette syndrome. *J Child Neurol* 2006; *21*:657–664.

Gelernter J, Vandenbergh D, Kruger SD et al. The dopamine transporter protein gene (SLC6A3): primary linkage mapping and linkage studies in Tourette syndrome. *Genomics* 1995; *30*:459–463.

George MS, Trimble MR, Ring HA et al. Obsessions in obsessive-compulsive disorder with and without Gilles de la Tourette's syndrome. *Am J Psychiatry* 1993; *150*:93–97.

Geurts HM, Grasman RP, Vertè S et al. Intra-individual variability in ADHD, autism spectrum disorders and Tourette's syndrome. *Neuropsychologia* 2008; *46*:3030–3041.

Geurts HM, Vertè S, Oosterlaan J et al. How specific are executive functioning deficits in attention deficit hyperactivity disorder and autism? *J Child Psychol Psychiatry* 2004; *45*:836–854.

Gillberg C, Wing L. Autism: not an extremely rare disorder. *Acta Psychiatr Scand* 1999; *99*:399–406.

Gilles de la Tourette, GAEB. Etude sur une affection nerveuse caracterisee par la incoordination motrice accompagnee d'echolalie et de coprolalie. *Archives Neurologiques* 1885; *19*–42, 158–200.

Goldman S, Wang C, Salgado MW et al. Motor stereotypies in children with autism and other developmental disorders. *Dev Med Child Neurol* 2009; *51*:30–38.

Gorman DA, Thomson T, Plessen KJ et al. Psychosocial outcome and psychiatric comorbidity in older adolescents with Tourette syndrome: controlled study. *Br J Psychiatry* 2010; *197*:36–44.

Grados MA, Mathews CA. Latent class analysis of Gilles de la Tourette syndrome using comorbidities: clinical and genetic implications. *Biol Psychiatry* 2008; *64*:219–225.

Green D, Charman T, Pickles A et al. Impairment in movement skills of children with autistic spectrum disorders. *Dev Med Child Neurol* 2009; *51*:311–316.

Hallahan DP, Kauffmann JM, Lloyd JW. *Introduction to learning disabilities*. Prentrice Hall, NJ, 1996.

Harris KM, Mahone EM, Singer HS. Nonautistic motor stereotypies: clinical features and longitudinal follow-up. *Pediatr Neurol* 2008; *38*:267–272.

An investigation of clinical records and subsequent telephone interviews to characterize the clinical features and long-term outcomes in children with motor stereotypies who do not manifest mental retardation or pervasive developmental disorder.

Hoekstra RA, Bartels M, Verweij CJ, Boomsma DI. Heritability of autistic traits in the general population. *Arch Pediatr Adolesc Med* 2007; *161*:372–377.

Hoeve M, Dubas JS, Eichelsheim VI et al. The relationship between parenting and delinquency: a meta-analysis. *J Abnorm Child Psychol* 2009; *37*:749–775.

Hornsey H, Banerjee S, Zeitlin H, Robertson MM. The prevalence of Tourette syndrome in 13–14-year-olds in mainstream schools. *J Child Psychol Psychiatry* 2001; *42*:1035–1039.

An epidemiological study on occurrence of TS in 13- to 14-year-old schoolchildren, which identified tics in 18.7% of the pupils. Seven adolescents out of 918 fulfilled the criteria for TS (0.76%).

Kanner L, Eisenberg L. Early infantile autism, 1943–1955. *Psychiatr Res Rep Am Psychiatr Assoc* 1957, 55–65.

Kerbeshian J, Burd L. Are schizophreniform symptoms present in attenuated form in children with Tourette disorder and other developmental disorders. *Can J Psychiatry* 1987; *32*:123–135.

Kessler RC, Coccaro EF, Fava M et al. The prevalence and correlates of DSM-IV intermittent explosive disorder in the National Comorbidity Survey Replication. *Arch Gen Psychiatry* 2006; *63*:669–678.

Khalifa N, von Knorring AL. Prevalence of tic disorders and Tourette syndrome in a Swedish school population. *Dev Med Child Neurol* 2003; *45*:315–319.

Khalifa N, von Knorring AL. Psychopathology in a Swedish population of school children with tic disorders. *J Am Acad Child Adolesc Psychiatry* 2006; *45*:1346–1353.

A population-based study showing the high prevalence of comorbidities in TS. About 90% of

children with TS also had psychiatric comorbid disorders, mostly ADHD.

Kirk SA. *Educating exceptional children*. Houghton Mifflin, Boston, 1962.

Kurlan R. Tourette's syndrome in a special education population: a pilot study involving a single school district. *Neurology* 1994; 44:699–702.

A pilot study showing that children with TS often require special education.

Kurlan R, Como PG, Miller B et al. The behavioral spectrum of tic disorders: a community-based study. *Neurology* 2002; 59:414–420.

Langen M, Durston S, Kas MJ et al. The neurobiology of repetitive behavior … and men. *Neurosci Biobehav Rev* 2011; 35:356–365.

Leckman JF, Walker DE, Cohen DJ. Premonitory urges in Tourette's syndrome. *Am J Psychiatry* 1993; 150:98–102.

Leckman JF, Zhang H, Vitale A et al. Course of tic severity in Tourette syndrome: the first two decades. *Pediatrics* 1998; 102:14–19.

Legg C, Penn C, Temlett J, Sonnenberg B. Language skills of adolescents with Tourette syndrome. *Clin Linguist Phon* 2005; 19:15–33.

Levitt JJ, McCarley RW, Dickey CC et al. MRI study of caudate nucleus volume and its cognitive correlates in neuroleptic-naive patients with schizotypal personality disorder. *Am J Psychiatry* 2002; 159:1190–1197.

Lewin AB, Murphy TK, Storch EA et al. A phenomenological investigation of women with Tourette or other chronic tic disorders. *Compr Psychiatry* 2011; 53:525–534.

A Web-based descriptive study on specific tic symptoms and tic severity, self-reported history of other psychiatric conditions, and impairment/lifestyle impact due to tics in a group of 275 men and 185 women.

Lewis C, Hitch GJ, Walker P. The prevalence of specific arithmetic difficulties and specific reading difficulties in 9- to 10-year-old boys and girls. *J Child Psychol Psychiatry* 1994; 35:283–292.

Lin H, Katsovich L, Ghebremichael M et al. Psychosocial stress predicts future symptom severities in children and adolescents with Tourette syndrome and/or obsessive-compulsive disorder. *J Child Psychol Psychiatry* 2007; 48:157–166.

A 2-year prospective study examining the relationship between psychosocial stress and fluctuations in tic, obsessive-compulsive, and depressive symptom severity, in children and adolescents with TS and/or OCD.

Mahler M. Psychoanalytic evaluation of tics: a sign and symptom in psychopathology. *Psychoanalytic Studies of the Child* 1949: 279–310.

Mason A, Banerjee S, Eapen V et al. The prevalence of Tourette syndrome in a mainstream school population. *Dev Med Child Neurol* 1998; 40:292–296.

Mathews CA, Bimson B, Lowe TL et al. Association between maternal smoking and increased symptom severity in Tourette's syndrome. *Am J Psychiatry* 2006; 163:1066–1073.

Muhle R, Trentacoste SV, Rapin I. The genetics of autism. *Pediatrics* 2004; 113: e472–e486.

Muller-Vahl K, Dodel I, Muller N et al. Health-related quality of life in patients with Gilles de la Tourette's syndrome. *Mov Disord* 2010; 25:309–314.

A study in 200 patients with TS on health-related quality of life. Reduced quality of life was found in association with severity of tics, depression, and age.

Neuner I, Ludolph A. [Tics and Tourette's syndrome throughout the life span]. *Nervenarzt* 2009; 80:1377–1387.

Olfson M, Crystal S, Gerhard T et al. Patterns and correlates of tic disorder diagnoses in privately and publicly insured youth. *J Am Acad. Child Adolesc Psychiatry* 2011; 50:119–131.

Ozonoff S, Strayer DL. Inhibitory function in nonretarded children with autism. *J Autism Dev Disord* 1997; 27:59–77.

Ozonoff S, Strayer DL, McMahon WM, Filloux F. Executive function abilities in autism and Tourette syndrome: an information processing approach. *J Child Psychol Psychiatry* 1994; 35:1015–1032.

The performance of nonretarded autistic children on tasks requiring global-local processing and inhibition was compared with that of TS subjects and controls. Autistic subjects, in contrast to TS subjects, were impaired on cognitive flexibility.

Palumbo D, Maughan A, Kurlan R. Hypothesis III. Tourette syndrome is only one of several causes of a developmental basal ganglia syndrome. *Arch Neurol* 1997; 54:475–483.

Pauls DL, Leckman JF. The inheritance of Gilles de la Tourette syndrome and associated behaviors. *N Engl J Med* 1986; 315:993–997.

Pauls DL, Leckman JF, Cohen DJ. Evidence against a genetic relationship between Tourette's syndrome and anxiety, depression, panic and phobic disorders. *Br J Psychiatry* 1994;*164*:215–221.

A large-scale controlled family study in TS, focussing on the relationship with anxiety disorders and depression.

Pauls DL, Raymond CL, Stevenson JM, Leckman JF. A family study of Gilles de la Tourette syndrome. *Am J Hum Genet* 1991; *48*: 154–163.

Pauls DL, Leckman JF, Cohen DJ. Familial relationship between Gilles de la Tourette's syndrome, attention deficit disorder, learning disabilities, speech disorders, and stuttering. *J Am Acad Child Adolesc Psychiatry* 1993; *32*:1044-1050.

Pennington BF. *Diagnosing learning disorders.* Guildford Press, New York, 1991.

Pennington BF. Genetics of learning disabilities. *J Child Neurol* 1995; *10* Suppl 1:S69–S77.

Pennington BF, Gilger JW, Pauls D et al. Evidence for major gene transmission of developmental dyslexia. *JAMA* 1991; *266*:1527–1534.

Pennington BF, Ozonoff S. Executive functions and developmental psychopathology. *J Child Psychol Psychiatry* 1996; *37*:51–87.

Peterson BS, Pine DS, Cohen P, Brook JS. Prospective, longitudinal study of tic, obsessive-compulsive, and attention-deficit/hyperactivity disorders in an epidemiological sample. *J Am Acad Child Adolesc Psychiatry* 2001; *40*:685–695.

A longitudinal prospective study in an epidemiological sample of 776 children and adolescents followed prospectively into early adulthood, with reassessments after 8, 10, and 15 years. Tics and OCD as well as OCD and ADHD were significantly associated in this sample.

Pollak Y, Benarroch F, Kanengisser L et al. Tourette syndrome-associated psychopathology: roles of comorbid attention-deficit hyperactivity disorder and obsessive-compulsive disorder. *J Dev Behav Pediatr* 2009; *30*:413–419.

Poyurovsky M, Koran LM. Obsessive-compulsive disorder (OCD) with schizotypy vs. schizophrenia with OCD: diagnostic dilemmas and therapeutic implications. *J Psychiatr Res* 2005; *39*:399–408.

Raine A. The SPQ: a scale for the assessment of schizotypal personality based on DSM-III-R criteria. *Schizophr Bull* 1991; *17*:555–564.

Rapin I. Autism spectrum disorders: relevance to Tourette syndrome. *Adv Neurol* 2001; *85*:89–101.

Riley WT, Treiber FA, Woods MG. Anger and hostility in depression. *J Nerv Ment Dis* 1989; *177*:668–674.

Rizzo R, Curatolo P, Gulisano M et al. Disentangling the effects of Tourette syndrome and attention-deficit/hyperactivity disorder on cognitive and behavioral phenotypes. *Brain Dev* 2007; *29*:413–420.

Rizzo R, Gulisano M, Calì PV, Curatolo P. Long-term clinical course of Tourette syndrome. *Brain Dev* 2011 [Epub ahead of print].

Robertson MM. Tourette syndrome, associated conditions and the complexities of treatment. *Brain* 2000; *123*:425–462.

Robertson MM. Mood disorders and Gilles de la Tourette's syndrome: An update on prevalence, etiology, comorbidity, clinical associations, and implications. *J Psychosom Res* 2006; *61*:349–358.

Robertson MM. The prevalence and epidemiology of Gilles de la Tourette syndrome. Part 1: the epidemiological and prevalence studies. *J Psychosom Res* 2008; *65*:461–472.

Robertson MM, Banerjee S, Hiley F, Tannock C. Personality disorder and psychopathology in Tourette's syndrome: a controlled study. *Br J Psychiatry* 1997; *171*:283–286.

A study using standardized rating scales and interviews on personality disorders, showing elevated rates in TS of all three clusters of personality disorders.

Robertson MM, Channon S, Baker J, Flynn D. The psychopathology of Gilles de la Tourette's syndrome: A controlled study. *Br J Psychiatry* 1993; *162*:114–117.

Roessner V, Becker A, Banaschewski T et al. Developmental psychopathology of children and adolescents with Tourette syndrome—impact of ADHD. *Eur Child Adolesc Psychiatry* 2007; *16* Suppl 1: S24–S35.

A cross-sectional study investigating various age groups of TS patients from a database including more than 3,500 cases, aiming to unravel the relationship between ADHD comorbidity in TS and internalizing and externalizing behaviors.

Rosenbaum JF, Fava M, Pava JA et al. Anger attacks in unipolar depression, Part 2: Neuroendocrine correlates and changes following fluoxetine treatment. *Am J Psychiatry* 1993; *150*:1164–1168.

Rosenberg LA, Brown J, Singer HS. Behavioral problems and severity of tics. *J Clin Psychol* 1995; 51:760–767.

Rutter M, Caspi A, Fergusson D et al. Sex differences in developmental reading disability: new findings from 4 epidemiological studies. *JAMA* 2004; 291:2007–2012.

A study providing evidence from four epidemiological studies that reading disabilities are clearly more common in boys than in girls.

Scahill L, Erenberg G, Berlin CM et al. Contemporary assessment and pharmacotherapy of Tourette syndrome. *NeuroRx* 2006; 3:192–206.

Sergeant JA, Geurts H, Oosterlaan J et al. How specific is a deficit of executive functioning for attention-deficit/hyperactivity disorder? *Behav Brain Res* 2002; 130:3–28.

Shapiro AK, Shapiro ES, Bruun RD, Sweet RD. *Gilles de la Tourette's syndrome*. Raven Press, New York, 1978.

Shaywitz SE, Shaywitz BA, Fletcher JM, Escobar MD. Prevalence of reading disability in boys and girls. Results of the Connecticut Longitudinal Study. *JAMA* 1990; 264:998–1002.

Simonoff E, Pickles A, Charman T et al. Psychiatric disorders in children with autism spectrum disorders: prevalence, comorbidity, and associated factors in a population-derived sample. *J Am Acad Child Adolesc Psychiatry* 2008; 47:921–929.

Singer HS. Motor stereotypies. *Semin Pediatr Neurol* 2009; 16:77–81.

Singer HS. Stereotypic movement disorders. *Handb Clin Neurol* 2011; 100:631–639.

Spencer T, Biederman J, Harding M et al. The relationship between tic disorders and Tourette's syndrome revisited. *J Am Acad Child Adolesc Psychiatry* 1995; 34: 1133–1139.

St Sauver JL, Katusic SK, Barbaresi WJ et al. Boy/girl differences in risk for reading disability: potential clues? *Am J Epidemiol* 2001; 154:787–794.

State MW. The genetics of child psychiatric disorders: focus on autism and Tourette syndrome. *Neuron* 2010; 68:254–269.

Stefl ME. Mental health needs associated with Tourette syndrome. *Am J Public Health* 1984; 74:1310–1313.

Stewart SE, Illmann C, Geller DA et al. A controlled family study of attention-deficit/

hyperactivity disorder and Tourette's disorder. *J Am Acad Child Adolesc Psychiatry* 2006; 45:1354–1362.

Sukhodolsky DG, Scahill L, Zhang H et al. Disruptive behavior in children with Tourette's syndrome: association with ADHD comorbidity, tic severity, and functional impairment. *J Am Acad Child Adolesc Psychiatry* 2003; 42:98–105.

A clinical study in four groups of children showing that TS-only children did not differ from normal controls in terms of psychopathology or behavior.

Tunmer W, Greaney K. Defining dyslexia. *J Learn Disabil* 2010; 43:229–243.

van den Hoofdakker BJ, Nauta MH, Dijck-Brouwer DA et al. Dopamine transporter gene moderates response to behavioral parent training in children with ADHD: A pilot study. *Dev Psychol* 2012; 48:567–574.

van den Hoofdakker BJ, Nauta MH, van der Veen-Mulders L et al. Behavioral parent training as an adjunct to routine care in children with attention-deficit/hyperactivity disorder: moderators of treatment response. *J Pediatr Psychol* 2010; 35:317–326.

van den Hoofdakker BJ, van der Veen-Mulders L, Sytema S et al. Effectiveness of behavioral parent training for children with ADHD in routine clinical practice: a randomized controlled study. *J Am Acad Child Adolesc Psychiatry* 2007; 46:1263–1271.

Verte S, Geurts HM, Roeyers H et al. Executive functioning in children with autism and Tourette syndrome. *Dev Psychopathol* 2005; 17:415–445.

A neuropsychological study examining four groups of children: high-functioning autism, TS, the two together, and a normal control group, indicating that executive function deficits are highly characteristic of children with high-functioning autism in comparison to children with TS and normal controls.

Volkmar FR, Cohen DJ. Current concepts: infantile autism and the pervasive developmental disorders. *J Dev Behav Pediatr* 1986; 7:324–329.

Walkup JT, Khan S, Schuerholz L et al. Phenomenology and natural history of tic-related ADHD and learning disabilities. In: Leckman JL & Cohen DJ (Eds.), *Tourette's syndrome: Tics, obsessions, compulsions— Developmental psychopathology and clinical care,* pp. 63–79. John Wiley & Sons Inc., New York, 1999.

Wanderer S, Roessner V, Freeman R et al. Relationship of obsessive-compulsive disorder to age-related comorbidity in children and adolescents with Tourette syndrome. *J Dev Behav Pediatr* 2012; 33: 124–133.

Wickramaratne PJ, Weissman MM. Using family studies to understand comorbidity. *Eur Arch Clin Neurosci* 1993; 243:150–157.

Yoshimasu K, Barbaresi WJ, Colligan RC et al. Gender, attention-deficit/hyperactivity disorder, and reading disability in a population-based birth cohort. *Pediatrics* 2010; 126: e788–e795.

5

Clinical Course and Adult Outcome in Tourette Syndrome

MICHAEL H. BLOCH

Abstract

This chapter summarizes the existing literature on the long-term course of Tourette syndrome. Tic symptoms typically reach their worst-ever severity between 10 and 12 years of age. One half to two thirds of children with Tourette syndrome experience a significant decline of tic symptoms that roughly coincides with adolescence. The impact of pharmacological or behavioral treatments upon the long-term prognosis remains an unexplored aspect. Some comorbid symptoms such as obsessive-compulsive symptoms in adulthood may also influence tic persistence into adulthood. Finally, potential predictors of tic outcome in adulthood include performance on some specific fine-motor skills and caudate volumes during childhood.

This illness is hereditary; it is characterized by motor incoordination in the form of abrupt muscular jerks that are often severe enough to make the patient jump; … the incoordination may be accompanied by articulated or inarticulated sounds. When articulated, the words are often repetitions of words which the patient may have just heard… Among the expressions which the patient may repeatedly utter … some may have the special character of being obscene (coprolalia); … the physical and mental health of these patients is otherwise basically normal. The condition seems *incurable and life long*, with onset in childhood.
—Gilles de la Tourette, 1884

GILLES DE la Tourette identified many of the cardinal characteristics of the syndrome that now bears his name in his original case series published in 1885 (Gilles de la Tourette, 1885). He observed the hereditary nature and childhood onset of Tourette syndrome (TS), the presence of motor and vocal tics, the presence of palilalia and coprolalia in some points, and, perhaps most importantly, the otherwise normal mental and physical health of these patients. However, Gilles de la Tourette erred in one important way in his original account: he suggested that the tics of TS are lifelong.

Although some adult patients with TS are among the most severely affected and treatment-refractory that we treat, decades of following children with TS has taught us that a majority of children with TS improve during adolescence, with greatly diminished tics in adulthood in the majority of cases (Bloch, Peterson et al., 2006; Leckman, Zhang et al., 1998). The purpose of this chapter is to outline the clinical course of individuals with TS. The chapter will begin by focusing on the course of tic symptoms in TS, then outline the clinical course of common comorbid conditions, and finish by discussing adult global functioning and psychosocial outcome of children with TS. We will additionally explore our knowledge about childhood predictors of prognosis in TS.

Lastly, we will examine the important clinical implications that our understanding of prognosis has for our treatment of individuals with tic disorders.

NATURAL HISTORY OF TICS IN TS

Tics in TS typically have an onset of around the age of 6 to 8 years. The vast majority (90–95%) of TS cases have an onset of tics between 4 and 13 years of age (Leckman et al., 1998). Tics typically begin as simple motor movements such as eye blinking, nose twitching, or facial grimaces (Leckman et al., 1998). Motor tics usually progress in a rostrocaudal direction with time. Vocal tics, when they appear, typically first manifest themselves a year or two after the onset of motor tics. Vocal tics begin as simple vocalizations such as throat clearing, sniffing, or fractions of words. With increasing age, both motor and vocal tics usually become more complex. Motor tics often evolve into more elaborate movements, and vocal tics often develop into words or phrases. Many TS patients experience

premonitory urges (Leckman et al., 1993). A premonitory urge is a sensory phenomenon that occurs immediately prior to a tic, similar to the need to sneeze or itch. Awareness of premonitory urges increases with age and is present in as many as 90% of adolescents with TS (Woods et al., 2005). Tic symptoms of TS generally occur in bouts and wax and wane in severity over time (Peterson & Leckman, 1998). Factors such as stress, anxiety, and fatigue are known to exacerbate tics in many individuals over the short term, whereas focused concentration, especially involving fine-motor movements such as playing a musical instrument, dancing, or playing sports, alleviates tics (Conelea & Woods, 2008). Heat sensitivity and infection (such as group A streptococcal infections) may exacerbate tics as well (Lin, Katsovich et al., 2007; Lombroso, Mack et al., 1991; Scahill, Lombroso et al., 2001). Chapters 1, 9, and 14 discuss short-term factors that exacerbate tic symptoms in greater detail. Many TS patients are able to temporarily suppress tics, but often at the expense of concentration and exhaustion (Himle, Woods et al., 2007) As children get older they typically develop a greater ability to suppress tics (Himle, Woods et al., 2007).

Tics in TS typically reach their worst severity between 10 and 12 years age. Roughly three quarters of children with tics experience their worst tics between 9 and 14 years of age (Bloch, Peterson et al., 2006). During adolescence half to two thirds of children with TS experience a drastic reduction in tics (Bloch, Peterson et al., 2006). Figure 5.1 demonstrates the clinical course of tic severity in a large cohort of 42 children with TS followed for an average of 7.3 years after initial evaluation (Leckman, Zhang et al., 1998). Figure 5.2 describes the adult tic outcome in a combined cohort of 82 children followed from initial evaluation (average age 11 years) to young adulthood (Bloch, Peterson et al., 2006; Leckman, Zhang et al., 1998;). As Figure 5.2 demonstrates, over one third of children with TS were completely tic-free at follow-up, slightly less than half had minimal to mild tics, and less than a quarter had moderate or greater tics at follow-up. These results contrast to their worst-ever period, where all individuals experienced at least moderate tics. Less than 5%

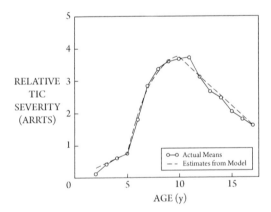

FIGURE 5.1 **Course of tic severity in childhood.** Plot of average tic severity in a cohort of 36 children from ages 2 to 18. Tics typically have an onset between ages 4 and 6 years, reach their worst between ages 10 and 12, and then decline in severity throughout adolescence. ARRTS, annual rating of relative tic severity. In the ARRTS, parents rate tic symptoms of their children on a six-point ordinal scale (absent [0], least severe, mild, moderate, severe, and most severe [6]).

(Adapted with permission from Leckman, Zhang et al., 1998.)

of individuals reported experiencing worse tics in young adulthood than they did in childhood. Similar results of tic improvement have been demonstrated in a large cohort of children with tics and comorbid attention-deficit/hyperactivity disorder (ADHD; Spencer, Biederman et al., 1999).

Although an uncommon outcome, the cases of TS that persist into adulthood are often the most severe (Cheung, Shahed et al., 2007). Coprolalia and self-injurious tics, which are present in a small minority of those experiencing tic symptoms, are much more common among adults with TS. Improved treatments are urgently needed for the minority of individuals with TS who experience a chronic and debilitating course.

NATURAL HISTORY OF COMMON COMORBID CONDITIONS IN TS

ADHD

In epidemiologic samples, greater than half of individuals with TS experience comorbid ADHD (Khalifa & von Knorring, 2006). The prevalence of ADHD in patients with TS who reach clinical attention may be even higher (Walkup, Khan et al., 1998). When ADHD

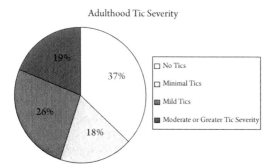

Adulthood Tic Severity

FIGURE 5.2   **Tic severity in adulthood.**   Adult tic severity in 82 children with significant childhood tic symptoms. Adult tic severity class is defined by Yale Global Tic Severity Total Tic Score (YGTSS): no tics (0), minimal tics (1–9), mild tics (10–19), moderate or greater tics (≥20). All individuals had moderate or greater severity tics in childhood. Less than 5% of individuals reported having worse tics as adults than in childhood. (See color insert.)

(Adapted with permission from Bloch & Leckman, 2009.)

is present in individuals with TS, the ADHD symptoms typically precede the onset of tic symptoms and are associated with greater social, behavioral, and academic problems than the tics themselves (Hoekstra, Steenhuis et al., 2004; Sukhodolsky, Scahill et al., 2003). Not surprisingly, comorbid ADHD symptoms in childhood have been associated with a decreased quality of life and global functioning in early adulthood for individuals with TS (Gorman, Thompson et al., 2010). Unfortunately, studies examining the clinical course of ADHD, specifically in individuals with comorbid tics, are lacking. In the general ADHD population, however, it has been shown that the hyperactivity symptoms of ADHD generally improve during adolescence, whereas the inattention symptoms of ADHD often persist into adulthood (Faraone, Biederman et al., 2006). Comorbid ADHD in children with TS often has a negative impact on concurrent social, academic, and behavioral function (Sukhodolsky, Scahill et al., 2003). Comorbid ADHD symptoms can also have a negative impact on future quality of life and global psychosocial functioning (Bernard, Stebbins et al., 2009). Chapter 2 provides a detailed overview of the various aspects of ADHD comorbidity in TS.

Obsessive-Compulsive Disorder

Roughly one third to one half of children with TS will experience comorbid obsessive-compulsive disorder (OCD) throughout their lifetime (Bloch, Peterson et al., 2006). OCD symptoms in patients with TS have an onset around the time that the tics reach their worst, but symptoms may also appear *de novo* in adulthood. OCD patients with comorbid tics tend to have greater rates of symmetry obsessions and counting, repeating, ordering, and arranging compulsions than OCD patients without comorbid tic symptoms (Leckman, Grice et al., 1994–95). In terms of pharmacotherapy, children with OCD and comorbid tics are likely to have a worse response to selective serotonin reuptake inhibitors (SSRIs) than children without comorbid tics (March, Franklin et al., 2007). While children with OCD and comorbid tics may not respond optimally to SSRIs, it has been shown that children with OCD, with and without comorbid tics, appear to have a similar response to cognitive-behavioral therapy (March, Franklin et al., 2007). Another treatment option for OCD patients with comorbid tics is antipsychotic medication. A meta-analysis of antipsychotic augmentation trials for treatment-refractory OCD suggests that OCD patients with comorbid tics may have an improved response to this intervention (Bloch, Landeros-Weisenberger et al., 2006). Chapter 3 provides a detailed overview of the various aspects of OCD comorbidity in TS.

Other Comorbid Conditions

Children with TS have higher rates of comorbid developmental disorders, learning disabilities, and disruptive behavior disorders than the general population (Kurlan, Whitmore et al., 1994). The symptoms of these comorbid conditions typically appear prior to the time that tics reach clinical attention. When present, aggressive treatment of these conditions is warranted. Currently, there is no evidence to suggest that the recommended treatment of these conditions should differ between individuals with and without comorbid tic disorders. Explosive rage attacks can be particularly challenging in individuals with TS, but therapies such as parent management training and anger management training, which are effective in the general population, are also effective in TS (Budman, Rockmore et al., 2003; Scahill, Sukhodolsky et al., 2006).

Children with TS experience comorbid depressive and anxiety disorders during adolescence and early adulthood more frequently than unaffected controls (Bloch, Peterson et al., 2006; Gorman, Thompson et al., 2010). Roughly 40% of children with TS will experience depression or a non-OCD anxiety disorder (Gorman, Thompson et al., 2010). Children with TS and their parents should be educated to recognize the signs and symptoms of these conditions. Chapter 4 provides a detailed overview of the various aspects of these comorbidities in TS.

PREDICTORS OF LONG-TERM OUTCOME

Clinical Assessment

Several prospective cohort studies have examined childhood predictors of long-term outcome in tic disorders (Bloch, Peterson et al., 2006; Corbett, Mathews et al., 1969; de Groot, Bornstein et al., 1994; Gorman, Thompson et al., 2010; Leckman, Zhang et al., 1998; Sandor, Musisi et al., 1990; Torup, 1962). Table 5.1 provides a detailed description of all prospective cohort studies that have examined long-term outcome (duration of follow-up greater than 5 years) in children with TS. These studies are fairly consistent in indicating that the vast majority of children with TS will improve during adolescence (range: 67–96%) (Bloch, Peterson et al., 2006; Corbett, Mathews et al., 1969; Leckman, Zhang et al., 1998; Sandor, Musisi et al., 1990; Torup, 1962). The average reduction in tics in adulthood from the worst-ever period is roughly two thirds (Bloch, Peterson et al., 2006; Leckman, Zhang et al., 1998). It is also clear from long-term follow-up studies that the likelihood of remission is much lower once children reach late adolescence and early adulthood (de Groot, Bornstein et al. 1994; Sandor, Musisi et al. 1990).

Few studies have examined clinical predictors of long-term outcome in children with TS. A couple of studies have associated childhood tic severity with adult outcome (Bloch, Peterson et al., 2006; de Groot, Bornstein et al., 1994). This finding, however, is at best a weak predictor that has not been replicated in all studies (Leckman, Zhang et al., 1998). Current tic severity likely has more prognostic value as children reach later adolescence. Isolated trials have associated more complex and vocal tics or a family history of persistent tics with persistence of symptoms into adulthood (de Groot, Bornstein et al., 1994; Torup, 1962). However, none of these findings have been replicated multiple studies. The current published literature suggests that traditionally evaluated clinical symptoms in childhood have limited value in terms of the long-term prognosis of tics.

Table 5.1 Prospective Long-Term Outcome Studies in Tourette Syndrome

Author (year)	N (Range or mean) (SD)	Baseline age (Range or mean) (SD)	Duration when available (Mean) (SD)	Age at follow-up (Range or mean) (SD)	ADHD (%)	OCD (%)	Average tic reduction from worst tic severity	% patients with tic remission	% patients with tic improvement	Predictors of outcome
Corbett (1969)	73	4–21	About 5 years on average (from <2 to >8 years)	6–29	Not available	Not available	Not available	40%	93%	Outcome associated with longer duration of follow-up and age of onset. Improved prognosis associated with age of onset between 6–8 years compared to earlier or later onset.
Gorman (2010)	65	10.8 (2.8)	7.3 (3.1)	18.1 (1.4)	66%	39%	Not available	Not available	Not available	Poorer psychosocial outcomes in the TS group correlated with greater tic severity, comorbid ADHD and OCD
Bloch (2006)	46	11.4 (1.6)	7.6 (2.7)	19 (1.8)	22%	41%	68%	33%	96%	Increased childhood tic severity weakly associated with adulthood tic severity
Sandor (1990)	33	19 (14)	7 (4)	25 (19)	Not available	Not available	Not available	Not available	67% by self-report	Not assessed

(Continued)

Table 5.1 (*Continued*)

Author (year)	N (Range or mean) (SD)	Baseline age (Range or mean) (SD)	Duration when available (Mean) (SD)	Age at follow-up (Range or mean) (SD)	ADHD (%)	OCD (%)	Average tic reduction from worst tic severity	% patients with tic remission	% patients with tic improvement	Predictors of outcome
De Groot (1994)	23	16.7	5	11–53 (mean 22.1)	Not available	60% had obsessive-compulsive symptoms	Not available	Not available	13%	Baseline complex motor tics predicted complex motor and vocal tics at follow-up; baseline obsessive-compulsive symptoms predicted obsessive-compulsive symptoms at follow-up
Leckman (1998)	36	11 (2.9)	7.5 (2.7)	18.4 (1)	69%	36%	73%	47%	88%	Childhood and worst tic severity not significantly associated with outcome
Torup (1962	220	13	5 (range 2–16)	18	Not available	Not available	Not available	50%	94%	Adult presence of tics in parents was associated with persistence of child's tics into adulthood

Previous research has not demonstrated that comorbid conditions in childhood such as ADHD and OCD are associated with increased tic severity in adulthood (Bloch, Peterson et al., 2006; Gorman, Thompson et al., 2010). However, lifetime comorbid ADHD and OCD symptoms have been associated with poorer adult psychosocial functioning in patients with TS (Gorman, Thompson et al., 2010). Nevertheless, current tic severity in adulthood is also associated with overall psychosocial functioning in longitudinal samples (Gorman, Thompson et al., 2010). Data have not demonstrated a link between worst-ever tic severity and adult psychosocial functioning.

Neuropsychological Assessment

Only one study, to our knowledge, has examined the association between neuropsychological testing in childhood and adult outcome in terms of tic severity (Bloch, Sukhodolsky et al., 2006). We evaluated a cohort of 32 children, aged 8 to 14, with TS and no comorbid ADHD who underwent clinical evaluation and a focused neuropsychological test battery consisting of the Purdue Pegboard, Beery Visual-Motor Integration (VMI) Test, and the Rey-Osterreith Complex Figure Task (RCFT). A follow-up clinical assessment was performed on these children an average of 7.5 years later. Poor performance with the dominant hand on the Purdue Pegboard test predicted worse adult tic severity and correlated with tic severity at the time of the childhood assessment. These results are consistent with previous studies that have demonstrated deficits in fine-motor coordination tests such as the Purdue Pegboard in patients with TS (Bornstein, 1991; Bornstein & Yang, 1991; Hagin, Beecher et al., 1982; Schultz, Carter et al., 1998). Purdue Pegboard performance deficiencies have been linked to poor social functioning in schizophrenia (Lehoux, Everett et al., 2003). There are at least two possible explanations for the ability of the Purdue Pegboard test to predict future tic and global psychosocial functioning in children with TS. First, poor Purdue Pegboard performance is a reflection of poor fine-motor skills in childhood. Fine-motor skill deficits make it difficult for these children to succeed in activities such as team sports, video games, and musical instruments that are instrumental to building self-esteem and social relationships in these pivotal developmental years. This experience of success is of increased importance in children with TS because of the social stigma that all too often accompanies their tics. Second, poor Purdue Pegboard performance is a sign of deficits in complex, visually guided or coordinated movements that are likely mediated by circuits involving the basal ganglia (Schultz, Carter et al., 1998). Deficits on Purdue Pegboard testing have been associated with reduced putamen volumes in Parkinson's disease patients (Alegret, Junque et al., 2001) and basal ganglia hyperperfusion in 99mTc-hexamethyl propylene amine oxime SPECT studies of patients with subclinical hepatic encephalopathy (Catafau, Kulisevsky et al., 2000). These findings are particularly of interest given the considerable evidence of basal ganglia abnormalities in TS patients. Reduced caudate volume has been previously demonstrated to be a morphological trait of TS on structural magnetic resonance imaging (MRI; Catafau, Kulisevsky et al., 2000; Peterson, Thomas et al., 2003). Fine-motor skills are also part of a series of neuropsychological deficits termed neurological "soft signs." Soft signs are motor, sensory, or integrative abnormalities found on neurological exams in individuals with no neurological lesion. Soft signs are thought to reflect complex patterns of deficits involving several systems (Anderson & Savage, 2004; Shaffer, Schonfeld et al., 1985). Increased neurological soft signs are associated with a diagnosis of ADHD, learning disorders, bipolar disorder, schizophrenia, chronic posttraumatic stress disorder, borderline personality disorders, and even externalizing and internalizing disorders in general (Chan, Xu et al., 2010; Dazzan & Murray, 2002; De la Fuente, Bobes et al., 2006; Dickstein, Garvey et al., 2005; Foodman & McPhillips, 1996; Gurvits, Gilbertson et al., 2000; Negash, Kebede et al., 2004; Pine, Wasserman et al., 1997). Other studies have associated the presence of neuropsychological soft signs with the persistence of schizophrenia and both internalizing and externalizing disorders in children (Mayoral, Bombin et al., 2008; Pine, Wasserman et al., 1997; Prikryl, Ceskova et al., 2007; Wilson, Pine et al., 2003). The presence of neurological soft signs is also correlated with the severity of visuospatial skill and nonverbal memory deficits in OCD patients (Mataix-Cols, Alonso et al., 2003). Further research is needed to determine the predictive validity of neurological soft signs in the persistence of OCD and psychiatric illness in general and to determine environmental risk factors associated with these deficits (Boks, Selten et al., 2007; Hertzig, 1991).

Neuroimaging

Only one study has examined the association between child neuroimaging data and long-term outcome in TS (Bloch, Leckman et al., 2005). We followed to young adulthood a cohort of 46 children with TS who underwent childhood volumetric imaging; they were largely overlapping with the clinical and neuropsychological samples described above. Subjects underwent initial childhood neuroimaging around the typical period when tics are at their worst severity (average age 11.4 years) and were followed to determine their clinical outcome an average of 7.5 years later. MRI scans were performed in childhood and acquired using a single 1.5-T scanner. Basal ganglia volumes were previously determined by investigators blinded to subject characteristics and hemisphere on UNIX workstations using ANALYZE 7.5 software. Hand tracing was used to define the basal ganglia after the images were enlarged eightfold to minimize mechanical tracing error (Peterson, Thomas et al., 2003).

Smaller childhood caudate volumes were associated with increased severity of tic and OCD symptoms in young adulthood. Figure 5.3 depicts a plot of the association between childhood caudate volume and adult tic severity in this TS cohort. This finding is consistent with other structural neuroimaging studies that have reported a reduction in caudate volume in subjects with TS compared to healthy controls. Large cross-sectional neuroimaging studies have demonstrated a small but significant 5% reduction in the caudate nucleus in TS subjects compared to controls (Peterson, Thomas et al.,

2003). Studies of monozygotic twins, discordant for tic severity, have demonstrated reduced caudate volumes in the more severely affected twin (Hyde, Stacey et al., 1995) These reductions in caudate volumes in children with TS have been further associated with the persistence of tic symptoms into adulthood (Bloch, Leckman et al., 2005).

These findings are also consistent of neuropathological research in TS. Postmortem neuro-stereological studies assessing neuronal density and numbers in five adults with severe, intractable TS and five healthy controls have suggested a possible mechanism for this caudate volume reduction (Kalanithi, Zheng et al., 2005; Kataoka, Kalanithi et al., 2010). TS subjects demonstrated a reduced overall number of two types of interneurons in the striatum (Kalanithi, Zheng et al., 2005; Kataoka, Kalanithi et al., 2010). Parvalbumin-positive interneurons and cholinergic interneurons were both reduced by over 50% in the caudate and putamen of TS patients (Kalanithi, Zheng et al., 2005; Kataoka, Kalanithi et al., 2010). Furthermore, adult TS patients showed the greatest decrease in cholinergic neurons in the anterior caudate, the area of prefrontal projections (Kataoka, Kalanithi et al., 2010). Cholinergic neurons were reduced to a lesser extent than in projection areas from the sensorimotor cortex (Kataoka, Kalanithi et al., 2010) The most posterior limbic projection areas demonstrated a similar density of cholinergic interneurons between TS subjects and controls (Kataoka, Kalanithi et al., 2010). These recent findings strongly implicate prefrontal and sensorimotor projection areas of the basal ganglia in the pathogenesis of TS. This focused loss of interneurons provides a mechanism by which TS patients have impairment of cognitive control or require increasing frontal activation to achieve normal levels of cognitive controls. This loss of interneurons in sensorimotor projection areas also suggests a possible mechanism of tic generation—abnormal firing of striatal projection neurons due to impaired inhibition. However, it is impossible to determine whether these striatal interneuron deficits are central to the pathogenesis of TS, a consequence of illness, or a compensatory mechanism for prolonged

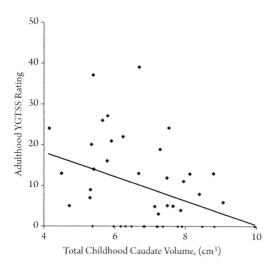

FIGURE 5.3 **Association of childhood caudate volume with adult tic severity.** Scatterplot of relative childhood caudate volume (adjusting for age, gender, and whole brain volume) and adult tic severity. Caudate volumes in childhood were associated inversely with tic and obsessive-compulsive symptom severity at follow-up in early adulthood (Bloch et al., 2005).

illness because postmortem studies (1) are all cross-sectional in nature and (2) exclusively rely on adults with prolonged disease because of the accessibility of data. More fine-grained, morphological neuroimaging studies, examining different areas in the basal ganglia in a longitudinal manner, can better put these neuropathological findings in context (see also Chapters 10 and 12 for detailed reviews of these aspects).

IMPLICATIONS FOR CLINICIANS

Box 5.1 highlights the key points for clinicians in this chapter. The natural developmental time course of tics in TS has profound implications for the treatment of individuals with this condition. Children with tics have a substantial probability of improvement and even the possibility of resolution of their tic symptoms during adolescence and young adulthood. Given the ephemeral nature of tics in many children, pharmacological treatment should be conservative and focused on reducing functional impairment. Psychoeducational interventions focused

on improving understanding of the nature and course of tic symptoms in parents, teacher, peers, and proband; improving family coping mechanisms to deal with tics; improving childhood resilience; and improving the classroom environment are particularly advisable (see also Chapter 22). Additionally, behavioral treatments for tics such as cognitive-behavioral interventions for tics (see Chapter 23) are favored by some compared to pharmacological options, given the particularly adverse side-effect profile of many of these agents in children.

By contrast, the treatment of an adult with significant and functionally impairing tics should be much more aggressive, as available data suggest that these symptoms are much less likely to improve naturally over time. Although the same psychoeducational, psychosocial, and behavioral treatments that are preferable in children are equally preferable in adults (for much the same reasons), a considerably lower threshold for adding pharmacological interventions (such as antipsychotics or alpha-2 agonists) exists, as the "tincture of time" is much less likely to be helpful in these patients.

Although some studies have suggested that some clinical predictors in childhood may predict long-term outcome such as poor fine-motor skills and worse and more complex tics, none of these potential predictors provide clinically meaningful information that would warrant substantially altering the prognosis of a patient with tics at any age. By contrast, pharmacological treatment of comorbid conditions such as ADHD and OCD is warranted, as these conditions are less likely to improve and more likely to cause significant long-term functional impairment. Furthermore, aggressive treatment of significantly harmful self-injurious tics or those leading to severe functional impairment (e.g., school refusal) is advisable at any age.

IMPLICATIONS FOR RESEARCHERS

Prospective cohort studies have established that a majority of children with tic symptoms experience a substantial reduction of tic symptoms during adolescence and young adulthood

(Bloch, Peterson et al., 2006; Leckman, Zhang et al., 1998). Research has suggested several possible predictors of long-term outcome, such as poor fine-motor skills, possibly worse tic severity, or the presence of more complex and vocal tics and smaller caudate volumes using volumetric neuroimaging. However, none of these possible predictors of long-term outcome have been replicated in multiple prospective longitudinal studies. Furthermore, it is not clear that any of

---

Box 5.1. Key Points

- Tic symptoms typically reach their worst severity between 10 and 12 years of age.
- Children with tics tend to become more aware of premonitory urges and display more complex tics as they get older.
- Half to two thirds of children with TS experience a significant decline of tic symptoms that roughly coincides with adolescence.
- There is no evidence to suggest that pharmacological or behavioral treatments for tics affect long-term prognosis.
- Comorbid ADHD symptoms, when they occur, typically precede the onset of tics, and comorbid OCD symptoms usually follow the onset of tics.
- The presence of OCD symptoms in adulthood is highly correlated with the persistence of tic symptoms into adulthood and is not strongly related to the presence of OCD symptoms in childhood.
- Poor fine-motor skills are associated with the persistence of tic symptoms into adulthood.
- Smaller caudate volumes are associated with the persistence of tic symptoms into adulthood.

Box 5.2. Questions for Future Research

Prognosis
- Does early medication treatment with antipsychotics or other tic-suppressing medications alter the long-term course of TS?
- Does early intervention with behavioral treatments for tics affect the long-term outcome or functional impairment?
- Do children with TS have a different prognosis based on the types of tics they present with (i.e., simple motor vs. complex vocal)?
- Does the clinical course of tics in parents inform the likely trajectory of tics in their offspring?
- Are particular genetic variations associated with long-term outcome?

Developmental Neurobiology of Tic Disorders
- How does brain morphology change during adolescence in patients whose tics improve during adolescence compared to those who don't improve?
- Which neuropsychological and neuroimaging abnormalities in TS are state or trait characteristics of the disorder?

these predictors, unless further refined, could meaningfully influence our understanding of prognosis for an individual child with TS or influence his or her treatment.

That being said, understanding how and why particular children with TS improve while others do not could greatly improve our understanding of the neuropathology of tics and related conditions and lead to novel and more personalized treatments. Additionally, many crucial and clinically salient questions about the prognosis of TS remain almost completely unexplored. Box 5.2 outlines several important questions for future research.

CONCLUSIONS

One half to two thirds of children with TS experience a diminishing of their tics during adolescence and young adulthood (Bloch, Peterson et al., 2006; Leckman, Zhang et al., 1998). Comorbid ADHD and OCD in TS often have a greater impact on adult functioning than the tics themselves. Poor fine-motor skills and reduced caudate volume in childhood have been associated with the persistence of tics into young adulthood. Further research is needed to (1) refine and confirm the moderators associated with symptom improvement during adolescence and (2) identify mediators associated with long-term outcome.

REFERENCES

Alegret M, Junque C, Pueyo R et al. MRI atrophy parameters related to cognitive and motor impairment in Parkinson's disease. *Neurologia* 2001; 16:63–69.

Anderson KE, Savage CR. Cognitive and neurobiological findings in obsessive-compulsive disorder. *Psych Clin North Am* 2004; 27:37–47.

Bernard BA, Stebbins GT, Siegel S et al. Determinants of quality of life in children with Gilles de la Tourette syndrome. *Mov Disord* 2009; 24:1070–1073.

Bloch MH, Landeros-Weisenberger A, Kelmendi B et al. A systematic review: antipsychotic augmentation with treatment refractory obsessive-compulsive disorder. *Mol Psychiatry* 2006; 11:622–632.

Bloch MH, Leckman JF. Clinical course of Tourette syndrome. *J Psychosom Res* 2009; 67:497–501.

Bloch MH, Leckman JF, Zhu H, Peterson BS. Caudate volumes in childhood predict symptom severity in adults with Tourette syndrome. *Neurology* 2005; 65:1253–1258.

The first prospective study to show that caudate volumes in children with TS predict the severity of tic and obsessive-compulsive symptoms in early adulthood. This study provides compelling evidence that morphological disturbances of the caudate nucleus within cortico-striatal-thalamo-cortical circuits are central to the persistence of both tics and obsessive-compulsive symptoms into adulthood.

Bloch MH, Peterson BS, Scahill L et al. Adulthood outcome of tic and obsessive-compulsive symptom severity in children with Tourette syndrome. *Arch Pediatr Adolesc Med* 2006; 160:65–69.

One of the first prospective studies showing that obsessive-compulsive symptoms in children with TS become more severe at a later age and are more likely to persist than tic symptoms.

Bloch MH, Sukhodolsky DG, Leckman JF, Schultz RT. Fine-motor skill deficits in childhood predict adulthood tic severity and global psychosocial functioning in Tourette's syndrome. *J Child Psychol Psychiatry* 2006; 47:551–559.

In this prospective study, fine-motor skill deficits appear to be a predictor of future tic severity and global psychosocial function in children with TS. The authors hypothesize that performance on the Purdue Pegboard test may serve as a useful endophenotype in the study of TS and provide a rough measure of the degree of basal ganglia dysfunction present in TS patients.

Boks MP, Selten JP, Leask S et al. Negative association between a history of obstetric complications and the number of neurological soft signs in first-episode schizophrenic disorder. *Psychiatry Res* 2007; 149:273–277.

Bornstein RA. Neuropsychological correlates of obsessive characteristics in Tourette syndrome. *J Neuropsychiatry Clin Neurosci* 1991; 3:157–162.

Bornstein RA. Neuropsychological performance in adults with Tourette's syndrome. *Psychiatry Res* 1991; 37:229–236.

Bornstein RA, Yang V. Neuropsychological performance in medicated and unmedicated patients with Tourette's disorder. *Am J Psychiatry* 1991; 148:468–471.

Budman CL, Rockmore L, Stokes J, Sossin M et al. Clinical phenomenology of episodic rage in children with Tourette syndrome. *J Psychosom Res* 2003; 55:59–65.

Catafau AM, Kulisevsky J, Bernà L et al. Relationship between cerebral perfusion in frontal-limbic-basal ganglia circuits and neuropsychologic impairment in patients with subclinical hepatic encephalopathy. *J Nucl Med* 2000; 41:405–410.

Chan RC, Xu T et al. Neurological soft signs in schizophrenia: a meta-analysis. *Schizophrenia Bull* 2010; 36:1089–1104.

Cheung MY, Shahed J, Jankovic J. Malignant Tourette syndrome. *Mov Disord* 2007; 22:1743–1750.

Conelea CA, Woods D. The influence of contextual factors on tic expression in Tourette's syndrome: a review. *J Psychosom Res* 2008; 65:487–496.

Corbett JA, Mathews MA, Connell PH, Shapiro DA. Tics and Gilles de la Tourette's syndrome: a follow-up study and critical review. *Br J Psychiatry* 1969; 115:1229–1241.

Dazzan P, Murray RM. Neurological soft signs in first-episode psychosis: a systematic review. *Br J Psychiatry* 2002; Suppl 43: s50–57.

de Groot CM, Bornstein RA, Spetie L, Burriss B. The course of tics in Tourette syndrome: a 5-year follow-up study. *Ann Clin Psychiatry* 1994; 6:227–233.

De la Fuente JM, Bobes J, Vizuete C et al. Neurologic soft signs in borderline personality disorder. *J Clin Psychiatry* 2006; 67:541–546.

Dickstein DP, Garvey M, Pradella AG et al. Neurologic examination abnormalities in children with bipolar disorder or attention-deficit/ hyperactivity disorder. *Biol Psychiatry* 2005; 58:517–524.

Faraone SV, Biederman J, Mick E. The age-dependent decline of attention deficit hyperactivity disorder: a meta-analysis of follow-up studies. *Psychol Med* 2006; 36:159–165.

Foodman A, McPhillips K. ADD and soft signs. *J Am Acad Child Adol Psychiatry* 1996; 35:841–842.

Gilles de la Tourette G. Etude sur une affection nerveuse caracterisee par de l'incoordination motrice accompagnee d'echolalie et de copralalie. *Archive Neurologie* 1885; 9:19–42, 158–200.

Gorman DA, Thompson N, Plessen KJ et al. Psychosocial outcome and psychiatric comorbidity in older adolescents with Tourette syndrome: controlled study. *Br J Psychiatry* 2010; 19:36–44.

Gurvits TV, Gilbertson MW, Lasko NB et al. Neurologic soft signs in chronic posttraumatic stress disorder. *Arch Gen Psychiatry* 2000; 57:181–186.

Hagin RA, Beecher R, Pagano G, Kreeger H. Effects of Tourette syndrome on learning. *Adv Neurol* 1982; 35:323–328.

Hertzig ME. Neurological 'soft' signs in low-birthweight children. *Dev Med Child Neurol* 1991; 23:778–791.

Himle MB, Woods DW, Conelea CA et al. Investigating the effects of tic suppression on premonitory urge ratings in children and adolescents with Tourette's syndrome. *Behav Res Ther* 2007; 45:2964–2976.

Hoekstra PJ, Steenhuis MP, Troost PW et al. Relative contribution of attention-deficit hyperactivity disorder, obsessive-compulsive disorder, and tic severity to social and behavioral problems in tic disorders. *J Dev Behav Pediatr* 2004; 25:272–279.

Hyde TM, Stacey ME, Coppola R et al. Cerebral morphometric abnormalities in Tourette's syndrome: a quantitative MRI study of monozygotic twins. *Neurology* 1995; 45:1176–1182.

Kalanithi PS, Zheng W, Kataoka Y et al. Altered parvalbumin-positive neuron distribution in basal ganglia of individuals with Tourette syndrome. *Proc Natl Acad Sci USA* 2005; 102:13307–13312.

Kataoka Y, Kalanithi PS, Grantz H et al. Decreased number of parvalbumin and cholinergic interneurons in the striatum of individuals with Tourette syndrome. *J Comp Neurol* 2010; 518:277–291.

Khalifa N, von Knorring AL. Psychopathology in a Swedish population of school children with tic disorders. *J Am Acad Child Adolesc Psychiatry* 2006; 45:1346–1353.

Kurlan R, Whitmore D, Irvine C et al. Tourette's syndrome in a special education population: a pilot study involving a single school district. *Neurology* 1994; 44:699–702.

Leckman JF, Grice DE, Barr LC et al. Tic-related vs. non-tic-related obsessive compulsive disorder. *Anxiety* 1994–1995; 1:208–215.

Leckman JF, Walker DE, Cohen DJ. Premonitory urges in Tourette's syndrome. *Am J Psychiatry* 1993; 150:98–102.

Leckman JF, Zhang H, Vitale A et al. Course of tic severity in Tourette syndrome: the first two decades. *Pediatrics* 1998; 102:14–19.

An influential birth-cohort study showing that the majority of TS patients display a consistent time course of tic severity. One of the earliest studies to suggest that the determination of the model parameters that describe each patient's course of tic severity may be of prognostic value and assist in the identification of factors that differentially influence the course of tic severity.

Lehoux C, Everett J, Laplante L et al. Fine motor dexterity is correlated to social functioning in schizophrenia. *Schizophr Res* 2003; 62:269–273.

Lin H, Katsovich L, Ghebremichael M et al. Psychosocial stress predicts future symptom severities in children and adolescents with Tourette syndrome and/or obsessive-compulsive disorder. *J Child Psychol Psychiatry* 2007; 48:157–166.

Lombroso PJ, Mack G, Scahill L et al. Exacerbation of Gilles de la Tourette's syndrome associated with thermal stress: a family study. *Neurology* 1991; 41:1984–1987.

March JS, Franklin ME, Leonard H et al. Tics moderate treatment outcome with sertraline but not cognitive-behavior therapy in pediatric obsessive-compulsive disorder. *Biol Psychiatry* 2007; 61:344–347.

Mataix-Cols D, Alonso P, Hernandez R et al. Relation of neurological soft signs to nonverbal memory performance in obsessive-compulsive disorder. *J Clin Exp Neuropsychol* 2003; 25:842–851.

Mayoral M, Bombin I, Zabala A et al. Neurological soft signs in adolescents with first episode psychosis: two-year followup. *Psychiatry Res* 2008; 161:344–348.

Negash A, Kebede D, Alem A et al. Neurological soft signs in bipolar I disorder patients. *J Affect Disord* 2004; 80:221–230.

Peterson BS, Leckman JF. The temporal dynamics of tics in Gilles de la Tourette syndrome. *Biol Psychiatry* 1998; 44:1337–1348.

An intriguing and inspiring work that provided initial evidence for the presence of a fractal, deterministic, and possibly chaotic process in the tic time series.

Peterson BS, Thomas P, Kane MJ et al. Basal ganglia volumes in patients with Gilles de la Tourette syndrome. *Arch Gen Psychiatry* 2003; 60:415–424.

Pine DS, Wasserman GA, Fried JE et al. Neurological soft signs: one-year stability and relationship to psychiatric symptoms in boys. *J Am Acad Child Adolesc Psychiatry* 1997; 36:1579–1586.

Prikryl R, Ceskova E, Kasparev T, Kucerova H. Neurological soft signs and their relationship to 1-year outcome in first-episode schizophrenia. *Eur Psychiatry* 2007; 22:499–504.

Sandor P, Musisi S, Moldofsky H, Lang A. et al. Tourette syndrome: a follow-up study. *J Clin Psychopharmacol* 1990; 10: 197–199.

Scahill L, Lombroso PJ, Mack G et al. Thermal sensitivity in Tourette syndrome: preliminary report. *Percept Mot Skills* 2001; 92:419–432.

Scahill L, Sukhodolsky DG, Bearss K et al. Randomized trial of parent management training in children with tic disorders and disruptive behavior. *J Child Neurol* 2006; 21:650–656.

Schultz RT, Carter AS, Gladstone M et al. Visual-motor integration functioning in children with Tourette syndrome. *Neuropsychology* 1998; 12:134–145.

Shaffer D, Schonfeld I, O'Connor PA et al. Neurological soft signs. Their relationship to psychiatric disorder and intelligence in childhood and adolescence. *Arch Gen Psychiatry* 1985; 42:342–351.

Spencer T, Biederman M, Coffey B et al. The 4-year course of tic disorders in boys with attention-deficit/hyperactivity disorder. *Arch Gen Psychiatry* 1999; 56:842–847.

Sukhodolsky DG, Scahill L, Zhang H et al. Disruptive behavior in children with Tourette's syndrome: association with ADHD comorbidity, tic severity, and functional impairment. *J Am Acad Child Adolesc Psychiatry* 2003; 42: 98–105.

Torup E. A follow-up study of children with tics. *Acta Paediatrica* 1962; 51:261–268.

Walkup JT, Khan S, et al. Phenomenology and natural history of tic-related ADHD and learning disabilities. In Leckman JF & Cohen DJ (Eds.), *Tourette's Syndrome: Tics, Obsessions, Compulsions—Developmental Psychopathology and Clinical Care.* John Wiley & Sones, New York, 1998, pp. 63–79.

Wilson JJ, Pine DS, Cargan A et al. Neurological soft signs and disruptive behavior among children of opiate dependent parents. *Child Psychiatry Hum Dev* 2003; 34:19–34.

Woods DW, Piacentini J, Himle MB, Chang S. Premonitory Urge for Tics Scale (PUTS): initial psychometric results and examination of the premonitory urge phenomenon in youths with Tic disorders. *J Dev Behav Pediatr* 2005; 26: 397–403.

6

The Prevalence of Tourette Syndrome and its Relationship to Clinical Features

LAWRENCE SCAHILL, SOREN DALSGAARD AND KATHRYN BRADBURY

Abstract

This chapter will summarize the results of and discuss the methodological issues related to the prevalence studies on Tourette syndrome conducted over the past 12 years. The best estimate for the prevalence of Tourette syndrome in school-age children is likely to fall between 5 and 7 cases per 1,000. The prevalence of chronic motor tic disorder in school-age children ranges from 3 to 8 per 1,000, whereas estimates of prevalence for chronic vocal tic disorder are less stable and await further study. Children with chronic tic disorders, even those with mild conditions, have a higher likelihood of other problems such as attention-deficit/hyperactivity disorder, disruptive behavior, and obsessive-compulsive disorder. The classic two-stage design seems an acceptable approach for prevalence studies of Tourette syndrome and related tic disorders; however, this requires sample sizes greater than 5,000 to ensure relatively narrow confidence intervals. From a public health perspective, chronic tics may serve as a marker of neurodevelopmental vulnerability. Community-based studies that improve case finding are likely to increase our understanding of the health impact of tic disorders in children.

INTRODUCTION

The study of the distribution and determinants of disease is the province of epidemiology. Central to these pursuits is the delineation of cases from non-cases. This classification is necessary for developing a trustworthy estimate of prevalence and is also essential for identifying associated features of cases compared to unaffected individuals. Accurate prevalence estimates and information on associations can provide valuable information on the public health impact of a given condition. For neuropsychiatric disorders such as Tourette syndrome (TS), there are no diagnostic laboratory tests or biological markers. Thus, the diagnosis is based on history and direct observation (whenever possible). Another potential contribution of epidemiological study is the documentation of the full syndrome from mild to severe. Mild cases of TS identified in community surveys may not come to clinical attention. These milder cases may show different associations and patterns of disability than more severe and obviously biased cases reaching clinical attention. Among the many challenges facing prevalence studies in TS are the ascertainment and assessment of a large, representative community sample. Prevalence studies in TS conducted over the past 12 years have used a range of sampling, sample size, assessment methods, and study designs. Large, well-crafted epidemiological studies are expensive, especially those involving in-person assessments (Hirtz et al., 2007).

Since 2000, 11 community surveys of various sizes have been designed and conducted to estimate prevalence. There have also been a handful of reviews on this topic (Hirtz et al., 2007; Knight et al., 2012; Robertson et al., 2009; Scahill et al., 2005). Collectively, these reviews reach differing conclusions about the prevalence of TS in children, with a range from 3 to 10 per thousand.

From a public health standpoint, however, this range is less than satisfactory. For example, 3 cases per 1,000 translates into approximately 150,000 cases of TS in school-age children in the United States, whereas 9 per 1,000 would translate into 450,000 children. This difference would presumably have dramatically different implications for health service needs (Centers for Disease Control and Prevention [CDC], 2009). The purpose of this chapter is to provide a critical review of community surveys conducted since 2000 in order to identify the best estimate of prevalence of TS in school-age children. We also examine the associated disability of TS in children to illustrate health service needs.

THE TWO-STAGE STUDY AS A MODEL DESIGN

The two-stage study is not the only rigorous approach to estimation of TS prevalence in a community sample of children, but this design illustrates several research elements and challenges facing investigators. A well-planned and well-funded two-stage study begins with ascertainment of a large community sample of children (Stage 1). In addition to the size of the sample, the source of the sample also warrants careful consideration. A detailed description of sampling, however, is beyond the scope of the current discussion.

In Stage 1, the full sample may be screened with a relatively brief parent questionnaire. The resulting screen-positive group is presumed to be enriched with true cases. These screen-positive cases are invited to participate in a full diagnostic assessment (Stage 2). A screen that does not miss many cases is said to have high *sensitivity*. On the other hand, if the screen is "overly" sensitive, the more detailed and expensive diagnostic assessment may be conducted on a large number of unaffected subjects. Thus, an efficient screen must somehow avoid missing cases and avoid the expense of conducting unnecessary diagnostic assessments on unaffected subjects (false positives). Because no screen is perfect, a small random sample of screen negatives should also be invited to return for a full assessment in Stage 2. The purpose of recruiting a random

sample of screen negatives is to identify *true cases* that were missed by the screening. This reflects the formula for the calculation of sensitivity for a screening test: True-positive cases ÷ (true positives on screening + false negatives on screening). Thus, the sensitivity of the screening test cannot be calculated without an estimate of false negatives from Stage 1. A large randomly selected screen-negative sample increases the likelihood of identifying true cases that were missed by the Stage 1 screening, but the yield may be low. Given that the full assessment at Stage 2 is costly, there is a need for balance in setting the percentage of randomly selected subjects among screen negatives.

The goal of Stage 2 is to classify true cases and non-cases; the full assessment includes a thorough evaluation of current and past tics as well as the presence of other psychiatric conditions, intellectual capacity, and overall development. This may be done by trained interviewers, who may not be experienced clinicians. Depending on the age of the sample, parents are likely to be key informants in this assessment. Past studies indicate that parents are reliable informants— but may be a source of false positives and false negatives. Therefore, the optimal study would also include face-to-face assessment of the child by an experienced clinician. Face-to-face assessment is also expensive and may not be possible, depending on the size of the study.

In addition to the source and size of the original sample and the diagnostic assessment methods used, another element that influences the reliability and validity of a prevalence estimate is response rate. A team of investigators may devise an elegant sampling strategy for Stage 1, only to have it undermined by a low response rate. Similarly, an accurate count of cases relies on a respectable rate of participation in Stage 2 (for both screen positives and screen negatives). A participation rate of 80% at each stage is considered optimal, but this rarely occurs in practice. As the participation rate goes down, the representativeness of the sample also goes down. For example, a large sample of 8,000 children at Stage 1 with a 40% response (n = 3,200) would raise questions about biased participation. If the estimated prevalence was higher than several prior studies, it might be that subjects with tics were more likely to participate.

THE PROBLEM OF THRESHOLD

Transient tics are relatively common in school-age children, ranging from 11% to 20% (Cubo et al., 2011; Kurlan et al., 2001; Linazasoro et al., 2006; Snider et al., 2002), with male-to-female ratios ranging from 2 to 1 to as high as 3.5 to 1. For most community-identified cases, the tics are mild and transient and may not constitute a disorder. The *Diagnostic and Statistical Manual—Fourth Edition—Revised* (American Psychiatric Association, 2000) defines three tic disorders that are relevant to the current discussion. Transient tic disorder consists of motor tics, vocal tics, or both lasting at least 2 weeks but less than 1 year. Chronic tic disorder is defined by the presence of motor or vocal tics (but not both) that persists for more than 1 year. TS includes multiple motor tics and at least one vocal tic lasting for more than 1 year (see Chapter 17 for a more detailed discussion of the differential diagnosis). Current diagnostic criteria specify that the onset of tics must occur before 18 years of age. Parents commonly report a fluctuating course for the tics over time. By age 10 years, most patients describe an ability to suppress tics for brief periods and the presence of an urge or warning before the execution of some or all of their tics (Leckman, 2002).

Community surveys conducted in various countries over the past 25 years provide an extraordinary range of prevalence estimates for TS in children, from 0.5 to 38 cases per 1,000 (Hirtz et al., 2007; Knight et al., 2012; Robertson, 2009; Scahill et al., 2005). The lowest estimate of 0.5 per 1,000 came from a survey of Israeli army inductees (Apter et al., 1993). This survey relied on self-reports from subjects between 16 and 18 years of age, when tics decline in many cases (Leckman, 2002). It is possible that a parent interview focused on lifetime diagnosis would have identified more cases. The upper bound came from a study of 1,255 schoolchildren (Kurlan et al., 2001). Due to the exceedingly low participation rate, this study does not offer a trustworthy prevalence estimate

(see below). If the estimates at the extremes are disregarded, the resulting range of prevalence from studies conducted over the past decade is 1 to 16 per 1,000. Although narrower than the extremely broad range of 0.5 to 38 per 1,000, 1 to 16 per 1,000 remains imprecise and insufficient to guide estimates of service needs for affected children. The variation in estimates across these community studies is likely due to differences in sampling method, sample size, rate of subject participation, assessment methods, and diagnostic threshold used to define cases.

It is clear that the estimate of prevalence of TS would be influenced by the symptom threshold used to define the disorder. Simply stated, if children with mild forms of TS are defined as true cases, the prevalence will increase. If the severity threshold is set higher, or if the diagnostic criteria require impairment, the prevalence will be lower. What may be less clear is the impact of case definition on associated features. For example, associations of tic disorders and other conditions such as attention-deficit/hyperactivity disorder (ADHD), anxiety disorders, or learning disability may vary across the range of severity from mild to more extreme.

Using Medline, we searched with several key words (Tourette syndrome, tic disorders, epidemiology, prevalence) to locate all studies published since 2000. We also consulted recent reviews to identify studies that may have been missed by the Medline search (Hirtz et al., 2007; Knight et al., 2012; Robertson et al., 2009; Scahill et al., 2005). To be included in the current review, the publication had to include a lifetime diagnosis of one or more chronic tic disorders. To facilitate comparison across studies, we calculated the 95% confidence interval (CI) from the data provided in each report (see formula in the legend of Table 6.1). The 95% CI expresses the range of possible prevalence estimates based on the observed prevalence and the study sample size. For example, consider two studies, one with a sample size of 1,000 and the other with 5,000. In each study, the observed prevalence was 7 cases per 1,000 children. The 95% CI for the sample size of 1,000 would be 2 to 12 cases per 1,000 compared to 5 to 9 cases per 1,000 in a sample of 5,000.

Table 6.1 Prevalence of TS in the Pediatric Population in Studies Conducted Between 2000 and 2012

Author/Year	N	Age	Design	Source of Sample	Diagnostic Assessment	Diagnostic Criteria	# of Cases	Prevalence (per 1,000)	95% CI (per 1,000)[a]
Kadesjo & Gillberg, 2000	435	10–11	Two stage	Birth cohort	In-person interview with parent, child, & teacher	DSM-IV	5	11	4–27
Kurlan et al., 2001	1255	8.5–17.5	Single stage	Randomly selected schools	In-person structured interview with parent & child	DSM-IVb	48	38c	27–49
Peterson et al., 2001	776	9–20	Single stage	Community cohort	In-person structured interview with parent & child	DSM-III	2	2.6	0–6.2
Hornsey et al., 2001	918	13–14	Three stage	Six schools; single mainstream class	In-person structured interview with parent & child	DSM-III-R	7	7.6	2–13.2
Khalifa & von Knorring, 2003	4479	7–15	Two stage	Community; all available in township	In-person structured interview with parent & child	DSM-IV	25	5.6	3.6–7.6
Wang & Kuo, 2003	2000	6–12	Three stage	School	In-person structured interview with parent & child	Tourette Syndrome Study Group	11	5.5	2.3–8.7
Jin et al., 2005	9742	7–16	Two stage	Community	In-person interview with parent & child	Chinese Diagnostic Standard for Psychiatric Disorders (3rd ed.)	42	4.3	3.0–5.6

Study	n	Age	Design	Setting	Method	Criteria	Cases	Prevalence	95% CI
Scahill et al., 2006	910	6–12	Two stage[d]	Community	In-person structured parent interview	DSM-IV	3	3.3	0–7
Kraft et al. (2012)	5974	9–15	Two stage	Birth cohort	Structured parent interview via telephone	DSM-IV	33	5.5	4.0–8.0
Cubo et al., 2011	741	5–17	Two stage	Regional community sample	Semistructured interview via telephone	DSM-IV	27	3.64	22.9–50[e]

a = Calculated from reported prevalence data and sample size 95% CI = estimate + 1.96 × square root of pq/n (where p = prevalence, q = 1 − p, n = sample size).

b = Did not use the "impairment" criterion

c = Regular education classes, and additional 24 cases from special education classes were identified.

d = Screening was for behavioral problems, not tics specifically.

e = Slightly different from the figures reported in the original paper, which used Poisson distribution rather than normal distribution

Table 6.1 presents the lifetime prevalence estimates for TS (per 1,000) from 11 community surveys. The countries represented in the table include Sweden, Denmark, Spain, the United States, Taiwan, China, and England. All but two of the studies listed in Table 6.1 used a multistage design (see description of two-stage design above). The variation in sample sizes across studies presented in Table 6.1 is striking (range 435–9,712). Studies with small sample sizes (e.g., less than 1,500) raise obvious questions about the representativeness of the sample. Because smaller samples in Stage 1 or low participation in Stage 2 may be enriched or deficient of true cases (due to sampling error), these studies are vulnerable to bias. For example, Kadesjo and Gillberg (2000) estimated a prevalence of 11 per 1,000, which is greater than the upper bound of the 95% CI for all but two studies presented in the table. This suggests that the sample of 435 in this study was enriched with TS cases. The 95% CI of 4 to 27 per 1,000 provided by these investigators indicates that 4 per 1,000 is equally plausible as 27 per 1,000. The 4 per 1,000 figure is relatively consistent with findings from 7 of the 10 studies presented in the table. The upper limit of 27 per 1,000 exceeds all studies but one listed in the table. Thus, these findings suggest that the estimate based on the sample of 435 is unstable, as another sample of 435 would likely yield a different result.

The sample size of 1,255 reported on by Kurlan and colleagues (2001) also raises fundamental questions about the representativeness of the sample. Although the sample size was nearly three times larger than the report by Kadesjo and Gillberg (2000), the study included only 11% of the invited participants. In the absence of information about the 89% of subjects who did not participate, the estimated prevalence is almost certainly biased. Taken together, the studies by Kadesjo and Gillberg (2000) and by Kurlan and colleagues (2001), which post the highest estimated prevalence of TS, appear to be biased toward a higher estimate of prevalence.

The study by Hornsey and colleagues (2001) reports a prevalence of 7.6 per 1,000 (95% CI = 2–13.2 per 1,000). This 95% CI includes the prevalence estimate reported by Kadesjo

and Gillberg (2000) but is still far below the estimate from Kurlan and colleagues (2001). Hornsey and colleagues (2001) began the survey with 1,012 potential subjects. Teachers provided screening results on more than 80% of the original sample, but parents completed the screening questionnaire on only 57% of subjects (574/1,012). Although parents were less likely than teachers to complete the screening questionnaire, teachers identified fewer possible cases in the screening phase. Of the 189 subjects who screened positive for a tic disorder, only 107 (57%) of the screen-positive cases participated in the diagnostic assessment. Despite the rigorous assessment procedures, the findings are difficult to interpret due to the problem of nonparticipation at each stage of the survey. Surprisingly, the authors adjusted the observed prevalence from 7.6 to 18.5 cases per 1,000. This recommendation was based on the unfounded assumption that 10 additional cases of TS would have been identified among the screen positives who did not participate in the diagnostic assessment. This assumption can be challenged on two grounds. First, the estimate of 18.5 per 1,000 is twofold greater or higher than most of the reports listed in Table 6.1 (notable exceptions are Kadesjo & Gillberg [2000] and Kurlan et al. [2001]). Second, nonparticipation is probably not random: parents concerned about a possible tic disorder in their child might have been more willing to participate in the study, not less. Thus, it is perilous to speculate on the number of true cases among the nonparticipants.

Cubo and colleagues (2011) surveyed children between 5 and 17 years of age from a small city and the surrounding area in Spain. The investigators randomly selected schools from urban and rural districts. Of the 1,047 children invited, 741 (71%) completed Stage 1. The screening included brief questionnaires completed by parents and teachers as well as direct observation in the classroom. Based on figure from the report, 179 children were screen positive. A sample of 145 children who screened negative was identified as a matched control sample. The diagnosis was made via phone interview by an experienced clinician.

The study identified 12 cases of TS (10 boys and 2 girls) with impairment and 27 cases (15 boys and 12 girls) if impairment was not part of the diagnosis. Based on the cases without the impairment criterion, this study provides a prevalence estimate of 36.4 per 1,000 (95% CI = 22.9–50 per 1,000). This prevalence estimate is larger than most of the surveys presented in Table 6.1. The CI overlaps with only two prior studies (Kadesjo & Gillberg, 2000; Kurlan et al., 2001). As noted above, each of these studies had flaws (small sample size and very low response rate) that threaten the trustworthiness of the prevalence estimates. The sample size of 741 in the study by Cubo and colleagues (2011) is larger than the report from Kadesjo and Gillberg (2000), but it is smaller than most studies listed in Table 6.1.

Only one study in Table 6.1 enrolled a subsample of screen negatives in the Stage 2 diagnostic assessment. Stefanoff and colleagues (2008) enrolled 1,579 sixth- and seventh-grade children in their two-stage prevalence study. The participation rate was excellent, with 88% participation at Stage 1 from the randomly selected schools. Of the 1,579 children, 611 (39%) were screened positive by parents or teachers. Of these, only 124 screen-positive cases were identified by both parent and teacher. Similar to the report by Hornsey and colleagues (2001), these results indicate that agreement on screen-positive status between parents and teachers is likely to be modest. This difference by informant reflects an important design decision. Including both parents and teachers in screening is likely to identify cases that might have been missed if only one informant was used for screening. On the other hand, if the screen-positive cases by parent and teacher are tallied, the rate of false-positive cases invited to participate in Stage 2 is likely to increase, which would increase the cost of the study.

At Stage 2, 531 (86.9%) of the screen-positive subjects and a random sample of 130 (13.4% of the Stage 1 sample) screen negatives participated (Stefanoff et al., 2008). Ninety-six subjects from the screen-positive group and 8 subjects from the screen-negative group were diagnosed with a tic disorder (i.e., transient tic disorder, chronic motor or vocal tic disorder, or TS). Of these, 9 cases were diagnosed with TS (whether any of these TS cases came from the screen-negative group was not reported). This suggests that the investigators did not use the screen-negative sample to estimate the rate of missed cases among the other 968 screen negatives (1,579 – 611 = 968). If even 1 case of TS came from the 130 randomly selected screen-negative subjects, there could be as many as 7 "missed cases" among the screen negatives (968/130 = 7.4). If none of the 9 identified cases of TS came from the randomly selected screen negatives, this would suggest that the screening method did not miss any cases and that the 9 cases per 1,579 (5.7 per 1,000, as listed in Table 6.1) is a plausible estimate of prevalence for TS.

Taken together, the findings from these studies suggest that the prevalence of TS is likely to fall between 3 and 8 cases per 1,000 in children between the ages of 6 and 18 years. Five of the 11 studies listed in Table 6.1 provide estimates of 4 to 6 per 1,000 (Jin et al., 2005; Khalifa & von Knorring, 2003; Kraft et al., 2012; Stefanoff et al., 2008; Wang & Kuo, 2003). This review suggests that estimates above 8 per 1,000 are questionable due to small sample size (Cubo et al., 2011; Kadesjo & Gillberg, 2000) and low participation rate (Kurlan et al., 2001). The studies by Hornsey (2001), Peterson (2001), and Scahill (2006) and their colleagues, which based their prevalence estimates on sample sizes of approximately 1,000 children, report a range from 2.6 to 7.6 per 1,000. The results reported by Peterson (2001; 2.6 per 1,000) and Scahill (2006; 3 per 1,000) and their colleagues appear to be low compared to the five larger studies with estimates of 4 to 6 per 1,000. These lower estimates may be due to the smaller sample sizes rather than design differences.

The previous discussion on the model two-stage design notwithstanding, only one study included a random sample of screen negatives. In that study, Stefanoff and colleagues (2008) did not use the identification of true cases in the randomly selected sample of screen negatives in the estimate of prevalence.

GENDER DISTRIBUTION OF TS

Reports from clinically ascertained samples of children with TS consistently show male-to-female ratios between 3 to 1 and 4 to 1 (CDC, 2009; Mol Debes et al., 2008). Community samples provide greater variation: 1 to 1 (Peterson et al., 2001), 1.25 to 1 (Cubo et al., 2011), 4 to 1 (Kraft et al., 2012), 9 to 1 (Khalifa & von Knorring, 2003), and 10 to 1 (Jin et al., 2005). The reason for this variability in community samples is not clear. In general, studies with larger sample sizes show higher male-to-female ratios. There are few estimates of male-to-female ratios for chronic motor or chronic vocal tic disorder and they are of uncertain reliability.

PREVALENCE OF TRANSIENT TIC DISORDER AND CHRONIC TIC DISORDERS

Table 6.2 presents the prevalence estimates for transient tic disorder, chronic motor tic disorder, and chronic vocal tic disorder available in six reports. Five studies presented in Table 6.1 did not provide useable estimates (Hornsey et al., 2001; Jin et al., 2005; Kadesjo & Gillberg, 2000; Peterson et al., 2001; Wang & Kuo, 2003). For example, in their sample of 776 youth between 9 and 20 years of age, Peterson and colleagues (2001) estimated a prevalence of 22 per 1,000 for motor tics and 2.6 per 1,000 for vocal tics. However, the study did not report on duration of tics, making it difficult to differentiate between transient and chronic tic disorders.

The range of estimates for transient, chronic motor, and chronic vocal tic disorders is wide within each category. Indeed, there are no clear patterns in these results. Khalifa and von Knorring (2003) reported a comparatively high rate of transient tic disorder compared to the other studies listed, and the rate of transient tic disorder is considerably higher than their estimates of chronic tic disorders. By contrast, Stefanoff and colleagues (2008) reported similar rates for transient tic disorder and chronic motor tic disorder. The rate of chronic motor tic disorder of 22.2 per 1,000 reported by Stefanoff and colleagues (2008) is threefold higher than the 6 to 8 cases per 1,000 estimated by Khalifa and von Knorring (2003), Scahill and colleagues (2005), and Kraft and colleagues (2012). The differentiation between transient tic disorder

and chronic motor tic disorder is based on the duration of the tic symptoms. It may be that the variation in the prevalence estimates for these disorders across these studies is due to differences in the methods used to elicit lifetime history and duration of tics.

Results from currently available studies on the prevalence of transient, chronic motor, and chronic vocal tic disorders are inconsistent, but a few tentative conclusions are possible. Based on the CIs for chronic motor tic disorder, a liberal estimate would be 8 to 40 cases per 1,000. If the estimates by Stefanoff (2008) and Cubo (2011) and their colleagues are regarded as outliers, the prevalence appears to range from 3 to 8 cases per 1,000. The estimate of chronic vocal tic disorder is less certain, but it may be as high as 8 cases per 1,000.

ASSOCIATED PROBLEMS

In clinically ascertained samples, high rates of ADHD, disruptive behavioral problems, obsessive-compulsive disorder (OCD), and anxiety in children with TS have been consistently observed. For example, Roessner and colleagues (2007) reported on 5,060 youth with TS (age range 5–17 years) from 65 sites in 22 countries. Participating clinicians completed a data entry form that included questions about TS and other psychiatric diagnoses. The rates of ADHD and OCD in this sample were 61% and 19%, respectively, which are consistent with previous clinical reports. Using data from a Danish health registry, Mol Debes and colleagues (2008) identified 376 cases of TS in children age 5 to 20. Of these, 36.9% were also diagnosed with ADHD, 39.8% with OCD, and 34.8% with disruptive behavior (groups were not mutually exclusive).

The CDC (2009) conducted a telephone survey of approximately 64,000 randomly selected households with children between 6 and 17 years of age. Parents were asked about the child's medical conditions (diabetes, asthma, seizures), psychiatric conditions (TS, ADHD, depression, autism), emotional and behavioral problems (anxiety and disruptive behavior), and health care utilization. Parents reported a prior diagnosis of TS in 3 children per 1,000 (for an estimated

Table 6.2 Prevalence of Transient, Chronic Motor, and Chronic Vocal Tic Disorders

Author/Year	Transient Tic Disorder			Chronic Motor Tic Disorder			Chronic Vocal Tic Disorder		
	# of Cases	Prevalence (per 1,000)	95% CI (per 1,000)	# of Cases	Prevalence (per 1,000)	95% CI (per 1,000)	# of Cases	Prevalence (per 1,000)	95% CI (per 1,000)
Kurlan et al., 2001	25[a]	20	12.2–27.6[a]	4	3	0.1–6.3[a]	6	5	1.0–8.6[a]
Khalifa & von Knorring, 2003	214	47.7	41.6–54.0	34	7.6	5.1–10.1	24	5.3	3.3–7.5
Scahill et al., 2006	7	7.7	2.0–13.4	7	7.7	2.0–13.4	4	4.4	0.1–8.7
Stefanoff et al., 2008	29	18.4	11.8–25.0	35	22.2	14.9–29.5	4	2.5	0–5.0
Kraft et al., 2012	18	3	1.6–4.4	37	6	4.2–8.2	NR	NR	NR
Cubo et al., 2011	20	27	16.5–38.5	37	50	34.2–66.6	7	9.4	2.5–16.3[b]

NR, not reported.

a = Estimated from Table 4 in the original report

b = Slightly different 95% CIs from the original paper due to use of normal distribution in calculation (present review) versus Poisson distribution (original report).

148,000 cases nationwide). The male-to-female ratio was 3 to 1. Compared to the estimated prevalence of 5 to 7 per 1,000 children (see Table 6.1), the finding of 3 cases per 1,000 suggests that many cases remain undetected. According to the parents, most TS cases were described as mild. Parents reported that 64% of the children with TS had a diagnosis of ADHD, 43% had a history of disruptive behavior, and 40% had a history of anxiety problems. These rates were significantly higher than the population of children without a history of TS.

Because clinic samples are vulnerable to ascertainment bias, we look to community samples to develop unbiased estimates on the frequency and patterns of co-occurring problems in children with TS. To date, only a handful of community surveys have examined the rates of co-occurring psychiatric disorders (Table 6.3).

Using teachers as informants, Gadow and colleagues (2002) collected data on a range of psychiatric symptoms in a community sample of 3,006 children (age 3–18 years). Using cutoff scores on a DSM-IV–based checklist to define the conditions of interest, the investigators defined four groups: tics alone, ADHD alone, tics plus ADHD, and unaffected controls. The survey did not include information on tic onset and course. Thus, differential diagnosis of tic disorders was not possible. The prevalence of tics (including all tic disorders without differential diagnosis) was 8.2%, with a 3-to-1 male-to-female ratio. Of the 246 children identified with tics, 128 (52%) were rated by teachers in the clinical range on ADHD compared to 7.3% in children without tics. In addition, children with tics and ADHD were more likely to have anxiety problems and disruptive behavior compared to those with ADHD alone, those with tics alone, or controls. These findings suggest that the combination of tics and ADHD is associated with greater disability than tics alone.

Kraft and colleagues (2012) also used a dimensional approach to examine co-occurring problems in a community sample of children with TS. The sample of 5,974 was ascertained from a birth cohort (total sample = 8,244). Subjects were screened for tics at Time 1 when the cohort was between 9 and 11 years of age. In subsequent waves of assessment, data were collected on a range of behavioral and emotional problems using the Strengths and Difficulties Questionnaire (SDQ, a validated 25-item parent survey). In the final stage of the study, when the sample was 13 to 15 years of age, parents of the subjects who screened positive at Time 1 were interviewed by telephone by an experienced clinician using a semistructured interview for the diagnosis of tic disorders. Seventy children were identified with a chronic tic disorder (33 with TS and 37 with chronic motor tic disorder). The investigators then defined four groups: chronic tic disorder alone, hyperactive (probable ADHD) alone, chronic tic disorder and hyperactive, and unaffected controls. On all dimensions of the SDQ, children in the chronic tic disorder plus hyperactive group were the most symptomatic and impaired, followed by the hyperactive group. On measures of disruptive behavior and peer problems, the chronic tic disorder alone group was essentially indistinguishable from controls.

Table 6.3 Prevalence of Co-occurring Psychiatric Conditions in Community Samples of Children with TS

Author/Year	N of Cases	Age Range	% ADHD	% OCD	% Disruptive Behavior
Kurlan et al., 2002	72	8.5– 17.5	38.4	10.9	17.4
Khalifa & von Knorring, 2006	25	7–15	68	16	44
Scharf et al., 2012	53	13	17.8	20.5	NR

The number of cases shown in Table 6.3 are those identified in regular education classes only

Kurlan and colleagues (2002) examined the co-occurrence of TS and psychiatric disorders in their community sample and identified a total of 72 cases of TS (48 in regular education classes and 24 in special education classes). As noted previously, the low participation rate in this study raises questions about the prevalence estimate. Nonetheless, the study used rigorous assessment methods and identified 38.4% and 10.9% of subjects with ADHD and OCD, respectively. Khalifa and von Knorring (2006) also used rigorous assessment methods. Although this was a much larger population sample than the survey by Kurlan and colleagues (2001), the number of cases of TS was smaller, at 25. Of these, two thirds had ADHD, 1 in 6 had OCD, and just under half had disruptive behavior problems (groups were not mutually exclusive).

Although the community survey by Scharf and colleagues (2012) was not informative for estimating the prevalence of tic disorders, it does provide useful information on the co-occurrence of ADHD and OCD. The sample consisted of a birth cohort of 6,678 children. The sample was surveyed at age 13 years. The investigators identified 290 children with a *possible* tic disorder. These subjects were classified into three groups: narrow (meeting full criteria for a chronic tic disorder), intermediate (slightly less strict in application of diagnostic criteria), and broad (presence of tic or tics but no requirement for persistent symptoms). These categories make it difficult to extract an estimate of prevalence for chronic tic disorders that is comparable to the studies presented in Table 6.1. Nonetheless, when the narrow and intermediate categories are combined, it is possible to estimate of the rates of co-occurring ADHD and OCD. As shown in Table 6.3, roughly 1 in 5 had ADHD and a similar number had OCD. These estimates are low for ADHD but consistent with other studies for OCD.

CONCLUSION AND DIRECTIONS FOR FUTURE RESEARCH

Tics are common in childhood, and in many cases they are isolated and transient. The best estimate for the prevalence of TS in school-age children is likely to fall between 5 and 7 cases per 1,000. The prevalence of 6 cases per 1,000 would translate into a count of 300,000 cases of TS among school-age children in the United States. The prevalence of chronic motor tic disorder appears to range from 3 to 8 per 1,000. The estimates of prevalence for chronic vocal tic disorder in school-age children are less stable and await further study. Although most cases have mild to moderate tic symptoms, children with chronic tic disorders, even those with mild conditions, have a higher likelihood of other problems, such as ADHD, disruptive behavior, and OCD. Children with tics alone, regardless of severity, appear to have only a slightly greater risk for impairment than children in the general population. Appropriate treatment requires recognition and diagnostic assessment. Findings from National Children's Health Survey suggest that many children with TS are missed. Given the potential for disability associated with tic disorders, improved recognition and appreciation for the impact of concurrent ADHD, OCD, and disruptive behavior is warranted.

The classic two-stage design is an acceptable approach for obtaining an estimate of the prevalence of TS and related tic disorders. To ensure relatively narrow CIs around the prevalence estimates, sample sizes of greater than 5,000 are needed. After establishing a valid sampling frame (e.g., Cubo et al., 2011; Khalifa & von Knorring, 2003; Kraft et al., 2012 Kurlan et al., 2001; Stefanoff et al., 2008), steps must be taken to ensure adequate participation—to avoid bias in the results. The screening tool in Stage 1 can be brief but should include motor and phonic tics. Available data suggest that teachers may be more responsive to screening requests, but parents are better informants. Because no screen is perfect, Stage 2 involves a random sampling of screen negatives to estimate the percentage of cases missed by the screen and to adjust the estimate of prevalence accordingly. The size of the screen-negative sample may be influenced by available resources.

The diagnosis of tic disorders requires a detailed history about the onset and course of tics. As suggested by the results in Table 6.2, imprecision on onset and course may contribute to variability in the estimates of transient tic disorder and chronic motor and vocal tic disorders. Face-to-face assessments may be considered the gold standard—although this increases the cost of the project. Finally, given the association of tic disorders with ADHD, OCD, disruptive behavior, and anxiety, rigorous assessment of concomitant problems is essential. From a public health perspective, chronic tics may serve as a marker of neurodevelopmental vulnerability. Community-based studies that improve case finding may also improve our comprehension about the public health impact of tic disorders in children.

REFERENCES

American Psychiatric Association. *Diagnostic and statistical manual of mental disorders.* 4th ed. rev. (DSM-IV-R). Washington, DC: American Psychiatric Association Press, 2000.

Apter A, Pauls DL, Bleich A et al. An epidemiological study of Gilles de la Tourette's syndrome in Israel. *Arch Gen Psychiatry* 731993; 50:734–8.

Centers for Disease Control and Prevention (CDC). Prevalence of diagnosed Tourette syndrome in persons aged 6–17 years – United States, 2007. *MMWR Morb Mortal Wkly Rep* 2009; 58:581–585.
From the National Survey of Child Health involving some 64,000 families in the U.S. Findings suggest that cases of TS are missed.

Cubo E, Gabriel y Galan JM, Villaverde VA et al. Prevalence of tics in school children in central Spain: a population-based study. *Pediatr Neurol* 2011; 45:100–108.

Gadow KD, Nolan EE, Sprafkin J, Schwartz J. Tics and psychiatric comorbidity and adolescents. *Dev Med Child Neurol* 2002; 44:330–338.

Hirtz D, Thurman DJ, Gwinn-Hardy K et al. How common are the "common" neurologic disorders? *Neurology* 2007; 68:326–337.

Hornsey H, Banerjee S, Zeitlin H, Robertson M. The prevalence of Tourette syndrome in 13–14 year olds in mainstream schools. *J Child Psychol Psychiatry* 2001; 42:1035–1039.

Jin R, Zheng RY, Huang WW et al. Epidemiological survey of Tourette syndrome in children and adolescents in Wenzhou of P.R. China. *Eur J Epidemiol* 2005; 20:925–927.
Largest community survey of TS to date. Study did not use DSM-IV criteria.

Kadesjo B, Gillberg C. Tourette's disorder: Epidemiology and comorbidity in primary school children. *J Am Acad Child Adolesc Psychiatry* 2000; 39:548–555.

Khalifa N, von Knorring AL. Prevalence of tic disorders and Tourette syndrome in a Swedish school population. *Dev Med Child Neurol* 2003; 45:315–319.

A model study in many ways, although it did not include a random sample of screen negatives in diagnostic assessment phase.

Khalifa N, von Knorring AL. Psychopathology in a Swedish population of school children with tic disorders. *J Am Acad Child Adolesc Psychiatry* 2006; 45:1346–1353.

Knight T, Steeves T, Day L et al. Prevalence of tic disorders: a systematic review and meta-analysis. *Pediatr Neurol* 2012; 47:77–90.

Kraft JT, Dalsgaard S, Obel C et al. Prevalence and clinical correlates of tic disorders in a community sample of school-age children. *Eur Child Adolesc Psychiatry* 2012; 21:5–13.

One of the few community-based studies that provides data on the course of tic disorders in children.

Kurlan R, Como PG, Miller B et al. The behavioral spectrum of tic disorders: a community-based study. *Neurology* 2002; 59:414–420.

Kurlan R, McDermott MP, Deeley C et al. Prevalence of tics in schoolchildren and association with placement in special education. *Neurology* 2001; 57:1383–1388.

Well-designed study, but interpretation of results limited by low participation rate.

Leckman JF. Tourette's syndrome. *Lancet* 2002; 360:1577–1586.

Linazasoro G, Van Blercom N, de Zarate CO. Prevalence of tic disorders in two schools in the Basque country: Results and methodological caveats. *Mov Disord* 2006; 21:2106–2109.

Mol Debes NM, Hjalgrim H, Skov L. Validation of the presence of comorbidities in a Danish clinical cohort of children with Tourette syndrome. *J Child Neurol* 2008; 23:1017–1027.

Peterson BS, Pine DS, Cohen P, Brook JS. Prospective, longitudinal study of tic, obsessive-compulsive, and attention-deficit hyperactivity disorders in an epidemiological sample. *J Am Acad Child Adolesc Psychiatry* 2001; 40:685–695.

Robertson MM, Eapen V, Cavanna AE. The international prevalence, epidemiology, and clinical phenomenology of Tourette syndrome: a cross-cultural perspective. *J Psychosom Res* 2009; 67:475–483.

Roessner V, Becker A, Banaschewski T, Freeman RD, Rothenberger A; Tourette Syndrome International Database Consortium. Developmental psychopathology of children and adolescents with Tourette syndrome—impact of ADHD. *Eur Child Adolesc Psychiatry* 2007; 16 Suppl 1:24–35.

Scahill L, Sukhodolsky DG, Williams SK, Leckman JF. Public health significance of tic disorders in children and adolescents. *Adv Neurol* 2005; 96:240–248.

Scahill L, Williams S, Schwab-Stone M et al. Disruptive behavior problems in a community sample of children with tic disorders. *Adv Neurol* 2006; 99:184–190.

Scharf JM, Miller LL, Mathews CA, Ben-Shlomo Y. Prevalence of Tourette syndrome and chronic tics in the population-based Avon longitudinal study of parents and children cohort. *J Am Acad Child Adolesc Psychiatry* 2012; 51:192–201.

Snider LA, Seligman LD, Ketchen BR. Tics and problem behaviors in schoolchildren: Prevalence, characterization, and associations. *Pediatrics* 2002; 110:331–336.

Stefanoff P, Wolanczyk T, Gawrys A et al. Prevalence of tic disorders among schoolchildren in Warsaw, Poland. *Eur Child Adolesc Psychiatry* 2008; 17:171–178.

Well-designed study. Prevalence estimate of TS consistent with other studies.

Wang HS, Kuo MF. Tourette's syndrome in Taiwan: an epidemiological study of tic disorders in an elementary school at Taipei County. *Brain Dev* 2003; 25 Suppl 1:S29–31.

SECTION 2

ETIOLOGY

7

Genetic Susceptibility in Tourette Syndrome

THOMAS V. FERNANDEZ AND MATTHEW W. STATE

Abstract

This chapter evaluates all the different approaches used so far to explore the complex genetic contribution to Tourette syndrome (TS). Whereas early twin and family studies suggested the important role of genes in the etiology of TS, the early segregation analyses failed to identify a single specific causative genetic locus and nonparametric linkage analyses could not identify common TS risk alleles. Similar to other areas of medicine, candidate gene association studies in TS have not yielded significant reproducible findings. Genome-wide association studies have proven valuable for identifying and replicating loci for common complex traits and disorders. The first study of this kind in TS identified the *COL27A1* gene as a possible contributing gene in a multi-ethnic TS cohort, but this finding requires replication. Some rare variant studies predating the era of genome-wide detection involved mapping *de novo* chromosomal abnormalities, yielding associations between a few candidate regions and TS. Only one mapping study so far led to the identification of a rare mutation in the *SLITRK1* gene, but subsequent human genetic studies provided conflicting evidence in favor of its involvement. Linkage analysis of an individual outlier TS family identified a deleterious mutation in the *HDC* gene, suggesting that histaminergic neurotransmission may be involved in the pathobiology of TS, as suggested also by pathway analysis of rare copy number variants. Finally, there seems to be a significant overlap of genes mapping within rare copy number variants in TS and those identified in autistic spectrum disorders.

INTRODUCTION

Tourette syndrome (TS) is a developmental neuropsychiatric disorder with onset in childhood, characterized by the presence of both motor and vocal tics that follow a waxing and waning course, often with improvement or remission in adulthood (Bloch et al., 2006; Leckman et al., 1998; Lin et al., 2002). There are multiple lines of evidence supporting an important contribution from genetic factors. However, in contrast to initial hypotheses that TS was a rare disorder resulting from a mutation in a single gene (Baron et al., 1981; Curtis, Robertson, & Gurling 1992; Kidd & Pauls, 1982; Pauls & Leckman, 1986), it is now clear that the syndrome is far more common than initially appreciated and that the genetics are anything but simple. Indeed, similar to other common neuropsychiatric disorders, it is clear that multiple variations in multiple genes, both within the individual and the population, are likely to be carrying risk, and the liability to develop TS appears to involve the interplay of both environmental and genetic factors (see Chapters 8 and 9). Moreover, the relevance of disorders such as autism and schizophrenia stretches beyond simply informing an understanding of the complex genetic architecture underlying TS; it is increasingly apparent that a wide range of clinically distinct developmental and neuropsychiatric disorders, including TS, may share specific genetic risk factors. This chapter summarizes the history of genetic studies in TS, focusing on the search for contributing variations in the structure and/or sequence of human DNA. It also reviews the most recent findings derived from high-throughput, high-resolution analyses of genetic variation. These rapidly evolving technologies, in conjunction with the development of very large patient cohorts, are driving tremendous progress in gene discovery across all of medicine.

HERITABILITY AND SEGREGATION ANALYSIS

The search for genes contributing to TS was preconditioned by a number of early twin and family studies. The former typically compare concordance, or the rate at which a pair of individuals share a diagnosis, in monozygotic twins (MZ) versus that in dizygotic twins (DZ). If genes play a significant role, one would expect to see a higher rate of concordance in twins who share all of their DNA (MZ) versus those twins who share about 50% of their genomes (DZ), the same amount of DNA as any sibling pair. Alternatively, if environment predominates, concordance rates should not significantly differ between MZ and DZ.

In the largest such TS study reported to date, Price and colleagues (1985) evaluated 43 twin pairs and found MZ concordance to be between 50% and 77%, compared to a concordance rate of 10% to 23% for DZ twins. These ranges reflected whether the authors considered only strictly defined TS or also included spectrum conditions (chronic tics, tics with obsessive-compulsive disorder) as an affected status. Similarly, in a study of 16 pairs of MZ twins, Hyde and colleagues (1992) reported that 56% were concordant for TS and 94% were concordant for tic disorders more broadly. Furthermore, MZ concordance has been shown to approximate 100% when study methodology has allowed for direct patient examination and included the diagnosis of chronic tics in addition to TS (Walkup et al., 1988).

These investigations consistently point to a significant genetic contribution to TS. It is also worth noting that the ability to precisely estimate the relative contributions of genes and environment has been, and continues to be, constrained both by a limited number of twin studies and the relatively small number of patients involved. However, consistent with the notion that genes play a major role, multiple investigations have found that TS and related tic disorders tend to aggregate within families and across multiple generations. Overall, the recurrence rate among siblings has been found to be on the order of 5% for females and more than 10% for males (Pauls et al., 1991), representing at least a 10-fold increase in risk for first-degree relatives compared to the overall prevalence of the disorder (Centers for Disease Control and Prevention, 2009; Robertson, 2008; Robertson, Eapen, & Cavanna, 2009).

In an effort to clarify precisely how genes might be contributing to TS, segregation analyses were undertaken assessing the transmission of related phenotypes in affected pedigrees and comparing these to known patterns of genetic inheritance. The earliest of these pointed to a so-called single-gene autosomal dominant inheritance pattern with partial penetrance (Baron et al., 1981; Curtis et al., 1992; Kidd & Pauls, 1982; Pauls & Leckman, 1986). In short, these studies suggested that most or all of TS cases would be explained by the inheritance of mutations in one gene, but that some people carrying a disorder-causing mutation would be expected to show subclinical symptoms or no relevant phenotype at all.

Nonetheless, despite intensive discovery efforts, no single TS genomic locus was identified and confirmed based on this hypothesis. Moreover, as the techniques for mapping Mendelian disorders improved throughout the 1990s, the failure to find a single gene responsible for TS became increasingly incompatible with this simple model of inheritance. In retrospect, the misapprehension that TS was a single-gene autosomal dominant disorder derived in part from an underestimation of the population prevalence of TS. In addition, when the large pedigrees upon which these inheritance models were developed were re-examined, it became clear that they exhibited a high rate of bilineal inheritance, an observation that has been confirmed in other clinical samples (Hanna et al., 1999; Kurlan et al., 1994; McMahon et al., 1996). This phenomenon involves individuals with TS having offspring with partners who also have TS, tics, or obsessive-compulsive disorder (OCD) and confounds the identification of a reliable Mendelian pattern of inheritance. Finally, recent segregation analyses have provided further support for the current characterization of TS as a complex, genetically heterogeneous disorder (Hasstedt et al., 1995; Seuchter et al., 2000; Walkup et al., 1996). In contrast to Mendelian inheritance, in which a single allele of large effect explains the phenotype, complex traits result from the interaction among multiple gene variants across one gene (allelic heterogeneity) or many genes (locus heterogeneity) and their environment, increasing the difficulty of discovering and confirming genetic risk factors.

LINKAGE STUDIES

Initial efforts at gene discovery utilized linkage analysis, based on the notion that TS is a genetically homogeneous disorder. This approach leverages the basic genetic principles of chromosomal crossover during meiosis and the random transmission of parental chromosomes to their offspring to determine the probability that a particular chromosomal segment (identified by evaluating genetic variations called markers) and a given phenotype are transmitted together from one generation to another. Two different types of linkage have been employed in the search for human disease genes in general and TS in particular: parametric and nonparametric analyses.

Parametric Linkage

Parametric linkage involves specifying a proposed model of transmission (e.g., dominant, recessive, or X-linked) and then calculating the odds of observing the data from a given pedigree or pedigrees under the proposed model versus the odds of observing the same pattern of transmission under the null hypothesis (the random assortment of chromosomes, or no linkage). Linkage results are reported as a logarithm of the odds (LOD). Approximately $10^3:1$ odds in favor of linkage at a genetic marker (LOD score of 3) is taken as the threshold for statistical significance in genome-wide parametric linkage

studies, roughly corresponding to a corrected p value of .05.

Parametric linkage analysis is a powerful approach to identify genes contributing to Mendelian disorders and has led to the discovery of genes for a very large number of simple genetic disorders across all of medicine (Collins, 1992; Lifton et al., 2001; Ropers & Hamel, 2005). Driven by the results of initial segregation analyses that were consistent with a single-gene autosomal dominant inheritance pattern, early linkage studies paid particular attention to large multigenerational pedigrees. These failed to identify a single specific genetic locus involved in the general etiology of TS. In fact, under a parametric model of autosomal dominant transmission and genetic homogeneity, linkage studies of very large families or combining pedigrees has eliminated any reasonable possibility that TS is, in fact, a genetically homogenous syndrome explained by mutations in one gene (Barr et al., 1999; Curtis et al., 2004; Heutink et al., 1992; McMahon et al., 1992; Pakstis et al., 1991; Pauls et al., 1990; Verkerk et al., 2006; Walkup et al., 1996).

Spurred by the substantial evidence supporting a genetic contribution to TS, the general lack of results from initial parametric linkage studies, and segregation analyses in the 1990s suggesting complex inheritance, the field experienced a general shift in thinking away from TS as single-gene Mendelian disorder and, consequently, toward alternative approaches to gene discovery.

Nonparametric Linkage

Nonparametric linkage analysis of related individuals began to supplant parametric linkage in large multigenerational pedigrees, based on this revised assumption that TS showed more complex inheritance than previously anticipated. This approach was favored as it does not require specification of a hypothesis about the mode of inheritance. Here, the objective is to identify regions of the genome that are shared among *affected* related individuals (or conversely not shared among phenotypically discordant relatives) more often than would be expected by chance. Similar to parametric linkage studies, results are presented as LOD scores, with the following generally accepted thresholds for statistical analysis: 2.3 to 3.5 is considered "suggestive" of linkage, 3.6 to 5.3 is statistically significant linkage, and more than 5.3 is highly significant linkage.

In 1999, the Tourette Syndrome Association International Consortium for Genetics (TSAICG) reported a nonparametric linkage study of 91 independent affected sibling pairs that resulted in multipoint maximum-likelihood scores of 2.3 on chromosome 4q and 2.0 on chromosome 8p (TSAICG, 1999). When the study was extended to 238 nuclear families, yielding 304 independent sibling pairs, and 18 large multigenerational families, evidence for linkage in these regions diminished. Instead, evidence for significant linkage was observed in a region on chromosome 2p (LOD = 4.4) when individuals with TS or chronic tics were considered affected (TSAICG, 2007).

Subsequently, several other nonparametric linkage studies in TS yielded LOD scores approaching or reaching statistical significance (Curtis et al., 2004; Paschou et al., 2004; Zhang et al., 2002). However, none have converged on a single region or led to the identification of mutations altering the structure or function of transcripts mapping within putative linkage intervals, generally considered the *sine qua non* of successful linkage efforts.

With the benefit of hindsight, the failure of these efforts to identify even one of potentially many TS risk genes can be traced to a number of factors: first, while the approach is theoretically capable of identifying alleles contributing to risk in a complex fashion, the technique is not particularly robust to extensive locus heterogeneity, especially if sample sizes are small. For example, if one imagines that 500 different genes contributed relatively equally to TS, the chances of identifying a statistically significant "excess of sharing" of any one region of the genome, even among 1,000 sibling pairs, would be very low. Compounding this problem was the fact that the cohorts available for these early studies were quite small, numbering in the low hundreds. More contemporary studies in other psychiatric disorders and across medicine more broadly have demonstrated that, in general, subject samples will need to be an order of magnitude larger than this to have a reasonable chance of identifying risk alleles that are common in the population (Altshuler et al., 2008).

CANDIDATE GENE ASSOCIATION STUDIES

In contrast to linkage studies that examine allele transmission within families, association studies assess allele frequencies within populations. Typically, these studies assess single nucleotide polymorphisms (SNPs) in biologically plausible candidate genes, using a case-control or transmission disequilibrium analytic design. Association methods are generally more powerful than linkage methods under a number of conditions that often prevail in complex disease. For example, they are considered more powerful in detecting common susceptibility variants of small effect. Association studies also have practical appeal in that they study affected individuals versus unrelated controls, or affected probands and their parents, allowing for recruitment of relatively large numbers of subjects from clinical samples compared to linkage, which requires identification of extended families or multiple affected siblings.

It should not seem surprising, then, that a large number of the TS genetic studies that followed on early linkage analyses focused on candidate gene SNP associations between cases and controls or transmission between parents and offspring. Based on a longstanding recognition that TS symptoms may be alleviated with administration of medications that block dopamine neurotransmission (see Chapter 24), candidate genes have included various dopamine receptor genes (*DRD2, DRD3, DRD4*) (Cruz et al., 1997; Díaz-Anzaldúa et al., 2004; Grice et al., 1996; Herzberg et al., 2010; Tarnok et al., 2007), the dopamine transporter (*DAT*) (Yoon et al., 2007), and the dopamine catabolizing enzyme catechol-O-methyltransferase (*COMT*) (Cavallini et al., 2000; Tarnok et al., 2007). Similarly, based on the reduction of TS symptoms with administration of adrenergic receptor agonists, clonidine and guanfacine (see Chapters 24 and 25), SNPs within noradrenergic transcripts (*ADRA1C, ADRA2A, ADRA2C*) (Chou et al., 2007; Xu et al., 2003) have also been examined for association. Other genes affecting neurotransmission, including dopamine beta hydroxylase (*DBH*) (Yoon et al., 2007), monoamine oxidase A (*MAO-A*) (Díaz-Anzaldúa et al., 2004), tyrosine hydroxylase (Comings et al., 1995), and several serotonergic genes (*TPH2, 5HT3, 5HTTLR*) (Brett et al., 1995; Cavallini et al., 2000; Mössner et al., 2007), have also been examined, as well as several genes involved in neurodevelopmental, neuroendocrine, and immunological function (Crane et al., 2011; Kindler et al., 2008; Laurin et al., 2009; Miranda et al., 2008).

In general, candidate gene association studies have not yielded significant reproducible findings in any area of medicine (Altshuler et al., 2008), and TS has not been an exception. Despite the popularity of the candidate gene association approach, there are several key limitations that seem to explain the inconsistent findings to date. First, the SNPs used in these studies are preordained and may not necessarily be the precise variations that influence TS. If this is the case, then the power to detect association relies on both the underlying structure of the genome in the region being tested as well as the similarity between the tested SNP frequencies and the frequencies of the unknown disease allele. Second, candidate gene association studies are notoriously vulnerable to false-positive results. One explanation can be found in the failure of many candidate gene association studies to control adequately for population stratification, which results from occult differences in ancestry between cases and controls. As the frequencies of certain genetic markers vary among differing ethnic groups, precise matching for these characteristics is essential for reliable and reproducible results. It has become strikingly clear that the practice of relying on self-reported ancestry is not an adequate protection against this confound. Third, based on the emerging picture of effect sizes for common alleles, the candidate gene association studies reported in TS have employed sample sizes that were not likely, in retrospect, to support the detection of common variant risks of plausible magnitude. Finally, given the presence of millions of SNPs and the very limited understanding of the cellular and molecular mechanisms underlying TS, there is an extremely low prior probability that any selected candidate gene or allele will be associated with the disorder, even when chosen based on plausible biological hypotheses (Altshuler et al., 2008; Manolio et al., 2009).

GENOME-WIDE ASSOCIATION STUDIES (GWAS)

The difficulties that attended candidate gene association studies, combined with rapidly advancing genomic technologies, motivated yet another methodological shift in the genetics of complex disorders, this time to the study of genome-wide association, testing hundreds of thousands to millions of common SNPs for association simultaneously, typically in cases versus controls. Results are presented as p values, with a significance threshold of 5×10^{-8}. This technique has revolutionized and brought renewed enthusiasm to the search for common genetic risk factors in complex disorders by using the power of association to detect small effects without the need for prior hypotheses regarding pathogenesis. Over the past several years, GWAS have identified SNPs implicating hundreds of robustly replicated loci for common complex traits and disorders (Hindorff et al.; Manolio, 2010).

Recently, the first GWAS of 1,496 cases and 5,249 controls was completed by the TSAICG. No loci reached the accepted threshold for statistical significance in the primary analysis of European-ancestry samples (1,285 cases and 4,964 controls) or in a secondary analysis combining all subjects, including Latin American population isolate samples. The locus with the lowest p value ($p = 1.85 \times 10^{-6}$) mapped to a single SNP within an intron of *COL27A1* (collagen, type XXVII, alpha 1) on chromosome 9q32 (Scharf et al., 2012). Replication efforts in larger cohorts are necessary to clarify the significance of this finding.

In other complex disorders, GWAS have identified mostly variants conferring relatively small increments of risk and explaining only a small proportion of familial clustering. The question of why so much heritability is unexplained by GWAS is one of several lines of evidence that has recently led to an increased focus on the contribution of rare and structural variants to complex disease (Manolio, 2010; Manolio et al., 2009).

RARE VARIATION IN TS

While the majority of efforts in TS genetics over the past decade have concentrated on the search for common alleles, there has also been a steady parallel effort to evaluate the contribution of rare variants. However, rather than investigating TS under the assumption that it is a genetically homogeneous entity, more recent rare-variant studies have conceptualized TS as a highly heterogeneous disorder. Under these circumstances, one pursues the hypothesis that rare variants carrying large effects may account for only a small fraction of the total population risk for TS but have the potential to highlight important biological mechanisms, as has been shown in a variety of other medical conditions (e.g., Ji et al., 2008; Johansen et al., 2010) (Fig. 7.1). Increasingly, as technology has advanced, it has also become possible to interrogate whether individually rare mutations in many genes may account for a considerable proportion of the total population risk (discussed in more detail below).

Chromosomal Alterations

Some of the rare-variant studies in TS predate the era of high-resolution genome-wide detection of structural or sequence variants and involved mapping *de novo* chromosomal abnormalities (i.e., deletions, duplications, translocations, inversions) using cytogenetic techniques such as karyotyping and fluorescence *in situ* hybridization (FISH). Beginning as early as the mid-1990s, a number of cytogenetic abnormalities were reported in TS probands or families that pointed to novel candidate genes or regions, including 2p12, 3p21.3, 7q35-36, 8q21.4, 9pter, 13q31, and 18q22.3 (Abelson et al., 2005; Boghosian-Sell et al., 1996; Cuker et al., 2004;

Petek et al., 2001; State et al., 2003; Verkerk et al., 2003).

Several of these findings reflected at least partially converging data from independent groups. For example, Boghosian-Sell and colleagues (1996) described a family in which TS segregated with a balanced 7;18 translocation. The breakpoint on chromosome 7 was mapped to within the chromosomal bands 7q22 and 7q31. Subsequently, Kroisel and colleagues (2001) described a *de novo* duplication on chromosome 7 (7q22.1-q31.1) observed in a 13-year-old boy with TS, moderate mental retardation, and minor physical anomalies. Both breakpoints were within or close to the breakpoint region described by Boghosian-Sell and colleagues (1996), suggesting that a gene located at or near this region may be involved in the pathogenesis of TS in some cases. Further molecular analysis of this same proband by Petek and colleagues (2001) revealed that the *de novo* abnormality was an inverted duplication that resulted in disruption of the *IMMP2L* gene, a human homologue of the yeast mitochondrial inner membrane peptidase subunit 2. This research group screened 39 TS patients and 95 multiplex autistic disorder (AD) families (due to the localization of *IMMP2L* in the critical region of an AD candidate locus on chromosome 7q, AUTS1) for sequence and copy number variation in *IMMP2L* (Petek et al., 2007) but found no coding mutations, and expression studies provided no evidence of parental imprinting at this gene locus. More recently, a patient with chronic tics and a 2;7 translocation and cryptic deletion at 7q31.1-7q31.2, including *IMMP2L*, has been reported, providing further evidence for the possible involvement of this gene in TS pathogenesis (Patel et al., 2011).

State and colleagues (2003) reported on a male proband with chronic tics and OCD who was found to carry a paracentric inversion involving chromosome 18q22, corresponding to the other breakpoint from the Boghosian-Sell report. The team mapped the telomeric end of the inversion to a genomic location that was within 1 Mb of the previously described breakpoint at 18q (Boghosian-Sell et al., 1996). Although no genes were structurally disrupted by this inversion, functional studies of two transcripts in the region showed replication timing dysregulation, suggesting that epigenetic influences might be altering gene expression in the region, and left open the possibility that genes in this region may serve as candidates in TS.

Subsequently, the same group reported a 14-year-old girl with severe OCD and a chronic tic disorder with a t(2;18)(p12;q22) translocation (Cuker et al., 2004). The patient's chromosome 18 breakpoint localized to the same chromosomal band as two previously reported rearrangements associated with TS, OCD, and chronic tic disorder (Boghosian-Sell et al., 1996; State et al., 2003) and mapped to a genomic position approximately 5 Mb from these rearrangements. The clustering of these three breakpoints within a relatively small genetic interval suggests that 18q22 may be a promising region for containing a gene or genes of etiological importance in the development of the TS/OCD phenotypic spectrum.

Two additional chromosomal mapping studies are notable because the regions implicated have also been identified with respect to other neurodevelopmental disorders. First, Verkerk and colleagues (2003) reported a shared complex rearrangement in a father with TS and his affected children, disrupting the *contactin-associated protein-like 2* gene (*CNTNAP2*) on chromosome 7q35. This gene encodes a membrane protein located peripherally in nodes of Ranvier that may be important for the distribution of potassium channels, which would affect signal conduction along myelinated neurons. *CNTNAP2* has been implicated in autism spectrum disorders, intellectual disability, and schizophrenia (Alarcón et al., 2008; Arking et al., 2008; Bakkaloglu et al., 2008; Friedman et al., 2008; Peñagarikano et al., 2011; Strauss et al., 2006; Zweier et al., 2009), is thought to be involved in glial neuronal interactions, and has been localized to synaptosomes in rat forebrain (Bakkaloglu et al., 2008). However, Belloso and colleagues (2007) subsequently described a familial balanced reciprocal translocation t(7;15)(q35;q26.1) in phenotypically normal individuals. In this family, the 7q35 breakpoint disrupted *CNTNAP2*, highlighting the phenomenon of partial penetrance

in which individuals with a risk variant do not express the phenotype. Second, Lawson-Yuen and colleagues (2008) reported a family transmitting a small exonic deletion of the *neuroligin 4, X-linked* (*NLGN4X*) gene from a mother (with learning disorder, anxiety, depression) to her two sons (with autism/motor tics and TS/attention-deficit/hyperactivity disorder, respectively). *Neuroligin 4* genes have previously been associated with autistic spectrum disorders (Jamain et al., 2003; Laumonnier et al., 2004; Marshall et al., 2008).

Slit and Trk-like family member 1 (SLITRK1). To date, only one cytogenetic mapping study has resulted in the identification of a deleterious rare mutation in a nearby gene. Abelson and colleagues (2005) reported a *de novo* chromosome 13 inversion in a family with a single case of TS. The gene *SLITRK1* mapped within 350 kb from the 13q31 breakpoint. Mutation screening of 174 unrelated TS probands of European ancestry identified an inherited single nucleotide frameshift deletion predicted to result in a prematurely truncated protein in a single family, in which one individual was affected with TS and another with trichotillomania. In addition, two independent occurrences of a very rare single base mutation (var321) were identified in a highly conserved base within the *SLITRK1* 3'UTR that corresponds to the binding site for the micro-RNA has-miR-189. Micro-RNAs (miRNAs) are short, 20 to 22 base, noncoding RNAs that typically suppress translation and destabilize messenger RNAs that bear complementary target sequences. Many miRNAs are expressed in a tissue-specific manner and may contribute to the maintenance of cellular identity. Screening for var321 in 4296 control chromosomes yielded a significant association with TS ($p = .0056$).

In vitro studies demonstrated that overexpression of *SLITRK1* in cortical neurons promotes dendritic growth, while the frameshift and the miRNA binding site variants have functional potential consistent with a loss-of-function mechanism. Studies of both *SLITRK1* and the miRNA predicted to bind in the variant-containing 3' region showed expression in basal ganglia and deep layers of cortex in both mouse and human, regions previously implicated in TS pathology (Stillman et al., 2009). A mouse knockout of *SLITRK1* was recently reported to show an anxiety phenotype and increased levels of noradrenergic neurotransmitters(Katayama et al., 2010), consistent with earlier findings in human studies of cerebrospinal fluid in TS (Leckman et al., 1995), which were attenuated by administration of clonidine, an alpha2-adrenergic agonist often used to treat TS patients (Katayama et al., 2010). Furthermore, a mouse knockout of a closely related molecule, *SLITRK5*, yields impaired corticostriatal dendritic morphology, an obsessive-compulsive and anxiety phenotype (Shmelkov et al., 2010).

Genetic studies attempting to verify the initial *SLITRK1* association have yielded inconsistent results. Several studies have investigated rare mutations: resequencing 334 TS subjects has not revealed additional pathogenic coding mutations (Chou et al., 2007; Deng et al., 2006; Zimprich et al., 2008). In contrast, Zuchner and colleagues (2006) reported several rare missense mutations that occurred in individuals with trichotillomania. Additional studies have evaluated common polymorphisms in the region, testing the hypothesis that the rare variant finding might point to the involvement of more common, lower-penetrance risk alleles. Here too, results have been mixed: Miranda and colleagues (2009) reported a positive association ($p = .04$) between a single SNP in *SLITRK1* and TS in a small candidate gene study (N = 154). More recently, haplotype analysis in a total of 376 nuclear families with TS revealed evidence of association with variation across *SLITRK1*, suggesting possible involvement of *SLITRK1* regulatory variants in TS etiology (Karagiannidis et al., 2012). However, in the first TS GWAS study by the TSAICG (Scharf et al., 2012), candidate gene analysis of all genotyped SNPs within and surrounding *SLITRK1* identified no nominally associated SNPs, including two SNPs previously reported to be associated with TS by Karagiannidis and colleagues (2012).

Finally, two separate groups specifically examined the rare variant var321 (Keen-Kim et al., 2006; Scharf et al., 2008) and did not find evidence for association. On balance, given the very low population frequency of this variant, neither study was well powered to confirm or refute an association with TS. Both reports expressed a concern that the original *SLITRK1* findings may have been a result of occult ethnic differences in cases versus controls (population stratification). However, genome-wide genotyping data and detailed haplotype analysis in individuals carrying var321 do not support this contention (O'Roak et al., 2010).

In sum, follow-up neurobiological studies of *SLITRK1* and related molecules have provided suggestive evidence for involvement in TS and related phenotypes. However, with regard to human genetic studies, the same types of constraints that have limited gene discovery in TS, namely small sample sizes and the related absence of studies employing the latest genomic technologies, have led to conflicting evidence and continued uncertainty about the role that variation in and around this locus may play in risk.

Parametric Linkage

As detailed above, initial linkage studies of large pedigrees failed to map a single gene mutation that explained most TS risk. Subsequently, parametric linkage efforts focused on studying smaller families to identify rare gene alleles of large effect. As noted above, the rationale for studying these so-called outlier families was not to identify a gene that would explain the etiology of the large majority of TS cases; rather, this approach seeks to identify rare variants that can help to elucidate the underlying biology of TS. The results of several such studies have reached or approached statistical significance (Breedveld et al., 2010; Curtis et al., 2004; Knight et al., 2010; Laurin et al., 2009; Mérette et al., 2000; Verkerk et al., 2006), but nearly all have not yet identified a rare mutation within the linkage intervals accounting for the statistical results.

The one exception is the report by Ercan-Sencicek and colleagues (2010) that utilized an outlier approach of investigating an individual interesting family (Fig. 7.1). The authors described a two-generation family with nine affected members with TS (Fig. 7.2). They identified a region on chromosome 15 that reached the maximum theoretical LOD score, given a model of dominant transmission in the pedigree. A heterozygous G-to-A transition at nucleotide position 951 in exon 9 of the *HDC* gene, resulting in a W317X substitution, was identified and predicted to result in a truncated protein lacking key segments of the active domain (Fig. 7.2). The loss of function for the enzyme carrying the mutation was confirmed biochemically. *In vitro* studies in *E. coli* indicated that the mutant protein might act in a dominant-negative manner, altering not only the mutation carrying protein but the function of the remaining normal allele as well. However, studies in mice that carry a highly similar version of the protein indicate that heterozygous HDC knockouts have approximately a 50% reduction in brain histamine (Ohtsu et al., 2001).

Histidine decarboxylase (HDC) is the rate-limiting enzyme in histamine biosynthesis, suggesting that histaminergic neurotransmission may be involved in the pathobiology of TS in this family. Histamine signaling in the central nervous system is mediated by four G protein-coupled receptors, located both presynaptically (predominantly H3 as well as H4) and postsynaptically (H1–H3). Presynaptic histamine receptors regulate the release of not only histamine but also a variety of other neurotransmitters, including dopamine. Several lines of evidence suggest that histamine acts in a counterregulatory fashion, with increased histamine resulting in decreased dopamine signaling and vice versa (Ferrada et al., 2008; Munzar et al., 2004). H2 and H3 receptors are enriched in the striatum and cortex, regions of the brain implicated in TS (Haas et al., 2008) (see Chapters 10 and 12), and studies of rodents with decreased brain histamine show increased sensitivity to stereotypies when administered dopamine agonists (Kubota et al., 2002).

Interestingly, recent *in vitro* studies of mouse brain demonstrate that histamine modulates many aspects of functional connectivity within the striatum. Histaminergic activity during increased attention and wakefulness affects the flow of excitatory inputs to the striatum and intrastriatal processing of those inputs, such that the net effect on striatal functioning is feed-forward inhibition and a suppressed excitatory drive (Ellender et al., 2011). Combined with the finding of a loss of function of HDC in an outlier family, these findings have the potential to lead to the development of animal models and eventually the development of novel therapeutics for TS (Fig. 7.1).

Copy Number Variation

Microarray technologies that can detect submicroscopic structural variation have revealed

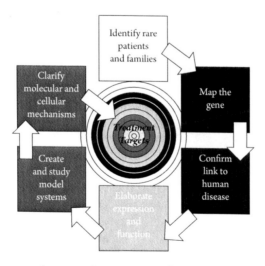

FIGURE 7.1 **An outlier approach to gene discovery.** Rather than seeking to identify a gene that will explain the etiology of a large majority of TS cases, the aim of this approach is to identify rare variants that can help elucidate the underlying biology of TS and point to novel treatment targets.

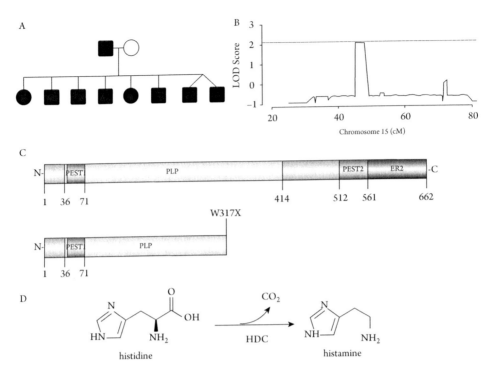

FIGURE 7.2 **Linkage analysis of an outlier pedigree identifies a mutation in *HDC*.**
(**A**) Two-generation pedigree with nine affected individuals. Squares indicate male and circles indicate female family members. Solid symbols indicate those with TS; the open circle is the unaffected mother. (**B**) Parametric linkage LOD scores for chromosome 15q. The horizontal line indicates the maximum theoretical LOD score (2.1) for this family. The affected father and all affected children have a G-to-A substitution at nucleotide position 951 of the *HDC* gene transcript. (**C**) The wild-type HDC protein (*top*) contains 662 amino acids with a pyridoxal 5'-phosphate (PLP) domain at the N-terminal end, two PEST domains (PEST1 and PEST2), and a C-terminal intracellular targeting domain (ER2). The mutant HDC protein (*bottom*) is predicted to be truncated at the site of the W317X mutation. The resulting product contains 316 amino acids and lacks a portion of the PLP domain, one of the two PEST domains, and the entire ER2 domain. (**D**) The HDC protein (L-histadine decarboxylase) is the rate-limiting enzyme in histamine biosynthesis. (See Ercan-Sencicek et al., 2010.)

extensive copy number variation (CNV) throughout the human genome (Conrad et al., 2010; Iafrate et al., 2004; Redon et al., 2006; Sebat et al., 2004) and provided new opportunities for genome-wide studies of such variation in TS and other neurodevelopmental disorders. Rather than examining only outlier cases and families for individual rare variants of large effect, CNV detection platforms have been used to pursue the "rare variant–common disease" hypothesis by high-throughput detection of rare CNVs across the genomes of cases and controls. Studies in schizophrenia (International Schizophrenia Consortium, 2008; McCarthy et al., 2009 Mulle et al., 2010; Stefansson et al.,

2008; Walsh et al., 2008; Wilson et al., 2006; Xu et al., 2008) and autistic spectrum disorders (Glessner et al., 2009; Marshall et al., 2008; Pinto et al., 2010; Sebat et al., 2007; Szatmari et al., 2007) demonstrated an increased burden of rare CNVs, particularly *de novo* gene variants (Marshall et al., 2008; Sanders et al., 2011; Sebat et al., 2007; Xu et al., 2008).

Results from studies examining structural variation in TS across the entire genome are just now beginning to emerge. An initial CNV study in 111 TS subjects and 73 controls identified several rare variants in TS and hypothesized an overlap of risk with both autistic spectrum disorders and schizophrenia, based on recurrent rare CNVs in the genes *neurexin 1* (*NRXN1*) and *catenin, alpha 3* (*CTNNA3*) (Sundaram et al., 2010). There was no detectable increase in occurrence of CNVs in cases versus controls, although the authors noted that the small sample size limited their ability to draw firm conclusions about the overall contribution of rare and *de novo* CNVs, or to show an association of particular structural variants with TS.

A subsequent larger study of rare CNVs in 460 TS subjects and 1,131 controls similarly found no statistically significant difference in rare CNV burden between cases and controls, although the burden of *de novo* rare exonic CNVs in 148 TS trios (2.7%) versus 436 control trios (0.7%) approached significance ($p = .07$) (Fernandez et al., 2012) (Fig. 7.3). Based on recent evidence from autistic spectrum disorders (Sanders et al., 2011), it is likely that a larger sample size of affected trios will be required

to detect a statistically significant difference of *de novo* CNVs between cases and controls. Interestingly, this more recent TS CNV study (Fernandez et al., 2012) found a significant overlap with genes mapping within rare CNVs in TS and those previously identified in autistic spectrum disorders, but not schizophrenia or intellectual disability (Fig. 7.3). In addition, pathway analyses using multiple algorithms revealed an enrichment of genes involved in histamine signaling, and three large, likely pathogenic *de novo* CNVs were identified, including one disrupting multiple gamma-aminobutyric (GABA) receptor genes (Fernandez et al., 2012).

Genome-Wide Sequencing

Next-generation sequencing is offering unprecedented opportunities to investigate genetic variation in large numbers of individuals. In other areas of medicine and other psychiatric

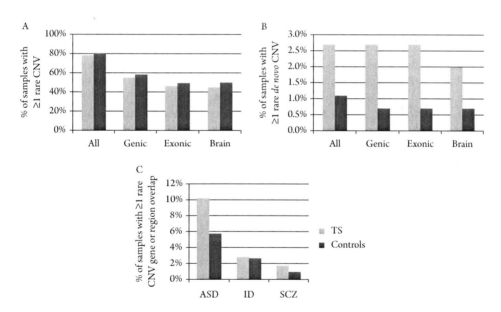

FIGURE 7.3   **Rare CNV in TS.**   (**A**) Proportion of 460 TS and 1,131 control subjects with at least one rare CNV. No comparisons reached statistical significance. (**B**) Proportion of 148 TS and 436 control parent–child trios with at least one rare *de novo* CNV. No comparisons reached statistical significance, despite an almost fourfold increase of genic *de novo* CNVs in TS versus controls (2.7% vs. 0.7%, $p = .07$). For each cohort in **A** and **B**, the following proportions were calculated: all rare CNVs, rare genic CNVs, rare exonic CNVs, and rare brain expressed CNVs. (**C**) Proportions of TS and controls with CNV overlap with genes implicated in autism spectrum disorders (ASD), intellectual disability (ID), and schizophrenia (SCZ). TS subjects show significantly more overlap with ASD genes compared to controls ($p = .002$), but no significant difference for ID ($p = .9$) or SCZ genes ($p = .4$). (See Fernandez et al., 2012.)

disorders, sequencing the human exome is allowing large-scale case-control studies of rare variation as well as mapping rare mutations in pedigrees that are too small to support traditional linkage analyses. To date, there has been only a single report of whole-exome sequencing in 10 members of a three-generation pedigree, with 7 affected by TS or chronic tics. Three novel, non-synonymous single nucleotide variants in three genes (*MRPL3, DNAJC13, OFCC1*) were found to segregate with the chronic tics phenotype and fell within linkage peaks approaching the maximum LOD score, although multiple additional regions also showed similar linkage intervals. Further studies are needed to clarify the importance of these variants in TS (Sundaram et al., 2010).

CLINICAL IMPLICATIONS

Similar to other common neuropsychiatric disorders, it is clear that multiple variations in multiple genes, both within the individual and the population, are likely to be carrying risk for TS. Furthermore, liability to develop the disorder appears to involve the interplay of both environmental and genetic factors (see Chapters 8 and 9). For these reasons, identification and confirmation of disease genes has been difficult, and it is not yet possible to determine or quantify whether carrying a specific genetic variant will modify the risk of developing TS in an individual. While we do know that this risk of developing TS in an individual is increased at least 10-fold if he or she has a first-degree relative (parent, sibling) with the disorder, there is currently no test for a gene variant that is able to determine relative risk. However, genetic studies to date have suggested potential novel therapeutic targets (e.g., GABA and histamine signaling pathways) that warrant further study. As demonstrated in other common, complex neuropsychiatric disorders such as autism spectrum disorders, the utilization of next-generation sequencing technologies in larger cohorts of affected individuals offers great promise to advance the field toward identifying, confirming, and quantifying specific gene variants and biological mechanisms that may confer risk.

CONCLUSIONS AND QUESTIONS FOR FURTHER RESEARCH

While the process of gene discovery in TS to date has been challenging, as it has been for all common genetically complex disorders, there remains both strong evidence that genes contribute to the disorder and real reason for optimism, given results in other neuropsychiatric and neurodevelopmental disorders (State, 2010; State & Levitt, 2011). First, twin and family studies, despite their small size and number, have consistently demonstrated that genetic factors play a role. Next, studies of rare variation utilizing an outlier approach have provided convincing, if not conclusive, evidence for the contribution of specific genes. Finally, early results from CNV analyses are largely consistent with those for autism spectrum disorders and schizophrenia. Large-scale studies in both of these disorders have resulted in dramatic advances in the understanding of their respective genomic architectures, findings that bode well for the future of TS genetics research.

In fact, results from other better-studied areas are an important touchstone for interpreting the current state of TS genetics. It has become clear that genome-wide investigations, including those of common as well as rare and *de novo* structural and single nucleotide variants, can be fruitful and that large sample sizes are a requirement. As noted throughout, such studies and approaches in TS are only beginning to emerge, and their current absence is sufficient to explain the relative lack of progress to date.

There is clearly a tremendous need and opportunity for further progress in this field of neuropsychiatric genetics. Limited patient resources have been an obstacle to adopting emerging technologies such as dense array genotyping and high-throughput sequencing. Large multisite collaborative efforts are needed to recruit sufficiently large sample cohorts that will provide adequate power to detect both common gene variants of small effect and rare gene variants of large effect, as both may account for a proportion of the genetic risk in TS. It is also likely that some of the uncertainty and inconsistency regarding current genetic findings in TS reflects a genetic architecture characterized by locus and allelic heterogeneity.

Box 7.1. Key Points

- Early twin and family studies point to a significant genetic contribution to TS.
- Informed by early segregation analyses in TS families pointing to single-gene autosomal dominant inheritance pattern with partial penetrance, initial efforts at gene discovery in TS utilized parametric linkage analysis in large multigenerational families but failed to identify a single specific genetic locus.
- Later segregation analyses support the current characterization of TS as a complex, genetically heterogeneous disorder.
- Nonparametric linkage analyses have yet to identify common TS risk alleles, likely owing to extensive locus heterogeneity and relatively small sample sizes.
- Similar to other areas of medicine, candidate gene association studies in TS have not yielded significant reproducible findings. Population stratification, small sample sizes, and low prior probability of selecting a relevant gene or allele are all likely contributing factors.
- GWAS have proven valuable for identifying and replicating loci for common complex traits and disorders across the medical field. The first GWAS study of TS yielded a positive finding involving *COL27A1* in a secondary analysis of a multi-ethnic TS cohort and requires replication.
- There has been an increasing effort to evaluate the contribution of rare allele variants toward TS, with the hypothesis that they have the potential to highlight important biological mechanisms even if they may account for only a small fraction of the total population risk.
- Some rare variant studies predating the era of genome-wide detection involved mapping *de novo* chromosomal abnormalities. Several findings from independent groups converged on novel candidate genes or regions: 7q31, *IMMP2L*, 18q22, *CNTNAP2*.
- To date, only one mapping study has resulted in the identification of a deleterious rare mutation in a nearby gene: *SLITRK1*. While neurobiological studies of this and related molecules are suggestive, human genetic studies so far have led to conflicting evidence and uncertainty about this gene's involvement in TS and related phenotypes.
- Linkage analysis of an individual outlier TS family identified a deleterious mutation in the *HDC* gene, suggesting that histaminergic neurotransmission may be involved in the pathobiology of TS in this family. Several lines of evidence, including animal findings and pathway analysis of rare CNVs in TS subjects, suggest that histamine neurotransmission warrants further study in TS and may be a promising therapeutic target.
- A recent study points to a significant overlap of genes mapping within rare CNVs in TS and those previously identified in autistic spectrum disorders, but not schizophrenia or intellectual disability.

The small size and number of twin studies obviously limits the precision of estimates of heritability in TS. This casts some doubt on the ultimate fraction of TS cases that need to be explained by genetic mechanisms. However, there is already evidence in TS that even a small number of well-characterized genetic findings have the potential to elucidate underlying biological mechanisms. While there is certainly more work to be done, several recent findings have already begun to steer the field in directions that were unforeseen no more than a few years ago, including suggesting a possible role for histamine in the etiology of some cases of TS the contribution of impaired dendritic growth in the striatum, and an overlap of genetic risks with a

- What are the relative contributions of genes and environment to TS? More twin studies with larger patient cohorts are needed to obtain more precise estimates of the relative contributions of genes and environment.
- What are the relative contributions of common versus rare variation to TS risk? Next-generation sequencing offers the opportunity to investigate both common and rare variation in large numbers of cases and controls.
- What are the relative contributions of inherited versus *de novo* sequence and structural variation to TS risk? Sequencing and genotyping studies of large cohorts are beginning to answer this question in autistic spectrum disorders and will likely illuminate this question in TS.
- What, if any, contribution to TS risk is conferred by variants in the "noncoding" genome? Falling costs of whole-genome sequencing will allow this question to be addressed in large cohorts of TS and controls in the near future.

range of other developmental disorders. There is reason for great optimism that the pace of genetic discovery in TS will accelerate and inform intervention strategies that will alleviate the suffering endured by those with TS and related disorders.

REFERENCES

Abelson JF, Kwan KY, O'Roak BJ et al. Sequence variants in SLITRK1 are associated with Tourette's syndrome. *Science* 2005; *310*:317–320.

The first paper to identify rare functional sequence mutations in individuals with TS. It also was the first to point to the SLITRK family of molecules in human developmental psychopathology and provided evidence for the relevance of micro-RNA-mediated regulation of gene expression in this process.

Alarcón M, Abrahams BS, Stone JL et al. Linkage, association, and gene-expression analyses identify CNTNAP2 as an autism-susceptibility gene. *Am J Hum Genet* 2008; *82*:150–159.

Altshuler D, Daly MJ, Lander ES. Genetic mapping in human disease. *Science* 2008; *322*:881–888.

Arking DE, Cutler DJ, Brune CW et al. A common genetic variant in the neurexin superfamily member CNTNAP2 increases familial risk of autism. *Am J Hum Genet* 2008; *82*:160–164.

Bakkaloglu B, O'Roak BJ, Louvi A et al. Molecular cytogenetic analysis and resequencing of contactin associated protein-like 2 in autism

spectrum disorders. *Am J Hum Genet* 2008; *82*:165–173.

Baron M, Shapiro E, Shapiro A, Rainer JD. Genetic analysis of Tourette syndrome suggesting major gene effect. *Am J Hum Genet* 1981; *33*:767–775.

Barr CL, Wigg KG, Pakstis AJ et al. Genome scan for linkage to Gilles de la Tourette syndrome. *Am J Med Genet* 1999; *88*:437–445.

Belloso JM, Bache I, Guitart M et al. Disruption of the CNTNAP2 gene in a t(7;15) translocation family without symptoms of Gilles de la Tourette syndrome. *Eur J Hum Genet* 2007; *15*:711–713.

Bloch MH, Peterson BS, Scahill L et al. Adulthood outcome of tic and obsessive-compulsive symptom severity in children with Tourette syndrome. *Arch Pediatr Adolesc Med* 2006; *160*:65–69.

Boghosian-Sell L, Comings DE, Overhauser J. Tourette syndrome in a pedigree with a 7;18 translocation: identification of a YAC spanning the translocation breakpoint at 18q22.3. *Am J Hum Genet* 1996; *59*:999–1005.

Breedveld GJ, Fabbrini G, Oostra BA et al. Tourette disorder spectrum maps to chromosome 14q31.1 in an Italian kindred. *Neurogenetics* 2010; *11*:417–423.

Highlights the potential for mapping of Mendelian forms of TS, which is sure to gain momentum with the rapid adoption of whole-exome and whole-genome sequencing approaches.

Brett PM, Curtis D, Robertson MM, Gurling HM. Exclusion of the 5-HT1A serotonin neuroreceptor and tryptophan oxygenase genes in a large British kindred multiply affected with Tourette's syndrome, chronic motor tics, and obsessive-compulsive behavior. *Am J Psychiatry* 1995; 152:437–440.

Cavallini MC, Di Bella D, Catalano M, Bellodi L. An association study between 5-HTTLPR polymorphism, COMT polymorphism, and Tourette's syndrome. *Psychiatry Res* 2000; 97:93–100.

Centers for Disease Control and Prevention (CDC). Prevalence of diagnosed Tourette syndrome in persons aged 6–17 years—United States, 2007. *MMWR Morb Mortal Wkly Rep* 2009; 58:581–585.

Chou IC, Tsai CH, Wan L et al. Association study between Tourette's syndrome and polymorphisms of noradrenergic genes (ADRA2A, ADRA2C). *Psychiatr Genet* 2007; 17:359.

Chou IC, Wan L, Liu SC et al. Association of the Slit and Trk-like 1 gene in Taiwanese patients with Tourette syndrome. *Pediatr Neurol* 2007; 37:404–406.

Collins FS. Positional cloning: let's not call it reverse anymore. *Nat Genet* 1992; 1:3–6.

Comings DE, Gade R, Muhleman D, Sverd J. No association of a tyrosine hydroxylase gene tetranucleotide repeat polymorphism in autism, Tourette syndrome, or ADHD. *Biol Psychiatry* 1995; 37:484–486.

Conrad DF, Pinto D, Redon R et al. Origins and functional impact of copy number variation in the human genome. *Nature* 2010; 464:704–712.

Crane J, Fagerness J, Osiecki L et al. Family-based genetic association study of DLGAP3 in Tourette syndrome. *Am J Med Genet B Neuropsychiatr Genet* 2011; 156B:108–114.
DLGAP3 (aka SAPAP3) is one of only only a few (also SLITRK5 and HoxB8) for which the mouse knockout demonstrates an excessive grooming phenotype that is responsive to treatment with a selective serotonin reuptake inhibitor.

Cruz C, Camarena B, King N et al. Increased prevalence of the seven-repeat variant of the dopamine D4 receptor gene in patients with obsessive-compulsive disorder with tics. *Neurosci Lett* 1997; 231:1–4.

Cuker A, State MW, King RA et al. Candidate locus for Gilles de la Tourette syndrome/ obsessive compulsive disorder/chronic tic disorder at 18q22. *Am J Med Genet A* 2004; 130A:37–39.

Curtis D, Brett P, Dearlove AM et al. Genome scan of Tourette syndrome in a single large pedigree shows some support for linkage to regions of chromosomes 5, 10 and 13. *Psychiatr Genet* 2004; 14:83–87.

Curtis D, Robertson MM, Gurling HM. Autosomal dominant gene transmission in a large kindred with Gilles de la Tourette syndrome. *Br J Psychiatry* 1992; 160:845–849.

Deng H, Le WD, Xie WJ, Jankovic J. Examination of the SLITRK1 gene in Caucasian patients with Tourette syndrome. *Acta Neurol Scand* 2006; 114:400–402.

Díaz-Anzaldúa A, Joober R, Rivière JB et al. Tourette syndrome and dopaminergic genes: a family-based association study in the French Canadian founder population. *Mol Psychiatry* 2004; 9:272–277.

Ellender TJ, Huerta-Ocampo I, Deisseroth K et al. Differential modulation of excitatory and inhibitory striatal synaptic transmission by histamine. *J Neurosci* 2011; 31:15340–15351.

Ercan-Sencicek AG, Stillman AA, Ghosh AK et al. L-histidine decarboxylase and Tourette's syndrome. *N Engl J Med* 2010; 362:1901–1908.
Reports on a rare nonsense mutation that provides the first evidence for a role for histaminergic neurotransmission in the etiology and modulation of TS and related disorders.

Fernandez TV, Sanders SJ, Yurkiewicz IR et al. Rare copy number variants in Tourette syndrome disrupt genes in histaminergic pathways and overlap with autism. *Biol Psychiatry* 2012; 71:392–402.
Reports a trend toward increased burden of de novo CNVs in TS versus controls, shows a significant overlap between genes overlapping TS CNVs and those implicated in autistic spectrum disorders, and provides further evidence supporting recent findings regarding the involvement of histaminergic and GABAergic mechanisms in the etiology of TS.

Ferrada C, Ferré S, Casadó V et al. Interactions between histamine H3 and dopamine D2 receptors and the implications for striatal function. *Neuropharmacology* 2008; 55:190–197.

Friedman JI, Vrijenhoek T, Markx S et al. CNTNAP2 gene dosage variation is associated with schizophrenia and epilepsy. *Mol Psychiatry* 2008; 13:261–266.

Glessner JT, Wang K, Cai G et al. Autism genome-wide copy number variation reveals ubiquitin and neuronal genes. *Nature* 2009; 459:569–573.

Grice DE, Leckman JF, Pauls DL et al. Linkage disequilibrium between an allele at the dopamine D4 receptor locus and Tourette syndrome, by the transmission-disequilibrium test. *Am J Hum Genet* 1996; 59:644–652.

Haas HL, Sergeeva OA, Selbach O. Histamine in the nervous system. *Physiol Rev* 2008; 88:1183–1241.

Hanna PA, Janjua FN, Contant CF, Jankovic J. Bilineal transmission in Tourette syndrome. *Neurology* 1999; 53:813–818.

Hasstedt SJ, Leppert M, Filloux F et al. Intermediate inheritance of Tourette syndrome, assuming assortative mating. *Am J Hum Genet* 1995; 57:682–689.

Herzberg I, Valencia-Duarte AV, Kay VA et al. Association of DRD2 variants and Gilles de la Tourette syndrome in a family-based sample from a South American population isolate. *Psychiatr Genet* 2010; 20:179–183.

Heutink P, van de Wetering BJ, Breedveld GJ, Oostra BA. Genetic study on Tourette syndrome in The Netherlands. *Adv Neurol* 1992; 58:167–172.

Hindorff LA, MacArthur J, Wise A et al. *A Catalog of Published Genome-Wide Association Studies.* Available from www.genome.gov/gwastudies.

Hyde TM, Aaronson BA, Randolph C et al. Relationship of birth weight to the phenotypic expression of Gilles de la Tourette's syndrome in monozygotic twins. *Neurology* 1992; 42:652–658.

Iafrate AJ, Feuk L, Rivera MN et al. Detection of large-scale variation in the human genome. *Nat Genet* 2004; 36:949–951.

International Schizophrenia Consortium (ISC). Rare chromosomal deletions and duplications increase risk of schizophrenia. *Nature* 2008; 455:237–241.

Jamain S, Quach H, Betancur C et al. Mutations of the X-linked genes encoding neuroligins NLGN3 and NLGN4 are associated with autism. *Nat Genet* 2003; 34:27–29.

Ji W, Foo JN, O'Roak BJ et al. Rare independent mutations in renal salt handling genes contribute to blood pressure variation. *Nat Genet* 2008; 40:592–599.

Johansen CT, Wang J, Lanktree MB et al. Excess of rare variants in genes identified by genome-wide association study of hypertriglyceridemia. *Nat Genet* 2010; 42:684–687.

Karagiannidis I, Rizzo R, Tarnok Z et al. Replication of association between a SLITRK1 haplotype and Tourette syndrome in a large sample of families. *Mol Psychiatry* 2012; 17:665–668.

Katayama K, Yamada K, Ornthanalai VG et al. Slitrk1-deficient mice display elevated anxiety-like behavior and noradrenergic abnormalities. *Mol Psychiatry* 2010; 15:177–184.

An animal model of SLITRK1 deficiency shows altered noradrenergic function and an anxiety phenotype that is rescued by alpha-agonists.

Keen-Kim D, Mathews CA, Reus VI et al. Overrepresentation of rare variants in a specific ethnic group may confuse interpretation of association analyses. *Hum Mol Genet* 2006; 15:3324–3328.

Raised the important issue of the potential confound of population stratification in studies of rare variants. The authors hypothesize that the reported association of SLITRK1 with TS by Abelson et al. is the result of occult overrepresentation of Ashkenazi cases versus controls.

Kidd KK, Pauls DL. Genetic hypotheses for Tourette syndrome. *Adv Neurol* 1982; 35:243–249.

Kindler J, Schosser A, Stamenkovic M et al. Tourette's syndrome is not associated with interleukin-10 receptor 1 variants on chromosome 11q23.3. *Psychiatry Res* 2008; 157:235–239.

Knight S, Coon H, Johnson M et al. Linkage analysis of Tourette syndrome in a large Utah pedigree. *Am J Med Genet B Neuropsychiatr Genet* 2010; 153B:656–662.

Another article that shows the potential for mapping of Mendelian forms of TS.

Kroisel PM, Petek E, Emberger W et al. Candidate region for Gilles de la Tourette syndrome at 7q31. *Am J Med Genet* 2001; 101:259–261.

Kubota Y, Ito C, Sakurai E et al. Increased methamphetamine-induced locomotor activity and behavioral sensitization in histamine-deficient mice. *J Neurochem* 2002; 83:837–845.

Kurlan R, Eapen V, Stern J et al. Bilineal transmission in Tourette's syndrome families. *Neurology* 1994; 44:2336–2342.

Laumonnier F, Bonnet-Brilhault F, Gomot M et al. X-linked mental retardation and autism are associated with a mutation in the NLGN4 gene, a member of the neuroligin family. *Am J Hum Genet* 2004; 74:552–557.

Laurin N, Wigg KG, Feng Y et al. Chromosome 5 and Gilles de la Tourette syndrome: Linkage in a large pedigree and association study of six candidates in the region. *Am J Med Genet B Neuropsychiatr Genet* 2009; 150B:95–103.

Another article that shows the potential for mapping of Mendelian forms of TS.

Lawson-Yuen A, Saldivar JS, Sommer S, Picker J. Familial deletion within NLGN4 associated with autism and Tourette syndrome. *Eur J Hum Genet* 2008; 16:614–618.

One of the first case reports to suggest an overlap between genes implicated in autistic spectrum disorders and those contributing to TS.

Leckman JF, Goodman WK, Anderson GM et al. Cerebrospinal fluid biogenic amines in obsessive compulsive disorder, Tourette's syndrome, and healthy controls. *Neuropsychopharmacology* 1995; 12:73–86.

Leckman JF, Zhang H, Vitale A et al. Course of tic severity in Tourette syndrome: the first two decades. *Pediatrics* 1998; 102:14–19.

Lifton RP, Gharavi AG, Geller DS. Molecular mechanisms of human hypertension. *Cell* 2001; 104:545–556.

Lin H, Yeh CB, Peterson BS et al. Assessment of symptom exacerbations in a longitudinal study of children with Tourette's syndrome or obsessive-compulsive disorder. *J Am Acad Child Adolesc Psychiatry* 2002; 41:1070–1077.

Manolio TA. Genome-wide association studies and assessment of the risk of disease. *N Engl J Med* 2010; 363:166–176.

Manolio TA, Collins FS, Cox NJ et al. Finding the missing heritability of complex diseases. *Nature* 2009; 461:747–753.

Marshall CR, Noor A, Vincent JB et al. Structural variation of chromosomes in autism spectrum disorder. *Am J Hum Genet* 2008; 82:477–488.

McCarthy SE, Makarov V, Kirov G et al. Microduplications of 16p11.2 are associated with schizophrenia. *Nat Genet* 2009; 41:1223–1227.

McMahon WM, Leppert M, Filloux F et al. Tourette symptoms in 161 related family members. *Adv Neurol* 1992; 58:159–165.

McMahon WM, van de Wetering BJ, Filloux F et al. *J Am Acad Child Adolesc Psychiatry* 1996; 35:672–680.

Miranda DM, Wigg K, Feng Y et al. Association study between Gilles de la Tourette syndrome and two genes in the Robo-Slit pathway located in the chromosome 11q24 linked/associated region. *Am J Med Genet B Neuropsychiatr Genet* 2008; 147B:68–72.

Miranda DM, Wigg K, Kabia EM et al. Association of SLITRK1 to Gilles de la Tourette Syndrome. *Am J Med Genet B Neuropsychiatr Genet* 2009; 150B:483–486.

Mulle JG, Dodd AF, McGrath JA et al. Microdeletions of 3q29 confer high risk for schizophrenia. *Am J Hum Genet* 2010; 87:229–236.

Munzar P, Tanda G, Justinova Z, Goldberg SR. Histamine h3 receptor antagonists potentiate methamphetamine self-administration and methamphetamine-induced accumbal dopamine release. *Neuropsychopharmacology* 2004; 29:705–717.

Mérette C, Brassard A, Potvin A et al. Significant linkage for Tourette syndrome in a large French Canadian family. *Am J Hum Genet* 2000; 67:1008–1013.

Mössner R, Müller-Vahl KR, Döring N, Stuhrmann M. Role of the novel tryptophan hydroxylase-2 gene in Tourette syndrome. *Mol Psychiatry* 2007; 12:617–619.

O'Roak BJ, Morgan TM, Fishman DO et al. Additional support for the association of SLITRK1 var321 and Tourette syndrome. *Mol Psychiatry* 2010; 15:447–450.

This paper rebuts the concerns raised in Keen-Kim et al. and Scharf et al. regarding the contribution of population stratification to the finding of association of the gene SLITRK1 with TS.

Ohtsu H, Tanaka S, Terui T et al. Mice lacking histidine decarboxylase exhibit abnormal mast cells. *FEBS Lett* 2001; 502:53–56.

Pakstis AJ, Heutink P, Pauls DL et al. Progress in the search for genetic linkage with Tourette syndrome: an exclusion map covering more than 50% of the autosomal genome. *Am J Hum Genet* 1991; 48:281–294.

Paschou P, Feng Y, Pakstis AJ et al. Indications of linkage and association of Gilles de la Tourette syndrome in two independent family samples: 17q25 is a putative susceptibility region. *Am J Hum Genet* 2004; 75:545–560.

Patel C, Cooper-Charles L, McMullan DJ et al. Translocation breakpoint at 7q31 associated with tics: further evidence for IMMP2L as a candidate gene for Tourette syndrome. *Eur J Hum Genet* 2011; 19:634–639.

Pauls DL, Leckman JF. The inheritance of Gilles de la Tourette's syndrome and associated behaviors. Evidence for autosomal dominant transmission. *N Engl J Med* 1986; 315:993–997.

Pauls DL, Pakstis AJ, Kurlan R et al. Segregation and linkage analyses of Tourette's syndrome and related disorders. *J Am Acad Child Adolesc Psychiatry* 1990; 29:195–203.

Pauls DL, Raymond CL, Stevenson JM, Leckman JF. A family study of Gilles de la Tourette syndrome. *Am J Hum Genet* 1991; 48:154–163.

Petek E, Schwarzbraun T, Noor A et al. Molecular and genomic studies of IMMP2L and mutation screening in autism and Tourette syndrome. *Mol Genet Genomics* 2007; 277:71–81.

Petek E, Windpassinger C, Vincent JB et al. Disruption of a novel gene (IMMP2L) by a breakpoint in 7q31 associated with Tourette syndrome. *Am J Hum Genet* 2001; 68:848–858.

Peñagarikano O, Abrahams BS, Herman EI et al. Absence of CNTNAP2 leads to epilepsy, neuronal migration abnormalities, and core autism-related deficits. *Cell* 2011; 147:235–246.

Pinto D, Pagnamenta AT, Klei L et al. Functional impact of global rare copy number variation in autism spectrum disorders. *Nature* 2010; 466:368–372.

Price RA, Kidd KK, Cohen DJ et al. A twin study of Tourette syndrome. *Arch Gen Psychiatry* 1985; 42:815–820.

Redon R, Ishikawa S, Fitch KR et al. Global variation in copy number in the human genome. *Nature* 2006; 444:444–454.

Robertson MM. The prevalence and epidemiology of Gilles de la Tourette syndrome. Part 1: the epidemiological and prevalence studies. *J Psychosom Res* 2008; 65:461–472.

Summarizes epidemiological TS data from around the world.

Robertson MM, Eapen V, Cavanna AE. The international prevalence, epidemiology, and clinical phenomenology of Tourette syndrome: a cross-cultural perspective. *J Psychosom Res* 2009; 67:475–483.

Ropers HH, Hamel BC. X-linked mental retardation. *Nat Rev Genet* 2005; 6:46–57.

Sanders S, Ercan-Sencicek AG, Hus V et al. Multiple recurrent de novo copy number variations (CNVs), including duplications of the 7q11.23 Williams-Buren syndrome region, are strongly associated with autism. *Neuron* 2011; 70:863–885.

Scharf JM, Moorjani P, Fagerness J et al. Lack of association between SLITRK1var321 and Tourette syndrome in a large family-based sample. *Neurology* 2008; 70:1495–1496.

Scharf JM, Yu D, Matthews CA et al. Genome-wide association study of Tourette syndrome. *Molecular Psychiatry* 2012 Aug 14 [Epub ahead of print].

First GWAS study in TS.

Sebat J, Lakshmi B, Malhotra D et al. Strong association of de novo copy number mutations with autism. *Science* 2007; 316:445–449.

Sebat J, Lakshmi B, Troge J et al. Large-scale copy number polymorphism in the human genome. *Science* 2004; 305:525–528.

Seuchter SA, Hebebrand J, Klug B et al. Complex segregation analysis of families ascertained through Gilles de la Tourette syndrome. *Genet Epidemiol* 2000; 18:33–47.

Shmelkov SV, Hormigo A, Jing D et al. Slitrk5 deficiency impairs corticostriatal circuitry and leads to obsessive-compulsive-like behaviors in mice. *Nat Med* 2010; 16:598–602.

A study of the SLITRK5 knockout mouse showing a behavioral phenotype of excessive grooming that responds to selective serotonin reuptake inhibitors. Furthermore, the authors show abnormal dendritic development on the striatum and altered glutamatergic activity in cortical striatal circuits.

State MW. The genetics of child psychiatric disorders: focus on autism and Tourette syndrome. *Neuron* 2010; 68:254–269.

State MW, Greally JM, Cuker A et al. Epigenetic abnormalities associated with a chromosome 18(q21-q22) inversion and a Gilles de la Tourette syndrome phenotype. *Proc Natl Acad Sci USA* 2003; 100:4684–4689.

State MW, Levitt P. The conundrums of understanding genetic risks for autism spectrum disorders. *Nat Neurosci* 2011; 14:1499–1506.

Stefansson H, Rujescu D, Cichon S et al. Large recurrent microdeletions associated with schizophrenia. *Nature* 2008; 455:232–236.

Stillman AA, Krsnik Z, Sun J et al. Developmentally regulated and evolutionarily conserved expression of SLITRK1 in brain circuits implicated in Tourette syndrome. *J Comp Neurol* 2009; 513:21–37.

Strauss KA, Puffenberger EG, Huentelman MJ et al. Recessive symptomatic focal epilepsy and mutant contactin-associated protein-like 2. *N Engl J Med* 2006; 354:1370–1377.

Sundaram SK, Huq AM, Wilson BJ, Chugani HT. Tourette syndrome is associated with recurrent exonic copy number variants. *Neurology* 2010; 74:1583–1590.

First study to report on the contribution of copy number variation in TS, and suggested an overlap of risks with other developmental neuropsychiatric disorders.

Szatmari P, Paterson AD, Zwaigenbaum L et al. Mapping autism risk loci using genetic linkage and chromosomal rearrangements. *Nat Genet* 2007; 39:319–328.

Tarnok Z, Ronai Z, Gervai J et al. Dopaminergic candidate genes in Tourette syndrome: association between tic severity and 3' UTR polymorphism of the dopamine transporter gene. *Am J Med Genet B Neuropsychiatr Genet* 2007; 144B:900–905.

Tourette Syndrome Association International Consortium for Genetics (TSAICG). A complete genome screen in sib pairs affected by Gilles de la Tourette syndrome. *Am J Hum Genet* 1999; 65:1428–1436.

Tourette Syndrome Association International Consortium for Genetics (TSAICG). Genome scan for Tourette disorder in affected-sibling-pair and multigenerational families. *Am J Hum Genet* 2007; 80:265–272.

Verkerk AJ, Cath DC, van der Linde HC et al. Genetic and clinical analysis of a large Dutch Gilles de la Tourette family. *Mol Psychiatry* 2006; 11:954–964.

Another article that shows the potential for mapping of Mendelian forms of TS.

Verkerk AJ, Mathews CA, Joosse M et al. CNTNAP2 is disrupted in a family with Gilles de la Tourette syndrome and obsessive compulsive disorder. *Genomics* 2003; 82:1–9.

First to identify Contactin Associated Protein 2 in human CNS pathology, and provided early evidence for an overlap in genetic risks between TS and other developmental neuropsychiatric disorders.

Walkup JT, LaBuda MC, Singer HS et al. Family study and segregation analysis of Tourette syndrome: evidence for a mixed model of inheritance. *Am J Hum Genet* 1996; 59:684–693.

Walkup JT, Leckman JF, Price RA et al. The relationship between obsessive-compulsive disorder and Tourette's syndrome: a twin study. *Psychopharmacol Bull* 1988; 24:375–379.

Walsh T, McClellan JM, McCarthy SE et al. Rare structural variants disrupt multiple genes in neurodevelopmental pathways in schizophrenia. *Science* 2008; 320:539–543.

Wilson GM, Flibotte S, Chopra V et al. DNA copy-number analysis in bipolar disorder and schizophrenia reveals aberrations in genes involved in glutamate signaling. *Hum Mol Genet* 2006; 15:743–749.

Xu B, Roos JL, Levy S et al. Strong association of de novo copy number mutations with sporadic schizophrenia. *Nat Genet* 2008; 40:880–885.

Xu C, Ozbay F, Wigg K et al. Evaluation of the genes for the adrenergic receptors alpha 2A and alpha 1C and Gilles de la Tourette syndrome. *Am J Med Genet B Neuropsychiatr Genet* 2003; 119B:54–59.

Yoon DY, Rippel CA, Kobets AJ et al. Dopaminergic polymorphisms in Tourette syndrome: association with the DAT gene (SLC6A3). *Am J Med Genet B Neuropsychiatr Genet* 2007; 144B:605–610.

Zhang H, Leckman JF, Pauls DL et al. Genome-wide scan of hoarding in sib pairs in which both sibs have Gilles de la Tourette syndrome. *Am J Hum Genet* 2002; 70:896–904.

Zimprich A, Hatala K, Riederer F et al. Sequence analysis of the complete SLITRK1 gene in Austrian patients with Tourette's disorder. *Psychiatr Genet* 2008; 18:308–309.

Zuchner S, Cuccaro ML, Tran-Viet KN et al. SLITRK1 mutations in trichotillomania. *Mol Psychiatry* 2006; 11:887–889.

Zweier C, de Jong EK, Zweier M et al. CNTNAP2 and NRXN1 are mutated in autosomal-recessive Pitt-Hopkins-like mental retardation and determine the level of a common synaptic protein in Drosophila. *Am J Hum Genet* 2009; 85:655–666.

8

Perinatal Adversities and Tourette Syndrome

PIETER J. HOEKSTRA

Abstract

This chapter provides a literature review and critical commentary on epidemiological works evaluating the association between pregnancy-related and birth-related adversities in Tourette syndrome. Perinatal risk factors for the development of Tourette syndrome include older paternal age, severe maternal psychosocial stress during pregnancy, maternal smoking during pregnancy, more and earlier prenatal care visits, delivery complications, and low Apgar score at 5 minutes after birth. Risk factors for more severe tics include older paternal age, maternal psychosocial stress during pregnancy, maternal severe nausea and/or vomiting during the first trimester, maternal smoking during pregnancy, maternal medication use during pregnancy, low birth weight, and delivery complications. Maternal smoking during pregnancy and low birth weight are risk factors for the presence of comorbid attention-deficit/hyperactivity disorder in individuals with a tic disorder. Older paternal age; maternal use of coffee, cigarettes, or alcohol during pregnancy; and forceps deliveries are risk factors for the presence of comorbid obsessive-compulsive disorder in individuals with a tic disorder.

INTRODUCTION

While twin and family studies have unequivocally pointed to a high heritability of Tourette syndrome (TS), they also have indicated that there is a substantial role for environmental factors in the etiology and expression of TS. The largest published twin study included 30 monozygotic and 13 dizygotic pairs of twins (Price et al., 1985), of which at least one member of the twin pairs was affected by TS. While much higher than for dizygotic twin pairs, concordance for tics for monozygotic twin pairs did not reach 100%. This was 53% for TS and 77% when diagnostic criteria were broadened to include any tic disorder in co-twins. Similar results were observed in a second study with 16 pairs of monozygotic twins (Hyde et al., 1992). Here, 56% of monozygotic twins were concordant for TS and 94% for any tic disorders. Thus, these twin studies indicate that, even in the case of monozygotic twin pairs, still sometimes the co-twin does not develop tics, despite being genetically identical to the co-twin with tics.

This can only be explained through a role of environmental factors. An intriguing possibility is that the role of these environmental factors can be understood through epigenetic mechanisms. Indeed, it has been found that approximately one third of monozygotic twins show epigenetic differences in DNA methylation and histone modification (Fraga et al., 2005).

Several environmental factors have indeed been implicated in the etiology of TS, including hormonal factors, psychosocial stress, and infections. A substantial body of evidence is available for prenatal and perinatal adverse events, including pregnancy, labor/delivery, and neonatal complications. Pregnancy complications may include maternal smoking, alcohol consumption, or use of medication, low intrauterine growth, premature or postterm delivery, and high levels of psychosocial maternal stress. Relevant labor/delivery complications are prolonged labor, abnormal presentation, premature rupture of membranes, umbilical cord around the baby's neck, a knotted cord, a prolapsed cord, placenta previa, and placental abruption or infarction. Common neonatal complications comprise cyanosis, delayed breathing or crying, aspiration, stained amniotic fluid, and decreased or increased fetal heart rate. Potential detrimental effects of birth complications on the immediate postbirth neonatal condition can be rated with the Apgar score, evaluating the newborn on five criteria (skin color, pulse rate, reflex irritability, muscle tone, and breathing). Each of these five criteria is to be rated on a scale from zero to two, and to be summed up, yielding total scores between zero and ten.

Pre- and perinatal adverse events are by no means uncommon. For example, almost a quarter of all expecting mothers in the United Kingdom continue to smoke at least 6 months into their pregnancy (Ward et al., 2007). The frequency of preterm births is about 13% in the United States and 5% to 9% in many other developed countries (Goldenberg et al., 2008). In the United States, premature rupture of membranes is reported to occur in 6% to 10% of pregnancies, 7% of all infants have low birth weight (<2,500 g; Kiely & Kleinman, 1993), and the incidence of breech presentation, the most common type of abnormal delivery presentation, is about 4%.

Although the mechanisms mediating the effects of these events remain undetermined, suboptimal degrees of oxygen and nutrient delivery to developing brain structures such as the basal ganglia and/or early trauma on the brain during crucial periods of development are thought to play an important role. Most studies have found that individuals with TS have on average higher rates of perinatal adversities than healthy subjects without tics. Studies have also consistently shown that perinatal adversities are associated with increased tic severity, a higher prevalence of comorbid disorders (including attention-deficit/hyperactivity disorder [ADHD] and obsessive-compulsive disorder [OCD]), and/or increased severity of comorbid symptoms. Less is known about the exact pathogenic mechanisms of the perinatal adversities involved, whether perinatal adversities operate independently or in interaction with genetic liability, or whether the consequences of perinatal adversities are greater for males than for females. In this chapter, the available studies in this area will be reviewed with an overview of current theories on the possible pathogenic pathways of perinatal adversities.

ASSOCIATION OF PERINATAL ADVERSITIES WITH THE PRESENCE OF TS

The most straightforward method of investigating a potential role of perinatal adversities in TS is to compare the frequencies of these events between children with TS (or tics in general) and healthy control children. A number of such case-control studies have been published. Although some, mostly small-scale, studies failed to identify differences in the frequency of pregnancy and delivery complications between children with tics and healthy controls, the overall picture emerging from the studies in this field is that of a clear association between the presence of tics or TS and perinatal adversities.

A pioneering, well-designed early study was that of Pasamanick and Kawi (1956), who studied the hospital obstetrical records of a cohort of 83 children of normal intelligence diagnosed as "tiqueurs" at Johns Hopkins Hospital, Baltimore, and compared these with the obstetrical record of the next newborn reported from the same birthplace as the child with tics, matched by race, sex, and maternal age group. The children with tics and their matched controls were also essentially similar with respect to socioeconomic status. A total of 21 birth complications occurred among the infants who would later develop tics versus 10 in the controls, a difference that reached significance. The percentage of mothers of children with tics with one or more complications was 33.3, compared with 17.6 for the controls; the percentage of those with two or more complications in the tic group was 7.8 versus only 2.0 in the healthy controls. The authors therefore tentatively placed the presence of tics on a "hypothesized continuum of reproductive casualty, consisting of brain damage incurred during the prenatal and paranatal periods as a result of abnormalities during these periods, leading to a gradient of injury extending from fetal and neonatal death through cerebral palsy, epilepsy, mental deficiency, reading disability, and behavior disorder." This referred to a then-emerging concept of minimal brain dysfunction thought to underlie behavior and attention disorders in children.

A study published more than 40 years later, but using a similar design, compared birth hospital records of 92 patients with TS with those of 460 controls (5 for each patient) matched by sex, year, and month of birth (Burd et al., 1999). There appeared to be three statistically significant differences between cases and controls. First, mothers of children who later developed TS tended to seek prenatal care earlier than controls and had also more prenatal visits. Only 15% of the cases sought prenatal care after the first trimester of pregnancy, whereas 27% of controls did not seek care until after the first trimester of pregnancy. Controls received prenatal care on average at 3 months whereas cases did at 2.4 months; controls had on average 8.5 prenatal visits and cases 10. Second, children who later developed TS had a lower Apgar score 5 minutes after birth compared to controls (8.4 vs. 8.8). Third, the father was older for children with a later diagnosis of TS compared to controls. Authors explained the higher number and earlier onset of prenatal care visits as an indication of a pregnancy with early problems apparent to both mother and doctor. These results, coupled with the higher Apgar scores reported in patients, support an association between perinatal adversities and the presence of TS.

A subsequent Italian case-control study (Saccomani et al., 2005) involving 48 referred children with TS, 48 with chronic tics, and 30 healthy control children found considerably more pre- or perinatal complications (based on parents' report) both in children with TS (54%) and in those with chronic tics (50%) than in controls (6%). A more recent case-control study (Motlagh et al., 2010) involving 45 individuals with TS alone, 52 individuals with ADHD alone, 60 individuals with TS+ADHD, and 65 unaffected control children aimed at investigating the potential role of four specific pre- and perinatal risk factors, based on maternal report date: heavy maternal smoking (>10 cigarettes per day at any point in the pregnancy); high levels of maternal stress (across a range of areas, including home environment, parental interpersonal relationship, availability of emotional support, parental employment, family's financial status, parents' physical health, and any legal issues); low birth weight (<2,500 g); and acute hypoxic–ischemic events (based on the presence of delivery or neonatal complications). Although a specific goal of the study was to investigate the role of these factors with regard to the presence of comorbid ADHD in children with TS, an aspect reviewed later on, this study provided further evidence of a role of perinatal adversities for TS as such. The rate of heavy maternal smoking in the group of children with TS+ADHD (11.6%) was slightly higher than the one for healthy controls (1.6%), whereas in patients with TS only this was intermediate (6.6%). Similarly, severe maternal psychosocial stress was judged to be 2.5 more frequent during the pregnancy of the offspring who later developed TS (TS only 22%; TS+ADHD 20%) than during pregnancies of healthy controls (8.1%). However, neither the proportion of children with low birth weight nor that of children with at least one delivery or neonatal complication differed between the TS group and the healthy control group. Finally, in another study, 25 children with TS, selected from a large population cohort, had a (non-significantly) reduced optimality score in the pre-, peri-, or neonatal periods compared to 25 controls without tics (Khalifa & von Knorring, 2005).

Some case-control studies, all involving small patient numbers, have failed to provide convincing evidence for an association between TS and perinatal adversities, probably due to low study power. Shapiro and colleagues (1972, 1973) reported a number of birth complications in a series of 34 TS patients that was not higher than the one expected in the general population; a similar conclusion was provided by Incagnoli and Kane (1983) in a series of 13 male patients with TS. Notwithstanding the results from these small case series, the overall evidence for a role of both pregnancy and delivery complications for TS is quite robust, including potentially avoidable factors such as heavy psychosocial stress and maternal smoking during pregnancy.

There is some indication that the male brain may be more vulnerable to the influence of pre- and perinatal insults than the female brain. Much more evidence of this is available in other neuropsychiatric disorders such as schizophrenia and ADHD. Interestingly, significantly more males than females with TS appeared to have a history of birth complications, both in a cohort of 91 consecutive adult TS subjects from a UK clinic (Eapen et al., 2004) and in a cohort of 60 patients with TS at the Yale Child Study Center (Santangelo et al., 1994). In the latter cohort, the frequency of delivery complications reported by mothers of boys with TS was more than nine times higher than that reported by mothers of girls with TS, largely due to more frequent forceps deliveries.

RELATIONSHIP BETWEEN PERINATAL ADVERSITIES AND TIC SEVERITY

Several studies that were overall well designed provided convincing evidence that children with TS with a history of pregnancy and/or birth complications have, on average, more severe tics than those without this history. A remarkable study involving 16 pairs of monozygotic twins in whom at least one twin had TS documented significantly different weight at birth between the two twins in 13 of the 16 pairs; the twin with the lower birth weight had higher tic scores in 12 of these 13 pairs (Hyde et al., 1992). Moreover, the magnitude of the intra-pair birth-weight difference was strongly related to the magnitude of the intra-pair difference in tic severity. This difference in tic severity could not be explained by any postnatal medical events. These results are remarkably similar to a previous report on seven monozygotic twin pairs who were fully discordant for TS, and in all of which the unaffected twin had a higher birth weight than the affected twin (Leckman et al., 1987). The primary causative factor for low birth weight is insufficient development of the placenta to meet the demands of the fetus. Thus, these findings suggest that crucial events affecting the phenotypic expression of TS occur *in utero*, during fetal development.

Another major cause for low birth weight is maternal smoking during pregnancy. Indeed, in one of the largest studies to date investigating the role of prenatal/perinatal complications, involving a cohort of 180 individuals with TS, prenatal maternal smoking was strongly associated with increased tic severity (Mathews et al., 2006). Other variables, such as paternal age, medication exposure *in utero*, and birth weight, were significantly, albeit less strongly, associated positively with tic severity; no association between symptom severity and hypoxia, forceps delivery, or hyperemesis during pregnancy was found. In contrast with these results, a recent study of 75 children and adolescents with tic disorder investigated the association of tic severity with pregnancy, delivery, and postnatal complications and with prenatal exposure to smoking and alcohol (Bos-Veneman et al., 2010a). In this cohort, the presence of delivery complications, but not of prenatal exposure to smoking, was related to higher tic severity. Thus, whereas the twin study by Hyde and colleagues (1992) and the large cohort study by Mathews and colleagues (2006) both point to a relevant role for pregnancy-related adverse events in increasing tic severity, delivery complications may also be involved.

Other relevant pregnancy-related factors potentially associated with increased tic severity are maternal life stress during pregnancy and severe nausea and/or vomiting during the first trimester, both of which were found to be significantly associated with tic severity in a cohort of 31 patients with TS (Leckman et al., 1990). Thus, as the authors of the study concluded, these findings suggest that common pregnancy phenomena such as morning nausea, often judged to be innocent, may have important long-term effects among vulnerable individuals. This finding fits well with the increased number of prenatal visits by mothers with future TS offspring, reported in the above-mentioned study by Burd and colleagues (1999). Moreover, as the authors speculate, life stressors during pregnancy may lead to long-term sensitizing effects on central neurochemical systems, perhaps including sensitivity of dopaminergic receptors within the basal ganglia, which could explain the increased expression of the TS vulnerability (see also Chapter 13).

RELATIONSHIP BETWEEN PERINATAL ADVERSITIES AND COMORBID CONDITIONS

More patients than not with TS are affected with comorbid neuropsychiatric disorders, which can often be more impairing than the tics themselves (see Chapters 2, 3, and 4). Therefore, it is not surprising that studies have also attempted to relate the presence of these comorbid disorders to a history of prenatal and perinatal adverse events. Most studies have investigated the two most common TS comorbidities, ADHD and OCD.

The first published study that looked at perinatal factors from this perspective came from investigators at the Yale Child Study Center (Santangelo et al., 1994). A comparison between 15 individuals with TS and comorbid OCD versus 34 patients with TS without OCD revealed some interesting differences: probands with comorbid OCD were nearly eight times more likely to have been delivered by forceps compared to those without OCD; this was highly statistically significant. Moreover, mothers of offspring who later developed comorbid OCD were significantly more likely to have used coffee, cigarettes, and alcohol during their pregnancy compared to mothers of children with TS without OCD. A subsequent smaller-scale study from Japan comparing 13 individuals with TS+OCD to 10 TS patients without comorbid obsessive-compulsive symptoms confirmed a higher frequency of perinatal adverse events in those with obsessive-compulsive symptoms compared to those without (Iida et al., 1996). Another small-scale study involving 38 referred patients with TS found that those with a lower birth weight had significantly more frequent comorbid conduct disorder and/or self-injurious behavior (Zelnik et al., 2002).

The first large-scale study, using the largest sample of patients TS ever reported (the Tourette Syndrome International Consortium database, comprising approximately 5,500 subjects with TS from different parts of the world), was aimed at investigating a possible role of perinatal adversities as risk factors for comorbid learning disability in TS. These turned out to be present in 27% of those with learning disability comorbidity and in 17% of those without, a statistically significant difference (Burd et al., 2005). The study failed, however, to provide information on the nature of these perinatal risk factors.

In the above-mentioned, well-designed cohort study (N = 180) by Mathews and colleagues (2006), maternal smoking during pregnancy was the strongest predictor of comorbid OCD, associated with an eightfold increase in risk. Increased paternal age was also associated with an increased risk of comorbid OCD, with an 8% higher risk for each year of paternal age, while no relationship between rates of OCD comorbidity and other prenatal/perinatal variables was seen. ADHD comorbidity was associated with lower birth weight and a higher number of prenatal problems. No relationship between pre- and perinatal factors and self-injurious behavior was found. Surprisingly, there was no significant association between maternal smoking during pregnancy and the presence of comorbid ADHD. The latter finding (that there was no relationship between prenatal exposure to tobacco and comorbid ADHD) is in remarkable contrast to later analyses from the Yale Child Study Center (Motlagh et al., 2010). This study, already briefly mentioned, compared maternal-report data on pre- and perinatal risk factors in a cohort of 222 children, including 45 individuals with TS alone, 52 with ADHD alone, 60 with TS+ADHD, and 65 unaffected control children. In this cohort, heavy maternal smoking and severe levels of psychosocial stress during pregnancy were independent risk factors for a comorbid diagnosis of ADHD in children with TS.

Perhaps the most definitive study so far into pre- and perinatal determinants of ADHD comorbidity, involving a comparison of 181 TS children with and 172 without comorbid ADHD, was quite convincingly supportive of the relevance of low birth weight and prenatal exposure to maternal smoking (Pringsheim et al., 2009). Exposure to pre- and perinatal adverse events was assessed using demographic information booklets completed by parents before

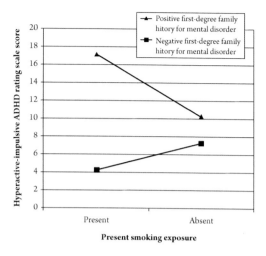

FIGURE 8.1   Role of prenatal smoking exposure regarding hyperactive-impulsive ADHD rating scale scores in patients with a tic disorder, with and without a relative mental disorder.

the diagnostic interview. Adjusted odds ratios for the comorbid diagnosis of TS and ADHD were 2.7 in children born with low birth weight and 2.4 for those exposed to maternal smoking. Thus, overall, studies that have investigated pre- and perinatal risk factors for the presence of the most common TS comorbidities seem to suggest that pregnancy factors (low birth weight and exposure to smoking) are mostly related to ADHD comorbidity and delivery complications to OCD comorbidity. Still, a role for maternal smoking during pregnancy with regard to ADHD comorbidity has not been consistent across studies, and it was strikingly absent in the study by Mathews and colleagues (2006). Currently, there is no obvious explanation for this discrepancy.

Other than searching for perinatal risk factors associated with the presence of a categorical comorbid diagnosis, an alternative approach is to consider the severity of comorbid symptoms, using a dimensional approach. We did this within our cohort of 110 children with tics from Groningen, the Netherlands, and found that pregnancy complications were associated with decreased comorbid obsessive-compulsive symptom severity, and prenatal smoking exposure with more severe comorbid depressive symptoms, autism spectrum symptoms, and symptoms of ADHD (Bos-Veneman et al., 2010a, 2010b; Fig. 8.1).

Finally, the relevance of lower birth weight, an important indicator of the quality of the environment *in utero*, to brain dysfunction beyond the motor circuits of the basal ganglia has been elegantly demonstrated in a study with conventional 18-channel electroencephalography (EEG) in 11 monozygotic twins where at least one member of the twin pair had TS (Hyde et al., 1994). In seven of the nine twin sets that differed in birth weight, the twin with the lower birth weight had EEG slowing. The authors speculate that the origin of this EEG slowing may lie in interactions between environmental insults to the central nervous system and the genetic component of TS, an interaction producing damage to the cortex, thalamus, or both. Interestingly, a worse overall EEG was related to lower global neuropsychological testing scores. Thus, this twin study confirms the relevance of pregnancy-related factors for overall functioning, beyond the mere presence of tics.

IS TS ASSOCIATED WITH PERINATAL ADVERSITIES LESS FAMILIAL?

Three independent case series have suggested that individuals with TS with a history of severe perinatal adversities tend to have a less familial form of TS. In a study of 52 Japanese probands with TS, it was observed that severe perinatal problems were associated with lower recurrence risks of TS and lower rates of TS comorbidities among their first-degree relatives when compared to the first-degree relatives of TS probands without these perinatal problems (Kano et al., 2001). A comparison of 39 first-degree relatives of 13 TS probands with severe perinatal problems and 126 first-degree relatives of 39 TS probands without such perinatal problems demonstrated that the first-degree relatives of TS probands with severe perinatal problems had obsessive-compulsive symptoms significantly less frequently than the first-degree relative of TS probands without perinatal problems. Also, the rate of tics in the first-degree relatives of TS probands with a history of severe perinatal problems was two times lower than that in first-degree relatives of TS probands without such perinatal problems.

A similar observation had previously been made in a small series of three TS patients with and five without a family history of TS; birth complications were primarily present in those without a positive family history (Párraga et al., 1998). Replication was also shown in a cohort recruited at the Yale Child Study Center in which 69 first-degree relatives of 23 TS probands with a history of severe perinatal problems were compared with 77 first-degree relatives of 23 TS probands without such perinatal problems in their history (Kano et al., 2002). The risk of TS was clearly increased among the relatives of probands without severe perinatal difficulties (11% vs. 4%). Thus, these observations seem to suggest that severe perinatal problems might in some cases be an independent causative factor for the later development of (nonfamilial) TS.

COMMENTARY ON AVAILABLE EVIDENCE

In this review, all published studies in the English language that addressed the role of prenatal and perinatal adverse events upon diagnosis of TS, tic symptom severity, and occurrence of TS comorbidities have been included. Table 8.1 summarizes the most salient findings of this review. The number of studies in this area has been relatively limited so far, and sample sizes

exceeding 100 were involved only occasionally. Despite this, published findings often reached statistical significance even in small cohorts, probably as a consequence of the relatively large effects of perinatal adversities. Also, findings were mostly in agreement across studies, with one notable exception: it is still unresolved whether maternal smoking during pregnancy is primarily related to ADHD comorbidity and not to tic symptom severity, as suggested by the analyses by Motlagh and colleagues (2010) and Pringsheim and colleagues (2009), or rather the other way around, as suggested by the study by Mathews and coworkers (2006). All three studies were well designed and involved relatively large sample sizes.

All reviewed studies merely reported associations between perinatal adversities and tics and/or comorbid conditions, and it should be emphasized that these do not necessarily indicate a causative role for pregnancy and delivery complications. Prenatal risk factors may also arise through confounders, including inherited ones. As a result, caution is required in assuming causation (Thapar & Rutter, 2009).

Although the relevance of perinatal adversities for the expression of TS vulnerability is beyond doubt, many areas remain neglected, compared to the wealth of studies published in relation to other childhood-onset neurodevelopmental disorders such as ADHD (see Nigg et al., 2010, for a comprehensive review on this topic). The most strikingly neglected research area is the study of gene–environment interactions. In child psychiatry, interest in gene–environment interactions has been fueled by findings regarding the interaction of life stressors with the serotonin transporter gene promoter polymorphism in depression (Risch et al., 2009) and the interaction of a functional promoter polymorphism in the monoamine oxidase A gene with child maltreatment in conduct disorder (Kim-Cohen et al., 2006). In the field of ADHD, a replicated pattern of findings has emerged from the growing literature: dopaminergic and serotonergic genotypes interact with environmental factors in influencing the severity of ADHD symptoms, with pre- and perinatal events primarily influencing hyperactivity and psychosocial events

Table 8.1 Pregnancy, Delivery, and Neonatal Complications Associated with the Diagnosis of TS, Tic Severity in Affected Individuals, and Presence or Severity of Comorbid ADHD and OCD

	Pregnancy Complications	Delivery Complications	Neonatal Complications
Presence of TS	More and earlier prenatal care visits (Burd et al., 1999) Older paternal age (Burd et al., 1999) Severe maternal psychosocial stress (Motlagh et al., 2010) Maternal smoking (Motlagh et al., 2010)	More frequent delivery complications (Pasamanick & Kawi, 1956; Saccomani et al., 2005)	Lower Apgar score at 5 min (Burd et al., 1999)
Tic severity	Lower birth weight (Hyde et al., 1992; Mathews et al., 2006) Maternal smoking (Mathews et al., 2006) Maternal medication use (Mathews et al., 2006) Older paternal age (Mathews et al., 2006) Maternal psychosocial stress (Mathews et al., 2006) Maternal severe nausea and/or vomiting during the first trimester (Leckman et al., 1990)	More frequent delivery complications (Bos-Veneman et al., 2010b)	
ADHD comorbidity	Lower birth weight (Pringsheim et al., 2009) Maternal smoking (Motlagh et al., 2010; Pringsheim et al., 2009; Bos-Veneman et al., 2010a)		
OCD comorbidity	Maternal use of coffee, cigarettes, or alcohol (Mathews et al., 2006; Santangelo et al., 1994) Older paternal age (Mathews et al., 2006)	More frequent forceps deliveries (Santangelo et al., 1994)	
Conduct disorder	Lower birth weight (Zelnik et al., 2002)		
Depressive symptoms	Maternal smoking (Bos-Veneman et al., 2010a)		
Autism spectrum symptoms	Maternal smoking (Bos-Veneman et al., 2010a)		

later in life showing a tendency to predominantly increase inattention (reviewed by Nigg et al., 2010).

Although the possibility of interactions between pregnancy and birth complications and genotypes was suggested as early as 1990 (Leckman et al., 1990), so far only one study involving gene–environment interactions in a cohort of patients with TS has been published (Bos-Veneman et al, 2010b). In this study, the interaction between dopamine receptor D4 (DRD4) gene 48-base pair variable number of tandem repeats and perinatal adversities and its effect on severity of tics and comorbid symptoms was investigated in 110 children with tics. In children without a DRD4 3-repeat allele, delivery complications were associated with more severe tics, but in children with a 3-repeat variant, an inverse relation between delivery complications and tic severity was found. Moreover, the relationship between delivery complications and internalizing symptom severity appeared to be most pronounced in children with a DRD4 2-repeat allele. Thus, the study provides preliminary evidence for interactions between common DRD4 polymorphisms with delivery complications regarding severity of tics and co-occurring internalizing symptoms. Future study of gene–environment interactions is likely to be promising and shed important new light on TS etiology.

This exciting field is expected to profit from future genetic findings and more sophisticated measures of the pre- and perinatal environment, leading to the possibility of mapping causal pathways with greater specificity.

Future, larger-scale studies could also try to more specifically investigate the timing, duration, magnitude, and type of prenatal and perinatal adverse events, including psychosocial stress, on neuronal long-term consequences. In rats it has been shown that elevated stress hormones during pregnancy adversely affect fetal development (Maccari & Morley-Fletcher, 2007; Weinstock, 2008), specifically during the last third of the gestational period, a critical time window for the development of prefrontal and limbic regions. These regions are critically involved in attention processing, working memory, decision making, impulse control, and modulation of emotional behaviors. Interestingly, some of these effects have been found to be male-specific (Martínez-Téllez et al., 2009). These preclinical findings fit well with the results of human studies that also suggested a greater sensitivity of the male brain to early insults.

CLINICAL IMPLICATIONS

A review with families of the role of perinatal adversities as a risk factor for tic disorders and

---

Box 8.1. Key Points

- Perinatal risk factors for the development of TS include older paternal age, severe maternal psychosocial stress during pregnancy, maternal smoking during pregnancy, more and earlier prenatal care visits, delivery complications, and low Apgar score at 5 minutes after birth.
- Risk factors for more severe tics include older paternal age, maternal psychosocial stress during pregnancy, maternal severe nausea and/or vomiting during the first trimester, maternal smoking during pregnancy, maternal medication use during pregnancy, low birth weight, and delivery complications.
- Maternal smoking during pregnancy and low birth weight are risk factors for the presence of comorbid ADHD in individuals with a tic disorder.
- Older paternal age; maternal use of coffee, cigarettes, or alcohol during pregnancy, and forceps deliveries are risk factors for the presence of comorbid OCD in individuals with a tic disorder.

associated comorbidities should be a routine part of any psychoeducational intervention (see Chapter 22 for an extensive overview on this topic). This should be done in a thoughtful manner, avoiding inducing feelings of guilt in the parents. On the one hand, this highlights the relevance of neurobiological factors to parents; on the other, a discussion with families might provide opportunities for prevention strategies. Although the usefulness of adhering to a healthy lifestyle during pregnancy for reducing the risk of tics in the offspring of genetically susceptible parents has not been formally studied, the promotion of healthy lifestyles during future pregnancies is likely to produce beneficial effects on the offspring and seems therefore advisable in any case.

REFERENCES

Bos-Veneman NG, Kuin A, Minderaa RB, Hoekstra PJ. Role of perinatal adversities on tic severity and symptoms of attention deficit/hyperactivity disorder in children and adolescents with a tic disorder. *J Dev Behav Pediatr* 2010a; 31:100–106.

Bos-Veneman NG, Minderaa RB, Hoekstra PJ. The DRD4 gene and severity of tics and comorbid symptoms: main effects and interactions with delivery complications. *Mov Disord* 2010b; 25:1470–1476.

Burd L, Freeman RD, Klug MG, Kerbeshian J. Tourette syndrome and learning disabilities. *BMC Pediatr* 2005; 5:34.

Burd L, Severud R, Klug MG, Kerbeshian J. Prenatal and perinatal risk factors for Tourette disorder. *J Perinat Med* 1999; 27:295–302.

Eapen V, Fox-Hiley P, Banerjee S, Robertson M. Clinical features and associated psychopathology in a Tourette syndrome cohort. *Acta Neurol Scand* 2004; 109:255–260.

Fraga MF, Ballestar E, Paz MF, et al. Epigenetic differences arise during the lifetime of monozygotic twins. *Proc Natl Acad Sci USA* 2005; 102:10604–10609.

Goldenberg RL, Culhane JF, Iams JD, Romero R. Epidemiology and causes of preterm birth. *Lancet* 2008; 371:75–84.

Hyde TM, Aaronson BA, Randolph C, et al. Relationship of birth weight to the phenotypic expression of Gilles de la Tourette's syndrome in monozygotic twins. *Neurology* 1992; 42:652–658.

This is an excellent, classic study involving 16 pairs of monozygotic twins in whom at least one member of the twin pairs had TS, thus enabling the researchers to study the influence of low birth weight as a marker of the quality of the environment in utero, ruling out genetic influences.

Hyde TM, Emsellem HA, Randolph C, et al. Electroencephalographic abnormalities in monozygotic twins with Tourette's syndrome. *Br J Psychiatry* 1994; 164:811–817.

Iida J, Sakiyama S, Iwasaka H, et al. The clinical features of Tourette's disorder with obsessive-compulsive symptoms. *Psychiatry Clin Neurosci* 1996; 50:185–189.

Incagnoli T, Kane R. Developmental perspective of the Gilles de la Tourette syndrome. *Percept Mot Skills* 1983; 57:1271–1281.

Kano Y, Leckman JF, Pauls DL. Clinical characteristics of Tourette syndrome probands and relatives' risks. *J Am Acad Child Adolesc Psychiatry* 2002; 41:1148–1149.

Kano Y, Ohta M, Nagai Y, et al. A family study of Tourette syndrome in Japan. *Am J Med Genet* 2001; 105:414–421.

Khalifa N, von Knorring AL. Tourette syndrome and other tic disorders in a total population of children: clinical assessment and background. *Acta Paediatr* 2005; 94:1608–1614.

Kiely JL, Kleinman JC. Birth-weight-adjusted infant mortality in evaluations of perinatal care: towards a useful summary measure. *Stat Med* 1993; 12:377–392.

Kim-Cohen J, Caspi A, Taylor A, et al. MAOA, maltreatment, and gene-environment interaction predicting children's mental health: new evidence and a meta-analysis. *Mol Psychiatry* 2006; 11:903–913.

Leckman JF, Dolnansky ES, Hardin MT, et al. Perinatal factors in the expression of Tourette's syndrome: an exploratory study. *J Am Acad Child Adolesc Psychiatry* 1990; 29:220–226.

Leckman JF, Price RA, Walkup JT, et al. Nongenetic factors in Gilles de la Tourette's syndrome. *Arch Gen Psychiatry* 1987; 44:100.

Although the sample size of the studied cohort of patients with TS was only modest (N = 31), the results of this study are intriguing. The severity of experienced maternal life stress during the pregnancy and severe nausea and/or vomiting during the first trimester were found to be significantly associated with tic severity. The authors for the first time mention the possibility of gene–environment interactions.

Maccari S, Morley-Fletcher S. Effects of prenatal restraint stress on the hypothalamus-pituitary-adrenal axis and related behavioural and neurobiological alterations. *Psychoneuroendocrinology* 2007; 32 (Suppl 1): 10–15.

Martínez-Téllez RI, Hernández-Torres E, Gamboa C, Flores G. Prenatal stress alters spine density and dendritic length of nucleus accumbens and hippocampus neurons in rat offspring. *Synapse* 2009; 63: 794–804.

Mathews CA, Bimson B, Lowe TL, et al. Association between maternal smoking and increased symptom severity in Tourette's syndrome. *Am J Psychiatry* 2006; 163:1066–1073.

Strengths of this excellent study include the large sample size (N = 180), the very comprehensive assessment of both tic symptomatology and a full range of comorbid conditions, the very detailed comprehensive assessment of pre- and perinatal adverse events, and the use of lifetime overall worst tic severity.

Motlagh MG, Katsovich L, Thompson N, et al. Severe psychosocial stress and heavy cigarette smoking during pregnancy: an examination of the pre- and perinatal risk factors associated with ADHD and Tourette syndrome. *Eur Child Adolesc Psychiatry* 2010; 19:755–764.

Nigg J, Nikolas M, Burt SA. Measured gene-by-environment interaction in relation to attention-deficit/hyperactivity disorder. *J Am Acad Child Adolesc Psychiatry* 2010; 49:863–873.

Párraga HC, Párraga MI, Spinner LR, et al. Clinical differences between subjects with familial and non-familial Tourette's syndrome: a case series. *Int J Psychiatry Med* 1998; 28:341–351.

Pasamanick B, Kawi A. A study of the association of prenatal and paranatal factors with the development of tics in children; a preliminary investigation. *J Pediatr* 1956; 48:596–601.

This classic and excellently designed study was the first to consider birth complications. Strengths include the relatively large sample size, the use of hospital obstetric records, and the elegant matching between cases and controls.

Price RA, Kidd KK, Cohen DJ, et al. A twin study of Tourette syndrome. *Arch Gen Psychiatry* 1985; 42:815–820.

Pringsheim T, Sandor P, Lang A, et al. Prenatal and perinatal morbidity in children with Tourette syndrome and attention-deficit hyperactivity disorder .*J Dev Behav Pediatr* 2009; 30:115–121.

The large sample size and good assessment of tics and ADHD comorbidity make this one of the most valuable studies on the role of pre- and perinatal adverse events with regard to ADHD comorbidity.

Risch N, Herrell R, Lehner T, et al. Interaction between the serotonin transporter gene (5-HTTLPR), stressful life events, and risk of depression: a meta-analysis. *JAMA* 2009; 301:2462–2471.

Saccomani L, Fabiana V, Manuela B, Giambattista R. Tourette syndrome and chronic tics in a sample of children and adolescents. *Brain Dev* 2005; 27:349–352.

Santangelo SL, Pauls DL, Goldstein JM, et al. Tourette's syndrome: what are the influences of gender and comorbid obsessive-compulsive disorder? *J Am Acad Child Adolesc Psychiatry* 1994; 33:795–804.

Shapiro AK, Shapiro E, Wayne H. Birth, developmental, and family histories and demographic information in Tourette's syndrome. *J Nerv Ment Dis* 1972; 155:335–344.

Shapiro AK, Shapiro E, Wayne HL, et al. Tourette's syndrome: summary of data on 34 patients. *Psychosom Med* 1973; 35:419–435.

Thapar A, Rutter M. Do prenatal risk factors cause psychiatric disorder? Be wary of causal claims. *Br J Psychiatry* 2009; 195:100–101.

Ward C, Lewis S, Coleman T. Prevalence of maternal smoking and environmental tobacco smoke exposure during pregnancy and impact on birth weight: retrospective study using Millennium Cohort. *BMC Public Health* 2007; 7:81

Weinstock M. The long-term behavioural consequences of prenatal stress. *Neurosci Biobehav Rev* 2008; 32:1073–1086.

Zelnik N, Newfield RS, Silman-Stolar Z, Goikhman I. Height distribution in children with Tourette syndrome. *J Child Neurol* 2002; 17:200–204.

9

Infections and Tic Disorders

TANYA K. MURPHY

Abstract

Several associations between infections, particularly Sydenham chorea and group A streptococcal (GAS) infections, and subsequent Tourette syndrome and obsessive-compulsive disorder (OCD) symptoms have been established, suggesting at least a nonspecific role of infections in a subgroup of patients with tics. In the late 1990s, researchers from the National Institute of Mental Health further characterized an entity they called "pediatric autoimmune neuropsychiatric disorders associated with streptococcus" (PANDAS). Children with PANDAS are more likely to have dramatic-onset, or "overnight," neuropsychiatric symptoms, remission of OCD or tic symptoms during antibiotic treatment, and evidence of GAS infections. The diagnosis of PANDAS requires more than laboratory evidence of exposure to streptococcal bacteria; it also requires evidence of a temporal association between repeated anti-streptolysin O titer elevation and the onset of OCD or tic symptoms. Although more evidence exists supporting the exacerbation of neuropsychiatric symptoms due to GAS infections, evidence also exists that *Mycoplasma pneumoniae*, respiratory infections, the common cold, and even stress have been linked to exacerbation of OCD and tic symptoms. The complex interaction of patient-specific attributes (neurochemical and immune vulnerability genes leading to maladaptive neuropsychiatric or immune function) with environmental attributes (psychosocial stress, injuries, substance exposures, and pathogen-specific properties) creates an interesting and ongoing research challenge.

If we were to confine ourselves to this description by Sydenham, which so far as typical cases of the disease are concerned is perfectly accurate, differentiation between tic and chorea would not be a matter of any complexity. Unfortunately, however, the varieties of this form of chorea are legion, and in practice one constantly meets with conditions suggesting alike the gesticulations of chorea and the convulsive reactions of tic. Moreover, it has been pointed out by Oddo that the fact of the habitual exaggeration of tic during the very years when chosen chorea is liable to appear is calculated to confuse the issue.
—Henry Meige and E. Feindel (1907)

This fixation on psychological theories of degeneration often led to ignoring clinical data that may have raised interesting alternative questions, especially in relation to the work of Koch and Pasteur, on the possible role of infection in these disorders.
—Howard Kushner (1999)

While the movements in the two diseases [tic and Sydenham's chorea] differ, one can pick out isolated movements in chorea identical with those of tic, and conversely in cases of tic some movements identical with chorea. It is true that chorea minor like rheumatic fever, is a self-limited disease, running a definite course, and as such differs from tic. There are cases of chorea, however, in which recurrences come so close together that the chorea minor goes over into a chorea intermittens, and even into a chorea permanens, in which the analogy to tic is very close.
—Laurence Selling (1929)

It is obvious that every sinus infection does not produce a tic any more than every tonsil infection produces nephritis, an arthritis or an endocarditis. There must be a definite specificity of the infection for certain tissues in tics, just as there is in other focal infections which one is familiar.
—Laurence Selling (1929)

Looking back over his [Edward E. Brown] years of practice and citing his previous publications, Brown found that most tickers had histories of frequent infections, sinusitis, and previous chorea.
—Howard Kushner (1999)

He [Yves Ranty] was convinced, as Langlois and Force had been two years earlier (1965), that the symptoms of Gilles de la Tourette's disease also should be connected with an "acute infection, [as] during Sydenham's chorea, in which the agent would be streptococcus or staphylococcus, and in which inflammatory phenomena of the brain stem can regress".
—Howard Kushner (1999)

INFECTIOUS AGENTS, whether bacteria, spirochetes, viruses, or prions, have been implicated in inciting many chronic illnesses, from peptic ulcers, diabetes, cancer, and multiple sclerosis (MS) to schizophrenia. Their role in neurological disorders has begun to garner much attention as research continues to show the integral role of immunological responses and disruption of immunological homeostasis in the pathology and clinical manifestations of these disorders. In MS, for example, immunological disruptions, such as irregularities in regulatory T-cell populations and function, have been shown to be a common clinical manifestation and to play a major role in the pathological mechanism in this disorder. Similarly in schizophrenia, neuroinflammation, believed to be the result of prenatal infection, is thought to precipitate the symptoms manifested clinically. Even more intriguing have been findings of an increased evidence of infection and viral titers in MS and schizophrenia (Pelonero et al., 1990;

Salvetti et al., 2009). Recently, findings in tic disorders have alluded to a similar etiology, with observations of a possibly causative link between group A streptococcal infection and symptom presentation. Despite the evidence, debate has continued for over 200 years about the role of infections in the presentation of tic disorders. Like the fable of the blind men examining the elephant in the dark, present-day observers are influenced by their biases and by differences in the clinical populations presenting to them. Rarely will a single factor explain why an individual will develop tics. Multiple etiologies are likely at play; none will act in isolation, but they will interact with the individual's unique mix of central nervous system (CNS) environmental insults, genetics, and immune challenges. In this chapter, historical observations, clinical presentations, and possible infectious triggers are reviewed. The dilemma of infectious markers is briefly discussed. Then assessment and considerations are discussed, followed by key points and unanswered questions.

ASSOCIATION OF INFECTIONS WITH TICS

Prior to the current predominant neurochemical theories to explain TS etiology, Langlois and Force described in 1965 a 6-year-old child who developed Tourette syndrome (TS) and Sydenham chorea (SC) symptoms after several infections (Langlois & Force, 1965). They successfully treated the child with antibiotics and neuroleptics. At the time, they did not view TS as incurable and separate from SC but as sequelae to acute chorea. Historically, this nosological as well as etiological confusion has existed between TS and SC (Kushner & Kiessling, 1996). In the mid-1980s, researchers noted that patients with SC often developed obsessive-compulsive disorder (OCD) symptoms, and some had tics as well (Kerbeshian et al., 1990; Swedo et al., 1989). Additional investigation found that some patients with group A streptococcal (GAS) infections, but without the neurological findings of SC, presented with acute OCD symptoms (Allen et al., 1995; Swedo, 1994). At the same time, Louise Kiessling and colleagues reported on the association of tics during GAS outbreaks in her developmental pediatric practice (Kiessling et al., 1993).

Based on these observations and reports, National Institute of Mental Health (NIMH) researchers further characterized these observation into an entity they called pediatric autoimmune neuropsychiatric disorders associated with streptococcus (PANDAS) in a 50-patient case series (Swedo et al., 1998). In this case series, GAS (44%) or pharyngitis (28%) was the inciting trigger and future exacerbations were associated with GAS infection in 31%, pharyngitis/upper respiratory illness in 42%, and GAS exposure in 4%. Another study examined streptococcal titers of 150 children at their initial evaluation for tics; results showed that 38% of those with tics had elevated antistreptolysin O (ASO) titers compared to 2% in the control group (Cardona & Orefici, 2001). In a prospective study of 25 youth with tics or OCD, those with an episodic or more acutely fluctuating presentation of tic/OCD symptoms were more likely to have chronically elevated streptococcal titers when compared to patients with remitting or stable symptoms (Murphy et al., 2004).

In a case-control study, 144 children aged 4 to 13 years old who received their first diagnosis of OCD, TS, or tic disorder between January 1992 and December 1999 (Mell et al., 2005) were matched to controls by birth date, sex, primary physician, and propensity to seek health care. Children with OCD or tic disorder were more likely than controls to have had streptococcal infection in the 3 months before onset date. The presence of multiple GAS infections within a 12-month period was associated with an increased risk of TS with an odds ratio of 13.6. A similar finding was reported in an examination of administrative claims data of many more cases and controls where subjects with newly diagnosed OCD, TS, or tic disorder (N = 742) were found to be more likely than controls (n = 3,647) to have had a diagnosis of streptococcal infection in the previous year (odds ratio: 1.54, 95% confidence interval: 1.29, 2.15). Prior streptococcal infection was also associated with incident diagnoses of attention-deficit/

hyperactivity disorder (ADHD; Leslie et al., 2008), suggesting that potential sequelae of frequent GAS infections are not limited to tic/OCD symptoms. Another database analysis did not support the relationship between streptococcal infection and postinfectious recurrences of OCD and TS (Schrag et al., 2009). The primary limitation of this study design was the lack of setting the analysis parameters to determine if an appropriate temporal proximity existed between the streptococcal infection and the onset of OCD or tics. Making this association at 2 and 5 years mitigates the detection of a temporal signal above the background GAS incidence in a typical pediatric population. The average age of onset for OCD was 16 years old in this study, well beyond the usual age of PANDAS presentation. In one study that prospectively examined 693 school-age children with monthly GAS cultures and behavioral observations, an increase in behavioral and motoric symptoms was seen especially in children who had repeated GAS infections (Murphy et al., 2007).

These results support that recent or chronic streptococcal infections may play a role in tic presentation. Another possibility is that patients with elevated titers may reflect a chronic immune response that then leaves patients more susceptible to exacerbations from other infections and stress (Benatar et al., 1988; Muller et al., 2004; Murphy et al., 2004; Read et al., 1986). Alternatively, perhaps a cumulative threshold of antibody is needed to trigger symptoms in some patients. Support for an exaggerated immune response to GAS was found in youth with tics compared to youth presenting with pharyngitis (Bombaci et al., 2009). In a study by Bombaci and colleagues, sera of tic patients with no clinical signs of infection, non-tic patients, and pharyngitis patients were compared for immunoreactivity to GAS antigens. The first major finding of this group was that tic patients presented with a serological profile significantly different from that of their non-tic counterparts. Additionally and possibly most relevant to the idea of infection-mediated symptomatology, was the increased reactivity of tic-patient sera to GAS antigens, being significant higher than non-tic patients and even pharyngitis patients.

Interestingly, this increased reactivity was seen even in tic patients with no signs of pharyngitis infection confirmed by ASO titer (Bombaci et al., 2009).

In a cross-sectional and prospective study by Martino and colleagues (2011), children and adolescents with TS (N = 168) were compared against youth with epileptic or sleep disorders without a history of TS (N = 177). In the cross-sectional study, higher severity ADHD, anxiety, and mood ratings were noted on children with TS versus the comparison group. A higher incidence of positive throat cultures were also noted, 8% of patients with TS versus 2% of the comparison group. The prospective study was limited to patients with TS only (N = 144). A psychometric assessment as well as collection of throat and blood specimens was performed. Positive throat cultures were identified in 7%, a rise in levels of ASO was found in 18%, and a rise in DNAseB titers was found in 18%. On the last two consecutive visits, persistently maintained elevated ASO titers were found in 57% of patients, while only 2% continued to have positive throat cultures. In 30% of the visits (369 total), a non–GAS-related sore throat was present. Youth with TS appeared more prone to develop GAS infections.

In a study by Leckman and colleagues (2011), children meeting the PANDAS criteria as specified by Dr. Swedo's 1998 criteria and a control group of non-PANDAS children with pediatric-onset TS and/or OCD were evaluated with raters unblinded to group assignment (however, laboratory results were blinded from clinical assessments). Subjects were compared on exacerbation type and incidence, laboratory findings, and the presence of GAS infection within a certain timeframe of exacerbation presentation versus children with similar demographic and clinical characteristics. Similar rates of exacerbations of tic and/or OCD were observed in both groups; however, changes in severity rating scores suggested that many exacerbations were of a mild nature. Additional exacerbations noted included anxiety, depression, and/or ADHD symptoms, with a slightly lower result in the non-PANDAS group. Similar rates were observed in both groups when examining newly diagnosed definite plus possible GAS infections. Furthermore, only 10.2% (6/59) of exacerbations linked to a GAS infection were noted within a 10-week period for both combined groups. All exacerbations were noted on children from the non-PANDAS group, three of which were from the same child. An increase in obsessive-compulsive symptoms was noted at each of his three exacerbations. One confound for this study was the way antibiotic prescribing was handled across groups. Of the 52 definite and possible new GAS infections, 21 were treated by the primary care clinician with a variety of appropriate antibiotics. In the PANDAS group, 60% (12/20) of the newly diagnosed GAS infections were treated compared with 28% (9/32) in the non-PANDAS group. Further, the study provided no information as to the number of days children received antibiotics in one group compared to the other group. Although limited by unblinded group assignments and imbalanced antibiotic treatment, the study concluded that there is a lack of temporal correlation between GAS infection and the presence of exacerbations in PANDAS patients.

In an exploration of the clinical factors associated with PANDAS, children with tics, OCD, or both (N = 109) were assessed by personal and family history, diagnostic interview, physical examination, medical record review, and measurement of baseline levels of streptococcal antibodies. Significant group differences were found on several variables, such that children with PANDAS (vs. those without PANDAS) were more likely to have had dramatic onset, definite remissions, remission of neuropsychiatric symptoms during antibiotic therapy, a history of tonsillectomies/adenoidectomies, evidence of GAS infection, and clumsiness (Murphy et al., 2012).

Although more support exists for GAS in pathogen-triggered neuropsychiatric symptoms, not all cases of infection-triggered OCD have been related to prior GAS infection. Probably one of the first examples in the literature to describe infection-precipitated tic disorders was by Selling in 1929 (Selling, 1929). He describes three cases where he attributes tic symptoms to a concurrent sinusitis, with improvement following sinus surgery. In 1931, von Economo documented several post-encephalitic syndrome patients whose clinical presentation was remarkable for hyperactivity, tics, and/or obsessive-compulsive symptomatology (von Economo, 1931). Researchers at NIMH (Allen et al., 1995) detailed four children who presented with sudden onset or worsening of OCD and/or tics following an infection (two viral, two GAS). This led to the coining of the term pediatric infection-triggered autoimmune neuropsychiatric disorders (PITANDS), which better captures the non-GAS triggers. In a retrospective examination of youth with tics, 53% were found to have an abrupt onset of symptoms; of this subset, 21% were shown to have the onset within 6 weeks of infection (Singer et al., 2000).

A study by Perrin and colleagues (2004) showed that both viral and GAS infections can lead to acute behavioral changes. However, this study's primary aim was to assess for a delayed response to GAS after removing from the analysis the acute behavioral group (those with concurrent behavior changes and GAS infection at baseline). However, GAS has been reported to induce behavioral changes concurrently with active infection (Murphy & Pichichero, 2002). In another series, tic exacerbations were noted to occur after a cold but a GAS association was not observed (Hoekstra et al., 2005). Another study found that a large percentage (87.5%) of symptom exacerbations among PANDAS patients cannot be definitively attributed to GAS infections, though GAS-related exacerbations did occur in 7.5% to 25% (Kurlan et al., 2008). The exacerbation rates (tics and/or OCD) were 0.56 per person-year for PANDAS case subjects and 0.28 per person-year for control subjects. A total of 43 definite or probable GAS infections were identified: 31 in the PANDAS group (in 22 subjects) and 12 in control subjects (in 9 subjects). The GAS (definite or probable) infection rates were 0.43 per person-year for PANDAS case subjects and 0.13 per person-year for control subjects.

Another respiratory pathogen, *Mycoplasma pneumoniae*, has been implicated in neurologic sequelae without a clearly understood pathophysiological mechanism (Yis et al., 2008). Muller and colleagues examined two children with tic exacerbations and found that both had evidence of Mycoplasma infection after extensive blood work (Muller et al., 2000). Both children were treated with erythromycin. Following 4 weeks of treatment, the boy no longer had tics and the girl had a marked improvement in her tics but not in her ADHD. In a study of 29 patients with TS compared to healthy controls, 59% of patients with TS but only 3% of the controls had positive or suspected positive antibody titers against *M. pneumoniae* via a microparticle agglutination assay. The results of the immunoblot technique demonstrated significantly more IgA-antibody positive results among TS patients than in the controls (31% vs. 3%), whereas the distributions of IgM and IgG antibody positivity were similar in both groups (Muller et al., 2004).

In an exploratory study by Krause and colleagues (2010), 32 subjects with TS (age 29.6 ± 15.1 years) were compared to 30 controls (age 33 ± 16.1 years) in an attempt to analyze the association between TS and intracellular infectious agents. *Chlamydia trachomatis, Chlamydia pneumoniae*, and *Toxoplasma gondii* IgA and IgG levels were assessed. The IgG levels of *C. trachomatis* were significantly elevated in the TS group, with *T. gondii* levels trending toward significance. A variety of limitations, such as an unbalanced gender distribution, effects of medication, and almost 20-year delay from time of onset to assessment, suggest that further exploration is necessary. Clearly not all symptom exacerbations are due solely to GAS, and case reports and studies support this possibility(Allen et al. 1995; Budman et al. 1997; Muller et al. 2004; Riedel et al. 1998) to include the common cold, sinusitis, and *M. pneumoniae*. Table 9.1 summarizes findings from the main studies exploring the association between infections and tic disorders.

Differentiating the role of stress from infections is not easily accomplished in many naturalistic clinical settings. Individuals with TS are frequently sensitive to psychosocial stress (Bornstein et al., 1990; Chappell et al., 1994; Charmandari et al, 2003; see also Chapter 14). Forty-five children with tic disorder and/or OCD were matched with 41 healthy control subjects and monitored over a 2-year period for GAS infections and the effect on psychological

Table 9.1 Examination of Infection Association with Tics

Reference	Sample Characteristics	Findings/Conclusions
Case Series		
Selling, 1929	(N = 3) Two 14-year-old boys and one 11-year-old boy	Tic disorders with evidence of sinus infection. Sinus surgery of the foci resulted in improvement of tics. Suggested tics are due to infectious origin, particularly of sinuses.
Kondo & Kabasawa, 1978	(N = 1) 11-year-old boy	Developed severe tics after illness with high fever. Treated with corticosteroid therapy and tics resolved.
Kerbeshian et al., 1990	(N = 1) 14-year-old girl	Following pharyngitis, preexisting motor tics were exacerbated by the onset of chorea. All movements improved after 8 months of antibiotic prophylaxis.
Allen et al., 1995	(N = 4) 4 boys aged 10–14 years	Infection-triggered OCD and tics treated with plasmapheresis (2) IVIG (1) and immunosuppressive doses of prednisone (1). All subjects had a clinically significant response immediately after treatment.
Tucker et al., 1996	(N = 1) 12-year-old girl; case study	Treatment-resistant OCD and chronic tics associated with strep infection treated multimodally. Significant improvement after plasmapheresis and prophylactic antibiotics.
Weiss & Garland, 1997	(N = 1) 10-year-old boy with infection-triggered severe OCD, chronic tics	Improvement of OCD/tics after antibiotic treatment. Argued for need of treatment guidelines in PANDAS cases.
Hansen & Bershow, 1997	(N = 2) Two boys with TS/OCD aged 2 and 9 years	IgA deficiency found in 10% of authors' patients with OCD/tics; recommend better understanding of immune status before initiating immune therapies.
Swedo et al., 1998	(N = 50) Children who met PANDAS criteria. Systematic clinical evaluation between 1991 and 1993.	111 of 144 symptom exacerbations suggested GAS infection as trigger.

(Continued)

Table 9.1 (*Continued*)

Reference	Sample Characteristics	Findings / Conclusions
Martinelli et al., 2002	(N = 1) 20-year-old female with adult-onset of tics and OC; case study following sore throat	Tics had abdominal muscle involvement. Except for age of onset, subject met all criteria for PANDAS.
Perlmutter et al., 1998	(N = 1) 5-year-old girl with sudden and dramatic onset of tics and OCD following a GAS throat infection	Subject improved after treatment with IVIG followed by antibiotic prophylaxis.
Orvidas & Slattery, 2001	(N = 2) Onset and exacerbations streptococcus-triggered OCD in 12-year-old girl and tics 8-year-old brother	Tonsillectomy performed with significant symptom improvement.
Segarra & Murphy, 2008	(N = 10) Children with PANDAS phenotype were studied for its relationship of GAS to OCD and/ or tic symptoms to possible development of cardiac involvement by color Doppler echocardiography evaluation.	All of the evidence suggests that the cardiac risk is low in youths with worsening tics or OCD temporally associated with a streptococcal infection.
Yis et al., 2008	(N = 5) Cases of *Mycoplasma pneumoniae* were discussed in terms of its effect on and damage to the CNS.	Pathogenesis of damage in the CNS by *M. pneumoniae* remains unknown. It is considered the major causes of encephalitis in children. Neurotoxicity and autoimmune mechanisms are still the most likely causable theories.
Lewin et al., 2011	(N = 3) Youth with PANDAS and their identical siblings (two sets of twins, one set of triplets)	Presentations showed marked variation across siblings from full PANDAS presentations to asymptomatic. Data highlight potential for environmental influences for discordant presentations in genetically identical siblings.

Lewin et al., 2011	26 youth with PANDAS, all with OCD; 19 with tics	Youth with PANDAS presented with marked impaired performance on tasks of visual-constructive and visual-spatial recall memory. Elevated GAS titers were associated with worse performance on tasks of neurocognitive and executive ability, fine motor speed, and elevated OCD symptom severity.
Antonelli et al., 2011	(N = 1) 43-year-old man with HIV-1 affected by TS after a sudden interruption of antiretroviral drugs	Patient had worsening of tics with viral load and significantly improved with antiviral treatment.
Case-Control		
Murphy et al., 1997	(N = 31) Patients with childhood-onset OCD and/or tics and HC (N = 21). GAS, ANeA, D8/17 levels measured.	No difference in GAS titer levels, trend toward increased ANeA binding.
Singer et al., 1999	ANeA study in 41 TS children and 39 control subjects	Children with TS have a higher median but not mean levels of ANeA. Assay failed to identify a relationship between antibodies and clinical phenotype or one-time markers for streptococcal infection.
Giedd et al., 2000	(N = 116) Volumetric MRIs in children \with PANDAS (N = 34) and HC children (N = 82)	BG volumes higher in PANDAS children than in healthy group.
Lougee et al., 2000	(N = 211) Proband = children with PANDAS (N = 54) and first-degree relatives (N = 157) interviewed	Rates of tic disorders and OCD in first-degree relatives of pediatric probands with PANDAS are higher than those reported in the general population.

(Continued)

Table 9.1 (*Continued*)

Reference	Sample Characteristics	Findings/Conclusions
Muller et al., 2000	Streptococcal titers studied in TS (N = 13) and HC children (N = 13); TS (N = 23) and HC adults (N = 23); schizophrenics (N = 17)	TS patients exhibited higher antistreptococcal titers than age-matched comparison groups of both children and adults.
Peterson et al., 2000	(N = 105) Subjects aged 7–55 years old with CTD, OCD, or ADHD and HC (N = 37). Antistreptococcal antibody titers and BG volumes measured.	ADHD was associated significantly with streptococcal titers. No significant association between antibody titers and CTD or OCD. BG volumes were significantly different in OCD and ADHD subjects compared to other groups.
Singer et al., 2000	(N = 80) Assessment of onset characteristics in TS children aged 5–17 years old	42 subjects had sudden, explosive onset or worsening of tic symptoms; 9 subjects had sudden, explosive onset or worsening of tic symptoms specifically associated with a streptococcal infection.
Cardona & Orefici, 2001	(N = 300) Children (150 with tics and 150 without tics) ASO titers compared for 11 seasons	ASO titers significantly higher compared to control subjects. Relationship exists between severity of tic disorder and magnitude of serologic response to GAS antigen.
Morshed et al., 2001	(N = 227) Autoantibody assessment of female (N = 103), male children (N = 124) and adults aged 8–85 years old. TS = 81, SC = 27, Autoimmune illness = 52, and HC = 67.	TS patients had significantly higher mean rank of total ANeA, ANA; streptococcal titers were higher in adults than did HC.

Muller et al., 2001	(N = 50) Antibodies against M proteins studied in 25 TS adults and 25 HC	Increased titers of antibodies against the streptococcal M12 and M19 proteins (RF associated serotypes) in TS patients compared with HC.
Loiselle et al., 2003	(N = 79) 41 TS children and 38 controls; ANeA, ANA antistreptococcal antibodies Measured	Inconclusive. Suggest that longitudinal measurements should be evaluated before definitive conclusions are drawn on associations between TS, ADHD, or OCD and ANeA, ANA streptococcal titers.
Cardona et al., 2004	(N = 23) Children (22 boys, 1 female) with tic disorder and possible strep were evaluated by echocardiography & GAS culture and ASO during a 5-yr period.	Of the 12 patients with echocardiographic abnormalities, 10 displayed very high antistreptolysin O (ASO) titers, 5 showed positive cultures for GAS, and 9 had abnormal ESR. The pathophysiology of GAS-infection related tic disorders is similar to that SC in some of the cases.
Muller et al., 2004	29 TS patients and 29 controls; M. pneumoniae titers were assessed via MAG and immunoblot.	Elevated titers and higher number of IgA-positive pts in the TS group were found, suggesting a role for M. pneumoniae in a subgroup of patients with TS.
Mell et al., 2005	(N = 318) Population-based data (1992–1999) from a West Coast health insurance organization. Children aged 4–13 years with OCD, TS, or tic disorder and matched controls were evaluated for an association between streptococcal infection and increased risk of new OCD, TS, or tic disorder.	Findings demonstrated PANDAS may arise as a result of postinfection autoimmunity response to childhood streptococcal infection.

(Continued)

Table 9.1 (*Continued*)

Reference	Sample Characteristics	Findings/Conclusions
Leslie et al., 2008	(N = 742) Insurance database used to compare occurrence of GAS infection (otitis media, sinusitis, and noninfectious condition [migraine] as control) in children aged 4–13 years with OCD, TS, other tic disorders, ADHD, or MDD newly diagnosed between Jan. 1998 and Dec. 2004. Matched controls (N = 3,647).	Subjects with newly diagnosed OCD, TS, tic disorder and ADHD, or MDD were more likely than controls to have had a diagnosis of streptococcal infection in the previous year or prior and therefore possibly establishing a temporal relationship.
Morer et al., 2008	32 prepubertal-onset OCD patients, N = 21 with TS, 19 controls ages 9–17 years	Anti-basal ganglia antibodies were not detected by immunohistochemistry in any sample. Data support the hypothesis of an autoimmune process underlying OCD or TS, although further research is needed.
Bombaci et al., 2009	Tic N = 21, GAS N = 239, and control N = 35. Antibody response to a representative panel of GAS antigens was compared in groups of patients with tic disorder, post-GAS pharyngitis and patients with neither tic disorder/overt GAS infection.	Tic patient sera exhibit immunological profiles that were broader and stronger than those of comparison groups but very similar to the post-GAS group.
Sanchez-Carpintero et al., 2009	22 children with non-comorbid ADHD and 22 controls	The frequency of ABGA in youth with non-comorbid ADHD does not differ from the control group. Those with ADHD were also found to have more recent GAS infections than controls, suggesting ABGA do not have a role in the pathogenesis of non-comorbid ADHD.

Study	Method	Findings
Schrag et al., 2009	Large primary care database was used to compare incidence of streptococcal infection in group with OCD, TS, and tics compared to a control group of matching age (2–25 yrs) and gender. N = 129 OCD patients and N = 2,211 matching controls; N = 126 TS/tic patients and N = 2,308 matching controls.	There was no overall increased risk of prior possible streptococcal infection in patients with a diagnosis of OCD, TS, or tics, but OCD patients had a slightly higher risk of history of possible streptococcal infection without prescription in the previous 2 yrs to the onset of OCD than the control population.
Krause et al., 2010	Association between neurotrophic agents, Chlamydia, Toxoplasma, and TS assessed in 32 TS patients and 30 healthy controls	Significantly higher rate of elevated antibody titers against *Chlamydia trachomatis* was found in TS patients compared to controls and may point to a possible role of Chlamydia and Toxoplasma in the pathogenesis of tic disorders.
Murphy et al., 2012	(N = 109) Children with tics and/or OCD assessed for medical history and three streptococcal antibodies; 41 considered "PANDAS"	Youth with PANDAS (vs. without PANDAS) were likely to have dramatic onset, definite remissions, remission of neuropsychiatric symptoms during antibiotic therapy, history of tonsillectomies/adenoidectomies, evidence of GAS infection, and clumsiness.

Prospective Longitudinal

Study	Method	Findings
Kiessling et al., 1994	IF staining to caudate in group of children referred for evaluation of neuropsychiatric disorders (N = 50, 24 with an associated movement disorder seen between June 1989 and June 1990). Replicated in children (N = 33, 21 with an associated movement disorder seen between June 1990 and November 1990).	In both samples, those with movement disorders were significantly more likely to have evidence of ANeA and to have at least one antistreptococcal titer elevated than were those without movement disorders. 44% were strongly positive for ANeA.

(Continued)

Table 9.1 (*Continued*)

Reference	Sample Characteristics	Findings/Conclusions
Murphy & Pichichero, 2002	(N = 12) School-aged children with new-onset PANDAS were assessed in relation to GABHS tonsillopharyngitis for a 3-yr period.	Exacerbations subsided after treatment with antibiotics after GABHS infections.
Luo et al., 2004	(N = 66) 47 Pediatric patients with TS and/or OCD and 19 controls were evaluated for newly acquired GABHS infections for 4 months.	The results suggest no clear relationship between new GAS infections and symptom exacerbations in an unselected group of patients with TS and/or OCD.
Murphy et al., 2004	(N = 25) Children with OCD and/or tic disorder (12 female, 13 male) evaluated for symptom severity and GAS antibody titers at 6-week intervals for up to 2 years.	In subjects with large symptom changes, positive correlations were found between ACHO and OCD severity rating changes. Patients with marked OCD/tic symptom changes may be characterized by prolonged GAS titer elevations and exhibit evidence of seasonal tic exacerbations.
Pavone et al., 2004	(N = 44) 22 PANDAS and 22 GABHS positive children were assessed by comparison of serum anti-brain antibody to human basal ganglia sections via indirect tissue IF.	14 PANDAS and 2 GABHS samples contained positive anti-basal ganglia staining. These results suggest that anti-brain antibodies are present in children with PANDAS that cannot be explained merely by a history of GABHS infection.
Perrin et al., 2004	(N = 814) Children aged 4 to 11 years seen for sore throat or well-child care to determine increase of symptom development among patients with strep evaluated for 12 weeks.	GAS infected, n = 411; GAS uninfected, n = 403. In GAS-infected individuals, PANDAS symptoms were more frequently noticed vs. the non-infected group, but no additional symptoms were noted in the following subsequent 12 weeks.

Study	Methods	Findings
Hoekstra et al., 2005	In a 24-week prospective longitudinal design study, two groups with tic disorder (children & adults) were evaluated to analyze the relationship between tic severity fluctuations and preceding infections.	In the pediatric group a strong association was noted but not in the adult group due to the limited number of streptococcal infections observed.
Murphy et al., 2007	(N = 693) Simultaneous throat cultures and relational analyses were made between GAS and movement/observation ratings for children (ages 3–12 years) for an 8-month period.	Combined behavior/GAS associations revealed a strong relationship; relative risk balance/swaying and non-tic grimacing were found to be responsible for a significant proportion of this association. Data identified a strong seasonal pattern, with significantly more GAS infections in autumn. Changes in motor function and behavior were identified in relationship to positive GAS culture with support that repeated GAS increases risk.
Kurlan et al., 2008	(N = 80) 40 matched PANDAS case-control pairs prospectively evaluated for GAS for a 2-year period	Symptom exacerbations in youth with PANDAS may be more vulnerable to GAS infections. GAS infection is not the only factor seen prior to exacerbations (accounted for 6/64 exacerbations) and therefore further studies will need to be conducted to determine the different subgroup factors.
Singer et al., 2008	(N = 12) Children with PANDAS, 8 boys and 4 girls; serum samples assessed at five time points	No correlation was identified between clinical exacerbations and autoimmune markers.
Lin et al., 2010	45 youth with TS and/or OCD compared to 41 controls over a 2-year period	A minority of youth with TS and early-onset OCD were sensitive to antecedent GAS infection. Infections also enhanced the predictive power of current psychosocial stress on future tic and OC symptom severity.
Leckman et al., 2011	31 subjects with PANDAS compared to 53 non-PANDAS assessed for clinical symptoms, throat cultures, and streptococcal antibody titers during a 25-month period	No group differences were found in the number of clinical exacerbations or the number of diagnosed GAS infections. Data suggest no evidence for a temporal association between GAS infections and tic/OCD symptom exacerbations in children with PANDAS.

(Continued)

Table 9.1 (*Continued*)

Reference	Sample Characteristics	Findings/Conclusions
Martino et al., 2011	168 youth with TS and 177 youth with epileptic or sleep disorders assessed for GAS infections, antistreptococcal, and anti-basal ganglia antibodies. Follow-up evaluations at 3-month intervals included 144 TS patients, assessing exacerbation of tics, OCD symptoms, and other psychiatric comorbidities.	TS patients exhibited higher frequency of GAS infections, higher ASO titers, and ABGA frequency than youth with epileptic or sleep disorders; may be a result of underlying immune dysregulation.
Randomized Control Trials		
Garvey et al., 1999	(N = 37) Double-blind, cross-over penicillin prophylaxis in PANDAS children enrolled for 8 months	Equal number of infections seen in both active and placebo phases. No significant change seen in OC or tic symptom severity between the two phases.
Perlmutter et al., 1999	(N = 29) Children with severe infection-triggered exacerbations of OCD or tic. 10 received plasma exchange, 9 received IVIG, and 10 got placebo. Children were recruited over a 4-year period for a 12-month study.	Plasma exchange and IVIG were both effective in lessening symptom severity for children with infection-triggered OCD and tic disorders.

Hallett et al., 2000	(N = 10) Animal study of subject rats (N = 5) and control rats (N = 5). Subject rats were infused with sera from TS children; control rats received sera from HC children. Rats observed for 10-day period.	Immunohistochemical analysis confirmed presence of IgG selectively bound to striatal neurons.
Taylor et al., 2002	(N = 36) Rats infused with sera from 12 TS patients with high levels of autoantibodies, 12 TS patients with low levels of autoantibodies, and 12 healthy controls. Rats' behavior was observed for 5 days after infusion.	Oral stereotypies significantly increased in rats infused with sera from patients with high levels of autoantibodies. The results are consistent with an autoimmune etiology in a subset of cases of TS.

Retrospective

Giulino et al., 2002	(N = 83) Onset assessment in children aged 6–17 years with primary diagnosis of OCD and primary caregivers	In URI-present versus URI-absent group, more patients experienced a sudden rather than insidious onset of symptoms. More patients with URI associated with sudden onset exhibited a comorbid tic disorder. Specific inquiry about OCD onset around time of URI should clue clinician to look prospectively for PANDAS.
Servello et al., 2011	(N = 272) Patients aged 17–77 years treated for various movement disorders, 39 were treated for treatment-refractory TS	In contrast to the overall rate of 3.7% for deep brain stimulation infection complications, those with TS receiving deep brain stimulation had a rate of 18%. It is unclear if this increase is due to disturbed immune function, inherent vulnerability to infections, or compulsive picking/touching the surgical site.

stress as a prediction of exacerbated symptom severity (Lin et al., 2010). Eleven of the 41 subjects were identified as meeting PANDAS criteria. The PANDAS group was at an increased risk for definite GAS infection compared to the normal control group and the non-PANDAS group. When analyzing the magnitude of worsening of tic symptoms, an increase in Yale Global Tic Severity Scale (YGTSS) scores was significantly greater in the infection group. A similar finding was noted in terms of obsessive-compulsive symptom severity. When analyzing the relationship between newly diagnosed GAS infections, measures of psychosocial stress, and future ratings of symptom severity within the patient group (using a pathway analysis of the relationships between longitudinally collected measures), it was concluded that a prior occurrence of definite or possible GAS infection and past levels of psychosocial stress were significantly associated with future worsening of tic severity. Similar results were noted when analyzing definite plus possible. Psychosocial stress and definite plus possible new diagnoses of GAS were significant predictors of future obsessive-compulsive symptom severity. The OCD severity was also a significant predictor of depressive symptoms. In an exploratory analysis of the data on the 11 PANDAS cases, the effect of definite or definite plus possible newly diagnosed GAS infections was even more significant in the PANDAS group. Based on these findings, it was concluded that GAS infections may cause a slight worsening of TS and OCD symptoms, and psychological stress continues to be a strong factor associated with future worsening of tic, obsessive-compulsive, and depressive symptoms.

Evidence of GAS relatedness will likely be a function of the acuity and characteristics of the clinical presentation. PANDAS, in its initial application, was intended to describe a child with a very severe and overnight onset of OCD, usually occurring a few days after or during a GAS infection. Tics were included due to the frequent co-occurrence with this presentation. Inconsistencies found across studies may have more to do with the selection of PANDAS cases, which varies across specialty clinics: a

tic specialty clinic may see fewer of these "classic" cases than an OCD specialty clinic. The possibility of other inciting agents was not on the forefront of initial studies. Furthermore, whereas GAS may be the instigating microbe at illness onset, the association may never be as evident in future exacerbations. This variability of presentation and triggers no doubt affects most biomarker studies. Even the acuity (also known as the duration of OCD/tic illness) can have profound effects on biomarker status as the individual moves from an acute inflammatory state to a chronic autoimmune state. These dilemmas were discussed at an NIH meeting in the summer of 2010 that resulted in a white paper on pediatric acute-onset neuropsychiatric syndrome (PANS) (Swedo et al., 2012) to describe this acute-onset subtype of OCD. As currently proposed, PANS is intended to be a broader phenotype (does not require a specific infectious trigger, no requirement to be prepubertal) but does move tics from a primary criterion to one of seven neuropsychiatric symptom categories, of which two categories are required to accompany the OCD primary category. Although further refinement of PANS is expected, these current criteria should aid in distinguishing this presentation from the typical waxing and waning of a chronic tic disorder.

INFECTION-RELATED RISKS

While not a novel observation, infection has become a major focus of neuropsychiatric research, with observations of immunological abnormalities and increased pathogen seroprevalence associated with several neuropsychiatric disorders. Other neurological disorders, such as MS and SC, have been the subject of similar observations, with significant immunological disruptions and serological evidence of infection that seem to correlate with symptom onset and/or exacerbations, particularly in SC. Strong genetic contributions have also been noted in these disorders, with evidence of strong familial associations with genetic polymorphisms that appear to confer increased disease susceptibility. Observations from tic disorders, once thought to be of the SC sequelae, have alluded to a similar etiology as there has been a strong causative association with infection and symptom onset and/or exacerbation as well as immunological irregularities similar to what is seen in SC and similar disorders. Although now a distinct clinical category, these similarities, which include neuropsychiatric comorbidities, an apparent infectious trigger, and an immune-mediated mechanism, may help to explain the role of infection in tics and similar disorders.

Genetic Susceptibility

While infection may serve as the precipitating event in tic disorders, genetic variability has been shown to play a major role in susceptibility, disease onset and progression, symptomatology, and severity. The role of genetics can be appreciated when one compares the clinical course of disorders characterized by single-gene etiologies to more complex disorders. While single-gene disorders such as fragile X syndrome often have well-defined etiologies and a homogeneous set of core symptoms, disorders such as MS and tics often have significant genetic variability and a heterogeneous phenotypic nature. In MS, for example, the high degree of heritability confirms a strong genetic etiology, although genetic variations within this population have made isolating a particular genetic culprit difficult. The major genetic variants observed in these individuals have been polymorphisms associated with immune regulation, which may account for the significant role immunological responses seem to play in these disorders. What seems to be most probable is the presence of genetic variants that confer increased susceptibility not only via alternations in neurochemical pathways but also via modulation of immunological responses to infection and other immune triggers. Polymorphisms in immune genes have been particularly prevalent within the MS population, particularly genes of the MHCII family, which correspond to regulation of T- and B-cell populations (Field et al., 2010; Haines et al., 1998). An example of this mechanism can be seen with Epstein-Barr virus (EBV) infection. Known to cause mononucleosis in adolescents and young adults, it is estimated that 90% of the population is infected with EBV, although only 30% to 50% of those infected develop the clinical illness (CDC, 2006). EBV has also been strongly associated with MS, evidenced by an increased seroprevalence of viral antibodies within this population (Salvetti et al., 2009; Vetsika & Callan, 2004). While immunological irregularities, particularly T-cell abnormalities, are a consistent finding in MS, there have also been findings of increased levels of EBV-specific CD8+ T-cell activation during the early course of the disease, suggesting a role for genetic susceptibility to disease development following infection and an altered immunological response to the pathogen in disease onset (Jilek et al., 2008). Similar observations have been made in GAS pharyngitis and the resulting sequelae such as rheumatic fever (RF), SC, and tics. Epidemiological studies indicate that the same streptococcal strain can cause infection of varying severity in different individuals, suggesting that host factors play an important role in determining the morbidity of GAS infections. Polymorphisms in Toll-like receptor (TLR) 4 have been found to be associated with vulnerability to recurrent GAS infection, while tumor necrosis factor alpha (TNF-α) polymorphisms have been implicated in conferring an increased susceptibility to the development of RF (Liadaki et al., 2011; Ramasawmy et al., 2007). Additionally, patients with a propensity to produce high levels of pro-inflammatory cytokines in response to GAS products are noted to exhibit severe clinical manifestations (Goldmann et al., 2003). For example, very young children or those with a mild immune deficiency may have atypical immune responses to GAS. This may be important when considering genetic susceptibility to infection-mediated disorders. In the case of bacterial pharyngitis infection, for example, GAS accounts for approximately 20% of infections, although only 2% to 3% of untreated GAS patients will develop RF, suggesting that genetic variability may play an important role in conferring infection and disease vulnerability (Murphy & Goodman, 2002). Additionally, elevations in B-cell antigen D8/17 have been a common observation and a suggested marker of disease susceptibility (Hoekstra et al., 2001).

Studies by several groups have found similar elevations TS and tic disorders, also thought to be GAS-mediated disorders (Hollander et al., 1999; Murphy et al., 1997). These findings further show how genetic variations, particularly in immune-related genes, can confer increased susceptibility to disease development. Within the tic population, only a subset of individuals will have an association with GAS at symptom onset, and of these, not all will show exacerbationswitheveryinfection.Howmuchthe individual's genetic composition versus the microbe's unique serotype contributes to susceptibility is unknown. These issues, coupled with conflicting research as to the severity and acuity of the studied populations, have contributed to the debate about the role of GAS infection in tics.

Compromised Blood–Brain Barrier

While genetics may play an important role in identifying individuals at risk for the development of infection-mediated neurological pathologies such as tics, it does little to explain the mechanism behind this connection. The propensity for immune-related genes to be implicated in these disorders, however, suggests a prominent role for the immune system and immune dysfunction in determining the course of these disorders and may hint at a potential pathological mechanism. The tendency for chorea or similar neurological pathologies to be associated with autoimmune disorders, or for chorea-like disorders to have "autoimmune"-type components, further suggests a strong connection between infection, immunological disruptions, and neurological disturbances. Disruptions in cell populations, which control immunological response, particularly those of an antigenic nature, as well as altered cytokine and inflammatory responses may contribute significantly to disease pathology. Autoantibody-mediated effects have been implicated in autoimmune disorders as well as chorea disorders (Baizabal-Carvallo & Jankovic, 2012; Park et al., 2012). In SC there have been observations of streptococcal antibodies against neuronal proteins in areas of the brain such as the basal ganglia. There is continued debate as to

plausibility of this mechanism, as it is not completely understood how autoantibodies would gain access to the CNS (Holman et al., 2011).

There are organs in the human body that enjoy immune privilege, most notably the brain, eye, testis, and fetal uterus. Due to a low level of complement, low MHC expression, tight junctions, and the relative lack of lymphatics, the cells of the immune system have great difficulty obtaining access to these tissues. Despite the lack of defined lymphatics in the brain, 14% to 47% of radiolabeled albumin injected into the CNS can be recovered in cervical lymph (Knopf et al., 1998), suggesting a connection between the CNS and the lymphatic system by which inflammatory cells could gain access to the CNS. In fact, studies have confirmed the presence of immune cells even under physiological conditions (Hickey, 1999; Miller, 1999), as Cserr and coworkers have demonstrated that elevated IgG to foreign, soluble proteins can be found in the cerebrospinal fluid of rats with an intact blood–brain barrier (BBB; Cserr & Knopf, 1992). These observations strengthen the role of aberrant production of autoreactive antibodies that can cross the BBB, allowing for reactive neuroimmunomodulation after microbial infections. It is known in other autoimmune diseases involving the CNS (MS, for example) that activation of the inflammatory cascade, with resultant production of cytokines and other immune factors, leads to increased BBB permeability and an influx of inflammatory cells (Abbott, 2000). This is an important consideration mechanistically given the immunological cascade following GAS infections.

The BBB may prove to be an important site in explaining the pathological mechanism behind GAS-mediated tic disorder. While the primary mechanism by which infection induces brain pathology is by viral entry or physical disruption of the BBB, secondary effects of infection, particularly the activation of neuroimmune pathways, may have a significant effect on BBB function and permeability. Microbes often affect innate and adaptive immune responses, resulting in immune activation that leads to cross-activation of neuroimmune pathways responsive to similar activating effectors that may not parallel their function in the periphery. BBB permeability is affected by several immunological factors, including cytokines such as TNF-α, and nitric oxide, a known vasodilator (McColl et al., 2008; Shukla et al., 1995). While streptococcus may not directly affect the BBB in the classical sense, its activation of the immune system may have a significant influence on the BBB and ultimately CNS function. Changes in cytokine expression, for example, may have a significant impact on BBB permeability. For example, the infusion of TNF-α into the circulation induces the activation of inflammatory cells on the CNS side of the BBB, including enhanced MHC expression and synthesis of eicosanoids, facilitating passage of lymphocytes through the BBB (Hickey, 1999; Tsuge et al., 2010). Likewise, soluble immune-activating factors such as interleukin (IL)-12, IL-6, and TNF-α released during GAS infection (Loof et al., 2008) may contribute to autoantibody production or affect transport of cytokines across the BBB via the circumventricular organs, activating the endothelium and leading to further vascular permeability (Banks et al., 1995). Cross-reactive B cells, possibly to a CNS epitope, could lead to intrathecal productivity of antibody (Knopf et al., 1998). Another important consideration is the role of the collective interaction of genetic vulnerabilities, their effect on immune function, and their reaction to pathogenic stimuli. A potential mechanism for these effects may lie in the collective interaction of genetic variants, which result in altered immunological responses. Altered responses in TNF-α, for example, whose polymorphisms have been shown to confer increased susceptibility to RF, can affect BBB permeability and antibody localization to brain regions. This in turn will affect disease onset and severity.

There is still the need for more research to address lingering questions concerning the mechanism linking GAS infection to tic pathology. The development of animal models continues to yield valuable insight; however, a true clinical representation is still elusive. Brimberg and colleagues (2012) inoculated rats with GAS antigen and showed that antibody production induced OCD behaviors. In these experiments, antibody penetration of the BBB was completely dependent on the injection of an additional bacterial adjuvant into the intraperitoneal cavity, which does not parallel what happens in children with tic disorders. Zhang and colleagues (2012) suggested that subcutaneous injections of monoclonal anti-streptococcus IgM induces stereotypies in a mouse, as well as Fos-like immunoreactivity in subregions of the caudate, nucleus accumbens, and motor cortex. While these studies do not answer all questions concerning the pathological mechanism of GAS infection in tics, they provide valuable insight into the relationship between GAS infection and autoantibody-mediated neuropsychiatric pathology. Particularly, antibody localization to the stratum, thalamus, and frontal cortex may help explain why specific neuropsychiatric symptoms have been associated with GAS infection and tic disorders.

Pathogen-Specific Attributes

While host factors seem to play the most critical role in determining disease progression in infection-related neurological disorders such as tics, pathogen characteristics may prove to play an equally important role. Characteristics such as virulence factors and antibiotic resistance are particularly important in determining postinfection prognosis. While host genetics will influence who may be at risk for infection and postinfection disorders, pathogenic factors may heavily influence host immunological responses, and in some instances may act in an almost synergistic manner to precipitate adverse outcomes. In the case of GAS, for example, host genetic variations may leave one patient at an increased risk for GAS sequelae such as RF and tics, while a particular GAS strain may be a genetic variant that confers increased virulence and antibiotic resistance. While it is clear that host genetics may determine which individuals are more susceptible to developing sequelae, bacterial attributes may determine how these pathogens behave in the clinical presentation of the disease and in the response to treatment. Virulent factors of particular importance include those that control immune suppression, immune evasion, and colonization. Interestingly, these factors are often controlled by genes readily mutated by pathogens to improve their survival. A key example of how these factors can influence the disease course and clinical presentation can again be illustrated with GAS. Although the majority of GAS infections lead to transient and non–life-threatening illnesses, some individuals develop more severe disorders such as necrotizing fasciitis as well as autoimmune sequelae such as RF and SC. Pathogenic factors that have been shown to contribute to these outcomes include improved immune evasion and immune suppression. In the case of necrotizing fasciitis, for example, several GAS strains have been shown to have transitioned from noninvasive to invasive, and to have improved colonization capabilities and the ability to evade host immunological attacks. This occurred by recombination of different strains and mutation in genes controlling DNase, superantigens, and other virulent factors (Lynskey et al., 2011). In the case of RF or tics, the ability of GAS to modulate immune function may be an important factor in determining disease course. In genetically vulnerable individuals, this may pave the way for sequelae. These mutations may also affect the clinical presentation via an indirect mechanism. Molecular mimicry, for example, is thought to be vital to the pathogenic mechanism in SC, tics, and other GAS-mediated disorders whereby antigenic interactions are implicated in disease pathology. M proteins, one of the major streptococcal virulence factors, have been shown to possess antigenic determinants that are shared with heart tissue, and are believed to be the main source of antigenic mimicry (Oehmcke et al., 2010). In RF, research has shown that specific GAS strains may be associated with a differential risk of the individual developing RF (Smoot et al., 2002) or necrotizing fasciitis (Cole et al., 2011). The same may be true of PANDAS. In the past decade, a greater degree of allelic and clinical diversity has been appreciated with respect to GAS infections (Musser & Shelburne, 2009). To date, over 80 serotypes of GAS have been described, with 150 alleles of the M protein, 89 alleles of speB, and 269 alleles of the Sic protein known to exist. In fact, 16 of the 44 known GAS proteins have been found to be immunogenic (Cunningham, 2012).

Some of these suspected virulence factors were not present in earlier strains of GAS—possibly due to the fact the GAS genome randomly reassorts over time or via horizontal gene transfer (Musser & Shelburne, 2009), increasing the chance of new virulence factors developing. One new virulence factor leads to the degradation of IL-8. This reassortment has also been used to explain the development of antibiotic resistance. The potential involvement for GAS superantigens in postinfection autoimmunity has been discussed (Williams et al., 2005). Clinical evidence that GAS may be changing is reflected in changes in the clinical manifestations of illnesses caused by GAS. In the outbreaks of RF in the mid-1980s, a higher representation of certain serotypes and mucoid strains of GAS was noted, and a large proportion of individuals had only mild or no history of prior pharyngitis. Reports suggest that the incidence of scarlet fever and necrotizing fasciitis has increased dramatically in the past few decades (Lynskey et al., 2011).

The relationship between tics and infection seems to be an interplay between pathogenic and host genetic variations, therefore, that ultimately determines not only which subset of the population becomes affected but also the clinical presentation. This can be appreciated in a clinical context when one considers the heterogeneity in symptom severity, presentation, and susceptibility in PANDAS patients and other diseases correlated with infection and/or immune dysfunction. Although it may be appealing to consider these in isolation, it is important to appreciate that host genetic variation and pathogenic genetic variation are two important components that alone may not be relevant but when considered together may explain clinical anomalies observed in these complex disorders.

INFECTION-RELATED MARKERS

The predominant theory at this time to explain the pathophysiology of PANDAS is molecular mimicry. Molecular mimicry occurs when antibodies intended to target the microbe also target self proteins. Many of the potential GAS antigens share or match human antigens such as cardiac and skeletal myosin, tropomyosin, vimentin, laminin, keratin, enolase, and so forth (Cunningham, 2009). Potential mechanisms by which autoantibodies cause clinical manifestations in CNS diseases include direct stimulation or blockade of receptors in the basal ganglia, or immune complexes promoting inflammation of these brain regions. In support of a CNS inflammatory response, basal ganglia enlargement was observed in volumetric neuroimaging of subjects with PANDAS (Giedd et al., 2000), and antineuronal antibody binding to basal ganglia tissue was found in both patients with PANDAS (Pavone et al., 2004) and patients with ADHD (Sanchez-Carpintero et al., 2009). In SC, anti-basal ganglia antibodies (ABGA) binding correlates with symptom severity (Church et al., 2002; Husby et al., 1976; Kotby et al., 1998).

Research by Kirvan and colleagues (2003) suggests a neuropsychiatric significance of N-acetyl-beta-D-glucosamine, the dominant epitope of GAS carbohydrate; moreover, anti-carbohydrate A antibody (ACHO) measures the immune response to this GAS epitope (Bloem et al., 1988) and has been shown to fluctuate with symptom changes (Murphy et al., 2004). Monoclonal antibodies in SC patients that were targeted to N-acetyl-beta-D-glucosamine were noted to also show specificity to mammalian lysoganglioside, a CNS ganglioside that influences neuronal signal transduction (Kirvan et al., 2003, 2006). However, brain cross-reactivity of ACHO from a nonclinical sample was not found (Sabharwal et al., 2006). The type of antibodies used (polyclonal vs. monoclonal) may contribute to the discrepant findings.

Related to the mechanism of stimulating autoantibodies (e.g., Graves' disease), binding of autoantibodies to neuronal cell surface antigens may promote signal transduction, leading to the release of excitatory neurotransmitters, and may explain mechanistically the symptoms of SC and PANDAS. Sera from these SC and PANDAS patients contained antibodies that targeted human neuronal cells and specifically induced calcium/calmodulin-dependent protein kinase II (CAMKII) activity, while sera from convalescing patients or from patients with other streptococcal-related diseases lacked activation of this enzyme. Patients with PANDAS were found to have an intermediate level of CAMKII activation relative to SC and healthy controls. CAMKII activity may demonstrate threshold effects on clinical presentation, as patients with PANDAS presenting with tics only showed the highest level of CAMKII activity, approaching that of SC. Activation of CAMKII has been shown to cause increased dopamine release in brain tissue, a potential mechanism by which clinical symptoms ensue (Kantor et al., 1999; Roberts-Lewis et al., 1986). In a large study, ABGA frequency was also higher in patients with TS (23%) versus a comparison group of youth with seizure or sleep disorders (8%). Within the TS group, no difference was noted in ABGA frequency whether the GAS culture was positive or negative (Martino et al., 2011).

In contrast, not all studies conducted have shown that anti-brain antibodies correlate with clinical exacerbations in PANDAS, and this is a topic of continued debate (Morer et al., 2008; Singer et al., 2008). For example, immunohistochemical techniques were used to identify serum anti-striatal antibody reactivity. In positive samples, double staining with anti-GFAP (glial) and anti-MAP2 (neuronal) was used to establish localization of the immunofluorescence (IF). No significant differences in IF or localization were identified in patients with PANDAS (N = 30) and TS (N = 30) compared to controls (N = 30). There was no correlation of IF with tic severity or elevated titers of antistreptococcal antibodies. However, the tic and the PANDAS groups had significantly elevated ASO and anti-DnaseB titers compared to the control group. Although this study did not find evidence of autoantibody-induced symptoms, it does not exclude a role for GAS in the pathophysiology of tics and PANDAS (Morris et al., 2009). Another study used SH-SY5Y cells, which possess many characteristics of dopaminergic neurons (Brilot et al., 2011). For example, these cells express tyrosine hydroxylase and dopamine-beta-hydroxylase, as well as the dopamine transporter. Using flow cytometry, serum IgG cell surface binding was measured in patients with SC (N = 11), PANDAS (N = 12), and TS (N = 11), and the results were compared to the findings in healthy controls (N = 11) and other neurologically affected controls (N = 11). The mean IgG cell surface binding was significantly higher in the SC group compared to all other groups (*p* < .001). By contrast, there was no difference between the PANDAS or TS groups and the controls. However, approximately half of SC group did not show increased binding, suggesting that sensitivity is low. In any case, this finding does not support an autoantibody mechanism for TS or PANDAS (tic-predominant presentation) for this specific assay.

While there has been disagreement as to the pathogenicity of antigenic mimicry or autoreactive autoantibodies, the adaptive immune system may yield other evidence of dysfunction of this arm of the immune system with the finding of T-cell, B-cell, and cytokine irregularities. A large proportion of current research into the pathophysiology of PANDAS has focused on the role of alterations in the adaptive and innate immune function of affected youth. Using flow cytometry techniques, Kawikova and colleagues (2007) found lower numbers of Tregs (CD4+/CD25+ T cells) in the peripheral blood of 37 children with TS and/or OCD compared to healthy children. The reduction of Tregs was most noticeable in TS patients with higher disease severity or during symptom exacerbations. This finding, if replicated, might be explained by a prolonged reaction to persisting foreign antigens, such as GAS, potentially leading to a compensatory loss. Weisz and colleagues (2004) found that the percentages of CD19-positive B cells was significantly elevated in RF and TS patients, as well as GAS pharyngitis patients, suggesting a role for inflammation and/or autoimmunity in the pathogenesis of these disorders. An increased frequency of activated B lymphocytes is also supported by a higher density of immunoglobulin receptors on the surface of B cells in these patients (Hoekstra et al., 2004).

Specific effector molecules, including cytokines, differentially modulate the activity of innate and adaptive immune systems. Leckman and colleagues (2005) measured plasma levels of a broad array of cytokines in 46 pediatric TS patients and 31 healthy controls, reporting increased baseline levels of TNF-α and IL-12 (Leckman et al., 2005). Of note, there was a 50% to 60% rise of these two cytokines, plus a general increase of all the main cytokines explored, during periods of tic symptom exacerbation. However, these combined cytokine and clinical fluctuations were more frequent in the non-PANDAS than in PANDAS cases. In contrast, Singer and colleagues (2008) found no association between clinical exacerbations in a very small prospective study. Serial serum samples were available on 12 children with PANDAS. Six subjects had a well-defined clinical exacerbation in association with a documented streptococcal infection, and six had a clinical exacerbation without an associated streptococcal infection. All of the serum samples were assayed for antibodies against human postmortem caudate, putamen, and prefrontal cortex; commercially prepared antigens; and complex sugars. Cytokines were measured by two different methodologies. No correlation was identified between clinical exacerbations and autoimmune markers.

ASSESSMENT AND TREATMENT

PANDAS diagnostic criteria are not always carefully applied in community settings (Gabbay et al., 2008), probably due to uncertainty about how to apply the course criteria and excessive emphasis on isolated elevations in streptococcal titers. In a tic specialty clinic, 31 (17.6%) of 176 patients received a diagnosis of PANDAS from community-based clinicians, and 19 of these subjects (61.3%) were judged as receiving a false-positive diagnosis of PANDAS (i.e., did not meet the full criteria described by Swedo and colleagues, 1998) by expert clinicians. The diagnosis was made for youth with OCD and/or tic symptoms who had only a single documented elevation in ASO titer; in some cases, the diagnosis was made without any documented laboratory evidence. A single documented elevation in ASO and/or anti-DNASeB indicates only previous exposure to streptococcal bacteria but does not give any indication of temporal association with the onset of tics and OCD. In 3.9% of the sample, the experts judged that a PANDAS classification was missed by community clinicians. Of the 31 subjects with community diagnoses of PANDAS, 27 (87%) were given antibiotics for either acute treatment of the index episode or prophylaxis. The duration of treatment ranged from brief courses (1 week) to long-term prophylaxis for up to 4 years, with 82% of these subjects receiving treatment without laboratory evidence of an infection. Certainly, the unwarranted use of antibiotics in children without objective laboratory evidence of infection could increase antibiotic resistance in the pediatric population. The gold standard for making the case for GAS relatedness would require either documentation of infection with a subtype that previously had not been present or, ideally, documentation of serial streptococcal titers showing a temporal relationship between the onset of symptoms and the titer rise. When compared to baseline levels, an increase of 0.2 log or greater in streptococcal titers following the onset of tic/OCD symptoms would be considered strong evidence for a correlation. Simply demonstrating the presence of elevated titers after the onset of OCD/tic symptoms is insufficient, as elevated titers are common in the 7- to 12-year-old group, even among children without symptoms of pharyngitis (Johnson et al., 2010).

In clinical settings, these lines of evidence are rarely obtained. It would be uncommon for a clinician to have baseline titers for a patient prior to or at the onset or exacerbation of tic/OCD symptoms. Further, in clinical practice, cultures are generally not subtyped for specific strains of GAS; rather, they are used to determine the presence or absence of an infection, which then guides treatment with an antibiotic. In one study of pediatricians, 79% reported that they would treat a presumed GAS infection with antibiotics without a positive culture (Paluck et al., 2001). Most children presenting with a PANDAS-like presentation do not have this level of documentation to support GAS infection. The frequency or dose of exposure and the clonotype of the infectious agent will also need to be considered. These difficulties in confirming a diagnosis of GAS infection lead to the ambiguity and skepticism in establishing the GAS relatedness to OCD/tic onset.

During the history-gathering process, careful attention should be given to reports of repeated, frequent infections, evidence of GAS in a young child (e.g., unexplained abdominal pain accompanied by fever), scarlet fever, brief episodes of tics, OCD or remitted compulsive urination, and especially sudden onset of OCD or tics accompanying an infectious illness. Males appear to be at a higher risk, as three quarters of PANDAS subjects are male (Swedo et al., 1998). Females have a slightly higher risk for developing SC, suggesting a gender dimorphic vulnerability to GAS. Another factor of susceptibility is age. If we use the RF model, RF and tic onset is rare in postpubertal subjects.

In patients with abnormal neurological findings such as muscle weakness, abnormal reflexes (slow return of patellar reflex [i.e., "hung-up"]) or chorea, further workup is indicated. In patients with new-onset OCD or tics, or recent symptom exacerbation, a throat culture is a relatively benign procedure that will help rule out the possibility of subclinical GAS infection-triggered symptoms. Streptococcal titers obtained at symptom onset should be repeated to examine for a rise in titers 4 to 6 weeks later. In patients with onset exceeding 4 weeks prior, streptococcal titers add some support but do not provide definitive proof of a streptococcal trigger. However, elevated titers may not be seen in very young patients. As many children who present with PANDAS are very young (3–6 years old), age-adjusted titer thresholds are recommended, since many laboratories use threshold values (e.g., elevation levels of an ASO of 200 IU/mL or DNAse of 400 IU/mL or higher) (Renneberg et al., 1989).

Proof that antimicrobial prophylaxis significantly reduces recurrence and/or exacerbation of tics would suggest a supportive role for infectious agents. By examining the scant literature on antibiotics used to prevent SC recurrences, the problems involved in determining efficacy become apparent. Although prophylactic antibiotic therapy in patients with SC appears successful in preventing neuropsychiatric exacerbations (Gebremariam, 1999), other investigators report that about a third of patients will continue to have a recurrence (Terreri et al., 2002). Studies in which SC patients received monthly prophylactic injections of benzathine penicillin G showed that not all SC recurrences appear to be triggered by GAS (Korn-Lubetzki et al., 2004), and that recurrences may occur after infections too mild or too brief to be easily detected (Berrios et al., 1985). While these studies suggest that some improvement in course occurs after prophylactic antibiotics, sample sizes were small, none of the studies were blinded, and since most patients with SC are encouraged to take prophylactic antibiotics until their late teens, no comparison data exist on the overall neuropsychiatric severity of those receiving treatment versus those who do not (Carapetis and Currie 1999); (Goldenberg et al. 1992); (Taranta 1959); (Gebremariam, 1999).

While the PANDAS hypothesis remains unsettled, the current treatment for patients meeting the PANDAS criteria continues to be the standard-of-care practices for patients with TS. Treatment studies have faced criticisms of study design and small sample size (Kurlan & Kaplan, 2004). A clinical trial involving the use of prophylactic oral penicillin in treating apparent episodes of PANDAS found no conclusive evidence that the antibiotic reduced clinical exacerbations (Garvey et al., 1999), likely due to the control group's frequent use of antibiotics. An active comparator trial comparing penicillin and azithromycin (Snider et al., 2005) was also considered inconclusive (Budman et al., 2005; Gilbert & Gerber, 2005). In this study, 11 subjects were maintained on penicillin and 12 on azithromycin during the 12-month study. Subjects randomized to both drugs had fewer streptococcal infections as well as fewer neuropsychiatric exacerbations during the study year, with no side effects or reports of adverse effects from the medications. The authors suggest that both antibiotics may be safe and effective in preventing GAS infection and in decreasing the number of neuropsychiatric exacerbations in these children. The main criticisms for this study were the comparison of retrospective data for the baseline year to prospective data of the treatment year and the use of an active comparator. Anecdotal reports by patients receiving antibiotics (in clinical settings) suggest that

some beta-lactam antibiotics are more effective than penicillin. Studies are needed first to establish antibiotic efficacy and second to determine which antibiotic is most efficacious in improving neuropsychiatric symptoms. Another issue to be addressed is that antibiotics may serve an additional, non-antimicrobial role in the treatment of some disorders (Rothstein et al., 2005), although this has not yet been supported by clinical studies for tic disorders. Anecdotal reports of tic symptom improvement after 2 to 6 weeks of antibiotic treatment suggest other possible mechanisms besides prevention of reinfection. One possible mechanism is that antibiotics decrease the antigenic load from undetected and asymptomatic intracellular GAS (Sela et al., 2000). Another possibility is via cytokine modulation. GAS is a potent inducer of interferon gamma (IFNγ) and most pro-inflammatory cytokines (Miettinen et al., 1998). Penicillin perhaps plays a synergistic role in symptom improvement by specifically conjugating to IFNγ and reducing IFNγ's activity (Brooks et al., 2003, 2005). Interesting but not fully explored parallels are that selective serotonin reuptake inhibitors (SSRIs), which are currently the pharmacological treatment of choice for OCD, have been found to exert anti-inflammatory effects by suppressing IFNγ (Kubera et al., 2001). GAS infections have been reported to also lead to tryptophan degradation, which may influence serotonin function (Murr et al., 2001). Antibiotic therapy, theoretically, could allow for normalization of tryptophan levels. Moreover, beta-lactam antibiotics may serve an additional, non-antimicrobial role in the treatment of some disorders. A screening of FDA-approved medications found that beta-lactam antibiotics such as ceftriaxone and penicillin promoted the expression of glutamate transporter GLT1 and demonstrated a neuroprotective role *in vivo* and *in vitro* when used in models of ischemic injury and motor neuron degeneration, both based in part on glutamate toxicity. These findings indicate that positive promoters of GLT1 expression may have a unique role in neuroprotection in neurological disorders such as amyotrophic lateral sclerosis (Rothstein et al., 2005), and the potential role of glutamatergic therapies in neuropsychiatric disorders

(Pittenger et al., 2006). Tic symptom improvement during antibiotic therapy may not only be secondary to antimicrobial effects but may also highlight the potential for multiple roles of antibiotics that would open the door for other mechanisms in tic pathophysiology and treatment.

The results of a plasmapheresis or intravenous immunoglobulin (IVIG) trial in the treatment of children with PANDAS add additional support for an immune-mediated pathology of OCD and tics (Perlmutter et al., 1999). These treatment gains, however, appear to be specific to children who *clearly* meet the criteria for PANDAS, as plasma exchange in four children with severe *chronic* OCD did not result in significant improvements (Nicolson et al., 2000), and IVIG did not show efficacy for patients with tic disorders (Hoekstra et al., 2004). For these patients, it is possible that a previous immune-mediated process resulted in a chronic neurological state that is less responsive to immune therapies or that this group represented patients with non–immune-mediated etiologies for their illness.

EVALUATING FOR SIMILAR PRESENTATIONS

Neurological sequelae, including myoclonus (DiFazio et al., 1998), poststreptococcal basal ganglia encephalopathy (Dale et al., 2001), and restless legs syndrome (Matsuo et al., 2004), have reported associations with GAS, suggesting that GAS may elicit a wide array of phenotypes that render varying degrees of overlap with RF. It is the absence of frank chorea and absence of carditis that differentiates PANDAS from SC. Subtle signs of neurological impairment have been reported to be associated with PANDAS (Swedo et al., 1998); however, neuropsychological dysfunction is commonly reported with tics/OCD (Bloch et al., 2006; Kuelz et al., 2004), and those with PANDAS may not have a differentiating neuropsychological profile when compared to youth with typical (non-PANDAS) OCD and TS (Hirschtritt et al., 2009). An evaluation of 26 children with PANDAS revealed an association between elevated GAS titers and neurocognitive deficits, with marked impairment in visuospatial recall memory (Lewin et al., 2011). It

---

Box 9.1. Key Points

- Several associations between infections, particularly SC and GAS infections, and subsequent TS and OCD symptoms have been established, suggesting at least a nonspecific role of infections in a subgroup of patients with tics.
- In the late 1990s, NIMH researchers further characterized an entity they called pediatric autoimmune neuropsychiatric disorders associated with streptococcus (PANDAS).
- Children with PANDAS are more likely to have dramatic-onset ("overnight") neuropsychiatric symptoms, remission of OCD or tic symptoms during antibiotic treatment, and evidence of GAS infections.
- Laboratory evidence of exposure to streptococcal bacteria does not confirm a PANDAS diagnosis and the absence of antibody elevations does not disprove the diagnosis.
- Although more evidence exists supporting the exacerbation of neuropsychiatric symptoms due to GAS infections, evidence also exists that Mycoplasma pneumonia, respiratory infections, the common cold, and even stress have been linked to exacerbation of OCD and tic symptoms.
- The complex interaction of patient-specific attributes (neurochemical and immune vulnerability genes leading to maladaptive neuropsychiatric or immune function) with environmental attributes (psychosocial stress, injuries, substance exposures, and pathogen-specific properties) creates an interesting and ongoing research challenge.

is estimated that rheumatic carditis is found in 30% to 64% of all SC patients, while data do not support a risk of developing rheumatic carditis for a child originally presenting with GAS-triggered OCD or tics (Cardona et al., 2004; Segarra & Murphy, 2008; Snider et al., 2004).

CONCLUSION AND FUTURE DIRECTIONS

Preliminary data suggest at least a nonspecific role of infections in a subgroup of patients with tics. In some cases, the findings have not been replicated. Since a widely accepted association between GAS and tics has yet to be established, the criteria for diagnosis of PANDAS will likely undergo iterative processing before reaching a final resolution.

From a nosologic viewpoint, the pathogenesis of PANDAS is postulated to be due to an infection by GAS that triggers an autoimmune state. The immune response to GAS could produce a misreading of self-epitopes, and it is this immunoreactivity that results in exacerbations with repeat GAS infections and possibly other infectious agents. Host susceptibility certainly contributes to the predisposition to develop PANDAS, and evidence supports familial risks for PANDAS, tics, and OCD. Genetic vulnerability to this type of immune response is supported by some documentation of PANDAS in multiple siblings (Dranitzki & Steiner, 2007); however, the presentation can also be notably discordant in identical siblings (Lewin et al., 2011).

The complex interaction of patient-specific attributes (neurochemical and immune

---

Box 9.2. Questions for Future Research

- What criteria should be used to determine if tics are triggered by infection? Spectrum presentations may not exclude an associated immune risk for tics/OCD. PANDAS criteria will need to undergo an iterative process to improve sensitivity and specificity.
- Is GAS unique in inciting tics/OCD or does another immune vulnerability exist regardless of the microbe that leads to tic presentation? Is GAS most often implicated due its high prevalence in children? Is the mechanism due to molecular mimicry or to a flawed immune/CNS communication during inflammatory events?
- How do various proposed infectious agents (e.g., GAS, Mycoplasma, influenza, perhaps Borrelia) differ in inciting tics? How are they the same?
- Do children with tic disorders have an innate overreaction to GAS?
- What will improvement in tics following immune treatment tell us about the pathophysiology of tics? Will this provide support for an infectious trigger or hint at aberrant immunological function? What role will treatment play to distinguish between those with PANDAS and those without?
- What phenotypic differences are needed to clearly delineate PANDAS from SC? Do children with PANDAS clearly differ in terms of genetic and environmental risks from those with RF?
- What is the course of PANDAS? Do these children remit, become chronic, or develop other disorders?
- If antibiotics or IVIG is found helpful, what is the optimal formulation, dose, and treatment duration?
- Will other immune therapies treat PANDAS/PANS? What role do the usual psychotherapeutic medications play in terms of altering immune function in a relevant manner for PANDAS? Does this subtype of children respond differently to tic evidence-based treatment?

vulnerability genes leading to maladaptive neuropsychiatric or immune function) with environmental attributes (psychosocial stress, injuries, substance exposures, and pathogen-specific properties) will certainly make this an interesting research challenge. Several studies are under way to examine immune-based therapies, susceptibility, triggers, host–pathogen interactions, and neuropathological process in PANDAS that may help in the understanding of not only PANDAS, but also pediatric tic disorders and other related neuropsychiatric presentations.

REFERENCES

Abbott NJ. Inflammatory mediators and modulation of blood–brain barrier permeability. *Cell Mol Neurobiol* 2000; *20*:131–147.

Allen AJ, Leonard HL, Swedo SE. Case study: a new infection triggered, autoimmune subtype of pediatric OCD and Tourette's syndrome. *J Am Acad Child Adolesc Psychiatry* 1995; *34*:307–311.

Antonelli F, Borghi V, Galassi G et al. Can HIV infection cause a worsening of tics in Tourette patients? *Neurol Sci* 2011; *32*:191–192.

Baizabal-Carvallo JF Jankovic J. Movement disorders in autoimmune diseases. *Mov Disord* 2012; *27*:935–946.

Banks WA, Kastin AJ, Broadwell RD. Passage of cytokines across the blood–brain barrier. *Neuroimmunomodulation* 1995; *2*:241–248.

Benatar A, Beatty DW, Human DG. Immunological abnormalities in children with acute rheumatic carditis and acute post-streptococcal glomerulonephritis. *Int J Cardiol* 1988; *21*:51–58.

Berrios X, Quesney F, Morales A et al. Are all recurrences of "pure" Sydenham chorea true recurrences of acute rheumatic fever? *J Pediatr* 1985; *107*:867–872.

Bloch MH, Peterson BS, Scahill L et al. Adulthood outcome of tic and obsessive-compulsive symptom severity in children with Tourette syndrome. *Arch Pediatr Adolesc Med* 2006; *160*:65–69.

Bloem A, Zenke G, Eichmann K, Emmrich F. Human immune response to group A streptococcal carbohydrate (A-CHO). II. Antigen-independent stimulation of IgM anti-A-CHO production in purified B cells by a monoclonal anti-idiotopic antibody. *J Immunol* 1988; *140*:277–282.

Bombaci M, Grifantini R, Mora M et al. Protein array profiling of tic patient sera reveals a broad range and enhanced immune response against group A streptococcus antigens. *PLoS One* 2009; *4*:e6332.

The first published study to provide evidence that sera from tic patients exhibit immunological profiles typical of those who elicited a broad, specific, and strong immune response to GAS.

Bornstein RA, Stefl ME, Hammond L. A survey of Tourette syndrome patients and their families: the 1987 Ohio Tourette Survey. *J Neuropsychiatry Clin Neurosci* 1990; *2*:275–281.

Brilot F, Merheb V, Ding A et al. Antibody binding to neuronal surface in Sydenham chorea, but not in PANDAS or Tourette syndrome. *Neurology* 2011; *76*:1508–1513.

Brimberg L, Benhar I, Mascaro-Blanco A et al. Behavioral, pharmacological, and immunological abnormalities after streptococcal exposure: A novel rat model of Sydenham chorea and related neuropsychiatric disorders. *Neuropsychopharmacology* 2012; *37*:2076–2087.

Brooks BM, Hart CA, Coleman JW. Differential effects of beta-lactams on human IFN-gamma activity. *J Antimicrob Chemother* 2005; *56*:1122–1125.

Brooks BM, Thomas AL, Coleman JW. Benzylpenicillin differentially conjugates to IFN-gamma, TNF-alpha, IL-1beta, IL-4 and IL-13 but selectively reduces IFN-gamma activity. *Clin Exp Immunol* 2003; *131*:268–274.

Budman C, Coffey B, Dure L et al. Regarding "Antibiotic prophylaxis with azithromycin or penicillin for childhood-onset neuropsychiatric disorders." *Biol Psychiatry* 2005; *58*:916–917.

Cardona F, Orefici G. Group A streptococcal infections and tic disorders in an Italian pediatric population. *J Pediatr* 2001; *138*:71–75.

Cardona F, Romano A, Cundari G et al. Colour Doppler echocardiography in children with group A streptococcal infection related tic disorders. *Indian J Med Res* 2004; *119*(Suppl):186–190.

CDC. *Epstein-Barr Virus and Infectious Mononucleosis* 2006. Available online at: http://www.cdc.gov/ncidod/diseases/ebv.htm.

Chappell P, Riddle M, Anderson G et al. Enhanced stress responsivity of Tourette syndrome patients undergoing lumbar puncture. *Biol Psychiatry* 1994; *36*:35–43.

Charmandari E, Kino T, Souvatzoglou E, Chrousos GP. Pediatric stress: hormonal mediators and human development. *Horm Res* 2003; 59:161–179.

Church AJ, Cardoso F, Dale RC et al. Anti-basal ganglia antibodies in acute and persistent Sydenham's chorea. *Neurology* 2002; 59:227–231.

Cole JN, Barnett TC, Nizet V, Walker MJ. Molecular insight into invasive group A streptococcal disease. *Nat Rev Microbiol* 2011; 9:724–736.

Cserr HF, Knopf PM. Cervical lymphatics, the blood-brain barrier and the immunoreactivity of the brain: a new view. *Immunol Today* 1992; 13:507–512.

Cunningham M, Perry H. *Autoimmunity and behavior: Sydenham's chorea and related disorders.* Paper presented at the 9th International Congress of Neuroimmunology Fort Worth, Texas (October 28, 2009).

Cunningham MW. Streptococcus and rheumatic fever. *Curr Opin Rheumatol* 2012; 24: 408–416.

Dale RC, Church AJ, Cardoso F et al. Poststreptococcal acute disseminated encephalomyelitis with basal ganglia involvement and auto-reactive antibasal ganglia antibodies. *Ann Neurol* 2001; 50:588–595.

DiFazio MP, Morales J, Davis R. Acute myoclonus secondary to group A beta-hemolytic streptococcus infection: A PANDAS variant. *J Child Neurol* 1998; 13:516–518.

Dranitzki Z, Steiner I. PANDAS in siblings: a common risk? *Eur J Neurol* 2007; 14:e4.

Field J, Browning SR, Johnson LJ et al. A polymorphism in the HLA-DPB1 gene is associated with susceptibility to multiple sclerosis. *PLoS One* 2010; 5:e13454.

Gabbay V, Coffey BJ, Babb JS et al. Pediatric autoimmune neuropsychiatric disorders associated with streptococcus: comparison of diagnosis and treatment in the community and at a specialty clinic. *Pediatrics* 2008; 122:273–278.

Garvey MA, Perlmutter SJ, Allen AJ et al. A pilot study of penicillin prophylaxis for neuropsychiatric exacerbations triggered by streptococcal infections. *Biol Psychiatry* 1999; 45:1564–1571.

Gebremariam A. Sydenham's chorea: risk factors and the role of prophylactic benzathine penicillin G in preventing recurrence. *Ann Trop Paediatr* 1999; 19:161–165.

Giedd JN, Rapoport JL, Garvey MA et al. MRI assessment of children with obsessive-compulsive disorder or tics associated with streptococcal infection. *Am J Psychiatry* 2000; 157:281–283.

Gilbert D, Gerber MA. Regarding "Antibiotic prophylaxis with azithromycin or penicillin for childhood-onset neuropsychiatric disorders." *Biol Psychiatry* 2005; 58:916.

Giulino L, Gammon P, Sullivan K et al. Is parental report of upper respiratory infection at the onset of obsessive–compulsive disorder suggestive of pediatric autoimmune neuropsychiatric disorder associated with streptococcal infection? *J Child Adolesc Psychopharmacol* 2002; 12:157–164.

Goldmann O, Chatwal GS, Medina E. Immune mechanisms underlying host susceptibility to infection with group A streptococci. *J Infect Dis* 2003; 187:854–861.

Haines JL, Terwedow HA, Burgess K et al. Linkage of the MHC to familial multiple sclerosis suggests genetic heterogeneity. The Multiple Sclerosis Genetics Group. *Hum Mol Genet* 1998; 7:1229–1234.

Hallett JJ, Harling-Berg CJ, Knopf PM et al. Anti-striatal antibodies in Tourette syndrome cause neuronal dysfunction. *J Neuroimmunol* 2000; 111:195–202.

Hansen CR Jr, Bershow SA. Immunology of TS/ OCD. *J Am Acad Child Adolesc Psychiatry* 1997; 36:1648–1649.

Hickey WF. Leukocyte traffic in the central nervous system: the participants and their roles. *Semin Immunol* 1999; 11:125–137.

Hirschtritt ME, Hammond CJ, Luckenbaugh D et al. Executive and attention functioning among children in the PANDAS subgroup. *Child Neuropsychol* 2009; 15:179–194.

Hoekstra PJ, Bijzet J, Limburg PC et al. Elevated D8/17 expression on B lymphocytes, a marker of rheumatic fever, measured with flow cytometry in tic disorder patients. *Am J Psychiatry* 2001; 158:605–610.

Hoekstra PJ, Manson WL, Steenhuis MP et al. Association of common cold with exacerbations in pediatric but not adult patients with tic disorder: a prospective longitudinal study. *J Child Adolesc Psychopharmacol* 2005; 15:285–292. **An association of viral infections and tic exacerbations in children was found, adding support to the role of the immune system in tic disorders.**

Hoekstra PJ, Minderaa RB, Kallenberg CG. Lack of effect of intravenous immunoglobulins on tics: a double-blind placebo-controlled study. *J Clin Psychiatry* 2004; 65:537–542.

Hollander E, DelGiudice-Asch G, Simon L et al. B lymphocyte antigen D8/17 and repetitive behaviors in autism. *Am J Psychiatry* 1999; *156*:317–320.

Holman DW, Klein RS, Ransohoff RM. The blood–brain barrier, chemokines and multiple sclerosis. *Biochim Biophys Acta* 2011; *1812*:220–230.

Husby G, van de Rijn I, Zabriskie JB et al. Antibodies reacting with cytoplasm of subthalamic and caudate nuclei neurons in chorea and acute rheumatic fever. *J Exp Med* 1976; *144*:1094–1110.

Jilek S, Schluep M, Meylan P et al. Strong EBV-specific CD8+ T-cell response in patients with early multiple sclerosis. *Brain* 2008; *131*:1712–1721.

Johnson DR, Kurlan R, Leckman J, Kaplan EL. The human immune response to streptococcal extracellular antigens: clinical, diagnostic, and potential pathogenetic implications. *Clin Infect Dis* 2010; *50*:481–490.

Kantor L, Hewlett GH, Gnegy ME. Enhanced amphetamine- and K+-mediated dopamine release in rat striatum after repeated amphetamine: differential requirements for Ca2+- and calmodulin-dependent phosphorylation and synaptic vesicles. *J Neurosci* 1999; *19*:3801–3808.

Kawikova I, Leckman JF, Kronig H et al. Decreased numbers of regulatory T cells suggest impaired immune tolerance in children with Tourette syndrome: a preliminary study. *Biol Psychiatry* 2007; *61*:273–278.

Kerbeshian J, Burd L, Pettit R. A possible post-streptococcal movement disorder with chorea and tics. *Dev Med Child Neurol* 1990; *32*:642–644.

Kiessling LS, Marcotte AC, Culpepper L. Antineuronal antibodies in movement disorders. *Pediatrics* 1993; *92*:39–43.

Results suggest prior GAS infections are associated with the presence of movement disorders.

Kiessling LS, Marcotte AC, Culpepper L. Antineuronal antibodies: tics and obsessive-compulsive symptoms. *J Dev Behav Pediatr* 1994; *15*:421–425.

Kirvan CA, Swedo SE, Heuser JS, Cunningham MW. Mimicry and autoantibody-mediated neuronal cell signaling in Sydenham chorea. *Nat Med* 2003; *9*:914–920.

Kirvan CA, Swedo SE, Kurahara D, Cunningham MW. Streptococcal mimicry and antibody-mediated cell signaling in the pathogenesis of Sydenham's chorea. *Autoimmunity* 2006; *39*:21–29.

Knopf PM, Harling-Berg CJ, Cserr HF et al. Antigen-dependent intrathecal antibody synthesis in the normal rat brain: tissue entry and local retention of antigen-specific B cells. *J Immunol* 1998; *161*:692–701.

Kondo K, Kabasawa T. Improvement in Gilles de la Tourette syndrome after corticosteroid therapy. *Ann Neurol* 1978; *4*:387.

Korn-Lubetzki I, Brand A, Steiner I. Recurrence of Sydenham chorea: implications for pathogenesis. *Arch Neurol* 2004; *61*:1261–1264.

Kotby AA, El Badawy N, El Sokkary S et al. Antineuronal antibodies in rheumatic chorea. *Clin Diagn Lab Immunol* 1998; *5*:836–839.

Krause D, Matz J, Weidinger E et al. Association between intracellular infectious agents and Tourette's syndrome. *Eur Arch Psychiatry Clin Neurosci* 2010; *260*:359–363.

Kubera N, Lin AH, Kenis G et al. Anti-inflammatory effects of antidepressants through suppression of the interferon-gamma/interleukin-10 production ratio. *J Clin Psychopharmacol* 2001; *21*:199–206.

Kuelz AK, Hohagen F, Voderholzer U. Neuropsychological performance in obsessive-compulsive disorder: a critical review. *Biol Psychol* 2004; *65*:185–236.

Kurlan R, Johnson D, Kaplan EL. Streptococcal infection and exacerbations of childhood tics and obsessive-compulsive symptoms: a prospective blinded cohort study. *Pediatrics* 2008; *121*:1188–1197.

Youth meeting published criteria for PANDAS were found to have increased symptom exacerbations and GAS infections compared with controls, along with a noted association between infections and exacerbations.

Kurlan R, Kaplan EL. The pediatric autoimmune neuropsychiatric disorders associated with streptococcal infection (PANDAS) etiology for tics and obsessive-compulsive symptoms: hypothesis or entity? Practical considerations for the clinician. *Pediatrics* 2004; *113*:883–886.

Kushner HI, Kiessling LS. The controversy over the classification of Gilles de la Tourette's syndrome, 1800–1995. *Perspect Biol Med* 1996; *39*:409–435.

Langlois M, Force L. Nosologic and clinical revision of Gilles de la Tourette disease evoked by the action of certain neuroleptics on its course. *Rev Neurol* (Paris) 1965; *113*:641–645.

Leckman JF, Katsovich L, Kawikova I et al. Increased serum levels of interleukin-12 and tumor necrosis factor-alpha in Tourette's syndrome. *Biol Psychiatry* 2005; *57*:667–673.

Leckman JF, King RA, Gilbert DL et al. Streptococcal upper respiratory tract infections and exacerbations of tic and obsessive-compulsive symptoms: a prospective longitudinal study. *J Am Acad Child Adolesc Psychiatry* 2011; *50*:108–118.

Found no evidence for a temporal association between GAS infections and tic/OCD exacerbations in children with published criteria for PANDAS.

Leslie DL, Kozma L, Martin A et al. Neuropsychiatric disorders associated with streptococcal infection: a case-control study among privately insured children. *J Am Acad Child Adolesc Psychiatry* 2008; *47*:1166–1172.

Neuropsychiatric disorders were found to be temporally related to prior streptococcal infections.

Lewin, AB, Storch EA, Murphy TK. Pediatric autoimmune neuropsychiatric disorders associated with Streptococcus in identical siblings. *J Child Adolesc Psychopharmacol* 2011; *21*:177–182.

Lewin, AB, Storch EA, Mutch PJ, Murphy TK. Neurocognitive functioning in youth with pediatric autoimmune neuropsychiatric disorders associated with streptococcus. *J Neuropsychiatry Clin Neurosci* 2011; *23*:391–398.

Liadaki K, Petinaki E, Skoulakis C et al. Toll-like receptor 4 gene (TLR4), but not TLR2, polymorphisms modify the risk of tonsillar disease due to *Streptococcus pyogenes* and *Haemophilus influenzae*. *Clin Vacc Immunol* 2011; *18*:217–222.

Lin H, Williams KA, Katsovich L et al. Streptococcal upper respiratory tract infections and psychosocial stress predict future tic and obsessive-compulsive symptom severity in children and adolescents with Tourette syndrome and obsessive-compulsive disorder. *Biol Psychiatry* 2010; *67*:684–691.

Loiselle CR, Wendlandt CR, Rohde CA, Singer HS. Antistreptococcal, neuronal, and nuclear antibodies in Tourette syndrome. *Pediatr Neurol* 2003; *28*:119–125.

Loof TG, Goldmann O, Medina E. Immune recognition of *Streptococcus pyogenes* by dendritic cells. *Infect Immun* 2008; *76*:2785–2792.

Lougee L, Perlmutter SJ, Nicolson R et al. Psychiatric disorders in first-degree relatives of children with pediatric autoimmune neuropsychiatric disorders associated with streptococcal infections (PANDAS). *J Am Acad Child Adolesc Psychiatry* 2000; *39*:1120–1126.

Luo F, Leckman JF, Katsovich L et al. Prospective longitudinal study of children with tic disorders and/or obsessive-compulsive disorder: relationship of symptom exacerbations to newly acquired streptococcal infections. *Pediatrics* 2004; *113*:e578–585.

Lynskey NN, Lawrenson RA, Sriskandan S. New understandings in *Streptococcus pyogenes*. *Curr Opin Infect Dis* 2011; *24*:196–202.

Martinelli P, Ambrosetto G, Minguzzi E et al. Late-onset PANDAS syndrome with abdominal muscle involvement. *Eur Neurol* 2002; *48*:49–51.

Martino D, Chiarotti F, Buttiglione M et al. The relationship between group A streptococcal infections and Tourette syndrome: a study on a large service-based cohort. *Dev Med Child Neurol* 2011; *53*:951–957.

Matsuo M, Tsuchiya K, Hamasaki Y, Singer HS. Restless legs syndrome: association with streptococcal or mycoplasma infection. *Pediatr Neurol* 2004; *31*:119–121.

McColl BW, Rothwell NJ, Allan SM. Systemic inflammation alters the kinetics of cerebrovascular tight junction disruption after experimental stroke in mice. *J Neurosci* 2008; *28*:9451–9462.

Mell LK, Davis RL, Owens D. Association between streptococcal infection and obsessive-compulsive disorder, Tourette's syndrome, and tic disorder. *Pediatrics* 2005; *116*:56–60.

This case-control study provided evidence suggesting that neuropsychiatric or behavioral disorders may arise as a result of a postinfectious autoimmune phenomenon.

Miettinen M, Matikainen S, Vuopio-Varkila J et al. Lactobacilli and streptococci induce interleukin-12 (IL-12), IL-18, and gamma interferon production in human peripheral blood mononuclear cells. *Infect Immun* 1998; *66*:6058–6062.

Miller DW. Immunobiology of the blood-brain barrier. *J Neurovirol* 1999; *5*:570–578.

Morer A, Lazaro L, Sabater L et al. Antineuronal antibodies in a group of children with obsessive-compulsive disorder and Tourette syndrome. *J Psychiatr Res* 2008; *42*:64–68.

Morris CM, Pardo-Villamizar C, Gause CD, Singer HS. Serum autoantibodies measured by immunofluorescence confirm a failure to differentiate PANDAS and Tourette syndrome from controls. *J Neurol Sci* 2009; *276*:45–48.

Morshed SA, Parveen S, Leckman JF et al. Antibodies against neural, nuclear, cytoskeletal, and streptococcal epitopes in children and adults with Tourette's syndrome, Sydenham's chorea, and autoimmune disorders. *Biol Psychiatry* 2001; 50:566–577.

Muller N, Kroll B, Schwarz MJ et al. Increased titers of antibodies against streptococcal M12 and M19 proteins in patients with Tourette's syndrome. *Psychiatry Res* 2001; 101: 187–193.

Muller N, Riedel M, Blendinger C et al. *Mycoplasma pneumoniae* infection and Tourette's syndrome. *Psychiatry Res* 2004; 129:119–125.

Muller N, Riedel M, Forderreuther S et al. Tourette's syndrome and *Mycoplasma pneumoniae* infection. *Am J Psychiatry* 2000; 157:481–482.

Muller N, Riedel M, Straube A et al. Increased anti-streptococcal antibodies in patients with Tourette's syndrome. *Psychiatry Res* 2000; 94:43–49.

Murphy ML, Pichichero ME. Prospective identification and treatment of children with pediatric autoimmune neuropsychiatric disorder associated with group A streptococcal infection (PANDAS). *Arch Pediatr Adolesc Med* 2002; 156:356–361.

Murphy T, Goodman W. Genetics of childhood disorders: XXXIV. Autoimmune disorders, part 7: D8/17 reactivity as an immunological marker of susceptibility to neuropsychiatric disorders. *J Am Acad Child Adolesc Psychiatry* 2002; 41:98–100.

Murphy T, Goodman WK, Fudge MW et al. B lymphocyte antigen D8/17: a peripheral marker for childhood-onset obsessive-compulsive disorder and Tourette's syndrome? *Am J Psychiatry* 1997; 154:402–407.

Murphy TK, Sajid M, Soto O et al. Detecting pediatric autoimmune neuropsychiatric disorders associated with streptococcus in children with obsessive-compulsive disorder and tics. *Biol Psychiatry* 2004; 55:61–68.

Murphy TK, Snider LA, Mutch PJ et al. Relationship of movements and behaviors to group A streptococcus infections in elementary school children. *Biol Psychiatry* 2007; 61:279–284.

Motor and behavioral changes were identified in relation to positive GAS cultures. Children with repeated GAS infections were found to have an increased risk for behavioral symptoms.

Murphy TK, Storch EA, Lewin AB et al. Clinical factors associated with pediatric autoimmune neuropsychiatric disorders associated with streptococcal infections. *J Pediatr* 2012; 160:314–319.

Clinical features associated with PANDAS were identified, advancing research support of a PANDAS subgroup by validating objective criteria compared with clinician impression.

Murr C, Gerlach D, Widner B et al. Neopterin production and tryptophan degradation in humans infected by *Streptococcus pyogenes*. *Med Microbiol Immunol* (Berl) 2001; 189:161–163.

Musser JM, Shelburne SA 3rd. A decade of molecular pathogenomic analysis of group A streptococcus. *J Clin Invest* 2009; 119:2455–2463.

Nicolson R, Swedo SE, Lenane M et al. An open trial of plasma exchange in childhood-onset obsessive-compulsive disorder without post-streptococcal exacerbations. *J Am Acad Child Adolesc Psychiatry* 2000; 39:1313–1315.

Oehmcke S, Shannon O, Morgelin M, Herwald H. Streptococcal M proteins and their role as virulence determinants. *Clin Chim Acta* 2010; 411:1172–1180.

Orvidas LJ, Slattery MJ. Pediatric autoimmune neuropsychiatric disorders and streptococcal infections: role of otolaryngologist. *Laryngoscope* 2001; 111:1515–1519.

Paluck E, Katzenstein D, Frankish CJ et al. Prescribing practices and attitudes toward giving children antibiotics. *Can Fam Physician* 2001; 47:521–527.

Park J, Kim JG, Park SP, Lee HW. Asymmetric chorea as presenting symptom in Graves' disease. *Neurol Sci* 2012; 33:343–345.

Pavone P, Bianchini R, Parano E et al. Anti-brain antibodies in PANDAS versus uncomplicated streptococcal infection. *Pediatr Neurol* 2004; 30:107–110.

Pelonero AL, Pandurangi AK, Calabrese V. Serum IgG antibody to herpes viruses in schizophrenia. *Psychiatry Res* 1990; 33:11–17.

Perlmutter SJ, Garvey MA, Castellanos X et al. A case of pediatric autoimmune neuropsychiatric disorders associated with streptococcal infections. *Am J Psychiatry* 1998; 155: 1592–1598.

Perlmutter SJ, Leitman SF, Garvey MA et al. Therapeutic plasma exchange and intravenous immunoglobulin for obsessive-compulsive disorder and tic disorders in childhood. *Lancet* 1999; 354:1153–1158.

Perrin EM, Murphy ML, Casey JR et al. Does group A beta-hemolytic streptococcal infection increase risk for behavioral and neuropsychiatric symptoms in children? *Arch Pediatr Adolesc Med* 2004; 158:848–856.

Peterson BS, Leckman JF, Tucker D et al. Preliminary findings of antistreptococcal antibody titers and basal ganglia volumes in tic, obsessive-compulsive, and attention deficit/hyperactivity disorders. *Arch Gen Psychiatry* 2000; 57:364–372.

Pittenger C, Krystal JH, Coric V. Glutamate-modulating drugs as novel pharmacotherapeutic agents in the treatment of obsessive-compulsive disorder. *NeuroRx* 2006; 3:69–81.

Ramasawmy R, Fae KC, Spina G et al. Association of polymorphisms within the promoter region of the tumor necrosis factor-alpha with clinical outcomes of rheumatic fever. *Mol Immunol* 2007; 44:1873–1878.

Read SE, Reid HF, Fischetti VA et al. Serial studies on the cellular immune response to streptococcal antigens in acute and convalescent rheumatic fever patients in Trinidad. *J Clin Immunol* 1986; 6:433–441.

Renneberg J, Soderstrom M, Prellner K et al. Age-related variations in anti-streptococcal antibody levels. *Eur J Clin Microbiol Infect Dis* 1989; 8:792–795.

Roberts-Lewis JM, Welsh MJ, Gnegy ME. Chronic amphetamine treatment increases striatal calmodulin in rats. *Brain Res* 1986; 384:383–386.

Rothstein JD, Patel S, Regan MR et al. Beta-lactam antibiotics offer neuroprotection by increasing glutamate transporter expression. *Nature* 2005; 433:73–77.

Sabharwal H, Michon F, Nelson D et al. Group A streptococcus (GAS) carbohydrate as an immunogen for protection against GAS infection. *J Infect Dis* 2006; 193: 129–135.

Salvetti M, Giovannoni G, Aloisi F. Epstein-Barr virus and multiple sclerosis. *Curr Opin Neurol* 2009; 22:201–206.

Sanchez-Carpintero R, Albesa SA, Crespo N et al. A preliminary study of the frequency of anti-basal ganglia antibodies and streptococcal infection in attention deficit/hyperactivity disorder. *J Neurol* 2009; 256:1103–1108.

Schrag A, Gilbert R, Giovannoni G et al. Streptococcal infection, Tourette syndrome, and OCD: is there a connection? *Neurology* 2009; 73:1256–1263.

Segarra AR, Murphy TK. Cardiac involvement in children with PANDAS. *J Am Acad Child Adolesc Psychiatry* 2008; 47:603–604.

Sela S, Neeman R, Keller N, Barzilai A. Relationship between asymptomatic carriage of *Streptococcus pyogenes* and the ability of the strains to adhere to and be internalised by cultured epithelial cells. *J Med Microbiol* 2000; 49:499–502.

Selling L. The role of infection in the etiology of tics. *Arch Neurol Psychiatry* 1929; 22: 1163–1171.

Servello D, Sassi M, Gaeta M et al. Tourette syndrome (TS) bears a higher rate of inflammatory complications at the implanted hardware in deep brain stimulation (DBS). *Acta Neurochir (Wien)* 2011; 153:629–632.

Shukla A, Dikshit M, Srimal RC. Nitric oxide modulates blood–brain barrier permeability during infections with an inactivated bacterium. *Neuroreport* 1995; 6:1629–1632.

Singer HS, Gause C, Morris C, Lopez P. Serial immune markers do not correlate with clinical exacerbations in pediatric autoimmune neuropsychiatric disorders associated with streptococcal infections. *Pediatrics* 2008; 121:1198–1205.

Singer HS, Giuliano JD, Hansen BH et al. Antibodies against a neuron-like (HTB-10 neuroblastoma) cell in children with Tourette syndrome. *Biol Psychiatry* 1999; 46:775–780.

Singer HS, Giuliano JD, Zimmerman AM, Walkup JT. Infection: a stimulus for tic disorders. *Pediatr Neurol* 2000; 22:380–383.

Smoot LM, McCormick JK, Smoot JC et al. Characterization of two novel pyrogenic toxin superantigens made by an acute rheumatic fever clone of *Streptococcus pyogenes* associated with multiple disease outbreaks. *Infect Immun* 2002; 70:7095–7104.

Snider LA, Lougee L, Slattery M et al. Antibiotic prophylaxis with azithromycin or penicillin for childhood-onset neuropsychiatric disorders. *Biol Psychiatry* 2005; 57:788–792.

Snider LA, Sachdev V, McKronis JE et al. Echocardiographic findings in the PANDAS subgroup. *Pediatrics* 2004; 114:e748–751.

Swedo SE. Sydenham's chorea. A model for childhood autoimmune neuropsychiatric disorders. *JAMA* 1994; 272:1788–1791.

Swedo SE, Leckman JF, Rose NR. From research subgroup to clinical syndrome: Modifying the PANDAS criteria to describe PANS (pediatric acute-onset neuropsychiatric syndrome). *Pediatr Therapeut* 2012; 2:2–8.

This article discusses the potential diagnostic criteria for PANS.

Swedo SE, Leonard HL, Garvey M et al. Pediatric autoimmune neuropsychiatric disorders associated with streptococcal infections: clinical description

of the first 50 cases. *Am J Psychiatry* 1998;
155:264–271.

This is the first report to identify and describe a subgroup of children meeting the working diagnostic criteria for PANDAS.

Swedo SE, Rapoport JL, Cheslow DL et al. High prevalence of obsessive-compulsive symptoms in patients with Sydenham's chorea. *Am J Psychiatry* 1989; 146:246–249.

Taylor JR, Morshed SA, Parveen S et al. An animal model of Tourette's syndrome. *Am J Psychiatry* 2002; 159:657–660.

Terreri MT, Roja SC, Len CA et al. Sydenham's chorea—clinical and evolutive characteristics. *Sao Paulo Med J* 2002; 120:16–19.

Tsuge M, Yasui K, Ichiyawa T et al. Increase of tumor necrosis factor-alpha in the blood induces early activation of matrix metalloproteinase-9 in the brain. *Microbiol Immunol* 2010; 54:417–424.

Tucker DM, Leckman JF, Scahill L et al. A putative poststreptococcal case of OCD with chronic tic disorder, not otherwise specified. *J Am Acad Child Adolesc Psychiatry* 1996; 35:1684–1691.

Vetsika EK, Callan M. Infectious mononucleosis and Epstein-Barr virus. *Expert Rev Mol Med* 2004; 6:1–16.

von Economo CV. *Encephalitis lethargica. Its sequelae and treatment.* Oxford, England: Oxford University Press, 1931.

Weiss M, Garland J. More on PANDAS [letter]. *J Am Acad Child Adolesc Psychiatry* 1997; 36:1163–1165.

Weisz JL, McMahon WM, Moore JC et al. D8/17 and CD19 expression on lymphocytes of patients with acute rheumatic fever and Tourette's disorder. *Clin Diagn Lab Immunol* 2004; 11:330–336.

Williams KA, Grant JE, Schlievert PM, Kim S. Exploring the pathophysiology of PANDAS, Streptococcus, Sydenham's, and superantigens. In S. H. Fatemi (Ed.), *Neuropsychiatric disorders and infection* (pp. 162–170), 2005. United Kingdom: Taylor & Francis.

Yis U, Kurul SH, Cakmakci H, Dirik E. *Mycoplasma pneumoniae*: nervous system complications in childhood and review of the literature. *Eur J Pediatr* 2008; 167:973–978.

Zhang D, Patel A, Zhu Y et al. Anti-streptococcus IgM antibodies induce repetitive stereotyped movements: cell activation and co-localization with Fcalpha/mu receptors in the striatum and motor cortex. *Brain Behav Immun* 2012; 26: 521–533.

SECTION 3

PATHOPHYSIOLOGY

10

Cellular and Molecular Pathology in Tourette Syndrome

FLORA M. VACCARINO, YUKO KATAOKA-SASAKI AND JESSICA B. LENNINGTON

Abstract

This chapter summarizes the available literature data on pathological findings in Tourette syndrome. In Tourette syndrome there are decreases in parvalbumin + gamma-aminobutyric (GABA)-ergic interneurons and cholinergic interneurons in the caudate and putamen. There is also loss of the normal distribution (highest in associative regions, intermediate in sensorimotor regions, and lowest in limbic regions) of cholinergic interneurons. There are no evident changes in choline acetyl-transferase distribution in striosomes versus matrix. There may also be changes in another interneuron population, the nitric oxide synthase (NOS)-containing interneurons. These findings are discussed in light of current views on the pathogenic mechanisms underlying tic disorders.

INTRODUCTION

The basal ganglia are considered a central station in the regulation of motor programs. Although the function of the basal ganglia is not entirely known, their circuitry has been extensively investigated. The basal ganglia are a set of nuclei situated deep within the cerebral cortical hemispheres. In the basal ganglia, a large number of cortical and subcortical excitatory inputs converge on a relatively small number of neurons whose firing represents complex temporal coincidence of neural activity in a vast number of afferent regions. Paradoxically, however, the main function of the basal ganglia is to exert negative regulation by tonically inhibiting ongoing neural activity in the thalamus. However, arousing stimuli that travel through the ascending reticular activating system, and those that, having been associated with the anticipation of rewards, activate the dopamine system, temporarily suppress the negative regulation of the basal ganglia, resulting in facilitation of sensory and motor functions. In this way the basal ganglia regulate the initiation of complex motor sequences and the execution of habits and in general facilitate the integration of voluntary and involuntary segments of cognitive and motor activity.

Patients with Tourette syndrome (TS) have a decreased volume of the caudate (CD) and putamen (PT) in the striatum (Peterson et al., 1993, 2003), the first station of the basal ganglia receiving inputs from the cerebral cortex, the thalamus, and midbrain dopamine neurons (Fig. 10.1). Although both cortical and cerebellar anatomical abnormalities have been described in subsequent neuroimaging studies of TS individuals (Frederiksen et al., 2002; Peterson et al., 2001; Sowell et al., 2008; Tobe et al., 2010; reviewed in Felling & Singer, 2011), the decrease in caudate volume has particular relevance since reduced volume of the caudate nucleus in childhood correlates significantly and inversely with the severity of tic and obsessive-compulsive disorder (OCD) symptoms in early adulthood (Bloch et al., 2005). Furthermore, in monozygotic twins discordant for severity of TS, the right CD was smaller in the most severely affected twin pair (Hyde et al., 1995). Overall, the neuroimaging studies suggest that the basal ganglia are a central component of the pathophysiology of TS (see also Chapter 12).

BASAL GANGLIA ANATOMY AND CIRCUITRY

The hypothesis that an inherited or developmentally acquired dysfunction of the basal ganglia causes TS is in agreement with studies in a variety of animal models suggesting that the basal ganglia are the main "integrators" of higher motor and cognitive functions (see also Chapter 15). One of their key functions is to select among ongoing sensorimotor activities based on their salience and motivational value, by integrating the activity of the dopamine system, which is activated by the anticipation of rewards, with sensory, motor, and attentional systems, which are channeled to the striatum via the thalamus and the cerebral cortex. Indeed, the CD and PT receive direct inputs from the cerebral cortex, the thalamus, and midbrain dopamine neurons. The final common output of the basal ganglia is the internal segment of the globus pallidus/substantia nigra reticulata (GPi/SNr), which tonically inhibits the ventral anterior and ventral lateral (VA/VL) and intralaminar (IL) thalamic nuclei, suppressing motor activity (Fig. 10.1A). It has been hypothesized that failure to integrate sensorimotor information within the basal ganglia may lead to the development of tics (see Chapter 11 on electrophysiology).

The medium spiny neurons (MSNs) of the CD and PT are projection neurons of the striatum that form two major pathways, the indirect and direct pathway, which have opposite effects on the GPi/SNr and behavior (Albin et al., 1989). The *direct pathway* inhibits the GPi/SNr, resulting in excitation of thalamic neurons and facilitation of motor behavior; conversely, the *indirect pathway* indirectly excites the GPi/SNr by inhibiting the subthalamic nucleus, inhibiting motor behavior (Fig. 10.1A).

The striatum, based on its cortical inputs, contains three major functional territories: the associative, sensorimotor, and limbic (Fig. 10.1B). These functional domains are largely segregated throughout the striatum. The associative territory

comprises almost the whole extension of the CD and the precommissural PT. The sensorimotor domain includes the dorsolateral aspect of the CD head, part of the dorsal precommissural PT, and the entire postcommissural PT. The main component of the limbic striatum is the nucleus accumbens, the deep layers of the olfactory tubercle, and the ventral part of both the CD and the PT (Parent, 1990). The corticostriatal projections terminate in the form of clusters of various sizes, whose distribution closely follows that of the two major striatal chemical compartments—the striosomes and the extrastriosomal matrix. Studies of the nonhuman primate have shown differential patterns of connectivity for the striosome and matrix compartments in the striatum (Eblen & Graybiel, 1995; Flaherty & Graybiel, 1993). Striosomes are interconnected with regions linked to limbic circuitry, and the matrix is interconnected with sensorimotor and associative cortical circuitry.

INTERNEURONS IN THE BASAL GANGLIA AND THEIR FUNCTIONAL IMPLICATIONS FOR DISORDERS

Recent evidence has shown important modulatory roles of striatal interneurons on these two pathways. There are four classes of interneurons within the striatum, identified by their expression of calcium binding proteins and co-transmitters: (1) parvalbumin (PV); (2) calretinin (CR); (3) somatostatin/nitric oxide synthase/neuropeptide Y (SST/NOS/NPY); and (4) cholinergic or choline acetyl transferase (ChAT)-positive neurons.

The fast-spiking, PV-positive interneurons form a non-habituating striatal inhibitory network (Kawaguchi et al., 1995; Kita et al., 1990), which is the main source of feed-forward inhibition from the cortex to the striatum. PV cells receive strong cortical synaptic input (Lapper et al., 1992) and respond with shorter latency than MSNs to cortical stimulation, preferentially suppressing the activity of MSNs of the *direct pathway* (Gittis et al., 2010, 2011; Mallet et al., 2005) (Fig. 10.1A).

The cholinergic interneurons have been long thought to play a role in associative

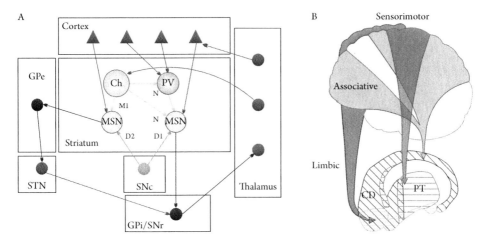

FIGURE 10.1 **The basal ganglia.** (**A**) Basal ganglia circuitry. *Red*, excitatory glutamatergic neurons; *blue*, inhibitory neurons; *green*, cholinergic neurons, *orange*, dopaminergic neurons. PV interneurons mediate the cortical feed-forward inhibition upon MSNs of the striatopallidal direct pathway, resulting in inhibition of voluntary movements. Cholinergic interneurons enhance the responsiveness of MSNs of the striatonigral indirect pathway, resulting in movement suppression. (**B**) Functional subdivisions of the basal ganglia projected on a lateral view of the basal ganglia and their cortical afferent systems. (See color insert.)

(Based upon Parent et al., 1990, and Bernacer et al., 2007.)

learning (Aosaki et al., 1994) and fire tonically with periodic pauses, which temporally coincide with burst firing in dopamine neurons. Cholinergic neurons receive a strong excitatory input from the median-parafascicular complex (IL) nuclei of the thalamus (Lapper & Bolam, 1992) (Fig. 10.1A). Cholinergic interneurons excite SST/NOS/NPY striatal interneurons, which in turn inhibit MSNs (English et al., 2012). Hence, MSNs can be inhibited directly by PV interneurons and indirectly by cholinergic neurons via the SST/NOS/NPY interneurons.

Most striatal MSNs are silent, except for those MSNs that are involved in the initiation of particular movements and related cognitive activity. This global suppression of MSN activity is caused by activation of the cortex and IL nuclei of the thalamus, which, in turn, feed upon two prominent inhibitory systems, the PV and SST/NOS/NPY GABAergic interneurons, respectively. Hence, any interference with striatal interneuron activity, or with their activation by their cortical and thalamic afferents, is expected to cause aberrant movement initiation, such as dyskinesias and tics.

BASAL GANGLIA INTERNEURONS IN TS

Our group reported the first unbiased and systematic neurological study of TS in 2005 (Kalanithi et al., 2005). It showed a disturbance in number or maturation of PV interneurons using stereology in postmortem basal ganglia tissue from three subjects with severe, persistent adult TS compared with age- and sex-matched normal controls (NCs). In this study, staining with cresyl violet, PV, met-enkephalin (enk), and substance P (SP) demonstrated a selective defect in striatal PV+ neurons but no demonstrable change in total neuron or glial cell numbers in the individuals examined. A follow-up study demonstrated a 50% to 60% decrease of PV and cholinergic interneurons in the CD and PT of five individuals with TS compared to matched NCs (Kataoka et al., 2010).

Our first study showed a decrease in PV+ cell densities in the CD (51%) and in the PT (37%) of the three subjects with TS, whereas an increase in PV+ cells was observed in the GPi (122%) in tissue from TS subjects. Immunostaining for SP and met-enk, neuropeptides contained within MSNs of the direct and indirect pathways, respectively, showed no differences in the apparent density or distribution between the NC and TS groups (Kalanithi et al., 2005).

Consistent with these preliminary results, in a subsequent more comprehensive study involving five cases of TS and matched NCs, we found a 55.7% decrease in the density of PV+ interneurons in the striatum of TS individuals (Fig. 10.2) (Kataoka et al., 2010). In this study, we also examined other classes of interneurons, CR and ChAT, as well as DARPP-32+ MSNs and cresyl violet-stained total neurons. There was no difference in the number of medium-sized CR+ interneurons (10–20 μm) between NC and TS individuals, whereas the density of large-sized CR+ interneurons (24–42 μm), 80% of which co-localize ChAT, was decreased by 52.9% in the TS group. This deficit of cholinergic interneurons was confirmed using ChAT immunostaining and stereology, showing a 49.4% decrease in ChAT+ neuron density in the TS striatum

(Fig. 10.2). Specifically, the overall density (cells/mm³, mean ± SEM) of ChAT+ cells in the NC and TS striatum was 213.6 ± 22.9 and 108.1 ± 22.9, respectively; the difference was highly significant by ANOVA [F $(1, 8)= 10.641$, $p = .011$] (Kataoka et al., 2010). Cholinergic cells represent less than 1% of the total number of neurons in the striatum; the density of cresyl violet-stained neurons in the striatum was not significantly different between the NC and TS groups, meaning that this combined decrease in PV+ and cholinergic interneurons in the striatum of TS patients is not attributable to a generalized neuronal loss. This specificity of changes in PV+ and cholinergic neuron density was also confirmed using DARPP-32 antibodies, demonstrating no significant change in MSNs.

We analyzed the distribution of cholinergic interneurons in the three main functional subdivisions of the striatum (the associative, sensorimotor, and limbic regions) to evaluate the

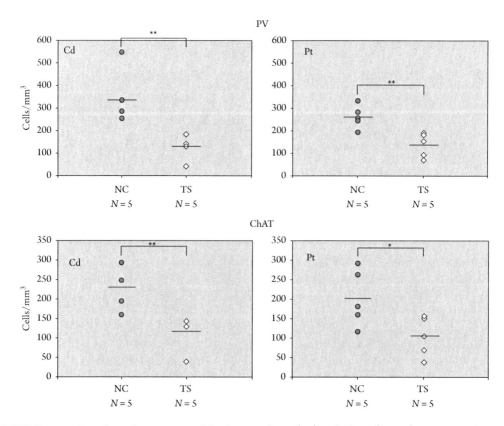

FIGURE 10.2 Stereological assessment of the density of PV+ (*top*) and ChAT (*bottom*) neurons in the caudate (Cd) and putamen (Pt), showing a significant reduction in patients with TS.

physiological implications of the above changes for cholinergic circuitry (Kataoka et al., 2010). ANOVA showed an overall significant effect of diagnosis (F $(1, 8)$ = 25.852; p = .001) and region (F $(2, 16)$ = 5.335; p = .017) and a significant interaction of diagnosis versus region (F $(2, 16)$ = 5.631; p = .014). Indeed, in NCs there was a gradient in the density of cholinergic neurons, with highest values in the associative and lowest in the limbic regions. Differences between associative and limbic and associative and sensorimotor neuron densities were both statistically significant in NC (Sidak post-hoc test, p = .016 and p = .031, respectively); in contrast, no significant difference was present among subregions in the TS striatum (Fig. 10.3). A comparison of the TS group with the NC group region by region by the Sidak post-hoc test indicated that the associative region showed the most pronounced decreases in cholinergic neuron density (60.0% decrease, p < .0005), followed by the sensorimotor region (44.7% decrease, p = .008), and that the limbic region was not significantly

different between TS and NC individuals (p = .402). In conclusion, cholinergic interneurons were decreased in TS patients in the associative and sensorimotor regions but not in the limbic regions of the striatum, such that the normal gradient in density of cholinergic cells (highest in associative regions, intermediate in sensorimotor, and lowest in limbic regions) was abolished (Fig. 10.3).

The remaining class of GABAergic interneurons, containing SST/NOS/NPY interneurons, was assessed using NOS immunostaining and stereology. There was a trend toward a decrease of NOS+ cell densities in the striatum of TS individuals (−45.4% in the CD, −53.2% in the PT), but it did not reach statistical significance (p = .0556 in the CD, p = .0542 in the PT). This trend is noteworthy since the SST/NOS/NPY interneurons are mediating the cholinergic-induced suppression of striatal activity, and thus act downstream of cholinergic cells in the striatal circuitry (English et al., 2012).

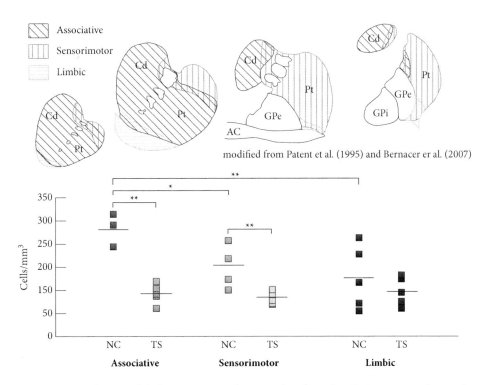

FIGURE 10.3 Distribution of cholinergic neuron density in basal ganglia of TS patients and normal controls (NC). *Red,* associative territory; *green,* somatosensory territory; *blue,* limbic territory. ** p < .001 by ANOVA. (See color insert.)

RNA-sequencing analyses performed on a total of 5 TS and 5 NC brains, of which only one TS brain overlapped with the previous immunocytochemical studies, suggested a significant decrease in ChAT at the transcript level (average fold change -27.2, $p = 5.42 \times 10^{-5}$). RT-PCR analyses done on a subset of these brains confirmed a strong trend toward the decrease in ChAT mRNA, although the RT-PCR values were not statistically significant due to sample variability. This parallel decrease in ChAT mRNA and protein suggests a possible loss of cholinergic neurons due to a developmental defect or a toxic or even neurodegenerative condition. However, it is also possible that the loss of neurons is only apparent, and that cholinergic cells are developmentally delayed or functionally altered and do not express ChAT message and protein at detectable levels. To approach this question, we looked at the expression of other cholinergic transcripts, using a dataset of cholinergic-enriched transcripts obtained by TRAP analyses in the mouse brain (Dougherty et al., 2010; Doyle et al., 2008). We found that, in addition to ChAT, five additional mRNAs enriched in cholinergic neurons (Ecel1, Lhx8, Slc18a3, Slc5a7, and TRPC3) are downregulated in the TS basal ganglia, lending support to the idea of an actual cell loss or widespread abnormality of the cholinergic system in TS. For example, the homeobox gene Lhx8, which controls the differentiation of cholinergic neurons, was decreased by -7.0 fold ($p = 9.17 \times 10^{-3}$); the vesicular acetylcholine transporter 3Slc18a3 was decreased by -5.2 fold ($p = 1.7 \times 10^{-2}$); and the choline transporter Slc5a7 was decreased by -148.1 fold ($p = 2.8 \times 10^{-7}$).

It was previously found that in an animal model of stereotypical behavior in which animals become sensitized by repeated cocaine administration, functional activation of basal ganglia neurons in the striosomes exceeded activation in the matrix, and this imbalance predicted the degree of motor stereotypy induced by the drug treatments (Canales & Graybiel, 2000). Thus, an imbalance in neuronal activity between these functional and neurochemical compartments (the striosomes and the matrix) may represent a neural correlate of motor stereotypy. Given the importance of the PV and cholinergic neurons for regulation of striatal activity, we mapped these cellular abnormalities within these functional territories to provide further insights into the circuitry that might function abnormally in TS given the presence of an inhibitory neuron defect in the striatum. In addition, a PV defect within the striosomes might secondarily affect the substantia nigra to which striosomes are interconnected and cause dopaminergic functional abnormalities (Minzer et al., 2004; for review see Felling & Singer, 2011).

We assessed the distribution of cholinergic and PV interneurons in the striosomes and matrix compartments of the striatum in both NC and TS subjects previously assessed for a global interneuron defect in the striatum. The results showed no significant changes in the compartmental distribution of both cholinergic and PV interneurons. In the middle portion of CD (from 7.2 mm anterior to the anterior edge of GPe to 7.2 mm posterior to the same edge), there was a trend toward an alteration in the PV+ neuron distribution (striosomes:matrix was 38%:62% in NC, whereas it was 20%:80% in TS), but it did not reach statistical significance ($p = .072$). In conclusion, there was a trend suggesting a lower number of PV cells within striosomes, in agreement with previous suggestions of a higher excitability of the striosomal compartment in connection to motor stereotypies in animals (Canales & Graybiel, 2000). However, this should be interpreted with caution given the low number of samples analyzed.

POTENTIAL ROLE OF THE CEREBRAL CORTEX IN TIC BEHAVIOR

In primates, somatosensory cortical areas, encompassing Brodmann areas 1–3 (BA 1–3) and motor/premotor cortical areas (BA 4–6), send projections primarily to the PT, whereas the dorsolateral prefrontal cortex (PFC) projects to the CD (Kemp & Powell, 1970; Kunzle, 1975; Parent & Hazrati, 1995; Selemon & Goldman-Rakic, 1985). There are at least four motor areas in humans: the primary motor (MI), premotor (PM), supplementary motor area (SMA), and cingulate motor area (CMA) (for a review, see Roland & Zilles, 1996). All these areas are activated bilaterally during the planning and execution of simple and complex movements, with the exception of primary motor cortex (BA4), which is predominantly activated contralaterally. It is thought that while the MI is involved in movement execution, the PM is activated by planning movements, and in general whenever movements are guided by sensory information, as in tracking or manipulating objects. In contrast, the SMA is activated by the performance of self-paced, overlearned (automatic) motor sequences, such as fluent speech, as well as by imagining or planning learned sequences; moreover, stimulation of the SMA can arrest movement.

Activity in this distributed sensorimotor circuit and in an additional set of territories was detected by positron emission tomography (PET) and functional magnetic resonance imaging (fMRI) before and during the occurrence of tics (see also Chapter 12). Tic-correlated activity was seen in the MI, PM, SMA, dorsolateral rostral prefrontal, Broca area and frontal operculum, anterior cingulate, insula, claustrum, PT, and CD (Bohlhalter et al., 2006; Hampson et al., 2009; Stern et al., 2000; Wang et al., 2011). While activity was stronger in the TS group in some of these regions, it appeared to be weaker in portions of the circuitry that exert negative control over motor pathways, notably the CD and anterior cingulate cortex, and less activity in these regions accompanied more severe tic symptoms (Wang et al., 2011). The tic-associated activation of the phylogenetically older insular cortex, which is involved in the integration of internal motivational states with executive functions, has been hypothesized to contribute to the uninhibited behavior of TS (Bohlhalter et al., 2006; Stern et al., 2000). Increased excitability of primary motor cortical areas has also been detected in a transcranial magnetic stimulation study of TS individuals (Ziemann et al., 1997; see also Chapter 11). Abnormal excitability of these cortical regions could be attributed to decreased intracortical inhibition or to increased excitability of thalamic afferents. Together, these studies suggest that increased activity in motor, somatosensory, and paralimbic areas may be involved in

tic generation and may account for the irresistible urge that accompanies tic behavior, whereas lower activity in prefrontal circuits subserving executive control may result in poor tic control. In addition to neuroimaging evidence, a neurochemical evaluation of frontal cortical regions from postmortem tissue in three cases of TS revealed neurotransmitter system dysfunctions in TS, notably dopamine, dopamine type 1 and 2 receptors, dopamine transporter, adenosine type 2 receptor, and vesicular monoamine transporter (Minzer et al., 2004; Yoon et al., 2007).

Stern and colleagues (2000) suggested the intriguing hypothesis that "tics may represent a paradoxical state in which brain regions … normally associated with a subjective experience of volition as they initiate action, are not operating under the volitional control of the patient." Although the neural substrate for the subjective experience of "lack of control" experienced by the patients is unclear, a reasonable hypothesis is that there is an abnormal integration between premotor and other brain regions in TS, particularly the PFC, a heterogeneous set of areas that are important for the voluntary control of motor routines (Bechara et al., 2000; Fuster, 2001). Dorsal PFC areas respond to temporal contingencies, evoke memories and emotions, monitor errors, and correct motor sequences (executive functions). This is consistent with the strong engagement of wide regions of PFC during tic suppression (Peterson et al., 1998) and with observations that increased alpha frequency band coherence (a measure of functional connectivity) was detected between prefrontal and sensorimotor areas in patients with TS in connection with the successful inhibition of unwanted movements (Serrien et al., 2005).

To assess whether the decrease in PV cells was specific to the striatum, we estimated their density in the insular and cingulate regions of the cerebral cortex, two areas that are prominently activated during tic behavior and are implicated in TS. We found a trend toward a decrease in the insular cortex, but overall no statistically significant decrease (Fig. 10.4). The low number of samples again precludes a definite conclusion; however, we note that in contrast to the clearly visible trend in the insular cortex, no such trend

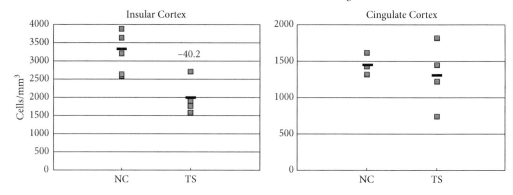

FIGURE 10.4   Density of PV+ neurons in the insular and cingulate regions of the cerebral cortex, assessed by unbiased stereological analyses. NC, normal controls.

was observed in the cingulate cortex. These data suggest the intriguing concept that TS individuals might exhibit differences in the number of inhibitory cortical interneurons in specific regions of the cortex. This is consistent with several transcranial magnetic stimulation (TMS) studies in which TS individuals have reduced short-interval cortical inhibition (SICI), a paradigm that assesses the functional recruitment of intracortical interneurons (see Chapter 11). Future analyses involving these as well as other cortical regions in a larger number of samples are required to rule out this possibility.

The neuroimaging analyses, our postmortem brain analyses, and the neurophysiology of the thalamo-cortical-striatal feed-forward circuit all implicate the basal ganglia and particularly the PV and cholinergic neurons in the pathophysiology of tic behavior.

CORTICOSTRIATAL FEED-FORWARD INHIBITION AND PV GABAERGIC NEURONS

Neurophysiological studies in striatal slices and whole-animal recording support the idea that PV striatal interneurons exert a strong inhibitory influence ("no-go") upon motor activity in response to cortical activation. PV cells receive direct, strong cortical synaptic input (Lapper et al., 1992) and respond with shorter latency than MSNs to cortical stimulation driving powerful feed-forward inhibition throughout the

striatum (Gittis et al., 2010; Mallet et al., 2005) (Fig. 10.1). PV cells also drive the synchronous oscillations in membrane potential and electrical activity involving the cortex and striatum (Berke et al., 2004). However, behavioral evidence for their implication in TS-related behaviors is still lacking. These cells are crucial for overall regulation of excitatory activity in multiple regions of the CNS, and thus animals with widespread loss of PV neuron activity develop seizures, confounding the overall picture.

Developing mice with selective PV neuron inactivation or loss is a promising strategy that may eventually yield insights into the roles of PV neurons in the basal ganglia and in TS. For example, the dt(sz) hamster develops paroxysmal dystonia at 30 to 40 days of life, concomitant to an increase in the activity of MSNs, which has been hypothesized to be based on a deficit of striatal (but not cortical) PV+ interneurons (Gernert et al., 2000). Interestingly, there is a spontaneous remission of paroxysmal dystonia in older dt(sz) hamsters, coinciding with a normalization of the density and increased arborization of striatal PV+ cells (Hamann et al., 2007). The data suggest that abnormal postnatal maturation or survival of striatal PV+ interneurons plays a critical role in the development of paroxysmal dystonia, but interestingly, this can be reversed later in life. While the data are still inconclusive given the possibility of other intervening factors in these mutants, a recent report suggests that a novel compound selectively inhibiting the firing of fast-spiking PV neurons infused into the sensorimotor striatum induces dystonic-like movements in mice (Gittis et al., 2011). Together with the physiological evidence, these animal models strongly suggest that a dysfunction of PV cells may cause a hyperkinetic movement disorder and that these cells represent a therapeutic target for TS. In general, these findings support the conclusion that PV cells are essential to avoid reverberant activity and obtain selective activation of MSNs in the striatal neuronal network.

THALAMOSTRIATAL FEED-FORWARD INHIBITION AND ChAT NEURONS

Cholinergic neurons of the striatum are activated by prominent projections from VA/VL and the centromedian-parafascicular (intralaminar) complex of the thalamus (McFarland & Haber, 2000, 2001) (Fig. 10.1). The VA/VL thalamic nuclei process sensorimotor information and, in turn, receive inhibitory projections from the GPi (Difiglia & Rafols, 1988; Hardman & Halliday, 1999). GPi projection neurons exhibit high-frequency tonic and oscillatory activity. Cholinergic neurons are also the main target of thalamostriatal afferent fibers originating from the intralaminar nuclei, which are the rostral component of the reticular activating system (Matsumoto et al., 2001). Thus, cholinergic neurons receive information about sensory stimulation and ongoing activity as well as the arousal state of the animal. In turn, cholinergic interneurons regulate the firing of the PV interneurons acting through nicotinic and muscarinic receptors (Koos & Tepper, 2002) and also excite SST/NOS/NPY interneurons through nicotinic receptors. Excitation of these inhibitory striatal interneurons results in a secondary prolonged GABA-mediated inhibition of MSNs (Carrillo-Reid et al., 2009; English et al., 2012; Galarraga et al., 1999). Other actions that have been attributed to cholinergic cells are a transient presynaptic inhibition of corticostriatal terminals impinging on MSNs of both pathways, and a direct facilitation of activity of MSNs of the indirect pathway via postsynaptic M1 class muscarinic receptors (Carrillo-Reid et al., 2009;

Ding et al., 2010; Galarraga et al., 1999). Hence, cholinergic interneurons exert complex actions on the striatal circuitry and their role is not completely understood. It would be interesting to know whether the inhibition of MSNs affects preferentially those of the *direct pathway*; if true, an inhibition of the direct pathway together with a facilitation of the *indirect pathway* would profoundly excite the GPi/SNr output neurons and thus inhibit motor behavior.

POSSIBLE CAUSES

Given the retrospective nature of our data, it is impossible to discern whether the observed changes in inhibitory and cholinergic interneurons are causally related to TS, represent long-term consequences of a remote pathophysiological event, or represent a secondary effect totally unrelated to the mechanism of disease. However, the defects in interneuron number are likely to compromise the overall ability of the striatum to organize ongoing behavior. The pattern of activation of striatal cholinergic and PV interneurons by cortical and thalamic afferents, respectively, may have an important role in the suppression of unwanted motor activity. For example, as discussed above, cholinergic cells within the striatum receive a "copy" of corticothalamic projections conveying sensorimotor information to the cerebral cortex; hence, a decrease in cholinergic neuron number will inevitably decrease the integration of multimodal information within the striatum. We hypothesize that a decrease in integrative ability may create a "disconnect" that facilitates tic behavior. This is dramatically demonstrated by neurosurgical experiments in which patients with intractable TS found partial relief from their symptoms after undergoing lesions of the intralaminar thalamic nuclei, or, more recently, when these nuclei were implanted with deep brain stimulation (DBS) electrodes (Temel & Visser-Vandewalle, 2004). As discussed above, the decrease in inhibitory and cholinergic striatal interneurons is likely to be attributable to a loss of cells rather than a downregulation in levels of specific transcripts or proteins. Potential causes of the striatal interneuron loss include developmental misspecification of neurons or toxic, degenerative, and inflammatory conditions affecting the survival of these cells in the postnatal period.

Developmental Defects

Inhibitory interneurons are generated within the basal telencephalon during embryonic development. This region encompasses three ganglionic eminences, the medial, lateral, and caudal eminence (MGE, LGE, and CGE, respectively). Cholinergic neurons are generated in the preoptic area, a more medial and caudal regions adjacent to the MGE. Neurons generated in these ventral regions migrate widely to the cerebral cortex, basal ganglia, and hippocampus to reach their final destination by the first postnatal week in rodents (Anderson et al., 2002; Flames et al., 2007; Xu et al., 2004). In humans, a large portion of cortical GABAergic interneurons might have a dorsal cortical origin, in addition to the common derivation from the basal telencephalon found in lower mammalian species (Letinic et al., 2002).

Genetic programs directed by series of divergent homeobox genes, including *Nkx2.1*, *Dlx1,2,5,6*, *Gbx1,2*, and *Lhx6*, control the specification, differentiation, and migration of GABAergic neurons (Long et al., 2009). This cascade is induced early in embryogenesis in ventral regions of the telencephalon by Sonic hedgehog (Shh), a secreted morphogen emanating from the rostral end of the notochord (Kobayashi et al., 2002). The homeobox gene *Nkx2.1*, the earliest gene required for interneuron specification, is activated by Shh in the prospective MGE (Sussel et al., 1999). Mice lacking Nkx2.1 do not form the globus pallidus, lack basal forebrain cholinergic neurons, and have reduced numbers of cortical GABAergic cells, including PV and STT neurons, that migrate from the MGE into the cortex. Interestingly, haploinsufficiency of *Nkx2.1* (also called TTF1) in humans has been reported in association with a dystonic movement disorder (Pohlenz et al., 2002). *Dlx* genes are downstream of *Nkx2.1*, are expressed by most interneurons, and are essential for many aspects of interneuron development. For example, *Dlx5*

and *Dlx6* are required for the migration, maturation, and function of PV cortical interneurons (Wang et al., 2010), whereas *Dlx1* is required for CR-, SST-, and NPY-positive interneurons (Cobos et al., 2005). All *Dlx* mutants have epilepsy. While *Dlx* genes mostly control cortical interneuron development, the homeobox genes *Gsh1* and *Gsh2* are required for the development of striatal interneurons by specifying the identity of LGE interneuron progenitors in cooperation with *Nkx2.1* (Corbin et al., 2003; Yun et al., 2003). Accordingly, Gsh1 and Gsh2 double mutant mice have severe hypoplasia of the striatum. In addition, Gsh genes are required for the development of olfactory bulb interneurons and telencephalic dopaminergic neurons (Yun et al., 2003). In contrast, the LIM-homeobox gene *Lhx8* is required for the development of cholinergic interneurons; Lhx8 mutants lack the nucleus basalis, a major source of the cholinergic input to the cerebral cortex, and exhibit a reduced number of cholinergic neurons in several other areas of the subcortical telencephalon, including the CD-PT, medial septal nucleus, nucleus of the diagonal band, and magnocellular preoptic nucleus (Zhao et al., 2003). Interestingly, *Lhx8* expression is reduced in the basal ganglia of TS individuals, suggesting a possible developmental origin for the cholinergic defects.

DEGENERATIVE AND NEUROINFLAMMATORY CONDITIONS

The role of neuroinflammation in TS is not fully understood (see also Chapters 9 and 14). In the normal brain, in addition to contemporary immune infiltration there are resident macrophages that enter the brain during embryonic development and remain in a resting form until activated during infection or inflammation events (Ginhoux et al., 2010; Hickey & Kimura, 1988; Rio-Hortega, 1919; for review see Engelhardt & Coisne, 2011; Saijo & Glass, 2011). Immune cells may also play a critical role in cell clearance and synaptic pruning during normal brain development (Tremblay et al., 2011).

In TS there is some evidence of involvement of the immune system, which traditionally stemmed from the hypothesis that an infection with group A β-hemolytic streptococcal infection (GABS) can trigger an autoimmune reaction involving the basal ganglia, a condition called pediatric autoimmune neuropsychiatric disorders associated with streptococcal infection (PANDAS) (Swedo et al., 1997) (for a review of the autoimmune hypothesis of TS, see Chapter 14). In support for such a hypothesis, TS individuals have shown increased levels of antineuronal and antinuclear antibodies, commonly expressed in autoimmune disorders (Kiessling et al., 1993; Morshed et al., 2001), decreases in regulatory T cells (Kawikova et al., 2007), increases in IL-12 and TNF-α serum levels, which were also found to positively correlate with tic severity (Gabbay et al., 2009; Leckman et al., 2005), as well as increases in IL-2 and monocyte chemotactic factor 1 (MCP-1, a marker of chronic inflammation) in brain tissue (Morer et al., 2010). These findings, however, have not always been replicated and remain controversial. Furthermore, there was a striking increase in the number of activated B lymphocytes among a group of unselected adult patients with TS compared with healthy subjects (Moller et al., 2008). Finally, a recent study found a significant increase in maternal self-reported history of autoimmune disorders in TS/OCD, and in a subset of PANDAS subjects, compared to the prevalence in the general population (Murphy et al., 2010).

Brain transcriptome analysis revealed that the expression of genes involved in several immune system pathways is upregulated in TS subjects, including genes involved in inflammatory response and immune cell trafficking (unpublished data). Some of the immune pathway-associated genes found to be upregulated in the brain of TS individuals have been previously been found to be upregulated in the blood of these patients (Tian et al., 2011a, 2011b), suggesting that changes in lymphocytes as well as myeloid-derived cells (monocytes/macrophages/microglia) may occur in this disorder. Interestingly, upregulation of several immunoglobulin genes was detected in the brain transcriptome of TS individuals, which agrees with evidence of abnormal oligoclonal bands of IgG in the cerebrospinal fluid of TS patients, suggestive of increased intrathecal IgG production (Wenzel et al., 2011).

How might these findings interface with the neuropathological findings? It is possible that the loss of interneurons in TS may be secondary to neuroinflammation. If aberrant immune-cell access to the brain is causal in TS, the noted decreases in PV+ and ChAT+ interneurons may be resulting from immune cell reactivity; however, such autoimmune-mediated cell loss is in contrast with the absence of increased loss of interneurons with age. Alternatively, the immune system may be acting in a stereotyped way, following some causal trigger that leads to a cascade of cues and ultimately to increased immune cell adhesion and infiltration into the striatum. Moving forward, the rapid onset of TS symptoms following an immunological challenge in PANDAS cases provides an interesting subset of subjects in which to

---

Box 10.1. Key Points

- In TS there are decreases in PV+ GABergic interneurons and cholinergic interneurons in the CD and PT.
- There is also loss of the normal distribution (highest in associative regions, intermediate in sensorimotor, and lowest in limbic regions) of cholinergic interneurons.
- There are no evident changes in ChAT distribution in striosomes versus matrix.
- There may also be changes in another interneuron population, the NOS-containing interneurons.

further explore the role of the immune system in TS.

Therapeutic Implications

Discovering the neurophysiological substrate for tics and other symptoms of TS is of paramount importance for treatment. Even in the case of developmental alterations, where the causes are likely to be remote, there is still hope that we could find treatments that compensate for brain circuitry dysregulation. In the case of cell losses or dysfunctions induced by immunological alterations, potential treatments could be tried similar to those employed in autoimmune disorders of the central nervous system. Finally, and similarly to what has been successfully tried in other basal ganglia disorders such as Parkinson's disease, neurotransmitter or cellular replacement therapy (locally delivered) represents a difficult but open area for therapeutics. It has been recently demonstrated in mouse models of seizures that transplantation of GABAergic interneuron precursors in the early postnatal mouse cortex results in diffuse cortical engraftment of exogenous GABAergic cells and reversal of epileptic symptoms (Alvarez-Dolado et al., 2006; Baraban et al., 2009).

REFERENCES

Albin RL, Young AB, Penney JB. The functional anatomy of basal ganglia disorders. *TINS* 1989; 12:366–375.

Alvarez-Dolado M, Calcagnotto ME, Karkar KM et al. Cortical inhibition modified by embryonic neural precursors grafted into the postnatal brain. *J Neurosci* 2006; 26:7380–7389.

Anderson SA, Kaznowski CE, Horn C et al. Distinct origins of neocortical projection neurons and interneurons in vivo. *Cereb Cortex* 2002; 12:702–709.

Aosaki T, Tsubokawa H, Ishida A et al. Responses of tonically active neurons in the primate's striatum undergo systematic changes during behavioral sensorimotor conditioning. *J Neurosci* 1994; 14:3969–3984.

Baraban SC, Southwell DG, Estrada RC et al. Reduction of seizures by transplantation of cortical GABAergic interneuron precursors into Kv1.1 mutant mice. *Proc Natl Acad Sci USA* 2009; 106:15472–15477.

Bechara A, Damasio H, Damasio AR. Emotion, decision making and the orbitofrontal cortex. *Cereb Cortex* 2000; 10:295–307.

Berke JD, Okatan M, Skurski J, Eichenbaum HB. Oscillatory entrainment of striatal neurons in freely moving rats. *Neuron* 2004; 43: 883–896.

Bloch MH, Leckman JF, Zhu H, Peterson BS. Caudate volumes in childhood predict symptom severity in adults with Tourette syndrome. *Neurology* 2005; 65:1253–1258.
This study reported that decreased caudate volume in childhood is inversely correlated with symptom severity in adulthood.

Bohlhalter S, Goldfine A, Matteson S et al. Neural correlates of tic generation in Tourette syndrome: an event-related functional MRI study. *Brain* 2006; 129:2029–2037.

Canales JJ, Graybiel AM. A measure of striatal function predicts motor stereotypy. *Nat Neurosci* 2000; 3:377–383.

Carrillo-Reid L, Tecuapetla F, Vautrelle N et al. Muscarinic enhancement of persistent sodium current synchronizes striatal medium spiny neurons. *J Neurophysiol* 2009; 102:682–690.

Cobos I, Calcagnotto ME, Vilaythong AJ et al. Mice lacking Dlx1 show subtype-specific loss of interneurons, reduced inhibition and epilepsy. *Nat Neurosci* 2005; 8:1059–1068.

Corbin JG, Rutlin M, Gaiano N, Fishell G. Combinatorial function of the homeodomain proteins Nkx2.1 and Gsh2 in ventral telencephalic patterning. *Development* 2003; 130:4895–4906.

Difiglia M, Rafols JA. Synaptic organization of the globus pallidus. *J Electron Microsc Tech* 1998; 10:247–263.

Ding JB, Guzman JN, Peterson JD et al. Thalamic gating of corticostriatal signaling by cholinergic interneurons. *Neuron* 2010; 67:294–307.

Dougherty JD, Schmidt EF, Nakajima M, Heintz N. Analytical approaches to RNA profiling data for the identification of genes enriched in specific cells. *Nucleic Acids Res* 2010; 38:4218–4230.

Doyle JP, Dougherty JD, Heiman M et al. Application of a translational profiling approach for the comparative analysis of CNS cell types. *Cell* 2008; 135:749–762.

Eblen F, Graybiel AM. Highly restricted origin of prefrontal cortical inputs to striosomes in the macaque monkey. *J Neurosci* 1995; 15:5999–6013.

Engelhardt B, Coisne C. Fluids and barriers of the CNS establish immune privilege by confining immune surveillance to a two-walled castle moat surrounding the CNS castle. *Fluids Barriers CNS* 2011; 8:4.

English DF, Ibanez-Sandoval O, Stark E et al. GABAergic circuits mediate the reinforcement-related signals of striatal cholinergic interneurons. *Nat Neurosci* 2012; 15:123–130.

Felling RJ, Singer HS. Neurobiology of Tourette syndrome: current status and need for further investigation. *J Neurosci* 2011; 31:12387–12395.

Flaherty AW, Graybiel AM. Output architecture of the primate putamen. *J Neurosci* 1993; 13:3222–3237.

Flames N, Pla R, Gelman DM et al. Delineation of multiple subpallial progenitor domains by the combinatorial expression of transcriptional codes. *J Neurosci* 2007; 27:9682–9695.

Frederiksen KA, Cutting LE, Kates WR et al. Disproportionate increase in white matter in right frontal lobe in Tourette syndrome. *Neurology* 2002; 58:85–89.

Fuster JM. The prefrontal cortex—an update: time is of the essence. *Neuron* 2001; 30:319–333.

Gabbay V, Coffey BJ, Guttman LE et al. A cytokine study in children and adolescents with Tourette's disorder. *Prog Neuropsychopharmacol Biol Psychiatry* 2009; 33:967–971.

Galarraga E, Hernandez-Lopez S, Reyes A et al. Cholinergic modulation of neostriatal output: a functional antagonism between different types of muscarinic receptors. *J Neurosci* 1999; 19:3629–3638.

Gernert M, Hamann M, Bennay M et al. Deficit of striatal parvalbumin-reactive GABAergic interneurons and decreased basal ganglia output in a genetic rodent model of idiopathic paroxysmal dystonia. *J Neurosci* 2000; 20:7052–7058.

Ginhoux F, Greter M, Leboeuf M et al. Fate mapping analysis reveals that adult microglia derive from primitive macrophages. *Science* 2010; 330:841–845.

Gittis AH, Leventhal DK, Fensterheim BA et al. Selective inhibition of striatal fast-spiking interneurons causes dyskinesias. *J Neurosci* 2011; 31:15727–15731.

Gittis AH, Nelson AB, Thwin MT et al. Distinct roles of GABAergic interneurons in the regulation of striatal output pathways. *J Neurosci* 2010; 30:2223–2234.

Hamann M, Richter A, Meillasson FV et al. Age-related changes in parvalbumin-positive interneurons in the striatum, but not in the sensorimotor cortex in dystonic brains of the dt(sz) mutant hamster. *Brain Res* 2007; 1150:190–199.

Hampson M, Tokoglu F, King RA et al. Brain areas coactivating with motor cortex during chronic motor tics and intentional movements. *Biol Psychiatry* 2009; 65:594–599.

Hardman CD, Halliday GM. The external globus pallidus in patients with Parkinson's disease and progressive supranuclear palsy. *Mov Disord* 1999; 14:626–633.

Hickey WF, Kimura H. Perivascular microglial cells of the CNS are bone marrow-derived and present antigen in vivo. *Science* 1988; 239:290–292.

Hyde TM, Stacey ME, Coppola R et al. Cerebral morphometric abnormalities in Tourette's syndrome: a quantitative MRI study of monozygotic twins. *Neurology* 1995; 45:1176–1182.

Kalanithi PS, Zheng W, Kataoka Y et al. Altered parvalbumin-positive neuron distribution in basal ganglia of individuals with Tourette syndrome. *Proc Natl Acad Sci USA* 2005; 102:13307–13312.

This was the first study to report a decrease in parvalbumin neuron number in the brain of TS patients.

Kataoka Y, Kalanithi PS, Grantz H et al. Decreased number of parvalbumin and cholinergic interneurons in the striatum of individuals with Tourette syndrome. *J Comp Neurol* 2010; 518:277–291.

This was the first report of a decrease in cholinergic neurons in the brain of TS patients.

Kawaguchi Y, Wilson CJ, Augwood SJ, Emson PC. Striatal interneurons: chemical, physiological and morphological characterization. *TINS* 1995; 18:527–535.

Kawikova I, Leckman JF, Kronig H et al. Decreased numbers of regulatory T cells suggest impaired immune tolerance in children with Tourette syndrome: a preliminary study. *Biol Psychiatry* 2007; 61:273–278.

Kemp JM, Powell TP. The cortico-striate projection in the monkey. *Brain* 1970; 93:525–546.

Kiessling LS, Marcotte AC, Culpepper L. Antineuronal antibodies in movement disorders. *Pediatrics* 1993; 92:39–43.

Kita H, Kosaka T, Heizmann CW. Parvalbumin-immunoreactive neurons in the rat neostriatum: a light and electron microscopy study. *Brain Res* 1990; 536:1–15.

Kobayashi D, Kobayashi M, Matsumoto K et al. Early subdivisions in the neural plate define distinct competence for inductive signals. *Development* 2002; 129:83–93.

Koos T, Tepper JM. Dual cholinergic control of fast-spiking interneurons in the neostriatum. *J Neurosci* 2002; 22:529–535.

Kunzle H. Bilateral projections from precentral motor cortex to the putamen and other parts of the basal ganglia. An autoradiographic study in *Macaca fascicularis*. *Brain Res* 1975; 88: 195–209.

Lapper SR, Bolam JP. Input from the frontal cortex and the parafascicular nucleus to cholinergic interneurons in the dorsal striatum of the rat. *Neuroscience* 1992; 51:533–545.

Lapper SR, Smith Y, Sadikot AF et al. Cortical input to parvalbumin-immunoreactive neurones in the putamen of the squirrel monkey. *Brain Res* 1992; 580:215–224.

Leckman JF, Katsovich L, Kawikova I et al. Increased serum levels of interleukin-12 and tumor necrosis factor-alpha in Tourette's syndrome. *Biol Psychiatry* 2005; 57:667–673.

This was the first study to report altered indices of innate immunity in the blood of TS individuals and the only replicated study of altered cytokine expression in TS.

Letinic K, Zoncu R, Rakic P. Origin of GABAergic neurons in the human neocortex. *Nature* 2002; 417:645–649.

Long JE, Cobos I, Potter GB, Rubenstein JL. Dlx1&2 and Mash1 transcription factors control MGE and CGE patterning and differentiation through parallel and overlapping pathways. *Cereb Cortex* 2009; 19 Suppl 1:i96–i106.

Mallet N, Le Moine C, Charpier S, Gonon F. Feedforward inhibition of projection neurons by fast-spiking GABA interneurons in the rat striatum in vivo. *J Neurosci* 2005; 25:3857–3869.

Matsumoto N, Minamimoto T, Graybiel AM, Kimura M. Neurons in the thalamic CM-Pf complex supply striatal neurons with information about behaviorally significant sensory events. *J Neurophysiol* 2001; 85:960–976.

McFarland NR, Haber SN. Convergent inputs from thalamic motor nuclei and frontal cortical areas to the dorsal striatum in the primate. *J Neurosci* 2000; 20:3798–3813.

McFarland NR, Haber SN. Organization of thalamostriatal terminals from the ventral motor nuclei in the macaque. *J Comp Neurol* 2001; 429:321–336.

Minzer K, Lee O, Hong JJ, Singer HS. Increased prefrontal D2 protein in Tourette syndrome: a postmortem analysis of frontal cortex and striatum. *J Neurol Sci* 2004; 219:55–61.

Moller JC, Tackenberg B, Heinzel-Gutenbrunner M et al. Immunophenotyping in Tourette syndrome—a pilot study. *Eur J Neurol* 2008; 15:749–753.

Morer A, Chae W, Henegariu O et al. Elevated expression of MCP-1, IL-2 and PTPR-N in basal ganglia of Tourette syndrome cases. *Brain Behav Immun* 2010; 24:1069–1073.

Morshed SA, Parveen S, Leckman JF et al. Antibodies against neural, nuclear, cytoskeletal, and streptococcal epitopes in children and adults with Tourette's syndrome, Sydenham's chorea, and autoimmune disorders. *Biol Psychiatry* 2001; 50:566–577.

Murphy TK, Storch EA, Turner A et al. Maternal history of autoimmune disease in children presenting with tics and/or obsessive-compulsive disorder. *J Neuroimmunol* 2010; 229:243–247.

Parent A. Extrinsic connections of the basal ganglia. *TINS* 1990; 13:254–258.

Parent A, Hazrati LN. Functional anatomy of the basal ganglia. I. The cortico-basal ganglia-thalamo-cortical loop. *Brain Res Brain Res Rev* 1995; 20:91–127.

Peterson BS, Riddle MA, Cohen DJ et al. Reduced basal ganglia volumes in Tourette's syndrome using three-dimensional reconstruction techniques from magnetic resonance images. *Neurology* 1993; 43:941–949.

Peterson BS, Skudlarski P, Anderson AW et al. A functional magnetic resonance imaging study of tic suppression in Tourette syndrome. *Arch Gen Psychiatry* 1998; 55:326–333.

Peterson BS, Staib L, Scahill L et al. Regional brain and ventricular volumes in Tourette's syndrome. *Arch Gen Psychiatry* 2001; 58:427–440.

Peterson BS, Thomas P, Kane MJ et al. Basal ganglia volumes in patients with Gilles de la Tourette syndrome. *Arch Gen Psychiatry* 2003; 60:415–424.

This was the first comprehensive study reporting decreased basal ganglia volume in a large cohort of TS individuals.

Pohlenz J, Dumitrescu A, Zundel D et al. Partial deficiency of thyroid transcription factor 1 produces predominantly neurological defects in humans and mice. *J Clin Invest* 2002; 109:469–473.

Rio-Hortega PD. El tercer elemento de los centros nerviosos. Poder fagocitario y movilidad de la microglia. *Biol Soc Esp Biol* 1919; 154:166.

Roland PE, Zilles K. Functions and structures of the motor cortices in humans. *Curr Opin Neurobiol* 1996; 6:773–781.

Saijo K, Glass CK. Microglial cell origin and phenotypes in health and disease. *Nat Rev Immunol* 2011; 11:775–787.

Selemon LD, Goldman-Rakic PS. Longitudinal topography and interdigitation of corticospinal projections in the rhesus monkey. *J Neurosci* 1985; 5:776–794.

Serrien DJ, Orth M, Evans AH et al. Motor inhibition in patients with Gilles de la Tourette syndrome: functional activation patterns as revealed by EEG coherence. *Brain* 2005; 128:116–125.

Sowell ER, Kan E, Yoshii J et al. Thinning of sensorimotor cortices in children with Tourette syndrome. *Nat Neurosci* 2008; 11:637–639.

Stern E, Silbersweig DA, Chee KY et al. A functional neuroanatomy of tics in Tourette syndrome. *Arch Gen Psychiatry* 2000; 57:741–748.

This was the first neuroimaging (PET) study exploring specific brain changes with tic occurrences.

Sussel L, Marin O, Kimura S, Rubenstein JL. Loss of Nkx2.1 homeobox gene function results in a ventral to dorsal molecular respecification within the basal telencephalon: evidence for a transformation of the pallidum into the striatum. *Development* 1999; 126:3359–3370.

Swedo SE, Leonard HL, Mittleman BB et al. Identification of children with pediatric autoimmune neuropsychiatric disorders associated with streptococcal infections by a marker associated with rheumatic fever. *Am J Psychiatry* 1997; 154:110–112.

This work defined PANDAS as a clinical and pathophysiological class of children with post-streptococcal infections predisposing to brain disorders.

Temel Y, Visser-Vandewalle V. Surgery in Tourette syndrome. *Mov Disord* 2004; 19:3–14.

Tian Y, Apperson ML, Ander BP et al. Differences in exon expression and alternatively spliced genes in blood of multiple sclerosis compared to healthy control subjects. *J Neuroimmunol* 2011a; 230:124–129.

Tian Y, Gunther JR, Liao IH et al. GABA- and acetylcholine-related gene expression in blood correlate with tic severity and microarray evidence for alternative splicing in Tourette syndrome: a pilot study. *Brain Res* 2011b; 1381:228–236.

Tobe RH, Bansal R, Xu D et al. Cerebellar morphology in Tourette syndrome and obsessive-compulsive disorder. *Ann Neurol* 2010; 67:479–487.

Tremblay ME, Stevens B, Sierra A et al. The role of microglia in the healthy brain. *J Neurosci* 2011; 31:16064–16069.

Wang Y, Dye CA, Sohal V et al. Dlx5 and Dlx6 regulate the development of parvalbumin-expressing cortical interneurons. *J Neurosci* 2010; 30:5334–5345.

Wang Z, Maia TV, Marsh R et al. The neural circuits that generate tics in Tourette's syndrome. *Am J Psychiatry* 2011; 168:1326–1337.

Wenzel C, Wurster U, Muller-Vahl KR. Oligoclonal bands in cerebrospinal fluid in patients with Tourette's syndrome. *Mov Disord* 2011; 26:343–346.

Xu Q, Cobos I, De La Cruz E et al. Origins of cortical interneuron subtypes. *J Neurosci* 2004; 24:2612–2622.

Yoon DY, Gause CD, Leckman JF, Singer HS. Frontal dopaminergic abnormality in Tourette syndrome: a postmortem analysis. *J Neurol Sci* 2007; 255:50–56.

Yun K, Garel S, Fischman S, Rubenstein JL. Patterning of the lateral ganglionic eminence by the Gsh1 and Gsh2 homeobox genes regulates striatal and olfactory bulb histogenesis and the growth of axons through the basal ganglia. *J Comp Neurol* 2003; 461:151–165.

Zhao Y, Marin O, Hermesz E et al. The LIM-homeobox gene Lhx8 is required for the development of many cholinergic neurons in the mouse forebrain. *Proc Natl Acad Sci USA* 2003; 100:9005–9010.

Ziemann U, Paulus W, Rothenberger A. Decreased motor inhibition in Tourette's disorder: evidence from transcranial magnetic stimulation. *Am J Psychiatry* 1997; 154:1277–1284.

11

Electrophysiology in Tourette Syndrome

MICHAEL ORTH

Abstract

Electrophysiological methods are noninvasive means to analyze qualitatively brain activation, and include electroencephalography (EEG) and event-related potentials, evoked potentials, transcranial magnetic stimulation (TMS), and magnetoencephalography (MEG). This chapter summarizes their contribution to the understanding of the pathophysiology of Tourette syndrome (TS). The TMS approach showed altered synaptic excitability and intracortical inhibition in these patients, with measures of motor cortical excitability associated with tic severity. At the same time, the reduced excitability of a measure of sensorimotor integration such as short-latency afferent inhibition suggests that sensory input has increased access to motor output in TS, consistent with a heightened sensitivity to sensory stimuli. Motor cortex excitability measures also differed between TS patients and control subjects during the preparation of voluntary movements and the suppression of undesired movements. The latter is associated with more widespread cortical activity in TS (increased cortico-cortical coupling on EEG and MEG coherence analysis). Recent evidence also suggests abnormal plasticity mechanisms in TS, but new studies are necessary to confirm this. Finally, using repetitive TMS as a treatment for tics has overall been disappointing, although some recent small studies without a placebo control arm suggest some effects of motor cortex inhibitory protocols.

INTRODUCTION

Chronic motor and phonic tics with childhood onset define Tourette syndrome (TS). Simple tics often relieve internal sensory urges felt in the area of the tic (i.e., premonitory sensations) (Bliss, 1980), while more complex tics, such as echophenomena, respond to the perception of external stimuli (see Chapter 1). Environmental factors, such as emotions or stressful situations, may also alleviate or exacerbate tics. These clinical observations suggest that TS is a sensorimotor disorder, where the sensitivity to external and internal stimuli might be increased and unwanted responses to sensory, motor, or emotional stimuli cannot be sufficiently suppressed (Greenberg et al., 2000; Ziemann et al., 1997). This may lead to tics and maybe to other types of habitual motor responses observed in TS patients, such as forced touching or compulsions, as described in detail in Chapters 1 and 3 (Leckman, 2002).

Pathophysiologically, the origins of tics very likely involve abnormal processing in cortico-basal ganglionic-thalamo-cortical circuits, in which information from many sources needs to be integrated with motor output (see Chapters 12 and 13 for further details on the pathobiology of TS). A glitch in this complex process may provide the driving force of a chain of events that culminates in unwanted behavior, such as tics, over which patients have incomplete control (Mink, 2006). Only a few brains of patients with TS have been studied postmortem (see Chapter 10), so that the understanding of the neurobiological underpinnings of tics must rely largely on *in vivo* studies (Kalanithi et al., 2005). Different methods help us to investigate brain structure, such as magnetic resonance imaging (MRI). This is complemented by functional analyses using new techniques such as functional MRI (fMRI), which allows us to study brain function *in vivo*, including areas deep within the brain such as the basal ganglia (see Chapter 12). fMRI assesses changes in blood flow when the brain is busy with a task compared to when it rests. Because an increase in blood flow equals an increase in brain activity, one can infer which brain areas are active during the task at hand. However, the type of activity remains uncertain: for instance, inhibitory and facilitatory activity may give rise to the same changes in blood flow. Electrophysiological methods, in contrast, can differentiate the quality of brain activation and can therefore add an important dimension to the noninvasive study of brain function.

For several reasons it may be challenging to study TS. Many TS patients have comorbid conditions, the most common of which are attention-deficit/hyperactivity disorder (ADHD) and obsessive-compulsive disorder (OCD) (see Chapters 2 and 3). In fact, "pure" TS may be the exception rather than the rule (Freeman et al., 2000). In addition to sensory urges and tics, persons with TS often act impulsively or have intrusive obsessions and compulsions, even when they do not meet threshold criteria for a clinical diagnosis of ADHD and/or OCD. When enrolling TS patients into studies it is therefore important to carefully assess these other problems. Studies involving TS patients with tics but few or no other symptoms, and ideally unmedicated, may contribute most to advance our understanding of tics in TS. However, this may not be representative of the majority of patients within the TS spectrum. A more detailed discussion of the complexities of studying TS can be found elsewhere (Gilbert, 2005).

In this chapter, first the different electrophysiological methods are briefly introduced before electrophysiological data from studies with TS patients are reviewed. For some time, studies have focused on tics or when patients were at rest; more recently, this has been extended to the physiology of voluntary movement control. Therefore, the focus is first on what is known about the electrophysiology of tics and the resting state before moving on to voluntary movement control—that is, the preparation and execution of voluntary movements and inhibiting movements. Next, repetitive transcranial

magnetic stimulation as a treatment option is discussed. The chapter closes with a synthesis of current electrophysiological thinking, including a number of unanswered questions.

METHODOLOGY

Several techniques have been used to study the electrophysiology of TS. These include electroencephalography and event-related potentials, evoked potentials, transcranial magnetic stimulation, and magnetoencephalography. In most instances, recordings have to be made from outside the brain. However, with the advent of deep brain stimulation (see Chapter 26) it is possible to record from electrodes placed into the basal ganglia. The following will give a brief overview of all these techniques, so that the reader gets a rough idea about how these techniques can be used and what their limitations are. This is not, of course, meant to be exhaustive: for more in-depth reviews of these methods the interested reader is referred to the relevant literature.

ELECTROENCEPHALOGRAPHY, MAGNETOENCEPHALOGRAPHY, AND EVENT-RELATED POTENTIALS

Electroencephalography (EEG) and magnetoencephalography (MEG) capture brain activity noninvasively and in real time, with a resolution in milliseconds. EEG records a map of postsynaptic synchronized activity of aligned neurons of the whole brain. Neurons within the cortex generate the largest potentials with the best resolution. The attenuation of recordings from deeper within the brain declines, so that the EEG is not the best tool for analysis of activity away from the cortex. However, synchrony between deeper brain structures (e.g., the thalamus and the cortex) is well known in different frequencies: delta (<2 Hz), theta (~2–7 Hz), alpha (~8–12 Hz), beta (12–30 Hz), and gamma (30–80 Hz) bands. MEG records from outside of the brain the magnetic fields that are produced by electrical activity within the brain. These magnetic fields are generated by postsynaptic current flows across neurons. One advantage of MEG compared to EEG is that the magnetic fields are not affected by the conductivity of the tissues of the head. This allows recording from deeper brain structures.

Event-related potentials (ERPs) refer to brain responses that reliably result from internal or external stimuli such as touch, smell, vision, or sound. The ERP is thought to reflect a higher cognitive response to a cognitively salient stimulus and requires processing of the physical stimulus. This is reflected in the evoked potential. Many trials (>100) need to be averaged so that the ERP stands out from the random background electrical brain activity. One example from clinical practice is the visual evoked potential (VEP), a potential recorded from the occipital lobe when focusing on, for example, a moving checkerboard.

One limitation is the susceptibility of these types of recording methodologies, especially of EEG, to movement artifacts. This is a particular problem in TS patients, given the presence of head and neck tics, so one needs to select either patients with less frequent and less severe head and neck tics, or those able to suppress them. It introduces a selection bias because the patient population studied may not be representative of the majority of TS patients. This makes the interpretation of results more difficult.

TRANSCRANIAL MAGNETIC STIMULATION

Transcranial magnetic stimulation (TMS) takes advantage of the principle of induction. Differently shaped coils of wire (e.g., round, figure-of-eight) encased in plastic are placed on the head. The coils are connected to a rapidly discharging large capacitator, which sends a strong current of about 8,000 A for about 1 ms through the windings of the induction coil. This in turn generates a magnetic field that is oriented perpendicularly to the plane of the coil. The magnetic field passes unimpeded through the skin and skull and induces a directed current in the surface of the brain that flows tangentially to the skull. If high enough, this current depolarizes nearby nerve cells in much the same way as if currents were applied directly to the cortical surface. Transcranial electrical stimulation (TES) of the brain had been used before TMS; however, electrical stimulation given to the scalp can be painful and is thus limited by the discomfort it produces. TMS has the advantage that the electrical current is induced in the brain and is therefore painless. TMS is also safe if the protocols adhere to the safety guidelines (Wassermann, 1998), so it can be used in awake human beings. There has been interest in using transcranial direct current stimulation (tDCS) (for a review see Nitsche et al., 2008). This technique uses currents that are too low to induce a neuronal action potential. It is thought that tDCS can hyper- or hypopolarize neurons and thus modify neuronal excitability. However, its effects may be more difficult to judge since, in contrast to TMS (see below), there is no clear output signal that helps to gauge the tDCS input.

Using TMS, there are currently two main ways of stimulation. Single- or paired-pulse TMS (for a review see Di Lazzaro et al., 2008; Pascual-Leone et al., 2002) can depolarize populations of neurons in the neocortex, resulting in an action potential. The effect of TMS depends on the coil position over the brain. If the coil is placed over the motor cortex, TMS induces a discharge in cortical motor neurons. This leads to a volley that descends the pyramidal tracts in the brain and spinal cord, and then the peripheral nerve. The peripheral nerve makes contact with a muscle; upon arrival of the descending volley a muscle twitch is visible and can be recorded as a motor-evoked potential (MEP). TMS can produce MEPs in various individual muscles or groups of muscles, depending where in the motor cortex the electrical current is induced. Commonly, one induces a twitch in a small hand muscle, such as the first dorsal interosseus (FDI). Flashes of light (phosphenes) might be experienced by the participant when the coil is placed on the occipital cortex. In most other areas of the cortex, the participant does not consciously experience any effect. However, TMS may influence behavior (e.g., reaction time on a cognitive task) or brain activity that can be detected using positron emission tomography (PET) or fMRI (Driver et al., 2009). These effects do not outlast the period of stimulation. One of the most widely used paired-pulse protocols investigates intracortical inhibition (short intracortical inhibition [SICI]) or intracortical facilitation (ICF). SICI and ICF are likely to be cortical in origin and probably reflect how intracortical interneurons influence the excitability of motoneurons (Kujirai et al., 1993).

Trains of stimuli can also be given with rTMS (for a review see Ridding & Ziemann, 2010; Thickbroom, 2007), or such trains can consist of paired stimuli with one stimulus given to a peripheral nerve and the other to the motor cortex (paired associative stimulation; Stefan et al., 2000). Depending on the frequency and intensity of stimulation, and coil orientation, rTMS can increase or decrease the excitability of corticospinal or cortico-cortical pathways. In contrast to single- or paired-pulse TMS, these effects can outlast the period of stimulation (usually for about 20–30 minutes). The participant usually does not consciously notice any effects; however, there may be subtle changes in behavior or brain activity similar to the single-pulse techniques described above (Driver et al., 2009).

ELECTROPHYSIOLOGICAL STUDIES OF TS

To understand what individual studies teach us about the pathophysiology of TS it is important to know in what state TS patients were studied. TS patients do not always tic. Tics tend to occur in bouts, with these bouts also occurring in bouts, and so on (see Chapter 1). There are truly tic-free intervals, and there may also be times when TS patients have no obvious tics but are not free of sensory urges, even though they can be resisted at these times. This indicates that the neural circuits driving tics, and helping to resist them, including the motor cortex, are not always in the same state. The following section reviews electrophysiological data when TS patients are at rest or tic; then the more recent interest in voluntary movement control is discussed. Finally, a section is dedicated to the use of rTMS for the treatment of tics.

Tics and Bereitschaftspotential

Tics appear volitional and yet cannot be fully controlled. Voluntary movements are usually preceded by a premovement potential (Bereitschaftspotential) in the EEG. Obeso and colleagues reported that in contrast to voluntary movements, tics were not preceded by a premovement potential (Obeso et al., 1981). This was confirmed later, but in some patients premovement negativity was also observed (Karp et al., 1996). The absence of a premovement potential before tics may indeed suggest that tics differ from purposeful movements. However, patients do report that at least some tics purposefully relieve premonitory sensations. This indicates that such tics may resemble planned movements and may explain why sometimes a premovement potential can be recorded.

Corticospinal Motor Neurons at Rest

When TS patients do not tic, several studies (Orth et al., 2005b; Ziemann et al., 1997) have shown that the intensity needed to induce an MEP (motor threshold) at rest and in a pre-activated state was similar in TS patients and controls. However, with higher stimulation intensity, TS patients recruited considerably fewer corticospinal neurons compared with controls (Fig. 11.1; Orth et al., 2008).

TMS activates axons of neurons in the cortex. The action potential travels along axons to then transsynaptically discharge, directly or indirectly, motor neurons in the spinal cord. Therefore, the threshold depends on the excitability of axon membranes at the site of stimulation and the membrane potential of postsynaptic neurons in motor cortex and spinal cord. When actively contracting a muscle, synaptic excitability is high so that changes in threshold usually are thought to reflect changes in axonal excitability. The active threshold was similar in TS and controls so that axonal excitability is probably normal. With muscles in a relaxed, or resting, state, synaptic excitability is less well specified than when active. Nevertheless, equal resting thresholds in patients and healthy controls suggest that the most excitable connections (i.e., those recruited at threshold) are in the same state in both groups (Heise et al., 2010; Orth et al., 2005b, 2008; Ziemann et al., 1997).

Above threshold, further neurons are recruited so that the resulting MEP becomes larger.

The slope of MEP recruitment depends on the difference in excitability between those neuronal elements in the corticospinal system that need higher intensities of stimulation and those activated at threshold. If there were little difference between the excitability of the most and least excitable members of this population, then a small increase in stimulus intensity would recruit many additional connections and create a large MEP: the gain of the input–output slope would be steep. In contrast, if the difference in excitability within the corticospinal neuron population were greater, then the same change in intensity would recruit only a small number

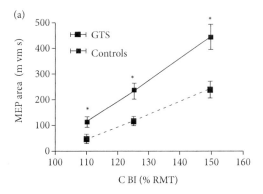

(a)

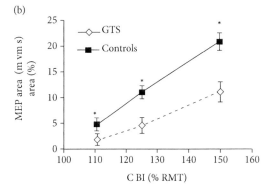

(b)

FIGURE 11.1 **Corticospinal system recruitment at rest.** (**A**) MEP size recorded from FDI after TMS shock to the M1 hand area with 110%, 125%, or 150% of resting motor threshold. Patients have smaller MEPs at all intensities (ANOVA, main effect of "group," *p = .001). (**B**) MEP size/M-wave ratios to control for differences in neuromuscular excitability. Patients have smaller ratios at all intensities (ANOVA, main effect of "group," *p = .001). Values are means ± SEM, n = 20 for TS patients, n = 24 for controls.

of extra connections and the MEP would remain small: the input–output relation would be shallow. Since TS patients recruited MEPs more gradually, there seems to be a greater difference between the most and the least excitable corticospinal neurons than normal (Orth et al., 2008). It is interesting to note that in a more recent study the recruitment slopes of controls and TS patients were similar (Heise et al., 2010). Assuming that this was not caused by a difference in the controls, this is not easily explained. One possible explanation is that the two TS cohorts were clinically different, and it may well be that the TS patients in our cohort had more tics than in the Heise and colleagues' (2010) cohort. It is well known that corticospinal excitability decreases when movements are inhibited (for a review see Stinear et al., 2009, and below). Thus, in patients with more tics there may be a greater need to inhibit movements in response to, for instance, sensory urges even though no movements are apparent during the experiments. If that were the explanation for the reduced corticospinal excitability in our patients (Orth et al., 2008), then one might want to speculate that our TS patients were in a state of (tic) movement inhibition rather than truly at rest. However, an argument against this assumption would be that with movement inhibition, at least in healthy controls, SICI probably increases. In TS, SICI is decreased (see below).

Inhibitory and Facilitatory Circuits at Rest

Several TMS studies in TS have demonstrated reduced SICI at rest (Gilbert et al., 2005; Orth et al., 2005a; Ziemann et al., 1997). While motor threshold and input–output curves described above examine corticospinal motor neurons, SICI and ICF assess intracortical interneurons. These interneurons contribute to the regulation of the excitability of corticospinal neurons within the motor cortex. In the SICI circuit the threshold intensity needed to produce SICI and the amount of SICI at suprathreshold intensities of conditioning shock can be distinguished (Orth et al., 2003). This showed that TS patients have normal thresholds for SICI, but that recruitment of inhibition at suprathreshold intensities was reduced (Orth et al., 2005a, 2008). Similar to the corticospinal neurons, it is thought that TMS pulses recruit SICI by exciting axons and that this then leads to synaptic release of inhibitory neurotransmitters such as GABA. Thus, normal thresholds in the presence of decreased recruitment would be compatible with the idea that in TS axonal excitability is normal, whereas the recruitment of synaptic inhibition in the SICI circuit is reduced. TS patients as a whole had increased ICF in one study (Orth & Rothwell, 2009), whereas others had not described any significant effects (Gilbert et al., 2005; Greenberg et al., 2000; Ziemann et al., 1997). This could simply be because of the well-recognized variability in measurements of ICF (Orth et al., 2003) but may also relate to varying intensities of the conditioning stimulus and the number of patients studied and/or their comorbidities.

A further inhibitory circuit can be examined when a TMS pulse is given to the motor cortex during tonic contraction of a target muscle; this produces an MEP followed by a period of EMG silence before the activity resumes its prestimulus baseline level of activity. This is the so-called cortical silent period. The duration of the cortical silent period may be shorter in patients than in controls (Orth et al., 2005a; Ziemann et al., 1997), or normal (Gilbert et al., 2004), especially when corrected for differences in absolute MEP amplitude between patients and controls (Orth et al., 2008). Thus, the relation between corticospinal excitability and the inhibitory mechanism responsible for the clinical silent period—presumably through corticospinal motor neuron recurrent collaterals (Orth & Rothwell, 2004)—is the same in patients and controls. This supports the notion that not all inhibitory systems are affected in TS. The above provides good evidence to suggest that the corticospinal system and the interneuron circuits that shape corticospinal output have in common a reduction of synaptic excitability.

Communication of cognitive, motor, and sensory information between the hemispheres involves the corpus callosum. Interhemispheric inhibition between the motor cortices can be investigated with TMS (Ferbert et al., 1992). In TS this was examined by Bäumer and colleagues (Baumer et al., 2010) based on the neuroimaging changes that have been observed in the morphology of the corpus callosum. They report that in a sample of pure, unmedicated TS patients left-to-right inhibition was weaker than right-to-left, and left-to-right inhibition also differed to controls. The asymmetry of interhemispheric inhibition was thus the opposite of what has been described by the same authors in normal controls (Baumer et al., 2007). Whether this reflects an abnormal development of these interhemispheric connections remains to be seen. However, in the same patients imaging revealed no evidence for any structural differences in the motor region of the corpus callosum (Baumer et al., 2007). The interpretation of these findings remains difficult; however, this illustrates that brain function and brain structure can be altered independently.

Sensory–Motor Integration at Rest

It is often crucial, for example to avoid injury, that sensory input such as painful stimulation translates into movement. Sensory afferent information traveling in sensory-afferent pathways (peripheral nerve, spinal cord, thalamus, sensory cortex) therefore needs to be linked to motor output. If some tics are an unsuppressed response to sensory urges, then we might expect to see abnormalities in inhibitory pathways that specifically link sensory input and motor output. Abnormal sensory motor gating has been proposed in studies assessing grip force behavior: TS patients employed higher grip forces to manipulate an object, while they were able to adjust grip force similar to controls when the load force changed (Nowak et al., 2005; Serrien et al., 2002). Interestingly, the sensorimotor cortex has also been implicated in the generation of tics in children (Sowell et al., 2008).

One sensory–motor integration pathway that can be tested in humans is sensory afferent inhibition (SAI; Tokimura et al., 2000). A transient sensory input leads to a rapid and short-lasting inhibition of motor cortex. SAI was reduced in the baseline state in patients (Orth et al., 2005a), consistent with the assumption of a reduced efficiency of synaptic inhibition. Given the possible influence of sensory inputs in triggering the release of tics, reduced SAI may be a direct physiological reflection of increased access of sensory input to motor output in TS. It is interesting that in TS patients but not in controls, a single dose of nicotine was able to strengthen the inhibitory effect measured with SAI and also SICI (Fig. 11.2; Orth et al., 2005a). This suggests that cholinergic stimulation can modulate the circuits underlying SAI and SICI.

ASSOCIATION OF TMS DATA WITH TIC RATINGS

If experimental data relate to the cause of the clinical phenotype of TS (i.e., motor and phonic tics), one would expect an association between the two, even though an association alone would, of course, not prove a causal relationship. Ziemann and colleagues showed that patients with distal tics (i.e., hand tics) and those not taking dopamine receptor antagonists had a shorter cortical silent-period duration and less SICI (Ziemann et al., 1997). In addition, Gilbert and colleagues demonstrated that less SICI was associated with greater motor tic severity as measured with rating scales, particularly in patients who did not take dopamine receptor antagonists and those who had comorbid ADHD (Gilbert et al., 2004). In untreated patients, we measured tic severity and distribution with standard clinical scales as well as detailed video analysis and correlated these with recruitment of corticospinal output and silent-period duration elicited by TMS (Orth et al., 2008). Our hypothesis was that clinically meaningful changes in cortical excitability would be specific to those tics that involve the cortical areas examined with TMS (e.g., hand and finger tics). Input–output measures were associated with video tic ratings for severity of complex tics, phonic tics, and hand/finger tics, while other tic ratings—scores on the Yale Global Tic Severity Scale (YGTSS; Leckman et al., 1989), the Modified Rush Video Scale (Goetz et al., 1999), or other raw tic video scores—were not (Fig. 11.3). This means that increased excitability of the motor cortex at

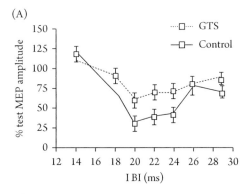

(A)

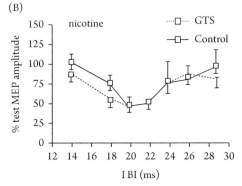

(B)

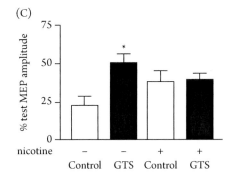

(C)

FIGURE 11.2 **Short interval afferent inhibition curves.** (**A**) In the absence of nicotine, both controls and TS patients showed significant inhibition at ISIs of 20, 22, and 24 ms (repeated measures ANOVA, $p = .001$). (**B**) In the presence of nicotine, the amount of inhibition was similar in controls and TS patients. (**C**) The analysis of the cortical inhibitory effects at maximum inhibition reveals that patients had less inhibition than controls (*$p = .006$). Nicotine had a different effect in controls and TS patients (repeated measures ANOVA, interaction between "group" and "time," $p = .012$). In the presence of nicotine, controls had less inhibition, while TS patients had more inhibition, but these effects were not significant. Values are means ± SEM, n = 9 for TS patients, n = 10 for controls.

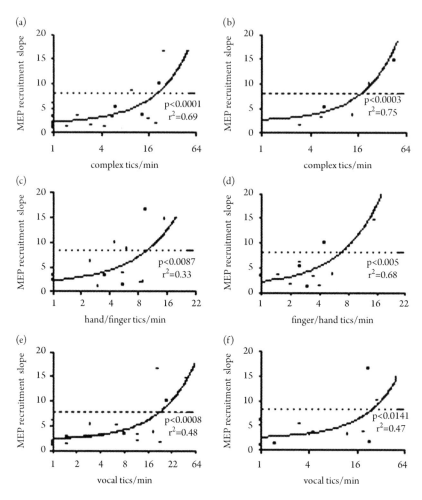

FIGURE 11.3 Linear regression analysis of tic frequency and MEP recruitment at rest. Compared with the mean slope of controls (*dotted line*), the majority of patients with tics had a shallower slope. In all patients taken together (**A, C, E**) there was a significant association of the slope of MEP size/M-wave ratios with complex tic frequency (**A**), hand/finger tic frequency (**C**), and vocal tic frequency (**E**). After preselecting patients for comorbidity, the association of the slope of MEP size/M-wave ratios with complex tic frequency (**B**), hand/finger tic frequency (**D**), and vocal tic frequency (**F**) was significant only in uncomplicated patients. Values are means ± SEM, n = 20 in A, C, D, and n = 12 in B, D, F. Note the logarithmic scale on the *x* axes.

rest was associated with more frequent tics. Predictions of complex tic, hand and finger tic, and phonic tic frequency were significant only in the subgroup of patients without comorbidity. Comorbidity such as ADHD very likely influences cortical excitability (Gilbert et al., 2004), with evidence suggesting that abnormalities in TS+ADHD may be more widespread than in TS alone (Orth & Rothwell, 2009); therefore, comorbidity may have introduced noise into the recordings from the whole group of patients.

Complex tics likely involve a large part of the motor cortex, including the M1 hand area, thus explaining the specific association of complex tic and hand/finger tic frequency with TMS measures from that area. Therefore, the specific association of electrophysiological measures from the M1 hand area of the motor cortex with movements originating from the same area (i.e., hand/finger tics in contrast to other body areas) suggests the difference in the excitability of the motor-neuron pool in a resting state could be clinically meaningful in patients. In contrast, in line with motor cortex excitability levels in a pre-activated state being similar to normal controls, there was no association of these measures with tic ratings.

Interestingly, Heise and colleagues observed an association of tic severity with the ability to normalize SICI when preparing a movement (see Heise et al., 2010, and below).

VOLUNTARY MOVEMENT CONTROL

Movement is an integral part of human life. Movements need to be planned and executed. This involves a choice of the appropriate movement or sequence of movements depending on the task at hand. In addition, one needs to get the timing right, so a movement has to be withheld until the right moment arrives. This means that movements may also have to be inhibited so they are not premature. The complex tasks of movement selection, initiation, and inhibition involve the prefrontal cortex, the basal ganglia, the supplementary motor area (SMA), and the pre-SMA, with subsequent integration of these inputs in the primary motor cortex (M1). In TS, the unwanted movements and their sensory prodromes add to this already complex process. Patients report that their tics or the sensory urges may interfere with planned movements or speech, something that is captured in the interference aspect of the YGTSS. On the other hand, it is a well-recognized phenomenon that engaging in a highly trained activity such as playing an instrument can virtually abolish sensory urges and tics. This illustrates that the forces driving tics compete with physiological frontostriatal network activity for access to the M1 as the main motor output effector.

Changes in the excitability of the motor cortex before a planned movement, or when movements have to be withheld, can be measured using TMS. In reaction-time paradigms involving "go/no go" tasks, a reduction of intracortical inhibition precedes an increase in corticospinal excitability (larger MEP amplitude; for a review see Stinear et al., 2009). Corticospinal excitability increases gradually from about 100 ms to 40 ms prior to muscle activation and then much more sharply from 40 ms to the actual movement (EMG activity; Starr et al., 1988). Reduced SICI and increased corticospinal excitability are maintained until about 50 ms before the end of muscle activation, when both measures return to their baseline excitability levels (Begum et al., 2005; Buccolieri et al., 2004). Motor cortex excitability may already change in a similar way when the need for a movement is imminent (expectation of an imperative cue in a reaction time task; van Elswijk et al., 2007). In contrast, corticospinal excitability decreases when a movement needs to be prevented (Hoshiyama et al., 1997; Nakata et al., 2006). This illustrates how movement selection, initiation, and prevention involve modulatory effects on motor cortex excitability of fronto-striato-cortical networks.

With movement preparation, cortical excitability increased less in TS subjects than in controls (Heise et al., 2010). Intracortical inhibition, in contrast, normalized quickly from the reduced levels of inhibition observed at rest (Heise et al., 2010). This increase in intracortical inhibition early on during movement preparation was particularly marked in those patients with fewer tics in whom corticospinal excitability was also lower. This suggests that tic control depends on the extent to which excitability of motor neurons can be reduced in line with an increase in the activity of intracortical interneurons.

By recording cortical activity simultaneously at several different cortical sites, EEG can help evaluate what happens across different cortical areas while movements are prepared or inhibited. Johannes and colleagues reported normal performance on this type of task but observed an increase in frontal cortex activity (Johannes et al., 2001). Serrien and colleagues combined a behavioral "go/no go" task with EEG recordings (Serrien et al., 2005) in nine unmedicated TS patients, one of whom had ADHD and one ADHD+OCD. Performance on the task was also normal. However, EEG revealed increased coherence between primary sensory motor (S1, M1), prefrontal, and frontomesial areas in the alpha frequency band when TS patients suppressed voluntary movements. TS patients thus needed to activate wider cortical areas than normal for the suppression of movements, including tics.

Using MEG, increased coherence was also found between SMA and M1 contralateral to the moving finger (Franzkowiak et al., 2012). These observations suggest that in TS the activation of wider cortical areas is necessary for planning and executing voluntary movements, but also for executing inhibitory control. It is conceivable that this represents efforts to compensate at a cortical level for the pathophysiology that causes TS.

Recently, an MEG study assessed cortical activity while TS patients moved a finger (Franzkowiak et al., 2010). In healthy individuals, voluntary movements are associated with a decrease of spontaneous oscillations at alpha (8–12 Hz) and beta (13–30 Hz) frequencies. This is called event-related desynchronization (ERD; Pfurtscheller & Aranibar, 1977). An increase of these oscillations is called event-related synchronization (ERS; Pfurtscheller & Lopes da Silva, 1999). Movement preparation and execution are associated with ERD in the contralateral S1/M1 area (Pfurtscheller & Berghold, 1989; Rau et al., 2003). With termination of the movement, a short burst of activity at beta frequencies, or ERS, occurs (Jurkiewicz et al., 2006). Beta-range ERD is thought to reflect M1 activation, while ERS most likely represents motor cortex inhibition. In TS patients, ERD at beta frequencies was higher than in controls in S1/M1 contralateral to the moving finger before finger movements and while the finger was moving. After movements ended, in both motor cortices ERS was higher in patients. In TS, this suggests increased motor cortex activation with movement planning and execution followed by increased inhibition (Franzkowiak et al., 2010). Since with voluntary movements there was no difference at alpha frequencies, in TS there is no evidence for any difference in processing sensory information at the cortical level (Salmelin et al., 1995). This means the main difference between TS patients and controls was in the motor system. Higher ERS in the ipsilateral motor cortex was associated with fewer tics, which lends further support to the hypothesis that increased motor cortex inhibition tries to put the brakes on the release of movements, including tics.

REPETITIVE TRANSCRANIAL MAGNETIC STIMULATION

Imaging studies revealed that during tic suppression and tics, activity was increased in premotor, prefrontal, and motor cortex, indicating increased activity in these brain areas (Eidelberg et al., 1997; Peterson et al., 1998; Stern et al., 2000). This led to the hypothesis that normalizing motor or premotor cortical excitability could be a potential treatment for tics in TS. Low-frequency rTMS has inhibitory effects on the stimulated brain area (Chen et al., 1997). This led to the rationale for small treatment trials with an rTMS protocol to inhibit the premotor or motor cortex (Munchau et al., 2002; Orth et al., 2005b). These trials involved a sham (i.e. placebo) condition, and the effects on tics were evaluated using the YGTSS (Leckman et al., 1989), video ratings, and self-ratings. No effects on tic severity were noted; even with higher stimulation intensities, and when given over longer time periods, tics did not improve consistently in TS in a further sham-controlled trial (Chae et al., 2004). These results do not support a role for motor or premotor rTMS at 1 Hz and 80% active motor threshold in the treatment of tics in TS.

Subsequently, Mantovani and colleagues reported that a different rTMS protocol using higher intensities of stimulation (100% resting motor threshold, bilateral supplementary motor area) given over 10 days had a beneficial effect on tics, OCD, and other measures, that lasted for 3 months (Mantovani et al., 2006). Similar effects were reported by Kwon and colleagues in 10 boys treated with 1-Hz rTMS at 100% resting motor threshold over the supplementary motor area (Kwon et al., 2011). rTMS may therefore have some promise as a potential treatment; however, the latter studies did not include a sham condition (i.e., placebo control), so it remains unclear how much of the effects were actually due to a placebo effect.

Recently, rTMS protocols have been used to examine plasticity in TS. Two studies observed no plasticity effects of inhibitory or facilitatory theta-burst rTMS in motor cortex or brainstem in TS patients (Suppa et al., 2011; Wu &

Gilbert, 2011). This suggests abnormal plasticity in TS. However, the effects of rTMS depend on several factors, including the state of the stimulated brain area before, during, and after stimulation, or medication (Ridding & Ziemann, 2010). Activity can have quite pronounced effects on the direction of plasticity effects. To induce the desired effects it is important that the participant is at rest before and during stimulation. The absence of any visible movement may not be synonymous with the motor cortex being at rest (Schieber, 2011). The motor cortex may be quite busy (e.g., dealing with sensory urges) even though the patient has no obvious movements. Therefore, the results of experiments addressing plasticity have to be interpreted with caution.

HOW SPECIFIC ARE THE ELECTROPHYSIOLOGICAL FINDINGS TO TS?

The electrophysiological findings described above are *not* specific to TS. Similarly altered motor cortex excitability has been found in other movement disorders, such as Parkinson's disease, atypical parkinsonian syndromes, or dystonia (for a review see Edwards et al., 2008). In Huntington's disease, reduced SAI and flatter input–output curves have been observed; data suggest that SAI might be a state marker, as it changed with proximity to motor onset, while input–output curves did not and might thus represent a trait marker of carrying the huntingtin gene expansion mutation (Schippling et al., 2009). It is thus clear that none of these electrophysiological paradigms can aid in the differential diagnosis of these movement disorders. However, they may have added value as biomarkers (e.g., in Huntington's disease). In TS, they may help delineate endophenotypes and thus be useful in the search of underlying genetic variants.

CONCLUSIONS AND PERSPECTIVES FOR FUTURE RESEARCH

What matters most to patients with TS is how bad their tics are and how much control they have over them. This reflects the balance between underlying deficits and adaptive, compensatory changes in different parts of cortico-subcortical networks involving the basal ganglia, motor and premotor cortex, thalamus, and prefrontal cortex. Much like tics take a waxing and waning course in intensity and can occur in bouts, the interactions between different parts of these cortico-subcortical networks, and ultimately their influence on shaping motor output, are not static but change continuously. This may be linked to the hypothesis that clusters of striatal neurons are active outside what is normally an orderly synchronized activity of the basal ganglia coupled with dysrhythmic thalamocortical projections (Leckman et al., 2006). Thus, studying something that is inherently fluid is challenging, and it may not always be possible to objectively control for the state of this system in the experimental setup. This introduces some uncertainty when interpreting data.

Bearing this in mind, in the resting state axonal excitability of corticospinal neurons and intracortical interneurons was consistently normal in TS. However, there is evidence that synaptic excitability in corticospinal neurons and the SICI circuit is lower than normal. In addition, an electrophysiological marker of sensory motor integration, SAI, was reduced in the baseline state in patients, consistent with the assumption of a reduced efficiency of synaptic inhibition. Given the possible influence of sensory inputs in triggering the release of tics, reduced SAI may be a direct physiological reflection of increased access of sensory input to motor output in TS. When reduced SICI was first noted in TS, it was conceivable that reduced inhibition in the cortex meant the motor cortex was more likely to release involuntary movements in TS. However, more recent evidence indicates that the gain of all motor cortex circuits may be reduced in TS, with the result that they become less sensitive to small changes in input from other areas. The more effectively the motor cortex can reduce its excitability, the more effectively tics can be controlled. Cortical inhibition may thus mirror an adaptive response to abnormal basal ganglia–motor cortex inputs that prevents the release of unwanted movements unless input signals are strong enough to overcome the reduced processing gain. A caveat to this interpretation is that, in the author's experience, many persons with TS who take part in research can sit still for the time the experiments take. This does not necessarily mean they are tic-free; sensory urges may still be present, so the situation in the laboratory may model a state of enhanced tic suppression. The data recorded in this state may well resemble those recorded when a normal movement is prepared but then has to be actively suppressed. Experiments examining control of voluntary movements revealed that in TS motor

---

Box 11.1. Key Points

- Electrophysiological methods can help differentiate the quality of brain activation and can therefore add an important dimension to the noninvasive study of brain function.
- Many TS patients have comorbid conditions, the most common of which are ADHD and OCD. It is therefore important to carefully assess these other problems when recruiting patients into studies.
- Several techniques have been used to study the electrophysiology of TS, including electroencephalography (EEG) and event-related potentials, evoked potentials, transcranial magnetic stimulation (TMS), and magnetoencephalography (MEG). These methods are painless but can be sensitive to movement artifacts.
- In TS, tic states, tic suppression states, and truly sensory urge and tic-free states alternate constantly. It may not always be possible to objectively control for the state of the motor system in the experimental setup. This introduces some uncertainty when interpreting data.
- In the resting state, axonal excitability of corticospinal neurons and intracortical interneurons was consistently normal in TS. However, there is evidence that synaptic excitability in corticospinal neurons and the SICI circuit is lower than normal.
- There is reduced excitability in a measure of sensory motor integration, SAI. This suggests that sensory input has increased access to motor output in TS and fits well with clinical observations of an increased sensitivity to sensory stimuli in TS.
- Measures of motor cortical excitability (SICI, input–output curves) are associated with tic severity. One study indicates that the electrophysiological measures from the M1 hand area of the motor cortex are specifically associated with movements originating from the same area (i.e., hand/finger tics) in contrast to other body areas.
- Cortical inhibition may mirror an adaptive response to abnormal basal ganglia–motor cortex inputs that prevents the release of unwanted movements unless input signals are strong enough to overcome the reduced processing gain.
- Experiments examining control of voluntary movements revealed that in TS, motor cortex excitability increases less than in controls when preparing a movement, even though intracortical inhibition (i.e., SICI) normalizes. At the same time, suppression of movement is associated with more widespread cortical activity in TS (increased cortico-cortical coupling on EEG and MEG coherence analysis).
- Using rTMS as a treatment for tics has been disappointing, even though some recent small studies without a placebo control arm suggest some effects of motor cortex inhibitory protocols.
- Recent evidence suggests abnormal plasticity in TS. However, the effects of plasticity-inducing protocols depend on the state of the stimulated brain area before, during, and after stimulation, or medication. Since it is difficult to accurately control for the state of brain activity (i.e., rest vs. active), results need to be interpreted with caution.

Box 11.2. Questions for Future Research

1. Can one distinguish better between a primary abnormality, which hence contributes to causing tics, and what may reflect secondary (e.g., compensatory) changes?
2. How do the circuits relevant for movement control and sensory gating develop from childhood to adulthood? Can we find experimental evidence for the hypothesis that tics persist and TS thus develops when the neuronal circuits responsible for sensory gating and movement control do not mature appropriately?
3. Do TS patients spend much more time than controls in a state of movement preparation because of tic-driving forces? Are they able to then suppress these movements so that from the outside they seem at rest? Is it possible to distinguish these states? How active is the motor cortex in TS in the absence of overt movements?
4. What can we learn from recordings from electrodes implanted for deep brain stimulation? How does the activity recorded from the stimulation site within the basal ganglia relate to recordings from the outside of the skull?
5. Is there a common electrophysiological signature for TS and its comorbidities? Or can TS be distinguished from its comorbidities? Is there an electrophysiological trait marker for TS?
6. What is the difference between chronic motor tics and TS? Do they differ just by degree, or are there more profound differences?

cortex excitability increases less than in controls when preparing a movement, even though intracortical inhibition (i.e., SICI) normalizes. At the same time, suppression of movement is associated with more widespread cortical activity in TS (increased cortico-cortical coupling on EEG and MEG coherence analysis).

It is interesting to speculate that TS patients may spend much more time than controls in a state of movement preparation because of tic-driving forces; they may be able to then suppress these movements so from the outside they seem at rest. To the researcher in the laboratory the challenge would be to distinguish these states, because the motor cortex can be quite active without any apparent movements (Schieber, 2011).

A key challenge remains the distinction between what may be a primary abnormality, which hence contributes to causing tics, and what may reflect secondary (e.g., compensatory) changes. It is difficult to draw any conclusions from cross-sectional designs, and longitudinal studies may take a long time and are also difficult

in a disorder that does not *per se* progress in adulthood. A further important question is how the circuits relevant for movement control and sensory gating develop from childhood to adulthood. The occurrence of tics in childhood suggests TS is a developmental disorder. Some tics are present for a short period of time in many healthy children as well but then disappear. This suggests that tics persist and TS thus develops when the neuronal circuits responsible for sensory gating and movement control do not mature appropriately. It is interesting to note in this regard that SICI was reduced in the motor cortex in healthy children, and to some degree in adolescents, while intracortical facilitation and conduction times along the corticospinal tract were normal (Fietzek et al., 2000; Walther et al., 2009). While being cautious about extrapolating from cross-sectional data, this may mean that reduced intracortical inhibition is necessary for motor learning in childhood and adolescence. Reduced SICI in TS could then be a sign of abnormal maturation of the motor brain.

The combination of a variety of techniques such as EEG, MEG, TMS, and imaging may also be helpful to inform us about effects at a network level after a well-defined challenge to the motor cortex. Such complementary assessments have already proven useful for the understanding of brain function (Driver et al., 2009). Some of the above techniques capture activity of the whole brain while TMS measures activity within the confines of the motor cortex or can manipulate excitability in that region. One could, for example, use one of the repetitive TMS protocols to manipulate motor cortex excitability and evaluate its effects on neuronal plasticity not only at the local level with TMS but also at the network level using imaging techniques. Recording from electrodes implanted for deep brain stimulation, so far an experimental new form of treatment for TS (e.g., Welter et al., 2008; see also Chapter 26), may also be valuable in this regard, similar to Parkinson's disease (Hammond et al., 2007).

REFERENCES

Baumer T, Dammann E, Bock F et al. Laterality of interhemispheric inhibition depends on handedness. *Exp Brain Res* 2007; *180*:195–203.

Baumer T, Thomalla G, Kroeger J et al. Interhemispheric motor networks are abnormal in patients with Gilles de la Tourette syndrome. *Mov Disord* 2010; 25:2828–2837.

Begum T, Mima T, Oga T et al. Cortical mechanisms of unilateral voluntary motor inhibition in humans. *Neurosci Res* 2005; 53:428–435.

Bliss J. Sensory experiences of Gilles de la Tourette syndrome. *Arch Gen Psychiatry* 1980; 37:1343–1347.

Buccolieri A, Abbruzzese G, Rothwell JC. Relaxation from a voluntary contraction is preceded by increased excitability of motor cortical inhibitory circuits. *J Physiol* 2004; 558: 685–695.

Chae JH, Nahas Z, Wassermann E et al. A pilot safety study of repetitive transcranial magnetic stimulation (rTMS) in Tourette's syndrome. *Cogn Behav Neurol* 2004; 17:109–117.

Chen R, Classen J, Gerloff C et al. Depression of motor cortex excitability by low-frequency transcranial magnetic stimulation. *Neurology* 1997; 48:1398–1403.

Di Lazzaro V, Ziemann U, Lemon RN. State of the art: Physiology of transcranial motor cortex stimulation. *Brain Stimul* 2008; 1:345–362.

Driver J, Blankenburg F, Bestmann S et al. Concurrent brain-stimulation and neuroimaging for studies of cognition. *Trends Cogn Sci* 2009; 13:319–327.

Edwards MJ, Talelli P, Rothwell JC. Clinical applications of transcranial magnetic stimulation in patients with movement disorders. *Lancet Neurol* 2008; 7:827–840.

Eidelberg D, Moeller JR, Antonini A et al. The metabolic anatomy of Tourette's syndrome. *Neurology* 1997; 48:927–934.

Ferbert A, Priori A, Rothwell JC et al. Interhemispheric inhibition of the human motor cortex. *J Physiol* 1992; 453:525–546.

Fietzek UM, Heinen F, Berweck S et al. Development of the corticospinal system and hand motor function: central conduction times and motor performance tests. *Dev Med Child Neurol* 2000; 42:220–227.

Franzkowiak S, Pollok B, Biermann-Ruben K et al. Altered pattern of motor cortical activation-inhibition during voluntary movements in Tourette syndrome. *Mov Disord* 2010; 25:1960–1966.

One of the first studies using magnetoencephalography in TS.

Franzkowiak S, Pollok B, Biermann-Ruben K et al. Motor-cortical interaction in Gilles de la Tourette syndrome. *PLoS One* 2012; 7: e27850.

Freeman RD, Fast DK, Burd L et al. An international perspective on Tourette syndrome: selected findings from 3,500 individuals in 22 countries. *Dev Med Child Neurol* 2000; 42:436–447.

Gilbert DL, Bansal AS, Sethuraman G et al. Association of cortical disinhibition with tic, ADHD, and OCD severity in Tourette syndrome. *Mov Disord* 2004; 19:416–425.

Gilbert DL, Sallee FR, Zhang J et al. Transcranial magnetic stimulation-evoked cortical inhibition: a consistent marker of attention-deficit/hyperactivity disorder scores in Tourette syndrome. *Biol Psychiatry* 2005; 57:1597–1600.

Goetz CG, Pappert EJ, Louis ED et al. Advantages of a modified scoring method for the Rush Video-Based Tic Rating Scale. *Mov Disord* 1999; 14:502–506.

Greenberg BD, Ziemann U, Cora-Locatelli G et al. Altered cortical excitability in obsessive-compulsive disorder. *Neurology* 2000; 54:142–147.

Hammond C, Bergman H, Brown P. Pathological synchronization in Parkinson's disease: networks, models and treatments. *Trends Neurosci* 2007; 30:357–364.

Heise KF, Steven B, Liuzzi G et al. Altered modulation of intracortical excitability during movement preparation in Gilles de la Tourette syndrome. *Brain* 2010; 133:580–590.

The authors show how motor cortical activity differs between TS and controls when preparing a normal movement.

Hoshiyama M, Kakigi R, Koyama S et al. Temporal changes of pyramidal tract activities after decision of movement: a study using transcranial magnetic stimulation of the motor cortex in humans. *Electroencephalogr Clin Neurophysiol* 1997; 105:255–261.

Johannes S, Wieringa BM, Mantey M et al. Altered inhibition of motor responses in Tourette syndrome and obsessive-compulsive disorder. *Acta Neurol Scand* 2001; 104:36–43.

Jurkiewicz MT, Gaetz WC, Bostan AC, Cheyne D. Post-movement beta rebound is generated in motor cortex: evidence from neuromagnetic recordings. *NeuroImage* 2006; 32: 1281–1289.

Kalanithi PS, Zheng W, Kataoka Y et al. Altered parvalbumin-positive neuron distribution in basal ganglia of individuals with Tourette syndrome. *Proc Natl Acad Sci USA* 2005; 102:13307–13312.

Important neuropathological examination of postmortem TS brains.

Karp BI, Porter S, Toro C, Hallett M. Simple motor tics may be preceded by a premotor potential. *J Neurol Neurosurg Psychiatry* 1996; 61:103–106.

Kujirai T, Caramia MD, Rothwell JC et al. Corticocortical inhibition in human motor cortex. *J Physiol* 1993; 471:501–519.

Kwon HJ, Lim WS, Lim MH et al. 1-Hz low frequency repetitive transcranial magnetic stimulation in children with Tourette's syndrome. *Neurosci Lett* 2011; 492:1–4.

Leckman JF. Tourette's syndrome. *Lancet* 2002; 360:1577–1586.

Leckman JF, Riddle MA, Hardin MT et al. The Yale Global Tic Severity Scale: initial testing of a clinician-rated scale of tic severity. *J Am Acad Child Adolesc Psychiatry* 1989; 28:566–573.

Leckman JF, Vaccarino FM, Kalanithi PS, Rothenberger A. Annotation: Tourette syndrome: a relentless drumbeat—driven by misguided brain oscillations. *J Child Psychol Psychiatry* 2006; 47:537–550.

Mantovani A, Lisanby SH, Pieraccini F et al. Repetitive transcranial magnetic stimulation (rTMS) in the treatment of obsessive-compulsive disorder (OCD) and Tourette's syndrome (TS). *Int J Neuropsychopharmacol* 2006; 9:95–100.

Mink JW. Neurobiology of basal ganglia and Tourette syndrome: basal ganglia circuits and thalamocortical outputs. *Adv Neurol* 2006; 99:89–98.

Munchau A, Bloem BR, Thilo KV et al. Repetitive transcranial magnetic stimulation for Tourette syndrome. *Neurology* 2002; 59:1789–1791.

Nakata H, Inui K, Wasaka T et al. Higher anticipated force required a stronger inhibitory process in go/no-go tasks. *Clin Neurophysiol* 2006; 117:1669–1676.

Nitsche MA, Cohen LG, Wassermann EM et al. Transcranial direct current stimulation: State of the art 2008. *Brain Stimul* 2008; 1:206–223.

Nowak DA, Rothwell J, Topka H et al. Grip force behavior in Gilles de la Tourette syndrome. *Mov Disord* 2005; 20:217–223.

Obeso JA, Rothwell JC, Marsden CD. Simple tics in Gilles de la Tourette's syndrome are not prefaced by a normal premovement EEG potential. *J Neurol Neurosurg Psychiatry* 1981; 44:735–738.

Orth M, Amann B, Robertson MM, Rothwell JC. Excitability of motor cortex inhibitory circuits in Tourette syndrome before and after single dose nicotine. *Brain* 2005a; 128:1292–1300.

Orth M, Kirby R, Richardson MP et al. Subthreshold rTMS over pre-motor cortex has no effect on tics in patients with Gilles de la Tourette syndrome. *Clin Neurophysiol* 2005b; 116:764–768.

Orth M, Munchau A, Rothwell JC. Corticospinal system excitability at rest is associated with tic severity in Tourette syndrome. *Biol Psychiatry* 2008; 64:248–251.

This study demonstrates an association of electrophysiological parameters with tic frequency.

Orth M, Rothwell JC. The cortical silent period: intrinsic variability and relation to the waveform of the transcranial magnetic stimulation pulse. *Clin Neurophysiol* 2004; *115*:1076–1082.

This study demonstrates electrophysiological differences between pure TS and TS with comorbidities, with more pronounced changes in the TS+ADHD group.

Orth M, Rothwell JC. Motor cortex excitability and comorbidity in Gilles de la Tourette syndrome. *J Neurol Neurosurg Psychiatry* 2009; *80*: 29–34.

Orth M, Snijders AH, Rothwell JC. The variability of intracortical inhibition and facilitation. *Clin Neurophysiol* 2003; *114*:2362–2369.

Pascual-Leone A, Davey NJ, Rothwell JC et al. *Handbook of transcranial magnetic stimulation*. London: Arnold, 2002.

Peterson BS, Skudlarski P, Anderson AW et al. A functional magnetic resonance imaging study of tic suppression in Tourette syndrome. *Arch Gen Psychiatry* 1998; *55*:326–333.

Pfurtscheller G, Aranibar A. Event-related cortical desynchronization detected by power measurements of scalp EEG. *Electroencephalogr Clin Neurophysiol* 1977; *42*:817–826.

Pfurtscheller G, Berghold A. Patterns of cortical activation during planning of voluntary movement. *Electroencephalogr Clin Neurophysiol* 1989; *72*:250–258.

Pfurtscheller G, Lopes da Silva FH. Event-related EEG/MEG synchronization and desynchronization: basic principles. *Clin Neurophysiol* 1999; *110*:1842–1857.

Rau C, Plewnia C, Hummel F, Gerloff C. Event-related desynchronization and excitability of the ipsilateral motor cortex during simple self-paced finger movements. *Clin Neurophysiol* 2003; *114*:1819–1826.

Ridding MC, Ziemann U. Determinants of the induction of cortical plasticity by non-invasive brain stimulation in healthy subjects. *J Physiol* 2010; *588*:2291–2304.

Salmelin R, Hamalainen M, Kajola M, Hari R. Functional segregation of movement-related rhythmic activity in the human brain. *Neuroimage* 1995; *2*:237–243.

Schieber MH. Dissociating motor cortex from the motor. *J Physiol* 2011; *589*:5613–5624.

Schippling S, Schneider SA, Bhatia KP et al. Abnormal motor cortex excitability in preclinical and very early Huntington's disease. *Biol Psychiatry* 2009; *65*:959–965.

Serrien DJ, Nirkko AC, Loher TJ et al. Movement control of manipulative tasks in patients with Gilles de la Tourette syndrome. *Brain* 2002; *125*:290–300.

Serrien DJ, Orth M, Evans AH et al. Motor inhibition in patients with Gilles de la Tourette syndrome: functional activation patterns as revealed by EEG coherence. *Brain* 2005; *128*:116–125.

Sowell ER, Kan E, Yoshii J et al. Thinning of sensorimotor cortices in children with Tourette syndrome. *Nature Neurosci* 2008; *11*:637–639.

Starr A, Caramia M, Zarola F, Rossini PM. Enhancement of motor cortical excitability in humans by non-invasive electrical stimulation appears prior to voluntary movement. *Electroencephalogr Clin Neurophysiol* 1988; *70*:26–32.

Stefan K, Kunesch E, Cohen LG et al. Induction of plasticity in the human motor cortex by paired associative stimulation. *Brain* 2000; *123*:572–584.

Stern E, Silbersweig DA, Chee KY et al. A functional neuroanatomy of tics in Tourette syndrome. *Arch Gen Psychiatry* 2000; *57*:741–748.

Stinear CM, Coxon JP, Byblow WD. Primary motor cortex and movement prevention: where Stop meets Go. *Neurosci Biobehav Rev* 2009; *33*:662–673.

Suppa A, Belvisi D, Bologna M et al. Abnormal cortical and brain stem plasticity in Gilles de la Tourette syndrome. *Mov Disord* 2011; *26*:1703–1710.

Thickbroom GW. Transcranial magnetic stimulation and synaptic plasticity: experimental framework and human models. *Exp Brain Res* 2007; *180*:583–593.

Tokimura H, Di Lazzaro V, Tokimura Y et al. Short latency inhibition of human hand motor cortex by somatosensory input from the hand. *J Physiol* 2000; *523*:503–513.

van Elswijk G, Kleine BU, Overeem S, Stegeman DF. Expectancy induces dynamic modulation of corticospinal excitability. *J Cogn Neurosci* 2007; *19*:121–131.

Walther M, Berweck S, Schessl J et al. Maturation of inhibitory and excitatory motor cortex pathways in children. *Brain Dev* 2009; *31*:562–567.

Wassermann EM. Risk and safety of repetitive transcranial magnetic stimulation: report and suggested guidelines from the International Workshop on the Safety of Repetitive Transcranial Magnetic Stimulation, June 5–7,

1996. *Electroencephalogr Clin Neurophysiol* 1998; *108*:1–16.

Welter ML, Mallet L, Houeto JL et al. Internal pallidal and thalamic stimulation in patients with Tourette syndrome. *Arch Neurol* 2008; 65:952–957.

Wu SW, Gilbert DL. Altered neurophysiologic response to intermittent theta burst stimulation in Tourette syndrome. *Brain Stimulation* 2011 May 1 [Epub ahead of print].

Ziemann U, Paulus W, Rothenberger A. Decreased motor inhibition in Tourette's disorder: evidence from transcranial magnetic stimulation. *Am J Psychiatry* 1997; *154*:1277–1284.

First study to demonstrate reduced activity of intracortical inhibitory interneurons in TS.

12

Neurobiology and Functional Anatomy of Tic Disorders

DEANNA J. GREENE, KEVIN J. BLACK AND BRADLEY L. SCHLAGGAR

Abstract

This chapter summarizes the highly valuable contribution of magnetic resonance imaging (MRI) to the understanding of the functional anatomy of tics and related disorders. Structural MRI studies have revealed reduced caudate volumes in children and adults with Tourette syndrome (TS), with a negative correlation between caudate volume in childhood and symptom severity later in life. Cortical thinning in sensorimotor cortices was detected in children and adults with TS, with a negative correlation between thickness and orofacial tic severity. Whereas adults with TS show cortical thinning and reduced gray matter volume in prefrontal regions, suggesting a failure in neural compensation to control tics into adulthood, results from children with TS are mixed. Measures of white matter have demonstrated larger volumes and reduced fractional anisotropy in the corpus callosum in TS. Results from functional MRI studies of motor control and cognitive control in TS are generally inconsistent. Putative cognitive control networks seem functionally immature and anomalous in TS, suggesting that functional anatomical abnormalities in TS may not be restricted to cortico-striato-thalamo-cortical circuits and involve cortical networks supporting cognitive control.

INTRODUCTION

Tourette syndrome (TS) is a developmental disorder of the central nervous system defined by the chronic presence of motor and vocal tics. While a clear neurobiological explanation for why tics occur remains unavailable, research has provided clues into the neurobiological dysfunctions that characterize the disorder. Understanding the neural underpinnings of TS will not only further our knowledge about the disorder, but can also help to inform targets for intervention and treatment.

The basal ganglia, a collection of subcortical nuclei, and its connections—specifically corticostriatal-thalamo-cortical (CSTC) circuits— have been the focus of most neurobiological research on TS. The basal ganglia are known to be involved in motor control and in other movement disorders (e.g., Parkinson's disease,

Huntington's disease). Further, CSTC circuits are involved in inhibitory control (Aron et al., 2007) and habit formation (Graybiel, 2008), both of which are implicated in TS. Inhibitory control is most obviously affected in TS within the motor domain, resulting in tics. Within the cognitive domain, inhibitory control is also altered, as there is evidence for atypical executive function in TS. In addition, the comorbidity rate with disorders of cognitive function, specifically obsessive-compulsive disorder (OCD) and attention-deficit/hyperactivity disorder (ADHD), is quite high. With regard to habit formation, there are several links between tics and habits. While habits are gradually learned stimulus–response associations, and tics are brief, nonrhythmic, stereotyped movements/vocalizations, they share several qualities. For one, both involve motor acts performed in response to sensory cues. In addition, some theories of

TS propose that tics are essentially inappropriate stimulus–response (sensory urge–tic) associations (Albin & Mink, 2006). Given the known involvement of CSTC circuits in habit formation, as well as in inhibitory control, these circuits have been highly implicated in TS and have been the primary focus of most studies concerning neuroanatomical functioning. More recently, studies have also interrogated the whole brain since other brain regions and large-scale brain networks may be important in TS, given the complex profile of the disorder.

This chapter will discuss magnetic resonance imaging (MRI) studies of children and adults with TS. MRI is a tool for noninvasive, *in vivo* investigation of brain structure and function, and as such, has grown in popularity for studying clinical disorders. We will first survey the MRI literature in TS, identify consistent results, and then discuss how such results fit with current models of CSTC dysfunction in TS.

STRUCTURAL MRI

To examine potential anatomical abnormalities in individuals with TS, many studies have applied structural MRI techniques. The most common approach has been to collect high-resolution structural MRI images and compute volumes of *a priori* regions of interest (ROIs). Volumes can be measured by manually tracing ROIs as well as by using automated tools to segment gray matter, white matter, and cerebral spinal fluid in order to define region borders. This volumetric technique has most often been applied to measure subcortical structures (e.g., basal ganglia, thalamus) as well as white matter tracts (e.g., corpus callosum). Automated segmentation and manual tracing of sulcal and gyral landmarks are used to identify cortical regions, and automated algorithms have been designed to quantify cortical thickness. Another approach for measuring volume, voxel-based morphometry (VBM), relies upon the local composition of brain tissue to estimate volume. VBM estimates the proportion of gray and white matter on a voxel-wise basis and takes into account the volume change needed to transform the corresponding part

of each individual's brain into standard space at that voxel. VBM has been applied to both cortical and subcortical regions. Finally, white matter tracts, and sometimes gray matter nuclei, have been imaged and measured using diffusion tensor imaging (DTI). DTI measures the diffusion value of water molecules in multiple directions, providing several quantitative measures of interest, including mean diffusivity (MD), which is an average of the diffusion in many different directions, and fractional anisotropy (FA), which is the degree of diffusion anisotropy. Since the diffusion of water molecules is likely anisotropic in fiber tracts, especially myelinated fiber tracts, DTI can be used to create maps of the anatomical connections in the brain.

It is important to note the heterogeneity in the groups of participants who have been studied across structural MRI studies of TS. While some studies have excluded participants with medication use and/or comorbidities, others have attempted to account for these variables in the statistical analyses, while yet others have not addressed these possible confounding factors at all. Also, various age ranges have been sampled, from young children to adolescents to adults. The differences among studies must be taken into account when interpreting the results. Table 12.1 summarizes the methods and results of the structural MRI studies in TS, allowing for a direct comparison of methodological differences. This section will review the results of many of these studies, organized according to the brain region of interest.

Basal Ganglia

The basal ganglia comprise a set of subcortical nuclei that include the caudate nucleus, putamen, globus pallidus (internal and external segments), subthalamic nucleus, and substantia nigra. Given the basal ganglia's known role in motor control and in other movement disorders, these structures have been the primary focus of many studies investigating the neurobiology of TS. In fact, one of the most consistent findings from structural neuroimaging of TS is reduced volumes of basal ganglia nuclei, particularly the caudate nucleus. One of the first studies to

Table 12.1 Structural MRI Studies in TS

Reference	N (TS sample size)	Age mean (SD) Range	Male: Female	Comorbid disorders	Medications	Controls (N) Age mean (SD) Age range	Hypotheses tested	Methodology	Main findings
Peterson et al. (1993)	N = 14	31.8 (8.5)	11:3	2 OCD, 4 OC-like symptoms, 3 ADHD in childhood	4 with past neuroleptic use	N = 14 32.4(8.8)	Volume of BG nuclei & lateral ventricles; asymmetry calculated	Manual tracing; ICC ranged 79–98%	↓ left lenticular volume & striatum; loss of asymmetry
Singer et al. (1993)	N = 37	11.5 7–16	29:8	18 ADHD	25 currently taking medication	N = 18 9.8 6–15	Volume of BG nuclei & lateral ventricles; asymmetry calculated	Manual tracing; ICC ranged 78–100%	↓ left GP in TS+ADHD; reduced and reversed asymmetry in Pu and lentiform in pure TS
Hyde et al. (1995)	N = 10 (more affected MZ twin with TS)	16.3 9–31 7.1–13.8	16:4	Not reported	Not reported	N = 10 (less affected MZ co-twin)	Volume of BG nuclei & ventricles; asymmetry calculated	Manual tracing; paired t-test to compare MZ twins	↓ right CN (trend in left) in more severely affected twin
Castellanos et al. (1996)	N = 14	10.4 (1.9) 7.1–13.8	14:0	All 14 ADHD	Neuroleptic-naïve	N = 31 10.9 (2.1) 6.7–13.9 ADHD only: N = 26	Volume of BG nuclei & anterior frontal cortex; asymmetry calculated	Semi-automated and manual tracing; ICC ranged 85–98%	Reversed asymmetry in GP in TS+ADHD vs. controls and in ADHD vs. controls

Study	N	Age	Sex (M:F)	ADHD	Medication	ADHD N/Age	Measure	Method	Findings
Baumgardner et al. (1996)	N = 37	11.8 (1.9)	32:5	21 ADHD	Not reported	N = 27 10.8 (2.6) ADHD only: N = 13	Volume of 5 CC subregions	Manual tracing; ICC = 98%	↑ CC in 4 of 5 subregions; one subregion ↓ in ADHD
Moriarty et al. (1997)	N = 16	35 (13) 17–62	11:6	Not reported	Medication-free for >3 mo.	N = 8 33 (10) 20–45	Volume of CN, CC & amygdala; asymmetry calculated	Manual tracing; ICC too low for amygdala, so not reported; ICC ranged 84–96% for other structures	Loss of CN asymmetry; ↑ CC
Zimmerman et al. (2000)	N = 19	10.9 7.6–15.2	0:19	8 ADHD	6 currently taking medication	N = 21 10.7 8–15	Volume of BG nuclei & lateral ventricles; asymmetry calculated	Manual tracing; ICC ranged 83–97%	↓ lateral ventricles; no difference in BG

(Continued)

Table 12.1 (*Continued*)

Reference	N (TS sample size)	Age mean (SD) Range	Male: Female	Comorbid disorders	Medications	Controls (N) Age mean (SD) Age range	Hypotheses tested	Methodology	Main findings
Peterson et al. (2001)	N = 155	18.7 (13.4) 6–63	114:41	62 OCD, 36 ADHD	72 currently taking medication	N = 131 20.8 (13.4)	Volume of 8 cortical regions per hemisphere, plus ventricles	Isointensity contour function & manual editing	Children: ↑ dorsal prefrontal & parieto-occipital cortex, ↓ premotor, orbitofrontal & subgenual cortex in boys; Adults: ↓ dorsal prefrontal & parieto-occipital cortex in women, ↑ premotor & parieto-occipital cortex in men; test of a neuroleptic-naive, pure TS subsample showed similar results
Hong et al. (2002)	N = 19	9.7 (2.7) 7–17	19:0	8 history of mild hyperactivity	Not reported	N = 17 9.8 (1.9) 7–13	Volume of GM, WM, CSF in cerebral lobes & cerebellum; asymmetry calculated	Semi-automated sterotactic-based parcellation; ICC >98%	↓ right and ↑ left frontal lobe gray matter; ↑ asymmetry; ↑ frontal white matter

Study	N	Age	Sex (M:F)	Diagnosis	Medication	Control	Measure	Method	Findings
Fredericksen et al. (2002)	N = 25	11.3 (2.3)	25:0	14 ADHD	Medication-free for >1 mo.	N = 26 10.6 (2.7) ADHD only: N = 12	Volume of GM, WM, CSF in cerebral lobes	Fuzzy segmentation protocol	↑ percentage of right frontal white matter; ↓ frontal volumes in ADHD
Peterson et al. (2003)	N = 154*	18.7 (13.4) 6–63	115:39	51 OCD, 41 ADHD	72 currently taking medications	N = 130 21 (13.5) 6–63	Volume of BG nuclei	Manual tracing; ICC > 90%	↓ CN in children and adults; ↑ CN in those taking neuroleptics; ↓ Pu & GP in adults; OCD associated with ↓ Pu overall and ↓ Pu, CN, GP in children
Plessen et al. (2004)	N = 158*	18.5 5–65	117:41	39 OCD, 32 ADHD, 10 OCD +ADHD	75 currently taking medication	N = 121 19.7	Volume of 5 CC subregions	Isointensity contour function & manual editing	↓ CC in children, ↑ CC in adults; CC size positively correlated with motor tic severity
Bloch et al. (2005)	N = 43	11.4 (1.6)	34:9	15 OCD, 8 ADHD	21 currently taking medications	None	Volume of BG nuclei; 7-year follow-up design	Manual tracing; ICC > 90%	↓ CN & Pu in childhood was associated with more severe tics on average 7 years later; ↓ CN in childhood associated with more severe OCD on average 7 years later

(Continued)

Table 12.1 (*Continued*)

Reference	N (TS sample size)	Age mean (SD) Range	Male: Female	Comorbid disorders	Medications	Controls (N) Age mean (SD) Age range	Hypotheses tested	Methodology	Main findings
Ludolph et al. (2006)	N = 14	12.5	14:0	Numbers not reported; not excluded	4 currently taking stimulants	N = 15 13.4	GM volume	VBM	Gray matter ↑ in ventral Pu and ↓ in hippocampus; both correlate with symptom severity
Lee et al. (2006)	N = 16	9.3 (2.3) 7–14	16:0	None	Medication-naïve	N = 16 10 (1.8) 7–13	Volume of thalamus	Manual tracing; ICC = 95%	↑ left thalamus; ↓ thalamic asymmetry
Amat et al. (2006)	N = 93	7–18	14:79	33 OCD and/or ADHD	Not reported	N = 32	Cerebral hyperintensities	2-rater consensus on proton-density & T2-weighted images	More hyperintensities in subcortical regions in TS and ADHD
Plessen et al. (2006)	N = 20	13.6 (1.9) 9–17	20:0	4 OCD, 5 ADHD	9 currently taking medication	N = 20 13.4 (2.4)	Area of CC; FA in CC	Isointensity contour function & manual editing; DTI (in-house software)	↓ FA in CC; when comorbidities and medications included as covariates of no interest, the results did not change

Study	N	Age	Sex (M:F)	Comorbidity	Medication	Comparison N & Age	Measures	Method	Results
Wang et al. (2007)	N = 15	33.4 (11.0)	10:5	3 OCD, 1 ADHD	Neuroleptic-naïve	N = 15 33.1 (11.6)	Volume and shape of BG nuclei & thalamus	Volumetric, large deformation high-dimensional brain mapping	No differences in volume or shape of the CN, Pu, NAc, & thalamus
Peterson et al. (2007)	N = 154*	18.7 (13.4) 6–63	114:40	Numbers not reported; not excluded	Numbers not reported; excluded	N = 128 20.2 (13.2)	Volume of amygdala & hippocampus	Manual tracing; ICC ranged 89–94%	↑hippocampus & amygdala; hippocampus & amygdala volumes negatively correlated with tic severity, OCD, & ADHD symptoms
Makki et al. (2008)	N = 23	11.8 (3.3) 5–17	19:4	Numbers not reported; not excluded	Numbers not reported; not excluded	N = 35 13.1 (3.2)	Volume; GM & WM volume; parallel & perpendicular diffusion, FA, MD of BG nuclei & thalamus	Manual tracing; VBM; DTI (DTI-Studio software)	↓left CN & bilateral thalamus; ↑MD in Pu; ↓MD in thalamus
Makki et al. (2009)	N = 18	11.3 (2.4) 6.9–17	14:4	Not reported	Not reported	N = 12 12.2 (4.1) 5.2–17.3	GM & WM volume; connectivity between caudate, thalamus, & 11 frontal regions	VBM; DTI analysis in FSL; connectivity estimate = probability of voxel in seed region to connect to a frontal target region	↓left CN (trend in right) & bilateral thalamus; ↓connectivity between CN & frontal regions

(Continued)

Table 12.1 (Continued)

Reference	N (TS sample size)	Age mean (SD) Range	Male: Female	Comorbid disorders	Medications	Controls (N) Age mean (SD) Age range	Hypotheses tested	Methodology	Main findings
Sowell et al. (2008)	N = 25	12.4 7–18	18:7	4 OCD, 5 ADHD	11 currently taking medication	N = 35 12.3 7–21	Cortical thickness in gray matter	Manual tracing of sulci	↓ thickness in sensorimotor, frontal and parietal cortex; thinning in sensorimotor and DLPFC associated with more severe tics
Muller-Vahl et al. (2009)	N = 19	30.4 18–60	19:0	1 mild OCD, 4 ADHD tendencies but did not meet diagnostic criteria	Medication-free for <5 mo.	N = 20 31.7 18–65	GM & WM volume over the whole brain	VBM; magnetization transfer imaging	↓ left CN, ACC, primary sensorimotor areas, middle frontal and medial frontal gyrus of right hemisphere; changes in white matter volume
Fahim et al. (2009)	N = 32 (16 sibling pairs)	17.2 (4.1)	22:10	10 OCD, 15 ADHD	Not reported	None	Cortical thickness & heritability of cortical thickness	Fully automated "CIVET" pipeline	High heritability in the motor-cingulate-insular cortices; thinning associated with increased tics and OCD symptoms in the cingulate and insula
Roessner et al. (2009)	N = 38	11.9 (1.3) 9.6–15.1	38:0	None	Medication-naïve	N = 38 12.2 (1.4)	GM & WM volume across the whole brain	VBM	No differences

Study	N	Age mean (SD) range	Sex (M:F)	Comorbidity	Medication	N	Age mean (SD) range	Measures	Method	Findings
Thomalla et al. (2009)	N = 15	34.5 (8.9)	13:2	None	None	N = 15		FA, eigenvalues, & MD of WM fibers	DTI analysis in FSL	↑ FA in somatosensory white matter; negative correlation with tic severity
Fahim et al. (2010)	N = 34	17.2 (4.1) 10–25	24:10	None	10 currently taking medication	N = 32	16.3 (3.6) 10–20	Cortical thickness	Fully automated "CIVET" pipeline	Cortical thinning in left somatosensory/motor and right orbitofrontal regions; thinning correlated with tic severity
Draganski et al. (2010)	N = 40	32.4 (11) 18–56	30:10	6 OCD, 11 ADHD, 8 OCD +ADHD	25 currently taking medication	N = 40	34.4 (9) 19–58	Cortical thickness; GM & WM volume; FA, MD	Voxel-based cortical thickness; VBM; DTI	↓ prefrontal and limbic volume; ↑ somatosensory volume; abnormalities in white matter
Worbe et al. (2010)	N = 60	30.3 (10.8)	41:19	17 OCD	28 currently taking medication	N = 30	29.1 (11)	Cortical thickness; volume of hippocampus	Cortical thickness = closest distance from GM/WM boundary to GM/CSF boundary at each vertex on tessellated surface; automated segmentation	Simple tics: thinning in premotor & sensorimotor areas; Complex tics: thinning in premotor, prefrontal, & parietal areas; Comorbid OCD: thinning in ACC & hippocampus

(Continued)

Table 12.1 (*Continued*)

Reference	N (TS sample size)	Age mean (SD) Range	Male: Female	Comorbid disorders	Medications	Controls (N) Age mean (SD) Age range	Hypotheses tested	Methodology	Main findings
Miller et al. (2010)	N = 149*	18.7 (13) 6–63	112:37	55 OCD, 42 ADHD, 10 OCD+ ADHD	87 currently taking medication	N = 134 22.9 (13.7)	Volume of thalamus	Isointensity contour function & manual editing; ICC > 90%	↑ thalamus
Tobe et al. (2010)	N = 163*	17.7 (12.5) 6–60	124:39	43 OCD, 34 ADHD, 14 OCD+ ADHD	85 currently taking medications	N = 147 22.5 (13.5)	Volume of cerebellum	Manual tracing	↓ lateral cerebellar hemispheres (crus I, lobules VI, VIIB, & VIIIA); associated with worse tics; less reduction when comorbid OCD
Neuner et al. (2010)	N = 19	30.1 (10.8) 18–55	13:6	1 OCD, 3 OCD+ ADHD	11 currently taking medication	N = 19 28.9 (8.5) 20–50	FA, MD, eigenvalues, eigenvectors, axial & radial diffusivity in WM tracts	DTI analysis in FSL	↓ FA & ↑ RD in corticospinal tract, CC, and non-motor association fiber pathways
Roessner et al. (2011a)	N = 55	12 (1.3)	55:0	None	None	N = 42 12.1 (1.3)	Volume of 5 CC subregions, BG nuclei, & thalamus	Automated segmentation & manual tracing; coefficient of variation ranged 0.9–4.7%	↑ Pu & callosal motor subregion 3

Study	N	Age mean (SD) range	Sex ratio	Comorbidity	Medication	N	Age mean (SD)	Measures	Method	Main findings
Neuner et al. (2011)	N = 15	29.4 (9.85) 18–48	11:4	None	8 currently taking medication	N = 15	28.2 (7.55)	FA, MD, eigenvalues, eigenvectors, axial & radial diffusivity of BG nuclei, NAc, thalamus, & amygdala	DTI analysis in FSL	Microstructural abnormalities in pallidum and Pu; increased abnormalities in NAc and amygdala associated with more severe symptoms
Jackson et al. (2011)	N = 14	15.3 10–18	12:2	None	7 currently taking medication	N = 14		FA, MD of WM tracts	DTI analysis in FSL	↓FA and/or ↑MD in CC and forceps minor; correlated with tic severity

Note: All main findings refer to the TS group vs. the control group and to regional volumes, unless otherwise specified.

*More or less the same sample as Peterson et al. (2001).

↓ = reduced/smaller; ↑ = increased/bigger.

ACC, anterior cingulate cortex; ADHD, attention-deficit/hyperactivity disorder; BG, basal ganglia; CC, corpus callosum; CN, caudate nucleus; DLPFC, dorsolateral prefrontal cortex; DTI, diffusion tensor imaging; FA, fractional anisotropy; GM, gray matter; GP, globus pallidus; ICC, intraclass correlation coefficient; MD, mean diffusivity; MZ, monozygotic; NAc, nucleus accumbens; OCD, obsessive-compulsive disorder; Pu, putamen; TS, Tourette syndrome; VBM, volumetric based morphometry; WM, white matter.

examine volumetric differences in TS reported smaller volumes in the left striatum (caudate and putamen) and left lenticular nucleus (globus pallidus and putamen) in a group of 14 adults with TS (Peterson et al., 1993). Further, control participants showed greater right than left caudate volume and greater left than right putamen and globus pallidus volume, while TS participants did not exhibit such asymmetries. Similarly, reduced volume in the left caudate has been reported in children (Makki et al., 2008), and loss of typical caudate asymmetry has been reported in adults (Moriarty et al., 1997), which was likely due to reduced volume in the right caudate (though not significant). In a group of monozygotic twin pairs with TS, smaller right caudate volume and a trend toward smaller left caudate volume were found in the identical co-twin with more severe symptoms compared to the identical co-twin with less severe symptoms (Hyde et al., 1995). Additionally, studies using VBM have reported reduced gray matter volume in the left caudate in adults with TS without comorbidities (i.e., so-called "pure TS") who are medication-free (Müller-Vahl et al., 2009), as well as in children (also showing a trend in the right caudate) (Makki et al., 2009). While these studies consistently report reduced caudate volumes in TS, the lateralization of the results varies across studies.

One of the largest volumetric studies of TS (n = 127) found smaller caudate volumes bilaterally in both children and adults with TS (Peterson et al., 2003). Interestingly, analyses of subgroups demonstrated that TS participants currently taking neuroleptic medications had larger basal ganglia volumes than both controls and neuroleptic-free TS participants, suggesting a corrective or over-corrective effect of the medication. Consistent with this suggestion, neuroleptics have been shown to increase striatal volumes in healthy rats (Chakos et al., 1998). Given the large sample in this volumetric TS study, the authors were also able to examine associations with comorbid diagnoses of OCD and/or ADHD. They found no effects of ADHD but a relationship between the presence of OCD and smaller putamen volume. Thus, smaller putamen volumes may be driven by the presence

of OCD, while smaller caudate volumes may be more specific to TS. Further, the bilateral findings in this study suggest that the lateralized findings in the previously discussed studies may be type II errors due to the smaller sample sizes examined, especially considering that several of those studies reported trends toward reduced caudate volumes in the other hemisphere.

Somewhat surprisingly, studies reporting reduced caudate volumes have failed to find a correlation between volume and symptom severity. However, longitudinal data have revealed a striking relationship between basal ganglia volume in childhood and symptom severity later in life. Bloch and colleagues (2005) collected symptom severity measures from 43 individuals with TS an average of 7.5 years (range 3.8–12.8) after their MRI scan sessions. Interestingly, those individuals with smaller caudate volumes in childhood had more severe tics at the follow-up assessment, along with more severe OCD symptoms. In addition, individuals with smaller putamen volumes also had more severe tics at the follow-up. These results suggest that caudate volume may serve as a promising predictor of adult prognosis in TS, consistent with the common findings of reduced caudate volumes in both children and adults with TS. Importantly, these results also demonstrate that the decrease in caudate volume is not only a consequence or adaptation of the brain to expressing or experiencing tics.

Compared to the caudate, the role of the putamen is less clear, as the results from Peterson and colleagues (2003) suggested that reduced putamen volume was due to OCD symptoms in TS, while Bloch and colleagues (2005) found an association between putamen volume in childhood and tic severity, but not OCD severity, later in life. Further complicating conclusions, two studies examining boys with TS reported *larger* putamen volumes compared to controls (Ludolph et al., 2006; Roessner et al., 2011a). Roessner and colleagues studied a large sample of boys with pure TS who were treatment-naïve, while Ludolph and colleagues studied a smaller sample, a subset of whom were taking stimulant medications, and did not report the incidence of OCD and ADHD. Another study reported reduced putamen asymmetry compared to controls in children with TS in the absence of significant volume differences (Singer et al., 1993). This reduction in the typical left > right putamen asymmetry was likely due to a complete reversal of the asymmetry in a subset of those children studied, which included children with and without comorbid ADHD. Thus, further investigation is necessary to discern whether or not there are reliable differences in putamen volume in TS and how such volume differences relate to comorbidities.

It is worth noting that not all studies investigating basal ganglia structure in TS have found differences when comparing to control participants. Unfortunately, the cause of the discrepant results across studies is not clear. For example, Wang and colleagues (2007) found no volumetric differences in any basal ganglia structures in 15 neuroleptic-naïve adults with TS (4 with comorbidities), while Zimmerman and colleagues (2000) found no differences in basal ganglia volume or asymmetry in 19 girls with TS, almost half of whom had comorbid ADHD. Thus, a comparison of age, presence of comorbidities, and medication use does not provide a clear explanation for the discrepant results, as can be further seen in Table 12.1.

Thalamus

The basal ganglia output nuclei, the globus pallidus internal segment (GPi) and substantia nigra pars reticulata (SNr), send projections primarily to the cortex and brainstem via the thalamus. Thus, the thalamus plays a major role in basal ganglia circuitry. Unfortunately, the structural imaging data on the thalamus in TS are largely inconsistent. Smaller thalamic volumes have been reported in children with TS (Makki et al., 2008, 2009); however, these studies did not control for or account for comorbidities or medication use. On the other hand, larger thalamic volumes have been reported in a study of treatment-naïve children with pure TS (Lee et al., 2006), as well as in a large-scale study of children and adults with TS (Miller et al., 2010). The results of Miller and colleagues did not change when examining subgroups of specific participants with pure TS, TS plus comorbidities, as

well as participants who were medication-free. Thus, it is possible that the findings of smaller thalamic volumes were due to the heterogeneity of the samples studied. However, another study that examined treatment-naïve boys with pure TS (Roessner et al., 2011a) as well as one that examined neuroleptic-naïve adults with pure TS (Wang et al., 2007) demonstrated no difference in thalamic volume compared to controls. Thus, further research is needed to reconcile the inconsistent findings regarding thalamic volumes in TS.

Medial Temporal Lobe

A few structural MRI studies in TS have reported differences in medial temporal lobe structures, including the hippocampus and amygdala. In one of the largest cohorts of children and adults with TS, Peterson and colleagues (2007) demonstrated larger hippocampus and amygdala volumes in children, and smaller volumes of both structures in adults. Consistent with those findings, Worbe and colleagues (2010) found smaller hippocampus volumes in adults with TS; however, this result was specific to the subgroup with comorbid OCD. In contrast to these results, Ludolph and colleagues (2006) showed decreased gray matter volume in the hippocampus in boys with TS. Given the connections between these limbic regions and the basal ganglia, it is worth further study to identify whether these limbic regions play an important role in TS.

Cerebral Cortex

The sensorimotor cortices are intuitive candidate cortical areas for investigation in TS due to the motor nature of tics and sensory disturbances that frequently accompany tics. Individuals with TS will typically describe a feeling of discomfort, known as a "premonitory urge" (a.k.a. sensory tic, premonitory sensation), that often precedes a tic and is briefly relieved by performance of the tic. Thus, TS involves both motor and sensory dysfunction. MRI studies that have measured cortical thickness and gray matter volume in sensorimotor cortices in TS are limited in number, but they have reached consistent results. Notably, Sowell and colleagues (2008) found cortical thinning in sensorimotor cortex, along with other regions (ventral frontal cortex, dorsal parietal cortex), in children with pure TS. Further, more severe facial tics were associated with increased thinning in ventral portions of primary motor and somatosensory cortices, regions that control orofacial muscles. Similarly, cortical thinning in left sensorimotor cortices was reported in a group of children and adults with pure TS, with increased thinning associated with increased tic severity (Fahim et al., 2010). A particularly striking study demonstrated specificity of cortical thinning depending on different TS phenotypes (Worbe et al., 2010). Adults with simple tics had cortical thinning in sensorimotor and premotor cortices; those with complex tics had cortical thinning in premotor, prefrontal, and parietal associative areas; and those with comorbid OCD had cortical thinning in the anterior cingulate cortex (ACC) and reduced volumes in the hippocampus. Thus, cortical thinning in sensorimotor cortices consistently relates to orofacial tics, which are often simple tics, and are among the most common symptoms in TS. It is worth noting that volume reduction, correlated with tic severity, has also been reported in another classic motor region, the cerebellum, in children and adults with TS (Tobe et al., 2010). However, in the TS literature, the cerebellum has received much less study than supratentorial motor regions. The morphometric approach taken by Tobe and colleagues deserves notice, as they examined shape in addition to volume. Inconsistent findings across studies may, therefore, be better understood by examining both shape and volume in order to identify specific portions within an ROI that "protrude" or "indent" in the patient population.

Differences in volume and thickness of other, nonprimary, frontal regions in TS have also been reported; these differences may be consistent with reports of atypical (whether improved or impaired) cognitive control in TS (e.g., Channon et al., 2003; Mueller et al., 2006). The results from adult studies of TS are fairly consistent, demonstrating cortical thinning and reduced gray matter volume in the prefrontal cortex (Draganski et al., 2010; Müller-Vahl et al., 2009; Peterson et al., 2001; Worbe et al., 2010), including the cingulate cortex (Draganski et al., 2010; Müller-Vahl et al., 2009; Worbe et al., 2010). In children, on the other hand, the results are more varied. Peterson and colleagues (2001) found that children with TS had larger dorsal prefrontal volumes and that, specifically, boys with TS had smaller premotor, orbitofrontal, and subgenual cortices. Sowell and colleagues (2008) found cortical thinning in ventral frontal regions, which correlated with symptom severity, in a group of boys and girls with TS. Hong and colleagues (2002) showed larger right frontal gray matter volume but smaller left frontal gray matter volume in boys with pure TS. This study also demonstrated larger frontal white matter volume in these children, a finding corroborated in another sample of boys with pure TS in which there was an increase in the proportion of white matter in the right frontal lobe (Fredericksen et al., 2002). Based on the consistent findings in adults with TS, several investigators have proposed that reduced prefrontal volume reflects a failure of the "more common" neural compensation that aids in controlling and ameliorating symptoms in adulthood (Peterson et al., 2001). If this theory is true, the inconsistent findings in children could reflect varied levels of compensation, and could perhaps predict which children will experience a relief in symptoms in adulthood. However, this hypothesis is based on the assumption that tics disappear in most adults who were diagnosed with TS as children. This assumption may not be well supported, as discussed further below in "Limitations and Future Directions."

Several studies described above also reported differences in cortical areas other than frontal and sensorimotor regions. Adults with TS have been reported to have reduced gray matter volume in parieto-temporo-occipital regions (Müller-Vahl et al., 2009) and thinning in right parietal cortex (Fahim et al., 2010), or larger parieto-occipital regions in men but smaller in women (Peterson et al., 2001). Children with TS have been shown to have cortical thinning in the dorsal parietal cortex (Sowell et al., 2008) and right parietal cortex (Fahim et al., 2010), and larger volumes in parieto-occipital regions (Peterson et al., 2001). Moreover, one study with a reasonably large sample of medication-naïve boys with TS reported no differences in gray matter volume in any cortical regions using VBM (Roessner et al., 2009). The implications of these results are unclear, but future studies will, we hope, start to shed light on the differences seen in other cortical regions.

White Matter

White matter structures have been interrogated to identify abnormalities in anatomical connections in TS. Much of this work has focused on the corpus callosum, the large white matter tract connecting the two cerebral hemispheres. Volumetric studies have generally found larger callosal volumes in several heterogeneous TS groups. Baumgardner and colleagues (1996) found larger volumes in four of five callosal subregions in children with TS compared to children with ADHD and to controls. Roessner and colleagues (2011a) found enlarged callosal motor subregion 3 (which connects the primary motor cortices) in a large sample of treatment-naïve boys with pure TS. Two groups reported larger cross-sectional area of the corpus callosum in adults with TS (Moriarty et al., 1997; Plessen et al., 2004). Further, Plessen and colleagues found that corpus callosum size was positively correlated with motor tic severity. However, they also found smaller callosal volumes in children with TS. It is possible that the results were confounded by comorbidities and medication use; however, assessments of these variables did not reveal any significant effects.

In addition to volumetric approaches, DTI has also been used to investigate, indirectly, the microstructural properties of the corpus callosum in TS. Reduced FA was reported in male children with TS (Plessen et al., 2006), in children with pure TS (Jackson et al., 2011), in adults with TS (Neuner et al., 2010), and in a monozygotic twin with TS compared to the co-twin with no tic symptoms (Cavanna et al., 2010). Thus, the most consistent findings within the corpus callosum are increased volume and

reduced FA. Smaller FA values could reflect reduced myelination, fewer axons, or atypical organization of axons within the white matter tract. Given the somewhat consistent finding of larger volumes, decreased FA in TS is relatively unlikely to reflect reduced myelination or fewer axons, as those microstructural differences would more likely coincide with smaller volumes. Thus, there may be atypical structural organization of axons in TS. However, studies that examine both volume and FA in the corpus callosum are necessary to investigate the relationship between these measures beyond speculation.

Other white matter tracts may also differ between TS and controls, although such studies are scarce to date. For example, probabilistic fiber tracking has revealed decreased structural connectivity between the caudate and the anterior dorsolateral prefrontal cortex (DLPFC) in children with TS, yet structural connectivity correlated with OCD behavior, not tic severity (Makki et al., 2009). DTI has shown increased FA in somatosensory white matter, which negatively correlated with tic severity, in medication-free adults with pure TS (Thomalla et al., 2009), as well as reduced FA in the forceps minor (which connects the lateral and medial surfaces of the prefrontal cortex via the genu of the corpus callosum) in children with pure TS (Jackson et al., 2011). While these studies provide interesting and potentially valuable information about white matter properties in TS, they merit replication and further study.

In sum, structural MRI has revealed some consistencies regarding the neuroanatomy of TS. First, caudate volumes are reduced in both children and adults with TS. Second, there is cortical thinning in sensorimotor cortices in children and adults with TS, along with a negative correlation between the thickness and the severity of orofacial tics. Third, adults with TS show cortical thinning and reduced gray matter volume in prefrontal cortical regions. Finally, the corpus callosum is larger and has reduced FA in TS.

It is worth keeping in mind that some inconsistencies among studies may be related to limitations in the methodologies. For instance, manual tracing of ROIs depends on the *a priori* choice of ROIs, requires blinding to prevent experimenter bias, and depends on the display scale (i.e., brightness can influence apparent anatomical edges). Moreover, manual tracing methods cannot easily exclude lacunae, unidentified bright objects (UBOs), or vascular space. While one benefit of VBM is the ability to compare structure across the whole brain simultaneously, that approach loses the benefits of testing a few *a priori* hypotheses and raises the risk of false positives due to the inherent multiple comparisons. Thus, different methodological decisions across studies may lead to inconsistent results.

FUNCTIONAL MRI

Functional neuroimaging studies in TS can provide information about the functional brain correlates of tic symptoms as well as other cognitive and motor functions. While there are studies that utilize radiotracer and perfusion imaging techniques, including single photon emission computed tomography (SPECT) and positron emission tomography (PET) (for comprehensive reviews, see Frey & Albin, 2006; Rickards, 2009), we will focus primarily on fMRI studies, which noninvasively measure brain function. fMRI indirectly measures neuronal activity using the ratio of oxyhemoglobin to deoxyhemoglobin as a contrast mechanism, resulting in a blood-oxygenation-level-dependent (BOLD) signal. Most commonly, BOLD activity is measured while participants perform a task, and this activity is contrasted to activity during a passive resting state or to activity during different task conditions. Thus, fMRI can be used to interrogate motor function and cognitive function, both of which may be affected in TS. Table 12.2 summarizes the methods and results of the fMRI studies in TS.

Tic-Related Activity

To study tic-related brain activity, several strategies have been employed. One approach identifies the timing of tics by documenting them with video and audio recordings. Then, using an event-related fMRI design, activity correlated with the performance of tics (taken as a measurement of "tic-related activity") can be compared to activity during which no tics occur. Using this approach, Gates and colleagues (2004) examined a single 15-year-old boy with coprolalia and compared his tic-related BOLD activity to a control participant's tic imitation-related BOLD activity. While both tics and imitations elicited increased activity in the precentral gyrus and middle frontal gyrus, only the TS participant's tics yielded increased activity in the caudate nucleus, cingulate cortex, cuneus, left angular gyrus, left inferior parietal gyrus, and occipital gyri. Also using tic recordings and a novel analysis method in a $H_2{}^{15}O$ PET study, Stern and colleagues (2000) found tic-related regional cerebral blood flow in a number of prefrontal, premotor, and primary motor cortical regions, and in the basal ganglia. In an fMRI study, Bohlhalter and colleagues (2006) studied a group of adults with TS and examined BOLD activity during the 2 seconds prior to tic onset and during tic onset. BOLD activity increased 2 seconds prior to tic onset in the supplementary motor area (SMA), lateral premotor cortex, parietal operculum, anterior cingulate cortex (ACC), insula, putamen, and ventrolateral thalamus. BOLD activity increased at tic onset in the sensorimotor cortices, cerebellum, superior parietal cortex, left DLPFC, and substantia nigra. The authors posited that the activity in paralimbic areas (ACC, insula) and the parietal operculum preceding tics may play a role in the premonitory urge, as these areas have also been shown to increase activity during unpleasant sensations. Interestingly, the ACC and insula are among the most common regions to show increased activity during virtually all fMRI studies that require general task control (Nelson et al., 2010). This finding suggests that prior to a tic, a task set or control mechanism comes online, perhaps in an attempt to control the impending tic. As a comparison condition, Bohlhalter and colleagues also instructed TS participants to imitate their own tics. Unfortunately, they were unable to analyze the imitation data for several reasons. First, there was more head movement during tic imitation than during actual tics in many participants. Secondly, the authors found it

Table 12.2 Functional MRI studies in TS

Reference	N (TS sample size)	Age mean(sd) range	Male: Female	Comorbid disorders	Medications	Controls N Age mean (sd) Age range	Task and design	Main findings
Peterson et al. (1998)	N = 22	35.7(10.9) 18–55	11:11	10 OCD, 3 childhood ADHD	7 currently taking medication	None	Tic suppression; block design	↓ activity during tic suppression vs. free tic blocks in ventral GP, Pu, thalamus, right PCC, left hippocampal area, cuneus, left sensorimotor cortex, left inferior parietal regions; ↑ symptom severity association with ↓ magnituded of suppression-related activity
Biswal et al. (1998)	N = 5	26.6(12.7) 17–49	4:1	2 OCD symptoms, 3 ADHD symptoms	Not reported	N = 5 30.2(14.5) 22–56	Bilateral finger tapping; block design	↑ area of activation in sensorimotor cortex during finger tapping
Serrien et al. (2002)	N = 3	24(8) 16–32	3:0	Not reported	None	N = 3	Motor lifting task; block design	↓ or no activity in secondary motor areas during motor task
Gates et al. (2004)	N = 1 (case study with coprolalia)	15	1:0	ODD	Medication naïve?	N = 1 (mimic tics)	Free tic; event-related design	↑ activity during tics in CN, cingulate, cuneus, left AG, left inferior parietal gyrus, and occipital gyri
Hershey et al. (2004)[a]	N = 8	35.5(13.5) 19–56	6:2	1 OCD, 3 ADHD, 1 OCD + ADHD	2 currently taking medication	N = 10 Age matched	Go/No-go task; block design; with and without levodopa infusion	No group differences

(Continued)

Table 12.2 (*Continued*)

Reference	N (TS sample size)	Age mean (sd) range	Male: Female	Comorbid disorders	Medications	Controls N Age mean (sd) Age range	Task and design	Main findings
Hershey et al. (2004)b	N = 8	35.5 (13.5) 19–56	6:2	1 OCD, 3 ADHD, 1 OCD + ADHD	2 currently taking medication	N = 10	2-back working memory task; block design; with and without levodopa infusion	↑ activity in medial frontal cortex, left parietal cortex, left thalamus during task; activity normalized with levodopa administration in TS
Bohlhalter et al. (2006)	N = 10	31 (11.2) 17–49	4:6	4 OCD, 2 ADHD	1 currently taking medication	None	Free tic and tic imitation sessions; event-related design	↑ activity 2 sec before tic-onset in SMA, lateral premotor, parietal operculum, ACC, insula, posterior Pu, thalamus; ↑ activity at tic-onset in motor regions
Marsh et al. (2007)	N = 66	24.4 (7.1) 8.4–52.6	47:19	25 OCD, 8 ADHD, 5 OCD + ADHD	Many currently taking medication	N = 70 26.7 (9.1) 7.1–57.2	Stroop task; block design	↑ activity in frontostriatal regions with increasing age in controls, but not in TS; ↓ activity in default mode regions with increasing age in controls, but not in TS; ↑ activity in left DLPFC associated with more severe symptoms
Baym et al. (2008)	N = 18 (6 excluded)	10.4 7–13	15:3	Numbers not reported; not excluded	16 were medication naïve	N = 19 (2 excluded) 10.3	Cognitive control (task-switching, response selection, rule manipulation) task; event-related design	↑ activity in PFC during task; ↑ activity in SN/VTA, BG, thalamus, NCa, and STN associated with increased tic severity

Study	N	Age (mean, range, M:F)	Comorbidity / Medication	Control N, Age	Task	Results
Hampson et al. (2009)	N = 16	30(9.7) 18–56 13:3	2 OCD, 2 ADHD 8 currently taking medication	N = 16 30(9)	Free tic in TS, tic imitation in controls, correlation with reference region	SMA differentiated tics and tic imitation before and after peak of tic activity
Raz et al. (2009)	N = 38	23.6(7.2) 22:16 8.9–64.6	1 OCD, 1 OCD + ADHD Numbers not reported; not excluded	N = 33 27(7.6) 8–59.2	Simon task; event-related design	↑ frontostriatal activity with ↑ age in controls, which was exaggerated in TS; ↑ frontostriatal activity associated with better performance in TS; ↑ tic severity associated with ↑ activity in inferior PFC & thalamus, and with ↓ activity in GP, Pu, & IFG
Church et al. (2009)a	N = 27	12.5 9.2–15.8 19:8	12 OCD and/or ADHD 19 currently taking medication	N = 27 12.5 10.4–15.8	Semantic judgement task; mixed block event-related design	Anomalous start-cue activity and adaptive control; functionally immature sustained control
Church et al. (2009)b	N = 33	12.7 9.9–15.8 25:8	17 OCD and/or ADHD 22 currently taking medication	N = 42 12.7 10.4–15.8	Rest looking at a blank screen with a fixation cross; rs-fcMRI	Functional immaturity in connections within the fronto-parietal control network and the cingulo-opercular control network; functionally anomalous connections were primarily in the fronto-parietal control network

(Continued)

Table 12.2 (*Continued*)

Reference	N (TS sample size)	Age mean(sd) range	Male: Female	Comorbid disorders	Medications	Controls N Age mean (sd) Age range	Task and design	Main findings
Mazzone et al. (2010)	N = 51	25.6(7.4)	36:15	21 OCD, 11 ADHD, 4 OCD + ADHD	21 currently taking medication	N = 69 25.9(8.6)	Blink suppression task; block design	↑ activity in dorsal ACC & right anterior temporal cortex, ↑ deactivation in SFG, ↓ deactivation in PCC during suppression; ↑ tic severity associated with ↑ activity in MFG & CN and ↓ activity in PFC, STG, and Pu; ↑ activity in right DLPFC & right inferolateral PFC with ↑ age
Roessner et al. (2011)b	N = 19	12.5(1.4)	19:0	Not reported	Treatment-naïve N = 16 12.9(1.6)	Finger tapping; block design	↓ activity in left precentral gyrus, right SPL, right IPL, right MTG, right; ↑ activity in left CN and medial frontal gyrus
Debes et al. (2011)	N = 39	13.9(2.1)	30:9	10 OCD, 5 ADHD, 2 OCD + ADHD	29 medication-naïve, 10 medication-free for > 6mo.	N = 37 13.8(2.5)	Stroop task, go/ no-go task, finger tapping; block design	No differences between groups in all 3 tasks; ↑ activity in right PCC & left STG during Go/no-go and in medial frontal gyrus during finger tapping associated with ↑ OCD; ↓ activity in cingulate associated with ↑ OCD

Study	N (TS)	Age, mean (SD)	M:F	Comorbidity	Medication	N (control)	Age, mean (SD)	Task	Main findings
Werner et al. (2011)	N = 19	34.3 (10.1)	13:6	2 OCD, 2 OCD + ADHD	9 currently taking medication	N = 18	37.5 (10.7)	Finger tapping (right hand, left hand, both hands); block design	↓ activity in brainstem & cerebellum for right hand; ↑ activity in PCC, precuneus, parietal cortex, right AG, left DLPFC for left hand; ↑ activity in left PFC for bimanual
Jackson et al. (2011)	N = 10	13.8 (1.8)	8:2	None	Some on medication	N = 15	14.3 (1.9)	Task-switching; event-related design	↓ activity in M1 in all conditions; ↑ activity in right PFC for incongruent-switch trials
Wang et al. (2011)	N = 13 (data available for 12)	33.5 (13.3)	8:5	6 OCD, 2 ADHD, 1 OCD + ADHD	6 currently taking medication	N = 21	32.5 (11.1)	TS group: free tic & self-paced tic imitation; Control group: self-paced tic imitation & cue-paced tic imitation; block design	Tics in TS vs. self-paced tic imitation in controls: ↑ activity & positive correlation with tic severity, in M1, PPC, SMA, left PFC, pallidum, thalamus, SN, & cerebellum; ↓ activity & negative correlation in ACC, CN, & parietal operculum; Granger causality revealed stronger effective connectivity among several cortical & subcortical regions in TS vs. controls.

Note: All main findings refer to the TS group vs. the control group, unless otherwise specified; ↓ = decreased, ↑ = increased, ACC = anterior cingulate cortex, ADHD = attention-deficit hyperactivity disorder, AG = angular gyrus, CN = caudate nucleus, DLPFC = dorsolateral prefrontal cortex, GP = globus pallidus, IFG = inferior frontal gyrus, IPL = inferior parietal lobule, M1 = primary motor cortex, MFG = middle frontal gyrus, MTG = middle temporal gyrus, NCa = nucleus accumbens, OCD = obsessive-compulsive disorder, PCC = posterior cingulate cortex, PFC = prefrontal cortex, PPC = posterior parietal cortex, Pu = putamen SFG = superior frontal gyrus, SMA = supplementary motor area, SN = substantial nigra, STG = superior temporal gyrus, STN = subthalamic nucleus, TS = Tourette syndrome, VTA = ventral tegmental area.

difficult to discriminate imitations from real tics. Finally, it is unlikely that imitating tics can be truly independent of actual tics, as tics are quite suggestible in TS (Robertson et al., 1999). For example, when individuals with TS talk about their tics aloud, they often perform the tic (Woods et al., 2001). Similarly, imitating one's own tics can lead to tic-related sensations and performance of an actual tic, such that a movement that begins as an imitation may end as a real tic. The authors suggest that such issues may be remedied by comparing real tics in TS patients to imitated tics in controls, as done in the case study by Gates and colleagues.

Hampson and colleagues (2009) followed the suggestion of Bohlhalter and colleagues and studied tic-related activity in a group of adults with TS and tic imitation in a group of controls. However, Hampson and colleagues used a different approach to identify the timing of tics: rather than using video and/or audio recordings, they relied upon the assumption that the occurrence of tics coincides with increased activity in primary motor cortex (M1). Accordingly, they utilized localizer scans to identify the specific portion of M1 related to each participant's tics (or imitations), which was used as the reference region. In separate experimental scans, they then identified those brain regions where activity was correlated with the activity in the reference region. This method identified similar regions for tics and tic imitation, with one notable exception: the SMA was more active for tics than for imitation, both before and after the peak of activity in the reference region. The authors suggest that increased activity in the SMA prior to a tic may be related to the premonitory urge. Consistent with this suggestion, electrical stimulation of the SMA has been shown to produce complex movements accompanied by an initial sensation or urge to perform the movement (Fried et al., 1991). Further, Bohlhalter and colleagues (2006) also report increased SMA activity 2 seconds prior to tic onset. Thus, activity in the SMA may be aberrant in TS, playing a role in the premonitory urge that often precedes tics.

Wang and colleagues (2011) compared tic imitation performed by both TS and control participants to TS participants' actual tics. Interrogating task-related regions that were identified by independent components analysis, they found greater activity for tics in TS than for tic imitation in controls in sensorimotor, premotor, supplementary motor, and prefrontal cortices as well as in the basal ganglia and thalamus. They observed positive correlations between activity and tic severity in these same regions. For the same contrast, there was less activity and negative correlations with tic severity in the ACC, parietal operculum, and caudate. They interpret their results to indicate that the findings in the former set of regions are likely to be related to the premonitory urge associated with tics in patients with TS, whereas the findings in the latter set of regions reflect relatively decreased top-down control in those same patients. Because the fMRI design was blocked, the timing of signals related to urge and control was not extracted specifically. Importantly, this study went a step further than task activation and tested effective connectivity between regions using Granger causality, a technique that assesses the directionality of interactions between regions. They demonstrated stronger effective connectivity among several cortical and subcortical regions in TS compared to controls. Thus, this study utilized a forward-thinking and potentially valuable approach for addressing issues of neural circuits with fMRI data.

Another approach for studying tic-related activity was implemented in a PET study (Lerner et al., 2007) in which "free-tic" sessions were compared to stage 2 sleep sessions in a group of adults with TS. In an age-matched control group, activity was compared during awake rest and stage 2 sleep. This method identified greater activity in the cerebellum, insula, putamen, thalamus, SMA, and motor cortex during tics in the TS group compared to awake rest in the control group. While these results are somewhat consistent with the results from fMRI studies, this block design did not allow the investigators to distinguish between activity related to the premonitory urge, the tics themselves, or resting periods between tics.

Tic Suppression

One of the earliest fMRI studies in TS compared BOLD activity during blocks in which participants were told to suppress their tics to blocks in which they were told to tic freely (Peterson et al., 1998). During tic suppression, BOLD activity varied (increased/decreased) in several basal ganglia nuclei, in the thalamus, and in cortical regions known to be involved in attention-demanding tasks. Notably, increased symptom severity was associated with decreased magnitude of suppression-related activity, whether it was increased activity in the cortex and caudate or decreased activity in the lenticular nucleus and thalamus. The authors speculated that the ability to inhibit tics might rely on the capacity to regulate subcortical activity. Therefore, the inability to suppress tics in TS may be due to impaired regulation, as less change in subcortical activity was related to more severe symptoms. These results should be viewed with some caution, however, as blocks of tics and blocks of tic suppression inherently differ in the amount of movement in the data, which can affect the BOLD signal. Furthermore, although the authors interpreted differences as relating to the presence or absence of active tic suppression, the blocks also differed (inversely) according to tic frequency. Decreased activity in the putamen during tic suppression may more simply be interpreted as increased activity in the putamen with movement.

One method for controlling for different amounts of movement in free tic and tic-suppression conditions is to include a control group. Of course, a control group will not have tics to suppress. However, blinks are present in both TS participants and controls and possess several similarities to tics. Blinking is a seemingly involuntary facial movement that can be under voluntary control, similar to tics. Blinks can be suppressed for a period of time, during which the urge to blink increases until a blink is performed, after which the urge is relieved, again akin to the premonitory urge that precedes many tics. Taking advantage of these similarities, Peterson's group revisited the examination of movement suppression with a more incisive experiment that measured the neural correlates of blink suppression in children and adults with TS and in matched controls (Mazzone et al., 2010). They found several differences between TS and control participants during blink suppression, including increased activation in the dorsal ACC and right anterior temporal cortex, more deactivation in the superior frontal gyrus, and less deactivation in the posterior cingulate cortex in TS. Increased tic severity was associated with decreased suppression-related activity in the right inferolateral prefrontal cortex, right superior temporal gyrus, and right putamen, and with increased task-related activity in the middle frontal gyrus and the caudate. In addition, there was an age-by-diagnosis interaction in the right DLPFC and right ventrolateral prefrontal cortex, driven by greater suppression-related activation with increasing age in TS as compared to controls. The authors posit that inhibitory control is amplified in adults with TS within both the motor domain (as seen in this blink-suppression study) and the cognitive domain (as seen in studies of cognitive control, which we discuss later in this section).

Motor Control

fMRI studies investigating motor control in TS have not yet converged on a consistent set of findings. Serrien and colleagues (2002) examined BOLD activity during object lifting and moving and found that activity in secondary motor areas (e.g., SMA, premotor cortex) was reduced or absent in TS compared to controls. In contrast, Biswal and colleagues (1998) found a larger area of activation in sensorimotor cortices during finger tapping in TS compared to controls. Both of the above studies had very small sample sizes and utilized different motor tasks, which may explain the discrepant results. However, recent studies implementing finger-tapping paradigms in larger sample sizes have also yielded inconsistent findings. Roessner and colleagues (2011b) reported less activity during finger tapping in the left precentral gryus, right superior parietal cortex, inferior parietal cortex, middle temporal gyrus, and middle frontal gyrus, as well as more activity during finger tapping in the left caudate and medial frontal gyrus, in boys with pure TS compared to controls. In contrast, a study of 39 children with TS found no difference in BOLD activity between

TS and controls during finger tapping (as well as during a Stroop task and a go/no-go task) (Debes et al., 2011). In fact, the only significant findings were correlations between OCD symptoms and task-related activity in the cingulate cortex and in the medial frontal gyrus. Werner and colleagues (2011) reported further conflicting results from a study of finger tapping in adults with TS. During an "easy" condition (finger tapping with the dominant hand), activity in the brainstem and cerebellum was attenuated, while during the "hard" conditions (tapping with the nondominant hand and with both hands), activity in the posterior cingulate, precuneus, parietal cortex, and left prefrontal regions increased. Thus, fMRI studies on motor control, most of which used finger-tapping paradigms, have not yet demonstrated convergent findings.

Executive Function

There is debate over whether executive function/cognitive control is affected in TS. Some studies have demonstrated impairments in several domains of executive function in TS, including response inhibition, selective attention, and cognitive flexibility (Bornstein et al., 1991; Channon et al., 2003; Watkins et al., 2005). Others have argued that such impairments are driven by comorbid conditions, showing that executive function is altered in TS only when comorbidities are present but does not differ between pure TS and controls (Brand et al., 2002; Ozonoff et al., 1998). Other studies have even shown evidence for enhanced executive function in TS, demonstrating better performance during tasks requiring high levels of cognitive control and task switching (Jackson et al., 2007; Mueller et al., 2006). While this debate continues, the increased focus on executive function in TS has led to a number of fMRI studies that have examined the neural correlates of different aspects of executive control in TS.

To study the neural correlates of response inhibition and selective attention in TS, Marsh and colleagues (2007) utilized a Stroop task, in which participants must name the color of a printed word. When the word itself spells out the name of a color but is printed in different color (e.g., the word "RED" printed in blue ink), participants must withhold the automatic response to read the word ("red") in order to correctly name the printed color (blue). Examining groups of children and adults with TS compared to controls, the authors found that while the TS and control groups performed similarly on the task, there were differences in brain activity. This divergence between behavioral performance and brain activity is important to note because the differences in brain activity cannot be attributed to variations in performance, but rather imply differences between groups in the neural mechanisms involved in the processes under study. This "behavioral phenocopy" (i.e., identical overt performance can be implemented by nonidentical functional neuroanatomy) demonstrates an important added value of functional neuroimaging to understanding group differences in information processing (Brown et al., 2005; Church et al., 2010; Palmer et al., 2004; Schlaggar et al., 2002). Marsh and colleagues found that in control participants, regions that are part of the "default mode network" (mesial prefrontal cortex, ventral ACC, posterior cingulate) were deactivated more with increasing age, and frontostriatal regions were activated more with increasing age. In contrast, TS participants showed no age-related change in these regions, except in the posterior cingulate, where the age-related change was opposite to that in controls (i.e., deactivations were reduced with increasing age). Investigating relationships with symptom severity revealed that greater DLPFC activity was associated with more severe tics. Further, greater activity in frontostriatal regions accompanied better performance in controls but poorer performance in TS; however, performance was measured outside the scanner rather than during the scan session itself. The results from this study demonstrate that the frontostriatal regions involved in response inhibition were more activated in those TS participants who had more difficulty with self-regulatory control, as reflected in both task performance and tic severity. The authors conclude that the development, severity, and continued presence of TS symptoms into adulthood may be due to disrupted maturation of the frontostriatal circuits involved in self-regulatory control.

While the results from Marsh and colleagues are compelling, they unfortunately have not been replicated. Another study tested the Stroop task in TS and found no differences in brain activity between children with TS and controls, even when the TS group was divided into subgroups with and without comorbidities (Debes et al., 2011). This study also implemented a go/no-go task, another approach for measuring response inhibition and selective attention. In this task, participants must press a button every time a letter appears on the screen, except when the letter "X" appears. Given that letters other than "X" appear a high percentage of the time, participants must withhold their responses during the rare "X" trials. Like with the Stroop, task-related activity during the go/no-go task did not differ between TS subjects and controls. Moreover, activity in the posterior cingulate and superior temporal gyrus was correlated with OCD symptoms, not tics, suggesting that brain dysfunction in response inhibition may be due to OCD comorbidities, rather than TS itself. Hershey and colleagues (2004a) also failed to find differences in brain activity during a go/no-go task between adults with TS and age-matched controls. In addition, they tested the effects of levodopa on BOLD activity during the task and found that activity was attenuated in the right parietal cortex and cerebellum during levodopa infusion. However, this drug effect did not differ significantly between groups.

Another task that measures response inhibition and selective attention is the Simon task, which measures the effect of stimulus location on responses to that stimulus. Generally, performance is better (i.e., faster, more accurate) when the location of the response is spatially congruent with the location of the stimulus to be acted upon, even when the location of the stimulus is irrelevant to the appropriate task response. In one version of the task, participants must respond to the direction of a leftward- or rightward-pointing arrow presented on the left or right of the screen. When the direction and location of the arrow are incongruent (e.g., a leftward arrow presented on the right side of the screen), participants must inhibit a response to the spatially congruent location of the stimulus. When this task was implemented in an fMRI study of children and adults with TS and matched controls, activity in frontostriatal regions increased with increasing age in controls, a pattern that was exaggerated in TS (Raz et al., 2009). The study also showed a positive correlation between tic severity and task-related activity in the inferior prefrontal cortex and the thalamus, and a negative correlation between tic severity and task-related activity in the globus pallidus, putamen, and inferior frontal gyrus. Finally, increased task-related frontostriatal activity was associated with better behavioral performance in TS. The relationship between tic severity and prefrontal increases in activity during the task is consistent with the findings of Marsh and colleagues (2007). However, the findings of exaggerated frontostriatal activity with age and the relationship between frontostriatal activity and performance are in contrast to the results from Marsh and colleagues. Thus, the evidence for impaired neural circuitry's involvement in response inhibition is inconsistent at present.

Other aspects of executive control have been investigated using fMRI in TS. Hershey and colleagues (2004b) demonstrated that adults with TS engage the medial frontal cortex, left parietal cortex, and thalamus more than controls while performing a working memory task. Interestingly, task-related activity in these regions normalized to control levels with administration of levodopa, suggesting that these regions are dysfunctional and are modulated by dopamine. Baym and colleagues (2008) developed a task to measure task switching, response selection, and rule manipulation in children with TS. They found increased activation in prefrontal regions, such that activity in the superior frontal gyrus was greater in TS compared to controls during all task conditions, while activity in the middle frontal gyrus was greater in TS compared to controls during rule manipulation and task switching. They also found that increased tic severity was accompanied by increased task-related activity in several subcortical regions, including the putamen, thalamus, subthalamic nucleus, and nucleus accumbens. These data suggest increased activity in frontal and subcortical regions in TS when cognitive flexibility is required.

Another interesting approach to studying executive control in TS involves examination of the integrity of previously identified control networks. Prior research has described two independent networks that support different aspects of cognitive control: a frontoparietal network involved in fast, adaptive, online task control, and a cingulo-opercular network involved in slower task maintenance (Dosenbach et al., 2007). Church and colleagues (2009b) interrogated these networks in adolescents with TS using fMRI during performance of a semantic judgment task. Using a mixed blocked/event-related design, they were able to separate BOLD activity related to a task start-cue and BOLD activity that was sustained throughout the task, in order to engage the frontoparietal and cingulo-opercular networks, respectively. Start-cue activity was attenuated in TS compared to controls in several regions, particularly those that are part of the previously identified frontoparietal network. To test whether this difference in TS represented anomalous activity or functional immaturity, the results were compared to changes over typical development. The attenuated start-cue activity differed entirely from typical developmental changes, suggesting anomalous adaptive task control in TS. Sustained activity also differentiated the TS group from the controls, in that the TS group showed a positive sustained signal in several regions of the frontal cortex, while the control group did not. This pattern was also found when comparing typical children and adults, suggesting functionally immature sustained control in TS. The authors reasoned that adolescents with TS have atypical and functionally immature control networks.

Functional networks can also be interrogated with functional connectivity methods. Recently, there has been increasing interest in examining functionally connected networks utilizing resting-state functional-connectivity MRI (rs-fcMRI). Using BOLD activity collected during rest (awake, and not performing a task), rs-fcMRI measures low-frequency, spontaneous fluctuations in the BOLD signal between brain regions. There has been one study implementing this technique to investigate brain networks in TS (Church et al., 2009a). Focusing on the two control networks previously identified by Dosenbach and colleagues (2007)—the frontoparietal network involved in adaptive online control, and the cingulo-opercular network involved in stable set maintenance—this TS study took advantage of findings demonstrating changes in connection strengths between regions in these networks over typical development (Fair et al., 2007). Church and colleagues investigated whether connections in these cognitive control regions in TS were functionally immature or anomalous compared to typical development. Results demonstrated functional immaturity in connections within both control networks, and functionally anomalous connections primarily in the frontoparietal network. Thus, both cognitive control networks are impaired in adolescents with TS, with adaptive online control experiencing the most anomalous dysfunction, corroborating the investigators' fMRI findings (Church et al., 2009b). Additional studies using rs-fcMRI to interrogate networks in TS will likely be conducted in the future and will provide valuable information that can be integrated with the fMRI and structural MRI data to gain additional insight into the neurobiological mechanisms involved in TS.

Overall, the fMRI data in TS are scarce and fairly inconsistent. However, the most compelling finding thus far is increased SMA activity just prior to tic onset, suggesting that the SMA plays a role in the premonitory urge. If future studies can continue to confirm this finding, the SMA may be a potential target for intervention, as relieving the premonitory urge has the potential to relieve tics. The other results from the fMRI studies just discussed are more mixed, potentially revealing altered activity in frontostriatal regions, but not consistently. Interestingly, the results from both studies by Church and colleagues demonstrate that differences in functional anatomy may go beyond CSTC circuits and also involve cortical networks that support cognitive control. TS is certainly a complex disorder in need of further well-designed large-scale fMRI studies in combination with other methodologies to better understand the underlying neurobiological mechanisms involved.

CSTC DYSFUNCTION IN TS

Mink (2001) proposed a compelling model of CSTC dysfunction in TS, built upon the notion that there is aberrant activity in a subset of striatal neurons. To understand how aberrant striatal activity might lead to tics, basic knowledge of basal ganglia circuitry is required. The caudate and putamen (striatum) are the main input nuclei of the basal ganglia, receiving excitatory input from the cortex. The GPi and SNr are the basal ganglia's output nuclei, sending inhibitory projections back to the cortex via the thalamus. More than one polysynaptic pathway conveys information from the striatum to the GPi and SNr, which have been referred to as the "direct" and "indirect" pathways of the basal ganglia (Alexander & Crutcher, 1990). The direct pathway involves inhibitory projections from the striatum directly to the GPi and SNr. The GPi and SNr send inhibitory axons to the thalamus, and the thalamus sends excitatory projections back to the cortex. Via this direct pathway, the cortex excites the striatum, which inhibits the GPi and SNr, releasing the thalamus from inhibition, allowing it to excite the cortex and therefore stimulating muscles and leading to the execution of a movement. On the other hand, the indirect pathway involves inhibitory projections from the striatum to the globus pallidus external segment (GPe). The GPe inhibits the subthalamic nucleus (STN), which sends excitatory projections to the GPi and SNr. Via this indirect pathway, the cortex excites the striatum, which inhibits the GPe, releasing the STN from inhibition and allowing it to excite the GPi and SNr. When stimulated, the GPi and SNr inhibit the thalamus from stimulating the cortex, resulting in less muscle movement. Thus, stimulation of the direct and indirect pathways results in opposing motor output. To make a desired movement, the cortex activates particular striatal neurons that lead to inhibition of the GPi and SNr, releasing the thalamus from inhibition and stimulating cortical neurons that control the desired movement. At the same time, the striatum inhibits the GPe, releasing the STN from inhibition and activating other surrounding GPi and SNr neurons. These neurons will then inhibit the thalamus and therefore inhibit competing undesired movements. Thus, the direct and indirect pathways work together to select the appropriate movement and inhibit others (for a thorough review of basal ganglia circuitry, see Mink, 1996).

Mink (2001) proposed that in TS, there is aberrant activity in a particular set of striatal neurons (Fig. 12.1). This activity ultimately results in the execution of an undesired movement (a tic). Striatal neurons that fire inappropriately will inhibit GPi and SNr neurons, releasing the thalamus from inhibition, which will excite cortical neurons involved in unwanted movements. In this model, distinct sets of striatal neurons correspond to different tics. Thus, aberrant activity in several different sets of striatal neurons will result in the common expression of multiple different tics. This model of tics is supported by postmortem data as well as microstimulation and microinjection data. Fewer parvalbumin-positive (PV+) interneurons have been reported in the striatum in postmortem TS brains (Kalanithi et al., 2005; Kataoka et al., 2010). Importantly, these PV+ interneurons inhibit the medium spiny neurons in the striatum, keeping the baseline firing rate of the striatum low. With fewer PV+ interneurons in the striatum in TS, there is less inhibition of the medium spiny neurons, and therefore an increased firing rate of these output neurons. This hyperactivity could be akin to the aberrant activity in the striatum proposed by Mink. Further evidence in support of the model comes from microstimulation in rhesus monkeys, as stimulating discrete regions of the putamen resulted in movements of specific body parts (Alexander & DeLong, 1985), while microstimulation of the SNr, GPi, and STN does not evoke movement (Basso & Liu, 2007; Horak & Anderson, 1984; Wichmann et al., 1994). Alexander and DeLong also demonstrated somatotopic organization in the putamen, supporting the idea that altered activity in discrete sets of striatal neurons correspond to tics involving particular body parts. Similarly, microinjection

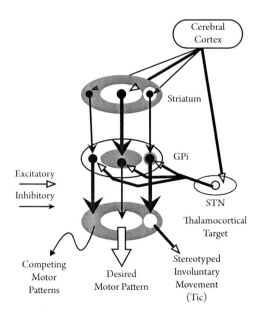

FIGURE 12.1 The diagram summarizes the model proposed by Mink (2001) to explain the generation of tics. A particular set of striatal neurons displays an aberrant activity. This leads to increased inhibition of neurons in the globus pallidus internal segment (GPi) and substantia nigra pars reticulata (SNpr); this will release the thalamus from inhibition and ultimately lead to excitation of cortical neurons involved in unwanted movements. The abnormal activity in several different sets of striatal neurons will lead to the expression of multiple different tics.

of bicuculline, a GABA-A antagonist, into the putamen of cynomolgus monkeys elicited stereotyped movements that resemble tics (Bronfeld et al., 2011; McCairn et al., 2009). Thus, externally administered excitation of the putamen results in tic-like movements, supporting the view that aberrant striatal activity, perhaps as a result of less inhibition from PV+ interneurons, gives rise to tics in TS.

How do the MRI data fit with this model of CSTC dysfunction? Overall, results from neuroimaging studies have revealed abnormalities in the structure and function of the subcortical and cortical components of the CSTC circuits. The most consistent finding has been reduced volume of the caudate nucleus, with Bloch and colleagues (2005) additionally demonstrating a relationship between caudate volume in children and symptom severity later in life. Thus, consistent abnormalities in the caudate implicate basal ganglia dysfunction in TS, although the relationship between volume and neural activity is unclear. Functionally, BOLD signal in the caudate was shown to increase during active suppression of tics. This increase in activity was attenuated in individuals with worse tic symptoms, suggesting impaired ability to regulate striatal activity in TS. PET and SPECT studies have demonstrated decreased activity and blood flow in the striatum (Braun et al., 1993; Eidelberg et al., 1997; Moriarty et al., 1995), which may relate to reduced striatal regulation. A similar relationship between BOLD signal during tic suppression and symptom severity was found in the lenticular nucleus and the thalamus, although activity in these regions decreased during tic suppression and the decrease in activity was attenuated in individuals with more severe symptoms. This relationship between BOLD activity in the basal ganglia and symptom severity fits with the idea of aberrant activity in the striatum. If such aberrant activity gives rise to tics, those individuals who can better regulate that activity will have less severe symptoms.

Cortical regions that receive input from and project to the basal ganglia have also shown some consistencies in the neuroimaging literature. Several studies showed cortical thinning in sensorimotor cortices in children and adults with TS, with a striking relationship between thinning in specific regions and TS subtypes. Simple tics were associated with cortical thinning in primary sensory, motor, and premotor regions; complex tics were associated with thinning in premotor, prefrontal, and parietal regions; and TS with obsessive-compulsive behaviors was associated with thinning in the ACC and reduced hippocampal volumes. Prior to these findings, Mink proposed that within the CSTC circuit, simple tics would be associated with altered activity in the motor cortex; complex tics would be associated with altered activity in the premotor, SMA, and cingulate motor areas; and compulsions would be association with altered activity in the orbitofrontal cortex. While the precise mapping of particular regions to specific symptoms found by Worbe and colleagues does not exactly coincide with Mink's proposal, it does provide support for the idea that altered function in different cortical regions gives rise to different variations of symptoms in TS. Another consistent finding regarding cortical structures is a reduction in prefrontal volume in adults with TS. This finding has been proposed to play a role in symptom regulation. With respect to Mink's model, prefrontal cortical regions may develop into adulthood in a way that increases control over the striatum and therefore can dampen aberrant striatal activity in TS and manage tics. In a child with TS, increased volume in prefrontal regions with development may allow for better regulation of striatal activity, resulting in a large reduction or disappearance of symptoms into adulthood. Thus, reduced prefrontal volume in adults with TS has been interpreted as reflecting a failure to develop the ability to regulate tics. Data both from adults with TS and from adults who had TS as children but whose symptoms have remitted would be very interesting and could be used to directly test this hypothesis.

The functional neuroimaging data, while inconsistent, provide some support for CSTC dysfunction in TS (cf. Wang et al., 2011). Increased activity in the SMA prior to tics has been suggested as reflecting the premonitory urge that precedes tics. Interestingly, the specific regions in the putamen where microinjection of bicuculline caused tic-like movements in monkeys (McCairn et al., 2009) likely receive input from the SMA. Given such projections, increased SMA activity may be a source of aberrant striatal activity, leading to tics. Many of the fMRI studies we discuss here did not find differences in BOLD activity between TS and controls during several different tasks. However, the studies of executive function in TS that did show differences, even when inconsistent with respect to the precise region or direction of signal change, found alterations primarily in frontal and striatal areas. Moving beyond measures limited to task activation, studies utilizing functional and effective connectivity methods have begun to examine the relationships between brain regions, and how such relationships may

be altered in TS (Church et al., 2009a; Wang et al., 2011). While these data are currently limited, future work that implements such recent advances in MRI methodology and analyses can directly test questions related to CSTC circuits and other neural circuitry.

Mink's model of CSTC dysfunction in TS is a nice platform from which to work. It is fairly straightforward, and variations of it have been proposed to explain other movement disorders as well. However, certain phenomenological characteristics of TS are not well explained by the model. For one, the model does not account for the influence of several internal and external modulators, including stress, fatigue, physical exercise, distraction, and social events, on tics. Heightened stress, fatigue, and social events, such as birthday parties, commonly amplify tic symptoms in TS (Conelea & Woods, 2008); however, a potential mechanism by which these factors lead to increased aberrant striatal activity is not addressed. By contrast, physical exercise and focused attention on other activities often reduce tic severity. Additionally, the model cannot explain why specific tics come and go and change with time. In TS, some tics will wax and wane, some will remain for years, while others will last for a time and then disappear, often replaced by another tic. The model does not provide a biological explanation for why discrete sets of striatal neurons may display aberrant activity for differing periods of time. These issues need to be explored and perhaps can inform modifications to the model over time.

LIMITATIONS AND FUTURE DIRECTIONS

Neuroimaging studies of TS, especially fMRI, are limited thus far, and many results are inconsistent. The inconsistencies could be due to the large heterogeneities in the samples that have been studied. For one, different studies have included varying age groups, many covering wide age ranges. Taking note of participants' ages across studies is important because TS can be thought of as a developmental disorder, as it has a fairly typical developmental course. The most common age of onset is 5 to 6 years old, with the peak in severity often occurring at about ages 9 to 11 (Leckman et al., 2006). Therefore, cross-sectional studies examining children and adolescents together, such as the group of 7- to 16-year-olds in the study by Singer and colleagues (1993), may be averaging together different developmental stages of the disorder. In addition, separate studies that sample different age ranges or means, even when they are all technically studying "children," may yield different results due to the developmental stage being sampled. Therefore, future studies with more restricted age ranges, larger sample sizes of wide age ranges, and longitudinal studies of a young cohort would be useful for capturing specific developmental stages of TS, and for comparing those stages across development. Additionally, understanding typical development is of the utmost importance for identifying atypical brain structure and function in developmental disorders. Direct comparisons to the typical course of development can help tease apart whether dysfunction in the brain represents actual abnormalities or developmental immaturity (Church et al., 2009a).

Similar concerns are evident in studies of adults with TS. In adulthood, tic symptoms often attenuate or disappear altogether, with some epidemiological studies reporting a significant reduction of symptoms in 50% of patients along with complete remittance in 40% of patients (e.g., Burd et al., 2001; Corbett et al., 1969). This observation has led some to propose that the persistence of TS into adulthood is the less common developmental trajectory, complicating the interpretation of results from studies of adults with TS (Peterson et al., 2001; Raz et al., 2009). However, most epidemiological studies relied upon self-report, which may not be the most reliable source. A compelling study that collected both self-report measures and video recordings found that 90% of adults who had TS as children still had tics, even though half of those with current tics reported no symptoms (Pappert et al., 2003). Thus, it is unclear whether TS in adulthood represents the most severe cases, the more self-aware patients, or simply the typical course of the disorder. To address this issue within the neuroimaging literature, studies comparing adults with active TS to adults who had childhood TS but whose symptoms have remitted or improved substantially would be quite useful. To our knowledge, such a design has not yet been implemented, and therefore this is an exciting direction for future research.

Another potential confounding factor in many of the neuroimaging studies surveyed in this chapter is the high rate of comorbidity in TS. Up to 50% of individuals with TS also have ADHD, and 20% to 60% also have OCD (Singer, 2005), both of which are associated with their own neurobiological abnormalities (Maia et al., 2008; Mana et al., 2010). In fact, only 10% to 12% of individuals with TS do not have any comorbidities at all (Freeman et al., 2000; Leckman et al., 1998). This high comorbidity rate presents several scientific and practical problems. First, investigators aim to be certain that neurobiological differences between participants with TS and healthy controls are attributable to TS itself and not to associated comorbid disorders. Thus, it is appealing to study a sample of individuals with pure TS so as not to confound the results. However, if pure TS represents only ~10% of the TS population, excluding participation for comorbidities will not only be difficult from a practical recruitment standpoint, but will also likely misrepresent the typical presentation of the disorder (Gilbert & Buncher, 2005). Therefore, it seems equally important, not to mention more feasible, to test an ecologically valid sample of individuals who will mostly present with comorbidities. While both approaches (testing pure TS, and testing TS with comorbidities) have been used and results from these studies can be compared, it is not clear which findings may be confounded by comorbidities. A close examination of Tables 12.1 and 12.2 shows that results from pure TS and TS with comorbidities are sometimes consistent and sometimes inconsistent, with no systematic pattern. Thus, the field is in need of studies with very large samples of subgroups (i.e., pure TS, TS+ADHD, TS+OCD, ADHD only, OCD only) to reveal the actual contributions of comorbid disorders. Further, longitudinal follow-ups of such studies are necessary to ensure accurate group assignment. For example, a child originally included in the pure TS group may present with OCD several years later. Thus, at the time of participation in the study, this child would more appropriately be categorized as TS with latent OCD, not pure TS. Therefore, cross-sectional collection of these subgroups could falsely assure investigators of the absence of underlying comorbidities, highlighting the importance of longitudinal designs.

Inconsistencies among studies in TS may also be due to the effects of psychoactive medications. Many participants recruited for TS research will be taking medications at the time of study participation or have taken medication for some period of time in their life to treat tics or comorbid symptoms. These medications, including neuroleptics, antidepressants, and stimulants, among others, have been shown to affect brain structure and function (Corson et al., 1999; Frazier et al., 1996; Gur et al., 1998; Peterson et al., 2003; Scherk & Falkai, 2006). Thus, treatment-naïve participants are ideal for understanding the neurobiology underlying the disorder and not the effects of medications. However, excluding treated patients may bias the sample (e.g., lower severity, lower access to care, different ethnic distribution). On a practical level, never-treated participants can be difficult to find, and excluding treated patients may limit the size of a study sample. These considerations have led many studies to include participants with past or current medication use. A number of these studies have attempted to account for medication use by testing whether a subgroup of medication-free participants yield similar results, or by including medication as a statistical covariate. Some have reported no change in results when accounting for medication use in post-hoc analyses (Church et al., 2009b; Peterson et al., 2001; Plessen et al., 2006; Tobe et al., 2010), while others have found more normalized structure or function in those subgroups currently taking medications (Church et al., 2009a; Peterson et al., 2003). Still, comparisons among studies that have included and excluded medication use do not completely disentangle whether certain effects are confounded by medication history or current use.

Another issue that must be considered when conducting and reviewing MRI studies on TS is movement. Head movement during image acquisition can cause motion artifacts because the brain shifts its location in space and the MR signal

Box 12.1. Key Points

- Structural MRI studies have revealed reduced caudate volumes in children and adults with TS, with a negative correlation between caudate volume in childhood and symptom severity later in life.
- There is cortical thinning in sensorimotor cortices in children and adults with TS, with a negative correlation between thickness and orofacial tic severity.
- Adults with TS show cortical thinning and reduced gray matter volume in prefrontal regions, suggesting a failure in neural compensation to control tics into adulthood. In children, results are mixed with regard to structural measures of prefrontal regions.
- Measures of white matter have demonstrated larger volumes and reduced FA in the corpus callosum in TS.
- Results from fMRI studies suggest that the SMA may be involved in the premonitory urge.
- Results from fMRI studies of motor control and cognitive control in TS are generally inconsistent.
- Putative cognitive control networks are functionally immature and anomalous in TS. Thus, differences in functional anatomy in TS may go beyond CSTC circuits and involve cortical networks supporting cognitive control.

can be disrupted. Such susceptibility to motion creates difficulty when using MRI to examine particular populations, including children as well as patients with movement disorders. Structural and functional MRI scans typically last 5 to 8 minutes. Holding still for the duration of the scan can be quite difficult in individuals with TS, as their tics will likely lead to some degree of head motion. Thus, it is critical to minimize motion during data acquisition, and to ensure that measured effects, particularly in fMRI studies, are not due to motion. While TS researchers generally do their best to minimize the effects of motion (e.g., by recruiting subjects whose tics do not involve head movement, or by accounting for motion in the analysis steps), some approaches to account for differences in motion may not completely remove movement-related biases. Further, some experimental designs, such as those in which head movement occurs in synchrony with task responses, and some analysis techniques, such as functional connectivity analyses, may be more susceptible to the effects of motion.

One final important point to consider is that results from cross-sectional neuroimaging studies in TS can have several alternative explanations. We will refer to the finding of smaller caudate volumes in TS as an illustration. One possible interpretation is that smaller caudate volume is an underlying neurobiological marker for the disorder. Accordingly, this neuroanatomical difference may serve as a predictor of TS, or could even be a biological cause of tics. Alternatively, reduced caudate volumes may result from having tics for years. To meet DSM-IV criteria for a diagnosis of TS, tics must persist for at least 1 year. Therefore, the participants in studies on TS have had tics for at least a year, and most often for many years. Thus, smaller caudate volumes may represent the brain's response to altered activity over time, or may be a compensatory response in an attempt to control tics. Unfortunately, cross-sectional studies cannot distinguish between these possible explanations. Longitudinal studies, like that by Bloch and colleagues (2005), and also those that collect neuroimaging data at later time points, are greatly needed to make more informed interpretations of neuroimaging results. In the example of smaller caudate volumes, the results

---

Box 12.2. Questions for Future Research

- What changes in neurobiology occur throughout development in TS? Are the neurobiological differences between TS and neurotypical groups specific to particular stages of development? Does atypical brain function indicate atypical and/or delayed development?
- What is the typical developmental course of tics into adulthood? What are the neurobiological factors that distinguish between adults with active TS and adults whose childhood TS symptoms have remitted or substantially improved?
- How do comorbidities contribute to the differences in brain structure and function found in TS? Which findings are more attributable to the presence of comorbidities rather than to the presence of TS itself, or does such a distinction even exist? How much do results from pure TS groups generalize to the TS population as a whole?
- How do psychoactive medications affect brain structure and function in TS? What is the best way to account for the effects of current or past medication use on brain data?
- What are the neurobiological mechanisms underlying differences found in brain structure or function in TS? Do such differences, as measured by MRI or other imaging techniques, represent the cause of tics or the effect of having tics for a period of time? Longitudinal studies, and critically, prospective longitudinal studies are greatly needed to better understand how to interpret result from brain imaging data.
- Does successful treatment normalize differences in brain structure or function in TS?

of Bloch and colleagues suggest that reduced caudate volume is *not* due to prolonged experience with tics.

Given the limitations just discussed, the field is in need of (1) studies that carefully consider stages of development within the TS population, (2) comparisons between adults with TS and adults whose childhood TS symptoms have attenuated or disappeared, (3) large samples of subgroups with and without comorbidities as well as with and without medication use, and (4) longitudinal studies. In addition, pharmacological aspects of TS have been prominent at least since the discovery of neuroleptic medications half a century ago, but surprisingly, pharmacological fMRI has seldom been applied to TS (Hershey et al., 2004b). Newer techniques, such as perfusion MRI, may encourage further work in this direction (Black et al., 2010). Further, with the advancement of MRI methods capable of interrogating brain networks and connections between regions, future studies can more directly address questions regarding circuitry (as in Church et al., 2009a; Wang et al., 2011).

Finally, the field is in need of prospective, longitudinal studies that capture tics right when they begin in childhood or even before they begin. This approach would enable investigators to answer many questions left hanging by cross-sectional designs. For example, do children who will go on to develop TS have neuroanatomical dysfunction when tics first begin? Or do neurobiological changes come from chronic ticcing or chronic tic suppression? The results from prospective longitudinal studies will address such questions, greatly advancing our knowledge of the neurobiological underpinnings of TS.

REFERENCES

Albin RL, Mink JW. Recent advances in Tourette syndrome research. *Trends Neurosci* 2006; 29:175–182.

Alexander GE, Crutcher MD. Functional architecture of basal ganglia circuits: neural substrates of parallel processing. *Trends Neurosci* 1990; 13:266–271.

Alexander GE, DeLong MR. Microstimulation of the primate neostriatum. II. Somatotopic organization of striatal microexcitable zones and their relation to neuronal response properties. *J Neurophysiol* 1985; 53:1417–1430.

Aron AR, Behrens TE, Smith S et al. Triangulating a cognitive control network using diffusion-weighted magnetic resonance imaging (MRI) and functional MRI. *J Neurosci* 2007; 27:3743–3752.

Basso MA, Liu P. Context-dependent effects of substantia nigra stimulation on eye movements. *J Neurophysiol* 2007; 97:4129–4142.

Baumgardner TL, Singer HS, Denckla MB et al. Corpus callosum morphology in children with Tourette syndrome and attention deficit hyperactivity disorder. *Neurology* 1996; 47:477–482.

Baym CL, Corbett BA, Wright SB et al. Neural correlates of tic severity and cognitive control in children with Tourette syndrome. *Brain* 2008; 131:165–179.

Biswal BB, Ulmer JL, Krippendorf RL et al. Abnormal cerebral activation associated with a motor task in Tourette syndrome. *AJNR* 1998; 19:1509–1512.

Black KJ, Koller JM, Campbell MC et al. Quantification of indirect pathway inhibition by the adenosine A2a antagonist SYN115 in Parkinson disease. *J Neurosci* 2010; 30:16284–16292.

Bloch MH, Leckman JF, Zhu H, Peterson BS. Caudate volumes in childhood predict symptom severity in adults with Tourette syndrome. *Neurology* 2005; 65:1253–1258.
This work stands out as including long-term clinical follow-up to help test the direction of causality in an association between a neuroimaging finding (here, decreased caudate volume) and symptom severity.

Bohlhalter S, Goldfine A, Matteson S et al. Neural correlates of tic generation in Tourette syndrome: an event-related functional MRI study. *Brain* 2006; 129:2029–2037.

Bornstein RA, Baker GB, Bazylewich T, Douglass AB. Tourette syndrome and neuropsychological performance. *Acta Psychiatr Scand* 1991; 84:212–216.

Brand N, Geenen R, Oudenhoven M et al. Brief report: cognitive functioning in children with Tourette's syndrome with and without comorbid ADHD. *J Pediatr Psychol* 2002; 27:203–208.

Braun AR, Stoetter B, Randolph C et al. The functional neuroanatomy of Tourette's syndrome: an FDG-PET study. I. Regional changes in cerebral glucose metabolism differentiating patients and controls. *Neuropsychopharmacology* 1993; 9:277–291.

Bronfeld M, Belelovsky K, Bar-Gad I. Spatial and temporal properties of tic-related neuronal activity in the cortico-basal ganglia loop. *J Neurosci* 2011; 31:8713–8721.

Brown TT, Lugar HM, Coalson RS et al. Developmental changes in human cerebral functional organization for word generation. *Cerebral Cortex* 2005; 15:275–290.

Burd L, Kerbeshian PJ, Barth A et al. Long-term follow-up of an epidemiologically defined cohort of patients with Tourette syndrome. *J Child Neurol* 2001; 16:431–437.

Cavanna AE, Stecco A, Rickards H et al. Corpus callosum abnormalities in Tourette syndrome: an MRI-DTI study of monozygotic twins. *J Neurol Neurosurg Psychiatry* 2010; 81:533–535.

Chakos MH, Shirakawa O, Lieberman J et al. Striatal enlargement in rats chronically treated with neuroleptic. *Biol Psychiatry* 1998; 44:675–684.

Channon S, Pratt P, Robertson MM. Executive function, memory, and learning in Tourette's syndrome. *Neuropsychology* 2003; 17:247–254.

Church JA, Fair DA, Dosenbach NU et al. Control networks in paediatric Tourette syndrome show immature and anomalous patterns of functional connectivity. *Brain* 2009a; 132:225–238.

This study innovatively used rs-fcMRI to study TS, and carefully tested whether group differences represented functional immaturities or abnormalities, an important step in understanding developmental disorders. Results demonstrated immature as well as anomalous functional connectivity within putative cognitive control networks in adolescents with TS.

Church JA, Petersen SE, Schlaggar BL. The "Task B Problem" and other considerations in developmental functional neuroimaging. *Hum Brain Mapp* 2010; 31:852–862.

Church JA, Wenger KK, Dosenbach NU et al. Task control signals in pediatric Tourette syndrome show evidence of immature and anomalous functional activity. *Front Hum Neurosci* 2009b; 3:38.

Conelea CA, Woods DW. The influence of contextual factors on tic expression in Tourette's syndrome: a review. *J Psychosom Res* 2008; 65:487–496.

Corbett JA, Mathews AM, Connell PH, Shapiro DA. Tics and Gilles de la Tourette's syndrome: a follow-up study and critical review. *Br J Psychiatry* 1969; 115:1229–1241.

Corson PW, Nopoulos P, Miller DD et al. Change in basal ganglia volume over 2 years in patients with schizophrenia: typical versus atypical neuroleptics. *Am J Psychiatry* 1999; 156:1200–1204.

Debes NM, Hansen A, Skov L, Larsson H. A functional magnetic resonance imaging study of a large clinical cohort of children with Tourette syndrome. *J Child Neurol* 2011; 26:560–569.

Dosenbach NU, Fair DA, Miezin FM et al. Distinct brain networks for adaptive and stable task control in humans. *Proc Natl Acad Sci USA* 2007; 104:11073–11078.

Draganski B, Martino D, Cavanna AE et al. Multispectral brain morphometry in Tourette syndrome persisting into adulthood. *Brain* 2010; 133:3661–3675.

Eidelberg D, Moeller JR, Antonini A et al. The metabolic anatomy of Tourette's syndrome. *Neurology* 1997; 48:927–934.

Fahim C, Yoon U, Das S et al. Somatosensory-motor bodily representation cortical thinning in Tourette: effects of tic severity, age and gender. *Cortex* 2010; 46:750–760.

Fair DA, Dosenbach NUF, Church JA et al. Development of distinct control networks through segregation and integration. *Proc Natl Acad Sci USA* 2007; 104:13507–13512.

Frazier JA, Giedd JN, Kaysen D et al. Childhood-onset schizophrenia: brain MRI rescan after 2 years of clozapine maintenance treatment. *Am J Psychiatry* 1996; 153:564–566.

Fredericksen KA, Cutting LE, Kates WR et al. Disproportionate increases of white matter in right frontal lobe in Tourette syndrome. *Neurology* 2002; 58:85–89.

Freeman RD, Fast DK, Burd L et al. An international perspective on Tourette syndrome: selected findings from 3,500 individuals in 22 countries. *Dev Med Child Neurol* 2000; 42:436–447.

Frey KA, Albin RL. Neuroimaging of Tourette syndrome. *J Child Neurol* 2006; 21:672–677.

Fried I, Katz A, McCarthy G et al. Functional organization of human supplementary motor cortex studied by electrical stimulation. *J Neurosci* 1991; 11:3656–3666.

Gates L, Clarke JR, Stokes A et al. Neuroanatomy of coprolalia in Tourette syndrome using functional magnetic resonance imaging. *Prog Neuropsychopharmacol Biol Psychiatry* 2004; 28:397–400.

Gilbert DL, Buncher CR. Assessment of scientific and ethical issues in two randomized clinical trial designs for patients with Tourette's syndrome: a model for studies of multiple neuropsychiatric diagnoses. *J Neuropsychiatry Clin Neurosci* 2005; 17:324–332.

Graybiel AM. Habits, rituals, and the evaluative brain. *Annu Rev Neurosci* 2008; 31:359–387.

Gur RE, Maany V, Mozley PD et al. Subcortical MRI volumes in neuroleptic-naive and treated patients with schizophrenia. *Am J Psychiatry* 1998; 155:1711–1717.

Hampson M, Tokoglu F, King RA et al. Brain areas coactivating with motor cortex during chronic motor tics and intentional movements. *Biol Psychiatry* 2009; 65:594–599.

The findings from this fMRI study revealed that the SMA differentiated tics in individuals with TS from tic imitations in control participants before and after the peak of "tic-related" activity, implicating the SMA in the premonitory urge that frequently precedes tics.

Hershey T, Black KJ, Hartlein J et al. Dopaminergic modulation of response inhibition: an fMRI study. *Brain Res Cogn Brain Res* 2004a; 20:438–448.

Hershey T, Black KJ, Hartlein J et al. Cognitive-pharmacologic functional magnetic resonance imaging in Tourette syndrome: a pilot study. *Biol Psychiatry* 2004b; 55:916–925.

Hong KE, Ock SM, Kang MH et al. The segmented regional volumes of the cerebrum and cerebellum in boys with Tourette syndrome. *J Korean Med Sci* 2002; 17:530–536.

Horak FB, Anderson ME. Influence of globus pallidus on arm movements in monkeys. II. Effects of stimulation. *J Neurophysiol* 1984; 52:305–322.

Hyde TM, Stacey ME, Coppola R et al. Cerebral morphometric abnormalities in Tourette's syndrome: a quantitative MRI study of monozygotic twins. *Neurology* 1995; 45:1176–1182.

Jackson GM, Mueller SC, Hambleton K, Hollis CP. Enhanced cognitive control in Tourette syndrome during task uncertainty. *Exp Brain Res* 2007; 182:357–364.

Jackson SR, Parkinson A, Jung J et al. Compensatory neural reorganization in Tourette syndrome. *Curr Biol* 2011; 21:580–585.

Kalanithi PS, Zheng W, Kataoka Y et al. Altered parvalbumin-positive neuron distribution in basal ganglia of individuals with Tourette syndrome. *Proc Natl Acad Sci USA* 2005; 102:13307–13312.

Kataoka Y, Kalanithi PSA, Grantz H et al. Decreased number of parvalbumin and cholinergic interneurons in the striatum of individuals

with Tourette syndrome. *J Comp Neurol* 2010; 518:277–291.

This follow-up to Kalanithi et al. (2005) included only five TS brains but is still the largest published autopsy study using modern methods. Results demonstrated a disproportionate loss of certain neurons in the striatum of individuals with TS.

Leckman JF, Bloch MH, King RA, Scahill L. Phenomenology of tics and natural history of tic disorders. *Adv Neurol* 2006; 99:1–16.

Leckman JF, Zhang H, Vitale A et al. Course of tic severity in Tourette syndrome: the first two decades. *Pediatrics* 1998; 102:14–19.

Lee JS, Yoo SS, Cho SY et al. Abnormal thalamic volume in treatment-naive boys with Tourette syndrome. *Acta Psychiatr Scand* 2006; 113:64–67.

Lerner A, Bagic A, Boudreau EA et al. Neuroimaging of neuronal circuits involved in tic generation in patients with Tourette syndrome. *Neurology* 2007; 68:1979–1987.

Ludolph AG, Juengling FD, Libal G et al. Grey-matter abnormalities in boys with Tourette syndrome: magnetic resonance imaging study using optimised voxel-based morphometry. *Br J Psychiatry* 2006; 188:484–485.

Maia TV, Cooney RE, Peterson BS. The neural bases of obsessive-compulsive disorder in children and adults. *Dev Psychopathol* 2008; 20: 1251–1283.

Makki MI, Behen M, Bhatt A et al. Microstructural abnormalities of striatum and thalamus in children with Tourette syndrome *Mov Disord* 2008; 23:2349–2356.

Makki MI, Govindan RM, Wilson BJ et al. Altered fronto-striato-thalamic connectivity in children with Tourette syndrome assessed with diffusion tensor MRI and probabilistic fiber tracking. *J Child Neurol* 2009; 24:669–678.

Mana S, Paillere Martinot ML, Martinot JL. Brain imaging findings in children and adolescents with mental disorders: a cross-sectional review. *Eur Psychiatry* 2010; 25:345–354.

Marsh R, Zhu H, Wang Z et al. A developmental fMRI study of self-regulatory control in Tourette's syndrome. *Am J Psychiatry* 2007; 164:955–966.

Mazzone L, Yu S, Blair C et al. An FMRI study of frontostriatal circuits during the inhibition of eye blinking in persons with Tourette syndrome. *Am J Psychiatry* 2010; 167:341–349.

McCairn KW, Bronfeld M, Belelovsky K, Bar-Gad I. The neurophysiological correlates of motor tics following focal striatal disinhibition. *Brain* 2009; 132:2125–2138.

Miller AM, Bansal R, Hao X et al. Enlargement of thalamic nuclei in Tourette syndrome. *Arch Gen Psychiatry* 2010; 67:955–964.

Mink JW. The basal ganglia: focused selection and inhibition of competing motor programs. *Prog Neurobiol* 1996; 50:381–425.

Mink JW. Basal ganglia dysfunction in Tourette's syndrome: a new hypothesis. *Pediatr Neurol* 2001; 25:190–198.

In this review, Mink discusses the organization and function of basal ganglia circuitry and proposes a useful model of aberrant striatal activity in TS.

Moriarty J, Costa DC, Schmitz B et al. Brain perfusion abnormalities in Gilles de la Tourette's syndrome. *Br J Psychiatry* 1995; 167: 249–254.

Moriarty J, Varma AR, Stevens J et al. A volumetric MRI study of Gilles de la Tourette's syndrome. *Neurology* 1997; 49:410–415.

Mueller SC, Jackson GM, Dhalla R et al. Enhanced cognitive control in young people with Tourette's syndrome. *Curr Biol* 2006; 16:570–573.

Müller-Vahl KR, Kaufmann J, Grosskreutz J et al. Prefrontal and anterior cingulate cortex abnormalities in Tourette syndrome: evidence from voxel-based morphometry and magnetization transfer imaging. *BMC Neuroscience* 2009; 10:47.

Nelson SM, Dosenbach NU, Cohen AL et al. Role of the anterior insula in task-level control and focal attention. *Brain Struct Funct* 2010; 214:669–680.

Neuner I, Kupriyanova Y, Stocker T et al. White-matter abnormalities in Tourette syndrome extend beyond motor pathways. *Neuroimage* 2010; 51:1184–1193.

Ozonoff S, Strayer DL, McMahon WM, Filloux F. Inhibitory deficits in Tourette syndrome: a function of comorbidity and symptom severity. *J Child Psychol Psychiatry* 1998; 39:1109–1118.

Palmer ED, Brown TT, Petersen SE, Schlaggar BL. Investigation of the functional neuroanatomy of single word reading and its development. *Scientific Studies of Reading* 2004; 8:203–223.

Pappert EJ, Goetz CG, Louis ED et al. Objective assessments of longitudinal outcome in Gilles de la Tourette's syndrome. *Neurology* 2003; 61:936–940.

Peterson B, Riddle MA, Cohen DJ et al. Reduced basal ganglia volumes in Tourette's syndrome using three-dimensional reconstruction techniques from magnetic resonance images. *Neurology* 1993; 43:941–949.

In one of the first volumetric studies of TS, this work revealed reduced volumes of the striatum and lenticular nucleus in adults with TS, a finding that has since been replicated.

Peterson BS, Choi HA, Hao X et al. Morphologic features of the amygdala and hippocampus in children and adults with Tourette syndrome. *Arch Gen Psychiatry* 2007; 64:1281–1291.

Peterson BS, Skudlarski P, Anderson AW et al. A functional magnetic resonance imaging study of tic suppression in Tourette syndrome. *Arch Gen Psychiatry* 1998; 55:326–333.

Peterson BS, Staib L, Scahill L et al. Regional brain and ventricular volumes in Tourette syndrome. *Arch Gen Psychiatry* 2001; 58, 427–440.

This study examined one of the largest TS cohorts in the literature; the same sample, more or less, is used in several other structural MRI studies from this group.

Peterson BS, Thomas P, Kane MJ et al. Basal ganglia volumes in patients with Gilles de la Tourette syndrome. *Arch Gen Psychiatry* 2003; 60:415–424.

Plessen KJ, Gruner R, Lundervold AJ et al. Reduced white matter connectivity in the corpus callosum of children with Tourette syndrome. *J Child Psychol Psychiatry* 2006; 47:1013–1022.

Plessen KJ, Wentzel-Larsen T, Hugdahl K et al. Altered interhemispheric connectivity in individuals with Tourette's disorder. *Am J Psychiatry* 2004; 161:2028–2037.

Raz A, Zhu H, Yu S et al. Neural substrates of self-regulatory control in children with adults with Tourette syndrome. *Can J Psychiatry* 2009; 54:579–588.

Rickards H. Functional neuroimaging in Tourette syndrome. *J Psychosom Res* 2009; 67:575–584.

Robertson MM, Banerjee S, Kurlan R et al. The Tourette syndrome diagnostic confidence index: development and clinical associations. *Neurology* 1999; 53:2108–2112.

Roessner V, Overlack S, Baudewig J et al. No brain structure abnormalities in boys with Tourette's syndrome: a voxel-based morphometry study. *Mov Disord* 2009; 24:2398–2403.

Roessner V, Overlack S, Schmidt-Samoa C et al. Increased putamen and callosal motor subregion in treatment-naive boys with Tourette syndrome indicates changes in the bihemispheric motor network. *J Child Psychol Psychiatry* 2011a; 52:306–314.

Roessner V, Wittforth M, Schmidt-Samoa C et al. Altered motor network recruitment during finger tapping in boys with Tourette syndrome. *Hum Brain Mapp* 2011b; 33:666–675.

Scherk H, Falkai P. Effects of antipsychotics on brain structure. *Curr Opin Psychiatry* 2006; 19:145–150.

Schlaggar BL, Brown TT, Lugar HM et al. Functional neuroanatomical differences between adults and school-age children in the processing of single words. *Science* 2002; 296:1476–1479.

Serrien DJ, Nirkko AC, Loher TJ et al. Movement control of manipulative tasks in patients with Gilles de la Tourette syndrome. *Brain* 2002; 125:290–300.

Singer HS. Tourette's syndrome: from behaviour to biology. *Lancet Neurol* 2005; 4:149–159.

Singer HS, Reiss AL, Brown JE et al. Volumetric MRI changes in basal ganglia of children with Tourette's syndrome. *Neurology* 1993; 43:950–956.

This was one of the first volumetric studies of TS, along with Peterson et al. (1993).

Sowell ER, Kan E, Yoshii J et al. Thinning of sensorimotor cortices in children with Tourette syndrome. *Nat Neurosci* 2008; 11:637–639.

This study examined cortical thickness in children with TS and demonstrated thinning in sensorimotor, frontal, and parietal cortices. Further, thinning in sensorimotor regions and DLPFC was associated with increased tic severity, providing a compelling link between cortical structure and TS symptoms.

Stern ER, Silbersweig D, Chee KY et al. A functional neuroanatomy of tics in Tourette syndrome. *Arch Gen Psychiatry* 2000; 57:741–748.

Thomalla G, Siebner HR, Jonas M et al. Structural changes in the somatosensory system correlate with tic severity in Gilles de la Tourette syndrome. *Brain* 2009; 132:765–777.

Tobe RH, Bansal R, Xu D et al. Cerebellar morphology in Tourette syndrome and obsessive-compulsive disorder. *Ann Neurol* 2010; 67:479–487.

Wang L, Lee DY, Bailey E et al. Validity of large-deformation high dimensional brain mapping of the basal ganglia in adults with Tourette syndrome. *Psychiatry Res* 2007; 154:181–190.

Wang Z, Maia TV, Marsh R et al. The neural circuits that generate tics in Tourette's syndrome. *Am J Psychiatry* 2011; 168; 1326–1337.

Watkins LH, Sahakian BJ, Robertson MM et al. Executive function in Tourette's syndrome and obsessive-compulsive disorder. *Psychol Med* 2005; 35:571–582.

Werner CJ, Stocker T, Kellermann T et al. Altered motor network activation and functional connectivity in adult Tourette's syndrome. *Hum Brain Mapp* 2011; 32:2014–2026.

Wichmann T, Bergman H, DeLong MR. The primate subthalamic nucleus. I. Functional properties in intact animals. *J Neurophysiol* 1994; 72:494–506.

Woods DW, Watson TS, Wolfe E et al. Analyzing the influence of tic-related talk on vocal and motor tics in children with Tourette's syndrome. *J Appl Behav Anal* 2001; 34:353–356.

Worbe Y, Gerardin E, Hartmann A et al. Distinct structural changes underpin clinical phenotypes in patients with Gilles de la Tourette syndrome. *Brain* 2010; 133:3649–3660.

This study revealed a compelling specificity in cortical thickness depending on TS phenotypes, such that individuals with simple tics, complex tics, and obsessive-compulsive behaviors demonstrated cortical thinning in distinct regions.

Zimmerman AM, Abrams MT, Giuliano J et al. Subcortical volumes in girls with Tourette syndrome: support for a gender effect. *Neurology* 2000; 54:2224–2229.

13

The Neurochemistry of Tourette Syndrome

HARVEY S. SINGER

Abstract

The pathobiology of Tourette syndrome (TS) involves the complex and integrated cortico-striatal-thalamo-cortical (CSTC) circuits. This chapter systematically analyzes the involvement in TS of all the neurotransmitter systems relevant to CSTC circuits. A major role for dopamine continues to be the most consistently observed neurotransmitter change in this condition. Of the various dopaminergic hypotheses proposed, an alteration of the tonic-phasic neurotransmitter release system appears most viable. However, it remains highly likely that TS patients exhibit dysfunction in several neurotransmitter systems, although new evidence is warranted to better understand the dysfunction of non-dopaminergic systems, particularly serotonergic, glutamatergic, and GABAergic ones.

INTRODUCTION

Tourette syndrome (TS) is an inherited, childhood-onset neuropsychiatric disorder characterized by a fluctuating course of multiple chronic motor and phonic tics. In addition, affected patients frequently have a variety of associated problems, including attention-deficit/hyperactivity disorder, obsessive-compulsive disorder, episodic outbursts, anxiety, depression, and school difficulties. Although the precise pathophysiological mechanism for TS remains undefined, neuroanatomical and neurophysiological studies (see Chapters 11 and 12) suggest the involvement of cortico-striato-thalamo-cortical (CSTC) circuits. In turn, neurotransmitters within these circuits have been proposed to have an etiological role based on their localization, known involvement in other movement disorders, measurement in postmortem samples, quantification using imaging protocols, and the clinical response to neurotransmitter-directed pharmacotherapy. Given the complex nature of tic symptoms and their frequent association with neuropsychological comorbidities,

it is highly possible that this disorder involves a dysfunction of more than one neurotransmitter or a focusing second messenger-like system. In addition, because many tic symptoms improve during the teenage and early adulthood years, a dynamic developmental alteration must be considered. This chapter provides a review of CSTC circuitry, its neurochemistry, and a discussion of evidence supporting the involvement of specific neurotransmitter systems in TS.

CSTC CIRCUITS

A series of parallel CSTC circuits link specific regions in the frontal cortex to subcortical structures (Fig. 13.1). Expanding evidence supports the role of CSTC pathways in the expression of tics and its accompanying neuropsychiatric problems (Berardelli et al., 2003; Bloch et al., 2005; Harris & Singer, 2006; Hoekstra et al., 2004; Singer & Minzer, 2003). Determining the specific site of abnormality within these circuits remains an area of active research. Knowledge of the neurotransmitter systems involved in these pathways is essential for understanding the proposed underlying effect of biochemical abnormalities in TS.

Cortex

Cortical pyramidal neurons provide the striatum with massive excitatory glutamatergic projections that make asymmetrical synaptic contact with the dendritic spines of GABAergic (gamma-aminobutyric acid) striatal medium-sized spiny neurons (MSNs) (Fig. 13.2). Five distinct but integrated parallel circuits (motor, oculomotor, dorsolateral prefrontal, lateral orbitofrontal, and anterior cingulate) connecting cortex to striatum have been described in primates (Alexander et al., 1986; Tekin & Cummings, 2002). Pyramidal neuron excitability is influenced by various inputs, including GABAergic interneurons, dopaminergic (DA) projections from the ventral tegmental area (VTA), serotonin (5HT) input from the median raphe, and norepinephrine (NE) from the locus coeruleus. Mesocortical DA inputs affect cortical pyramidal neurons directly and indirectly via modulation of GABAergic interneurons. Dopamine D1, D2, and D4 receptors are present on cortical GABAergic interneurons (Mrzljak et al., 1996; Smiley et al., 1994). Dopaminergic stimulation of receptors on cortical interneurons is generally regarded as promoting a GABA-mediated inhibition of pyramidal cells (Del Arco & Mora, 2000; Gorelova et al., 2002; Seamans et al., 2001b). The direct effect of D1 receptor stimulation on prefrontal neurons, however, is more complex, dependent on the functional status of these neurons at the time of receptor stimulation (Yang et al., 1999). For example, cortical D1 receptor augmentation is most effective when the neuron is already activated (depolarized) by excitatory input (Seamans et al., 2001a).

Striatum

The striatum, long considered the major pathophysiological site in TS, is divided into two major regions: the dorsal (caudate and putamen) and ventral "limbic" (nucleus accumbens) striatum. Functionally, the dorsal striatum is primarily involved in motor behaviors and the ventral

striatum in motivational processes (Clithero et al., 2011; Groenewegen et al., 2003; Nestler, 2005; Richard & Berridge, 2011). Striatal neurons are divided into two main subtypes:

1. Projection neurons. These neurons are also called MSNs because of their size and the presence of numerous dendritic spines. MSNs represent approximately 95% of total striatal neurons, and virtually all use GABA as their main neurotransmitter, but subsets coexpress a number of neuroactive peptides and enkephalin (Fig. 13.1). Direct pathway (striatum to globus pallidus interna [GPi]/substantia nigra pars reticulata [SNpr]) MSNs express dopamine D1 receptors, M1 and M4 muscarinic acetylcholine receptors, and the neuropeptide substance P. Indirect pathway MSNs (striatum to globus pallidus externa [GPe]) express dopamine D2 receptors, M1 receptors, adenosine A2A receptors, and enkephalin.

2. Interneurons. Striatal interneurons (Fig. 13.3) consist of giant aspiny cholinergic interneurons and several subtypes of medium-sized GABAergic interneurons: a fast-spiking interneuron that expresses the calcium binding protein parvalbumin; an electrophysiologically unidentified interneuron expressing the calcium binding protein calretinin; an interneuron that exhibits both low threshold spiking and plateau potentials and coexpresses the peptides somatostatin and neuropeptide Y (NPY) as well as the enzyme neuronal nitric oxide synthase (Tepper & Bolam, 2004); and a newly identified additional NPY-expressing interneuron (Ibanez-Sandoval et al., 2011). Cholinergic interneurons exert a neuromodulatory effect on MSN and GABAergic interneurons exert powerful, fast feed-forward effects on MSNs (Gittis et al., 2010; Tepper et al., 2008).

Corticostriatal Pathways

Cortical pyramidal neuronal inputs to the striatum release glutamate, which via AMPA receptors elicits excitatory postsynaptic potentials. N-methyl-D-aspartate (NMDA) receptors, acting via voltage-gated ion channels, are also capable of modulating striatal activity. In addition to the glutamatergic cortical input, MSNs also

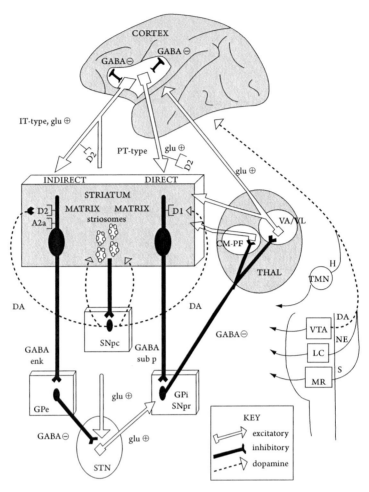

FIGURE 13.1 The CSTC pathway and ascending cortical inputs. Hypothesized abnormalities have included disorders of excess excitation or diminished inhibition, disruptions in frontal cortex, striatum, or striosomes, and abnormalities of various synaptic neurotransmitters. A2a, adenosine 2a receptor; DA, dopamine; GABA, gamma-aminobutyric acid; GLU, glutamate; GPe, globus pallidus externa; GPi, globus pallidus interna; H, histamine LC, locus coeruleus; MR, median raphe; NE, norepinephrine; S, serotonin; STN, subthalamic nucleus; VTA, ventral tegmental area; CM-PF, centromedian-parafascicular complex; enk, enkephalins; SNpc, substantia nigra pars compacta; SNpr, substantia nigra pars reticulate; sub P, substance P; THAL, thalamus; TMN, tuberomammillary nucleus; VA/VL, ventral anterior/ventral lateral nuclei. (Modified from Harris & Singer, 2006.)

receive glutamate input from the intralaminar nuclei of the thalamus; dopamine from the substantia nigra pars compacta (SNpc) and ventral tegmental area (VTA); GABA, substance P, and enkephalin from other MSNs; acetylcholine, GABA, or peptides from striatal interneurons; and histamine from the tuberomammillary nucleus of the posterior hypothalamus.

Dopamine has potent modulatory effects on MSNs, dependent on the receptor type (D1 or D2)

located on dendritic shafts and spines. D2 stimulation inhibits NMDA-mediated glutamate transmission, the excitability of MSN, and long-term potentiation, thereby decreasing neuronal excitability. In contrast, D1 stimulation facilitates glutamate transmission and promotes NMDA function, MSN excitability, and long-term potentiation (Centonze et al., 2001; Cepeda et al., 2001; Cepeda & Levine, 1998; Levine et al., 1996; Nicola et al., 2000; Onn et al., 2000; West & Grace, 2002).

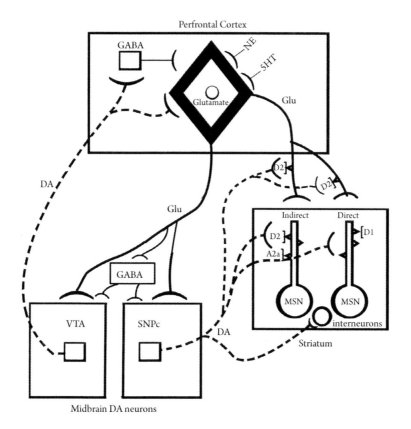

FIGURE 13.2   Interactions between glutamate and the dopaminergic system. 5HT, serotonin; A2a, adenosine 2a receptor; NE, norepinephrine; VTA, ventral tegmental area; SNPc, substantia nigra pars compacta; GABA, gamma-aminobutyric acid; Glu, glutamate; D1, dopamine D1 receptor; D2, dopamine D2 receptor; DA dopamine; MSSN, medium-sized spiny neurons. (Modified from Singer et al., 2010.)

D1 receptor stimulation is most effective when the cells are in a depolarized state due to the convergence of excitatory inputs (Marti et al., 2002; West & Grace, 2002). Dopamine also influences cortical input via D2 receptors located on presynaptic glutamatergic corticostriatal terminals. Activation of these presynaptic receptors reduces the release of glutamate, a mechanism speculated to explain some of the pharmacotherapeutic action of neuroleptics (Daly & Moghaddam, 1993; Morari et al., 1994). Large aspiny cholinergic and GABAergic interneurons in the dorsal striatum and nucleus accumbens also possess dopaminergic receptors (Alcantara et al., 2003).

Striatothalamic Pathways

The typical simplified expression of striatothalamic projections shows two separate striatal output pathways, referred to as "direct" and "indirect." The direct pathway transmits striatal information monosynaptically to the GPi and SNpr, whereas the indirect system conveys information to these same regions via a disynaptic relay from GPe to the subthalamic nucleus (STN). GABAergic outputs from GPi/SNpr project to mediodorsal thalamic nuclei, the centromedian-parafascicular thalamic complex, the peduculopontine tegmental nucleus, and habenula. The SNpr also projects to the superior colliculus. The parallel direct and indirect pathways have opposing effects on GABAergic GPi/SNpr output neurons; the direct pathway inhibits and the indirect pathway stimulates. In turn, these pathways have a reverse effect on thalamocortical (VA-VL) neurons and facilitation of motor activity; that is, activation of the direct pathway facilitates motor activity

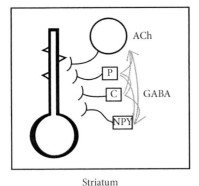

Striatal interneurons

Striatum

FIGURE 13.3 Striatal MSNs and interneurons. ACh, acetylcholine; P, parvalbumin; C, calretinin; NPY, neuropeptide Y; MSN, medium-sized spiny neuron; GABA, gamma-aminobutyric acid.

via disinhibition of thalamocortical neurons, whereas activation of the indirect pathway reduces motor activity by increasing inhibition of thalamocortical neurons. In addition to the two-pathway model, movement disorders may also result from imbalances between striatal striosomal and matrix components; the matrix contains the direct and indirect pathways' MSNs, whereas striosomes contain MSNs that receive input from parts of the limbic cortex with projections directly or indirectly to the SNpc (Crittenden & Graybiel, 2011).

Thalamocortical and Thalamostriatal Pathways

The thalamic targets of GPi/SNpr, in turn, project to the frontal lobe, with the VA-VL thalamic complex providing excitatory innervation to motor-related cortical areas. The topographic representation noted in the striatum and globus pallidus is maintained within the thalamus and subsequent projections to the premotor and motor cortex.

LOCATION OF ABNORMALITY?

The identification of the underlying neurochemical abnormality in TS would benefit from knowledge of the precise anatomical abnormality in TS. There is consensus, with both direct and indirect evidence, for involvement of the CSTC pathway (Berardelli et al., 2003; Hoekstra et al., 2004; Singer & Minzer, 2003). Identification of the primary site, however, remains an area of active research (Felling & Singer, 2011; Harris & Singer, 2006). The major candidates include:

1. Striatum: Evidence for the striatal component is based on associations between basal ganglia dysfunction and movements in other disorders and numerous, but variable, abnormalities on neuroimaging studies (Felling & Singer, 2011). Additional support comes from neuroanatomical studies showing abnormalities of striatal interneurons, as highlighted in Chapter 10 (Kalanithi et al., 2005; Kataoka et al., 2010).

2. Cortex: Other researchers have focused on a primary cortical dysfunction in TS, based on the presence of executive dysfunction (Harris et al., 1995; Schuerholz et al., 1998), cognitive inhibitory deficits (Stern et al., 2008), anatomical regional abnormalities (Ludolph et al., 2008; Peterson et al., 2001, 2007; Sowell et al., 2008), alterations in size of the corpus callosum (Baumgardner et al., 1996; Plessen et al., 2004), immature functional connectivity (Church et al., 2009), functional imaging suggesting that tic suppression involves increased frontostriatal activity (Mazzone et al., 2010), transcranial magnetic stimulation studies demonstrating prominent tic-related activity in primary motor and Broca's areas (Moll et al., 1999; Ziemann et al., 1997), and others (see Felling & Singer, 2011). Direct evidence also comes from semiquantitative immunoblot investigations on postmortem tissue, which showed a greater number of changes in prefrontal centers (BA9) than in caudate, putamen, or ventral striatum (Minzer et al., 2004; Yoon et al., 2007a).

3. Other: In the original circuit hypothesis the emphasis was placed on the cortex and striatum. Subsequent iterations, however, have emphasized the possibility of convergence and a greater involvement of the cerebellum (DeLong & Wichmann, 2009). For example, cerebellar output via the thalamus influences the striatum and output from the STN synapses in the cerebellum (Bostan et al., 2010; Bostan & Strick, 2010; Hoshi et al., 2005).

NEUROTRANSMITTER ABNORMALITIES

As discussed in the CSTC section, numerous neurotransmitters (dopamine, glutamate, GABA, serotonin, acetylcholine, norepinephrine, opiates) are involved in the transmission of messages through these pathways, and each has been proposed as a potential TS pathophysiological mechanism (Singer & Minzer, 2003). Which, if any, of these neurotransmitters is the primary pathological factor remains to be definitively determined. Neurochemical hypotheses tend to be based on extrapolations from several areas, including clinical trials evaluating the response to specific medications (see also Chapter 24); cerebrospinal fluid, blood, and urine studies; neurochemical assays on postmortem brain tissues (see also Chapter 10); positron emission tomography (PET) and single photon emission tomography (SPECT) studies; and genetic analyses (see also Chapter 7). Recognizing the difficulty in obtaining fresh postmortem samples and the potential interaction of drugs on different systems (Daly & Moghaddam, 1993; Morari et al., 1994), more recent efforts have probed specific neurotransmitters using SPECT and PET.

In each of the following individual neurotransmitter sections, the discussion will include the mechanism by which the synaptic messengers could influence tics, results of transmission-altering pharmacological trials, and existing confirmatory laboratory and imaging support. Each of these confirmatory approaches has its limitations. Although recent investigations emphasize imaging abnormalities, it is essential to recognize that spatial resolutions need to be improved, better "time-locking" is required between tics and imaging, and regions of the brain other than the basal ganglia need evaluation (see also Chapter 12; Rickards, 2009). In addition, there are concerns in neurochemically oriented protocols involving compensatory changes, the role of associated symptoms, prior medication use, the age and gender of subjects, and other confounding factors.

DOPAMINE

Dopamine plays a major role in the control of motor function, temporal processing, reward learning, and response inhibition (Liang et al., 2008; Jones & Jahanshahi, 2011; Richard & Berridge, 2011; Hershey et al., 2004). In proposed dopaminergic hypotheses for TS, the primary pathological abnormality could be at the level of the striatum or cortex and could be the result of supersensitive dopamine receptors, dopamine hyperinnervation, abnormal presynaptic terminal function, or excess dopamine release. Each of these possibilities will be discussed in greater detail with the suggestion that evidence favors the dopamine release hypothesis. It is also possible, but never investigated, that TS could be associated with proteins (e.g., serine/threonine protein phosphatases; Walaas et al., 2011) that regulate dopamine signaling.

In the striatum, activation of MSN D1 receptors (direct pathway) results in enhanced thalamocortical movement-stimulating activity, whereas activation of D2 receptors (indirect pathway) results in reduced thalamocortical glutamate activity and diminished movement. In addition to short-term effects, dopamine can modulate corticostriatal transmission by the mechanism of long-term depression or potentiation (Centonze et al., 1999; Groves et al., 1995; Wickens et al., 1995). This modulation either strengthens or weakens the efficacy of corticostriatal synapses and can, in turn, mediate reinforcement of specific discharge patterns (Mink, 2001). DA-induced fluctuating abnormalities in the resting potential of striatal neurons have been hypothesized to influence tic waxing and waning and also to explain the lack of identifiable abnormality in DA transmission (Mink, 2001). In the cortex, dopamine innervation from the VTA both directly and indirectly influences pyramidal neuron activity. In a rodent model, lesioning VTA dopaminergic neurons alters motor skill learning (Hosp et al., 2011). Thus, tic activity could be due to excess corticostriatal pathway glutamate stimulation secondary to D1 receptor augmentation in prefrontal cortical neurons.

In general, the dopamine hypothesis implies increased signal transduction due to either an increased amount of dopamine (high tonic levels or increased phasic release) or an increased sensitivity to the neurotransmitter (e.g., increased number or affinity of dopamine receptors). Initial confirmation of excess dopamine was sought by measurements of cerebrospinal fluid homovanillic acid (HVA), the major metabolite of dopamine; an elevation of HVA would imply that its precursor dopamine was similarly elevated. Basal and turnover levels of cerebrospinal fluid HVA, however, were statistically reduced, not elevated, in TS subjects (Butler et al., 1979; Cohen et al., 1978; Singer et al., 1982b), and levels were restored to normal after the administration of haloperidol (Singer et al., 1982a). Further, unconjugated plasma HVA did not correlate with tic severity scores (Riddle et al., 1988b). Subsequent findings of normal concentrations of dopamine, HVA, and 3,4-dihydroxyphenylacetic acid (DOPAC) in postmortem striatal samples also corroborated that there was no excessive production or prolonged (tonic) release of dopamine. As will be discussed, however, these early studies did not eliminate the possibility of altered dopamine innervations or phasic dopamine release.

Based solely on clinical experience with tic-suppressing pharmacotherapy, the preponderance of evidence supports the involvement of dopamine. Dopaminergic antagonists, such as pimozide, fluphenazine, haloperidol, risperidone, and aripiprazole, suppress motor and vocal tics in the majority of affected patients (Singer, 2010). Symptomatic improvement has also been reported following the administration of agents that block dopamine synthesis (e.g., α-methyl-para-tyrosine) or prevent the accumulation of dopamine in presynaptic storage vesicles (e.g., tetrabenazine) (Porta et al., 2008; Sweet et al., 1974). Conversely, tics may be exacerbated following treatment with agents that increase central dopaminergic activity (e.g., L-dopa and central stimulants) and have appeared after withdrawal of neuroleptic drugs (Karagianis & Nagpurkar, 1990; Klawans et al., 1978).

Although the dopaminergic system has been proposed to play a part in TS pathogenesis, no consistent linkage or association could be demonstrated between patients with TS and candidate genes (O'Rourke et al., 2009), such as the dopamine D2–D5 receptor alleles (Barr et al., 1997; Devor et al., 1998; Diaz-Anzaldua et al., 2004; Hebebrand et al., 1997), mutations in the D1 receptor (Thompson et al., 1998), or dopamine beta hydroxylase gene (Ozbay et al., 2006). Some association studies or mutation screenings also yielded negative results for the dopamine and norepinephrine transporters (Diaz-Anzaldua et al., 2004; Stober et al., 1999). In contrast, a significant association has been reported between TS and a dopamine transporter polymorphism (DAT1 *Ddel*) (Yoon et al., 2007b). Linkage has not been demonstrated between TS and the glycine, GABA, glutamate, α- and β-adrenergic, or glucocorticoid receptor alleles (Barr et al., 1999a; Brett et al., 1997) or between TS and a functional polymorphism in the catechol-O-methyltransferase gene (Barr et al., 1999b).

Postulated Dopamine Abnormalities

SUPERSENSITIVE POSTSYNAPTIC DOPAMINE RECEPTORS?

Because levels of HVA were not increased in cerebrospinal fluid, investigators initially focused on a potential abnormality of postsynaptic receptors, either an increased number or greater affinity of dopamine receptors. A limited number of single-point binding assays in postmortem striatum for D1 ([3H] SCH 23390) and D2 ([3H] spiperone) receptors were not significantly different in control and TS membrane preparations (Singer et al., 1991). Mean values for D2 receptors were slightly increased in the caudate and putamen, but most likely represented upregulation associated with chronic haloperidol therapy. Investigations of D2 dopamine receptors by PET and SPECT have produced inconsistent findings in studies comparing TS patients and controls (George et al., 1994; Singer et al., 2002; Turjanski et al., 1994; Wolf et al., 1996; Wong et al., 1997, 2008). Several studies do support the hypothesis that the dopamine receptor is involved in the neurobiology of TS. In a study of five sets of identical twins, increased binding of

[^{123}I]iodobenzamide ([^{123}I]-IBZM) was observed in the head of the caudate nucleus in association with increased tic severity (Wolf et al., 1996). In a PET study using a spiperone derivative, 3-N [^{11}C]-methylspiperone, B_{MAX} levels above the 95th percentile prediction limit (normal regressed against age) were observed in 4 of 20 adult subjects, and multiple linear regression analyses revealed a trend between the severity of vocal tics and B_{MAX} values (Wong et al., 1997). In a study of 14 adults with TS, D2 binding was increased in the left ventral striatum (Wong et al., 2008). In contrast to these studies, others using [^{123}I] IBZM or [^{11}C] raclopride did not show differences in D2 receptors (George et al., 1994; Singer et al., 2002; Turjanski et al., 1994). One study using the ligand ([^{123}I]-IBZM suggested that dopamine receptors were significantly different in medicated but not neuroleptic-naïve patients (Muller-Vahl et al., 2000b). In the cortex, two small studies have suggested reduced extrastriatal D2/D3 dopamine binding potentials as measured by the high-affinity D2/D3 receptor antagonists [11C] FLB 457 and [F18] fallypride (Gilbert et al., 2006; Steeves et al., 2010). Fallypride imaging data results differ from a report of increased cortical dopamine receptors assayed in postmortem tissues (Minzer et al., 2004; Yoon et al., 2007a), possibly due to the limitation of PET binding to externalized surface receptors.

DOPAMINE HYPERINNERVATION?

A second hypothesis suggests a dopaminergic hyperinnervation within the striatum of affected individuals. Investigators have used two approaches in attempt to confirm excess dopamine terminals: binding to the DA transporter (DAT) or the vesicular monoamine transporter type 2.

DAT Binding.

Measurement of 3H-mazindol binding in a small number of postmortem samples from subjects with TS showed a significant increase in the number of striatal presynaptic dopamine carrier sites (Singer et al., 1991). Attempts to provide support for postulated dopamine hyperinnervation, using as a marker the number of dopamine terminals measured by PET or SPECT binding, have generally identified higher levels of binding. A study of five adults with TS studied with [^{123}I]β-CIT SPECT found that striatal DAT binding was higher than in controls, but the reported correlations in the midbrain and thalamus could be influenced by serotonin binding (Malison et al., 1995). In a study using a similar technique, the mean striatal activity ratio was significantly higher in TS patients, and 5 of the 12 TS subjects showed striatum/occipital cortex ratios more than 2 standard deviations above the normal mean (Muller-Vahl et al., 2000a). Dopamine transporter binding using higher-resolution scanning with [^{123}I] FP-CIT showed increased striatal binding but no association with TS-related behaviors (Serra-Mestres et al., 2004). This finding was confirmed in another small study (Choen et al., 2004). Several studies have also used a (99m) Tc-TRODAT-1 SPECT/CT imaging methodology and obtained varying results: in 10 TS patients there was a marked increase in DAT (Mena et al., 2004); in 10 there was no difference (Hwang et al., 2008); and 18 drug-naïve TS patients showed significantly higher uptake in the striatum (Liu et al., 2010). In contrast, some investigators using SPECT or PET techniques in adult patients with TS showed no difference in DAT binding compared to controls (Heinz et al., 1998; Stamenkovic et al., 2001). In summary, most studies support increased levels of striatal DAT binding.

VMAT2 Binding.

Evaluation of dorsal striatal dopaminergic innervation has also been evaluated by use of *in vivo* measures of vesicular monoamine transporter type 2 (VMAT2) binding using the ligand (+)—alpha- [^{11}C] dihydrotetrabenazine. In general, these studies have shown little differences between TS subjects and controls: in 8 adults with TS there was no change (Bohnen et al., 1999); in 19 there was an increase in ventral striatal binding (Albin et al., 2003), but in a repeat investigation by the same authors there were no differences between 33 TS adults and controls (Albin et al., 2009). Hence, in contrast to DAT binding, these results suggest that there is no increased striatal innervation, but rather a potential abnormality in the regulation of dopamine reuptake.

PRESYNAPTIC DA ABNORMALITY?

A presynaptic dopamine abnormality involving dopa decarboxylase activity has been proposed. In a small PET study, 11 adolescents with TS accumulated [^{18}F]-fluorodopa at a level 25% higher in the left caudate nucleus and 53% higher in the right midbrain compared with levels in control subjects (Ernst et al., 1999). The authors suggest that upregulation of dopa decarboxylase activity could explain these alterations and that the process reflects deficits in a variety of functional elements of the dopamine system. Other investigators have postulated an abnormality in central nervous system neuronal membrane based on a decreased dopamine uptake into platelet storage granules (Rabey et al., 1995).

ELEVATED INTRASYNAPTIC DOPAMINE RELEASE?

On the basis of electrophysiological and neurochemical data, dopamine release has both a homeostatic (tonic) and spike-dependent (phasic) component. A proposed abnormality of the phasic and/or tonic dopamine release system model in TS could exist in either the cortex or striatum.

Tonic Release.

Tonic dopamine, which exists extracellularly in low concentration, determines long-term dopamine homeostasis, including regulation of postsynaptic receptors. The tonic (or basal) level of dopamine is defined primarily as an extrasynaptic measure and is calculated by use of microdialysis and electrophysiological measurements. Dopamine autoreceptors (D2 and D3 subtypes) are proposed as regulators of tonic dopamine control. A reduction in tonic dopamine levels would result in an upregulation of postsynaptic

dopamine receptors. Possible reasons for a lower tonic dopamine level could include an overactive dopamine transporter system or altered autoregulator. Hence, in TS, suggestions of a possible tonic dopamine abnormality are supported by several imaging studies showing a significant increase in the number of presynaptic dopamine transporter carrier sites in the postmortem striatum (Singer et al., 1991) and frontal cortex (Minzer et al., 2004) and increased SPECT/PET binding of dopamine transporters in pediatric and adult imaging protocols (Choen et al., 2004; Liu et al., 2010; Malison et al., 1995; Mena et al., 2004; Muller-Vahl et al., 2000a; Serra-Mestres et al., 2004).

Phasic Release.

Phasic dopamine, in contrast, is spike-dependent dopamine released into the synaptic cleft. With sufficient stimulation or when an uptake blocker is given in high concentrations, phasic dopamine can escape this region. A surrogate measure of phasic dopamine is the intrasynaptic dopamine release induced by the use of stimulant challenges, such as with amphetamine. A hyperresponsive spike-dependent (phasic) dopaminergic system could be the result of an alteration in afferent cortical inputs with or without a coexisting abnormality of dopamine transporters.

Several studies have demonstrated an increased release of dopamine in striatum following amphetamine stimulation (Singer et al., 2002; Wong et al., 2008). In one study, seven adults with TS and five age-matched controls each received two PET scans with high-specific-activity [11C]raclopride. The first scan followed an intravenous injection of saline; the second followed an intravenous injection of amphetamine. After the amphetamine challenge, the mean value of intrasynaptic dopamine in the putamen (as determined by true equilibrium bolus estimation) increased by 21% in the subjects with TS and did not change in the comparison subjects (Singer, Szymanski, et al. 2002). In a second study, as compared with controls, DA release was significantly increased in the ventral striatum in subjects with TS (Wong,

Brasic, et al. 2008). Further, an [11C]-FLB457 PET study in conjunction with an amphetamine challenge showed that TS subjects had regions of increased dopamine release involving medial frontal gyri and anterior cingulate cortex (Steeves et al., 2010). A smaller reduction of the 99mTC TRODAT-1 dopamine transporter binding ratio, after a methylphenidate challenge, in the caudate of TS patients was also interpreted as further evidence for a phasic dysfunction (Yeh et al., 2007). The phasic dopamine hypothesis is further supported by clinical findings, including (1) the exacerbation of tics by stimulant medications, likely secondary to enhanced dopamine release from the axon terminal; (2) tic exacerbation by environmental stimuli, such as stress, anxiety, and medications; events shown to increase phasic bursts of dopamine; (3) tic suppression with very low doses of dopamine agonists, likely owing to a presynaptic reduction in phasic dopamine release; and (4) PET studies in TS patients following improvement of symptoms after deep brain stimulation (DBS) of the centomedian-parafascicular complex of the thalamus. In two preliminary DBS reports the suggested mechanism of improvement is an upregulation of dopamine receptors associated with a decrease in dopamine release (Kuhn et al., 2012; Vernaleken et al., 2009). More specifically, in a small number of patients with thalamic stimulators and clinical improvement, [18F] fallypride PET scans were obtained about 6 months after surgery. D2/3 receptor availability was measured under anesthesia, 1 day apart, during "stimulator-on" and "stimulator-off" conditions and showed a dramatic decrease in binding potential from the "on" to "off" condition, suggesting an increased release of endogenous dopamine in the "off" condition, and a dramatic elevation of D2/3 receptor availability (thalamus, caudate, putamen, and temporal cortex) in the baseline "on" condition as compared to healthy subjects.

GLUTAMATE

Glutamate is the primary excitatory neurotransmitter of approximately 60% of neurons in the mammalian brain (Nieuwenhuys, 1994). It is the excitatory neurotransmitter of corticostriatal neurons, output neurons from the subthalamic nucleus, and thalamostriatal and thalamocortical projections. Descending glutamate frontal afferents also modulate mesocortical (VTA) and midbrain (SNpc) dopamine neurons via an activating ("accelerator") and inhibitory ("brake") pathway (Carlsson et al., 1999; Kegeles et al., 2000). The model of dual modulation of the mesolimbic DA system by the prefrontal cortex has been confirmed in studies showing that extracellular DA concentrations in the nucleus accumbens are increased or decreased following high- or low-frequency cortical stimulation, respectively (Jackson et al., 2001; Taber & Fibiger, 1995).

Several lines of evidence suggest that a dysfunction of the glutamatergic system may have a role in TS (Singer et al., 2010). Reduced levels of this amino acid were detected in four postmortem TS samples in GPi, GPe, and SNpr (Anderson et al., 1992a, 1992b). Since, in the same study, levels of glutamate and aspartate were normal in a variety of cortical regions, further studies are necessary to clarify the meaning of glutamate changes. Based on the reduction of glutamate in pallidal areas and MRI volumetric studies showing reduction in the size of the left globus pallidus, a role for reduced subthalamic nucleus glutamate output (either excessive inhibition from GPe projections or a primary developmental abnormality of the STN) has been proposed (Anderson et al., 1992a, 1992b). In the latter, reduced STN glutamate would result in diminished excitation of the inhibitory GPi/SNpr and ultimately increased thalamocortical excitation.

Brain imaging has identified altered morphology of the corpus callosum (Baumgardner et al., 1996; Mostofsky et al., 1999; Peterson et al., 1994; Plessen et al., 2004) and abnormal functional interhemispheric connectivity in TS (Baumer et al., 2010). Whether this anatomical alteration, however, translates into altered cortical glutamate neurotransmission requires further investigation. In addition, neural activity in primary motor cortex GABA-mediated intracortical circuits, as measured by transcranial magnetic stimulation, is decreased in children and adults with TS. Hence, diminished cortical GABAergic activity would be expected to result in increased glutamatergic excitation.

Gene-based studies in TS patients have provided additional links to glutamate. A large multigenerational family genome scan and a genome scan using sibling pairs and multigenerational families have identified evidence for linkage to 5p13, an area that overlaps with the genomic region for the glial glutamate transporter1 (*SLC1A3* or *EAAT1*) gene (Barr et al., 1999a; TSAICG, 2007). A missense variant involving a highly conserved residue, E219D, has been identified in a small number of individuals with TS, and a 3H-glutamate uptake assay showed that E219D conveys a significant increase in EAAT1-mediated glutamate uptake (Adamczyk et al., 2010). DLGAP3, the gene for the postsynaptic scaffolding protein (SAP90/PSD95-associated protein 3), which is highly expressed in glutamatergic synapses in the striatum, is a promising candidate gene (Crane et al., 2011). Other factors supporting a potential role for glutamate in TS include its essential role in pathways involved with CSTC circuits, the extensive interaction between the glutamate and dopamine neurotransmitter systems, and preliminary reports demonstrating that glutamate-altering medications have a beneficial therapeutic effect on obsessive-compulsive symptoms (Coric et al., 2005; Grant et al., 2007).

ACETYLCHOLINE

A dopaminergic–cholinergic balance is important for the maintenance of normal movements. Cholinergic interneurons influence both MSNs and other interneurons within the striatum. Cholinergic fibers also project from the basal forebrain to the cortex and from the lateral tegmental area to the locus coeruleus. The effects of cholinergic and anticholinergic agents in the treatment of tics are conflicting. The administration of cholinergic precursors, including choline, lecithin, and dimethylaminoethanol (deanol), had little effect on motor tics (Barbeau, 1980; Polinsky et al., 1980; Stahl & Berger, 1981; Tanner et al., 1982). In contrast, anticholinergic agents (physostigmine)

reduced the frequency of motor tics but exacerbated vocal tics (Tanner et al., 1982). Mecamylamine, a nicotinic acetylcholine antagonist, has had variable effects in relieving motor and vocal tics (Shytle et al., 2002; Silver et al., 2000), and transdermal nicotine has unconvincing effects (Scahill et al., 2006). Using circulating lymphocytes as a peripheral means to measure changes in central nervous system muscarinic receptors, [3H]-QNB binding was reduced in untreated TS patients (Tanner et al., 1982). Other laboratory investigations, however, have not provided support for an abnormality of the cholinergic system. In cerebrospinal fluid, acetylcholinesterase and butyrylcholinesterase activities did not differ from controls (Singer et al., 1984). In postmortem brain samples, the activity of choline acetyltransferase (ChAT), the synthesizing enzyme for acetylcholine, as well as muscarinic receptors, as measured by QNB binding, were

similar to controls (Singer et al., 1990). In contrast to the above neurochemical analyses, the regional density of ChAT-containing interneurons in postmortem TS samples was reduced in the caudate and putamen (see also Chapter 10; Kataoka et al., 2010).

GABA

GABAergic MSNs are the primary projection neurons from the striatum for both striato-GPi (direct) and striato-GPe (indirect) pathways. GABA is also the neurotransmitter for several striatal interneurons. Several GABAergic hypotheses have been proposed for the production of tics: an alteration of GABAergic projections from the striatum and the impairment of either cortical or striatal GABAergic interneurons. A deficiency of cortical inhibitory interneurons, suggested by reduction of short-interval intracortical inhibition measured by double-pulse TMS (Gilbert et al., 2004; Heise et al., 2010; Orth et al., 2008; Ziemann et al., 1997), would have a direct enhancing effect on glutamate activity (see also Chapter 11). In the striatum, a profound imbalance in the number of parvalbumin-positive neurons has been identified—increased in the GPi and decreased in the striatum (see Chapter 10; Kalanithi et al., 2005).

A second anatomical study confirmed the reduction of parvalbumin-containing interneurons in postmortem TS caudate and putamen (Kataoka et al., 2010). Since parvalbumin-containing interneurons are GABAergic and have projections to MSNs as well as other interneurons, their reduction would likely result in a neurochemical imbalance. Recent studies have suggested that fast-spiking interneurons may preferentially target direct over indirect pathway MSNs (Gittis et al., 2010). From a developmental perspective, both GABAergic MSNs and many cortical GABAergic interneurons migrate from similar embryonic regions in the ganglionic eminence (Anderson et al., 1997). It has therefore been postulated in TS that a single adverse event during development could affect both striatal and cortical inhibitory function (Leckman, 2002).

Despite the described anatomical abnormalities, there are limited additional data to support an abnormality of GABA in TS. A recent PET study provided support for the hypothesis of disinhibition of circuits involving the basal ganglia and thalamus (Lerner et al., 2012). Eleven TS patients and 11 healthy volunteers were studied using [(11C)] flumazenil, showing decreased binding of $GABA_A$ receptors in TS patients bilaterally in the ventral striatum, globus pallidus, thalamus, amygdala, and right insula, as well as increased $GABA_A$ binding in the substantia nigra bilaterally, in the left periaqueductal gray, right posterior cingulated cortex, and bilateral cerebellum. Benzodiazepines, which enhance the inhibitory effect of GABA, have some efficacy in tic suppression (Gonce & Barbeau, 1977). Several studies have evaluated the therapeutic effect of baclofen, a $GABA_B$ receptor agonist. Results in two open-label protocols were variable (Awaad, 1999; Shapiro, 1988), and a small double-blind placebo-controlled crossover study showed statistical improvement in an overall impairment score, but not reduction of tics (Singer et al., 2001). The activity of glutamate decarboxylase, the highly specific presynaptic marker for GABAergic interneurons in the cerebral cortex, is normal in postmortem cortex (Singer et al., 1990), as are levels of GABA in various brain regions, whole blood, and cerebrospinal fluid (Anderson et al., 1992b).

NORADRENERGIC SYSTEM

Noradrenergic (NA) fibers project widely to the cerebral cortex from the locus coeruleus and may modulate frontal subcortical circuits implicated in TS. Sensorimotor gating abnormalities, suggested in TS (Swerdlow et al., 2006), are associated with altered NA regulation within distinct thalamocortical and ventral forebrain networks (Alsene et al., 2011). NA projections could also influence tic activity via indirect influences on other neurotransmitter systems (e.g., dopamine). Firm evidence for an NA mechanism in TS is limited and partly based on the therapeutic effect of the alpha-adrenergic agonists clonidine and guanfacine (Bloch et al., 2009; Singer, 2010). Although primarily viewed as a selective α2-adrenoceptor agonist active presynaptically, clonidine also decreases the release of glutamate (Jellish et al., 2005; Shinomura et al., 1999) and has been shown to regulate spontaneous and glutamate-modulated firing activity in medial frontal cortical pyramidal neurons (Wang et al., 2011). Adults with TS do have increased levels of cerebrospinal fluid norepinephrine (NE), 55% greater than healthy controls (Leckman et al., 1995a), and excrete elevated levels of urinary NE in response to the stress involved with having a lumbar puncture (Chappell et al., 1994). Measurements of NE are normal in plasma; levels of its metabolite, 3-methoxy-4-hydroxyphenylethylene glycol (MHPG), are normal in plasma and cerebrospinal fluid and variable in urine (Ang et al., 1982; Bornstein & Baker, 1990; Baker et al., 1990; Butler et al., 1979; Leckman et al., 1995a; Riddle et al., 1988a, 1988b; Singer et al., 1982a). Platelet α2-adrenoceptors are normal in TS (Silverstein et al., 1985). NE levels were normal in postmortem cerebral cortex and basal ganglia (Singer et al., 1990, 1991). Alpha-receptor densities have been variable in postmortem cortex, either normal (Singer et al., 1990) or increased in BA10 and BA11 (Yoon et al., 2007a). The latter, if confirmed, could lead to a reduction in the basal release of dopamine, since activation of α2A receptors has been shown to inhibit dopamine release in the prefrontal cortex (Gobert et al., 1998).

SEROTONIN

Serotoninergic fibers project from the medial raphe to the striatum, SNpc, VTA, nucleus accumbens, and prefrontal cortex. The mechanism by which serotonin could influence tics is speculative and likely via its effect on other neurotransmitters. Serotonin does alter the release of dopamine via several mechanisms, including presynaptic 5-hydroxytryptamine heteroceptors, inhibitory and stimulatory somatodendritic receptors, and 5-hydroxytryptamine-2 receptor action on the dopamine receptor site (Kuroki et al., 2003; Sershen et al., 2000; Smythies, 2005). It has also been suggested that serotonin promotes dopamine release via a mechanism that occurs in the absence of a stimulating ligand (Cobb & Abercrombie, 2003). Lastly, serotonin may suppress glutamatergic neurotransmission by reducing glutamate release via the activation of presynaptic 5HT1B receptors (Guo & Rainnie, 2010).

In obsessive-compulsive disorder, a comorbid clinical problem in many TS subjects, pharmacological studies strongly support an association with serotonin. Ondansetron, a 5-hydroxytyrptamine antagonist, has been suggested to have tic-suppressing effects (Toren et al., 2005), although selective serotonin reuptake inhibitors have not suppressed tics effectively. Serotonin receptor genes HTR3A and HTR3B are normal (Niesler et al., 2005); however, polymorphic variants of tryptophan hydroxylase 2 have been postulated to be associated with TS (Mossner et al., 2007).

In cerebrospinal fluid studies, 5-hydroxyindoleacetic acid (5-HIAA), the principal metabolite of serotonin, is reduced in some, but not all, patients with TS (Butler et al., 1979; Cohen et al., 1978; Leckman et al., 1995a; Singer et al., 1982b). Levels of this metabolite in the cerebral cortex are normal (Singer et al., 1990), whereas tryptophan and 5-HIAA may be globally decreased in basal ganglia regions (Anderson et al., 1992a, 1992b). Plasma tryptophan, whole blood serotonin, and the 24-hour excretion of serotonin have also been reported to be reduced in TS subjects (Comings, 1990; Leckman et al., 1995b). The relative density of 5HT-1A receptors in postmortem frontal and occipital cortex from a small number of TS subjects was normal (Yoon et al., 2007a). A SPECT binding study showed a negative correlation between vocal tics and [123I]-b-CIT binding to the serotonin transporter in the midbrain and thalamus, indicating that serotoninergic neurotransmission in the midbrain and serotoninergic or noradrenergic neurotransmission in the thalamus can be important factors in the expression of TS (Heinz et al., 1998). Other [123I]-b-CIT and SPECT studies investigating serotonin transporter binding capacity in patients with TS have also shown reduced binding, but findings appeared in association with the presence of obsessive-compulsive disorder (Muller-Vahl et al., 2005). Results measuring binding ([18F] altanserin) to 5-hydroxytryptamine-2A receptors have been variable, ranging from unchanged (Wong et al., 2005) to increased in multiple brain regions (Haugbol et al., 2007; Wong et al., 2005). PET of tryptophan metabolism (alpha-[11C]-methyl-L-tryptophan) has demonstrated decreased uptake in dorsolateral prefrontal cortical regions and increased uptake in the thalamus (Behen et al., 2007). The findings of increased dopamine release, decreased serotonin transporter (SERT) binding potential, and possible elevation of 5-HT2A receptor binding in individuals with TS plus obsessive-compulsive disorder have suggested a condition of increased phasic dopamine release modulated by low 5-HT in subjects with TS plus obsessive-compulsive disorder (Wong et al., 2008).

OPIATES AND ENDOCANNABINOIDS

Opiate systems, including dynorphin and metenkephalin, are localized within the basal ganglia, interact with dopamine neurons, and may have important influences on the control of movements. The distribution of neuropeptides differentiates distinct output pathways from the striatum: GPe is rich in enkephalin, the GPi is rich in dynorphin, and the ventral striatum contains a mixed distribution.

In a postmortem study, dynorphin A [1–17] immunoreactivity was decreased in striatal fibers projecting to the GPe in a severely affected TS patient (Haber et al., 1986; Haber & Wolfer, 1992). Another dynorphin, dynorphin A [1–8], was increased in the cerebrospinal fluid of TS patients, and the concentration of this opiate correlated with the severity of obsessive-compulsive symptoms but not with tic severity (Leckman et al., 1988). The use of the opiate antagonist naloxone in the treatment of tics has produced conflicting results. For example, some investigators have found a dramatic improvement in symptoms (Kurlan et al., 1991; Sandyk, 1987), whereas others have found only a rare responder (Erenberg & Lederman, 1992) or a significant dose-related effect (van Wattum et al., 2000). The finding that withdrawal of a patient from opiates unmasked TS-like symptoms has been cited as further evidence for their role in TS (Lichter et al., 1988). Several studies have suggested that cannabinoids (smoking marijuana or using oral delta-9-tetrahydrocannabinol) has a beneficial effect on tics (Muller-Vahl, 2009). Only limited SPECT studies analyzing the cannabinoid CB1 receptor with [123I]AM281 have been published (Berding et al., 2004). TS is not associated with mutations in the central cannabinoid receptor (CNR1) gene (Gadzicki et al., 2004).

HISTAMINE

Histaminergic neurons are located in the tuberomammillary nucleus (TBN) of the posterior hypothalamus and send fibers to most brain regions, including the cortex, striatum, GP, VTA, and SN (Nuutinen & Panula, 2010). These neurons exhibit a diurnal rhythm, with high activity during wakefulness and reduced activity during sleep. In an analysis of linkage in a two-generation autosomal dominant fashion pedigree, a rare functional mutation was identified in the HDC gene that encodes L-histidine decarboxylase, the rate-limiting enzyme in histamine biosynthesis (Ercan-Sencicek et al., 2010).

Four types of histamine receptors have been identified. H1 and H2 are expressed both peripherally and postsynaptically in the central nervous system, H3 nearly exclusively in the brain, and H4 mainly in the immune system but also in the brain (Flik et al., 2011). H3 receptors, found in high concentration in the cortex, striatum, and hippocampus, are located on both histamine nerve terminals and on postsynaptic cells (Haas et al., 2008). Histamine 1, 2, and 3 receptors are members of the G-protein-coupled receptor family; H1 and H2 are activators of cyclic AMP and lead to neuronal excitation, whereas H3 stimulation inhibits cAMP and neuronal activity. Prefrontal cortex H3 receptors play an important role in the autoregulation of histamine neurotransmission (Flik et al., 2011). In the striatum, H3 receptors are located postsynaptically on MSNs and have an important role in modulating dopamine neurotransmission (Ferrada et al., 2008; Moreno et al., 2011; Pillot et al., 2002).

Based upon their multiple proposed interactions, the histaminergic system could have a significant role in the pathogenesis of tics via several possible mechanisms: (1) histamine 3 receptor postsynaptic stimulation of (a) cortical pyramidal neurons would inhibit glutamate output to the striatum and TBN (Flik et al., 2011) or (b) MSNs would counteract the motor activation induced by D1 and D2 stimulation (Ferrada et al., 2008); (2) stimulation of H3 heteroreceptors could reduce the release of dopamine, glutamate, serotonin, or other neurotransmitters (Brown et al., 2001; Hashemi et al., 2011; Leurs et al., 2005; Molina-Hernandez et al., 2000; Schlicker et al., 1994); (3) stimulation of H2 receptors could depolarize direct and indirect MSNs (Ellender et al., 2011) or excite GP neurons (Chen et al., 2005); and (4) histaminergic neurons have the ability to serve as an alternative source of dopamine, via their ability to take up and convert levodopa to dopamine (Yanovsky et al., 2011). The activity of fast-spiking GABAergic interneurons on MSNs does not appear to be affected by histamine (Ellender et al., 2011).

In rodents, ciproxifan, an H3 antagonist/inverse agonist, modulates locomotor sensitization induced by methamphetamine (Motawaj & Arrang, 2011). In a single patient with TS and cataplexy, the medication pitolisant, an inverse agonist of the H3 receptor, did not decrease tics (Hartmann et al., 2012).

ADENOSINE

Adenosine A2a receptors in the striatum are localized postsynaptically on MSNs that also have a high density of D2 receptors. A2a and D2 receptors form heteromers, and by means of an allosteric interaction, adenosine receptor stimulation counteracts D2 receptor modulation of glutamate (NMDA) excitatory input (Ferre et al., 2011). A second type of interaction between A2a and D2 receptors takes place at the level of adenylyl cyclase. In an animal model of spontaneous stereotypies, the coadministration of an A2a and A1 receptor agonist attenuated movements in a dose-dependent fashion (Tanimura et al., 2010).

SECOND MESSENGER SYSTEM ABNORMALITY

Identification of a postreceptor defect involving a second messenger system could potentially explain the presence of reported abnormalities within a variety of neurotransmitter systems in TS. For example, for several neurotransmitters an interaction exists with adenosine 3′,5′-monophosphate (cAMP); D1 and α-adrenergic receptors activate adenylate cyclase activity, whereas opiate (μ and δ), α-2-adrenergic, D2, serotonergic (5-HT_{1A}), and muscarinic (M4) receptors inhibit cyclase activity. Activation of cAMP signaling increases the activity of the cAMP-dependent protein kinase A and the dopamine- and cAMP-dependent phosphoprotein of 32 kDa (DARPP-32). In TS postmortem brain samples, cAMP levels were 34% to 56% of normal in frontal, temporal, and occipital cortices and 23% of normal in the putamen (Singer et al., 1991). A follow-up postmortem study of frontal and occipital lobes investigated the production and catabolism of cAMP as well as receptor binding activities for [3H]-inositol 1,4,5-triphosphate (IP_3) to IP_3 receptors and [3H]-phorbol ester to protein kinase C (Singer et al., 1995). Results suggested that alterations in the cAMP and phosphoinositide second messenger generating systems were not major contributing factors in the development of TS. More specifically, there were no significant differences in adenylyl cyclase activity whether assayed under basal conditions or after stimulation with a nonhydrolyzable guanine triphosphate analogue, a selective enzyme stimulator, or a β-adrenergic agonist. Further, D2 receptor activation, the inhibitory guanine nucleotide protein, and cAMP phosphodiesterase were not altered in TS samples (Singer et al., 1995).

In addition to cAMP and phosphoinositide systems, some investigators have suggested a potential role for other striatal signaling components in the causation of movement disorders:

Box 13.1. Key Points

- An expanding body of evidence indicates that the pathological mechanism in TS involves the complex and integrated CSTC circuits. Although an initial focus was on the striatum, increasing data support a significant role for cortical involvement as well.
- Neurochemically, proposals for the underlying synaptic mechanism have included virtually all of the neurotransmitter systems involved in CSTC circuits, and the precise abnormality remains speculative. The strongest evidence, however, continues to favor a major role for dopamine.
- Of the various proposed dopaminergic hypotheses, an alteration of the tonic-phasic neurotransmitter release system appears most viable. Nevertheless, given the complex interactions between potential agents, it remains likely that several transmitter systems are involved. This author looks forward to the development of new biological concepts and the application of innovative techniques in the study of this complex disorder.

---

the dopamine-regulated striatal signaling system (e.g., regulator of calmodulin signaling, AARP-16, serine/threonine protein phosphatases); extracellular signal-related kinases (ERK); and the mammalian target of rapamycin complex 1 (mTORC1) (Feyder et al., 2011; Walaas et al., 2011). These systems have not been investigated in TS.

REFERENCES

Adamczyk A, Gause CD, Sattler R et al. Genetic and functional studies of a missense variant in a glutamate transporter, SLC1A3, in Tourette syndrome. *Psychiatric Genetics* 2010; 21:90–97.

Albin RL, Koeppe RA, Bohnen NI et al. Increased ventral striatal monoaminergic innervation in Tourette syndrome. *Neurology* 2003; 61:310–315.

Albin RL, Koeppe RA, Wernette K et al. Striatal [11C]dihydrotetrabenazine and [11C]methylphenidate binding in Tourette syndrome. *Neurology* 2009; 72:1390–1396.

Alcantara AA, Chen V, Herring BE et al. Localization of dopamine D2 receptors on cholinergic interneurons of the dorsal striatum and nucleus accumbens of the rat. *Brain Res* 2003; 986:22–29.

Alexander GE, DeLong MR, Strick PL. Parallel organization of functionally segregated circuits linking basal ganglia and cortex. *Ann Rev Neurosci* 1986; 9:357–381.

Alsene KM, Rajbhandari AK, Ramaker MJ, Bakshi VP. Discrete forebrain neuronal networks supporting noradrenergic regulation of sensorimotor gating. *Neuropsychopharmacology* 2011; 36:1003–1014.
Discusses noradrenergic regulation of distinct thalamocortical and ventral forebrain networks.

Anderson GM, Pollak ES, Chatterjee D et al. Brain monoamines and amino acids in Gilles de la Tourette's syndrome: a preliminary study of subcortical regions. *Arch Gen Psychiatry* 1992a; 49:584–586.

Anderson GM, Pollak ES, Chatterjee D et al. Postmortem analysis of subcortical monoamines and amino acids in Tourette syndrome. *Adv Neurol* 1992b; 58:123–133.

Anderson SA, Eisenstat DD, Shi L, Rubenstein JL. Interneuron migration from basal forebrain to neocortex: dependence on Dlx genes. *Science* 1997; 278:474–476.

Ang L, Borison R, Dysken M, Davis JM. Reduced excretion of MHPG in Tourette syndrome. Adv Neurol 1982; 35:171–175. Awaad Y. Tics in Tourette syndrome: new treatment options. *J Child Neurol* 1999; 14: 316–319.

Baker GB, Bornstein RA, Douglass AB, Carroll A, King G. Urinary excretion of metabolites of norepinephrine in Tourette's syndrome. *Mol Chem Neuropathol* 1990; 13:225–232.

Barbeau A. Cholinergic treatment in the Tourette syndrome. *N Engl J Med* 1980; 302: 1310–1311.

Barr CL, Wigg KG, Pakstis AJ et al. Genome scan for linkage to Gilles de la Tourette syndrome. *Am J Med Genet* 1999a; 88:437–445.

Barr CL, Wigg KG, Sandor P. Catechol-O-methyltransferase and Gilles de la Tourette syndrome. *Mol Psychiatry* 1999b; 4:492–495.

Barr CL, Wigg KG, Zovko E et al. Linkage study of the dopamine D5 receptor gene and Gilles de la Tourette syndrome. *Am J Med Genet* 1997; 74:58–61.

Baumer T, Thomalla G, Kroeger J et al. Interhemispheric motor networks are abnormal in patients with Gilles de la Tourette syndrome. *Mov Disord* 2010; 25:2828–2837.

Baumgardner TL, Singer HS, Denckla MB et al. Corpus callosum morphology in children with Tourette syndrome and attention deficit hyperactivity disorder. *Neurology* 1996; 47:477–482.

Behen M, Chugani HT, Juhasz C et al. Abnormal brain tryptophan metabolism and clinical correlates in Tourette syndrome. *Mov Disord* 2007; 22:2256–2262.

Berardelli A, Curra A, Fabbrini G et al. Pathophysiology of tics and Tourette syndrome. *J Neurol* 2003; 250:781–787.

Berding G, Muller-Vahl K, Schneider U et al. [123I]AM281 single-photon emission computed tomography imaging of central cannabinoid CB1 receptors before and after delta-9-tetrahydrocannabinol therapy and whole-body scanning for assessment of radiation dose in Tourette patients. *Biol Psychiatry* 2004; 55:904–915.

Bloch MH, Leckman JF, Zhu H, Peterson BS. Caudate volumes in childhood predict symptom severity in adults with Tourette syndrome. *Neurology* 2005; 65:1253–1258.

Bloch MH, Panza KE, Landeros-Weisenberger A, Leckman JF. Meta-analysis: treatment of attention-deficit/hyperactivity disorder in children with comorbid tic disorders. *J Am Acad Child Adolesc Psychiatry* 2009; 48:884–893.

Bohnen NI, Minoshima S, Kilbourn MR et al. Presynaptic monoaminergic vesicular transporter imaging in Tourette syndrome using (+)-[alpha]-[11C]DTBZ PET. *Neurology* 1999; 52:A176.

Bornstein RA, Baker GB. Urinary amines in Tourette's syndrome patients with and without phenylethylamine abnormality. *Psychiatry Res* 1990; 31:279–286.

Bostan AC, Dum RP, Strick PL. The basal ganglia communicate with the cerebellum. *Proc Natl Acad Sci USA* 2010; 107:8452–8456.

Bostan AC, Strick PL. The cerebellum and basal ganglia are interconnected. *Neuropsychol Rev* 2010; 20:261–270.
Reviews the substantial interactions between the cerebellum and basal ganglia.

Brett PM, Curtis D, Robertson MM, Gurling HM. Neuroreceptor subunit genes and the genetic susceptibility to Gilles de la Tourette syndrome. *Biol Psychiatry* 1997; 42:941–947.

Brown RE, Stevens DR, Haas HL. The physiology of brain histamine. *Prog Neurobiol* 2001; 63:637–672.

Butler IJ, Koslow SH, Seifert WE et al. Biogenic amine metabolism in Tourette syndrome. *Ann Neurol* 1979; 6:37–39.

Carlsson A, Waters N, Carlsson ML. Neurotransmitter interactions in schizophrenia—therapeutic implications. *Biol Psychiatry* 1999; 46:1388–1395.

Centonze D, Gubellini P, Picconi B et al. Unilateral dopamine denervation blocks corticostriatal LTP. *J Neurophysiol* 1999; 82:3575–3579.

Centonze D, Picconi B, Gubellini P et al. Dopaminergic control of synaptic plasticity in the dorsal striatum. *Eur J Neurosci* 2001; 13:1071–1077.

Cepeda C, Hurst RS, Altemus KL et al. Facilitated glutamatergic transmission in the striatum of D2 dopamine receptor-deficient mice. *J Neurophysiol* 2001; 85:659–670.

Cepeda C, Levine MS. Dopamine and N-methyl-D-aspartate receptor interactions in the neostriatum. *Dev Neurosci* 1998; 20:1–18.

Chappell P, Riddle M, Anderson G et al. Enhanced stress responsivity of Tourette syndrome patients undergoing lumbar puncture. *Biol Psychiatry* 1994; 36:35–43.

Chen K, Wang JJ, Yung WH et al. Excitatory effect of histamine on neuronal activity of rat globus pallidus by activation of H2 receptors in vitro. *Neurosci Res* 2005; 53:288–297.

Choen KA, Ryu YH, Namkoong K et al. Dopamine transporter density of the basal ganglia assessed with [123I]IPT SPECT in drug-naive children with Tourette's disorder. *Psychiatry Res* 2004; *130*:85–95.

Church JA, Fair DA, Dosenbach NU et al. Control networks in paediatric Tourette syndrome show immature and anomalous patterns of functional connectivity. *Brain* 2009; *132*:225–238.

Clithero JA, Smith DV, Carter RM, Huettel SA. Within- and cross-participant classifiers reveal different neural coding of information. *Neuroimage* 2011; *56*:699–708.

Cobb WS, Abercrombie ED. Differential regulation of somatodendritic and nerve terminal dopamine release by serotonergic innervation of substantia nigra. *J Neurochem* 2003; *84*:576–584.

Cohen DJ, Shaywitz BA, Caparulo B et al. Chronic, multiple tics of Gilles de la Tourette's disease. CSF acid monoamine metabolites after probenecid administration. *Arch Gen Psychiatry* 1978; *35*:245–250.
Initial investigation of cerebrospinal fluid monoamine metabolites in TS.

Comings DE. Blood serotonin and tryptophan in Tourette syndrome. *Am J Med Genet* 1990; *36*:418–430.

Coric V, Taskiran S, Pittenger C et al. Riluzole augmentation in treatment-resistant obsessive-compulsive disorder: an open-label trial. *Biol Psychiatry* 2005; *58*:424–428.

Crane J, Fagerness J, Osiecki L et al. Family-based genetic association study of DLGAP3 in Tourette syndrome. *Am J Med Genet B Neuropsychiatr Genet* 2011; *156*:108–114.

Crittenden JR, Graybiel AM. Basal ganglia disorders associated with imbalances in the striatal striosome and matrix compartments. *Front Neuroanat* 2011; 5:59.

Daly DA, Moghaddam B. Actions of clozapine and haloperidol on the extracellular levels of excitatory amino acids in the prefrontal cortex and striatum of conscious rats. *Neurosci Lett* 1993; *152*:61–64.

Del Arco A, Mora F. Endogenous dopamine potentiates the effects of glutamate on extracellular GABA in the prefrontal cortex of the freely moving rat. *Brain Res Bull* 2000; *53*:339–345.

DeLong M, Wichmann T. Update on models of basal ganglia function and dysfunction. *Parkinsonism Relat Disord* 2009; *15*(Suppl 3):S237–240.
Provides an update on circuit models of basal ganglia function and dysfunction.

Devor EJ, Dill-Devor RM, Magee HJ. The Bal I and Msp I polymorphisms in the dopamine D3 receptor gene display, linkage disequilibrium with each other but no association with Tourette syndrome. *Psychiatr Genet* 1998; 8:49–52.

Diaz-Anzaldua A, Joober R, Riviere JB et al. Tourette syndrome and dopaminergic genes: a family-based association study in the French Canadian founder population. *Mol Psychiatry* 2004; 9: 272–277.

Ellender TJ, Huerta-Ocampo I, Deisseroth K et al. Differential modulation of excitatory and inhibitory striatal synaptic transmission by histamine. *J Neurosci* 2011; 31: 15340–15351.

Ercan-Sencicek AG, Stillman AA, Ghosh AK et al. L-histidine decarboxylase and Tourette's syndrome. *N Engl J Med* 2010; 362:1901–1908.
Linkage analysis identifying a functional mutation in a gene encoding L-histidine decarboxylase, the rate-limiting enzyme in histamine biosynthesis.

Erenberg G, Lederman RJ. Naltrexone and Tourette's syndrome. *Ann Neurol* 1992; *31*:574.

Ernst M, Zametkin AJ, Jons PH et al. High presynaptic dopaminergic activity in children with Tourette's disorder. *J Am Acad Child Adolesc Psychiatry* 1999; *38*:86–94.

Felling RJ, Singer HS. Neurobiology of Tourette syndrome: current status and need for further investigation. *J Neurosci* 2011; *31*: 12387–12395.
A review discussing the clinical problem, etiology, and neurobiology of Tourette syndrome with emphasis on animal models and structural and functional abnormalities.

Ferrada C, Ferre S, Casado V et al. Interactions between histamine H3 and dopamine D2 receptors and the implications for striatal function. *Neuropharmacology* 2008; *55*:190–197.

Ferre S, Quiroz C, Orru M et al. Adenosine A(2A) receptors and A(2A) receptor heteromers as key players in striatal function. *Front Neuroanat* 2011; 5:36.

Feyder M, Bonito-Oliva A, Fisone G. L-DOPA-induced dyskinesia and abnormal signaling in striatal medium spiny neurons: focus on dopamine D1 receptor-mediated transmission. *Front Behav Neurosci* 2011; 5:71.

Flik G, Dremencov E, Cremers TI et al. The role of cortical and hypothalamic histamine-3 receptors in the modulation of central histamine neurotransmission: an in vivo electrophysiology and microdialysis study. *Eur J Neurosci* 2011; 34:1747–1755.

Gadzicki D, Muller-Vahl KR, Heller D et al. Tourette syndrome is not caused by mutations in the central cannabinoid receptor (CNR1) gene. *Am J Med Genet* 2004; 127B:97–103.

George MS, Robertson MM, Costa D et al. Dopamine receptor availability in Tourette's syndrome. *Psychiatry Res* 1994; 55: 193–203.

Gilbert DL, Bansal AS, Sethuraman G et al. Association of cortical disinhibition with tic, ADHD, and OCD severity in Tourette syndrome. *Mov Disord* 2004; 19:416–425.

Gilbert DL, Christian BT, Gelfand MJ et al. Altered mesolimbocortical and thalamic dopamine in Tourette syndrome. *Neurology* 2006; 67:1695–1697.

Gittis AH, Nelson AB, Thwin MT et al. Distinct roles of GABAergic interneurons in the regulation of striatal output pathways. *J Neurosci* 2010; 30:2223–2234.

Gobert A, Rivet JM, Audinot V et al. Simultaneous quantification of serotonin, dopamine and noradrenaline levels in single frontal cortex dialysates of freely-moving rats reveals a complex pattern of reciprocal auto- and heteroreceptor-mediated control of release. *Neuroscience* 1998; 84:413–429.

Gonce M, Barbeau A. Seven cases of Gilles de la Tourette's syndrome: partial relief with clonazepam: a pilot study. *Can J Neurol Sci* 1977; 4:279–283.

Gorelova N, Seamans JK, Yang CR. Mechanisms of dopamine activation of fast-spiking interneurons that exert inhibition in rat prefrontal cortex. *J Neurophysiol* 2002; 88:3150–3166.

Grant P, Lougee L, Hirschtritt M, Swedo SE. An open-label trial of riluzole, a glutamate antagonist, in children with treatment-resistant obsessive-compulsive disorder. *J Child Adolesc Psychopharmacol* 2007; 17:761–767.

Groenewegen H, van der Heuvel O, Cath D, Voon P, Veltman D. Does an imbalance between the dorsal and ventral striatopallidal systems play a role in Tourette's syndrome? A neuronal circuit approach. *Brain and Development* 2003; 25:S3–S14.

Groves P, Garcia-Munoz M, Linder J et al. Elements of the intrinsic organization and information processing in the neostriatum. In: Houk J, Davis J, Beiser D (Eds.), *Models of information processing in the basal ganglia*. Cambridge, MA: MIT Press, 1995, pp. 51–96.

Guo JD, Rainnie DG. Presynaptic 5-HT(1B) receptor-mediated serotonergic inhibition of glutamate transmission in the bed nucleus of the stria terminalis. *Neuroscience* 2010; 165:1390–1401.

Haas HL, Sergeeva OA, Selbach O. Histamine in the nervous system. *Physiol Rev* 2008; 88:1183–1241.

Haber SN, Kowall NW, Vonsattel JP et al. Gilles de la Tourette's syndrome. A postmortem neuropathological and immunohistochemical study. *J Neurol Sci* 1986; 75:225–241.

Haber SN, Wolfer D. Basal ganglia peptidergic staining in Tourette syndrome. *A follow-up study*. *Adv Neurol* 1992; 58:145–150.

Harris EL, Schuerholz LJ, Singer HS et al. Executive function in children with Tourette syndrome and/or attention deficit hyperactivity disorder. *J Int Neuropsychol Soc* 1995; 1:511–516.

Harris K, Singer HS. Tic disorders: neural circuits, neurochemistry, and neuroimmunology. *J Child Neurol* 2006; 21:678–689.

Hartmann A, Worbe Y, Arnulf I. Increasing histamine neurotransmission in Gilles de la Tourette syndrome. *J Neurol* 2012; 259:375–376.

Hashemi P, Dankoski EC, Wood KM et al. In vivo electrochemical evidence for simultaneous 5-HT and histamine release in the rat substantia nigra pars reticulata following medial forebrain bundle stimulation. *J Neurochem* 2011; 118:749–759.

Haugbol S, Pinborg LH, Regeur L et al. Cerebral 5-HT2A receptor binding is increased in patients with Tourette's syndrome. *Int J Neuropsychopharmacol* 2007; 10:245–252.

Hebebrand J, Nothen MM, Ziegler A et al. Nonreplication of linkage disequilibrium between the dopamine D4 receptor locus and Tourette syndrome. *Am J Hum Genet* 1997; 61:238–239.

Heinz A, Knable MB, Wolf SS et al. Tourette's syndrome: [I-123]beta-CIT SPECT correlates of vocal tic severity. *Neurology* 1998; 51:1069–1074.

Heise KF, Steven B, Liuzzi G et al. Altered modulation of intracortical excitability during movement preparation in Gilles de la Tourette syndrome. *Brain* 2010; 133:580–590.

Hershey T, Black KJ, Hartlein JM et al. Cognitive-pharmacologic functional magnetic resonance imaging in Tourette syndrome: a pilot study. *Biol Psychiatry* 2004; 55: 916–925.

Hoekstra PJ, Anderson GM, Limburg PC et al. Neurobiology and neuroimmunology of Tourette's syndrome: an update. *Cell Mol Life Sci* 2004; 61:886–898.

Hoshi E, Tremblay L, Feger J et al. The cerebellum communicates with the basal ganglia. *Nat Neurosci* 2005; 8:1491–1493.

Hosp JA, Pekanovic A, Rioult-Pedotti MS, Luft AR. Dopaminergic projections from midbrain to primary motor cortex mediate motor skill learning. *J Neurosci* 2011; 31:2481–2487.

Hwang WJ, Yao WJ, Fu YK, Yang AS. [99mTc] TRODAT-1/[123I]IBZM SPECT studies of the dopaminergic system in Tourette syndrome. *Psychiatry Res* 2008; 162:159–166.

Ibanez-Sandoval O, Tecuapetla F et al. A novel functionally distinct subtype of striatal neuropeptide Y interneuron. *J Neurosci* 2011; 31:16757–16769.

Jackson ME, Frost AS, Moghaddam B. Stimulation of prefrontal cortex at physiologically relevant frequencies inhibits dopamine release in the nucleus accumbens. *J Neurochem* 2001; 78:920–923.

Jellish WS, Murdoch J, Kindel G et al. The effect of clonidine on cell survival, glutamate, and aspartate release in normo- and hyperglycemic rats after near complete forebrain ischemia. *Exp Brain Res* 2005; 167:526–534.

Jones CR, Jahanshahi M. Dopamine modulates striato-frontal functioning during temporal processing. *Front Integr Neurosci* 2011; 5:70.

Kalanithi PS, Zheng W, Kataoka Y et al. Altered parvalbumin-positive neuron distribution in basal ganglia of individuals with Tourette syndrome. *Proc Natl Acad Sci USA* 2005; 102:13307–13312.

Karagianis JL, Nagpurkar R. A case of Tourette syndrome developing during haloperidol treatment. *Can J Psychiatry* 1990; 35:228–232.

Kataoka Y, Kalanithi PS, Grantz H et al. Decreased number of parvalbumin and cholinergic interneurons in the striatum of individuals with Tourette syndrome. *J Comp Neurol* 2010; 518:277–291.

TS postmortem anatomical study showing a reduction of acetylcholine- and parvalbumin-containing neurons in the caudate and putamen.

Kegeles LS, Abi-Dargham A, Zea-Ponce Y et al. Modulation of amphetamine-induced striatal dopamine release by ketamine in humans: implications for schizophrenia. *Biol Psychiatry* 2000; 48: 627–640.

Klawans HL, Falk DK, Nausieda PA, Weiner WJ. Gilles de la Tourette syndrome after long-term chlorpromazine therapy. *Neurology* 1978; 28:1064–1066.

Kuhn J, Janouschek H, Raptis M et al. In vivo evidence of deep brain stimulation-induced dopaminergic modulation in Tourette's syndrome. *Biol Psychiatry* 2012; 71: e11–e13.

Kurlan R, Majumdar L, Deeley C et al. A controlled trial of propoxyphene and naltrexone in patients with Tourette's syndrome. *Ann Neurol* 1991; 30:19–23.

Kuroki T, Meltzer HY, Ichikawa J. 5-HT 2A receptor stimulation by DOI, a 5-HT 2A/2C receptor agonist, potentiates amphetamine-induced dopamine release in rat medial prefrontal cortex and nucleus accumbens. *Brain Res* 2003; 972:216–221.

Leckman JF. Tourette's syndrome. *Lancet* 2002; 360:1577–1586.

Leckman JF, Goodman WK, Anderson GM et al. Cerebrospinal fluid biogenic amines in obsessive-compulsive disorder, Tourette's syndrome, and healthy controls. *Neuropsychopharmacology* 1995a; 12:73–86.

Leckman JF, Pauls DL, Cohen DJ. Tic disorders. In: Bloom FE, Kupfer DJ (Eds.), *Psychopharmacology: fourth generation of progress*. New York: Raven Press, 1995b, pp. 1665–1674.

Leckman JF, Riddle MA, Berrettini WH et al. Elevated CSF dynorphin A [1–8] in Tourette's syndrome. *Life Sci* 1988; 43:2015–2023.

Lerner A, Bagic A, Simmons JM et al. Widespread abnormality of the gamma-aminobutyric acid-ergic system in Tourette syndrome. *Brain* 2012; 135:1926–1936.

Leurs R, Bakker RA, Timmerman H, de Esch IJ. The histamine H3 receptor: from gene cloning to H3 receptor drugs. *Nat Rev Drug Discov* 2005; 4:107–120.

Levine MS, Li Z, Cepeda C et al. Neuromodulatory actions of dopamine on synaptically-evoked neostriatal responses in slices. *Synapse* 1996; 24:65–78.

Liang L, DeLong MR, Papa SM. Inversion of dopamine responses in striatal medium spiny neurons and involuntary movements. *J Neurosci* 2008; 28:7537–7547.

Lichter D, Majumdar L, Kurlan R. Opiate withdrawal unmasks Tourette's syndrome. *Clin Neuropharmacol* 1988; 11:559–564.

Liu H, Dong F, Meng Z et al. Evaluation of Tourette's syndrome by (99m)Tc-TRODAT-1 SPECT/CT imaging. *Ann Nucl Med* 2010; 24:515–521.

Ludolph AG, Pinkhardt EH, Tebartz van Elst L et al. Are amygdalar volume alterations in children with Tourette syndrome due to ADHD comorbidity? *Dev Med Child Neurol* 2008; 50:524–529.

Malison RT, McDougle CJ, van Dyck CH et al. [123I]beta-CIT SPECT imaging of striatal dopamine transporter binding in Tourette's disorder. *Am J Psychiatry* 1995; 152:1359–1361.

Marti M, Mela F, Bianchi C et al. Striatal dopamine-NMDA receptor interactions in the modulation of glutamate release in the substantia nigra pars reticulata in vivo: opposite role for D1 and D2 receptors. *J Neurochem* 2002; 83:635–644.

Mazzone L, Yu S, Blair C et al. An FMRI study of frontostriatal circuits during the inhibition of eye blinking in persons with Tourette syndrome. *Am J Psychiatry* 2010; 167:341–349.

Mena I, Miranda M, Hernandez M et al. Dopamine transporter imaging in Tourette syndrome: evaluation by neuroSPECT of Trodat 1-Tc99m. *Mov Disord* 2004; 19:1282.

Mink JW. Basal ganglia dysfunction in Tourette's syndrome: a new hypothesis. *Pediatr Neurol* 2001; 25:190–198.

Minzer K, Lee O, Hong JJ, Singer HS. Increased prefrontal D2 protein in Tourette syndrome: a postmortem analysis of frontal cortex and striatum. *J Neurol Sci* 2004; 219:55–61.

Molina-Hernandez A, Nunez A, Arias-Montano JA. Histamine H3-receptor activation inhibits dopamine synthesis in rat striatum. *Neuroreport* 2000; 11:163–166.

Moll GH, Wischer S, Heinrich H et al. Deficient motor control in children with tic disorder: evidence from transcranial magnetic stimulation. *Neurosci Lett* 1999; 272:37–40.

Morari M, O'Connor WT, Ungerstedt U, Fuxe K. Dopamine D1 and D2 receptor antagonism differentially modulates stimulation of striatal neurotransmitter levels by N-methyl-D-aspartic acid. *Eur J Pharmacol* 1994; 256:23–30.

Moreno E, Hoffmann H, Gonzalez-Sepulveda M et al. Dopamine D1-histamine H3 receptor heteromers provide a selective link to MAPK signaling in GABAergic neurons of the direct striatal pathway. *J Biol Chem* 2011; 286: 5846–5854.

Mossner R, Muller-Vahl KR, Doring N, Stuhrmann M. Role of the novel tryptophan hydroxylase-2 gene in Tourette syndrome. *Mol Psychiatry* 2007; 12:617–619.

Mostofsky SH, Wendlandt J, Cutting L et al. Corpus callosum measurements in girls with Tourette syndrome. *Neurology* 1999; 53:1345–1347.

Motawaj M, Arrang JM. Ciproxifan, a histamine H-receptor antagonist/inverse agonist, modulates methamphetamine-induced sensitization in mice. *Eur J Neurosci* 2011; 33:1197–1204.

Mrzljak L, Bergson C, Pappy M et al. Localization of dopamine D4 receptors in GABAergic neurons of the primate brain. *Nature* 1996; 381: 245–248.

Muller-Vahl KR. Tourette's syndrome. *Curr Top Behav Neurosci* 2009; 1:397–410.
Cannabinoids have a beneficial effect on TS. A role for opiates is also suggested.

Muller-Vahl KR, Berding G, Brucke T et al. Dopamine transporter binding in Gilles de la Tourette syndrome. *J Neurol* 2000a; 247:514–520.

Muller-Vahl KR, Berding G, Kolbe H et al. Dopamine D2 receptor imaging in Gilles de la Tourette syndrome. *Acta Neurol Scand* 2000b; 101:165–171.

Muller-Vahl KR, Meyer GJ, Knapp WH et al. Serotonin transporter binding in Tourette syndrome. *Neurosci Lett* 2005; 385:120–125.

Nestler EJ. The neurobiology of cocaine addiction. *Sci Pract Perspect* 2005; 3:4–10.

Nicola SM, Surmeier J, Malenka RC. Dopaminergic modulation of neuronal excitability in the striatum and nucleus accumbens. *Annu Rev Neurosci* 2000; 23:185–215.

Niesler B, Frank B, Hebebrand J, Rappold G. Serotonin receptor genes HTR3A and HTR3B are not involved in Gilles de la Tourette syndrome. *Psychiatr Genet* 2005; 15:303–304.

Nieuwenhuys R. The neocortex. An overview of its evolutionary development, structural organization and synaptology. *Anat Embryol (Berl)* 1994; *190*:307–337.

Nuutinen S, Panula P. Histamine in neurotransmission and brain diseases. *Adv Exp Med Biol* 2010; *709*:95–107.

Onn SP, West AR, Grace AA. Dopamine-mediated regulation of striatal neuronal and network interactions. *Trends Neurosci* 2000; *23*:S48–56.

O'Rourke JA, Scharf JM, Yu D, Pauls DL. The genetics of Tourette syndrome: a review. *J Psychosom Res* 2009; *67*:533–545.

Orth M, Munchau A, Rothwell JC. Corticospinal system excitability at rest is associated with tic severity in Tourette syndrome. *Biol Psychiatry* 2008; *64*:248–251.

Ozbay F, Wigg KG, Turanli ET et al. Analysis of the dopamine beta hydroxylase gene in Gilles de la Tourette syndrome. *Am J Med Genet B Neuropsychiatr Genet* 2006; *141*:673–677.

Peterson BS, Choi HA, Hao X et al. Morphologic features of the amygdala and hippocampus in children and adults with Tourette syndrome. *Arch Gen Psychiatry* 2007; *64*:1281–1291.

Peterson BS, Leckman JF, Duncan JS et al. Corpus callosum morphology from magnetic resonance images in Tourette's syndrome. *Psychiatry Res* 1994; *55*:85–99.

Peterson BS, Staib L, Scahill L et al. Regional brain and ventricular volumes in Tourette syndrome. *Arch Gen Psychiatry* 2001; *58*:427–440.

Pillot C, Ortiz J, Heron A et al. Ciproxifan, a histamine H3-receptor antagonist/inverse agonist, potentiates neurochemical and behavioral effects of haloperidol in the rat. *J Neurosci* 2002; *22*:7272–7280.

Plessen KJ, Wentzel-Larsen T, Hugdahl K et al. Altered interhemispheric connectivity in individuals with Tourette's disorder. *Am J Psychiatry* 2004; *161*:2028–2037.

Polinsky RJ, Ebert MH, Caine ED et al. Cholinergic treatment in the Tourette syndrome. *N Engl J Med* 1980; *302*:1310.

Porta M, Sassi M, Cavallazzi M et al. Tourette's syndrome and role of tetrabenazine: review and personal experience. *Clin Drug Investig* 2008; *28*:443–459.

Rabey JM, Oberman Z, Graff E, Korczyn AD. Decreased dopamine uptake into platelet storage granules in Gilles de la Tourette disease. *Biol Psychiatry* 1995; *38*:112–115.

Richard JM, Berridge KC. Nucleus accumbens dopamine/glutamate interaction switches modes to generate desire versus dread: D(1) alone for appetitive eating but D(1) and D(2) together for fear. *J Neurosci* 2011; *31*:12866–12879.

Rickards H. Functional neuroimaging in Tourette syndrome. *J Psychosom Res* 2009; *67*:575–584.
A review discussing the strengths and weaknesses of functional imaging and a synthesis of data in TS.

Riddle MA, Leckman JF, Anderson GM et al. Plasma MHPG: within- and across-day stability in children and adults with Tourette's syndrome. *Biol Psychiatry* 1988a; *24*:391–398.

Riddle MA, Leckman JF, Anderson GM et al. Tourette's syndrome: clinical and neurochemical correlates. *J Am Acad Child Adolesc Psychiatry* 1988b; *27*:409–412.

Sandyk R. Opioid receptor differentiation and Gilles de la Tourette syndrome. *Int J Neurosci* 1987; *32*:995–996.

Scahill L, Erenberg G, Berlin CM, Jr. et al. Contemporary assessment and pharmacotherapy of Tourette syndrome. *NeuroRx* 2006; *3*:192–206.

Schlicker E, Malinowska B, Kathmann M, Gothert M. Modulation of neurotransmitter release via histamine H3 heteroreceptors. *Fundam Clin Pharmacol* 1994; *8*:128–137.

Schuerholz LJ, Singer HS, Denckla MB. Gender study of neuropsychological and neuromotor function in children with Tourette syndrome with and without attention-deficit hyperactivity disorder. *J Child Neurol* 1998; *13*:277–282.

Seamans JK, Durstewitz D, Christie BR et al. Dopamine D1/D5 receptor modulation of excitatory synaptic inputs to layer V prefrontal cortex neurons. *Proc Natl Acad Sci USA* 2001a; *98*:301–306.

Seamans JK, Gorelova N, Durstewitz D, Yang CR. Bidirectional dopamine modulation of GABAergic inhibition in prefrontal cortical pyramidal neurons. *J Neurosci* 2001b; *21*:3628–3638.

Serra-Mestres J, Ring HA, Costa DC et al. Dopamine transporter binding in Gilles de la Tourette syndrome: a [123I]FP-CIT/SPECT study. *Acta Psychiatr Scand* 2004; *109*:140–146.

Sershen H, Hashim A, Lajtha A. Serotonin-mediated striatal dopamine release involves the dopamine uptake site and the serotonin receptor. *Brain Res Bull* 2000; *53*:353–357.

Shapiro AK. *Gilles de la Tourette syndrome.* New York: Raven, 1988.

Shinomura T, Nakao S, Adachi T, Shingu K. Clonidine inhibits and phorbol acetate activates glutamate release from rat spinal synaptoneurosomes. *Anesth Analg* 1999; 88:1401–1405.

Shytle RD, Silver AA, Sheehan KH et al. Neuronal nicotinic receptor inhibition for treating mood disorders: preliminary controlled evidence with mecamylamine. *Depress Anxiety* 2002; 16:89–92.

Silver AA, Shytle RD, Sanberg PR. Mecamylamine in Tourette's syndrome: a two-year retrospective case study. *J Child Adolesc Psychopharmacol* 2000; 10:59–68.

Silverstein F, Smith CB, Johnston MV. Effect of clonidine on platelet alpha 2-adrenoreceptors and plasma norepinephrine of children with Tourette syndrome. *Dev Med Child Neurol* 1985; 27:793–799.

Singer HS. Treatment of tics and Tourette syndrome. *Curr Treat Options Neurol* 2010; 12:539–561.

Singer HS, Butler IJ, Tune LE et al. Dopaminergic dsyfunction in Tourette syndrome. *Ann Neurol* 1982a; 12:361–366.

Singer HS, Dickson J, Martinie D, Levine M. Second messenger systems in Tourette's syndrome. *J Neurol Sci* 1995; 128:78–83.

Singer HS, Hahn IH, Krowiak E et al. Tourette's syndrome: a neurochemical analysis of postmortem cortical brain tissue. *Ann Neurol* 1990; 27:443–446.

Postmortem study of TS brains suggesting an abnormality of cAMP and a role for a second messenger system abnormality.

Singer HS, Hahn IH, Moran TH. Abnormal dopamine uptake sites in postmortem striatum from patients with Tourette's syndrome. *Ann Neurol* 1991;30: 558–562.

Singer HS, Minzer K. Neurobiology of Tourette syndrome: concepts of neuroanatomical localization and neurochemical abnormalities. *Brain and Development* 2003; 25(Suppl):S70–S84.

Singer HS, Morris C, Grados M. Glutamatergic modulatory therapy for Tourette syndrome. *Med Hypotheses* 2010; 74:862–867.

Discusses evidence in support of a role for glutamate in TS.

Singer HS, Oshida L, Coyle JT. CSF cholinesterase activity in Gilles de la Tourette's syndrome. *Arch Neurol* 1984; 41:756–757.

Singer HS, Szymanski S, Giuliano J et al. Elevated intrasynaptic dopamine release in Tourette's syndrome measured by PET. *Am J Psychiatry* 2002; 159: 1329–1336.

Demonstrated an increased release of dopamine in the striatum following amphetamine stimulation.

Singer HS, Tune LE, Butler IJ et al. Clinical symptomatology, CSF neurotransmitter metabolites, and serum haloperidol levels in Tourette syndrome. *Adv Neurol* 1982b; 35:177–183.

Singer HS, Wendlandt J, Krieger M, Giuliano J. Baclofen treatment in Tourette syndrome: a double-blind, placebo-controlled, crossover trial. *Neurology* 2001; 56:599–604.

Smiley JF, Levey AI, Ciliax BJ, Goldman-Rakic PS. D1 dopamine receptor immunoreactivity in human and monkey cerebral cortex: predominant and extrasynaptic localization in dendritic spines. *Proc Natl Acad Sci USA* 1994; 91:5720–5724.

Smythies J. Section V. Serotonin system. *Int Rev Neurobiol* 2005; 64:217–268.

Discusses interactions between serotonin and dopamine.

Sowell ER, Kan E, Yoshii J et al. Thinning of sensorimotor cortices in children with Tourette syndrome. *Nat Neurosci* 2008; 11:637–639.

Stahl SM, Berger PA. Physostigmine in Tourette syndrome: evidence for cholinergic underactivity. *Am J Psychiatry* 1981; 138:240–242.

Stamenkovic M, Schindler SD, Asenbaum S et al. No change in striatal dopamine re-uptake site density in psychotropic drug naive and in currently treated Tourette's disorder patients: a [(123)I]-beta-CIT SPECt-study. *Eur Neuropsychopharmacol* 2001; 11:69–74.

Steeves TD, Ko JH, Kideckel DM et al. Extrastriatal dopaminergic dysfunction in Tourette syndrome. *Ann Neurol* 2010; 67:170–181.

Stern ER, Blair C, Peterson BS. Inhibitory deficits in Tourette's syndrome. *Dev Psychobiol* 2008; 50:9–18.

Stober G, Hebebrand J, Cichon S et al. Tourette syndrome and the norepinephrine transporter gene: results of a systematic mutation screening. *Am J Med Genet* 1999; 88:158–163.

Sweet RD, Bruun R, Shapiro E, Shapiro AK. Presynaptic catecholamine antagonists as treatment for Tourette syndrome. Effects of alpha methyl para tyrosine and tetrabenazine. *Arch Gen Psychiatry* 1974; 31:857–861.

Swerdlow NR, Bongiovanni MJ, Tochen L, Shoemaker JM. Separable noradrenergic and dopaminergic regulation of prepulse inhibition in rats: implications for predictive validity and Tourette syndrome. *Psychopharmacology (Berl)* 2006; *186*:246–254.

Taber MT, Fibiger HC. Electrical stimulation of the prefrontal cortex increases dopamine release in the nucleus accumbens of the rat: modulation by metabotropic glutamate receptors. *J Neurosci* 1995; *15*:3896–3904.

Tanimura Y, Vaziri S, Lewis MH. Indirect basal ganglia pathway mediation of repetitive behavior: attenuation by adenosine receptor agonists. *Behav Brain Res* 2010; *210*:116–122.

Demonstrated that the administration of adenosine receptor agonists can attenuate spontaneous stereotypies in an animal model.

Tanner CM, Goetz CG, Klawans HL. Cholinergic mechanisms in Tourette syndrome. *Neurology* 1982; *32*:1315–1317.

Tekin S, Cummings JL. Frontal-subcortical neuronal circuits and clinical neuropsychiatry: an update. *J Psychosom Res* 2002; *53*:647–654.

Tepper JM, Bolam JP. Functional diversity and specificity of neostriatal interneurons. *Curr Opin Neurobiol* 2004; *14*:685–692.

Tepper JM, Wilson CJ, Koos T. Feedforward and feedback inhibition in neostriatal GABAergic spiny neurons. *Brain Res Rev* 2008; *58*: 272–81.

Thompson M, Comings DE, Feder L et al. Mutation screening of the dopamine D1 receptor gene in Tourette's syndrome and alcohol dependent patients. *Am J Med Genet* 1998; *81*:241–244.

Toren P, Weizman A, Ratner S et al. Ondansetron treatment in Tourette's disorder: a 3-week, randomized, double-blind, placebo-controlled study. *J Clin Psychiatry* 2005; *66*:499–503.

TSAICG. Genome scan for Tourette disorder in affected-sibling-pair and multigenerational families. *Am J Hum Genet* 2007; *80*:265–272.

Turjanski N, Sawle GV, Playford ED et al. PET studies of the presynaptic and postsynaptic dopaminergic system in Tourette's syndrome. *J Neurol Neurosurg Psychiatry* 1994; *57*: 688–692.

van Wattum PJ, Chappell PB, Zelterman D et al. Patterns of response to acute naloxone infusion in Tourette's syndrome. *Mov Disord* 2000; *15*:1252–1254.

Vernaleken I, Kuhn J, Lenartz D et al. Bithalamical deep brain stimulation in Tourette syndrome is associated with reduction in dopaminergic transmission. *Biol Psychiatry* 2009; *66*:e15–17.

Walaas SI, Hemmings HC, Jr., Greengard P, Nairn AC. Beyond the dopamine receptor: regula-tion and roles of serine/threonine protein phosphatases. *Front Neuroanat* 2011; *5*:50.

Wang Y, Liu J, Gui ZH et al. alpha2-Adrenoceptor regulates the spontaneous and the GABA/glutamate modulated firing activity of the rat medial prefrontal cortex pyramidal neurons. *Neuroscience* 2011; *182*:193–202.

West AR, Grace AA. Opposite influences of endogenous dopamine D1 and D2 receptor activation on activity states and electrophysiological properties of striatal neurons: studies combining in vivo intracellular recordings and reverse microdialysis. *J Neurosci* 2002; *22*:294–304.

Wickens JR, Kotter R, Alexander ME. Effects of local connectivity on striatal function: stimulation and analysis of a model. *Synapse* 1995; *20*:281–298.

Wolf SS, Jones DW, Knable MB et al. Tourette syndrome: prediction of phenotypic variation in monozygotic twins by caudate nucleus D2 receptor binding. *Science* 1996; *273*: 1225–1227.

Early study of dopamine receptors in identical twins showing increased binding in the head of the caudate in association with tic severity.

Wong D, Brasic J, Kuwabara H et al. *Abnormalities of dopamine and serotonin neuroreceptors with PET in Tourette syndrome.* Society for Neuroscience. Vol Program No. 1012.15.2005. Washington, DC, 2005.

Confirmed an abnormality of dopamine release and suggested an interaction between dopamine and serotonin in concomitant obsessive-compulsive disorder.

Wong DF, Brasic JR, Singer HS et al. Mechanisms of dopaminergic and serotonergic neurotransmission in Tourette syndrome: clues from an in vivo neurochemistry study with PET. *Neuropsychopharmacology* 2008; *33*: 1239–12351.

Wong DF, Singer HS, Brandt J et al. D2-like dopamine receptor density in Tourette syndrome measured by PET. *J Nucl Med* 1997; *38*:1243–1247.

Yang CR, Seamans JK, Gorelova N. Developing a neuronal model for the pathophysiology of schizophrenia based on the nature of electrophysiological actions of dopamine in the prefrontal cortex. *Neuropsychopharmacology* 1999; *21*:161–194.

Yanovsky Y, Li S, Klyuch BP et al. L-Dopa activates histaminergic neurons. *J Physiol* 2011; *589*:1349–1366.

Yeh CB, Lee CS, Ma KH et al. Phasic dysfunction of dopamine transmission in Tourette's syndrome evaluated with 99mTc TRODAT-1 imaging. *Psychiatry Res* 2007; *156*:75–82.

Yoon DY, Gause CD, Leckman JF, Singer HS. Frontal dopaminergic abnormality in Tourette syndrome: A postmortem analysis. *J Neurol Sci* 2007a; 255:50–56.

Yoon DY, Rippel CA, Kobets AJ et al. Dopaminergic polymorphisms in Tourette syndrome: association with the DAT gene (SLC6A3). *Am J Med Genet B Neuropsychiatr Genet* 2007b; 144:605–610.

Ziemann U, Paulus W, Rothenberger A. Decreased motor inhibition in Tourette's disorder: evidence from transcranial magnetic stimulation. *Am J Psychiatry* 1997; 154:1277–1284.

14

Immunity and Stress Response in Tourette Syndrome

DAVIDE MARTINO

Abstract

This chapter summarizes the evidence in favor of dysfunctional immune responses and stress responses in Tourette syndrome (TS). A generalized activation of immune-inflammatory mechanisms at a systemic level is supported by the analysis of lymphocyte subpopulations and peptide markers, such as neopterin. Co-variations between systemic levels of pro- and anti-inflammatory cytokines and clinical severity in TS suggests an interplay between immunity and behavioral abnormalities in these patients. Moreover, preliminary evidence supports a possible liability to autoimmunity in TS patients (e.g., decreased numbers of T-regulatory lymphocytes and abnormal immunoglobulin profiles). The transcriptome approach is likely to provide new evidence in favor of the contribution of immune-regulatory genes in TS. Finally, patients with TS exhibit an enhanced reactivity of the hypothalamic-pituitary-adrenal axis to external stressors, despite a preserved diurnal cortisol rhythm and normal restoration of the baseline activity of the axis following the acute stress response.

INTRODUCTION

The relationship between immune responses and Tourette syndrome (TS) and related disorders has been an object of interest for clinical and basic researchers in recent times. The possibility of an immunological connection for TS is suggested by different factors. First of all, group A ß-hemolytic streptococcus (GABHS), *Mycoplasma pneumoniae*, *Borrelia burgdorferi*, viral agents such as varicella zoster virus, and other pathogens have been reported as potential causes of "postinfectious tourettism" in anecdotal reports as well as in larger observational clinical series (see Chapter 9). Second, there is increasing evidence of abnormal immune responses in other common neurodevelopmental disorders, particularly autistic spectrum disorders (Goines & Van de Water, 2010). Third, many proteins first identified in the immune system are also expressed in the developing and adult nervous system. Some of these proteins

(e.g., pro-inflammatory cytokines, proteins of the innate immune system, and components of the major histocompatibility complex and their receptors) play essential roles in the establishment and modulation of synaptic connections during development (Boulanger, 2009; Yirmiya & Goshen, 2011). A better comprehension of neural–immune interactions and neuroimmunomodulation could provide important advances in the understanding of normal brain development and of the core mechanisms of neurodevelopmental disorders, including TS and related disorders. The first part of this chapter will provide an overview of immune response regulation in TS.

Similar to the involvement of the immune system, a possible involvement of the hypothalamic-pituitary-adrenal (HPA) axis in TS is suggested by clinical observations of worsening of tic severity during socially challenging stressful periods. The second part of this chapter critically reviews the available evidence on the stress response in TS, and contextualizes these hormonal effects with genetic, social, and cognitive influences on the mechanisms of disease in this condition.

GENERAL CONCEPTS OF IMMUNE RESPONSE

There is a huge interplay between two arms of the immune system, the innate and the adaptive (Medzhitov, 2009). The innate immune system is the first line of inflammatory defense and recognizes a limited number of pathogen-associated molecular patterns through a limited number of pattern-recognition receptors (Janeway, 1989). The main innate immune effector cells include dendritic cells (DCs), phagocytes, and natural killer (NK) cells, all capable of killing intracellular and extracellular infectious agents. The adaptive immune system recognizes many more antigens compared to the innate immune system, which are presented by specialized antigen-presenting cells (APCs), thus developing an antigen-specific response in a more delayed fashion. T and B lymphocytes are the main effector cells of adaptive immunity, supporting cell-mediated and antibody-mediated immune responses.

Two main T-cell populations have been described, which differ by expression of CD4 or CD8 on the cell surface. CD8+ (cytotoxic) T cells directly recognize tumor or infected cells by expressing foreign antigens forming complexes with major histocompatibility complex (MHC) molecules. After recognition, CD8+ T cells mediate killing of those cells by secreting cytotoxic granules; moreover, CD8+ T cells may modulate the function of immune cells of the innate system (e.g., phagocytes and NK cells).

CD4 (or T-helper [Th]) cells orchestrate the function of both adaptive (CD8+ T cells, B cells) and innate (NK cells, phagocytes) effector cells. Th cells may differentiate toward distinct subsets, secondary to signals provided by DCs during antigen presentation. These subsets comprise Th1, Th2, Th3, and Th17 cells. The differentiation toward Th1 cells is facilitated by the secretion of interleukin (IL)-12; this subset promotes cellular immunity against intracellular pathogens and tumor cells. Th2 cells instead secrete IL-4 and facilitate the elimination of extracellular pathogens. The Th17 subset is promoted by the secretion of transforming growth factor-beta (TGF-β) and IL-6 by DCs and is involved in the protection against extracellular bacteria, as well as in the pathogenesis of autoimmune diseases.

Th cells may also differentiate into T-regulatory cells (Tregs or CD4+CD25+), which suppress several functions of effector antigen-specific T cells and protect against the development of autoimmunity. Autoimmune diseases result from the breakdown of immune tolerance processes, which suppress the activity of potentially self-reactive T and B lymphocytes, thus limiting immune responses towards the "self." One of the mechanisms of peripheral tolerance involves Tregs, which are potent inhibitors of B, CD4+, and CD8+ T lymphocytes. The polarization of Th cells toward a specific phenotype is therefore crucial for the precise modulation of the ongoing immune response: abnormalities of this regulatory aspect may lead to pathological downstream effects, such as enhanced cancer growth or severe autoimmune responses.

IMMUNOPHENOTYPING: IMMUNE CELL SUBPOPULATIONS

Abnormalities in the regulation of immune response can be reflected by a skewed quantitative distribution of the various immune cell subpopulations in favor of specific phenotypes, with relative increases or decreases of immune competent cell subpopulation counts in the peripheral blood. Kawikova and colleagues (2007) used fluorescence-activated cell sorting (FACS) to compare the relative count of specific immune cell subpopulations between 37 children with tic and/or obsessive-compulsive disorder (OCD) and 9 healthy children matched by age and parent education status. Cross-sectional comparisons between groups yielded a 62% lower percentage of *naïve* CD4+CD25+ T cells (i.e., Tregs) on the total number of *naïve* CD4+ T cells (i.e., Th cells) in children with moderate to severe symptoms, compared to healthy subjects. Tregs tended to decrease particularly during symptom exacerbations, but this finding was based on only six exacerbation events and did not reach statistical significance. These authors also looked for differences in the Vß-repertoire of T-cell receptors (TCRs) of CD4+ and CD8+ T cells. The TCR of about 95% of T cells is composed of two different protein chains, α and β; the variable region of the chains is crucial for antigen recognition and accounts for the great diversity in specificity of the TCR for the processed antigen. In the organization of the adaptive immune response, each antigen is recognized by a specific segment of the Vß region on the TCR. Given the hypothesized link between streptococcal infection and immune activation in a subgroup of patients with tics and OCD (see Chapter 9), specific attention was given to Vß subsets recognized by streptococcal superantigens (e.g., pyrogenic exotoxins). Superantigens are antigens concentrated on the surface of antigen-presenting cells by binding to MHC class II molecules and cross-linking multiple TCR molecules, which results in strong TCR signaling, nonspecific activation of a large number of T cells, and secretion of large amounts of cytokines. Interestingly, the patients' frequency of CD8+ Vß18+ T cells, which bind to streptococcal pyrogenic exotoxin I, was 40% that of healthy subjects, suggesting either a functional exhaustion of this subpopulation, secondary to prolonged exposure to this superantigen or to other antigens, or an abnormal genetic rearrangement of variable regions on the TCR.

Another exploratory pilot study by Moller and colleagues (2008) used the same methodology to compare 20 adults with TS to 20 age-matched healthy volunteers (mean age of the whole population, 37 years). The most statistically significant results of this study were a 65% to 75% higher percentage of CD69+ B cells, and an approximately 65% higher percentage of CD4+CD95+ and CD8+CD95+ T cells among TS patients compared to healthy subjects. These differences coherently indicate an increased number of activated lymphocytes in the peripheral blood of TS patients, since CD69 is a general marker of activation for B cells, whereas CD95 (or Fas) is involved in the induction of apoptosis of T cells, which might be enhanced to compensate for the abnormal number of activated T cells. Overall, these results support the hypothesis of a generalized overactivation of lymphocytes in TS but do not provide insight into the causal link between immune activation and the tic disorder.

A number of reports have explored the role of a lymphocyte surface antigen, the D8/17 ligand, as a possible diagnostic marker of tic disorders and pediatric OCD (Chapman et al., 1998; Hoekstra et al., 2004a; Murphy et al., 1997; Weisz et al., 2004). The monoclonal IgM antibody D8/17 reacts with antigens found to be significantly more expressed on the surface of B cells from patients with acute rheumatic fever or rheumatic heart disease, thus representing a potential marker for poststreptococcal autoimmune sequelae. The measurement of D8/17-bound B cells from peripheral blood was performed using different methods, including immunofluorescence and flow cytometry. These studies provided highly different estimates of the frequency of D8/17 binding among children with tics or obsessive-compulsive symptoms, as well as insufficient interrater reliability of this test with either of the two techniques. Moreover, Hoekstra and colleagues (2004a) showed that, compared to healthy control subjects, patients with tics exhibit a higher percentage of positive binding of B cells not only to D8/17, but also to a control monoclonal IgM targeting a neuroendocrine antigen expressed by small cell lung cancer cells. This finding was interpreted as nonspecific overexpression of the receptor for IgM on the surface of peripheral B cells, potentially indicating a generalized functional activation of B cells. Consistent with this, another report documented a significantly higher percentage of CD19+ B cells in the peripheral blood of a small group of patients with TS (Weisz et al., 2004). The poor reliability of the D8/17 marker in tic disorders can also be inferred by the results of a prospective longitudinal study that found no clear relationship between the amplification of D8/17-bound B cells and tic symptom exacerbations (Luo et al., 2004).

Finally, the examination of human leukocyte antigen (HLA) types is broadly used for immunophenotyping in human disease. Preliminary reports have produced contradictory findings on the association between distinct HLA serotypes measured on peripheral lymphocytes and TS (Caine et al., 1985; Min et al., 1991). A more recent report (Schoenian et al., 2003) performed a genotype analysis of the HLA-DRB subtypes (which are involved in antigen presentation mechanisms) in 83 TS trios, formed by the affected index child and both parents, using a nonparametric genotyping method (transmission disequilibrium test). Although this study could have been underpowered, its results do not suggest a link between the HLA-DRB locus and TS. Further studies assessing HLA genotype distribution, as well as polymorphisms in the TCR loci, in tic disorders are necessary to exclude the possibility to predict TS occurrence based on genetic factors linked to immune regulation.

A number of limitations can be pointed out for studies on immunophenotyping in patients with tic disorders. All of these reports were based on relatively small clinical samples, which were heterogeneous in terms of age, exposure to medications, and degree of psychiatric comorbidities. A confirmation of these findings on new, larger clinical populations is warranted to replicate these data and measure the effect of potential confounding factors. Patients were always compared to healthy subjects; the use of pathological control groups might be useful to understand whether these immune changes are specific to the tic disorder or are, instead, nonspecifically associated with a chronic behavioral disorder. Finally, the existence of a cause-and-effect relationship between tics and the frequency of immune cell subpopulations has not been clearly demonstrated to date using available prospective data.

Overall, there is initial evidence of a skewed quantitative distribution of lymphocyte subpopulations in patients with tic disorders in comparison to healthy subjects of similar age. Patients with tics exhibit a generalized, apparently nonspecific, overactive immune response, involving T, B, and possibly also NK cells. Moreover, the reduced relative count of Tregs, which needs to be confirmed by larger studies, may indicate a predisposition to autoimmune processes. Reduced numbers of Tregs are detected in autoimmune conditions like lupus erythematosus, rheumatoid arthritis, type 1 diabetes, and multiple sclerosis, whereas increased levels occur in hepatitis B and C viruses and cytomegalovirus infections, and in several types of cancer (Cools et al., 2007). It is poorly understood whether these immunophenotype changes are related to environmental triggers, such as streptococcal or other infections, or stress. Finally, the immunophenotyping analyses conducted so far in tic disorders are not exhaustive. The functional differentiation of Th cells into Th1, Th2, Th3, or Th17 subtypes, which plays a major role in orchestrating the immune response at a systemic level, has not been directly explored in patients with tics.

FUNCTIONAL MEASURES OF IMMUNE CELLS: EFFECTOR MOLECULES AND GENE EXPRESSION PROFILES

Effector molecules (cytokines, chemokines, adhesion molecules) modulate the activity of innate and adaptive immune-competent cells. Adaptive responses are regulated by Th1, Th2, Th3, and Th17 lymphocytes, which promote and control cell-mediated and antibody-mediated responses. Cytokines are polypeptides released at sites of inflammation by various cell types, ranging from fibroblasts to macrophages, T cells, and astrocytes, and have a wide variety of effects on the immune system, from activation and recruitment to suppression of immune cells. Within adaptive responses, different cytokines convey the regulatory effect of different T-cell subpopulations: some cytokines are considered pro-inflammatory, whereas others are considered anti-inflammatory. Moreover, in many circumstances, there is a cascade of cytokine secretion within the responding T cell, such that one cytokine triggers the release of another cytokine. Chemokines are inflammatory mediators that modulate the recruitment of different lymphocyte subpopulations toward the site of inflammation, through their chemoattractant properties. Adhesion molecules are surface molecules (of which soluble isoforms can be measured in biological fluids) mediating the extravasation and entry of circulating lymphocytes into an area of inflammation. The variation in serum concentration of these effector molecules may provide important insight into the pattern of regulation of the immune response in both healthy and diseased individuals.

Only a handful of studies have compared, using a cross-sectional design, the serum concentrations of immune effector molecules in patients with tic disorders to those in control groups. These studies differ in sample size, comorbidity profile, exposure to psychotropic medications, detection method, and type of effector molecules measured. The only finding that has been replicated in at least two of these studies is the presence of higher serum concentrations of IL-12, an activator of Th1 and NK cells, in patients compared to control subjects (Gabbay et al., 2009; Leckman et al., 2005). However, in Leckman and colleagues' study (2005), the patient group included 46 children with a tic disorder and/or OCD, but details on the specific subgroups (i.e., patients with a tic disorder alone, OCD alone, or tic disorder plus OCD) were not available. In the study by Gabbay and colleagues (2009), IL-12 serum concentrations were significantly higher than in healthy subjects only in the subgroup of children with TS plus OCD, but not in children with TS without OCD; there was a statistical trend ($p < .06$) for higher IL-12 concentrations in the whole group of 32 TS patients compared to the 16 healthy control subjects. However, Bos-Veneman and colleagues (2010), in the largest-to-date cross-sectional study on cytokine levels in children with TS, found no difference in IL-12 levels between 66 patients and 71 healthy volunteers. Although the previous studies suggest the possibility that increased IL-12 serum levels are associated with OCD comorbidity rather than with the tic disorder itself, this is not supported by data from Bos-Veneman and colleagues (2010), who detected an inverse association between this marker and the severity of obsessive-compulsive symptoms. Other effector molecules have been explored in these cross-sectional works, which provided inconsistent, and therefore inconclusive, results. These

include the cytokines IL-2 and tumor necrosis factor-α (TNF-α), and the soluble isoform of adhesion molecules like soluble vascular cell adhesion molecule-1 (sVCAM-1; Bos-Veneman et al., 2010; Martino et al., 2005).

Prospective longitudinal observations evaluating the association between exacerbations of symptoms in patients with tic disorders and serum levels of effector molecules are very limited. Leckman and colleagues (2005) studied cytokine fluctuations in respect to rigorously defined clinical exacerbations of tics and obsessive-compulsive symptoms, observing a significant effect of Visit, due to a 49% and 58% increase of IL-12 and TNF-α levels, respectively, at the exacerbation compared to the pre-exacerbation visits. In this study, worsening of symptoms in these patients was however accompanied by a general increase of serum levels of a wide array of both pro-inflammatory and anti-inflammatory cytokines; there was also a significant relationship between tic severity and TNF-α levels, which was not observed for obsessive-compulsive or depressive symptom severity measures. These concurrent fluctuations of severity and immune markers could not be observed in children with the putatively "poststreptococcal" Tourette-like illness named PANDAS, described in Chapter 9 (Leckman et al., 2005; Singer et al., 2008).

Available data on the relationship between markers of acute inflammation and diagnosis and severity of tic disorders are also inconclusive. Erythrocyte sedimentation rate and C-reactive protein (CRP) did not differ at baseline in two relatively large prospective studies (Luo et al., 2004; Martino et al., 2011), and CRP did not co-vary with symptom severity when this was measured prospectively (Luo et al., 2004). Luo and colleagues (2004) measured also serum neopterin, a pteridine produced by human monocytes/macrophages particularly during cell-mediated Th1-type immune responses. Neopterin levels may be raised in several autoimmune diseases, including systemic lupus erythematosus, rheumatoid arthritis, and multiple sclerosis. At baseline, 22% of the TS/OCD children had an elevated serum level of neopterin, compared to none of the control subjects; conversely, when determinations at the 23 exacerbation events identified in the cohort were compared to those from their respective pre-exacerbation period (separated by a mean interval of 3.2 months), there was no significant difference in neopterin serum levels between pre-exacerbation and exacerbation. This was consistent with a subsequent, larger case-control cross-sectional study that reported increased neopterin levels in TS patients in the absence of correlation with tic severity (Hoekstra et al., 2007).

Finally, another approach to explore the activity of immune cells is to analyze their gene expression using microarray profiling. This technique allows the assessment of genome-wide expression changes (transcriptomics), and subsequently the measurement of the activity of dysregulated molecular pathways within the same cells. Two pilot studies initially applied cluster analyses to these methodologies to compare children and adults with TS to age-matched healthy control subjects (Lit et al., 2007; Tang et al., 2005). Interestingly, 14 NK cell genes were overexpressed in 10 of 16 familial cases of TS compared to 16 control subjects (Lit et al., 2007). A subsequent study from the same group (Lit et al., 2009) used an expression microarray of more advanced generation on a larger population sample in which 28 case and 30 control children/adolescents were more carefully matched for age, sex, and race. These authors also assessed expression pathway changes throughout age. Although no overall differences were found between TS and control subjects, the expression of a number of genes and multiple pathways differed between TS and control subjects within different age strata (5–9 years, 10–12 years, 13–16 years). With respect to genes involved in immune regulatory pathways, there was a significant age-related difference in the expression of interferon response, viral processing, and NK and CD8+ T-cell genes. NK cell genes, including the cytotoxic granule proteins granzyme A, granzyme B, and perforin, were mostly overexpressed in youngsters of approximately 13 years of age. These proteins constitute a shared killing pathway between NK cells and CD8+ T cells, highly relevant to the destruction of virally infected cells. Age-related changes in viral response pathways also included changes in B-cell immunoglobulin genes. A possible explanation for these differences could be the presence of an abnormal immune recognition of pathogens, mediated, among other molecules, by interferon regulatory factors. These factors were upregulated in younger children with TS (5–9 years), and this could partially account for an increased synthesis of cytokines such as TNF-α in these patients.

Many of the limitations highlighted for studies on immunophenotyping are also applicable to studies addressing effector molecules in TS, including the use of small and heterogeneous clinical samples, the lack of pathological control groups, and important methodological discrepancies in the design of the two available prospective studies. In addition, the intriguing finding of an age-dependent change in expression of immune regulatory proteins (Lit et al., 2009) was obtained through age stratification of a clinical sample collected cross-sectionally, and therefore needs verification in truly longitudinal cohorts.

Future work should focus on elucidating the association between the organization of the immune response and clinical course in well-characterized subgroups of patients within the TS spectrum. This should be achieved through frequent longitudinal observation of adequately sized clinical samples. Further attention should be given to other immune regulatory molecules that are differentially expressed in other neurodevelopmental disorders, such as transforming growth factor-ß (Vargas et al., 2005), involved in development, cell migration and apoptosis, and regulatory aspects in both immune and the central nervous systems, and macrophage inhibitory factor (Grigorenko et al., 2008), a crucial pro-inflammatory molecule that is constitutively expressed in the brain, where it exerts important effects on both nervous and endocrine systems. The study of proteins functionally bridging the different regulatory systems of the human body might provide very important data on the involvement of immune regulatory molecules in neural development and maintenance, as well as clarifying whether these proteins exert harmful or beneficial influences over brain maturation in patients with neurodevelopmental disorders. Finally, some of the data summarized above suggest that TS patients might respond abnormally to pathogens. It is unclear whether the abnormally regulated expression of genes involved in viral response leads to inadequate defense against viral infections in children with TS; likewise, whether an abnormal immune response to common pathogens might contribute to tic onset and/or exacerbation needs to be addressed in future studies.

NEUROINFLAMMATION

The presence of immune cell activation within the brain of TS patients is still uncertain. Brain biopsies and lumbar punctures are invasive procedures, often not ethically justifiable in patients with TS, and postmortem specimens from adults with this condition are very limited in number, are often of poor quality, and do not come from representative clinical samples. For these reasons, data on neuroinflammatory changes in TS are extremely limited.

Two studies used microarray analysis to quantify mRNA of a number of candidate peptides in the brains of three and four adults with TS respectively, comparing them to control brains from subjects who did not suffer from neurological disease. The transcriptomics approach was the only feasible one in these specimens, since prior tissue processing hindered immunohistochemical analysis that could have directly shown lymphocyte infiltration or microglial activation. A series of selected markers of lymphocyte recruitment and activation were assessed. Interestingly, Morer and colleagues (2010) showed a 2.3-fold elevation of IL-2 gene transcript expression in the basal ganglia of TS brains compared to control brains, whereas Hong and colleagues (2004) reported a 2.9-fold increase of IL-2 receptor ß gene transcript expression in postmortem putamen of TS patients. These results are suggestive of increased synthesis and receptor activation of IL-2, a major T-cell-derived growth factor, in the basal ganglia of TS patients. An additional finding from Morer and colleagues' study (2010) was a 6.5-fold elevated expression of monocyte chemotactic factor-1 (MCP-1) in postmortem specimens of TS cases. MCP-1, a chemokine linked to neuroinflammation originating from a variety of causes, may increase the blood–brain barrier permeability, allowing the infiltration of leukocytes and antibodies in the nervous tissue. Interestingly, it also seems to be involved in the differentiation of neural stem cells into neurones, astrocytes, and oligodendrocytes (Lawrence et al., 2006); this seems particularly intriguing with respect to the observed abnormal distribution of interneurons in the basal ganglia of TS patients, and, again, suggests the possibility of neural–immune interactions within the mechanisms of neural development. These sample sizes of these postmortem studies are unfortunately too small to allow any clear conclusion. Chapter 10 provides an update on pathological and transcriptomics studies in postmortem specimens from TS patients.

An important recent work (Wenzel et al., 2011) analyzed the cerebrospinal fluid (CSF) of 21 TS patients of different ages (mean age 29 years, range 9–51). The albumin quotient, expressing the state of the blood–CSF barrier, showed minor alterations in only three patients, indicating the absence of noteworthy changes of the barrier in the vast majority of TS patients. Although quantitative intrathecal IgG production was normal, isoelectric focusing analyses of oligoclonal bands found positive (>4 bands) or borderline (2 or 3 bands) intrathecal IgG production in 8 of the 21 patients (38%); another 2 patients displayed a mirrored oligoclonal band pattern. Although a control group specifically collected for this study was lacking, a standard CSF examination performed in the same laboratory of 99 healthy volunteers detected CSF oligoclonal bands in only 3% of this population. This finding suggests intrathecal antibody synthesis occurring in a subgroup of TS patients.

Overall, although proofs of ongoing neuroinflammation in TS are still very preliminary due to the paucity of studies addressing this aspect, the initial evidence is promising and encourages researchers to look into this in greater detail. The role of microglia also deserves further exploration. Microglia can act as APCs and develop into brain macrophages, thus performing immunological functions within the brain. However, the expression of immune proteins by microglia is not necessarily synonymous with inflammation, because these molecules can have roles specific to the central nervous system. Importantly, microglia may have a role in maintaining synaptic integrity and the activity of specific pathways (Graeber, 2010). A mutation of the *Hoxb8* gene induces a loss of function in a microglia lineage of hematopoietic origin in mice (Chen et al., 2010). These mice showed excessive grooming leading to trichotillomania (i.e., compulsive hair removal), homologous to OCD spectrum behaviors in humans. This lineage of microglia is specifically expressed in regions relevant to the syntactic groom chain (cortex, striatum, and brainstem). A challenging goal of future research is therefore to elucidate the role of microglia in the pathogenesis of tics and other stereotyped behaviors, and to understand better how this relates to peripheral changes in the regulation of the immune response.

IMMUNOGLOBULINS

Antibody production has attracted wide interest in clinical and basic research of TS. This was related to the hypothesis of antibody-mediated autoimmunity in the putatively "poststreptococcal" subgroup of patients with tic and OCD. Recent evidence has shown that antibody response to pathogens like GABHS may be constitutively enhanced in the general population of children with a tic disorder (Bombaci et al., 2009). This might certainly be the consequence of the demonstrated higher exposure to this pathogen in tic disorders (see Chapter 9) but may also suggest a higher reactivity of the immune system in building up an antibody response against GABHS.

A more in-depth examination of the regulatory aspects of the immune response has, in fact, shown that patients with TS might have an abnormal profile of immunoglobulin production, possibly as a consequence of an altered pattern of immune regulation. Bos-Veneman and colleagues (2011) presented a cross-sectional comparison of plasma levels of total IgG1, IgG2, IgG3, IgG4, IgM, IgA, and IgE between children/adolescents with chronic tic disorders (the majority of whom had TS) and healthy peers from two independent cohorts, one from the Netherlands (53 patients vs. 53 healthy) and another from the United States (21 patients vs. 21 healthy). The only consistent between-group differences across the two cohorts were a reduced level of IgG3 and of IgM; however, the lower IgM levels in the Dutch cohort might have been due to a confounding effect of gender, whereas in the U.S. cohort this difference reached only the level of a statistical trend. All other comparisons did not yield differences that could be detected in both cohorts.

Another work published by the same U.S. group mainly focused on PANDAS, comparing total levels of IgG, IgM, and IgA between 24 youngsters with TS/OCD (19 of whom fulfilled the Swedo criteria for PANDAS) and 22 healthy age-matched control subjects (Kawikova et al., 2010). Interestingly, the PANDAS subgroup had significantly lower levels of total IgA, whereas total IgG and IgM did not differ from healthy subjects. This finding had already been highlighted, although not adequately underscored, by other authors (Hansen & Bershow, 1997). Moreover, this was the first study highlighting a potential immunological marker, other than antistreptococcal antibody titers, differentiating the PANDAS subgroup from the general population of TS patients, although a direct comparison between PANDAS and non-PANDAS TS patients is necessary to verify this.

Even if based on relatively small sample sizes of medicated patients, the findings from these two studies suggest a number of considerations. IgG3 represents 4% to 8% of the total IgG produced by the immune system. This subclass of IgG is a potent activator of the classical component cascade, leading to the formation of membrane attack complexes and to the elimination of a variety of microbial pathogens through different mechanisms (neutralization, opsonization, sensitization for killing by NK cells). A reduction of IgG3 blood levels, like that observed in two independent cohorts of TS patients, might therefore lead to a higher proneness of these patients to infections, mainly upper and lower respiratory tract infections. Interestingly, TS patients are more exposed to some forms of upper respiratory tract infections, primarily those caused by GABHS. PANDAS patients were found to have lower total IgA levels compared to healthy children (Kawikova et al., 2010): if systemic IgA levels mirror the expression level of IgA secreted at mucosal surfaces, which are important to prevent microbial attachment and neutralize bacterial exotoxins at the mucosal surface, then this IgA dysgammaglobulinemia might also predispose to microbial colonization of these epithelia, and explain, at least in part, the higher exposure to GABHS. On the other hand, IgA downregulates cell-mediated immune responses and may predispose to autoimmunity: interestingly, about one fifth of patients with IgA immunodeficiency manifest comorbid autoimmune disorders (Jacob et al., 2008). Although the exact meaning for these changes in the immunoglobulin profile of TS patients is still uncertain, it represents an additional, intriguing proof of altered immune regulation in this condition. Table 14.1

provides a broad overview of immune regulatory aspects of TS.

AUTOIMMUNITY

Some of the abnormalities of immune regulation reported in patients with tic disorders, such as reduced percentage of Tregs or decreased IgA production, are potentially predisposing to autoimmunity. However, if and how autoimmune mechanisms play a role in the pathophysiology of TS remains under investigation (Martino et al., 2009), and the relevance of cell-mediated or antibody-mediated autoimmune mechanisms remains undefined.

Most pathogenic autoantibodies in neurological disorders bind to proteins or receptors on the cell surface of neurons, axons, or endothelium. Given that a pathogenic self-antigen–autoantibody binding generally involves surface proteins or lipids whose conformation is well preserved *in vivo*, it is likely that conformational epitopes are

Table 14.1 Evidence for Immunological Changes in TS

	References
Level 1 findings	
Increased concentration of neopterin in serum	Luo et al., 2004; Hoekstra et al., 2007
Decreased concentration of IgG$_3$ in serum	Bos-Veneman et al., 2010
Level 2 findings	
Increased number of CD4+CD95+ and CD8+CD95+ T cells	Moller et al., 2008
Increased number of CD69+ B cells	Moller et al., 2008
Increased concentration of interleukin-12 and tumor necrosis factor-α in serum during symptom exacerbations	Leckman et al., 2005 Kawikova et al., 2007
Decreased number of Tregs in peripheral blood and increased concentration of interleukins 4, 5, 6, and 10 in serum during symptom exacerbations (only statistical trend)	Leckman et al., 2005
Overexpression of NK cell genes in peripheral blood mononuclear cells in adolescents with TS of interferon regulatory factors in children with TS aged 5–9 years	Lit et al., 2009
Oligoclonal bands synthesized intrathecally in the CSF	Wenzel et al., 2011*
Decreased concentration of IgA in serum in TS children with PANDAS	Kawikova et al., 2010

*Historical control group
From case-control cross-sectional or case-only prospective studies with at least 10 subjects per group. Level 1 findings are defined as results obtained in at least two independent cohorts and not contradicted by any adequately powered study. Level 2 findings are defined as results obtained in only one study and not contradicted by any adequately powered study.

more relevant than linear ones (i.e., characterized by the basic amino acid sequence of a protein antigen) in autoantibody-mediated human pathology. Most of the immunological methods used so far in the investigation of tic disorders are methods that alter protein structure, and thus could be misleading. For example, Western blotting and enzyme-linked immunosorbent assay (ELISA) involve homogenization and detergents that release cytoplasmic antigens, unravel proteins, and disrupt disulphide bonds. Both these two methods and indirect immunofluorescence methods have provided very contrasting findings in patients with TS and PANDAS (for a critical review of these works, see Martino et al., 2009). By contrast, recent discoveries of pathogenic autoantibodies have used live cell systems that express candidate self-antigens in their natural conformational state on the cell surface. For instance, the quantification of antibody binding to neuroblastoma or animal brain-derived live cell lines has theoretical advantages over methods that disrupt cell and protein structure. Two small studies applied this technology (Kirvan et al., 2006; Singer et al., 1999), showing that TS and PANDAS sera all contained autoantibodies that bound to the cell surface of neuroblastoma cell lines or rat striatal neurons. However, a recent study by Brilot and colleagues (2011) performed a more accurate quantitative measurement of IgG cell surface binding to live differentiated cells from the SH-SY5Y cell line, as well as to a nonneuronal control cell line, using the FACS flow cytometry method. There was no significant difference in IgG cell surface binding between sera from 12 patients with PANDAS, 11 patients with TS, and two groups of control subjects. Although this does not rule out the possibility that TS and PANDAS patients produce specific antibodies to conformational epitopes that are not expressed by the SH-SY5Y cell line, the findings from this study are not supportive of relevant autoantibody-mediated mechanisms in TS or PANDAS.

In addition to employing methods that preserve the native structure of antigens, more research is warranted to assess the pathogenic effects of autoantibodies identified in these disorders on cell function and animal behavior.

Following this line, preliminary work on the putative self-antigens targeted by these antineuronal antibodies has been published in recent years. Self-antigens of 40, 45, and 60 kDa have been identified in patients and Sydenham's chorea, other poststreptococcal neuropsychiatric disorders, and TS by Church and colleagues (2003, 2004), and were subsequently identified (Dale et al., 2006) as glycolytic enzymes (aldolase C, neuron-specific enolase, nonneuronal enolase, and pyruvate kinase M1). These glycolytic enzymes are present in the neuronal cytoplasm and on the cell surface of neurons and are involved in energy metabolism and ion channels support. The same enzymes exist on the cell surface of streptococcal bacteria; interestingly, nonneuronal enolase has been previously proposed as a self-antigen in rheumatic fever (Fontan et al., 2000). Pyruvate kinase M1 was subsequently identified as a self-antigen in TS by Kansy and colleagues (2006), who found elevated anti-pyruvate kinase antibodies during streptococcal-induced exacerbations of tics. Martino and colleagues (2007, 2011) reported that between 20% and 25% of children with TS from two large cohorts expressed antineuronal glycolytic enzyme antibodies, which were not associated with basal ganglia volumes (Martino et al., 2008) or tic severity when patients were followed up prospectively (Martino et al., 2007). These findings were not, however, confirmed by Singer and colleagues (2005, 2008), and the pathogenic potential of these autoantibodies has not been demonstrated to date.

Kirvan and colleagues (2003, 2006) found cross-reactivity of autoantibodies between streptococcal N-acetyl-glucosamine and brain lysoganglioside GM1, a neuronal cell-surface molecule; antibodies against lysoganglioside GM1 and tubulin (Kirvan et al., 2007) were elevated in poststreptococcal disorders, including Sydenham's chorea and PANDAS. Furthermore, these autoantibodies increased the activity of calcium-calmodulin–dependent protein kinase II (CaM kinase II), possibly upregulating tyrosine hydroxylase (and therefore dopamine synthesis), which could theoretically result in involuntary movements and abnormal behaviors. However, the above-mentioned work by

Kawikova and colleagues (2010) does not support the relevance of anti-lysoganglioside GM1 antibodies in patients with TS or PANDAS: 24 patients with TS/OCD (80% of whom fulfilled PANDAS criteria) did not differ from healthy subjects in their serum level of IgM and IgG against ganglioside GM1, lysoganglioside, and other antigens previously identified in multiple sclerosis (myelin basic protein and myelin-associated glycoprotein).

Even if future research should confirm that one or more autoantibodies are present in a subgroup of patients with tic disorders, the mere presence of autoantibodies in the bloodstream is not sufficient to prove their role in disease causation. For autoantibodies to be considered pathogenic, they should be present in the target organ, passive transfer of autoantibodies should induce disease in animals, and patients' symptoms should improve after removal of autoantibodies. Due to the relative paucity of postmortem data, the presence of autoantibodies in the brain of TS patients has never been explored. Induction of disease in animals after patients' antibody infusion was attempted with inconsistent results (see Martino et al., 2009, for a review). A recent animal model of Sydenham's chorea and PANDAS showed anti-human D1/D2 dopamine receptor antibodies in sera of rats immunized with GABHS, suggesting that this class of autoantibodies may play an important role in the molecular mimicry of "poststreptococcal" neuropsychiatric disorders (Brimberg et al., 2012). Future, stronger evidence supporting the role of this new class of autoantibodies is needed to evaluate their relevance to a subgroup of patients with chronic tic disorders.

Finally, no human studies demonstrated that removal of specific antineural autoantibodies improves patient symptoms. Hoekstra and colleagues (2004b) found no benefit of intravenous immunoglobulins in TS adult patients, whereas Perlmutter and colleagues (1999) demonstrated 1-month and 1-year benefit of plasma exchange and intravenous immunoglobulins compared to placebo in children and adolescent patients with PANDAS. However, in the absence of more robust and consistent evidence, current recommendations do not support the use of these agents in TS.

In conclusion, at present we lack a clear autoantibody marker showing a diagnostic and/or a pathogenic relevance in patients with tic disorders, including those with the potentially immune-mediated PANDAS syndrome. Novel research using conservative approaches on live cells should be performed, in line with the current paradigm supporting conformational epitopes as the pathogenically relevant antigenic determinants in central nervous system autoantibody-mediated disorders. If and when a clear epidemiological association between one or more autoantibodies targeting conformational epitopes and tic disorders will be demonstrated, this will certainly constitute a solid rationale for investigating the role of autoantibodies in disease causation in these patients.

Beyond the discussed relevance of antineural antibodies, additional evidence in favor of an ongoing autoimmune process in tic disorders is also limited. Antinuclear antibodies, commonly found in a number of autoimmune diseases and particularly in systemic lupus erythematosus, have been found to be elevated in a population of 81 children and adolescents with TS compared to control subjects (Morshed et al., 2001). This marker was in equivocal relation to antistreptococcal markers, antineural antibodies, and clinical characteristics in this study, whereas a subsequent work failed to replicate this finding (Loiselle et al., 2003). Although tics may occasionally occur in patients with antiphospholipid antibody syndrome (Martino et al., 2006; Seijo-Martinez et al., 2008), systematic analyses have shown antiphospholipid antibodies to be a coincidental or epiphenomenal occurrence in the general population of TS patients (Singer et al., 1997; Toren et al., 1994). Other markers of systemic autoimmune diseases, such as other autoantibodies not directed to neural tissue or complement factors, have not been explored in detail in tic disorders.

Finally, an interesting report from Murphy and colleagues (2010) in the United States explored the maternal risk for an autoimmune response in 107 children with tics and/or OCD compared to population norms, using a structured interview. Autoimmune disorders were reported in approximately 18% of study mothers; despite the lack of a control population, it is likely that this percentage is greater than the general prevalence of autoimmune diseases in women from the United States. An additional finding of this study was that the frequency of self-report of autoimmune diseases was relatively higher in mothers of children with "likely PANDAS" versus "unlikely PANDAS." A higher familial risk of autoimmune diseases has also been reported in other neurodevelopmental illnesses, such as autistic spectrum patients (Sweeten et al., 2003), in whom 47.5% of patients have a family member with an autoimmune disease (approximately fivefold more than control populations). Maternal autoimmunity, in particular, may on the one hand indicate a genetic predisposition to the development of autoimmune mechanisms; on the other hand, it might directly damage the offspring by producing antibodies to fetal brain tissue during pregnancy that might alter normal brain development, as increasingly suggested by clinical and animal model studies of autism (Goines & Van der Water, 2010). Whether antibodies to fetal tissue are produced by mothers of children with TS or OCD needs to be investigated. Table 14.2 summarizes the evidence in favor of and against the involvement of autoimmunity in TS.

ALLERGY

The association between allergic illnesses and TS has been investigated only in epidemiological studies conducted in the population of Taiwan. An older retrospective study compared the reactivity to multiple allergens in 72 TS patients to a historical control population from the same area, showing clinical evidence of allergy was significantly more common in TS patients (Ho et al., 1999). This prompted Chang and collaborators (2011) to perform a longitudinal retrospective case-control study that used a very large health insurance national database comparing 845 youngsters (aged 18 or less) with newly diagnosed TS to 3,378 control subjects who were frequency-matched to cases by age, gender, and level of urbanization. These authors showed that all four allergic diseases explored (allergic rhinitis,

Table 14.2 Autoimmunity in TS

	References
Pro-autoimmunity	
Decreased number of T-regulatory cells in peripheral blood (preliminary)	Kawikova et al., 2007
Intrathecal synthesis of oligoclonal bands in CSF	Wenzel et al., 2011
Decreased concentration of IgA in serum (only in PANDAS subgroup)	Kawikova et al., 2010
Maternal family history of autoimmune diseases	Murphy et al., 2010
Concurrent fluctuations of cytokines and clinical severity	Leckman et al., 2005
Synthesis of antineural antibodies (controversial)	See Martino et al., 2009, for a detailed review.
Con-autoimmunity	
No association with HLA subtypes	Schoenian et al., 2003
No increase in IgG index	Wenzel et al., 2011
No autoantibodies to nuclear proteins (controversial)	Morshed et al., 2001; Loiselle et al., 2003
No TS-specific antibodies	See Martino et al., 2009, for a detailed review.

asthma, allergic dermatitis, and allergic conjunctivitis) were associated with a higher risk of TS, with adjusted odds ratios of 2.18, 1.82, 1.61, and 1.33, respectively. When age and comorbidities were included in the logistic regression model, both increased the association between allergic diseases and diagnosis of TS.

Although this type of retrospective longitudinal study based on health insurance databases may be susceptible to a certain degree of information bias due to limited accuracy in data collection, this finding interestingly suggests that TS patients may indeed be more prone to allergy, as they seem to be toward some types of infectious illnesses and to autoimmunity.

GENERAL CONSIDERATIONS ON IMMUNITY AND PATHOPHYSIOLOGY OF TS

What is the link, if any, between the abnormalities of immune response summarized herein and current views on the pathogenesis of TS? Although most of the immune changes detected so far need to be substantiated by further research, it is tempting to speculate on possible ways in which nervous and immune systems might interact in patients with TS. Three potential mechanisms of interaction are proposed below, which should not be seen as mutually exclusive.

First, abnormalities of neural transmission and immune response may be interconnected. Central dopamine systems have always been considered to play an important etiological role in TS (see Chapter 13 for a detailed review on neurotransmitter systems in TS). There is compelling evidence of a hyperdopaminergic state in some cases of TS, with increased ventral striatal dopaminergic innervation and elevated intrasynaptic dopamine release in the striatum following amphetamine administration. Also, dopamine receptor blocking agents are among the most effective and frequently used drugs in the treatment of tics (see Chapter 24).

Dopamine is a very important bridge between the nervous and immune systems. It modulates the function of immune cells in an autocrine/paracrine fashion by acting through receptors present on the surface of these cells (Sarkar et al.,

2010). Furthermore, dopaminergic innervation of lymphoid tissues through sympathetic nerves has clearly been described, as well as brain dopamine-mediated regulation of peripheral immune functions. Other diseases with abnormal dopaminergic systems, such as Parkinson's disease and schizophrenia, are associated with altered immune function. If abnormal dopamine release is not restricted to the brain but also involves the peripheral innervation of immune cells, it might also contribute to abnormal immune effector responses like those seen in TS patients. Of note, dopamine has unique and opposite effects on T-cell function: it may activate naïve T cells in the absence of any additional stimulating agent, but it may also inhibit the activation of stimulated T cells. This complex modulation may play a role in the generalized activation of different T- and B-cell subtypes observed in TS. Tregs, which may be inhibited in TS patients, can be downregulated by dopamine through D1/D5 receptors present on the surface of these cells. In this respect, a small study intriguingly reported increased expression of D5 receptors on peripheral lymphocytes of TS patients, which might be related to downregulation of Tregs (Ferrari et al., 2008). Dopamine is also reported to induce cytokine secretion by naïve T cells. The stimulation of dopamine D3 and D1/D5 receptors increases the secretion of TNF-α and the stimulation of D2 receptors induces IL-10 secretion, both of which were shown to be increased in the plasma of children with exacerbations of tics and/or obsessive-compulsive symptoms.

In conclusion, part of the immune abnormalities observed in TS patients might be related to abnormal dopaminergic modulation of immune cells. Other neurotransmitters, such as serotonin, glutamate, and acetylcholine, also show immunoregulatory properties, and their role in the pathogenesis of tic disorders is being increasingly investigated.

Second, immunological triggers such as infections might enhance immune responses and lead to functional damage of the brain networks involved in action selection and monitoring. According to a previously published pathogenic model, the increased exposure of TS patients to GABHS (or other) infections might induce the synthesis of cross-reactive antineural antibodies. The relevance of antibodies binding to dopamine receptors has recently been advocated to play a role in neuropsychiatric disorders, including tics, associated with group A streptococcal infections (Brimberg et al., 2012). Among these receptors, D2 autoreceptors located on presynaptic membranes are a potentially very interesting target of autoimmunity in these disorders, given their inhibitory modulation on dopamine release. Antiglycolytic enzyme antibodies might theoretically modify neuronal excitability and affect neurotransmitter release, although evidence to support this hypothesis is currently lacking. At the same time, an increased exposure to GABHS infections might promote first-line inflammatory responses or trigger cytokine release via a superantigen-mediated mechanism. In line with this, a subtype of T cells expressing TCR binding to a common streptococcal superantigen may be reduced in number in TS patients (Kawikova et al., 2007); functional exhaustion or apoptosis secondary to prolonged superantigenic exposure is a possible explanation for this finding.

On the other hand, the increased exposure to GABHS might itself be a consequence of immune dysregulation. Decreased concentrations of IgG3 and IgA (the latter reported in PANDAS children) might facilitate the invasion of respiratory tract pathogens, thus potentially initiating a vicious circle leading to chronically enhanced activation of immune/ inflammatory responses (Bos-Veneman et al., 2010; Kawikova et al., 2010). Future work will clarify whether prophylactic measures against GABHS or other pathogens will have an effect on the risk of onset or exacerbation of tics and related behaviors. Figure 14.1 proposes a model of immune-mediated basal ganglia dysfunction in tics and obsessive-compulsive symptoms.

Third, immune cells and effector molecules contribute to abnormal brain development, eventually leading to tics and associated behavioral abnormalities. Like autism and schizophrenia, TS seems to be caused by a combination of genetic changes and environmental insults during early development. Like autism and schizophrenia, TS may be associated with a predisposition to enhanced immune activity, autoimmunity, and allergies. In contrast to autism and schizophrenia, though, evidence is only preliminary for TS, and the associations with specific genetic variants in cytokines, cytokine receptors, and MHC genes that have been reported in autistic and schizophrenic patients have not been adequately investigated so far in TS patients. A large body of evidence supports the integral role of immune molecules in modulating neurogenesis, neuronal migration, axon guidance, synapse formation, and activity-dependent shaping of circuits and synaptic plasticity (Garay & McAllister, 2010). Whereas evidence in favor of the contribution of altered immune regulation to neurodevelopmental disorders like autism and schizophrenia is increasing at an outstanding pace, the "neurodevelopmental" approach to immune dysregulation in TS is only beginning.

THE STRESS RESPONSE IN TS: GENERAL CONSIDERATIONS

An involvement of endocrine modulation of stress in TS is suggested by the strong relationship between stress and anxiety levels and severity of TS symptoms. Several clinical reports indicate that acute physical and social stress, fatigue, and anxiety are relevant contextual factors leading to worsening of tics and related symptoms (see also Chapter 1). A small study on four children with TS evaluated the effects of emotional stimuli on the severity of tics to determine whether these effects were mediated through autonomic responses; videotaped rating of tics and electrophysiological monitoring of heart and respiratory rate and pattern were performed while children were watching a movie known to induce age-appropriate emotional stimulation (Wood et al., 2003). Whereas there was a relationship between the emotional context and tic severity, the latter did not correlate with cardiac or respiratory function, suggesting that stress-related severity changes in TS are not directly linked to autonomic responses. On rare occasions, an emotional or physical trauma may be temporally linked to the onset of tics in patients with TS (Carney, 1977). Also, medication requirements may change based on exposure to stress (Surwillo et al., 1978), and intervening stress may be a confounding factor hindering

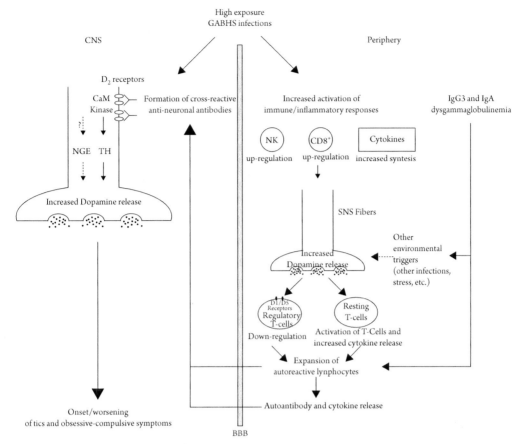

FIGURE 14.1   **Proposed model of immune-mediated basal ganglia dysfunction in tics and obsessive-compulsive symptoms.**   *Periphery.* Infections such as GABHS infections might contribute to the activation of inflammatory responses in the periphery, leading to NK and cytotoxic T-cell functional upregulation, and to increased synthesis of pro-inflammatory cytokines. Enhanced dopamine regulation of T cells in the periphery might also contribute to downregulation of regulatory T cells (Tregs) and to the amplification of pro-inflammatory cytokine release. Such enhanced dopamine modulation of peripheral immune cells may be consequential to overactive sympathetic responses induced by higher exposure to stressors. The downregulation of Tregs might lead to expansion of autoreactive lymphocytes and the development of autoimmunity. Autoimmunity might also be facilitated by dysgammaglobulinemia of undefined origin, which might also increase susceptibility to infections in these patients, generating a vicious circle. *Brain.* Clonal selection and expansion of autoreactive lymphocytes in the periphery, possibly facilitated by molecular mimicry between microbial and host antigens, might induce the formation of cross-reactive antineuronal antibodies. Candidate target self-antigens include D2 presynaptic dopamine receptors (autoreceptors), modulating calcium-calmodulin dependent (CaM) kinase II activity and ultimately presynaptic dopamine release, and membrane-bound neuronal glycolytic enzymes (NGE), which might modulate membrane excitability. These antibody-driven functional changes might play a role in the onset and worsening of tics and obsessive-compulsive symptoms (Based on Martino et al., 2009).

the objective evaluation of response to a treatment for tics. Prospective studies clearly showed a short-term predictive effect of psychosocial stress levels upon the future severity of tics and obsessive-compulsive symptoms in youngsters with TS/OCD (Lin et al., 2007, 2010). Finally, the functional activity of the HPA axis may be involved in the generation of animal models of stereotyped behaviors possibly showing face validity for TS.

EPIDEMIOLOGICAL RESEARCH ON PSYCHOSOCIAL STRESS AND TS

A very limited number of studies investigated the relationship between psychosocial stress and the diagnosis and symptom severity of TS. Most of these studies concentrated on exploring longitudinally if and how life stressors predicted the future severity of tics and other related symptoms in the short term. Hoekstra and colleagues (2004c) analyzed the correlation between scores from questionnaires on small life events and self-rating scores of tic severity in 24 youngsters aged 7 to 16 years and 28 adults with TS. The study revealed only a small, albeit significant, positive correlation between negative events and tic severity; however, it was not replicated in the pediatric group. This study was limited by the small sample size, the lack of healthy controls, and the use of a life event questionnaire rather than a rating instrument directly measuring stress levels. These limitations were overcome in a subsequent study in which consecutive ratings of tic and obsessive-compulsive and depressive symptom severity were obtained for 45 youngsters with TS and/or OCD and 41 healthy control subjects over 2 years (Lin et al., 2007). Measurements of psychosocial stress were made prospectively in both groups using parent report (Parent Perceived Stress Scale [PSS-P]), youth self-report (Daily Life Stressors Scale [DLSS]), and a clinician-rated measure of long-term contextual threat (Yale Children's Global Stress Index [YCGSI]). All longitudinal measures were obtained based on monthly ratings. A structural equation modeling framework for unbalanced repeated measures was employed to assess the temporal sequence of psychosocial stress with symptom severity. The underlying true stress levels manifested by the three available longitudinal stress measures was modeled in a latent time-varying stress construct; in this construct, the effect of time lag was studied using the nearest recorded past reading of a longitudinal measure as a covariate for a current reading. The results showed higher psychosocial stress in case than in control subjects. Current levels of psychosocial stress and depression were independent and significant predictors of future

tic severity after controlling for the effect of age (inversely associated with tic severity), although this predictive effect was small. Importantly, current tic severity did not predict psychosocial stress or depressive symptoms. Current stress levels were stronger predictors of future obsessive-compulsive and depressive symptoms severity, whereas only current ratings of depressive symptoms were modestly predictive of future ratings of psychosocial stress. In these models, PSS-P proved to be the most robust predictor of stress-related outcomes, followed by DLSS and YCGSI. A subsequent study from the same group (Lin et al., 2010) analyzed in the same population the interaction between GABHS infections and psychosocial stress and their impact on future symptom severity. Although definite newly diagnosed GAS infections had a modest predictive effect upon future tic severity, the inclusion of this variable in the model increased the predictive power of the stress construct defined above by a factor of almost 3 (i.e., from 0.13 to 0.37); the effect of both environmental factors remained significant when both definite and possible newly diagnosed GABHS infections were entered into the model. The interaction between the two factors exerted an even stronger impact upon future obsessive-compulsive symptom severity. Definite or possible newly diagnosed GABHS infections robustly increased the current psychosocial stress levels but did not exert any predictive effect upon future depressive symptoms. Overall, these two studies indicate that psychosocial stress levels influence the future severity of obsessive-compulsive symptoms and to a lesser extent of tics, suggesting the involvement of stress response mechanisms in the pathogenesis of these behavioral symptoms. The potential interaction with GABHS infections suggests also the interplay of immune and endocrine mechanisms, although this needs to be explored in further detail.

As mentioned above, the role of stress in promoting the onset of tics is based mainly on anecdotal reports. The effect of maternal stress during pregnancy has been explored in a case-control study by Motlagh and colleagues (2010), already summarized in Chapter 8, which included 45 individuals with TS only, 52 with attention-deficit/hyperactivity disorder (ADHD) only, 60 with TS+ADHD, and 65 without major neuropsychiatric disorders. This study investigated several prenatal and perinatal risk factors. Severe psychosocial stress during pregnancy was identified when events occurring during pregnancy were sufficiently severe to disrupt existing patterns of family life, such as severe marital conflict with separation or a threat of separation, death or serious injury to a relative, or periods of unemployment. There was a trend for higher levels of severe maternal psychosocial stress during pregnancy in both offspring with TS alone and offspring with TS+ADHD, whereas the association was strongly significant (odds ratio 6.8, 95% CI 2–23.3) with the diagnosis of ADHD alone. This association with ADHD alone was even stronger, although at a lower degree of significance, when severe maternal stress during pregnancy was combined with limited coping abilities in the family in a single variable (odds ratio 16.3, 95% CI 1.5–135.1); as in severe maternal stress alone, there was only a trend for an association of the combined variable and diagnoses of TS only or TS+ADHD. Despite the obvious limitations of retrospective data collection and limited sample size, these results suggest an effect of pregnancy-related maternal stress upon the risk for neurodevelopmental disorders like ADHD and, possibly, TS.

GENERAL CONCEPTS ON THE HPA AXIS IN HUMAN PHYSIOLOGY AND DISEASE

The HPA axis is the major, evolutionarily conserved part of the neuroendocrine system, involved in the control of reactions to stress and in the regulation of various physiological processes, including gastrointestinal function, energy storage and expenditure, immune response, mood and emotions, and sexual behavior. It consists of a system of direct influences and feedback interactions among the paraventricular nucleus (PVN) of the hypothalamus (synthesizing corticotrophin-releasing hormone [CRH]), the anterior lobe of the pituitary gland (producing adrenocorticotropic hormone [ACTH]), and the adrenal cortices, which produce glucocorticoid hormones (mainly cortisol in humans). From the PVN, CRH is transported to the anterior pituitary, stimulating ACTH release; the latter induces the synthesis and release of cortisol from the adrenal gland. In addition, the HPA axis is strongly influenced by limbic structures (Fig. 14.2). Anatomical connections between brain areas such as the amygdala, hippocampus, and hypothalamus facilitate the activation of the HPA axis. Specific sensory information related to threats is processed by the basolateral and central nuclei of the amygdala and conveyed as fear-signaling impulses both to the sympathetic nervous system and the HPA axis. The alarm reaction to stress is then triggered by a sudden increase in cortisol production, which facilitates a subsequent phase of adaptation during which the previous alarm reactions are suppressed, thus allowing the body to tune up appropriate countermeasures. The hippocampus, on the other hand, expresses high levels of glucocorticoid receptors and plays a significant role in negative feedback regulation of the HPA axis.

The regulation of the HPA axis comprises three interrelated processes: the maintenance of a diurnal (circadian) rhythm, the stress response (i.e., the activation in response to a challenge or threat), and the restoration of basal activity by means of negative feedback mechanisms. Cortisol is one of the main effectors of the alarm stress response and has a very important role in the maintenance of the homeostasis of body systems. CRH release and subsequent HPA axis activity are influenced by the sleep/wake cycle. In healthy individuals, cortisol rises rapidly in the morning after awakening, gradually falls throughout the day, rises again in late afternoon, and then falls again in late evening, reaching the lowest levels during the middle of the night. This circadian rhythm is already well developed by the third month of postnatal life (Price et al., 1983), and its maintenance has a relevant role for cognitive and social functioning during development (Bartels et al., 2003). CRH release is also deeply influenced by exposure to social and physical stressors, consisting of novel, threatening, and unpredictable situations or stimuli. Finally, the release of CRH from the hypothalamus is influenced by blood levels of cortisol, which exerts a negative feedback over the PVN and the anterior pituitary, leading to restoration of the baseline activity of the axis. Several monoamine neurotransmitters are also involved in the regulation of the HPA axis, particularly dopamine, noradrenaline, serotonin, and histamine, as well as other hypothalamic peptides such as oxytocin.

A dysfunctional HPA axis is associated with a number of neuropsychiatric and medical diseases. For example, HPA hyperreactivity can be observed in major depression (Stetler & Miller, 2011) and could be associated also with higher susceptibility to infections (Mason, 1991) and cardiovascular disease (McEwen, 1998). Autoimmune illnesses, such as lupus (Weiner, 1991), rheumatoid arthritis (Tsigos and Chrousos, 2002), and multiple sclerosis (Heesen et al., 2007), are, instead, associated with HPA hyporeactivity. Overall, the functioning of the HPA axis may be an index of the cumulative stress toll on the body, which might be abnormally high if stress responses are chronically overactive (McEwen, 1988).

HPA AXIS FUNCTIONING IN TS

Early reports focused on the modulation of HPA axis regulation by drugs with a therapeutic potential for TS, acting on the noradrenergic (clonidine) or opiatergic (naloxone) systems (Sandyk & Bamford, 1988). These reports did not investigate the HPA axis with the aim of acquiring novel information on its regulation in TS, but rather explored the regulation of the HPA axis as an indirect measure of dysfunction of specific neurotransmitter systems. In particular, Sandyk and Bamford (1988) explored the relevance of a dysfunction of opioid and noradrenergic systems in TS by evaluating the effect of a low-dose naloxone challenge on the HPA axis. Given that opioids can depress HPA axis activity via a tonic inhibition upon the noradrenergic pathway originating in the locus coeruleus, these authors hypothesized and observed that

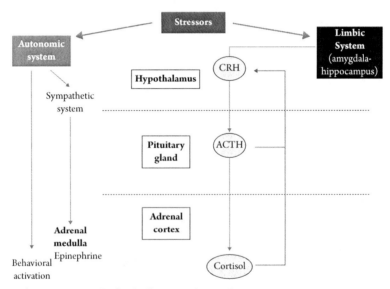

FIGURE 14.2 **The HPA axis is the final effector pathway of acute stress responses.** External stressors play a crucial role in activating the axis via limbic structures. Cells in the hypothalamus produce CRH, which in turn binds to specific receptors on pituitary cells, producing ACTH. ACTH will eventually target the adrenal gland, stimulating the production of adrenocortical hormones, especially cortisol. Cortisol will then initiate metabolic effects related to the stress response, and at the same time exert negative feedback (*red lines and arrows*) to both hypothalamus and anterior pituitary, leading to compensatory decrease of CRH and ACTH production. Autonomic responses, particularly related to sympathetic activation, represent an alternative set of effector pathways of the acute stress response.

low doses of an opioid antagonist (i.e. naloxone), generally ineffective in healthy individuals, produce a significant rise in cortisol secretion in TS patients, suggestive of a chronic reduction in opiatergic control over the HPA axis. However, this finding is very difficult to interpret, since this study involved only six individuals with TS, lacked control participants, and has never been replicated.

More recent studies analyzed in larger detail the three main processes of HPA axis regulation in TS (i.e., maintenance of the diurnal cortisol rhythm, acute stress response, restoration to basal activity). An abnormally flattened circadian cortisol cycle has been linked to chronic stress. Corbett and colleagues (2008b) conducted the only study to date that assessed rigorously the circadian profile of cortisol secretion in children with TS. Twenty unmedicated children with a diagnosis of TS (17 boys) between 7 and 13 years of age were compared to 16 age-matched, typically developing subjects (11 boys). TS patients had higher scores than typical individuals on OCD, ADHD, and anxiety scales. Basal levels of salivary cortisol were collected three times per day (morning, mid-afternoon, and evening) for three diurnal cycles. Of note, cortisol levels measured in saliva correlate very well with the amount of free cortisol in blood but show only moderate correlations with total cortisol levels (i.e., cortisol bound to binding proteins in blood plus biologically active, unbound, "free" cortisol). Corbett and colleagues (2008b) did not detect differences in the natural cortisol circadian pattern, although there was a trend for lower cortisol values in the evening in the TS group compared to the typical group. Moreover, the first morning cortisol sample was highly positively correlated with the number of motor tics, while evening cortisol values were negatively correlated with the number, intensity, or interference of motor tics, global impairment, and overall tic severity. Surprisingly, lower diurnal cortisol levels were associated with greater scores on the Multidimensional Anxiety Scale for Children (MASC-C), whereas parents' stress was not associated with their children's cortisol levels. These authors explained the trend for lower cortisol values in the evening as a possible consequence of chronic stress. It is, however, unclear whether this chronic exposure to stress is related predominantly to the presence of tics. If this is the case, a deeper evening trough of cortisol could be the consequence of a prolonged and stressful inhibitory effort to suppress tics throughout the day or, conversely, the consequence of an "anxiolytic" effect of tic release, given the negative correlation of evening cortisol levels to tic severity. Also, the opposite diurnal pattern (i.e., higher cortisol levels in the evening) detected in autistic patients using a similar experimental design is striking (Corbett et al., 2008a).

During the second process of HPA axis regulation—acute stress response—stressors of variable nature, posing a challenge or threat to the individual and potentially deranging homeostasis, activate CRH release. A few studies have analyzed the HPA axis response to different stressors in individuals with TS. The stressors employed in these studies are related to the anticipation of a physical threat. Chappell and colleagues (1994) examined the stressful effects of a lumbar puncture on plasma ACTH and cortisol, urinary catecholamines, and self-ratings and clinician ratings of anxiety in 13 unmedicated TS adults and 10 age-matched normal subjects (age range, 17–41 years). Plasma ACTH and cortisol levels were measured at 8 a.m., 11:30 a.m. noon, 12:25 p.m. (immediately prior to lumbar puncture), 12:45 p.m., 1 p.m., 1:30 p.m., 2:00 p.m., and 2:30 p.m. Although the plasma cortisol levels peaked just after the lumbar puncture for both the adult TS subjects and the matched control subjects, the TS patients exhibited a significantly higher ACTH secretion throughout the day both before and after the lumbar puncture. Depression and anxiety levels could not be held responsible for this difference. This abnormal response was also accompanied by a significantly higher excretion of noradrenaline prior to the lumbar puncture, and a correlation of urinary noradrenaline excretion with clinician ratings of tic severity among TS patients. This latter finding is consistent with a previous study from the same group that found 55% higher levels of noradrenaline in the CSF of an overlapping group of 33 unmedicated TS patients compared to a matched control group of healthy volunteers (Leckman et al., 1995). The same group (Chappell et al., 1996) used a very similar experimental protocol to analyze concentrations of CRH at the time of lumbar puncture in 21 TS patients (age range 13–44 years, 15 males), 20 OCD patients (age range 19–61 years, 8 males), and 29 normal subjects (age range 19–58 years, 17 males). TS patients had approximately 30% higher levels of CSF CRH than the other two groups ($p < .04$), whereas OCD patients did not differ from healthy subjects, regardless of their tic comorbidity. Age, gender, height, body weight, tic severity, obsessive-compulsive symptom severity, depression and anxiety scores, and lifetime history of major depression or generalized anxiety disorder did not influence these results. However, there were no significant correlations between CSF CRF levels and the CSF concentration of noradrenaline (which is known to activate the HPA axis through locus coeruleus projections to the PVN) or of its major metabolite, 3-methoxy-4-hydroxyphenylglycol. The above-mentioned study by Corbett and colleagues (2008b) challenged TS and typically developing children with a mock scanning procedure (i.e., a MRI simulation), obtaining salivary samples before and after the exposure, as well as before and after a real MRI scan session. Although this stressor may be regarded as of milder intensity than the lumbar puncture procedure, it can still be conceptualized as a model of environmental stress, given that it consists of a novel event involving mild restraint and exposure to unpleasant noises. Mock scanning sessions occurred between 1 and 3 p.m., and salivary samples were collected upon arrival, 20 minutes after exposure to the mock scan, 40 minutes after exposure to the mock scan and immediately prior to the real scan, and 1 hour after the beginning of the real scan. TS children exhibited a significantly higher cortisol response compared to typically developing children at all four time points, except for the post-real MRI time point, for which there was only a statistical trend. Although this finding differs from that seen in adults with TS, where there was no differential increase in plasma cortisol levels relative to controls from before to after the lumbar puncture,

the results from the available studies consistently suggest a higher responsiveness of the HPA axis to stressors in TS patients (increased levels of CSF CRH and plasma ACTH in adults and higher levels of cortisol in children). Of note, no study to date has employed the Trier Social Stress Test, and its version for children, in TS. This test seems particularly accurate in measuring the acute response to stressors characterized by social-evaluative threat, in that it is a highly standardized laboratory stress task comprising a preparation period and a free speech and mental arithmetic task in front of an audience. This experimental setting seems particularly valid to reproduce the naturalistic scenario of psychosocial stress known to act as an aggravating contextual factor in patients with tic disorders. Moreover, novel studies should control more accurately for a number of variables (e.g., sex, general health status, smoking habits, female menstrual cycle phase, personality factors, time of day, social support, genetic factors, etc.) that might introduce additional interindividual variability in HPA axis stress responses.

The third process of HPA axis regulation, the restoration of the basal activity of the system, is mainly determined by negative feedback mechanisms exerted by circulating cortisol over the hypothalamic and pituitary levels. Direct evidence of this regulatory aspect is lacking in TS. Indirect evidence is available from Corbett and colleagues' study (2008b), in which the decrease in cortisol value between the post-mock and the pre-real MRI time points may indicate efficient negative feedback of cortisol over the axis. Thus, the results of this study might indeed reflect enhanced reactivity rather than abnormal restoration of baseline activity. On the other hand, the lower evening cortisol values might also be caused by an abnormally enhanced negative feedback mechanism, as has also been proposed for posttraumatic stress disorder (Yehuda et al., 1995). The direct way to address this issue is by using the dexamethasone suppression test (DST). Dexamethasone is an exogenous steroid that provides negative feedback to the pituitary to suppress the secretion of ACTH, whereas it is ineffective over the hypothalamus because it cannot pass the blood–brain barrier. A low dose of dexamethasone suppresses cortisol in normal individuals. A pathological nonsuppression response on the DST has been observed in other neurodevelopmental disorders like ADHD or autism (Kaneko et al., 1993), further creating the rationale to explore in greater depth this aspect of HPA axis regulation also in TS patients.

GENERAL CONSIDERATIONS ON STRESS RESPONSE AND PATHOPHYSIOLOGY OF TS

Although with some methodological limitations, including small sample size, studies exploring stress responses in TS patients overall suggest increased susceptibility to stress and possibly higher chronic exposure to stressors. Although this has been shown in both youngsters and adults with TS, the peak of symptom severity of TS in early adolescence coincides with a developmental phase proposed to represent a time of increased susceptibility to stress. Recent work from a rat model shows that younger adolescent animals might be protected from the effect of chronic stress, whereas late adolescent animals are more likely to manifest an increased HPA response to stress (Jankord et al., 2011). Although HPA axis functioning may differ substantially between rodents and primates, this finding suggests the possibility that the physiological window of vulnerability to stress encountered during adolescence might

---

Box 14.1. Key Points

- The analysis of lymphocyte subpopulations in TS suggests a possible systemic activation of several T- and B-cell subtypes. There is preliminary evidence in favor of decreased numbers of Tregs, a predisposing factor to ongoing autoimmunity. Increased D8/17 binding to B cells may be epiphenomenal to the generalized activation of B cells.
- Neopterin, a nonspecific marker of systemic inflammation, is increased in youngsters with TS. Two pro-inflammatory cytokines (IL-12 and TNF-α) may co-vary with the severity of tics and obsessive-compulsive symptoms in pediatric patients. Preliminary evidence suggests that this co-variance involves a wide array of both pro-inflammatory and anti-inflammatory cytokines. A number of genes related to both cell- and antibody-mediated immune responses may be overexpressed at specific ages in youngsters with TS. Albeit limited, data from cytokine measurements and transcriptomics profiles in TS patients are coherent with the systemic immune activation detected by studies on lymphocyte subpopulations.
- TS patients have a decreased level of IgG3 immunoglobulins. This suggests less efficient mechanisms of neutralization of pathogens via complement-mediated mechanisms or phagocytosis. Children with PANDAS may have reduced levels of IgA, which could predispose them to microbial invasion, and even to autoimmunity.
- Intrathecal antibody synthesis may occur in a subgroup of TS patients, although there is no current evidence of blood–brain barrier breakdown. New research is needed to demonstrate the presence of neuroinflammation in this condition.
- To date, the association between TS and autoantibodies has not been demonstrated. Interestingly, however, there is a higher degree of maternal family history of autoimmune diseases among TS patients.
- TS patients could be prone to the most common allergic illnesses (asthma, atopic dermatitis, rhinitis, conjunctivitis), but more work is needed in this area.
- Patients with TS exhibit an enhanced reactivity of the HPA axis to external stressors, despite preserved diurnal cortisol rhythm and normal restoration of the baseline activity of the axis following the acute stress response

be disrupted in TS patients, leading to earlier, and possibly more prolonged, presentation of the "vulnerability" period, with a relative shortening of the "protected" period. Also, it has been clearly shown that limbic structures play a significant role in the regulation of the HPA axis, and their involvement in the processing of emotions and motor output in TS might also lead to altered regulation of stress responses. However, the direct link between the limbic system and the HPA axis has never been studied in these patients to date.

An additional consideration on the HPA axis should take into account that the development of this system might be dependent on some environmental features during very early stages, starting from the prenatal period (Gatzke-Kopp, 2011). An evolutionary model suggests that maternal cortisol serves to "prime" or program offspring to increase sensitivity to postnatal threat cues (Crespi & Denver, 2005). It is tempting to hypothesize that the hyperreactivity of the HPA axis observed in TS patients is, at least in part, the organizational effect of an increased exposure to maternal cortisol *in utero* (O'Donnell et al., 2012). As highlighted above, a recent case-control study reported a trend for an association between severe levels of psychosocial stress during pregnancy and a diagnosis of TS, whereas high pregnancy-related stress significantly predicted a diagnosis of ADHD (Motlagh et al., 2010). This hypothesis becomes even more intriguing

---

Box 14.2. Questions for Future Research

- T-helper cells are the main regulator of immune responses: is there a pattern of functional differentiation of T-helper cells that is typical of TS and related disorders?
- Do markers of immune activation (e.g., frequency of lymphocyte subpopulations, cytokine levels, immunoglobulin levels) co-vary with the severity of tics and other abnormal behaviors in patients? If yes, is this co-variation suggestive of a cause-and-effect relationship, or is it purely epiphenomenal?
- What is really happening beyond the blood–brain barrier in TS patients? Is there ongoing neuroinflammation? Is there a temporal relationship between intrathecal synthesis of antibodies and the clinical course in this condition? What is the role of microglia in the pathogenesis of tics and other stereotyped behaviors?
- What is the true relationship between infections and increased immune activity in TS? Is the latter a consequence of exposure to pathogens? Or, instead, are TS patients made more vulnerable to pathogens as a consequence of an abnormal organization of immune responses? Are both of these scenarios true, and occurring within a vicious circle?
- Could more appropriate antibody screening methodologies (e.g., based on live cells) finally identify autoantibodies associated with a subgroup of TS patients, and what could their pathogenic role be?
- Is there a true predisposition of TS patients to allergies, and what are the underlying mechanisms for this?
- Does the HPA axis of TS patients undergo early priming, eventually leading to HPA hyperreactivity during postnatal life and enhanced acute response to stressors? Are TS patients truly more exposed to chronic stress than typically developing subjects? Is this enhanced acute response to stressors in TS detectable also with more socially challenging types of stressor? What is the role of limbic structures (hippocampus, amygdala, lateral septum) in modulating the response to acute stress in TS patients? Are TS patients exposed to increased glucocorticoids *in utero*, and how does this influence the development of the dopaminergic system?

if one considers that also the dopamine system is especially sensitive to indicators of adversity via the maternal stress response system. In rat models, an increased exposure to glucocorticoids *in utero* may enlarge midbrain dopamine nuclei (McArthur et al., 2007) and alter the expression of genes related to dopamine transmission (e.g., the dopamine transporter gene; Son et al., 2007). Moreover, the presence of glucocorticoid receptors in the nucleus accumbens makes dopamine neurons especially reactive to stressors across the lifespan (Piazza & Moal, 1996). Therefore, the possibility that an increased intrauterine exposure to cortisol, secondary to maternal stress, might contribute to both a hypersensitive HPA axis and to a hyperresponsive dopaminergic mesolimbic system suggests a possible common denominator for motor, behavioral, and HPA-related changes in TS.

REFERENCES

Bartels M, de Geus EJ, Kirschbaum C, et al. Heritability of daytime cortisol levels in children. *Behav Genet* 2003; 33:421–433.

Bombaci M, Grifantini R, Mora M, et al. Protein array profiling of tic patient sera reveals a broad range and enhanced immune response against Group A Streptococcus antigens. *PLoS One* 2009; 4:e6332.

An important work presenting a sophisticated comparative analysis of antibody response profile in children with tics, children with acute pharyngitis, and normal children.

Bos-Veneman NG, Bijzet J, Limburg PC, et al. Cytokines and soluble adhesion molecules in children and adolescents with a tic disorder. *Prog Neuropsychopharmacol Biol Psychiatry* 2010; 34:1390–1395.

The largest-to-date cross-sectional study assessing cytokine levels in tic disorders; did not support major changes in cytokine levels in these conditions but suggested a possible relationship of cytokine release to disease expression.

Bos-Veneman NG, Olieman R, Tobiasova Z, et al. Altered immunoglobulin profiles in children with Tourette syndrome. *Brain Behav Immun* 2011; 25:532–538.

A well-conducted cross-sectional case-control study on two independent cohorts demonstrating abnormal immunoglobulin concentrations in TS children.

Boulanger LM. Immune proteins in brain development and synaptic plasticity. *Neuron* 2009; 64:93–109.

Brilot F, Merheb V, Ding A, et al. Antibody binding to neuronal surface in Sydenham chorea, but not in PANDAS or Tourette syndrome. *Neurology* 2011; 76:1508–1513.

An influential work challenging the presence of circulating antineuronal antibodies in tic disorders.

Brimberg L, Benhar I, Mascaro-Blanco A, et al. Behavioral, pharmacological, and immunological abnormalities after streptococcal exposure: a novel rat model of Sydenham chorea and related neuropsychiatric disorders. *Neuropsychopharmacology* 2012 Apr 25 [Epub ahead of print].

The first report highlighting a possible pathogenic role of antibodies targeting dopamine receptors in putatively "poststreptococcal" tic disorders.

Caine ED, Weitkamp LR, Chiverton P, et al. Tourette syndrome and HLA. *J Neurol Sci* 1985; 69:201–206.

Carney PA. Recurrence of Gilles de la Tourette syndrome. *Br Med J* 1977; 1:884.

Chang YT, Li YF, Muo CH, et al. Correlation of Tourette syndrome and allergic disease: nationwide population-based case-control study. *J Dev Behav Pediatr* 2011; 32:98–102.

Chapman F, Visvanathan K, Carreno-Manjarrez R, Zabriskie JB. A flow cytometric assay for D8/17 B cell marker in patients with Tourette's syndrome and obsessive-compulsive disorder. *J Immunol Methods* 1998; 219:181–186.

Chappell PB, Riddle M, Anderson G, et al. Enhanced stress responsivity of Tourette syndrome patients undergoing lumbar puncture. *Biol Psychiatry* 1994; 36:35–43.

The first work directly exploring and identifying increased reactivity of the HPA axis and related noradrenergic sympathetic systems in adults with TS measuring hormonal and behavioral effects of the stress induced by lumbar puncture.

Chappell PB, Leckman JF, Goodman W, et al. Elevated cerebrospinal fluid corticotrophin-releasing factor in Tourette's syndrome: comparison to obsessive-compulsive disorder and normal controls. *Biol Psychiatry* 1996; 39:776–783.

This study completes the previous one by measuring corticotrophin-releasing factor in the CSF of TS patients, differentiating them from OCD patients.

Chen SK, Tvrdik P, Peden E, et al. Hematopoietic origin of pathological grooming in Hoxb8 mutant mice. *Cell* 2010; *141*:775–785.

Church AJ, Dale RC, Giovannoni G. Anti-basal ganglia antibodies: a possible diagnostic utility in idiopathic movement disorders? *Arch Dis Childhood* 2004; 89:611–614.

Church AJ, Dale RC, Lees AJ, et al. Tourette's syndrome: a cross sectional study to examine the PANDAS hypothesis. *J Neurol Neurosurg Psychiatry* 2003; 74:602–607.

Cools N, Ponsaerts P, Van Tendeloo VFI, Berneman ZN. Regulatory T cells and human disease. *Clin Devel Immunol* 2007; 2007:89195.

Corbett BA, Mendoza SP, Baym CL, et al. Examining cortisol rhythmicity and responsivity to stress in children with Tourette syndrome. *Psychoneuroendocrinology* 2008b; 33: 810–820.

Corbett BA, Mendoza S, Wegelin JA, et al. Variable cortisol circadian rhythms in children with autism and anticipatory stress. *J Psychiatry Neurosci* 2008a; 33:227–234.

One of the most methodologically rigorous studies exploring the HPA axis in patients with TS, and the first exclusively involving children. For the first time the diurnal rhythmicity of the axis and the return to baseline following acute stress are explored, using exposure to mock and real MRI.

Crespi EJ, Denver RJ. Ancient origins of human developmental plasticity. *Am J Hum Biol* 2005; 17:44–54.

Dale RC, Candler PM, Church AJ, et al. Neuronal surface glycolytic enzymes are autoantigen targets in post-streptococcal autoimmune CNS disease. *J Neuroimmunol* 2006; 172:187–197.

Ferrari M, Termine C, Franciotta D, et al. Dopaminergic receptor D5 mRNA expression is increased in circulating lymphocytes of Tourette syndrome patients. *J Psychiat Res* 2008; 43:24–29.

The only work to date exploring dopamine receptors on the surface of lymphocytes in TS, providing a possible explanation for immunophenotyping changes in this condition.

Fontan PA, Pancholi V, Nociari MM, Fischetti VA. Antibodies to streptococcal surface enolase react with human alpha-enolase: implications in poststreptococcal sequelae. *J Infect Dis* 2000; 182:1712–1721.

Gabbay V, Coffey BJ, Guttman LE, et al. A cytokine study in children and adolescents with Tourette's disorder. *Prog Neuropsychopharmacol Biol Psychiatry* 2009; 33:967–971.

An interesting case-control cross-sectional study supporting the association between increased IL-12 serum levels and TS, and suggesting the possibility of different neuroimmunological functioning between TS with and without comorbid OCD.

Garay PA, McAllister K. Novel roles for immune molecules in neural development: implications for neurodevelopmental disorders. *Front Synaptic Neurosci* 2010; 2:136.

Gatzke-Kopp LM. The canary in the coalmine: the sensitivity of mesolimbic dopamine to environmental adversity during development. *Neurosci Biobehav Rev* 2011; 35:794–803.

Goines P, Van de Water J. The immune system's role in the biology of autism. *Curr Opin Neurol* 2010; 23:111–117.

Graeber MB. Changing face of microglia. Science 2010; 330:783-788.

Grigorenko EL, Han SS, Yrigollen CM, et al. Macrophage migration inhibitory factor and autism spectrum disorders. *Pediatrics* 2008; 122:e438–445.

Hansen CR Jr, Bershow SA. Immunology of TS/OCD. *J Am Acad Child Adolesc Psychiatry* 1997; 36:1648–1649.

Heesen C, Gold SM, Huitinga I, Reul JM. Stress and hypothalamic-pituitary-adrenal axis function in experimental autoimmune encephalomyelitis and multiple sclerosis – a review. *Psychoneuroendocrinology* 2007; 32:604–618.

Ho CS, Shen EY, Shyur SD, Chiu NC. Association of allergy with Tourette's syndrome. *J Formos Med Assoc* 1999; 98:492–495.

Hoekstra PJ, Anderson GM, Troost PW, et al. Plasma kynurenine and related measures in tic disorder patients. *Eur Child Adolesc Psychiatry* 2007; 16 Suppl 1:71–77.

Hoekstra PJ, Bijzet J, Limburg PC, et al. Elevated binding of D8/17-specific monoclonal antibody to B lymphocytes in tic disorder patients. *Am J Psychiatry* 2004a; 161:1501–1502.

Hoekstra PJ, Minderaa RB, Kallenberg CG. Lack of effect of intravenous immunoglobulins on tics: a double-blind placebo-controlled study. *J Clin Psychiatry* 2004b; 65:537–542.

Hoekstra PJ, Steenhuis MP, Kallenberg CG, Minderaa RB. Association of small life events with self reports of tic severity in pediatric and adult tic disorder patients: a prospective longitudinal study. *J Clin Psychiatry* 2004c; 65:426–431.

Hong JJ, Loiselle CR, Yoon DY, et al. Microarray analysis in Tourette syndrome post-mortem putamen. *J Neurol Sci* 2004; 225:57–64.

Although based on a very small number of specimens, this report showed for the first time abnormal expression of immune molecules in the brain of TS patients.

Jacob CM, Pastorino AC, Fahl K, et al. Autoimmunity in IgA deficiency: revisiting the role of IgA as a silent housekeeper. *J Clin Immunol* 2008; 28 Suppl 1:S56–S61.

Janeway CA Jr. Approaching the asymptote? Evolution and revolution in immunology. *Cold Spring Harb Symp Quant Biol* 1989; 54:1–13.

Jankord R, Solomon MB, Albertz J, et al. Stress vulnerability during adolescent development in rats. *Endocrinology* 2011; 152:629–638.

Kaneko M, Hoshino Y, Hashimoto S, et al. Hypothalamic-pituitary-adrenal axis function in children with attention-deficit hyperactivity disorder. *J Autism Dev Disord* 1993; 23: 59–65.

Kansy JW, Katsovich L, McIver KS, et al. Identification of pyruvate kinase as an antigen associated with Tourette syndrome. *J Neuroimmunol* 2006; 181:165–176.

Kawikova I, Leckman JF, Kronig H, et al. Decreased numbers of regulatory T cells suggest impaired immune tolerance in children with Tourette syndrome: a preliminary study. *Biol Psychiatry* 2007; 61:273–278.

The first report on the distribution of immune cell subpopulations in TS, providing preliminary evidence of downregulation of T-regulatory lymphocytes in this condition.

Kawikova I, Grady BP, Tobiasova Z, et al. Children with Tourette's syndrome may suffer immunoglobulin A dysgammaglobulinemia: preliminary report. *Biol Psychiatry* 2010; 67:679–683.

The first systematic report of IgA dysgammaglobulinemia in a subgroup of children with TS/OCD, suggesting an increased predisposition to respiratory infections in these patients.

Kirvan CA, Cox CJ, Swedo SE, Cunningham MW. Tubulin is a neuronal target of autoantibodies in Sydenham's chorea. *J Immunol* 2007; 178:7412–7421.

Kirvan CA, Swedo SE, Heuser JS, Cunningham MW. Mimicry and autoantibody-mediated neuronal cell signaling in Sydenham chorea. *Nat Med* 2003; 9:914–920.

Kirvan CA, Swedo SE, Snider LA, Cunningham MW. Antibody-mediated neuronal cell signaling in behavior and movement disorders. *J Neuroimmunol* 2006; 179:173–179.

Lawrence DM, Seth P, Durham L, et al. Astrocyte differentiation selectively upregulates CCL2/monocyte chemoattractant protein-1 in cultured human brain-derived progenitor cells. *Glia* 2006; 53:81–91.

Leckman JF, Goodman WK, Anderson GM, et al. CSF biogenic amines in obsessive-compulsive disorder, Tourette's syndrome, and healthy controls. *Neuropsychopharmacology* 1995; 12:73–86.

Leckman JF, Katsovich L, Kawikova I, et al. Increased serum levels of tumour necrosis factor-alpha and IL-12 in Tourette's syndrome. *Biol Psychiatry* 2005; 57:667–673.

The only prospective study on children/adolescents with TS/OCD to explore the correlation between cytokine serum levels and clinical severity in TS.

Lin H, Katsovich L, Ghebremichael M, et al. Psychosocial stress predicts future symptom severities in children and adolescents with Tourette syndrome and/or obsessive-compulsive disorder. *J Child Psychol Psychiatry* 2007;48:157–166.

A seminal work confirming the short-term predictive value of psychosocial stress upon the future severity of tics and obsessive-compulsive symptoms in TS.

Lin H, Williams KA, Katsovich L, et al. Streptococcal upper respiratory tract infections and psychosocial stress predict future tic and obsessive-compulsive symptom severity in children and adolescents with Tourette syndrome and obsessive-compulsive disorder. *Biol Psychiatry* 2010;67:684–691.

Lit L, Enstrom A, Sharp FR, Gilbert DL. Age-related gene expression in Tourette syndrome. *J Psychiat Res* 2009; 43:319–330.

Lit L, Gilbert DL, Walker W, Sharp FR. A subgroup of Tourette's patients overexpress specific natural killer cell genes in blood: a preliminary report. *Am J Med Genet B* 2007; 144B:958–963.

A very interesting study using a transcriptomics approach to show age-related changes in the expression of genes related to NK cell function and regulation of viral response in youngsters with TS.

Loiselle CR, Wendlandt JT, Rohde CA, Singer HS. Antistreptococcal, neuronal, and nuclear antibodies in Tourette syndrome. *Pediat Neurol* 2003; 28:119–125.

Luo F, Leckman JF, Katsovich L, et al. Prospective longitudinal study of children with tic disorders and/or obsessive-compulsive disorder: relationship of symptom exacerbations to newly acquired streptococcal infections. *Pediatrics* 2004; 113:e578–585.

A well-conducted prospective study that showed for the first time increased baseline plasma concentrations of neopterin in TS.

Martino D, Chew NK, Mir P, et al. Atypical movement disorders in antiphospholipid syndrome. *Mov Disord* 2006; 21:944–949.

Martino D, Church AJ, Defazio G, et al. Soluble adhesion molecules in Gilles de la Tourette's syndrome. *J Neurol Sci* 2005; 234:79–95.

Martino D, Defazio G, Church AJ, et al. Antineuronal antibody status and phenotype analysis in Tourette's syndrome. *Mov Disord* 2007; 22:1424–1429.

Martino D, Draganski B, Cavanna A, et al. Anti-basal ganglia antibodies and Tourette's syndrome: a voxel-based morphometry and diffusion tensor imaging study in an adult population. *J Neurol Neurosurg Psychiatry* 2008; 79:820–822.

The latter two articles showed the lack of any association between antistriatum antibodies and clinical presentation and brain volumetry in unselected patients with TS.

Martino D, Dale RC, Gilbert DL, Giovannoni G, Leckman JF. Immunopathogenic mechanisms in Tourette syndrome: a critical review. *Mov Disord* 2009; 24:1267–1279.

Martino D, Chiarotti F, Buttiglione M, et al. The relationship between group A streptococcal infections and Tourette syndrome: a study on a large service-based cohort. *Dev Med Child Neurol* 2011; 53:951–957.

Although based on a long average intervisit interval, this is the largest prospective study to date to analyze antineural autoantibodies, in addition to markers of streptococcal infection, in an unselected population of children with TS.

Mason D. Genetic variation in the stress response: susceptibility to experimental allergic encephalomyelitis and implications for human inflammatory disease. *Immunol Today* 1991; 12:57–60.

McArthur S, McHale E, Gillies GE. The size and distribution of midbrain dopaminergic populations are permanently altered by perinatal glucocorticoid exposure in a sex-, region-, and time-specific manner. *Neuropsychopharmacology* 2007; 32:1462–1476.

McEwen BS. Protective and damaging effects of stress mediators. *N Engl J Med* 1998; 338:171–179.

Medzhitov R. Approaching the asymptote: 20 years later. *Immunity* 2009; 30:766–775.

Min SK, Lee H, Park KI, et al. Tourette disorder and HLA typing. *Yonsei Med J* 1991; 32:315–318.

Moller JC, Tackenberg B, Heinzel-Gutenbrunner M, et al. Immunophenotyping in Tourette syndrome—a pilot study. *Eur J Neurol* 2008; 15:749–753.

An interesting report showing upregulation of activated T and B lymphocytes in adults with TS.

Morer A, Chae W, Henegariu O, et al. Elevated expression of MCP-1, IL-2 and PTPR-N in basal ganglia of Tourette syndrome cases. *Brain Behav Immun* 2010; 24:1069–1073.

An interesting postmortem study detecting elevated expression of monocyte chemotactic factor-1 and interleukin-2 in the brains of TS patients, supporting the existence of chronic inflammatory processes in the basal ganglia.

Morshed SA, Parveen S, Leckman JF, et al. Antibodies against neural, nuclear, cytoskeletal, and streptococcal epitopes in children and adults with Tourette's syndrome, Sydenham's chorea, and autoimmune disorders. *Biol Psychiatry* 2001; 50:566–577.

Motlagh MG, Katsovich L, Thompson N, et al. Severe psychosocial stress and heavy cigarette smoking during pregnancy: an examination of the pre- and perinatal risk factors associated with ADHD and Tourette syndrome. *Eur Child Adolesc Psychiatry* 2010; 19:755–764.

Murphy TK, Goodman WK, Fudge MW, et al. B lymphocyte antigen D8/17: a peripheral marker for childhood-onset obsessive-compulsive disorder and Tourette's syndrome? *Am J Psychiatry* 1997; 154:402–407.

Murphy TK, Storch EA, Turner A, et al. Maternal history of autoimmune disease in children presenting with tics an/or obsessive-compulsive disorder. *J Neuroimmunol* 2010; 229:243–247.

A very intriguing work showing familial predisposition to autoimmune diseases in tic disorders.

O'Donnell KJ, Bugge Jensen A, Freeman L, et al. Maternal prenatal anxiety and downregulation of placental 11β-HSD2. *Psychoneuroendocrinology* 2012; 37:818–826.

Perlmutter SJ, Leitman SF, Garvey MA, et al. Therapeutic plasma exchange and intravenous immunoglobulin for obsessive-compulsive disorder and tic disorders in childhood. *Lancet* 1999; 354:1153–1158.

Piazza PV, Moal ML. Pathophysiological basis of vulnerability to drug abuse: role of an interaction between stress, glucocorticoids, and dopaminergic neurons. *Ann Rev Pharmacol Toxicol* 1996; 36:359–378.

Price DA, Close GC, Fielding BA. Age of appearance of circadian rhythm in salivary cortisol values in infancy. *Arch Dis Child* 1983; 58:454–456.

Sandyk R, Bamford CR. Heightened cortisol response to administration of naloxone in Tourette's syndrome. *Int J Neurosci* 1988; 39:225–227.

Sarkar C, Basu B, Chakroborty D, et al. The immunoregulatory role of dopamine: an update. *Brain Behav Immun* 2010; 24:525–528.

Schoenian S, Konig I, Oertel W, et al. HLA-DRB genotyping in Gilles de la Tourette patients and their parents. *Am J Med Genet B Neuropsychiatr Genet* 2003; 119B:60–64.

Seijo-Martinez M, Mosquera-Martinez JA, Romero-Yuste S, Cruz-Martinez J. Ischemic stroke and epilepsy in a patient with Tourette's syndrome: association with the antiphospholipid syndrome and good response to levetiracetam. *Open Neurol J* 2008; 2:32–34.

Singer HS, Gause C, Morris C, et al. Serial immune markers do not correlate with clinical exacerbations in pediatric autoimmune neuropsychiatric disorders associated with streptococcal infections. *Pediatrics* 2008; 121:1198–1205.

Singer HS, Giuliano JD, Hansen BH, et al. Antibodies against a neuron-like (HTB-10 neuroblastoma) cell in children with Tourette syndrome. *Biol Psychiatry* 1999; 46:775–780.

Singer HS, Hong JJ, Yoon DY, Williams PN. Serum autoantibodies do not differentiate PANDAS and Tourette syndrome from controls. *Neurology* 2005; 65: 1701–1707.

Singer HS, Krumholz A, Giuliano J, Kiessling LS. Antiphospholipid antibodies: an epiphenomenon

in Tourette syndrome. *Mov Disord* 1997; 12:738–742.

Son GH, Chung S, Geum D, et al. Hyperactivity and alteration of the midbrain dopaminergic system in maternally stressed male mice offspring. *Biochem Biophys Res Commun* 2007; 352:823–829.

Stetler C, Miller GE. Depression and hypothalamic-pituitary-adrenal activation: a quantitative summary of four decades of research. *Psychosom Med* 2011; 73: 114–126.

Surwillo WW, Shafti M, Barrett CL. Gilles de la Tourette: a 20-month study of the effects of stressful life events and haloperidol on symptom severity. *J Nerv Ment Dis* 1978; 166:812–816.

Sweeten TL, Bowyer SL, Posey DJ, et al. Increased prevalence of familial autoimmunity in probands with pervasive developmental disorders. *Pediatrics* 2003; 112:e420.

Tang Y, Gilbert DL, Glauser TA, et al. Blood gene expression profiling of neurologic diseases: a pilot microarray study. *Arch Neurol* 2005; 62:210–215.

Toren P, Toren A, Weizman A, et al. Tourette's disorder: is there an association with the antiphospholipid syndrome? *Biol Psychiatry* 1994; 35:495–498.

Tsigos C, Chrousos GP. Hypothalamic-pituitary-adrenal axis, neuroendocrine factors and stress. *J Psychosom Res* 2002; 53:865–871.

Vargas DL, Nascimbene C, Krishnan C, et al. Neuroglial activation and neuroinflammation in the brain of patients with autism. *Ann Neurol* 2005; 57:67–81.

Weiner H. Social and psychosocial factors in autoimmune disease. In: Ader A, Felten DL, Cohen N (eds.), *Psychoneuroimmunology*. 1991. Academic Press, San Diego, pp. 955–1012.

Weisz JL, McMahon WM, Moore JC, et al. D8/17 and CD19 expression on lymphocytes of patients with acute rheumatic fever and Tourette's disorder. *Clin Diagn Lab Immunol* 2004; 11:330–336.

Wenzel C, Wurster U, Muller-Vahl KR. Oligoclonal bands in cerebrospinal fluid in patients with Tourette's syndrome. *Mov Disord* 2011; 26:343–346.

The first demonstration of intrathecal synthesis of antibodies in unselected patients with TS;

however, does not provide clear evidence of blood–brain barrier breakdown.

Wood BL, Klebba K, Gbadebo O, et al. Pilot study of effect of emotional stimuli on tic severity in children with Tourette's syndrome. *Mov Disord* 2003; *18*:1392–1395.

Yehuda R, Boisoneau D, Lowy MT, Gillel EL Jr. Dose-response changes in plasma cortisol and lymphocyte glucocorticoid receptors following dexamethasone administration in combat veterans with and without posttraumatic stress disorder. *Arch Gen Psychiatry* 1995; 52:583–593.

Yirmiya R, Goshen I. Immune modulation of learning, memory, neural plasticity and neurogenesis. *Brain Behav Immun* 2011; 25:181–213.

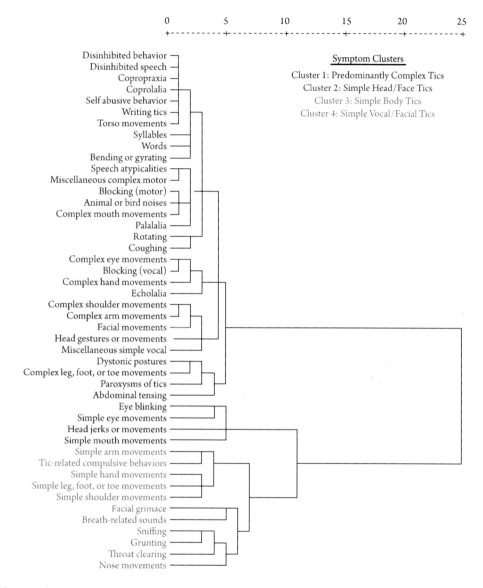

FIGURE 1.2 **Tic symptom dimensions** This figure presents the rescaled dendrogram of agglomerative hierarchical cluster analysis using Ward's method of 46 YGTSS symptom checklist items. Text colors indicate clustered symptoms.

(From Kircanski K, Woods DW, Chang SW, Ricketts EJ, Piacentini JC. Cluster analysis of the Yale Global Tic Severity Scale (YGTSS): Symptom dimensions and clinical correlates in an outpatient youth sample. *J Abnorm Child Psychol* 2010; 38:777–788.)

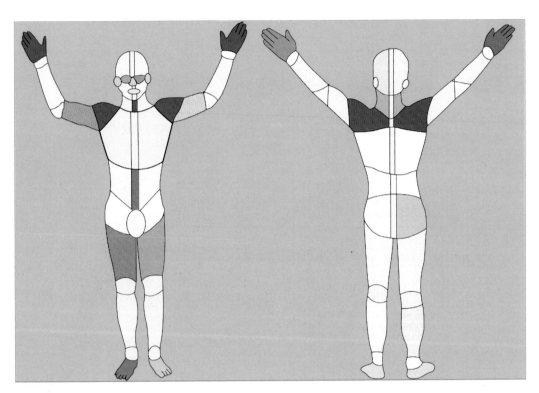

FIGURE 1.3   **Density of premonitory urges**   The densities of premonitory urges for each of 89 anatomical regions are depicted, indicating the proportion of cases that identify that body region as a site of premonitory urges. The highest density (intensity of the red color) on the scale represents the total premonitory urges per region per person, the lowest represents 0 urges per region per person, and the midpoint represents 20 urges per region per person. These data are based on current premonitory urges ever experienced as assessed in a self-report questionnaire (N = 135).

(From Leckman JF, Walker DE, Cohen DJ. Premonitory urges in Tourette syndrome. *Am J Psychiatry* 1993; *150*:98–102.)

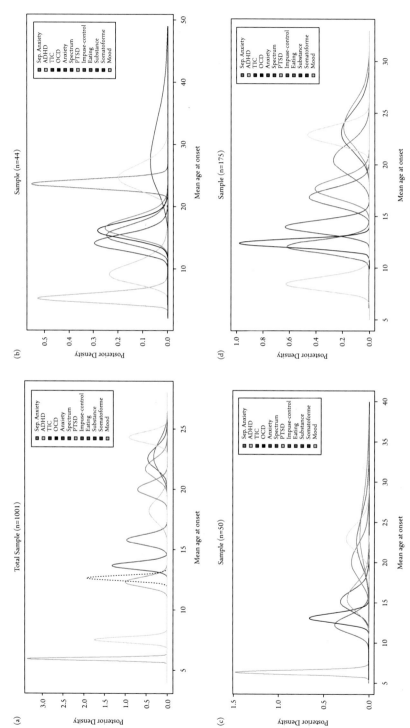

FIGURE 3.3   Psychiatric comorbidities distribution throughout the lifespan and when OCD is preceded by specific psychiatric comorbidities. Sep Anxiety, separation Anxiety; ADHD, attention-deficit/hyperactivity disorder; TIC, tic disorders; OCD, obsessive-compulsive disorder; Anxiety, generalized anxiety disorder; Spectrum, other obsessive-compulsive spectrum disorders; PTSD, posttraumatic stress disorder; impulse-control, impulse-control disorders; eating, eating disorders; Substance, substance dependence; somatoform, somatoform disorders; Mood, mood disorders; n, absolute values.

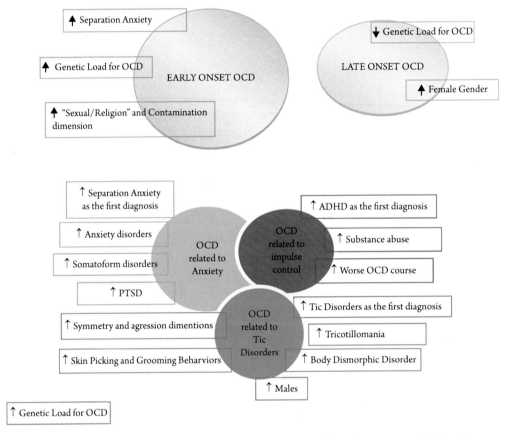

FIGURE 3.4 Models of OCD subtypes according to age at onset and psychiatric comorbid disorders. ADHD, attention-deficit/hyperactivity disorder; OCD, obsessive-compulsive disorder; PTSD, posttraumatic stress disorder.

(Adapted from de Mathis et al., personal communication).

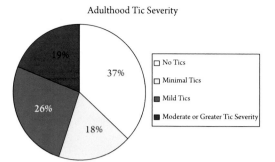

Adulthood Tic Severity

19%

37%

26%

18%

☐ No Tics
☐ Minimal Tics
■ Mild Tics
■ Moderate or Greater Tic Severity

FIGURE 5.2   **Tic severity in adulthood**   Adult tic severity in 82 children with significant childhood tic symptoms. Adult tic severity class is defined by Yale Global Tic Severity Total Tic Score (YGTSS): no tics (0), minimal tics (1–9), mild tics (10–19), moderate or greater tics (≥20). All individuals had moderate or greater severity tics in childhood. Less than 5% of individuals reported having worse tics as adults than in childhood.

(Adapted with permission from Bloch & Leckman, 2009.)

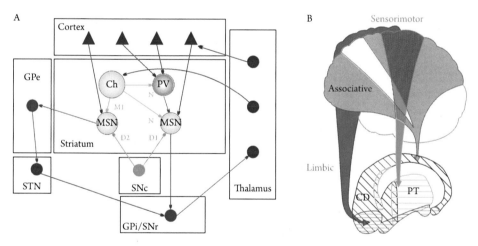

FIGURE 10.1   **The basal ganglia**   (**A**) Basal ganglia circuitry. *Red*, excitatory glutamatergic neurons; *blue*, inhibitory neurons; *green*, cholinergic neurons, *orange*, dopaminergic neurons. PV interneurons mediate the cortical feed-forward inhibition upon MSNs of the striatopallidal direct pathway, resulting in inhibition of voluntary movements. Cholinergic interneurons enhance the responsiveness of MSNs of the striatonigral indirect pathway, resulting in movement suppression. (**B**) Functional subdivisions of the basal ganglia projected on a lateral view of the basal ganglia and their cortical afferent systems.

(Based upon Parent et al., 1990, and Bernacer et al., 2007.)

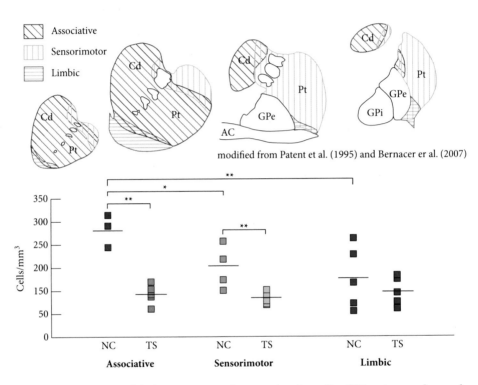

FIGURE 10.3   Distribution of cholinergic neuron density in basal ganglia of TS patients and normal controls (NC). *Red*, associative territory; *green*, somatosensory territory; *blue*, limbic territory. ** *p* < .001 by ANOVA.

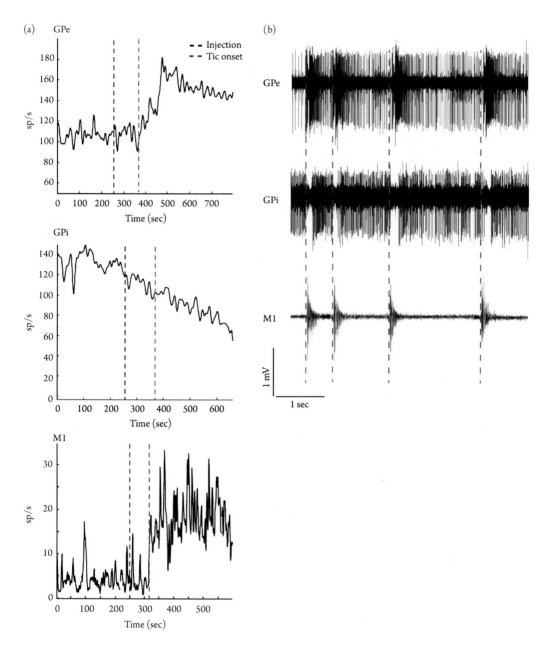

FIGURE 15.3   **Examples of tic-related neuronal activity in the globus pallidus (GP) following bicucul-line injection**   (**A**) Examples of mean firing rates from continuously recorded single primary motor cortex (M1), GP external and internal segment neurons, before and after injection, which show firing rate changes consistent with theoretical models of TS. (**B**) Examples of raw neuronal traces from M1 and both segments of the GP, which illustrate how the rate changes are phasic and locked to the appearance of tics (*red lines*).

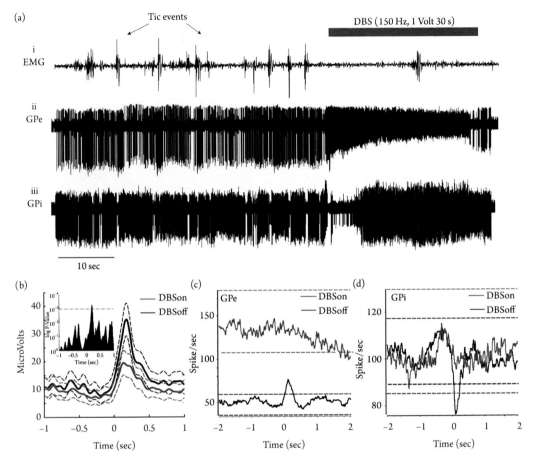

FIGURE 15.5 **EMG and neuronal data during tics with GPi HF-DBS** (**A**) Examples of raw data from EMG and neuronal activity in the pallidum after administration of bicuculline and during HF-DBS. The top trace shows EMG recorded from the orofacial region, in which the large voltage transients are tic events. The bottom two traces are simultaneous recordings from both segments of the globus pallidus (GPe and GPi) during expression of the above tics. (**B**) Quantification of the reduction in tic-related EMG peak voltage amplitude. The histogram shows the EMG signals aligned to tic onset. The inset shows a graphical representation of the *t*-test across bins between the two experimental conditions and the reduction in peak amplitude of the tic-related EMG ($p < .001$). (**C**) Modulation of activity in a GPe neuron by tics (black trace) and HF-DBS (red trace). Neuronal activity is aligned to tic onset. Note that the large increase in activity under the off-stimulation condition was abolished by HF-DBS. The *dashed lines* represent confidence intervals of 99% and are color-coded to each condition. (**D**) Modulation of activity in a GPi neuron by tics (black trace) and HF-DBS (red trace). The activity is aligned to tic onset. Note that the decrease in activity under the off-stimulation condition was abolished during HF-DBS.

From McCairn et al. High-frequency pallidal stimulation blocks tic-related neuronal activity in a non-human primate model of Tourette syndrome. *NeuroReport* 2012)

15

Animal Models of Tics

KEVIN W. MCCAIRN, YUKIO IMAMURA AND MASAKI ISODA

Abstract

This chapter summarizes the different approaches used in the development of valid animal models of tic disorders, which represent important platforms to explore pathobiological mechanisms, as well as to test and validate experimental treatments. Rodent genetic and pharmacological models have been developed throughout the years, providing useful insight into the neuroanatomy and neurochemistry of tics and related behaviors. In particular, focal microinjections of gamma-amino-butyric acid (GABA)-ergic antagonists have helped identify the role of specific structures and pathways in the basal ganglia and how they relate to discrete behaviors associated with Tourette syndrome. Immune-based models are instead aiming at identifying specific disease-causing agents and antigens, in light of the contribution of immune mechanisms to the generation of tics. Sensorimotor gating models are beginning to address the phenomenon of the premonitory urge and provide a generalized testing protocol that can be applied across the different experimental platforms that have been developed for Tourette syndrome. Continuing to combine empirical and theoretical data from the clinic and the laboratory will allow greater understanding of Tourette syndrome.

INTRODUCTION

The development of animal models of Tourette syndrome (TS) and tic disorders has been a continuing direction and goal of medical research for many years. The assumption that TS is an inherited genetic abnormality with diffuse neuroanatomical pathology influenced by environmental factors, leading to a complex profile of motor and neuropsychiatric abnormalities, has proved to make the disorder a difficult condition to model. Several animal models of TS have been reported in the scientific literature. These models primarily include both rodent and nonhuman primate (NHP) platforms, and each has been able to mimic various symptoms of the disorder through a number of different experimental manipulations. Owing to the complex etiology of TS, a single, specific model representative of all the underlying pathologies and symptom profiles has proved elusive. The purpose of this review will be to summarize the major advances in the development of TS experimental models, and to compare and contrast their relative strengths and weaknesses, with a view to suggesting future refinements and research directions.

As a clinical condition, the symptoms of TS are wide-ranging and include both motor and neuropsychiatric abnormalities. The involuntary movements associated with the disorder, generally termed tics, vary in form, severity, and anatomical position on a patient-by-patient basis. Tics range from short "myoclonus-like" jerks that involve only one or a few muscles, to complex motor or vocal tics that involve sequential activation of several muscle groups that overlap with neuropsychiatric abnormalities. The neuropsychiatric comorbidities associated with TS are generally considered to involve obsessive-compulsive disorder (OCD), attention-deficit/hyperactivity disorder (ADHD), learning difficulties, and sleep perturbations, with patients also at risk for depression and anxiety (Gilles de la Tourette, 1885; Obeso et al., 1982; Tourette Syndrome Classification

Study Group, 1993). The current state of the art strongly suggests that TS is a disorder of cortico–basal ganglia–thalamic circuits (CBTCs), with some studies emphasizing the structures of the basal ganglia (Albin & Mink, 2006; Mink, 2001; Peterson, 2001) and others suggesting structural changes in the cortex, specifically the frontal, anterior cingulate, parietal, and temporal regions (Peterson, 2001; Sowell et al., 2008; Worbe et al., 2010). The underlying reasons for the disorder, however, remain obscure, with evidence linking both genetic and environmental factors (Abelson et al., 2005; Kurlan, 1998; Paschou et al., 2004).

In this chapter, we first summarize the anatomical and functional organization of CBTCs, with particular emphasis on the three functional subdivisions in each node (motor, associative, and limbic) and two parallel pathways in each subdivision (direct and indirect). This basic concept is of particular importance in understanding the pathophysiology of TS and thus developing its animal models. We then outline three validity criteria that a TS animal should satisfy to be a clinically desirable model. Finally, we review five major categories and techniques of animal models. These include transgenic intervention in rodents, systemic injections of pharmacological compounds, exposure to TS-related immunoreactive sera, local and site-specific microinjections of pharmacological substances, and sensory gating models.

CORTICO–BASAL GANGLIA–THALAMIC CIRCUITS

CBTCs are found in the central nervous system (CNS) of all vertebrates. The anatomical connections of these nuclei and their pharmacology appear to be relatively conserved across species, thus allowing translational research from a number of different experimental platforms. To understand the contribution of animal models to TS and tic research, it is necessary to clarify the anatomy of the basal ganglia, the role of neurotransmitters at each critical node, and the influence of the "indirect" and "direct" pathways. Further discussion on the neural circuits believed to be involved in TS symptoms can be found in Chapters 12 and 13.

Striatum

It has been shown that the principal input node (striatum) to the basal ganglia receives a large, segregated projection from the cortical mantle. When examining the results of gross histological analysis, using anatomical tracers, it can be seen that the projections from each cortical area terminate in longitudinal bands within the striatum (Selemon & Goldman-Rakic, 1985). The projections from the cortex to the striatum are glutamatergic and excitatory (Kemp & Powell, 1970), and have been described as a functional tripartite division of motor, associative, and limbic projections (Francois et al., 2004; Parent & Hazrati, 1995; Percheron & Filion, 1991). This tripartite division has been proposed to further consist of five functional circuits (two motor, two associative, and one limbic), as demonstrated by transneuronal transport of viral vectors (Alexander et al., 1986; Hoover & Strick, 1993). For example, the data from transneuronal viral studies show that the motor circuits originate from the primary (M1), premotor (PM), and supplementary motor area (SMA) cortices, they project primarily to the putamen (a subdivision of the striatum) and then to the pallidal/nigral complex, and, from there, they terminate in the ventrolateral regions of the thalamus. A schematic of the topography of the principal circuits is shown in Figure 15.1A. Although in the scientific literature there is a consensus that a topographical relationship exists between the functional areas of the cortex and the striatum, it is also acknowledged that there is a great deal of convergence/divergence—that is, inputs from more than one cortical area project onto the same area of the striatum, or inputs from one area of the cortex spread to innervate several patches of striatum (Flaherty & Graybiel, 1991, 1994).

The striatum is further anatomically divided into striosomal (patch) and extrastriosomal (matrix) compartments (see also Chapters 10 and 13). The heterogeneity of the two compartments is clear from both the macroscopic and molecular (neurotransmitter) perspectives. The gross morphological differences can be observed after staining for choline acetyltransferase activity, with the striosomal compartments staining weakly compared with the matrix (Graybiel & Ragsdale Jr., 1978, 1980). The striosomal compartments are also characterized by low levels of expression of D2 dopamine receptor binding sites, and low enkephalin, substance P (neurokinin 1) receptors, and diacylglycerol n-regulated guanine nucleotide exchange factor 1 (CalDAG-GEF1) immunoreactivity. The matrix compartment, by contrast, is characterized by high levels of D2 dopamine receptors and high enkephalin and calbindin immunoreactivity (Graybiel, 1990; Jakab et al., 1996; Kawasaki et al., 1998).

Direct and Indirect Pathways

The principal efferent target of the striatum is the globus pallidus (Szabo, 1967). Numerous studies have implied the presence of two pathways for each of the functional circuits described previously, which pass from the striatum to the globus pallidus (Albin et al., 1989, 1995; DeLong, 1990). In these early "box-and-arrow" models it is assumed that the pathways through the basal ganglia influence behavior by reducing or facilitating overall cortical excitability, through changes in tonic activity at the output of the basal ganglia. These pathways are referred to on the basis of their anatomical and physiological properties as the "direct" and "indirect" pathways (Fig. 15.1B). It has been proposed that the direct pathway has an overall excitatory effect on a particular area of the cortex that sends projections to the basal ganglia, whereas the indirect pathway produces a net inhibitory effect. The underlying physiology of these two opposite effects has been proposed to lie in the distribution, phenotype, and efferent targets of the cells at each functional layer of the direct and indirect pathway within the basal ganglia.

In summary, the direct pathway receives glutamatergic projections from the cortex, which form synapses onto gamma-aminobutyric acid (GABA) medium dense spiny neurons (MSNs) within the striatum (Wilson & Groves, 1980). These cells predominantly express D1 dopamine subtype receptors and also express the neuropeptides substance P and dynorphin as co-transmitters with GABA. The MSNs of the direct pathway are believed to project preferentially to the output nucleus of the basal ganglia, the globus pallidus internus (GPi) and substantia nigra pars reticulata (SNr) (Albin et al., 1989; Parent et al., 1989). The physiological consequence of GABAergic projections from the striatum onto the GPi/SNr is inhibition of tonically active GPi/SNr cells when MSNs are activated by excitatory cortical inputs. This inhibition of GPi cells disinhibits downstream pallidal receiving ventral anterior (VA) and ventral lateral thalamic (VL) neurons. The increase in the activity of thalamic neurons then facilitates the corresponding area of the cortex. The SNr also projects to the thalamus but has large efferents to the superior colliculus and mesopontine tegmentum (Carpenter et al., 1976; Hikosaka & Wurtz, 1983; Mehler & Nauta, 1974).

The indirect pathway also receives glutamatergic excitatory inputs from the cortex. These excitatory projections then synapse onto MSNs that predominantly express D2 dopamine subtype receptors and utilize GABA and enkephalin as their co-transmitters. The principal difference between D1 and D2 MSNs is their efferent targets. The cells that predominantly express D2 receptors project preferentially to the external segment of the globus pallidus (GPe), which in turn projects to the subthalamic nucleus (STN) (Szabo, 1967). The STN in turn sends excitatory glutamatergic projections to the output nuclei of the basal ganglia (Nauta & Cole, 1974, 1978; Parent et al., 1989). The effect of these inhibitory projections to the STN from the GPe is to increase tonic STN activity when indirect pathway MSNs are activated by cortical inputs, thus reducing inhibitory outflow from the GPe to the STN. The reduction of inhibition to the STN has a net effect of inhibiting the pallidal receiving areas of the thalamus by increasing the level of tonic inhibitory output from the GPi. The contribution of the STN to the indirect pathway is further complicated by direct cortical projections to the STN, often referred to as the "hyper-direct" pathway (Kitai & Deniau, 1981; Nambu et al., 1997; Rouzaire-Dubois & Scarnati, 1985). Studies in NHPs have shown that activation of the hyper-direct pathway induces an early and late excitation in the external segment of the globus pallidus (Nambu et al., 1990, 2000). For the purpose of this review, specific attention will be focused on the internal pathways of the basal ganglia, the indirect and direct pathways, and their roles in generating tics and other associated symptoms of TS.

Globus Pallidus

The globus pallidus plays a major role in processing neuronal information that passes through the different pathways of the striatum. The pallidal complex is divided into two major nuclei, the GPe and GPi. Classical organizational schemes of the GPe view this nucleus as a principal relay of the indirect pathway (Gerfen & Wilson, 1996; Smith et al., 1998). As well as a large efferent projection to the STN, the GPe also sends projections to the GPi (Hazrati et al., 1990; Smith et al., 1994), the thalamic reticular nucleus (Hazrati & Parent, 1991), and back to the striatum (Beckstead, 1983; Kita et al., 1999). Golgi studies of GPe neurons have shown the cells as having large dendritic trees that are orthogonal to the incoming striatal inputs (Francois et al., 1984b; Yelnik et al., 1984), suggesting that large regions of the striatum converge onto pallidal cells. Similarly to the striatum, the globus pallidus is believed to be composed of functional territories that are dependent on the principal striatal inputs that they receive. These territories are described as limbic for the anterior ventral component of the nucleus, with the dorsolateral region receiving projections from the dorsolateral/associative territories of the striatum, whereas the posterior regions are believed to be primarily involved in sensorimotor function (Francois et al., 1984a; Haber et al., 1990; Hedreen & DeLong, 1991; Parent et al., 1984; Smith & Parent, 1986). Additional evidence for the distribution of the pallidum into functional territories has been obtained by calbindin (Cb) immunohistochemical staining. This staining technique has shown a gradient of Cb staining that correlates closely to the striatal inputs to the pallidum; high Cb intensity is found in areas that receive projections from the limbic territories, and progressively weaker staining is found toward the sensorimotor territories (Francois et al., 1994; Kita, 2007). Similar to the GPe, the GPi/SNr complex also has cells with large dendritic trees orthogonal to the lateral border and efferent projections entering the nucleus (Francois et al., 1984b; Yelnik et al., 1984). Like the GPe, the GPi has been proposed to have a functional segregation into "motor," "limbic," and "sensorimotor" territories (Baron et al., 2001; Shink et al., 1997; Sidibe et al., 1997). Recent studies, however, have suggested a more divergent pattern for the efferents that project from the GPi (Parent & Parent, 2004).

Under normal conditions, the firing properties of the majority of globus pallidus cells can be described as a semi-Poisson process in which cells fire at a high frequency. The GPe is characterized by having a slightly lower mean firing rate than the GPi, with intermittent pausing activity. However, small subpopulations of cells within the pallidal complex have been identified and are classified by their low frequency of firing and their ability to fire bursts of action potentials (DeLong, 1971, 1972; Gardiner & Kitai, 1992; Magill et al., 2000). Encoding of behavioral parameters in neuronal activity is also dependent on the context of the action (i.e., whether the task being performed is guided by sensory cues or memory) (Turner & Anderson, 2005). Normal globus pallidus firing activity is also characterized by the absence of any significant low-frequency oscillatory and correlated behavior between neighboring and distant neurons in the spectral and temporal domains (Bergman et al., 1998; Nini et al., 1995). For a review and discussion on the implications of the latest findings relating to pallidal anatomy and physiology, see Parent and colleagues (2001) and Nambu (2008).

Beyond the Static Box-and-Arrow Model

The proposed reason for the distribution of excitatory and inhibitory effects converging onto the pallidal/output nuclei of the basal ganglia is that the basal ganglia are actively selecting motor programs and behavioral routines while suppressing others. In early models, these findings were used to construct a hypothesis of

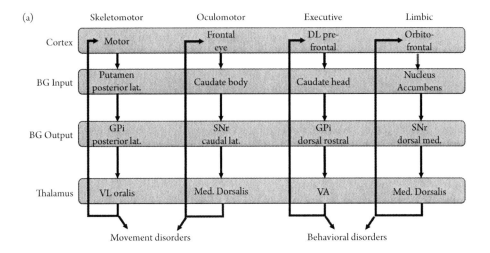

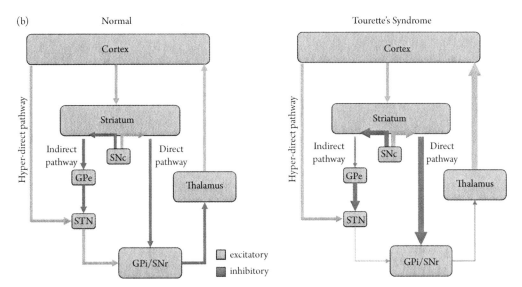

FIGURE 15.1   The cortico–basal ganglia–thalamic loop.   (A) The parallel organization of proposed CBTCs and their distribution into the tripartite functional divisions of motor, associative/executive, and limbic circuits. Movement disorders are believed to manifest as dysfunctions of the sensorimotor circuits and behavioral disorders as abnormal functioning within the associative and limbic circuits. (Adapted from Alexander et al., 1986.) **(B)** Examples of inhibitory and excitatory pathways underlying basal ganglia function in the normal and the hyperkinetic TS condition. Under the normal condition, interplay between the intrinsic pathways of the CBTC is hypothesized to allow for normal execution of behavior. In TS, the manifestation of a hypothesized focal abnormality at the level of the striatum leads to an imbalance between the indirect and direct pathways, such that inhibitory outflow from the basal ganglia is reduced. This leads to disinhibition of the thalamocortical circuits and release of pathological behavior.

(Adapted from Albin et al., 1989.)

basal ganglia dysfunction leading to hypo- and hyperkinetic disorders in the context of the "box-and-arrow" model (Albin et al., 1989; DeLong, 1990). In this model, it is assumed that the basal ganglia influence behavior by changing (reducing or facilitating) overall cortical excitability through the interplay of the direct (striatum → GPi) and indirect (striatum → GPe → STN → GPi) pathways. According to this model, hyperkinetic disorders are a result of increased excitability of the cortex owing to a reduction in GPi activity, caused either by a loss of excitatory drive from the STN or by an increase in the level of inhibitory signaling from the GPe and/or striatum (Albin et al., 1989; DeLong & Wichmann, 2007). These models, however, do not differentiate between different hyperkinetic disorders and do not address the specific pathophysiology underlying TS; they are also limited by the assumption that tonic activity in each principal node of the CBTCs is the important factor in symptom generation. More details with respect to the underlying pathophysiology of TS can be found in Chapters 12 and 13.

Addressing the specific temporal and spatial properties of both normal behavior and abnormal symptoms associated with basal ganglia disorders requires more detailed models. Network-level models were based on the basic concepts of the box-and-arrow model, and extended them to incorporate interactions within the nuclei to view the basal ganglia as performing a process of "action selection." In these models, the basal ganglia are viewed as initiating or modulating behavior by choosing one or more actions out of a multitude of actions presented to them by the cortex (Beiser & Houk, 1998; Isoda & Hikosaka, 2007, 2008; Redgrave et al., 1999; Tepper et al., 2004). Thus, in the normal state, increased activity in a small group of striatal neurons leads to a focused inhibition of a group of pallidal neurons. This is accompanied by diffuse activation of the rest of the nucleus via opposing signals through the direct and indirect pathways. This activation pattern in the basal ganglia output structure leads in turn to the disinhibition or release of a specific cortical-driven behavior, while suppressing all other competing behaviors (Mink, 1996). In the context of basal ganglia-related hyperkinetic disorders, on the basis of these models it is predicted that a dysfunction within the basal ganglia circuit could lead to the impaired inhibition of competing actions (Mink, 2003). In particular, the expression of tics is viewed as a focal excitatory abnormality in the striatum. This abnormality causes the formation of an erroneously inhibited group of neurons in the GPi that leads to disinhibition of cortical neurons that release a tic (Fig.

15.1B). It is then presumed from these models that a similar perturbation in the associative and limbic regions of the striatum would lead to the neuropsychiatric/complex motor abnormalities associated with TS (Albin & Mink, 2006; Mink, 2001). A major goal for animal models is to determine whether the theoretical models based on known anatomy and physiology are germane to the clinical condition of TS.

VALIDITY CRITERIA FOR DEVELOPING ANIMAL MODELS

Development of preclinical animal models requires that the experimental platform satisfy one of three major validity criteria: face, predictive, and construct criteria. The number of criteria that the model satisfies is generally considered to be a marker of the relevance of the model to a clinical condition, and the robustness of the findings that can be extrapolated from the model (Swerdlow & Sutherland, 2006). Face validity is reached when the model in question demonstrates phenomenological behavioral symptoms that are similar to the clinical condition. Predictive validity is dependent on data from the model validating clinical observation, for example the effect of different drugs or treatments on symptom profiles. Construct validity requires that the theoretical basis underlying the model matches pathophysiological observations in patients. An example of a basal ganglia preclinical model with a very high validity is the NHP 1-methyl-4-phenyl-1,2,3,6-tetrahydropyridine (MPTP) model for Parkinson's disease. In this model, systemic administration of MPTP, a dopaminergic neuron-specific toxin, induces a hypokinetic syndrome, which mimics many of the behavioral and neurophysiological characteristics of the clinical disorder. This hypokinetic syndrome is also responsive to many of the same treatment modalities that are used to treat the disorder, for example drugs and surgical interventions, and thus satisfies each of the validity criteria expected from an animal model. Any animal model of simple and complex motor tics should, like the MPTP model, be able to satisfy all the expected criteria for a clinically relevant model.

Currently, the major animal models of tics can be classed into five different categories: systemic challenge with psychomotor stimulants, systemic challenge with TS-related immunoreactive sera, transgenic models in rodents, sensorimotor gating models, and circuit-specific intracerebral microinjection of drugs and immunoreactive sera into rodents and primates. Due to the complex etiology of TS, it has been suggested that each of the preclinical models currently available to researchers lacks some degree of accepted validity that would be desirable in an animal model of TS (for discussion see Swerdlow & Sutherland, 2006). This does not mean, though, that insights into the disorder cannot be gained by careful utilization of existing methods and theoretical insights into cortico–basal ganglia function.

ANIMAL MODELS OF TICS

Genetic Models

Genetic abnormalities have long been postulated to play a causal role in TS, and further discussion with specific relevance to the genetic basis of TS can be found in Chapter 7. A number of rodent genetic platforms have been proposed as putative models for TS. Many of these models have focused on the "dopamine hypothesis" and include dopamine (DA)-transporter knockout mice, in which a hyperdopaminergic state is induced (Berridge et al., 2005), transgenic mice in which D1 receptors are targeted (McGrath et al., 2000; Nordstrom & Burton, 2002), and a D3 receptor gene knockout mouse (Accili et al., 1996). These rodent models are hypothesized to mimic the biochemical abnormalities in TS patients and show TS-like behaviors, including complex stereotypy and disorders of attention (for review, see Comings, 2001). Although clinical, pharmacological, and animal studies point to DA abnormalities as a causative factor in TS, the role of DA in TS would appear to be complicated further by interactions with other neurotransmitters (i.e., glutamate, serotonin [5-HT], and histamine). The use of transgenic models is beginning to elucidate these interactions and

how these interactions may be compromised in TS.

As discussed in the introduction, cortical inputs to the basal ganglia predominantly utilize glutamate, an excitatory neurotransmitter. It has been demonstrated that activation of corticolimbic neurotransmission by glutamate exacerbates the TS- and OCD-like symptoms in an animal model of TS, whereas a glutamate antagonist alleviates such symptoms (McGrath et al., 2000). In addition to the effects of glutamatergic neurotransmission itself on TS, glutamate is also modulated by DA receptor activity. To clarify the pathogenesis of TS from DA-modified glutamate receptor activation, Nordstrom and Burton (2002) generated transgenic mice that show potentiation of glutamate receptor activity via induction by a cholera neurotoxin in D1 receptor-expressing neurons. In these mice, when D1 receptors are activated by the toxin, glutamatergic synaptic transmission is activated. These transgenic mice show OCD-like behavior and other typical symptoms of TS.

Another potential genetic model with relevance to TS is the discovery of the *Slit and Trk-like family member (SLITRK1)* gene (Aruga & Mikoshiba, 2003), with *SLITRK1* genes having been identified as a candidate responsible for TS (Abelson et al., 2005; Deng et al., 2006). The *Slit and Trk-like* family consists of six members that encode a number of leucine-rich transmembrane proteins. It has been suggested that *SLITRK* genes are responsible for cell migration, axonal targeting, and neuronal differentiation. Overexpression of *SLITRK1* induces neuronal outgrowth extension, whereas *SLITRK2-6* inhibits that extension (Aruga & Mikoshiba, 2003). *TRK* encodes a neurotrophin that regulates synaptic plasticity and affects neuronal survival and differentiation. *SLITRK* genes are predominantly expressed in the cortex, thalamus, and basal ganglia in the embryonic and postnatal mouse brain. A number of rodent models with putative symptom profiles similar to TS, focusing on the SLITRK genes, have recently been published, thus further implicating this family of genes in the pathogenesis of TS. A rodent/mouse TS model deficient in *SLITRK1* has recently been developed and proposed to show abnormalities in behavior. The SLITRK1-deficient mice exhibit elevated anxiety and immobility (Katayama et al., 2010); however, the SLITRK1 knockout mouse model lacks a certain degree of face validity in terms of the type of symptoms they express. A more phenotypically relevant model is the SLITRK5 knockout rodent; this particular model does display behavioral abnormalities that are more analogous to the symptoms expressed in TS, and include excessive self-grooming and elevated anxiety levels. In conjunction with the behavioral abnormalities, SLITRK5-deficient mice show selective overactivation of the orbitofrontal cortex (a key node in the limbic circuitry), with concurrent abnormalities in striatal cell morphology and deviations in glutamate receptor composition, which are partially recovered by administration of fluoxetine (Shmelkov et al., 2010). The identification of specific polymorphisms and mutations is an important development in the field of TS animal models, and opens research directions with respect to how developmental abnormalities contribute to the symptoms associated with TS. For a review on the emerging role of the SLITRK gene family in TS, see Proenca and colleagues (2011).

There are also a number of other genetic models that model OCD-like behavior and are of direct relevance to TS. The first of these is the SAPAP3 mutant mouse (SAP90/PSD95-associated protein); this model emphasizes the importance of corticostriatal projections and CBTC networks in TS. SAPAP family proteins are molecules that are associated with postsynaptic density components of excitatory neuronal synapses, and are believed to be scaffolding complexes vital for trafficking and targeting neurotransmitter receptors and signaling molecules. The SAPAP3 knockout mouse shows obsessive-type grooming, electrophysiological, biochemical, and structural abnormalities, which are rescued by lentiviral-mediated expression of SAPAP3 (Welch et al., 2007).

The Hoxb8 mutant mouse is another model relevant to TS, and can be considered an atypical model, as the underlying pathology of the platform differs from common theoretical models of the disorder. Hox genes are normally associated with embryonic development and the establishment of core body plans along the axis of the embryo (Capecchi, 1997). They are also involved in the development of multiple tissues and organs and, of particular relevance to this model, the hematopoietic system and its role in maintenance and differentiation of myeloid progenitor cells, which are precursors of microglia (Perkins & Cory, 1993). Hoxb8 mutant mice show pathological stereotypical behavior, which manifests as excessive grooming. What is of particular importance from this model is that it removes the emphasis from abnormalities in projection neurons that form part of the CBTCs and brainstem circuits that have been identified for grooming behavior and form the basis of current models, and instead highlights the importance of microglia (Chen et al., 2010).

Recent studies have begun to implicate histamine as a neurotransmitter, which may be implicated in the pathogenesis of TS. These studies suggest that low levels of histamine within the basal ganglia may cause the symptoms associated with the disorder (Collins, 2011; Ercan-Sencicek et al., 2010). Histamine has been identified as a key basal ganglia neurotransmitter after high levels of the rate-limiting enzyme for histamine synthesis, L-histidine decarboxylase (HDC), were found in the striatum of rodents (Krusong et al., 2011). HDC knockout mice do show behavioral abnormalities, which might be of relevance to modeling TS, including abnormalities in locomotion, and interestingly hypersensitivity to challenge with DA agonists (Kubota et al., 2002; Ohtsu & Watanabe, 2003).

Another genetic model of relevance to TS is the dtsz hamster, which is a model of non-kinesiogenic paroxysmal dystonia (Loscher et al., 1989; Richter & Loscher, 1998). Although dystonia is a distinct neurological condition that presents differently from TS, there is a class of tics that do have a dystonic nature (see Chapter 1); these tics, like dystonia, involve repetitive gyrating, bending, and twisting movements. As a consequence of both disorders theoretically being hyperkinetic basal ganglia-mediated conditions, there are several interesting pathological correlates between the model and idiopathic TS that bear closer scrutiny. A recent groundbreaking study on postmortem TS brains has emphasized abnormalities in the distribution of inhibitory GABAergic fast-spiking neurons within the basal ganglia of TS patients, suggesting that the underlying cause may not be a disorder of monoamines, but instead a consequence of abnormal GABAergic processing (Kalanithi et al., 2005; Kataoka et al., 2010; see also Chapter 10). It has been reported that the *dtsz* hamster possesses a similar anatomical abnormality of reduced GABAergic fast-spiking neurons (Gernert et al., 2000), and, like in TS patients, the presentation of symptoms seems to follow the same time course, with gradual worsening and peak severity at early adolescence, and improvements as the subjects mature and reach adulthood (Hamann et al., 2005; Loscher et al., 1989). The *dtsz* hamster also displays electrophysiological abnormalities in the output nuclei of the basal ganglia consistent with hyperkinetic disorder predictions from the box-and-arrow models (Gernert et al., 2000; Leblois et al., 2010). This lends support to the hypothesis that decreased and aberrant output from the basal ganglia is a key feature of hyperkinetic basal ganglia-mediated pathologies. Obviously more research needs to be done with respect to the *dtsz* model to determine if it does satisfy validity criteria as a model for TS, but the parallel pathologies that have been identified would appear to suggest that the model warrants further study.

Systemic Administration of Pharmacological Compounds

There are a number of different compounds that when administered systemically (i.e., intramuscularly) can induce repetitive stereotyped behavior in test subjects—the principal drugs among these are those that modulate monoamines, especially DA and 5-HT. In TS, the hypothesis that DA plays an integral part of TS pathophysiology has been a central tenet of theories to explain the pathophysiology of tic behavior (for review see Albin & Mink, 2006; Albin, 2006). Changes in DA transmission have reportedly been observed in TS patients using positron emission tomography (PET; Singer et al., 2002; see also Chapter 13), and DA antagonists

(e.g., haloperidol, a postsynaptic D2 receptor antagonist) are routinely given to TS patients and those suffering from tic disorders to control their symptoms (Ross & Moldofsky, 1978; Seignot, 1961; Shapiro et al., 1983). A number of experiments have provided evidence for the role of DA in TS and have demonstrated that a hyperdopaminergic tone induced by systemic administration of DA agonists (e.g., amphetamine) can induce stereotypic behaviors, a form of complex motor tic (Randrup et al., 1963; for review see Randrup & Munkvad, 1974). Recent work has shown that induction of stereotypy through the use of systemically administered DA agonists is accompanied by specific genetic activation of the striatum and cerebral cortex, in particular upregulation of the *fos-jun* family in striatal striosomes, which are markers of early gene transcription (Canales & Graybiel, 2000a, 2000b; Graybiel et al., 1990). Importantly, these groundbreaking studies show that the ratio of striosomal to matrix early gene expression increases and is tightly correlated to the intensity of the stereotypies. Striosomes have been shown to receive inputs from limbic networks in the cortex (i.e., anterior cingulate and orbitofrontal cortex) and project to the dopaminergic substantia nigra (Bolam et al., 2000; Gerfen, 1992; Haber et al., 1995). This anatomical configuration and enhancement of striosomal activity are hypothesized to induce complex motor tics, because an increased DA level alters normal processing of reward saliency and behavioral reinforcement, thus decreasing the range of expressed behaviors and increasing the number of repetitions of selected behaviors.

These studies provided a valuable insight into the circuitry of complex motor and simple tics, and have emphasized the role of DA and the striosomes in TS and OCD spectrum disorders. It is, however, not clear, owing in part to the lack of specificity of the manipulation (i.e., systemic administration of the DA agonist), whether the abnormal activity or recruitment of cortical areas that project preferentially to the striosomes leads to the increased activity in this particular striatal compartment, or if an intrinsic plastic change within the striosomes is responsible for the abnormal behavior. Also, DA receptors are present in other critical nodes of the basal ganglia complex and can thus directly or indirectly affect each of the nuclei in an unpredictable manner (Smith & Kieval, 2000). There have been recent attempts in rodents to address this question; however, the method of administration was not through a systemic route. Stereotypies were induced by co-activating D1 and D2 striatal receptors using focal microinjection of DA agonists, and single-cell activity was monitored in the basal ganglia output nuclei SNr. The results of this series of investigations showed that the level of basal ganglia inhibitory output following focal activation of the striatal DA system becomes highly variable, with a general net increase of inhibitory output. These observations would appear to question the validity of decreased pallidal output as a requirement for the induction of tic states (Waszczak et al., 2001, 2002) and stand in contrast to the obvious decreases observed in studies utilizing focal administration of GABA antagonists (see later discussion).

Recent work utilizing systemic delivery of DA agonists and antagonists has identified differential stereotypic behavioral profiles depending on whether D1 receptors are stimulated through direct D1 specific agonists, or are upregulated through chronic exposure to specific D1 antagonists (Taylor et al., 2010). When animals are acutely exposed to D1 agonists they engage in sequential super-stereotypy, whereby they overexpress complete grooming chains. In contrast, sudden withdrawal of D1 antagonists, which leads to a rapid upregulation of D1 receptors, induces simple stereotypies that include intense scratching and biting behaviors. As OCD behavior in TS can range from complex sequential movements to short simple tics, this model may provide insights into the different nature and heterogeneity of OCD behavior and simple tics associated with the disorder.

In addition to systemic administration of DA as a method for inducing tics, other work has focused on 5-HT. Similar to DA, 5-HT is a monoamine neurotransmitter that mediates synaptic transmission in a number of key CNS regions, including the basal ganglia, hypothalamus, and brainstem. Pharmacological evidence from clinical studies suggests that several compounds that modulate 5-HT activity are effective for tic treatment. These include ondansetron, a 5-HT3 antagonist (Rizzo et al., 2008; Toren et al., 1999); tetrabenazine, an inhibitor of the 5-HT vesicular neurotransmitter transporter (Gros & Schuldiner, 2010; Jankovic & Orman, 1988); and olanzapine, a neuroleptic drug that functions as an antagonist of 5-HT-2A/2C and D2 receptors (Budman et al., 2001). In addition, serotonin reuptake inhibitors (SSRIs) have been utilized for the treatment of TS and tic disorders (Jimenez-Jimenez & Garcia-Ruiz, 2001; Silay & Jankovic, 2005).

It has been known for some time that systemic exposure to 2,5-dimethoxy-4-iodophenyl-2-aminopropane (DOI), a 5-HT receptor agonist, induces head twitches (Colpaert & Janssen, 1983; Peroutka et al., 1981), which are believed to be phenomenologically similar to the motor tics seen in TS patients (Handley & Dursun, 1992; Tizabi et al., 2001). The tics induced by DOI have been shown to be modulated by co-administration of cholinergic agonists (e.g. donepezil, an acetylcholine esterase inhibitor, or nicotine, an agonist of nicotinic acetylcholine receptors (nAChR)), and DA antagonists e.g. haloperidol. Correlated with the amelioration of DOI-induced head twitches, nicotine was found to increase 5-HT receptor expression in the striatum and cerebellum, but caused no change in midbrain receptor levels (Hayslett & Tizabi, 2005; Tizabi et al., 2001). Conversely, donepezil- and haloperidol-induced attenuation of DOI-induced head twitches was correlated with decreased 5-HT levels in the frontal cortex (Hayslett & Tizabi, 2005). This specific animal model has thus emphasized that the relative levels of relevant neurotransmitters in relation to each other, and their effects on the upregulation and downregulation of receptors at anatomically distinct sites, are important factors to consider in the development of TS symptoms. The behavioral profile and transmitter distribution reported with this model, would benefit from an analysis of the fast electrophysiological responses associated with the changes in each of the key nuclei of the CBTCs.

Exposure to TS-Related Immunoreactive Sera

Immune-related pathophysiology in the etiology of TS has been suggested for many years (Leonard et al., 1992; Swedo et al., 1998; see also Chapter 14). Available evidence suggests that in some susceptible individuals, TS may result from exposure to group A β-hemolytic streptococcal infection (GABHS), an entity known as pediatric autoimmune neuropsychiatric disorders associated with streptococcal infections (PANDAS; for a broad discussion on this topic, see Chapter 9). Recent studies from several groups (Hallett et al., 2000; Liu et al., 2008; Taylor et al., 2002) have shown that sera from TS patients are capable of inducing complex motor tics when infused into the striatum of rodents. These symptoms included excessive licking/grooming, head shaking, and vocalizations. A recent study utilizing immunohistochemical staining and ELISA methods (i.e., detection of subtle changes in protein expression) indicated that in the TS serum-infused rat model, the DA expression level in the striatum is significantly higher than that in the sham-operated control group (i.e., surgical operation without the TS serum infusion), and the 5-HT level in the striatum is significantly lower (Jijun et al., 2010).

Other studies using intrastriatal infusion of TS sera, however, have shown a lack of behavioral abnormalities following infusion of sera/basal ganglia-specific antibodies from TS patients (Loiselle et al., 2004; Singer et al., 2005). Obviously, a TS model that is reproducible using intrastriatal infusion of TS sera would lead to a greater understanding of the disorder and the underlying pathology; however, until the results are replicable, the contributions such models make are going to be limited. Specifically, if the models do become reproducible, the neurophysiological and pathological correlates of the induced symptoms (electrophysiological, molecular, genetic, and anatomical) need to be explored at a network level through CBTCs.

Another immunoreactive model with relevance to TS utilizes systemic administration of GABHS homogenate delivered subcutaneously (Hoffman et al., 2004), or passive transfer of antibodies reactive to GABHS delivered intravenously (Yaddanapudi et al., 2010). These studies have shown that anti-CNS antibodies that bind to key brain areas associated with TS, specifically the globus pallidus, thalamus, and also regions of the cerebellum, are present systemically within the model. Behaviorally, the model develops abnormalities of motor control that present as excessive and repetitive rearing, and the mice show disorders of social interaction, learning, and memory. As with all the models of TS, there are caveats that need to be taken into account with respect to the relevance of the model. In this particular case, it should be recognized that mice are not natural hosts to GABHS, and as such the underlying immune response may differ to what happens in pediatric patients. Also the basis of this model, unlike the intrastriatal models, does not use sera from TS or PANDAS patients.

Microinjection into Basal Ganglia as an Investigational Tool for TS

Intracerebral focal microinjection of pharmacological agents targeted to either the striatum or the GPe, has opened new avenues of study with respect to the clarification of the clinical condition of TS. Previous studies in rodents and NHPs established that focal disruption of GABAergic transmission within the motor cortex, striatum, and GPe can lead to the expression of hyperkinetic motor abnormalities, which are described in the literature as "brief repetitive myoclonic type actions/tics" or "choreic-like movements," typically involving single muscle pairs in the orofacial region and upper limbs (Crossman et al., 1984, 1988; Marsden et al., 1975; Tarsy et al., 1978). Utilization of microinjection techniques, specifically the blockade of GABA using bicuculline, has a long history in the field of medical research for investigating movement disorders. The use of bicuculline has several advantages when studying movement disorders: there is a relatively rapid onset of symptoms following drug delivery (typically 2 to 10 minutes); the effect is reversible, with symptoms lasting about 2 hours; and the response is repeatable by visiting the same injection site at a later date. These established techniques have now been expanded to develop a robust model of the complex motor/neuropsychiatric symptoms associated with TS. Importantly for conceptual models of simple and complex tics, this method has shown that disruption of GABAergic processing in areas of the basal ganglia (striatum and GPe) that receive projections from nonmotor territories (i.e., associative and limbic regions) could induce abnormal behaviors that present as a reorganization of an animal's normal repertoire of behaviors without abnormal movement such as simple tics or chorea, and can be considered as forms of complex tics (Francois et al., 2004; Grabli et al., 2004; Worbe et al., 2009).

EFFECT OF BICUCULLINE MICROINJECTIONS IN THE PUTAMEN AND GPE ON SPONTANEOUS BEHAVIOR

Following the disinhibition of the sensorimotor circuit with bicuculline, depending on the site of injection, disorders of movement become apparent. These movements are defined as abnormal because they are not observed within the normal repertoire of movements expressed by the animals. If the injections are targeted into the sensorimotor putamen, then the principal effect of relevance to TS is one of brief myoclonic-like tics, which are typically expressed in the orofacial region or upper limbs and are highly periodic, typically expressing a 0.5- to 5-Hz rhythm (Fig. 15.2A). If the injections are targeted into the GPe, the typical response is a choreic-like movement, which consists of irregular and sustained flexion movements involving either one or two contiguous joints. However, in a minority of cases chorea can be induced from putamen injections and tic-like contractions can be induced by GPe injections, depending on the site of the microinjection. Importantly for TS research, the appearance of TS-like symptoms after a focal disruption in the striatum gives the model construct validity, as one of the major theoretical models of TS hypothesizes that symptoms arise owing to an as-yet-undefined focal abnormality (probably involving dopamine) within the striatum (Albin & Mink, 2006; Mink, 2001). Furthermore, face validity is achieved, as shown by the observation that when the same focal manipulation of GABA blockade is carried out in the different functional territories of the striatum and GPe, a number of other behavioral abnormalities are expressed. The responses induced by these injections into nonmotor territories can be defined as global perturbations of the natural behavioral organization in an animal, in the absence of dyskinesia or alteration of basic movement control or execution. One of these effects, which occurs when the injection is placed into the limbic territories of the striatal or pallidal complex, is the intense expression and persistent repetition of a particular behavior belonging to the animal's normal repertoire; this response is stereotypical in nature and is analogous to OCD-like behavior. The stereotypies induced by microinjection of bicuculline consist predominantly of manipulating or licking a part of the body (often the tail or fingers). The other behavioral effect, which occurs when the injection is targeted into associative regions, is a hyperactive state in which the animals overexpress several behaviors from among their normal repertoire; this abnormal behavior typically involves arm as well as leg movements, but with frequent changes between movements, which are analogous to the symptoms of ADHD.

These groundbreaking results obtained from NHPs show that, depending on the site of microinjection with respect to hypothesized functional territories, microinjection of bicuculline can produce either movement or behavioral disorders, even though in both cases the same alteration of neuronal activity is presumably produced by microinjection of the GABA antagonist. Thus, each of the fundamental symptom types of TS (i.e., motor tics and neuropsychiatric abnormalities/complex motor tics [OCD and ADHD]) can be induced by the same underlying manipulation of GABA processing, with the only difference between the appearance of different symptoms being the anatomical position of the perturbation in relation to the functional territories of CBTCs.

ELECTROPHYSIOLOGY OF TICS

A recent advance of the microinjection methodology has been the observation of rapid network

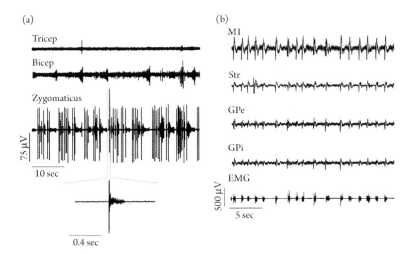

FIGURE 15.2   **Tic-related EMG and LFP activity.**   (**A**) Multiple EMG traces recorded during a typical microinjection experiment using bicuculline targeted to the sensorimotor striatum. The figure demonstrates that the induced tics are focal in space and restricted to the orofacial region: note the periodicity of tic events. (**B**) Simultaneous recordings of LFP activity in primary motor cortex, striatum, and globus pallidus external and internal segments with EMG activity in the orofacial region: note the highly synchronous nature of the LFP voltage transients at anatomically segregated regions and the appearance of tics in the EMG.

changes along the cortico–basal ganglia axis during the expression of simple motor tics. By injecting bicuculline into the sensorimotor striatum and simultaneously recording in the cortex, striatum, and GPe/GPi, it has been possible to gain insights into how the activities in the basal ganglia and cortex may be altered during the expression of symptoms in TS. Following induction of motor tics in NHPs, changes in local field potential activity have been reported (McCairn et al., 2009). Delivery of bicuculline to the striatum induces stereotypic changes in local field potential activity (LFP). These "LFP spikes" are typically a few hundred milliseconds long and appear in conjunction with electromyographic (EMG) events produced by the tics. The LFP spikes appear simultaneously at all the recorded nodes: the cortex, striatum, and both segments of the globus pallidus (Fig. 15.2B). Similar results of synchronous LFP activity in the striatum and cortex have been reported following GABA modulation in felines, in rodents (McKenzie & Viik, 1975; Tarsy et al., 1978), and recently in NHPs (Darbin & Wichmann, 2008). Low-frequency LFP signals are classically regarded as the sum of synaptic activity in

a small area around the recording electrode, and are considered to represent the total inputs to a system (Rasch et al., 2007). Therefore, a large voltage deflection as noted in the LFP spikes might represent the synchronized activity of a large population of cells in the upstream nucleus of the recording site. If this is the case, then the LFP spikes represent a time-locked recruitment and activation of large populations of neurons propagating along the cortico–basal ganglia axis. Support for this hypothesis can be found in the large proportion of neurons showing major changes in their firing rate time-locked to the LFP spikes and the generation of motor tics, which are discussed below.

SINGLE-CELL ACTIVITY FOLLOWING BICUCULLINE MICROINJECTION AND ITS RELATIONSHIP TO TICS

One of the principal predictions made on the basis of theoretical models of tic disorders, is that tic states should be accompanied by changes in the rate of firing of the neurons at key nodes of the CBTCs. The results of microinjection experiments confirmed this to be the case, with neurons in the GPe showing an increased firing rate, those in the GPi showing a decreased firing rate, and those in the primary motor cortex showing an increased mean firing rate—in line with theoretical models (Fig. 15.3A). However, the changes were phasic in both the pallidum and cortex, so the observed rate changes were not tonic in nature (Fig. 15.3B).

With respect to the prevalence of responses in each of the CBTC critical nodes, the microinjection protocol caused large numbers of cells (70–80%) in each region to display tic-related activity (Fig. 15.4). An interesting caveat to this observation is that pallidal responses were highly prevalent across each of the functional territories, suggesting that the focal abnormality in the striatum caused by the injection caused a loss of anatomical specificity in downstream neurons (for further discussion of this phenomenon see Bronfeld & Bar-Gad, 2011). Another interesting observation with respect to the neuronal correlates of tic behavior in this model was that the phasic changes were highly periodic in the low-frequency range (Fig. 15.4). The manifestation of low-frequency periodic activity in CBTCs has been proposed to be a causative factor for tic generation (Leckman et al., 2006). In a recent study, low-frequency, oscillatory bursting activity in pallidal receiving areas of the thalamus in TS patients undergoing surgery for deep brain stimulation was observed (Marceglia et al., 2010). This observation lends credence to the model being a clinically relevant platform.

The opposite phasic and periodic changes in firing rates of the GPe and GPi in response to the disinhibition of the striatum are difficult to reconcile with known anatomy and physiology of the normal basal ganglia, particularly if it's assumed that the pallidal responses are a consequence of disinhibition (i.e., increased activity in both pathways originating from within the striatum, which initiates tics). There are several plausible explanations for this phenomenon; bicuculline could induce a phasic reduction of inhibitory outflow from the striatum caused by lateral inhibition within the striatum itself, which increases GPe activity, and this activity directly inhibits GPi. Support for this hypothesis can be found in the work of Darbin and Wichmann (2008), who showed that fast-spiking inhibitory neurons in the striatum, which form a lateral inhibitory network, show a tight coupling of activity with LFP spikes following striatal microinjection of GABA antagonists. More recent studies, however, have demonstrated that bicuculline can cause differential effects on striatal projection neurons during tic states depending on their distance from the site of the microinjection (Bronfeld et al., 2011; Worbe et al., 2009), which could potentially underlie the observed changes. Further studies should be completed to assess the role of all key nuclei of the basal ganglia in the tic propagation mechanism, including the STN, SNr, thalamus, and recently discovered functional connections to non-basal ganglia nuclei such as the cerebella dentate nucleus (Hoshi et al., 2005) and cerebellar cortex (Bostan & Strick, 2010).

Another potentially important insight obtained from the bicuculline microinjection methodology, is the emphasis on GABAergic transmission and how its disruption can lead to TS-like symptoms. In light of the observation that TS patients show reduced expression of fast-spiking inhibitory GABAergic neurons (Kalanithi et al., 2005; Kataoka et al., 2010), it is possible that the underlying cause of TS may not be a disorder of monoamines, but instead a consequence of abnormal GABAergic processing. This hypothesis is also supported by the observation that GABA agonists such as clonazepam and baclofen can ameliorate symptoms of TS (Goetz, 1992; Singer et al., 2001).

A key feature of the bicuculline TS model is that it provides an ideal platform in which to test the neurosurgical intervention of high-frequency deep brain stimulation (HF-DBS). This neurosurgical intervention is being increasingly used as a treatment for intractable TS; further discussion on the role of HF-DBS for TS can be found in Chapter 26. Theoretical models and clinical reports suggest that this treatment modality should be and is effective. Currently there are two published reports that have used the bicuculline model to study different symptoms and stimulation targets related to TS. The first showed that stereotypy induced by focal injection of bicuculline into the limbic territory of the GPe is reduced by STN stimulation (Baup et al., 2008).

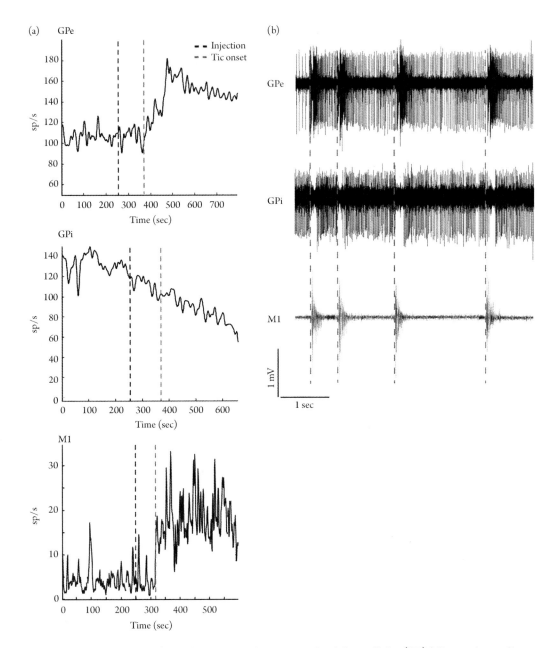

FIGURE 15.3   Examples of tic-related neuronal activity in the globus pallidus (GP) following bicuculline injection.   (**A**) Examples of mean firing rates from continuously recorded single primary motor cortex (M1), GP external and internal segment neurons, before and after injection, which show firing rate changes consistent with theoretical models of TS. (**B**) Examples of raw neuronal traces from M1 and both segments of the GP, which illustrate how the rate changes are phasic and locked to the appearance of tics (*dashed lines*). (See color insert.)

Although this study provided behavioral correlates of a therapeutic response, there were no direct studies of the neurophysiological response to stimulation. A more recent study has identified how pallidal tic-related physiology is disrupted by DBS targeted to the GPi (McCairn et al., 2012). Importantly for TS, this study showed that DBS abolished tic-related phasic responses in GP neurons and was capable of reducing the amplitude of tic events (Fig. 15.5).

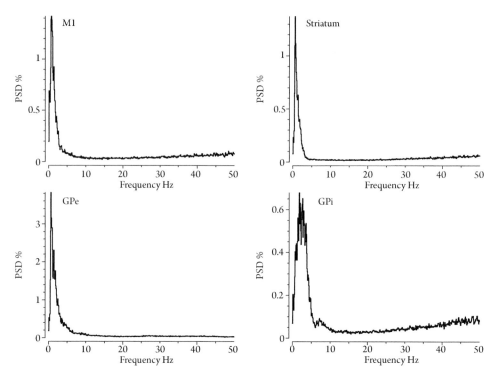

FIGURE 15.4 **Examples of tic-related low-frequency oscillations in CBTCs following bicuculline microinjection.** Power spectral density plots for typical primary motor cortex, striatum and pallidal neurons during tic states: note the significant low-frequency peaks. These peaks are a consequence of the periodic phasic alterations in each critical node, both increases and decreases in firing rates, which underlie the appearance of tics.

DEFICIENT SENSORIMOTOR GATING TESTS AND TS ANIMAL MODELS

A principal feature of the majority of TS animal models is that they emphasize face validity and have thus focused on explicit motor abnormalities that present in a number of ways, such as simple myoclonic-like tics, simple behavioral tics, and complex OCD-like behavior such as sequential super-stereotypies. A major criticism of these models is that they do not address one of the major symptoms of TS—the phenomenon of the premonitory urge (see Chapter 1 for detailed description). The premonitory urge can be described as an uncomfortable physical sensation that may feel like an itch or crawling sensation (Bliss, 1980; Leckman et al., 1993). These uncomfortable sensory phenomena are relieved by performing a tic-related behavior in the locality of the sensation—for example, a phonic tic

in response to uncomfortable sensations in the throat. There is, however, a testing protocol that could be used as a standalone platform or with established TS animal models that may address this issue. This testing paradigm is generally referred to as a "deficient sensorimotor gating test" and utilizes prepulse inhibition (PPI) as a methodology for testing impaired sensorimotor responses to a startle stimulus (Swerdlow & Sutherland, 2005, 2006). The PPI paradigm is a generalized testing protocol, and therefore it is a test that can be used across different experimental platforms that have been manipulated in a multitude of ways, thereby enhancing the utility of each model as a dependent measure.

Briefly, in a PPI experimental paradigm, the startle reflex to an unexpected sensory event such as a puff of air is reduced if it is paired with a similar but smaller-amplitude event just prior to delivery of the larger startle event. It has been demonstrated that TS patients have a deficiency

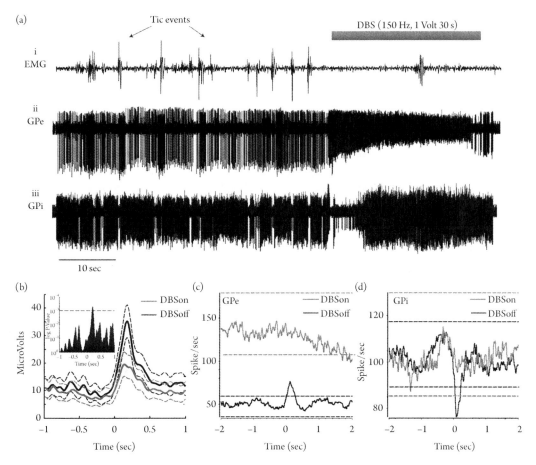

FIGURE 15.5 **EMG and neuronal data during tics with GPi HF-DBS.** (**A**) Examples of raw data from EMG and neuronal activity in the pallidum after administration of bicuculline and during HF-DBS. The top trace shows EMG recorded from the orofacial region, in which the large voltage transients are tic events. The bottom two traces are simultaneous recordings from both segments of the globus pallidus (GPe and GPi) during expression of the above tics. (**B**) Quantification of the reduction in tic-related EMG peak voltage amplitude. The histogram shows the EMG signals aligned to tic onset. The inset shows a graphical representation of the *t*-test across bins between the two experimental conditions and the reduction in peak amplitude of the tic-related EMG ($p < .001$). (**C**) Modulation of activity in a GPe neuron by tics (black trace) and HF-DBS (red trace). Neuronal activity is aligned to tic onset. Note that the large increase in activity under the off-stimulation condition was abolished by HF-DBS. The *dashed lines* represent confidence intervals of 99% and are color-coded to each condition. (**D**) Modulation of activity in a GPi neuron by tics (black trace) and HF-DBS (red trace). The activity is aligned to tic onset. Note that the decrease in activity under the off-stimulation condition was abolished during HF-DBS. (See color insert.)

From McCairn et al. High-frequency pallidal stimulation blocks tic-related neuronal activity in a non-human primate model of Tourette syndrome. *NeuroReport* 2012

in their ability to gate sensory phenomena when measured using PPI (i.e., the expected inhibition that should be present with a paired stimulus is absent). In addition to the abnormal responses to external stimuli such as the air puff test, TS patients are also shown to have impaired cortical inhibition when utilizing paired pulses via transcranial magnetic stimulation (Castellanos et al., 1996; Swerdlow et al., 2001; Ziemann et al., 1997). This deficiency of sensorimotor gating has been hypothesized to underlie the phenomenon of the premonitory urge (i.e., an inability to filter out extraneous sensory stimuli leading to hypersensitivity, which is relieved by the action of the tic). An important feature of the PPI testing paradigm is that there are a number of known neurochemical pathways that affect PPI performance, including and of particular relevance to TS DA, norepinephrine, glutamate, and 5-HT. As a consequence of these well-studied pathways, the PPI test is favored for its ability to screen compounds that might be of clinical value in treating symptoms associated with TS that target these pathways. For example, it has been demonstrated that DA agonists disrupt PPI responses in rodents and the response is recovered using DA antagonists, which are also used to treat symptoms of TS. The PPI model might also be useful for nonpharmacological interventions such as DBS, where targeting of critical nodes in the CBTC might be useful for restoring gating functions.

Although the PPI paradigm would appear to provide valuable insights into the gating mechanisms that may be disrupted in TS, there is a fundamental weakness in most neurodevelopmental models utilizing PPI. This flaw stems from the observation that PPI deficits in rodent neurodevelopmental models tend to appear in adulthood, whereas TS-related symptoms and PPI deficits emerge in childhood. For an in-depth review and discussion of the PPI model and its relevance to TS, see Swerdlow and Sutherland, 2006.

CONCLUDING REMARKS AND FUTURE PERSPECTIVES

We have reviewed five major platforms for animal models of TS, which are summarized in Table 15.1. As has been discussed, the complex profile of motor and neuropsychiatric abnormalities in TS makes it difficult for those models to satisfy all the validity criteria. The complexity of TS manifestations is partly because structural and functional alterations in the TS brain can reflect causes or consequences of the disorder. Indeed, it has been suggested that children with TS may follow unique developmental trajectories whereby they undergo compensatory neuroplastic changes and gain control over their symptoms (Jackson et al., 2011; Plessen et al., 2004;

Serrien et al., 2005). In light of this, acute and reversible models with circuit-specific microinjections of bicuculline have advantages over other models in that they have little compensatory impacts on underlying processes. On the other hand, such models do not allow in-depth investigations of long-term changes in structure and function that are associated with TS symptoms. Future work should be carried out to consolidate experimental findings obtained from acute and chronic TS models in a complementary manner to gain insights into the etiology and pathophysiology of TS.

In recent years DBS has received considerable attention as a potential therapeutic option for patients with severe TS refractory to medication (Hariz & Robertson, 2010; Mink et al., 2006). Importantly, DBS has also been proposed as a surgical treatment for intractable cases with comorbid OCD (Haynes & Mallet, 2010) and depression (Hamani et al., 2010; Mayberg et al., 2005). This parallel implies similar neuronal network mechanisms underlying these behavioral disorders. Use of appropriate animal models and experimental techniques may allow clarification of the network abnormalities commonly involved in TS and comorbid neuropsychiatric disorders. This would, in turn, lead to a better understanding of the mechanisms of DBS action in a range of neurological and psychiatric illnesses.

From a motor control perspective, an interesting aspect of TS resides in the potentially "semivoluntary" nature of tic generation. TS patients often report an urge preceding tic onset, an uncomfortable bodily sensation that drives the individual to perform the tic (Kwak et al., 2003). Moreover, tics can be temporarily suppressed against such a premonitory urge (Serrien et al., 2005). These observations lead to a hypothesis that the tic movement *per se* is under some intentional control. In support of this hypothesis, neuroimaging studies have shown that the generation of tics is associated with premovement activation of voluntary motor structures, such as the supplementary motor area and the anterior cingulate cortex (Bohlhalter et al., 2006; Hampson et al., 2009). Tics might be equivalent to voluntary movements in their physiological

Table 15.1 Summary of Key Animal Models of Tic Disorders

Category	Platform	Description of manipulation	Key features	References
Genetic	D1CT-7 mouse	Insertion of cholera toxin A1 subunit into cortical-basal ganglia D1 receptor-expressing cells	Tics and OCD-like behaviors induced by cortical excitability following exposure to cholera toxin	McGrath et al., 2000 Nordstrom & Burton, 2002
	DAT-KD mouse D3 knockout mouse	Reduced DAT expression Reduced expression of D3 receptors	Reduced reuptake of endogenous DA leading to stereotypy Animals show hyperactivity.	Berridge et al., 2005 Accili et al., 1996
	Slitrk mouse	Knockout of Slitrk1 & Slitrk5 gene	Models potential candidate genes for the cause of TS. Slitrk1 animals show elevated anxiety and noradrenergic abnormalities. Slitrk5 animals display stereotyped behavior, increased anxiety, and abnormalities in striatal cell morphology and glutamate receptor composition.	Katayama et al., 2010 Shmelkov et al., 2010
	SAPAP3 mutant mouse	SAP90/PSD95-associated protein knockout	Animals show obsessive-type grooming with associated abnormalities in electrophysiological, biochemical, and structural abnormalities in CBTCs.	Welch et al., 2007
	Hoxb8 mutant mouse	Modulation of Hoxb8 allele through IRES-Cre recombinase knock-ins	The models show excessive grooming, while the only reported abnormalities within neural circuits responsible for grooming are related to microglia.	Chen et al., 2010
	HDC knockout	Knockout of rate-limiting enzyme for histamine production	Histamine identified as an important transmitter in the striatum. HDC knockout causes a hypersensitivity to dopamine and abnormalities of locomotion.	Kubota et al., 2002 Ohtsu & Watanabe,, 2003

(Continued)

Table 15.1 (*Continued*)

Category	Platform	Description of manipulation	Key features	References
	dtsz hamster	Recessive gene expressed in inbred Syrian hamsters	Animals develop paroxysmal dystonia and show abnormalities of fast-spiking inhibitory GABAergic neurons in the striatum. The model also shows similarity to TS in the developmental time course of symptoms.	Loscher et al., 1998 Gernert et al., 2000
Systemic drug administration	Rodent	Systemic administration of DA agonists & antagonists	In response to agonists animals develop intense stereotypies that are believed to be analogous to OCD. The intensity of stereotypy is reflected in striosomal to matrix upregulation of markers for early gene transcription. Sudden withdrawal of D1 antagonists can induce simple motor tics. These studies are providing insights into the heterogeneity of OCD behaviors.	Randrup et al., 1963 Graybiel et al., 1990 Canales & Graybiel, 2000 Taylor et al., 2010
	Rodent	Systemic administration of 5-HT agonist—DOI	Induces repetitive head twitches and implicates 5-HT abnormalities in TS.	Handley & Dursun, 1992 Tizabi et al., 2001
Focal administration of immunoreactive sera	Rodent	Microinjection of sera from TS patients targeted to the striatum and systemic administration of GABHS	Induces stereotypies and vocalizations with upregulation of DA levels in the striatum. Anti-CNS antibodies are often found systemically.	Hallett et al., 2000 Taylor et al., 2002 Hoffman et al., 2004 Yaddanapudi, 2010

Focal administration of pharmacological agents	Rodent, feline, NHP	Microinjection of GABA antagonists targeted to functional territories of CBTCs	Selectively induces each of the fundamental symptom types, motor & neuropsychiatric, and allows quantification of fast network changes in CBTCs. Also provides a platform to test deep brain stimulation.	Marsden et al., 1975 Grabli et al., 2004 Baup et al., 2008 Worbe et al., 2009 McCairn et al., 2009 McCairn et al., 2012
Sensory gating models	Rodent	Utilizes prepulse inhibition (PPI) testing paradigm as a correlate of the premonitory urge	Clinical studies have demonstrated that TS patients suffer a deficiency in sensory gating when tested with a paired stimulus. PPI testing paradigm is well established and can be used to screen for therapeutic compounds and interventions that might be of benefit to TS.	Swerdlow & Sutherland, 2005 Swerdlow & Sutherland, 2006

Box 15.1. Key Points

- Although TS is a complex disorder comprising both motor and neuropsychiatric symptoms, a number of different experimental platforms have been developed with which to investigate the different symptoms and their etiologies.
- Animal models provide a platform from which to test and validate experimental treatments.
- Rodent genetic models are providing insights into TS by investigating suspected candidate genes and the role of different neurotransmitters and neural pathways/circuits through either upregulation or knockout of neurotransmitters and candidate genes.
- Systemic pharmacological challenge using specific agonists and antagonists has provided a means to reproduce behavioral symptoms similar to those expressed in TS. This work has helped localize specific structures in CBTCs that may contribute to TS-like behavior and have highlighted the importance of different receptor activations for discrete behaviors.
- Immune-based models are helping to identify specific disease-causing agents and antigens that may cause TS.
- Focal microinjection of GABAergic antagonists has helped identify the role of specific structures and pathways in the basal ganglia and how they relate to discrete behaviors associated with TS. Disruption of sensorimotor regions tends to induce classic motor tics, while the same perturbation in limbic structures leads to OCD-like behavior. This model has also demonstrated the fast latency network changes that occur with motor tics in the CBTC and how they are modified by HF-DBS.
- Sensorimotor gating models are beginning to address the phenomenon of the premonitory urge and provide a generalized testing protocol that can be applied across the different experimental platforms that have been developed for TS.
- Continuing to combine empirical and theoretical data from the clinic and laboratory will allow greater understanding of TS.

Box 15.2. Questions for Future Research

- Progress with respect to identifying specific etiologies for TS points to multiple factors that may cause the condition. Is it therefore possible to develop a single animal model that has true face, construct, and predictive validity?
- Animal models continue to provide data leading to increasingly complicated theoretical models of CBTC function in TS. In light of the expanding knowledge base provided by animal studies, and the types of invasive methodology often required to obtain the data, will it be possible to validate these observations directly from TS patients?
- Genetic models have implicated several causative genes, anatomical pathways/networks, and neurotransmitters that can induce TS-like behaviors. Will it be possible to link each of the variants in these models to specific subtypes of TS?
- Similar TS-like behavioral abnormalities across different platforms and experimental manipulations (i.e., stereotypic grooming) and the ability to induce each of the subtypes of TS-like

behavior with the same manipulation but targeted to different functional areas imply common neural mechanisms for behavioral execution. Is it possible to identify an underlying pathophysiology (i.e., abnormal oscillations) or key regions in the brain that link all the different experimental manipulations and common symptom expression?
- Focal manipulations of GABAergic processing appear to provide a powerful technique for investigating the anatomical pathways of different TS behaviors and the fast latency network changes that underlie them. Is it possible to extend this methodology so that longer-term genetic, biochemical, and proteomic changes in response to the manipulation can be studied?

substrate yet be somehow misperceived as involuntary owing to an abnormal experience of volition (Moretto et al., 2011). Successfully developing animal models of TS might offer a unique opportunity to address issues on the neuronal underpinnings of volition and voluntary motor control.

To conclude, the pathophysiology of TS remains a mystery. However, as reviewed in this chapter, a large body of evidence has revealed characteristic abnormalities of the anatomy, chemistry, and physiology of the CBTCs of the TS brain. The continuing effort to advance and refine animal models of TS with integrative approaches—both empirical and theoretical—would provide new insights into the etiology of TS. This focused research may open up new therapeutic strategies for patients with TS and related behavioral disorders.

REFERENCES

Abelson JF, Kwan KY, O'Roak BJ et al. Sequence variants in SLITRK1 are associated with Tourette's syndrome. *Science* 2005; *310*: 317–320.

Accili D, Fishburn CS, Drago J et al. A targeted mutation of the D3 dopamine receptor gene is associated with hyperactivity in mice. *Proc Natl Acad Sci USA* 1996; *93*:1945–1949.

Albin RL. Neurobiology of basal ganglia and Tourette syndrome: striatal and dopamine function. *Adv Neurol* 2006; *99*:99–106.

Albin RL, Mink JW. Recent advances in Tourette syndrome research. *Trends Neurosci* 2006; *29*:175–182.

Albin RL, Young AB, Penney JB. The functional anatomy of basal ganglia disorders. *Trends Neurosci* 1989; *12*:366–375.

Albin RL, Young AB, Penney JB. The functional anatomy of disorders of the basal ganglia. *Trends Neurosci* 1995; *18*:63–64.

Alexander GE, DeLong MR, Strick PL. Parallel organization of functionally segregated circuits linking basal ganglia and cortex. *Annu Rev Neurosci* 1986; *9*:357–381.

Aruga J, Mikoshiba K. Identification and characterization of Slitrk, a novel neuronal transmembrane protein family controlling neurite outgrowth. *Mol Cell Neurosci* 2003; *24*:117–129.

Baron MS, Sidibe M, DeLong MR, Smith Y. Course of motor and associative pallidothalamic projections in monkeys. *J Comp Neurol* 2001; *429*:490–501.

Baup N, Grabli D, Karachi C et al. High-frequency stimulation of the anterior subthalamic nucleus reduces stereotyped behaviors in primates. *J Neurosci* 2008; *28*:8785–8788.

Beckstead RM. A pallidostriatal projection in the cat and monkey. *Brain Res Bull* 1983; *11*:629–632.

Beiser DG, Houk JC. Model of cortical-basal ganglionic processing: encoding the serial order of sensory events. *J Neurophysiol* 1998; *79*:3168–3188.

Bergman H, Feingold A, Nini A et al. Physiological aspects of information processing in the basal ganglia of normal and parkinsonian primates. *Trends Neurosci* 1998; *21*:32–38.

Berridge KC, Aldridge JW, Houchard KR, Zhuang X. Sequential super-stereotypy of an instinctive fixed action pattern in hyper-dopaminergic mutant mice: a model of obsessive compulsive disorder and Tourette's. *BMC Biol* 2005; 3:4.

Bliss J. Sensory experiences of Gilles de la Tourette syndrome. *Arch Gen Psychiatry* 1980; 37:1343–1347.

Bohlhalter S, Goldfine A, Matteson S et al. Neural correlates of tic generation in Tourette syndrome: an event-related functional MRI study. *Brain* 2006; 129:2029–2037.

Bolam JP, Hanley JJ, Booth PA, Bevan MD. Synaptic organisation of the basal ganglia. *J Anat* 2000; 196:527–542.

Bostan AC, Strick PL. The cerebellum and basal ganglia are interconnected. *Neuropsychol Rev* 2010; 20:261–270.

Bronfeld M, Bar-Gad I. Loss of specificity in basal ganglia-related movement disorders. *Front Syst Neurosci* 2011; 5:38.

Bronfeld M, Belelovsky K, Bar-Gad I. Spatial and temporal properties of tic-related neuronal activity in the cortico-basal ganglia loop. *J Neurosci* 2011; 31:8713–8721.

Budman CL, Gayer A, Lesser M et al. An open-label study of the treatment efficacy of olanzapine for Tourette's disorder. *J Clin Psychiatry* 2001; 62:290–294.

Canales JJ, Graybiel AM. A measure of striatal function predicts motor stereotypy. *Nat Neurosci* 2000a; 3:377–383.

Canales JJ, Graybiel AM. Patterns of gene expression and behavior induced by chronic dopamine treatments. *Ann Neurol* 2000b; 47:S53–S59.
A seminal study that highlighted the importance of relative activity between striatal striosomes and matrix compartments as markers of stereotypic activity.

Capecchi MR. Hox genes and mammalian development. *Cold Spring Harb Symp Quant Biol* 1997; 62:273–281.

Carpenter MB, Nakano K, Kim R. Nigrothalamic projections in the monkey demonstrated by autoradiographic technics. *J Comp Neurol* 1976; 165:401–415.

Castellanos FX, Fine EJ, Kaysen D et al. Sensorimotor gating in boys with Tourette's syndrome and ADHD: preliminary results. *Biol Psychiatry* 1996; 39:33–41.

Chen SK, Tvrdik P, Peden E et al. Hematopoietic origin of pathological grooming in Hoxb8 mutant mice. *Cell* 2010; 141:775–785.
Emphasizes that stereotypic behavior could originate from abnormalities in microglia within CBTCs.

Collins S. Treating Tourette's. A gene mutation that causes low histamine levels may be behind some tic disorders. *Sci Am* 2011; 304:22.

Colpaert FC, Janssen PA. The head-twitch response to intraperitoneal injection of 5-hydroxytryptophan in the rat: antagonist effects of purported 5-hydroxytryptamine antagonists and of pirenperone, an LSD antagonist. *Neuropharmacology* 1983; 22:993–1000.

Comings DE. Clinical and molecular genetics of ADHD and Tourette syndrome. Two related polygenic disorders. *Ann NY Acad Sci* 2001; 931:50–83.

Crossman AR, Mitchell IJ, Sambrook MA, Jackson A. Chorea and myoclonus in the monkey induced by gamma-aminobutyric acid antagonism in the lentiform complex. The site of drug action and a hypothesis for the neural mechanisms of chorea. *Brain* 1988; 111:1211–1233.

Crossman AR, Sambrook MA, Jackson A. Experimental hemichorea/hemiballismus in the monkey. Studies on the intracerebral site of action in a drug-induced dyskinesia. *Brain* 1984; 107:579–596.

Darbin O, Wichmann T. Effects of striatal GABA-A receptor blockade on striatal and cortical activity in monkeys. *J Neurophysiol* 2008; 99:1294–1305.

DeLong MR. Activity of pallidal neurons during movement. *J Neurophysiol* 1971; 34:414–427.

DeLong MR. Activity of basal ganglia neurons during movement. *Brain Res* 1972; 40:127–135.

DeLong MR. Primate models of movement disorders of basal ganglia origin. *Trends Neurosci* 1990; 13:281–285.

DeLong MR, Wichmann T. Circuits and circuit disorders of the basal ganglia. *Arch Neurol* 2007; 64:20–24.

Deng H, Le WD, Xie WJ, Jankovic J. Examination of the SLITRK1 gene in Caucasian patients with Tourette syndrome. *Acta Neurol Scand* 2006; 114:400–402.

Ercan-Sencicek AG, Stillman AA, Ghosh AK et al. L-histidine decarboxylase and Tourette's syndrome. *N Engl J Med* 2010; 362:1901–1908.

Flaherty AW, Graybiel AM. Corticostriatal transformations in the primate somatosensory system. Projections from physiologically mapped body-part representations. *J Neurophysiol* 1991; 66:1249–1263.

Flaherty AW, Graybiel AM. Input-output organization of the sensorimotor striatum

in the squirrel monkey. *J Neurosci* 1994;
14:599–610.

Francois C, Grabli D, McCairn K et al. Behavioural
disorders induced by external globus pallidus
dysfunction in primates II. Anatomical study.
Brain 2004; 127:2055–2070.

Francois C, Percheron G, Yelnik J. Localization
of nigrostriatal, nigrothalamic and nigrotectal
neurons in ventricular coordinates in macaques.
Neuroscience 1984a; 13:61–76.

Francois C, Percheron G, Yelnik J, Heyner S.
A Golgi analysis of the primate globus pallidus. I.
Inconstant processes of large neurons, other neuronal types, and afferent axons. *J Comp Neurol*
1984b; 227:182–199.

Francois C, Yelnik J, Percheron G, Tande D.
Calbindin D-28k as a marker for the associative
cortical territory of the striatum in macaque.
Brain Res 1994; 633:331–336.

Gardiner TW, Kitai ST. Single-unit activity in the
globus pallidus and neostriatum of the rat during
performance of a trained head movement. *Exp
Brain Res* 1992; 88:517–530.

Gerfen CR. The neostriatal mosaic: multiple levels
of compartmental organization. *Trends Neurosci*
1992; 15:133–139.

Gerfen CR, Wilson CJ. The basal ganglia. In:
Swanson LW, Bjorklund A, Hokfelt T (eds.),
*Handbook of Chemical Neuroanatomy, Vol 12:
Integrated Systems of the CNS, Part III*. 1996,
pp. 371–468. Elsevier Science.

Gernert M, Hamann M, Bennay M et al. Deficit
of striatal parvalbumin-reactive GABAergic
interneurons and decreased basal ganglia
output in a genetic rodent model of idiopathic paroxysmal dystonia. *J Neurosci* 2000;
20:7052–7058.

**Abnormalities in GABAergic interneurons
have been identified in TS patients; this
model appears to have a similar anatomical
pathology and symptom time course as TS
patients.**

Goetz CG. Clonidine and clonazepam in
Tourette syndrome. *Adv Neurol* 1992;
58:245–251.

Grabli D, McCairn K, Hirsch EC et al. Behavioural
disorders induced by external globus pallidus
dysfunction in primates: I. Behavioural study.
Brain 2004; 127:2039–2054.

**Groundbreaking study that showed that the same
pertubation of GABAergic processing via GABA
antagonists could induce each of the fundamental behavioral phenotypes associated with
TS depending on the functional territory it was
injected into in the CBTCs.**

Graybiel AM. Neurotransmitters and neuromodula-
tors in the basal ganglia. *Trends Neurosci* 1990;
13:244–254.

Graybiel AM, Moratalla R, Robertson HA.
Amphetamine and cocaine induce drug-specific
activation of the c-fos gene in striosome-matrix
compartments and limbic subdivisions of
the striatum. *Proc Natl Acad Sci USA* 1990;
87:6912–6916.

Graybiel AM, Ragsdale CW, Jr. Histochemically
distinct compartments in the striatum of
human, monkeys, and cat demonstrated by
acetylthiocholinesterase staining. *Proc Natl
Acad Sci USA* 1978; 75:5723–5726.

Graybiel AM, Ragsdale CW, Jr. Clumping of
acetylcholinesterase activity in the developing
striatum of the human fetus and young infant.
Proc Natl Acad Sci USA 1980; 77:1214–1218.

Gros Y, Schuldiner S. Directed evolution reveals
hidden properties of VMAT, a neurotransmitter
transporter. *J Biol Chem* 2010; 285:5076–5084.

Haber SN, Kunishio K, Mizobuchi M, Lynd-Balta E.
The orbital and medial prefrontal circuit through
the primate basal ganglia. *J Neurosci* 1995;
15:4851–4867.

Haber SN, Lynd E, Klein C, Groenewegen HJ.
Topographic organization of the ventral striatal
efferent projections in the rhesus monkey: an
anterograde tracing study. *J Comp Neurol* 1990;
293:282–298.

Hallett JJ, Harling-Berg CJ, Knopf PM et al.
Anti-striatal antibodies in Tourette syndrome
cause neuronal dysfunction. *J Neuroimmunol*
2000; 111:195–202.

**The first study to show that TS-related antibod-
ies could induce TS-like behavior in animal
models.**

Hamani C, Nobrega JN, Lozano AM. Deep brain
stimulation in clinical practice and in animal
models. *Clin Pharmacol Ther* 2010; 88:559–562.

Hamann M, Sander SE, Richter A. Age-dependent
alterations of striatal calretinin interneuron
density in a genetic animal model of primary
paroxysmal dystonia. *J Neuropathol Exp Neurol*
2005; 64:776–781.

Hampson M, Tokoglu F, King RA et al. Brain areas
coactivating with motor cortex during chronic
motor tics and intentional movements. *Biol
Psychiatry* 2009; 65:594–599.

Handley SL, Dursun SM. Serotonin and Tourette's
syndrome: movement such as head-shakes and

wet-dog shakes may model human tics. *Adv Biosci* 1992; 85:235–253.

This study highlighted the role of monoamines other than dopamine in inducing tic-like behavior.

Hariz MI, Robertson MM. Gilles de la Tourette syndrome and deep brain stimulation. *Eur J Neurosci* 2010; 32:1128–1134.

Haynes WI, Mallet L. High-frequency stimulation of deep brain structures in obsessive-compulsive disorder: the search for a valid circuit. *Eur J Neurosci* 2010; 32:1118–1127.

Hayslett RL, Tizabi Y. Effects of donepezil, nicotine and haloperidol on the central serotonergic system in mice: implications for Tourette's syndrome. *Pharmacol Biochem Behav* 2005; 81:879–886.

Hazrati LN, Parent A, Mitchell S, Haber SN. Evidence for interconnections between the two segments of the globus pallidus in primates: a PHA-L anterograde tracing study. *Brain Res* 1990; 533:171–175.

Hazrati LN, Parent A. Projection from the external pallidum to the reticular thalamic nucleus in the squirrel monkey. *Brain Res* 1991; 550:142–146.

Hedreen JC, DeLong MR. Organization of striatopallidal, striatonigral, and nigrostriatal projections in the macaque. *J Comp Neurol* 1991; 304:569–595.

Hikosaka O, Wurtz RH. Visual and oculomotor functions of monkey substantia nigra pars reticulata. IV. Relation of substantia nigra to superior colliculus. *J Neurophysiol* 1983; 49:1285–1301.

Hoffman KL, Hornig M, Yaddanapudi K et al. A murine model for neuropsychiatric disorders associated with group A beta-hemolytic streptococcal infection. *J Neurosci* 2004; 24:1780–1791.

Hoover JE, Strick PL. Multiple output channels in the basal ganglia. *Science* 1993; 259:819–821.

Hoshi E, Tremblay L, Feger J et al. The cerebellum communicates with the basal ganglia. *Nat Neurosci* 2005; 8:1491–1493.

Isoda M, Hikosaka O. Switching from automatic to controlled action by monkey medial frontal cortex. *Nat Neurosci* 2007; 10:240–248.

Isoda M, Hikosaka O. Role for subthalamic nucleus neurons in switching from automatic to controlled eye movement. *J Neurosci* 2008; 28:7209–7218.

Jackson SR, Parkinson A, Jung J et al. Compensatory neural reorganization in Tourette syndrome. *Curr Biol* 2011; 21:580–585.

Jakab RL, Hazrati LN, Goldman-Rakic P. Distribution and neurochemical character of substance P receptor (SPR)-immunoreactive striatal neurons of the macaque monkey: accumulation of SP fibers and SPR neurons and dendrites in "striocapsules" encircling striosomes. *J Comp Neurol* 1996; 369:137–149.

Jankovic J, Orman J. Tetrabenazine therapy of dystonia, chorea, tics, and other dyskinesias. *Neurology* 1988; 38:391–394.

Jijun L, Zaiwang L, Anyuan L et al. Abnormal expression of dopamine and serotonin transporters associated with the pathophysiologic mechanism of Tourette syndrome. *Neurol India* 2010; 58:523–529.

Jimenez-Jimenez FJ, Garcia-Ruiz PJ. Pharmacological options for the treatment of Tourette's disorder. *Drugs* 2001; 61:2207–2220.

Kalanithi PS, Zheng W, Kataoka Y et al. Altered parvalbumin-positive neuron distribution in basal ganglia of individuals with Tourette syndrome. *Proc Natl Acad Sci USA* 2005; 102:13307–13312.

Kataoka Y, Kalanithi PS, Grantz H et al. Decreased number of parvalbumin and cholinergic interneurons in the striatum of individuals with Tourette syndrome. *J Comp Neurol* 2010; 518:277–291.

Katayama K, Yamada K, Ornthanalai VG et al. Slitrk1-deficient mice display elevated anxiety-like behavior and noradrenergic abnormalities. *Mol Psychiatry* 2010; 15:177–184.

The identification of Slitrk genes as a possible candidate for TS means that this particular genetic model could help identify some of the underlying causes for TS.

Kawasaki H, Springett GM, Mochizuki N et al. A family of cAMP-binding proteins that directly activate Rap1. *Science* 1998; 282:2275–2279.

Kemp JM, Powell TP. The cortico-striate projection in the monkey. *Brain* 1970; 93:525–546.

Kita H. Globus pallidus external segment. *Prog Brain Res* 2007; 160:111–133.

Kita H, Tokuno H, Nambu A. Monkey globus pallidus external segment neurons projecting to the neostriatum. *Neuroreport* 1999; 10:1467–1472.

Kitai ST, Deniau JM. Cortical inputs to the subthalamus: intracellular analysis. *Brain Res* 1981; 214:411–415.

Krusong K, Ercan-Sencicek AG, Xu M et al. High levels of histidine decarboxylase in the striatum of mice and rats. *Neurosci Lett* 2011; 495:110–114.

Kubota Y, Ito C, Sakurai E et al. Increased methamphetamine-induced locomotor activity and behavioral sensitization in histamine-deficient mice. *J Neurochem* 2002; 83:837–845.

Kurlan R. Tourette's syndrome and `PANDAS': will the relation bear out? Pediatric autoimmune neuropsychiatric disorders associated with streptococcal infection. *Neurology* 1998; 50:1530–1534.

Kwak C, Dat VK, Jankovic J. Premonitory sensory phenomenon in Tourette's syndrome. *Mov Disord* 2003; 18:1530–1533.

Leblois A, Reese R, Labarre D et al. Deep brain stimulation changes basal ganglia output nuclei firing pattern in the dystonic hamster. *Neurobiol Dis* 2010; 38:288–298.

Leckman JF, Vaccarino FM, Kalanithi PS, Rothenberger A. Annotation: Tourette syndrome: a relentless drumbeat—driven by misguided brain oscillations. *J Child Psychol Psychiatry* 2006; 47:537–550.

Leckman JF, Walker DE, Cohen DJ. Premonitory urges in Tourette's syndrome. *Am J Psychiatry* 1993; 150:98–102.

Leonard HL, Lenane MC, Swedo SE et al. Tics and Tourette's disorder: a 2- to 7-year follow-up of 54 obsessive-compulsive children. *Am J Psychiatry* 1992; 149:1244–1251.

Liu X, Wang Y, Li D, Ju X. Transplantation of rat neural stem cells reduces stereotypic behaviors in rats after intrastriatal microinfusion of Tourette syndrome sera. *Behav Brain Res* 2008; 186:84–90.

Loiselle CR, Lee O, Moran TH, Singer HS. Striatal microinfusion of Tourette syndrome and PANDAS sera: failure to induce behavioral changes. *Mov Disord* 2004; 19:390–396.

Loscher W, Fisher JE, Jr., Schmidt D et al. The sz mutant hamster: a genetic model of epilepsy or of paroxysmal dystonia? *Mov Disord* 1989; 4:219–232.

Magill PJ, Bolam JP, Bevan MD. Relationship of activity in the subthalamic nucleus-globus pallidus network to cortical electroencephalogram. *J Neurosci* 2000; 20:820–833.

Marceglia S, Servello D, Foffani G et al. Thalamic single-unit and local field potential activity in Tourette syndrome. *Mov Disord* 2010; 25:300–308.

Marsden CD, Meldrum BS, Pycock C, Tarsy D. Focal myoclonus produced by injection of picrotoxin into the caudate nucleus of the rat. *J Physiol* 1975; 246:96P.

Mayberg HS, Lozano AM, Voon V et al. Deep brain stimulation for treatment-resistant depression. *Neuron* 2005; 45:651–660.

McCairn KW, Bronfeld M, Belelovsky K, Bar-Gad I. The neurophysiological correlates of motor tics following focal striatal disinhibition. *Brain* 2009; 132:2125–2138.

An important study demonstrating the fast latency network changes that occur throughout the CBTC in the generation of motor tics.

McCairn KW, Iriki A, Isoda M. High-frequency pallidal stimulation blocks tic-related neuronal activity in a non-human primate model of Tourette syndrome. *Neuroreport* 2012; 23:206–210.

The first study to directly record tic-related neuronal activity in the output nucleus of the CBTC and how it is modulated by deep brain stimulation.

McGrath MJ, Campbell KM, Parks CR, Burton FH. Glutamatergic drugs exacerbate symptomatic behavior in a transgenic model of comorbid Tourette's syndrome and obsessive-compulsive disorder. *Brain Res* 2000; 877:23–30.

An important model for emphasizing the role of cortical hyperactivity for the generation of TS-like behavior, especially OCD-like symptoms.

McKenzie GM, Viik K. Chemically induced chorieform activity: antagonism by GABA and EEG patterns. *Exp Neurol* 1975; 46:229–243.

Mehler WR, Nauta WJ. Connections of the basal ganglia and of the cerebellum. *Confin Neurol* 1974; 36:205–222.

Mink JW. The basal ganglia: focused selection and inhibition of competing motor programs. *Prog Neurobiol* 1996; 50:381–425.

Mink JW. Basal ganglia dysfunction in Tourette's syndrome: a new hypothesis. *Pediatr Neurol* 2001; 25:190–198.

Mink JW. The basal ganglia and involuntary movements: impaired inhibition of competing motor patterns. *Arch Neurol* 2003; 60: 1365–1368.

Mink JW, Walkup J, Frey KA et al. Patient selection and assessment recommendations for deep brain stimulation in Tourette syndrome. *Mov Disord* 2006; 21:1831–1838.

Moretto G, Schwingenschuh P, Katschnig P et al. Delayed experience of volition in Gilles de la

Tourette syndrome. *J Neurol Neurosurg Psychiatry* 2011; *82*:1324–1327.

Nambu A. Seven problems on the basal ganglia. *Curr Opin Neurobiol* 2008; *18*: 595–604.

Nambu A, Tokuno H, Hamada I et al. Excitatory cortical inputs to pallidal neurons via the subthalamic nucleus in the monkey. *J Neurophysiol* 2000; *84*:289–300.

Nambu A, Tokuno H, Inase M, Takada M. Corticosubthalamic input zones from forelimb representations of the dorsal and ventral divisions of the premotor cortex in the macaque monkey: comparison with the input zones from the primary motor cortex and the supplementary motor area. *Neurosci Lett* 1997; *239*:13–16.

Nambu A, Yoshida S, Jinnai K. Discharge patterns of pallidal neurons with input from various cortical areas during movement in the monkey. *Brain Res* 1990; *519*:183–191.

Nauta HJ, Cole M. Efferent projections of the subthalamic nucleus. *Trans Am Neurol Assoc* 1974; *99*:170–173.

Nauta HJ, Cole M. Efferent projections of the subthalamic nucleus: an autoradiographic study in monkey and cat. *J Comp Neurol* 1978; *180*:1–16.

Nini A, Feingold A, Slovin H, Bergman H. Neurons in the globus pallidus do not show correlated activity in the normal monkey, but phase-locked oscillations appear in the MPTP model of parkinsonism. *J Neurophysiol* 1995; *74*:1800–1805.

Nordstrom EJ, Burton FH. A transgenic model of comorbid Tourette's syndrome and obsessive-compulsive disorder circuitry. *Mol Psychiatry* 2002; *7*:617–625, 524.

Obeso JA, Rothwell JC, Marsden CD. The neurophysiology of Tourette syndrome. *Adv Neurol* 1982; *35*:105–114.

Ohtsu H, Watanabe T. New functions of histamine found in histidine decarboxylase gene knockout mice. *Biochem Biophys Res Commun* 2003; *305*:443–447.

Parent A, Bouchard C, Smith Y. The striatopallidal and striatonigral projections: two distinct fiber systems in primate. *Brain Res* 1984; *303*:385–390.

Parent A, Hazrati LN. Functional anatomy of the basal ganglia. I. The cortico-basal ganglia-thalamo-cortical loop. *Brain Res Brain Res Rev* 1995; *20*:91–127.

Parent A, Levesque M, Parent M. A re-evaluation of the current model of the basal ganglia. *Parkinsonism Relat Disord* 2001; *7*:193–198.

Parent A, Smith Y, Filion M, Dumas J. Distinct afferents to internal and external pallidal segments in the squirrel monkey. *Neurosci Lett* 1989; *96*:140–144.

Parent M, Parent A. The pallidofugal motor fiber system in primates. *Parkinsonism Relat Disord* 2004; *10*:203–211.

Paschou P, Feng Y, Pakstis AJ et al. Indications of linkage and association of Gilles de la Tourette syndrome in two independent family samples: 17q25 is a putative susceptibility region. *Am J Hum Genet* 2004; *75*:545–560.

Percheron G, Filion M. Parallel processing in the basal ganglia: up to a point. *Trends Neurosci* 1991; *14*:55–59.

Perkins AC, Cory S. Conditional immortalization of mouse myelomonocytic, megakaryocytic and mast cell progenitors by the Hox-2.4 homeobox gene. *EMBO J* 1993; *12*:3835–3846.

Peroutka SJ, Lebovitz RM, Snyder SH. Two distinct central serotonin receptors with different physiological functions. *Science* 1981; *212*:827–829.

Peterson BS. Neuroimaging studies of Tourette syndrome: a decade of progress. *Adv Neurol* 2001; *85*:179–196.

Plessen KJ, Wentzel-Larsen T, Hugdahl K et al. Altered interhemispheric connectivity in individuals with Tourette's disorder. *Am J Psychiatry* 2004; *161*:2028–2037.

Proenca CC, Gao KP, Shmelkov SV et al. Slitrks as emerging candidate genes involved in neuropsychiatric disorders. *Trends Neurosci* 2011; *34*:143–153.

Randrup A, Munkvad I. Pharmacology and physiology of stereotyped behavior. *J Psychiatr Res* 1974; *11*:1–10.

Randrup A, Munkvad I, Udsen P. Adrenergic mechanisms and amphetamine induced abnormal behaviour. *Acta Pharmacol Toxicol (Copenh)* 1963; *20*:145–157.

Rasch MJ, Gretton A, Murayama Y et al. Inferring spike trains from local field potentials. *J Neurophysiol* 2007; *99*:1461–1476.

Redgrave P, Prescott TJ, Gurney K. The basal ganglia: a vertebrate solution to the selection problem? *Neuroscience* 1999; *89*:1009–1023.

Richter A, Loscher W. Pathology of idiopathic dystonia: findings from genetic animal models. *Prog Neurobiol* 1998; *54*:633–677.

Rizzo R, Marino S, Gulisano M, Robertson MM. The successful use of ondansetron in a boy with both leukemia and Tourette syndrome. *J Child Neurol* 2008; 23:108–111.

Ross MS, Moldofsky H. A comparison of pimozide and haloperidol in the treatment of Gilles de la Tourette's syndrome. *Am J Psychiatry* 1978; 135:585–587.

Rouzaire-Dubois B, Scarnati E. Bilateral corticosubthalamic nucleus projections: an electrophysiological study in rats with chronic cerebral lesions. *Neuroscience* 1985; 15:69–79.

Seignot JN. A case of tic of Gilles de la Tourette cured by R 1625. *Ann Med Psychol (Paris)* 1961; 119:578–579.

Selemon LD, Goldman-Rakic PS. Longitudinal topography and interdigitation of corticostriatal projections in the rhesus monkey. *J Neurosci* 1985; 5:776–794.

Serrien DJ, Orth M, Evans AH et al. Motor inhibition in patients with Gilles de la Tourette syndrome: functional activation patterns as revealed by EEG coherence. *Brain* 2005; 128:116–125.

Shapiro AK, Shapiro E, Eisenkraft GJ. Treatment of Gilles de la Tourette's syndrome with clonidine and neuroleptics. *Arch Gen Psychiatry* 1983; 40:1235–1240.

Shink E, Sidibe M, Smith Y. Efferent connections of the internal globus pallidus in the squirrel monkey: II. Topography and synaptic organization of pallidal efferents to the pedunculopontine nucleus. *J Comp Neurol* 1997; 382:348–363.

Shmelkov SV, Hormigo A, Jing D et al. Slitrk5 deficiency impairs corticostriatal circuitry and leads to obsessive-compulsive-like behaviors in mice. *Nat Med* 2010; 16:598–602.

An especially important study that correlates Slitrk5 abnormalities with pathology in corticostriatal circuits and TS-like behavior.

Sidibe M, Bevan MD, Bolam JP, Smith Y. Efferent connections of the internal globus pallidus in the squirrel monkey: I. Topography and synaptic organization of the pallidothalamic projection. *J Comp Neurol* 1997; 382:323–347.

Silay YS, Jankovic J. Emerging drugs in Tourette syndrome. *Expert Opin Emerg Drugs* 2005; 10:365–380.

Singer HS, Mink JW, Loiselle CR et al. Microinfusion of antineuronal antibodies into rodent striatum: failure to differentiate between elevated and low titers. *J Neuroimmunol* 2005; 163:8–14.

Singer HS, Szymanski S, Giuliano J et al. Elevated intrasynaptic dopamine release in Tourette's syndrome measured by PET. *Am J Psychiatry* 2002; 159:1329–1336.

Singer HS, Wendlandt J, Krieger M, Giuliano J. Baclofen treatment in Tourette syndrome: a double-blind, placebo-controlled, crossover trial. *Neurology* 2001; 56:599–604.

Smith Y, Kieval JZ. Anatomy of the dopamine system in the basal ganglia. *Trends Neurosci* 2000; 23:S28–S33.

Smith Y, Parent A. Differential connections of caudate nucleus and putamen in the squirrel monkey (*Saimiri sciureus*). *Neuroscience* 1986; 18:347–371.

Smith Y, Shink E, Sidibe M. Neuronal circuitry and synaptic connectivity of the basal ganglia. *Neurosurg Clin North Am* 1998; 9:203–222.

Smith Y, Wichmann T, DeLong MR. Synaptic innervation of neurones in the internal pallidal segment by the subthalamic nucleus and the external pallidum in monkeys. *J Comp Neurol* 1994; 343:297–318.

Sowell ER, Kan E, Yoshii J et al. Thinning of sensorimotor cortices in children with Tourette syndrome. *Nat Neurosci* 2008; 11:637–639.

Swedo SE, Leonard HL, Garvey M et al. Pediatric autoimmune neuropsychiatric disorders associated with streptococcal infections: clinical description of the first 50 cases. *Am J Psychiatry* 1998; 155:264–271.

Swerdlow NR, Karban B, Ploum Y et al. Tactile prepuff inhibition of startle in children with Tourette's syndrome: in search of an "fMRI-friendly" startle paradigm. *Biol Psychiatry* 2001; 50:578–585.

Swerdlow NR, Sutherland AN. Using animal models to develop therapeutics for Tourette Syndrome. *Pharmacol Ther* 2005; 108: 281–293.

Swerdlow NR, Sutherland AN. Preclinical models relevant to Tourette syndrome. *Adv Neurol* 2006; 99:69–88.

Szabo J. The efferent projections of the putamen in the monkey. *Exp Neurol* 1967; 19:463–476.

Tarsy D, Pycock CJ, Meldrum BS, Marsden CD. Focal contralateral myoclonus produced by inhibition of GABA action in the caudate nucleus of rats. *Brain* 1978; 101:143–162.

Taylor JL, Rajbhandari AK, Berridge KC, Aldridge JW. Dopamine receptor modulation of repetitive grooming actions in the rat: potential relevance for Tourette syndrome. *Brain Res* 2010; *1322*:92–101.

Intriguing study that may provide insights into the causes of the different types of stereotypic behavior associated with TS.

Taylor JR, Morshed SA, Parveen S et al. An animal model of Tourette's syndrome. *Am J Psychiatry* 2002; *159*:657–660.

Tepper JM, Koos T, Wilson CJ. GABAergic microcircuits in the neostriatum. *Trends Neurosci* 2004; *27*:662–669.

Tizabi Y, Russell LT, Johnson M, Darmani NA. Nicotine attenuates DOI-induced head-twitch response in mice: implications for Tourette syndrome. *Prog Neuropsychopharmacol Biol Psychiatry* 2001; *25*:1445–1457.

Toren P, Laor N, Cohen DJ et al. Ondansetron treatment in patients with Tourette's syndrome. *Int Clin Psychopharmacol* 1999; *14*:373–376.

Turner RS, Anderson ME. Context-dependent modulation of movement-related discharge in the primate globus pallidus. *J Neurosci* 2005; *25*:2965–2976.

Waszczak BL, Martin L, Boucher N et al. Electrophysiological and behavioral output of the rat basal ganglia after intrastriatal infusion of d-amphetamine: lack of support for the basal ganglia model. *Brain Res* 2001; *920*:170–182.

Waszczak BL, Martin LP, Finlay HE et al. Effects of individual and concurrent stimulation of striatal D1 and D2 dopamine receptors on electrophysiological and behavioral output from rat basal ganglia. *J Pharmacol Exp Ther* 2002; *300*:850–861.

Welch JM, Lu J, Rodriguiz RM et al. Cortico-striatal synaptic defects and OCD-like behaviours in Sapap3-mutant mice. *Nature* 2007; *448*:894–900.

Wilson CJ, Groves PM. Fine structure and synaptic connections of the common spiny neuron of the rat neostriatum: a study employing intracellular inject of horseradish peroxidase. *J Comp Neurol* 1980; *194*:599–615.

Worbe Y, Baup N, Grabli D et al. Behavioral and movement disorders induced by local inhibitory dysfunction in primate striatum. *Cereb Cortex* 2009; *19*:1844–1856.

Worbe Y, Gerardin E, Hartmann A et al. Distinct structural changes underpin clinical phenotypes in patients with Gilles de la Tourette syndrome. *Brain* 2010; *133*:3649–3660.

Yaddanapudi K, Hornig M, Serge R et al. Passive transfer of streptococcus-induced antibodies reproduces behavioral disturbances in a mouse model of pediatric autoimmune neuropsychiatric disorders associated with streptococcal infection. *Mol Psychiatry* 2010; *15*:712–726.

Yelnik J, Percheron G, Francois C. A Golgi analysis of the primate globus pallidus. II. Quantitative morphology and spatial orientation of dendritic arborizations. *J Comp Neurol* 1984; *227*:200–213.

Ziemann U, Paulus W, Rothenberger A. Decreased motor inhibition in Tourette's disorder: evidence from transcranial magnetic stimulation. *Am J Psychiatry* 1997; *154*:1277–1284.

SECTION 4

DIAGNOSIS AND ASSESSMENT

16

Whither the Relationship Between Etiology and Phenotype in Tourette Syndrome?

MARY M. ROBERTSON AND VALSAMMA EAPEN

Abstract

The Tourette syndrome (TS) phenotype is not unitary but heterogeneous. This chapter offers a critical commentary on available research on the definition of the phenotype of TS, analyzed from different perspectives, and provides an update on the nosography of tic disorders. Endophenotype studies indicate that there are indeed a few correlations between etiology and phenotype, and this is an exciting area. Gender and other behavioral differences may indicate different etiological factors, and there is some evidence to suggest the existence of obsessive-compulsive behavior/disorder endophenotpyes. Early neuroimaging studies suggest that this may be due to prenatal and perinatal difficulties, which influence the phenotypic expression of the TS gene(s). Thus, replication studies are required with similar methods and with the TS patients subdivided into phenotypes. The clinical phenotype and the severity of symptoms, as well as the associated psychopathology observed in TS, may be influenced by the nature and extent of involvement of the above circuitry based on both genetic and nongenetic factors as well as the developmental period in question. There may be shared molecular genetic pathways affecting development across diagnostic boundaries mediated through neurodevelopmental genes.

INTRODUCTION

This chapter will focus on the etiological theories of TS with regard to the individual phenotypes. We will briefly discuss current etiologies and phenotype, as well as relevant predisposing factors that have an impact on phenotype but are seldom mentioned in the TS literature. We will consider endophenotypes and how they may pave the way for TS and allied disorders as well as how they may be expanded in the future. We will briefly mention possible reasons for the lack of clarity of etiology when compared to other disorders that were once thought to be unitary conditions but have turned out to be genetically heterogeneous (dystonia, Huntington's disease). Finally, we will make some suggestions for possible future research and nomenclature for TS, citing relevant examples.

WHAT IS TS? A HISTORICAL PERSPECTIVE AND NOSOLOGY

The definition and diagnosis of TS have changed over time, from the time of its original description in 1825 by Itard and further characterization by Gilles de la Tourette in 1885 and 1889. Although it appears that the notion of phenotype, the comorbid conditions, and the psychiatric illnesses associated with TS are often assumed to be recent discoveries, they were actually noted in nearly all the early descriptions (Guinon, Grasset, and Gilles de la Tourette; see Robertson & Reinstein, 1991). It is important to note that most experts now acknowledge (as did the early writers) that (1) TS is a heterogeneous syndrome, and one for which there is currently no definitive test; (2) TS has many phenotypes; and (3) at the end of the day, TS is currently a "committee-specified diagnosis" that some individuals in our opinion erroneously call a *disorder.*

Some Problems with the Nosology and Diagnosis of TS and How It Affects the Phenotype

It has been shown that TS is common (Robertson, 2008a, 2008b; see also Chapter 6). As it will be shown (vide infra) that the etiology and its relationship to the TS phenotypes are complex, as is the psychopathology, one must ask: *What is TS?* Are there different types of TS? Since Dr. Georges Gilles de la Tourette originally described the disorder in 1885, emphasizing the "core" symptoms of motor tics, minor motor incoordination, coprolalia, and echolalia, the phenotypic definitions of TS have changed. In addition, coprolalia has never been required in any diagnostic categorization. Finally, both the DSM (2000) and World Health Organization (1992) criteria have stipulated that TS is a unitary condition. In addition to the motor and vocal (phonic) tics that are the hallmarks of TS, several comorbid conditions (e.g., attention-deficit/hyperactivity disorder [ADHD]; obsessive-compulsive behaviors [OCB], obsessive-compulsive symptoms, and disorder [OCD]; and self-injurious behaviors) and psychopathologies (e.g., depression, anxiety) have been described (see Chapters 2, 3, and 4), but it is unclear as to whether and how these are linked to TS etiologies and phenotypes.

The various definitions of TS will continue to change and affect phenotype, and possibly vice versa. For instance, the Chinese have their own diagnostic system, CCMD III (Chinese Criteria of Mental Disorder III). This results in the Chinese prevalence figures being somewhat lower, even though some Chinese TS studies use DSM criteria (Robertson, 2008a). In addition, DSM criteria have changed substantially over time: for example, with regard to the upper age limit for age at onset (15, 18, 21 years), distress and impairment criteria, the duration of tics (usually >1 year), and whether or not there should be tic-free intervals, and how long they should be.

Robertson (2008a, 2008b) pointed out that in the WHO (1992) criteria there has never been an age of onset stipulation, with the result that some "adult-onset tic disorders" may be included in the TS umbrella in some studies in Europe, while similar cases will be excluded in the United States and other countries employing DSM criteria. These "adult-onset tic disorders" have indeed been documented from Canada (Chouinard & Ford, 2000) and the United Kingdom (Eapen et al., 2002), but they often had different etiologies, such as being secondary to infections, trauma, or noxious agents. In other words, they were different from "pure or primary" TS. Furthermore, others have described TS as commencing before 1 year of age (Burd & Kerbeshian, 1987). These data highlight the complexity of diagnosis of TS and related tic disorders even further. In addition, many erroneously believe that coprolalia must be present for the diagnosis because this was highlighted by Gilles de la Tourette (1885) in his original cohort and due to the media characterization of the syndrome.

The Varying Phenotypes of TS: The Current Status—TS Is Suggested Not to Be a Unitary Condition

Few attempts have been made to formally classify TS patients on the basis of their tic phenomenology, and one must also consider the effects of comorbidity and psychopathology when considering phenotype. In addition to the complex etiology of TS with genetic heterogeneity, it appears that TS is not a unitary condition, as shown by phenomenological studies (Robertson, Trimble & Lees, 1988) and by those employing hierarchical cluster analyses (HCA), principal-component factor analyses (PCFA), and latent class analysis (LCA) (e.g., Alsobrook & Pauls, 2002; Cavanna et al., 2011; Eapen et al., 2004; Grados et al., 2008; Mathews et al., 2007; Robertson & Cavanna, 2007; Robertson, Althoff, Hafez et al., 2008; Storch et al., 2004), all of which reported many factors/classes. All these studies add to the growing body of evidence that TS is not a unitary condition and can be disaggregated into more homogeneous symptom components. In all studies that directly have specifically examined for it, one factor has included simple motor and phonic/vocal tics. Table 16.1 summarizes the studies suggesting

Table 16.1 Studies Showing Different Phenotypes (Factors, Classes, Clusters) in Tourette Syndrome and Their Etiological Suggestions

Authors	Year of publication	Country of study	Number of subjects in study	Results showing variables obtained	Methods of analysis	Number of phenotypes	Factors and clusters and/or phenotypes found	Aetiological Suggestions from authors	Other aetiological suggestions
Alsobrook & Pauls	2002	USA	85	26 (clusters of tic symptoms)	HCA + PCFA	4	Aggression Tics Compulsions Tapping + absence of grunting	¾ = heritable aggressive compulsions tapping+no grunting	OBS/OCB/OCD related to TS genetically and an integral part of TS (see Table 2)
Eapen et al.	2004	UK	91	11 (behavioral symptoms only)	PCFA	2	Obsessionality Anxiety/ depression	n/a	
Storch et al.	2004	USA	67	15 (tic symptoms + behavioral symptoms)	PCFA	4	Aggression ADHD OCD Tics	n/a	Martino et al ADHD not linked to ABGA. OBS/OCB/OCD related to TS genetically and an integral part of TS (see Table 2)
Mathews et al.	2007	USA	254	38 (tic symptoms + tic-related symptoms)	HCA	2	Simple tics Complex tics + OCD symptoms		OBS/OCB/OCD related to TS genetically and an integral part of TS (see Table 2)

(Continued)

Table 16-1 (*Continued*)

Authors	Year of publication	Country of study	Number of subjects in study	Results showing variables obtained	Methods of analysis	Number of phenotypes	Factors and clusters and/or phenotypes found	Aetiological Suggestions from authors	Other aetiological suggestions
Robertson & Cavanna	2007	UK	69 from 1 large pedigree	18 (clusters of tic symptoms + behavioral symptoms)	HCA + PCFA	4	Tics ADHD + aggression Anxiety/depression/obsessionality + self-injurious behaviors	One large Pedigree—so All heritable	Martino et al ADHD not linked to ABGA. OBS/OCB/OCD related to TS genetically and an integral part of TS (see Table 2)
Grados et al.	2008	International	952 subjects from 222 families	3 (diagnosis of TS + OCD + ADHD)	LCA	5	TS + OCD symptoms/behavior TS + OCD TS + OCD + ADHD Minimally affected class Complex motor tics + OCD	Only TS+ ADHD+ OCD Heritable	Martino et al ADHD not linked to ABGA. OBS/OCB/OCD related to TS genetically and an integral part of TS (see Table 2)

Robertson et al.	2008	UK	410	20 (clusters of tic symptoms + tic-related symptoms)	HCA + PCFA	5	Non-obscene socially inappropriate behaviors + complex vocal tics Complex motor tics Simple tics Compulsions Self-touching	n/a	OBS/OCB/OCD related to TS genetically and an integral part of TS (see Table 2)
Cavanna et al. 2011		UK	639		PCFA	3	Complex motor tics + echo-pali-phenomena ADHD symptoms + aggressive behaviors Complex vocal tics + coprophenomena	n/a	Martino et al ADHD not linked to ABGA

Updated and modified from Cavanna et al., 2011.

more than one factor (i.e., phenotype) in TS. In addition, what is interesting is that ADHD and OCD/OCB are usually considered comorbid with TS, while other psychopathology is not. Eapen and colleagues (2004), in a PCFA study, reported two factors: one was obsessionality and the other was anxiety and depression, which is somewhat counterintuitive (given that depression and anxiety are not usually considered either comorbid with [Robertson, 2006] or genetically related [Pauls et al., 1994] to TS).

Many clinicians pragmatically separate TS into types that make clinical sense, namely "pure" TS (motor and vocal/phonic tics only), "full-blown TS" (with copro-, echo-, and paliphenomena; Robertson & Baron-Cohen, 1998), and "TS plus," coined by Packer (1987) to describe patients with a "full house" of comorbid and psychiatric conditions. Whether further such analytic studies, along with concomitant genetic studies, will echo these subdivisions is eagerly awaited. For "TS plus," there are suggestions from neuropsychological (Channon et al., 2006; Marsh et al., 2004), neuroradiological (Peterson et al., 2003), and behavioral (Carter et al., 2000; Peterson et al., 2001) data that it is the comorbidities that seem to predict current and future outcome, both in terms of the tic symptoms and the functional status more broadly.

Analytic Studies and the TS Phenotype

Although 90% of patients with TS have tics as well as other phenomena in both clinical (Freeman et al., 2000) and community (Khalifa & von Knorring, 2003, 2005) settings, few studies (Robertson & Cavanna, 2007) have examined the phenotype and included all these aspects in the analysis. In particular, what has not occurred is a study examining PCFA, HCA, or LCA plus comorbid conditions and psychopathology in a consecutive clinical TS cohort: it is hoped that one will soon be undertaken and that this will also include etiological factors such as genetic analysis, perinatal disorders (PNDs), and neuroimmunology. When such an analytic study along with a concomitant genetic study is

undertaken, one wonders at the conclusions and hopes that it and subsequent studies will echo the phenotypic divisions already discussed.

NATURAL HISTORY: PROGNOSIS, ENVIRONMENTAL EFFECTS, AND THE CHANGING PHENOTYPES OF TS OVER LIFE

Chapter 5 has been devoted to this, but in the interest of demonstrating how time and age alter phenotype, brief mention will be made of this aspect. Robertson (2008a, 2008b) has discussed in detail the lifetime prognosis of TS. It was initially thought that TS was life-long, but then Erenberg and colleagues (1987) first suggested that TS symptoms decreased with age. Leckman and colleagues (1998) subsequently highlighted the natural course of the disorder, suggesting that the prognosis was better, with the onset of TS at 5.6 years, the worst severity being at 10 years, and the majority of symptoms disappearing in half of the patients by 18 years. Coffey and colleagues (2004) reported a similar age at onset and found that, although tics persisted, impairment reduced with time. Bloch and colleagues (2006a) also reported a reduction in tics during adolescence (average age at worst tic severity being 10.6 years): only increased tic severity in childhood was associated with increased tic severity at follow-up. However, worst-ever obsessive-compulsive symptoms occurred approximately 2 years later than worst tic severity; increased childhood IQ was associated with increased OCD severity at follow-up.

Studies reviewed by Coffey and colleagues (2000, 2004) showed that the course of TS is remitting. Pappert and colleagues (2003) reviewed their TS patients (aged 8–14 years) using a 5-minute videotape at first visit and then at follow-up between 1978 and 1991 using video and blinded rating, and showed that 90% of the adults still had tics. Despite many adults suggesting that they were tic-free, no less than 50% had objective evidence of tics on video. The mean tic disability score decreased significantly with age: all tic domains improved with age, and this was not related to medication. Garcia-Ribes and colleagues (2003) studied clinical factors predicting the initial remission of tics in TS children (51% comorbidity [34% ADHD, 17% OCD]) and 26% school underachievement) over 5 years. Regardless of treatment, remission was determined by tic-related factors such as later age at onset and shorter time of evolution of tics. Further, while OCD or ADHD was significantly related to school failure, this did not relate to the evolution or remission of tics. Altman and colleagues (2009) examined the effects of TS on prognosis from a different point of view in 180 adults with TS, using a mailed questionnaire survey. "Personal acceptance" and "medication use" were the most important factors in coping with TS, while the severity of vocal tics had a much greater influence on adult functioning than that of motor tics. Although TS continued to interfere with their lives into adulthood, the impact was relatively modest, and they were able to cope using family and medical support.

Lin and colleagues (2010) undertook a longitudinal study on 45 TS cases who had had group A beta-hemolytic streptococcal infections (GABHS) and compared them with 41 matched controls over a 2-year period using blind ratings. Results showed that only a minority of children with TS and early-onset OCD were sensitive to antecedent GABHS infections. The most recent study is that by Leckman and colleagues (2011), who conducted a blinded, prospective, longitudinal study with a group of children who had had GABHS infections and who also met criteria for PANDAS (pediatric autoimmune neuropsychiatric disorder associated with streptococcus; n = 31) and a group of children with TS and/or OCD but without a PANDAS history (n = 53). Results showed no evidence for a temporal association between GABHS infections and tic/obsessive-compulsive symptom exacerbation in those who met the PANDAS diagnostic criteria, and there were no group differences in the number of clinical exacerbations or the number of newly diagnosed GABHS infections. The results of this study, as well as those of others (Lin et al., 2010; Mell et al., 2005), suggest that in fact GABHS is associated with a particular TS phenotype, and it may be the one that excludes ADHD as a comorbid diagnosis (Martino et al., 2007).

The previous studies and Box 16.1 suggest that the phenotype changes with time and age, and that, when older, these mildly impaired and/or no longer impaired individuals will still have TS, albeit mild. This is an intriguing echo of Gilles de la Tourette (1889), who stated over 120 years ago that "Once a ticcer, always a ticcer."

Box 16.1. Key Points

- The TS phenotype is not unitary, but heterogeneous.
- Endophenotype studies indicate that there are indeed a few correlations between etiology and phenotype, and this is an exciting area.
- Gender and other behavioral (OCB) differences may indicate different etiological factors, and there is some evidence to suggest the existence of OCD/OCB endophenotypes.
- Early neuroimaging studies suggest that this may be due to prenatal and perinatal difficulties, which influence the phenotypic expression of the TS gene(s). Thus, replication studies are required with similar methods and with the TS patients subdivided into phenotypes.
- The clinical phenotype and the severity of symptoms, as well as the associated psychopathology observed in TS, may be influenced by the nature and extent of involvement of the above circuitry based on both genetic and nongenetic factors as well as the developmental period in question.
- There may be shared molecular genetic pathways affecting development across diagnostic boundaries mediated through neurodevelopmental genes.

ETIOLOGICAL FACTORS

It is now recognized that the etiology of TS is multifactorial: genetic, environmental, immunological, and hormonal factors interact to establish vulnerability (Martino et al., 2009a, and also Chapters 7, 8, 9, and 14). One may well ask: What is the current status as to the relationship between these factors and the phenotype? In addition, one may ask: When etiologies are definitive in subgroups (almost certainly in certain phenotypes), what will the etiology (or etiologies) and phenotype (or phenotypes) be? Despite several decades of genetic research, and more recently other etiologies such as infections (e.g., Swedo et al., 1998) and prenatal/perinatal events (Leckman et al., 1987, 1990), it is surprising that relatively little is known about etiology and phenotypes. Whether or not the various phenotypes are associated with different etiologies has not been widely studied, but Table 16.1 presents a few such studies that examined phenotypic manifestations in the light of presumed etiological factors.

Phenotype: Current Theories and Suggestions

Having briefly discussed current knowledge about TS diagnostic criteria and prognosis, as well as how the phenotype changes with time, let us explore other factors affecting the phenotype.

One of the earliest hints at genetic factors influencing phenotype came from the authors' group using clinical (Robertson, Trimble & Lees, 1988) and segregation analysis studies (Eapen et al., 1993). The latter study found that OCB is an alternative phenotypic expression of the putative TS gene(s), and that there may be gender-dependent differences in the expression of phenotypes, with female members having more obsessive-compulsive symptoms and male members exhibiting more tic symptoms. Further, the presence of certain characteristic obsessive-compulsive symptoms and earlier age of onset in the proband suggest that this is a familial form linked to TS (Eapen et al., 1997a). However, the issue of familial phenotypic expression is complicated by the phenomenon of bilineality. McMahon and colleagues (1996) observed bilineal transmission in a large TS pedigree of four generations, with evidence of some disorder in 67% of the descendants and 44% of the married-in spouses. The offspring of two parents with tic disorders had significantly more lifetime tics, more severe tics, and earlier age at onset of TS compared to those with one or no affected parents. In another study, Kurlan and colleagues (1994) observed that among 39 high-density families in which five or more relatives were reported to have TS, bilineal transmission was evident in 33% (considering tics) and 41% (considering tics or OCB), which was confirmed by examination in 77% of the kindreds. Both parents of the proband were affected (tics or OCB) in 38% of high-density TS pedigrees, and the frequency of bilineal transmission was related to the proband's severity of TS, supporting the contention that bilineal transmission and homozygosity are common in TS and that these phenomena might play a role in determining severity of illness.

In addition to bilineality, parent-of-origin effects caused by genomic imprinting have also been suggested to influence the phenotypic expression in TS. Thus, Eapen and colleagues (1997b), in a study of 437 first-degree relatives, found that 16.7% had matrilineal inheritance and 13.9% had patrilineal inheritance, and that the maternally transmitted offspring showed a significantly earlier age at onset. This points to a parent-of-origin effect on the putative TS gene that could be explained by meiotic events or even intrauterine environmental influences. These findings may help explain the hitherto conflicting reports about the nature of genetic transmission in TS, and suggest a need to re-examine family data separately for maternally and paternally transmitted cases.

Social factors affect births, babies, and subsequent development (Blumenshine et al., 2010; Brown et al., 2011; Liu, 2011; Metcalfe et al., 2011; Vettore et al., 2010). As a more specific example, low birth weight has been associated with disadvantage measured at multiple levels and has been shown to be associated with a high risk of executive function deficit, including impulse control (Ni et al., 2011), behavioral, and psychiatric problems (Elgen et al., 2002).

Although detailed already in Chapter 8, let us briefly examine what PNDs have been invoked as specifically affecting the TS phenotype. While numerous studies have documented PND in TS patients, few have been specific, and social factors that are important in generic maternity care have not been studied in TS. The first study to link phenotype and etiology was that by Leckman and colleagues (1987), who reported that nongenetic factors (PNDs— intrauterine) were at play in TS: in 23% of 30 monozygotic twin pairs who were discordant for TS, and in all of the discordant pairs (n = 6), the unaffected co-twin had a higher birth weight than the twin affected with TS. Leckman and colleagues (1990) continued investigating PND in 31 TS patients, demonstrating that the severity of maternal life stress during pregnancy, the gender of the child, and the presence of severe nausea and/or vomiting during the first trimester were significantly associated with current tic severity. Thereafter, Hyde and colleagues (1992, 1994, 1995) and Randolph and colleagues (1993) demonstrated that in monozygotic twins in whom at least one twin had TS, and who were concordant for tic diagnosis but not for severity, those with more severe tics had lower birth weights, more abnormal EEGs, reduced right caudate nucleus volumes, and significantly poorer neuropsychological performance, all of which they suggested were as a result of the PNDs. Relatively recently, maternal smoking has been studied in TS patients, and it appears that maternal smoking is associated with different phenotypes, including increased tic severity (Mathews et al., 2006; Motlagh et al., 2010), low birth weight (Pringsheim et al., 2009), and psychosocial stress (Motlagh et al., 2010). While these results are encouraging, it is unclear whether the difficulties are generic (resulting in neurodevelopmental problems) or more specific to TS, and further controlled studies are needed examining for possible PNDs as contributing etiological factors as well as the actual etiological effects specific to TS.

It is generally accepted that TS occurs more in males (Robertson, 2000). Although this may well be due to genetic factors, the frequent male-to-male transmission observed in large pedigrees appears to rule out the presence of an X-linked vulnerability gene (Leckman, 2003), and has led to the hypothesis (Peterson et al., 1992) that androgenic steroids may act at certain key developmental periods to influence the natural history of TS and related disorders. It has been suggested that androgenic steroids may be responsible for these effects, or they may well act indirectly through estrogens formed in key brain regions by the aromatization of testosterone (Leckman 2003).

In this context, there have been some suggestions with regard to symptomatology differences within the genders. Thus, several authors (Debes et al., 2010a; Eapen et al., 1993; Pauls et al., 1991; Robertson & Gourdie, 1990) demonstrated that males are more likely to have tics, while females are more likely to have OCD, OCB, or obsessive-compulsive symptoms. Further, significantly more males have an earlier age at onset of TS and a history of birth complications (Eapen et al., 2004). It has also been shown that boys are more likely than girls to demonstrate disruptive behaviors (Comings & Comings, 1987a). It has further been suggested that ADHD is more common in second-degree relatives of females (Debes et al., 2010a). Lewin and colleagues (2012) described the tic and TS phenomenology in 185 women and 275 men (18–79 years) using identical schedules. Sixty-eight percent of women had severe motor tics and 40% had severe vocal tics: many of the women with persistent tics suffered from psychiatric comorbidity and psychosocial consequences (underachievement, social distress). The authors suggested that tic severity in women may be associated with lifestyle interference as well as anxiety and depression, and these may be more common in women.

Swedo and colleagues (1998) set the scene for the possible link between streptococcal infection and TS to be investigated. She described youngsters with PANDAS (see Chapter 9), and thereafter many laboratories also found increased streptococcal infections in patients with TS. The epidemiological data on the relationship between GABHS infections and TS are summarized in Chapter 9 and the immunological features of TS in Chapter 14. The only study to examine phenotype and etiology in this area was that by Martino and colleagues (2007), who examined phenotypic features of anti-basal ganglia antibodies (ABGA)-positive and -negative patients among 53 children and 75 adults with TS: 23% of children and 25% of adults were ABGA-positive. On multivariate logistic regression analysis, only ADHD remained inversely correlated with ABGA. This suggests that immunity might be abnormal in a subgroup of people with TS, possibly those who do not have ADHD. However, before any conclusions can be definitively drawn, further studies are needed.

Although early researchers referred to tic disorders as "stress-sensitive" (Jagger et al., 1982; Shapiro et al., 1988; Silva et al., 1995), it is only relatively recently that the area of stress and stressful life events has been formally investigated in TS, with interesting results from the point of view of phenotype. Chapter 14 provides further details on this aspect. In one of the earliest studies, Surwillo and colleagues (1978) noted that during stressful life events, tics were helped by haloperidol, but they wondered whether or not the waxing and waning of tics could be caused by life events. Hoekstra and colleagues (2004a) found that, contrary to expectations, life events affected tics in only a minority of TS patients. Horesh and colleagues (2008) then documented that the onset of TS was not related to life events. Unfortunately, with the relatively small number of studies and conflicting anecdotal findings, traditional views, and evidence, little more can be deduced other than that further research is necessary. It has been noted in a review that stressful psychosocial life events may be associated with subsequent worse severity of depression, with lesser effects on tics and obsessionality (Stern & Robertson, 1997).

Few studies have been on the effects of cultural factors on phenotype, but interesting findings have emerged from the few that have, suggesting that while the core symptoms of motor and vocal tics remain consistent universally, there may well be cultural differences in the extended phenotype.

In an international registry of 430 case reports compiled by Abuzzahab and Anderson (1976), consisting mainly of North American and European populations, some cross-cultural symptom differences were noted, but other subsequent independent studies on separate TS cohorts have failed to replicate such differences (Lees et al., 1984; Shapiro & Shapiro, 1982). Although studies have suggested that the "core" TS symptoms are similar across cultures (Eapen & Robertson, 2008; Robertson et al., 1994), there may be some variations in the presentation with regard to associated features. For example, a study from Korea observed fewer OCD symptoms and behaviors compared to the Western population (Min & Lee, 1986), while a greater male preponderance and lower rates of coprolalia were noted by Japanese investigators (Nomura et al., 1992). The presence of coprolalia has shown considerable variation across cultures, with rates as low as 4% to 11% in Japan (Nomura & Segawa, 1979, 1982), 46% in New Zealand (Robertson et al., 1994), and 60% in Hong Kong (Lieh-Mak et al., 1982). In addition, the lower rates of coprolalia observed among the middle class and those from strict religious backgrounds (Butler, 1984), as well as a case report from China that reported the vocalization of a young girl that translated as "down with Chou En-lai," has led to the suggestion that some of these features with social connotations may be modified by cultural and psychosocial factors (Earls, 1992). On the other hand, a high rate of 74% for coprolalia reported from cross-cultural case reports (Staley et al., 1997) and 50% from another Japanese cohort (Kano et al., 1998) may be indicative of the differences in sample selection and diagnostic criteria used by different authors.

A review of TS symptoms and associated features by Staley and colleagues (1997) reported 39 cases from cross-cultural sources and concluded that the pattern is similar between that observed in North American and European samples and that from other regions and cultures around the world. However, minor differences were also noted, including the fact that the percentage of males in Eastern and Asiatic samples exceeded that found in Western studies

(Nomura et al., 1982). This may be attributed at least in part to the sample-selection methods or help-seeking patterns of patients in certain cultures where females are more reluctant than males to seek help. In addition, the methodological differences in the diagnostic criteria, as well as the instruments used to ascertain associated features, would mean that the differences observed need not necessarily be a true reflection of the situation.

The only study to directly compare TS symptomatology and phenotype across two different cultures using identical methods did indeed report significant differences in the TS "behavioral phenotype." The study compared consecutive cohorts of 35 age- and sex-matched young Arab patients with TS from the United Arab Emirates (UAE) with Caucasians from the United Kingdom (UK). In the main, the phenomenology of the motor and vocal tics and the rates of occurrence of OCD and ADHD were similar in the two cohorts. Coprolalia was higher in the UK cohort (25.7%) than the UAE sample (8.6%), while the rates for copropraxia were 11.4% and 2.9% respectively: coprolalia was noted to correlate with the severity of TS. However, oppositional defiant disorder (ODD) and conduct disorder (CD) were also more common in the UK cohort (19 [54.3%] and 7 [20%] respectively) than to the UAE cohort (4 [11.4%] and 2 [5.7%] respectively), but this was not linked to any other clinical feature or severity of TS. The rate of aggression was also much higher in the UK than UAE patients (20% and 2.9%, respectively). The high rates of disruptive behaviors, aggression, ODD, and CD in the UK cohort deserve comment in the context of culture affecting phenotype. The authors suggested that sociocultural/religious factors and differences between the two populations/countries account for this. For example, in the UAE, family stability is high, with both parents present and often a large supportive family network; there is also a strongly embedded religious discipline, a strong patriarchal presence, and strictly enforced moral and legal codes. Thus, some of the potentially complex and challenging conditions, such as behavioral and conduct disturbances, that are often encountered among TS patients in the Western population seem to be the result of environmental and other modulating factors.

One study tried specifically to determine whether or not the presence of several putative etiological factors influenced TS severity. Neave and colleagues (2008) assessed 104 consecutive TS patients using the schedules Yale Global Tic Severity Scale (YGTSS) and the Motor tic, Obsessions and compulsions, Vocal tic Evaluation Survey (MOVES) (see Chapter 19): a positive family history was present in 91%, prenatal or perinatal difficulties were present in 48%, and recurrent throat infections were present in 35%. Results showed that there were no significant differences in tic severity between groups with and without a positive family history, prenatal or perinatal adversities, or recurrent throat infections. The results were also not influenced by examining subsets with varying strength of family history nor number of possible etiological factors. The authors concluded that tic severity was not related to any of the three possible etiological factors: this could be confounded by the heterogeneity of TS, by overreporting of mild birth difficulties, and/or by nonspecificity of throat infections (Neave et al., 2008). There have been several other suggestions as to the etiology of the various TS phenotypes (Table 16.2): these have been either supported by evidence-based studies (with references given) or deduced by the authors' personal clinical and research experience.

PHENOTYPES WITHIN TS THAT ARE AFFECTED BY COMORBID CONDITIONS: ADHD AS AN EXAMPLE

It is well known that ADHD is present in about 60% of individuals with TS (e.g., Freeman et al., 2000, 2007). In addition, ADHD occurs in half the factors (phenotypes) in the studies undertaken using PCFA, HCA, and/or LCA (Table 16.1). However, the precise relationship between TS and ADHD is unclear (see also Chapter 2). Numerous studies in youngsters comparing children with TS alone, TS+ADHD, ADHD alone, and/or unaffected controls (Carter et al.,

Table 16.2 Current TS Phenotypes (Including Comorbidities and Psychopathologies) and Suggested Etiologies

Phenotype (s)	Reported prevalence of symptoms	Etiology	References
Factors	n/a	Heritable	Alsobrook & Pauls, 2002
Aggression			
Compulsion			
Tapping + no grunting			
Factor TS + OCD + ADHD	n/a	Heritable	Grados et al., 2008
Increased tic severity	n/a	Smoking in pregnancy	Mathews et al., 2006;Motlagh et al., 2010
		Stress	Lin et al., 2007
		Stress in pregnancy	Motlagh et al., 2010
		Anxiety	Woods et al., 2005
		ADHD	Marsh et al., 2004
		Stress & GABHS infection	Lin et al., 2010
		Lower birth weight	Pringsheim et al., 2009Leckman et al., 1987, 1990
		PNDs + Lower birth weight	Hyde et al., 1992, 1994, 1995
		Cortical thinning associated with increased tic severity	Numerous—see text
ADHD	60 %	-	Freeman et al., 2000,2007
	75%	-	Kurlan et al., 1996
		Not straightforward	Pauls et al., 1984, 1986
		Not genetic	Eapen & Robertson, 1996
			Stewart et al., 2006
		Genetic	Comings & Comings, 1984, 1990
		Probably genetic	Knell & Comings, 1993
		Negative ABGA	O'Rourke et al., 2011
		Maternal smoking	Bloch et al., 2011
		Separate entity	

Obsessive-compulsive behaviors and disorder	30–40% 69%		Martino et al., 2007 Mathews et al., 2006 Motlagh et al., 2010 Yordanova et al., 1997 Freeman et al., 2000 Kurlan et al., 1996 Pauls et al., 1986 Comings & Comings, 1987b
		Genetic Integral part of TS	Eapen et al., 1997a Leckman et al., 2003
Depressive symptomatology	13–76%	Multifactorial stigmatizing bullying at school, neuroanatomical substrates similar	Robertson, 2006 Pauls et al., 1994 Robertson et al., 1988
		not genetic	Robertson, 2003
		More in females, older patients, & those with echo-phenomena	Snijders et al., 2006
		Correlates: age, tic severity, ADHD, OCD, childhood conduct disorder	
Dysphoria	Unknown	Side effects medication	Robertson, 2000
Personality disorder	Many in clinic populations	Only 2 studies	Shapiro et al., 1973, 1988
		Healthy controls	Robertson et al., 1997
		All types personality disorders	Robertson, 2003
		As a result of childhood ADHD, ODD, CD, & not TS *per se*	Robertson, 2003
		Referral bias	

(Continued)

Table 16.2 (*Continued*)

Phenotype(s)	Reported prevalence of symptoms	Etiology	References
Oppositional defiant disorder & conduct disorder	15%	As a result of childhood ADHD Possible cultural influences	Freeman et al., 2000 Robertson, 2003 Eapen & Robertson, 2008
Anxiety disorder	18%	Secondary to having TS (e.g., as a result of tics in public) Part of TS School phobia/separation anxiety	Freeman et al., 2000 Robertson, 2003 Linet, 1985
Self-injurious behaviors	14%	Obsessional Impulsive	Freeman et al., 2000 Robertson et al., 1989 Mathews et al., 2004
Non-obscene socially inappropriate behaviors	22% (behavior) 30% (urge)	Linked to impulsivity Not related to obsessionality	Kurlan et al., 1996
Sexually inappropriate behaviors	6%	Due to comorbidity & impulsivity	Freeman et al., 2000 Freeman et al., 2000 Present author
Aggression Anger control problems	Approximately 30% 37%	Significantly related to forced to touch copropraxia Related to comorbidity	Robertson et al., 1988 Freeman et al., 2000
Rage & impulsivity	Common	More research needed	Budman et al., 1998 Present author
Alcoholism & substance abuse		Reduces tics (? self-medication) Linked to ADHD	Robertson et al., 1988 Present author Haddad et al., 2009 Charach et al., 2011

Condition	Prevalence	Comment	References
Mania & bipolar affective disorder	Very uncommon	Possibly related to OCD / More research needed	Burd & Kerbeshian, 1984 / Berthier et al., 1998 / Robertson, 2003 / Present author
Autism, Asperger's syndrome & social communication disorder	6–11%	Unknown & more research required / Suggest neurodevelopmental disadvantage > vulnerable	Baron-Cohen et al., 1999a / Baron-Cohen et al., 1999b / Canitano & Vivanti, 2007
Pervasive developmental disorder	4.5%	As immediately above—more research required	Freeman et al., 2000 / Present author
Learning disability & mental retardation	3.9%	Suggested due to shared general neurodevelopmental problems	Freeman et al., 2000 / Present author
Dyslexia & dyspraxia	Uncommon	Possibly due to general neurodevelopmental problems	Present author
Epilepsy	Rare	No relationship, chance occurrence, both common / Possibly subgroup with GTS, ADHD, & epilepsy	Present author / Rizzo et al 2010
Schizophrenia	Rare	No relationship at all; both disorders are common, so chance occurrence	Present author
Cognitive impairment (subjective "dulling")	Common with early (previous) treatments (e.g., haloperidol)	Secondary to medications such as older neuroleptics (haloperidol & pimozide)	Robertson et al., 1988
Slightly lower IQ	> controls	Unknown	Debes et al., 2011
Dementia	Does not exist	No relationship at all. TS begins early & improves with age & there is no cognitive decline. If a patient with TS develops cognitive decline, must consider dementia (e.g., Huntington's disease)	Present author

Modified, adapted, and updated from Robertson, 2003.

2000; Hoekstra et al., 2004b; Pierre et al., 1999; Rizzo et al., 2007; Spencer et al., 1998; Stephens & Sandor, 1999; Sukhodolsky et al., 2003; Termine et al., 2006) have shown that TS-alone patients did not differ from unaffected controls on many ratings, apart from having more internalizing symptoms. In contrast, children with TS+ADHD had higher ratings on disruptive behaviors, internalizing behavior problems, and poorer social adaptation than children with TS alone or controls. Similarly in adults, Haddad and colleagues (2009) compared adults with TS alone with those with TS+ADHD. TS+ADHD patients had significantly more depression, anxiety, OCB, and maladaptive behaviors (e.g., aggression to property, attacking other people, forensic encounters, alcohol/drug abuse). In contrast, Spencer and colleagues (2001) studied ADHD patients and compared them to "healthy" control subjects. Results showed that 12% of ADHD patients but only 4% of controls had tics. The tic disorders had a remitting course, were not associated with stimulant use and, importantly, had little impact on the functional abilities of the patients with ADHD (Spencer et al., 2001). A recent study undertaken on patients with "primary ADHD" (Charach et al., 2011) involved a comparative meta-analysis of 13 studies examining alcohol and substance abuse in ADHD. They showed that childhood ADHD is associated with alcohol and drug use in adults and with nicotine use in adolescence. Thus, taken on their own, both age and ADHD affect other diagnoses as an individual grows up. This illustrates the complexity that exists when more than one diagnosis (TS and ADHD), other conditions (alcohol or substance abuse), and other variables, such as age, are present simultaneously. Adding further complexity is the etiology of the ADHD found in people with TS. As has been shown, it is unlikely that all cases of ADHD in TS are genetically linked, but indeed recent studies have suggested that other nongenetic factors such as maternal smoking during pregnancy may be associated with the development of ADHD in TS children (Mathews et al., 2006; see Chapter 8 for further discussion). One could say that ideally each of the comorbidities found in TS should be examined in such detail as this, but this may lead us astray in the main quest—for TS phenotype and etiology.

Thus, although ADHD occurs commonly in TS (about 60–75%), there has been much debate as to whether or not they are genetically related. Comings and colleagues (Table 16.2) have always suggested a genetic relationship between TS and ADHD, whereas Pauls and colleagues (Table 16.2) disputed this, while Eapen and Robertson (1996) have suggested that there are subsets with and without a genetic link to ADHD. In addition, Bloch and colleagues (2011) showed in a meta-analysis that alpha-2 agonists work best for tics in individuals with ADHD but hardly at all for individuals with tics and no ADHD.

OCD (and OCB and obsessive-compulsive symptoms) and TS, on the other hand, were always shown to be genetically related (Table 16.2), with no dissenting reports. Most of the other relationships between TS and psychopathology are complex and, for instance in the case of depression, multifactorial (Robertson et al., 2006a). Rizzo and colleagues (2010) reported eight youngsters (median age 14.6 years) with triple comorbidity of TS, epilepsy, and ADHD, in whom the seizures were well controlled. They noted three other cases of triple comorbidity involving TS, ADHD, and behavioral disturbance, while the coexistence of TS, epilepsy, and emotional difficulties had also been previously reported (Eapen et al., 1997c). They suggested further that this may be a nosological entity and that increased dopamine- and glutamate-mediated excitatory activity could explain the co-occurrence of the symptoms (Rizzo et al., 2010). In this context, it must be noted that Yordanova and colleagues (1997, 2006; see also Chapter 2) have also suggested, on the basis of neurophysiological studies, that TS+ADHD may well be a separate nosological entity.

ENDOPHENOTYPES: WHAT DO THEY TELL US ABOUT TS ETIOLOGY AND PHENOTYPE?

Before we embark on the discussion of endophenotypes and TS, it may be best to remind the reader what indeed is an endophenotype; this has been well summarized by Gottesman and Gould (2003) as "measurable components unseen by the unaided eye along the pathway between disease and distal genotype." They may be neurophysiological, biochemical, endocrinal, neuroanatomical, cognitive, or neuropsychological. This proposed "biomarker" must be associated with illness in the population, must be heritable, and is essentially state-independent (i.e., is manifest whether or not disease/illness is active); within families, it co-segregates with illness (Gershon & Goldin, 1986; Gottesman & Gould, 2003). Gottesman and Gould (2003) discuss schizophrenia as an example, with the "illness" being "psychosis" and the endophenotypes being defective sensorimotor gating (i.e., difficulty in filtering information from multiple sources and measured by prepulse inhibition [PPI]) and a decline in working memory, both of which have a clear genetic component. Examples of genes that underlie these endophenotypes include RELN (coding for Reelin, which has been associated with performance in working memory tests [Wedenoja et al., 2008, 2010]) and CHRNA7 (coding the nicotinic acetylcholine receptors [alpha7 nAchRs], which normalize the P50 auditory evoked potential gating deficits and, to a lesser extent, improve the PPI of the acoustic startle response; Leiser et al., 2009]). These examples not only illustrate the meaning of endophenotype but also pave the way for examining this in the context of TS, which is as yet a "syndrome" (cluster of symptoms) rather than a disease with a clearly defined etiology.

Neurophysiological Studies Showing Possible Endophenotypes in TS

The Bereichtschaftspotential (normal premovement EEG potential) was probably the first endophenotype in TS. Thus, Obeso and colleagues (1981) studied six patients with TS and showed that tics were not preceded by the normal premovement EEG or Bereichtschaftspotential in five of the six patients, whereas when the subjects mimicked their own tics, the voluntary jerks were prefaced by the potential, and the authors concluded that tics in TS are physiologically different from normal self-paced willed human movements. Subsequently, Karp and colleagues (1996) found that, in three of five patients, tics were not preceded by the normal premovement EEG or Bereichtschaftspotential. However, premotor negativity was present in two, and the authors suggested that this could be due to internal triggering stimuli. Thus, three independent centers found similar results, and this absence of Bereichtschaftspotential could represent the first TS endophenotype, albeit probably nonspecific (i.e., the same would probably be found with other nonwilled movements).

Yordanova and colleagues (1997) examined patients with TS+ADHD, looking at the effect of the combined diagnosis on the amplitude of the postimperative negative variation (PINV) as an indicator of frontal lobe functioning and self-regulation of behavior in three groups: TS alone, ADHD alone, and controls. Their results only partially supported the notion of a separate entity, but paved the way for their later study (Yordanova et al., 2006), which showed that there was spontaneous theta activity and increased event-related theta activity in patients with the combined nosological disorder TS+ADHD. They suggested that this was a psychophysiological marker (endophenotype) of this entity.

Cognitive and Neuropsychological Abnormalities as Possible Endophenotypes in TS

As stated above, it is known that the PPI of the acoustic startle response is a measure of sensorimotor gating in some neuropsychiatric disorders, such as schizophrenia, OCD, Huntington's disease (HD), posttraumatic stress disorder, and also TS, and experimentally induced PPI deficits in rats are regarded as an endophenotype to study the biological mechanisms in such disorders (Alsene et al., 2011; Freudenberg et al., 2007; Gottesman & Gould, 2003). Subsequent research has shown that selectively breeding rats for high and low PPI levels, respectively, leads to groups with different PPI performance, which remains stable from the second generation onward (Freudenberg et al., 2007). The same group then examined whether the low PPI is accompanied by other behavioral deficits. They examined learning and memory abilities, behavioral flexibility, and perseveration in these animals. Rats with low PPI showed increased perseveration during switching between an egocentric and allocentric radial maze task. Enhanced perseveration was also found in an operant behavioral task. Other abnormalities in perseveration suggested that rats selectively bred for low PPI showed cognitive deficits that are apparent in a number of disorders with deficient information processing (Freudenberg et al., 2007). There is a clinical parallel between perseveration and palilalia and palipraxia (both seen in TS), and hence this is relevant to our discussion.

A few encouraging studies have now been published examining the possibility of sensorimotor gating as a TS endophenotype. These studies have examined both patients with TS and compared them to controls as well as using animal models. For example, Sutherland Owens and colleagues (2011) studied 18 subjects with TS, many of whom had premonitory urges before their tics, and compared them with 22 healthy control subjects to examine the relationship between premonitory urge scores and measures of sensory gating, as well as symptom severity scales. Results showed that, in subjects with TS, the Sensory Gating Inventory (SGI) score, but not the Structured Interview for Assessing Perceptual Anomalies (SIAPA) score, was highly significantly elevated in TS individuals. Neither premonitory urge scores nor sensory gating scales correlated significantly with symptom severity. The authors suggested that TS subjects endorse difficulties with sensory gating and that the SGI may be valuable for further research in the area (Sutherland Owens et al., 2011).

Bloch and colleagues (2006b) examined 32 children (aged 8–14 years) clinically and then administered a focused neuropsychological testing battery and performed a follow-up assessment an average of 7.5 years later (aged approximately 15–21 years). Ordinal logistic regression analysis was used to correlate neuropsychological testing at Time 1 with tic severity, OCD severity, and global psychosocial functioning at Time 2. Results showed that poor performance with the Purdue Pegboard test predicted worse adulthood tic severity and correlated with tic severity at the time of the childhood assessment. Poor performance on the Visual Motor Integration (VMI) and Purdue Pegboard tests (both dominant and nondominant hand) also predicted worse adult global psychosocial functioning. None of the neuropsychological battery of tests was useful in predicting obsessive-compulsive symptoms. The authors suggested that fine-motor skills could be a predictor of future tic severity and global psychosocial functioning in youngsters with TS. They also hypothesized that performance on the Purdue Pegboard test may serve as a useful endophenotype in the study of TS and may provide a high measure of the degree of basal ganglia dysfunction present in patients with TS. It is recognized that TS is characterized by dysfunctional connectivity between prefrontal cortex and subcortical structures and altered mesocortical and/or mesostriatal dopamine release. Since time processing is also regulated by frontostriatal circuits and modulated by dopaminergic transmission, Vicario and colleagues (2010) investigated time processing in children with TS, with a view to establish a functional endophenotype. They compared time-processing abilities between 9 children with TS alone and 10 age- and gender-matched control subjects, employing a time reproduction task in which subjects had to judge whether a test interval is longer or shorter than a given reference interval. In addition, IQ, sustained and divided attention, and working memory were assessed in both groups. Results demonstrated that the TS subjects were "supernormal" in the tasks, in the sense that they reproduced in an overestimated fashion supra-second, but not sub-second, time intervals. The precision of supra-second time interval reproduction correlated with tic severity: the lower the tic severity, the closer the reproduction of supra-second time intervals to their real duration. Time reproduction performance did not significantly correlate with IQ, attention, and working memory in either group; in addition, no differences between groups were documented in the time comparison task. Thus, the improvement in time processing in TS children appeared specific for the supra-second range of intervals, consistent with an enhancement in the "cognitively controlled" timing system, which mainly processes longer-duration intervals, and depends upon dysfunctional connectivity between the basal ganglia and the dorsolateral prefrontal cortex. Furthermore, the absence of between-group differences on time comparison suggests that TS subjects manifest a selective impairment of "motor" timing abilities, rather than of perceptual time abilities. The authors suggested that their data supported an enhancement of cognitive control processes in TS youngsters, probably facilitated by effortful tic suppression (Vicario et al., 2010). This is somewhat reminiscent of an early study by Channon and colleagues (1992), who observed attentional deficits in a TS group attributed to tic suppression. Another study demonstrated lower IQ in TS than controls (but less than one standard deviation below), but interestingly an earlier age at onset of tics and presence of comorbidities were associated with these specific deficits on cognitive performance (Debes et al., 2010b).

In summary, a few possible endophenotypes have been reported in TS, including abnormal sensorimotor gating (via PPI), performance of the Purdue Pegboard test, and enhancement of cognitive control processes in TS youngsters, the latter probably facilitated by effortful tic suppression.

Neurochemical Abnormalities as Possible TS Endophenotypes

Alsene and colleagues (2011) documented that emerging evidence suggests that norepinephrine regulates PPI, but that the neuronal circuitry has, to date, been unknown. They demonstrated that stimulation of the locus ceruleus, the primary source of norepinephrine to the forebrain, induces a PPI deficit that is a result of downstream norepinephrine release. They undertook studies in Sprague Dawley rats and showed new pathways in the regulation of PPI, suggesting that norepinephrine transmission within distinct thalamocortical and ventral

forebrain networks may subserve the sensorimotor gating deficits in disorders, including TS. There have also been studies linking small caudate nucleus volume (see below) and a reduction in parvalbumin-expressing fast-spiking GABAergic and cholinergic interneurons in the dorsal striatum, and poor outcome in TS (Kalanithi et al., 2005; Kataoka et al., 2010), an interesting and only recently investigated area.

Neuroimaging Showing Possible Endophenotypes in TS

With regard to the occurrence of psychopathology in TS, it could be suggested that, rather than genetic specificity for TS, the behavioral and/or neuropsychiatric abnormalities may be due to common brain endophenotypic mechanisms shared by TS and related disorders. The search for brain endophenotypes in TS is currently gaining momentum. It is now agreed that the underlying pathophysiology in TS is dysfunction of cortical-striato-thalamo-cortical circuits, and at least 10 studies have observed structural and diffusion changes in these areas, many of which may be TS endophenotypes.

As has been mentioned earlier, the Weinberger group (Hyde et al., 1992, 1994, 1995; Randolph et al., 1993) showed that in monozygotic twins in whom at least one twin had TS, and who were concordant for tic diagnosis but not for severity, those with more severe tics had lower birth weight, more abnormal EEG abnormalities, reduced right caudate nucleus volumes, and significantly poorer neuropsychological performance, all of which were attributed to prenatal developmental problems. Hyde and colleagues (1992) demonstrated that, within the 16 pairs of monozygotic twins (12 male and 4 female pairs; 56% concordant for diagnosis of TS and 94% for diagnosis of tic disorder), the twins with more severe tics had lower birth weights; in addition, the magnitude of the intra-pair birth weight difference strongly predicted the magnitude of the intra-pair tic score difference. The authors further stated that the difference in tic severity could not be explained by any postnatal medical events, but suggested that the events affecting the phenotypic expression of TS occur *in utero* and that the factors causing birth weight difference are also related to tic severity (Hyde et al., 1992). The group then demonstrated that global neuropsychological performance was significantly worse in the twins with more severe tics, with significant differences emerging on attention, visuospatial perception, and motor function tests (Randolph et al., 1993). Also, the twins with the more severe tics had significantly more abnormal EEGs by qualitative visual analysis; most of the differences were due to excessive frontocentral theta activity, suggesting dysfunction outside the basal ganglia. There was also a significant relationship between a lower global neuropsychological testing score and a worse overall EEG. A similar relationship was found between birth weight and EEG abnormality in that the twin with lower birth weight had a worse EEG in seven of the nine pairs with different intra-pair birth weight (Hyde et al., 1994). The same authors then investigated cerebral morphometric analyses of MRIs in 10 twin pairs discordant for severity and showed significantly reduced right caudate volumes (particularly in the anterior part of the nucleus) in the more severely affected twins. In addition, the mean volume of the left lateral ventricle was 16% smaller in the more severely affected twin, and the normal asymmetry of the lateral ventricles (left greater than right) was not present in the more severely affected twins, who had a trend toward a larger right lateral ventricle. Moreover, the difference within a pair in the degree of loss of the normal asymmetry correlated with the difference within a pair in the severity of the tic disorder (Hyde et al., 1995). Wolf and colleagues (1996) continued investigating the twin sets, demonstrating significant differences in D2 dopamine receptor binding in the head of the caudate nucleus, which predicted differences in phenotypic severity.

Moriarty and colleagues (1997) used HMPAO SPECT studies in 25 people from large families with both TS and OCB (with no tics), expecting that TS individuals would show more striatal and frontal hypoperfusion while patients with OCD would show more hyperperfusion. The results, however, showed hypoperfusion in the striatal, frontal, and temporal regions in affected individuals in TS families regardless of whether they had TS, tics, or OCB. This is different from the finding of hypoperfusion that is observed in individuals with primary OCD in the absence of a family history of tics. Thus, the finding of a shared cerebral blood flow pattern abnormality among affected TS family members with tics or OCB suggest a common underlying pathophysiology linking TS and OCB phenotypes, and raise the possibility of a neuroimaging endophenotype.

Heinz and colleagues (1998) used [1-123] beta-CIT SPECT imaging to examine *in vivo* the density of brain monoaminergic transporters in the basal ganglia, midbrain, and thalamus in 10 patients with TS and 10 age- and gender-matched healthy controls. Results showed a significant negative correlation between a measure of overall tic severity and beta-CIT binding in the midbrain and thalamus: when examined *post hoc*, these correlations were determined largely by vocal tic severity. Peterson and colleagues (2001) used MRI to study 155 individuals with TS and 131 controls (children and adults in both groups). Results showed that in people with TS, larger volumes were identified in the dorsal prefrontal regions and the parieto-occipital regions, while there were smaller inferior occipital volumes. In patients with TS there were significant associations of cerebral volumes with age, and the differences between sexes in the parieto-occipital regions were reduced: the age-related findings were most evident in children and the sex differences were most obvious in adults. These changes were not demonstrated in healthy controls. The authors concluded that the pathophysiology was broadly distributed in the cortical systems in TS patients.

Sowell and colleagues (2008) studied TS children using MRI and demonstrated cortical thinning in the frontal and parietal lobes in TS group when compared to healthy controls. Interestingly, the thinning was most prominent in ventral parts of the sensory and motor homunculi that control the facial, orolingual, and laryngeal musculature, areas that are commonly involved in tic symptoms. There were correlations between tic symptoms and cortical thickness in the sensorimotor regions, suggesting their involvement in tic pathophysiology.

Makki and colleagues (2009) used diffusion tensor MRI and probabilistic fiber tracking to study brain changes in 18 TS children compared with 12 age-matched healthy controls. Tractography of the fronto-striatal-thalamic circuit was achieved using probability distribution function of individual voxels. They demonstrated that the TS group had a significantly lower probability of connection between caudate nucleus and anterior dorsolateral frontal cortex of the left. In addition, they showed that OCB was negatively associated with connectivity score of the left caudate and anterior dorsolateral frontal cortex and was positively associated with connectivity score for the subcallosal gyrus and for the lentiform nucleus. Peterson and colleagues (2003), in a study of basal ganglia volume using high-resolution magnetic resonance images in 154 children and adults with TS and 130 healthy control subjects, observed that caudate nucleus volumes were significantly smaller in children and adults with TS, and that lenticular nucleus volumes were smaller in adults with TS and in children with TS who were diagnosed as having comorbid OCD. These authors suggested that reduced caudate nucleus volumes may be a good candidate marker for a trait abnormality in the structure of the basal ganglia in persons with TS, and that smaller lenticular nucleus volumes may be an additional marker for the presence of comorbid OCD and for the persistence of tic symptoms into adulthood.

Thomalla and colleagues (2009) used diffusion tensor MRI imaging in 15 unmedicated adults with TS alone and 15 healthy age- and sex-matched controls. They also used voxel-based morphometry of regional fractional anisotropy to examine regional differences in white matter between groups. In patients with TS there were bilateral fractional anisotropy increases in white matter, in the postcentral and precentral gyri, below the left supplementary area, and in the right ventro-posterolateral thalamus, suggesting microstructural changes in the somatosensory system that correlated with tic severity. Draganski and colleagues (2010) employed multispectral brain morphometry to study 40 TS adult patients and compare them to 40 matched controls. Results showed that

in the TS patients there was a reduction in gray matter volume in cortices bilaterally (especially the orbitofrontal, anterocingulate, and ventrolateral prefrontal areas), extending into the limbic mesial temporal lobe. In addition, the prefrontal cortical thinning correlated negatively with tic severity and the volume increase in the primary somatosensory cortex was dependent on the intensity of the premonitory sensations. Other studies that have conducted voxel-based morphometry have also suggested gray matter reduction and cortical thinning (Ludolph et al., 2006; Muller-Vahl et al., 2009), while midbrain involvement in the form of increased gray matter has also been reported (Garraux et al., 2006). However, the only study to account for age, treatment status, and homogeneity of clinical symptoms (by Roessner et al., 2009) revealed no difference between treatment-naïve boys with TS alone and healthy controls. This raises the question as to whether the previous findings and the inconsistencies noted could be due to the confounding effects of age, gender, medication, comorbidity, methods used, severity, presence of premonitory sensation, as well as compensatory mechanisms due to tic suppression, especially in adults with long duration of symptoms.

Neuner and colleagues (2010) used fMRI to examine the implicit discrimination of six emotional facial expressions in 19 TS adults and compared them to matched healthy controls. Results showed that the TS patients had significantly higher amygdala activation, which was most pronounced with fearful, angry, and neutral expressions. In addition, the activity of the left amygdala correlated negatively with the personality trait extraversion. They concluded that this was either due to deficient frontal inhibition (as a result of structural change), or due to desynchronization in the interaction of the cortico-striatal-thalamo-cortical network within structures of the limbic system. They further suggested that their data showed an altered pattern of implicit emotion discrimination.

Fahim and colleagues (2010) conducted MRI scans on 34 patients with TS (age range 10–25 years; mean 17.2 years) and 32 normal age-matched controls (10–20 years; mean 16.30 years), and brain morphometry was assessed using the fully automated CIVET pipeline at the Montreal Neurological Institute. Results showed several significant differences between TS individuals and controls, and also gender differences. They found that male TS patients had thinner cortices in frontoparietal cortical areas than TS females, and reported a significant negative correlation between tic severity and sensorimotor cortical thickness.

Worbe and colleagues (2010) studied 60 adults with TS and 30 matched controls, assessing cortical thickness measurement and 3T high-resolution T1-weighted images. Patients with TS were divided into three groups: (i) simple tics, (ii) simple and complex tics, and (iii) tics and OCD. Results showed that patients with TS had reduced cortical thickness in the motor, premotor, prefrontal, and lateral orbitofrontal cortices, and also that tic severity correlated negatively with cortical thinning in the parietal and temporal cortices. The groups were able to be differentiated as follows: (i) those with simple tics had thinning in the primary motor regions; (ii) those with both simple and complex tics had thinning that extended to the premotor, prefrontal, and parietal areas; and (iii) those with tics and OCD showed a trend to thinning of the anterior cingulate cortex and hippocampus. In addition, there was a negative correlation with thickness in the anterior cingulate cortex and a positive correlation with thickness in medial premotor areas (Worbe et al., 2010).

Pourfar and colleagues (2011) used [(18) F]-fluorodeoxyglucose PET to examine metabolic brain networks in 12 unmedicated TS patients, some of whom also had OCD, and 12 age-matched controls. They used a spatial covariance analysis to identify two disease-related metabolic brain networks, one associated with TS in general (distinguishing TS from controls) and another correlating with OCD severity (within the TS group alone). Results showed that TS patients and controls were significantly different ($p < .0001$), with an abnormal spatial covariance pattern. The TS-related pattern was characterized by reduced resting metabolic activity of striatum and the orbitofrontal cortex, and was also associated with relative increases in the premotor cortex and cerebellum. Analysis

of the TS cohort alone revealed the presence of a second metabolic pattern that correlated with OCD in these patients. This OCD-related pattern was characterized by reduced activity of the anterior cingulate and dorsolateral prefrontal cortical regions and increased activity in the primary motor cortex and precuneus; it correlated with obsessive-compulsive symptom severity. These findings suggested that different manifestations of TS are associated with the expression of two distinct abnormal metabolic brain networks, and that these, and potentially other disease-related spatial covariance patterns, may prove useful as biomarkers for assessing treatments for TS and its various comorbidities (Pourfar et al., 2011).

Genetic Abnormalities and Possible TS Endophenotypes

Robertson and Trimble (1993) reported chromosomal analysis of a cohort of 68 consecutive TS patients. Only 3 were abnormal: one case of XYY chromosome, one case of heterochromatin of chromosome 1 (through duplication of a band [1qh+]), and one of heterochromatin of chromosome 9 with structural rearrangement ([inv 9 qh], [p11q13]). Subsequently, patients with TS and the chromosome 22q11 deletion syndrome (previously called Catch-22 syndrome [Robertson et al., 2006b]) and patients with TS and Smith Magenis syndrome (17p11.2 deletion syndrome [Shelley et al., 2007]) were reported, showing phenotypic features of both disorders. It was suggested that both regions hold promise for containing a gene(s) of importance in TS. Finally, a cohort of cases with the phenotype of TS and fragile X were documented (Schneider et al., 2008), as well as TS and Down syndrome phenotypes (e.g., Barabas et al., 1986; Collacott & Ismail, 1988; Karlinsky & Berg, 1987; Karlinsky et al., 1986; Kerbeshian & Burd, 2000). It was, however, suggested that these comorbid cases of TS and Down syndrome (5 cases of TS in 425 cases of Down syndrome [1.2%]) were more likely to be "tardive" TS cases, as these patients with TS plus Down syndrome had no typical family history of TS, had a relatively late onset, and had been previously treated with neuroleptics and/ or stimulants (Myers & Pueschel, 1995). While all these results are interesting, there have been few replications, and these have not brought us closer to identifying the putative TS genes.

CRITICAL COMMENTARY

The most common clinical characteristic studied in TS has been tic severity. This has been associated with, or positively correlated with, maternal smoking (Mathews et al., 2006; Motlagh et al., 2010), low birth weight (Pringsheim et al., 2009), low birth weight and PNDs (Hyde et al., 1992, 1994, 1995; Randolph et al., 1993; Wolf et al., 1996), psychosocial stress (Motlagh et al., 2010), anxiety (Woods et al., 2005), stress (Lin et al., 2007), stress and GABHS (Lin et al., 2010), presence of ADHD (Marsh et al., 2004), and adverse life events (Hoekstra et al., 2004a). With regard to endophenotypes, most of the information has been obtained on tic severity, which has been correlated with cortical thinning. A poor outcome/prognosis has also been linked with a reduced caudate nucleus volume, and a reduction in parvalbumin-expressing fast-spiking GABAergic and cholinergic interneurons in the dorsal striatum. In addition, a poor outcome (in this case increased tic severity) has been associated with poor fine-motor skills and enhancement of cognitive control processes, probably facilitated by effortful tic suppression. Of interest is that absence of Bereichtschaftspotential may well have been the first TS endophenotype to identify tics versus willed movement (albeit somewhat nonspecific). Further, it appears that TS individuals endorse difficulties with sensory motor gating and have abnormal Purdue Pegboard test results.

An increase in prevalence of TS over the years has been suggested: What does this say about current diagnosis and phenotype? It is now recognized that TS is common. The most convincing evidence comes from a large review in which all raw data were used; it showed that 3,992 of 420,761 children aged 4 to 18 years studied in the community in 15 international studies had a diagnosis of TS (1%, although the percentage ranged between 0.4% and 3.8% in the studies;

Robertson, 2008a). However, tics and TS are much more common in special education populations and those with learning disabilities (Eapen et al., 1997d) and, in particular, in children with autism (Baron-Cohen et al., 1999a), which suggests the involvement of overlapping neurodevelopmental pathways with distinct clinical phenotypes (Eapen & Črnčec, 2009). In this regard, Burd and colleagues (2005) identified phenotype differences between the TS without learning disabilities group and the children with both TS and learning disabilities. The "etiology" in these subgroups of TS may be different and in part due to compromised neural development. However, prevalence rates are also affected by the age of the cohort, and up to 20% of children exhibit tics as a developmental phenomenon: "all that tics may not be Tourette's" (Eapen et al., 1994).

Simple tics are one of only many possible suggested TS clinical phenotypes, but it is as yet unclear which phenotypes are genetically distinct. In addition, different phenotypes may not only be different etiological/clinical entities, but could also represent the same disorder at different developmental stages (i.e., phenotypical heterochronia). It is well known that, when following a child with TS, we often find that ADHD is present before tic onset, and that often OCD follows some years later. Thus, this would also clearly alter the prevalence rate. In addition, TS may not represent a unitary phenotype, and could instead represent multiple phenotypes, as yet not delineated by endophenotypes, which may also be a confounder of prevalence rates. The prevalence of the "maladies des tics" or "true" TS, as described by Dr. Georges Gilles de la Tourette in 1885 and including multiple tics, coprolalia, and echolalia, is unknown, but it is certain to be far less common than the disorder consisting of motor and vocal tics, possibly 10% to 15% of 1%.

Robertson (2008a, 2008b) has previously discussed that having TS or some of its phenotypes (e.g., OCB) may well be positively advantageous to the species (e.g., these people are meticulous, accurate, punctual, clean, and tidy). There have been great historical figures with TS, such as Dr. Samuel Johnson, Peter the Great, and Tolstoy's brother: clearly to carry any of these genes would be advantageous for humankind (see Robertson, 2008a, 2008b; Robertson & Cavanna, 2008). In this context other scholars have argued that both the "thrifty phenotype" (Wells, 2007) and anxious-depressive-cyclothymic phenotypes (Akiskal & Akiskal, 2005) may be adaptive. Other authors have suggested that the increase in prevalence in type 2 diabetes has occurred because our species' original adaptation to glucose metabolism has now been superseded by a sedentary lifestyle, resulting in more illness (Lipsitch & Sousa, 2002). Another suggestion is that assortative mating (Kurlan et al., 1994; McMahon et al., 1996) has been increasingly documented in TS, and this will lead to an increase in the numbers of TS individuals. A final suggestion is that the number of people with TS will increase as the population grows. However, although the number of TS cases will increase, they are highly likely to represent the same percentage of the total population, and thus the prevalence should remain the same. In this context, what is extraordinary is that a study from the United States published in 2007, which estimated the incidence and prevalence of 12 neurological disorders all supposed to be "common," reported that "for Tourette Syndrome, the data were insufficient" (CDC, 2009). This highlights the fact that, although TS is common, it is still considered uncommon by many clinicians, and further epidemiological studies with stringent methods are needed (Robertson, 2008a, 2008b).

Whither TS?

It is now recognized that TS has many varied phenotypes, as well as contributory etiological factors including familial as well as perinatal, hormonal, and immunological influences. Although TS was described in 1825, and since 1885 it has been recognized as an entity, the etiological factors identified so far are far from being conclusive. Its pathophysiology is as yet not well understood, and the environmental factors outlined above probably modify genetic effects. In addition, no causative genes have been found yet, and there is almost certainly going to

be genetic heterogeneity in TS; whether or not this will be specific to a particular phenotype is unknown. Some TS cases may turn out to be due to rare variants such as SLITRKI (e.g., Abelson et al., 2005; O'Roak et al., 2010), the L-histidine decarboxylase gene affecting histamine biosynthesis (Ercan-Senecicek et al., 2010), or the IMMP2L gene (Patel et al., 2011; Petek et al., 2001), although it has been emphasized that overrepresentation of rare variants (e.g., SLITRK1) in a specific ethnic group may confuse the interpretation of association analyses (Keen-Kim et al., 2006). It is likely that TS, in the main, will *not* be due to a single gene (much like type 2 diabetes and multiple sclerosis). The situation is further complicated by the fact that TS is probably the only neuropsychiatric disorder to have such wide, characteristic, and common varieties of phenotypes, comorbidities, and other psychiatric disorders, as described earlier and in Chapters 2, 3, and 4.

The scientific history of TS has been hampered by the relatively small numbers of patients in clinical cohorts. In addition, until relatively recently the prevalence data suggested that TS was rare to uncommon, and some still argue that TS is uncommon. Further, TS is not a disorder that brings in much funding for research, which may be due to the fact that it has been thought to be rare and that it may improve with age rather than being life-threatening or worsening with age. The way that TS is diagnosed and classified is also an area of potential difficulties. Thus, more research is required with replication of previous results (confirmation of or disagreement with).

Criticisms of DSM and ICD

The current diagnostic criteria are those specified by the American Psychiatric Association (APA, currently DSM-IV-TR, 2000) and the World Health Organisation (currently ICD 10, 1992). The DSM criteria have changed substantially over time—for example, with regard to the upper age limit for age at onset (15, 18, 21 years), distress and impairment criteria, duration of tics (usually >1 year), and whether or not there are tic-free intervals and how long they should be. WHO has never had an age stipulation.

DSM-V and ICD-11 are about to be published, and although websites are able to supply tentative suggestions as to the diagnostic criteria and classifications of the various syndromes and disorders, nothing will be set in stone until the final publication. The international criteria (DSM and ICD) have, in our opinion, not been particularly useful, in that the changes have not been based on empirical data and seem to have no evidence base. Take, for example, DSM-IV: it has been shown that impairment and distress were included as diagnostic criteria; one need only be a clinical member of a TS clinic over many years to understand that the majority of individuals (e.g., family members of probands/patients) are mildly affected and do not have any impairment or distress. The upper age at onset allowed changed from 15, to 18, to 21 years: this made no sense at all. We ask whether DSM-V and ICD-11 will be helpful in our quest for a marriage of etiology and phenotype. Having perused the available websites, we suggest that both the DSM-V and ICD-11 criteria will not change substantially and thus will not be more helpful than they have been to date. It is suggested that research groups undertake more studies using specific research diagnostic criteria and always examine for differences between, for example, TS alone and TS+ADHD, TS+OCD, TS+ADHD+OCD, and so on. Only then will we be able to determine the underlying etiologies that underpin the various phenotypes.

A nomenclature change has occurred in many disorders that were at first considered to be unitary or homogeneous and that are now realized to be heterogeneous and divided into subtypes, as is the case with dystonia, Parkinson's disease, Huntington's disease, and motor neuron disease. Once the etiology of TS is better understood, we will be in a better position to link this to clinical phenotypes and be able to subdivide what is now subsumed under the TS umbrella from an etiological and phenotypic standpoint.

It is suggested that TS may well be divided into a variety of subtypes. These will be designated according to the replicated factors from the factor analytic studies (highly likely to also make clinical sense) and linked to etiological bases. The only factor (phenotype) that has been replicated, several times in fact, is that of a "pure simple motor and phonic tic factor," which all specialist clinicians treating patients with TS are able to identify clinically (and which occurs in about 10% of both community and clinical samples). However, as can be seen in this chapter, currently relatively few "causes" can be inextricably linked to a particular phenotype in TS. Robertson (2008b) suggested that, with regard to the nomenclature of TS, type 1 TS would comprise patients with simple motor and phonic/vocal tics only (as this is seen clinically and has been replicated many times). Other subtypes (types 2, 3, 4, etc.) may follow, and it is likely that these will mirror the clusters and factors and ideally the etiologies identified by future studies (Tables 16.1 and 16.2). In future studies we hope that these clinically determined factors and subtypes will be assigned different etiological bases, such as genetic, immunological, and perinatal-related, to name just a few. We suggest that only when the TS genes are identified and other etiological mechanisms are fully understood will we understand more clearly what constitutes the TS phenotypes. It will also become clearer what psychopathologies and tic phenomena are important in the various phenotypes, and whether or not these are related to the various etiologies. An example in this context would be the dementias (particularly Pick's disease), and how their nosology has changed over the years via an iterative process (see Robertson, 2008b).

This suggested future nomenclature for TS could allow more precise clinical and/or etiological descriptions of TS. We realize that these suggestions are perhaps slightly premature based on the available information. For example, there are no clearly delineated genetic factors or age-distinct differences in TS. Hence, a definition based solely on phenomenology and comorbidity may be ultimately misleading. Nevertheless, in the future, when etiologies and phenomenological subtypes will become more established, a subtype nomenclature may be appropriate (Robertson, 2008b). Clearly, these differing phenotypes would affect much of the research into TS, including prevalence and possibly medication response in the first instance.

CONCLUSIONS

Despite enormous efforts, the journeys into phenotype and etiology in the world of TS have only just begun. We should remember the long and difficult journeys that have been traveled in other conditions like dystonia, Parkinson's disease, Huntington's disease-like syndrome, and motor neuron diseases: now that these have defined causes and phenotypes, much more can be discovered, and importantly more appropriate treatments can also be identified. In our opinion one of the reasons we have not identified any major gene, and no other definitive other causative agent, is that we have been (i) examining and researching the incorrect phenotype, (ii) asking the wrong questions, and (iii) using incorrect prevalence data. Many clinicians pragmatically separate TS into types that make clinical sense, namely "pure" TS (motor and vocal/phonic tics only), "full-blown TS" (plus copro-, echo-, and pali- phenomena) (Robertson & Baron-Cohen, 1998), and "TS-plus," coined by Packer (1987) to describe those patients with a full house of comorbid conditions (ADHD, OCD, OCB, self-injurious behaviors) and psychopathology (e.g., depression, personality disorders). Whether further factor analytic studies, along with concomitant genetic and environmental studies, will echo these subdivisions, is eagerly awaited.

Endophenotype studies indicate that there are indeed a few correlations between etiology and phenotype, and this is an exciting area. Furthermore, gender and other behavioral (OCB) differences may indicate different etiological factors, and there is some evidence to suggest the existence of OCD/OCB endophenotypes. However, early neuroimaging studies suggest that this may be due to prenatal and perinatal difficulties, which influence the phenotypic expression of the TS gene(s). Thus, replication studies are required with similar methods and with the TS patients subdivided into phenotypes. Future research should address these issues (Box 16.2).

Finally, we suggest that new research nomenclature based on etiology and endophenotype be devised. In TS, it has been proposed that the involvement of the dopaminergic striatal pathways results in tics, while that of the serotonergic striatal-limbic minicircuits results in OCD, the involvement of dopamine/noradrenergic frontal cortical circuits results in ADHD and socially inappropriate behaviors, and the involvement of the entire cortical striatal–pallidothalamic–cortical circuitry results in a number of comorbidities and psychopathology. Thus, the clinical phenotype and the severity of symptoms as well as the associated psychopathology observed in TS may be influenced by the nature and extent of involvement of the above circuitry based on both genetic and nongenetic factors as well as the developmental period in question. It seems that there may be shared molecular genetic pathways affecting development across diagnostic

---

Box 16.2. Directions for Future Research

- Study etiological factors (genetic, prenatal and perinatal factors, gender, environmental and immunological factors) alongside phenotypes.
- Using different phenotypic definitions (e.g., motor and vocal tics only, tics with comorbid OCD, ADHD, etc.), examine how the different definitions and phenotypic groupings affect etiological theories.
- Using endophenotypes, explore the relationship between clinical features, course, and outcomes.
- Explore the link between specific genotypes, neurocognitive profiles as endophenotypes, and clinical phenotypic characteristics.

boundaries mediated through neurodevelopmental genes (Eapen, 2011). Examples of this include neurexin and CNTNAP2 genes, both implicated in TS and autism. Thus, defects in synaptic development may result in abnormal development across disorders and broad domains and distinct phenotypic patterns may be the final endpoint of divergent but overlapping developmental trajectories. It may well be that a large part of the genetic susceptibility for TS may be shared with other comorbid disorders, especially OCD, ADHD, and even autism spectrum disorders, suggesting the notion of a general genetic susceptibility for neurodevelopmental problems rather than specific genes as a cause of specific disorders. Future studies should elucidate the genetic underpinnings of the developmental processes involved in the TS circuitry and the corresponding neurocognitive profiles, which in turn would pave the way for better phenotypic characterization.

ACKNOWLEDGMENTS

The authors thank Dr. Jeremy Stern for his helpful suggestions and comments on the manuscript.

REFERENCES

Abelson JF, Kwan KY, O'Roak BJ et al. Sequence variants in SLITRK1 are associated with Tourette's syndrome. *Science* 2005; *310*:317–320.

Abuzzahab FS, Anderson FO. Gilles de la Tourette's syndrome: cross-cultural analysis and treatment outcome. In FS Abuzzahab, FO Anderson (Eds.), *Gilles de la Tourette's Syndrome: International Registry* (pp. 71–79). St. Paul, MN: Mason Publishing Co., 1976.

Akiskal KK, Akiskal HS. The theoretical underpinnings of affective temperaments: implications for evolutionary foundations of bipolar disorder and human nature. *J Affect Disord* 2005; *85*:231–239.

Alsene KM, Rajbhandari AK, Ramaker MJ et al. Discrete forebrain neuronal networks supporting noradrenergic regulation of sensorimotor gating. *Neuropsychopharmacology* 2011; *36*:1003–1014.

Alsobrook JP 2nd, Pauls DL. A factor analysis of tic symptoms in Gilles de la Tourette's syndrome. *Am J Psychiatry* 2002; *159*:291–296.

Altman G, Staley JD, Wener P. Children with Tourette disorder: a follow-up study in adulthood. *J Nerv Ment Dis* 2009; *197*:305–310.

American Psychiatric Association. *Diagnostic and statistical manual of mental disorders: DSM-IV-TR.* 4th ed. Washington, DC: American Psychiatric Association, 2000.

Barabas G, Wardell B, Sapiro M et al. Coincident Down's and Tourette syndromes: three case reports. *J Child Neurol* 1986; *1*:358–360.

Baron-Cohen S, Mortimore C, Moriarty J et al. The prevalence of Gilles de la Tourette's syndrome in children and adolescents with autism. *J Child Psychol Psychiatry* 1999b; *40*:213–218.

Baron-Cohen S, Scahill L, Izaguirre J et al. The prevalence of Gilles de la Tourette syndrome in children and adolescents with autism: a large scale study. *Psychol Med* 1999a; *29*:1151–1159.

Berthier ML, Kulisevsky J, Campos VM. Bipolar disorder in adult patients with Tourette's syndrome: a clinical study. *Biol Psychiatry* 1998; *43*:364–370.

Bloch MH, Peterson BS, Scahill L et al. Adulthood outcome of tic and obsessive-compulsive symptom severity in children with Tourette syndrome. *Arch Pediatr Adolesc Med* 2006a; *160*:65–69.

Bloch M, State M, Pittenger C. Recent advances in Tourette syndrome. *Curr Opin Neurol* 2011; *24*:119–125.

Bloch MH, Sukhodolsky DG, Leckman JF et al. Fine-motor skill deficits in childhood predict adulthood tic severity and global psychosocial functioning in Tourette's syndrome. *J Child Psychol Psychiatry* 2006b; *47*:551–559.

Blumenshine P, Egerter S, Barclay CJ et al. Socioeconomic disparities in adverse birth outcomes: a systematic review. *Am J Prev Med* 2010; *39*:263–272.

Brown SJ, Yelland JS, Sutherland GA et al. Stressful life events, social health issues and low birthweight in an Australian population-based birth cohort: challenges and opportunities in antenatal care. *BMC Public Health* 2011; *11*:196.

Budman CL, Bruun RD, Park KS et al. Rage attacks in children and adolescents with Tourette's disorder: a pilot study. *J Clin Psychiatry* 1998; *59*:576–580.

Burd L, Freeman RD, Klug MG et al. Tourette syndrome and learning disabilities. *BMC Pediatr* 2005; *5*:34.

Burd L, Kerbeshian J. Gilles de la Tourette's syndrome and bipolar disorder. *Arch Neurol* 1984; *41*:1236.

Burd L, Kerbeshian J. Onset of Gilles de la Tourette's syndrome before 1 year of age. *Am J Psychiatry* 1987; *144*:1066–1067.

Butler IJ. Tourette's syndrome. Some new concepts. *Neurol Clin* 1984; *2*:571–580.

Canitano R, Vivanti G. Tics and Tourette syndrome in autism spectrum disorders. *Autism* 2007; *11*:19–28.

Carter AS, O'Donnell DA, Schultz RT et al. Social and emotional adjustment in children affected with Gilles de la Tourette's syndrome: associations with ADHD and family functioning. *J Child Psychol Psychiatry* 2000; *41*:215–223.

Cavanna AE, Critchley HD, Orth M et al. Dissecting the Gilles de la Tourette spectrum: a factor analytic study on 639 patients. *J Neurol Neurosurg Psychiatry* 2011; *82*:1320–1323.

Centers for Disease Control and Prevention (CDC). Prevalence of diagnosed Tourette syndrome in persons aged 6–17 years — United States, 2007. *Morbidity and Mortality Weekly Report* 2009; *58*:581–606.

Channon S, Flynn D, Robertson MM. Attentional deficits in the Gilles de la Tourette syndrome. *Neuropsychiatry Neuropsychol Behav Neurol* 1992; *5*:170–177.

Channon S, Gunning A, Frankl J et al. Tourette's syndrome (TS): cognitive performance in adults with uncomplicated TS. *Neuropsychology* 2006; *20*:58–65.

Charach A, Yeung E, Climans T et al. Childhood attention-deficit/hyperactivity disorder and future substance use disorders: comparative meta-analyses. *J Am Acad Child Adolesc Psychiatry* 2011; *50*:9–21.

Chouinard S, Ford B. Adult onset tic disorders. *J Neurol Neurosurg Psychiatry* 2000; *68*: 738–743.

Coffey BJ, Biederman J, Geller D et al. The course of Tourette's disorder: a literature review. *Harv Rev Psychiatry* 2000; *8*:192–198.

Coffey BJ, Biederman J, Geller D et al. Reexamining tic persistence and tic-associated impairment in Tourette's disorder: findings from a naturalistic follow-up study. *J Nerv Ment Dis* 2004; *192*:776–780.

Collacott RA, Ismail IA. Tourettism in a patient with Down's syndrome. *J Ment Defic Res* 1988; *32*:163–166.

Comings DE, Comings BG. Tourette's syndrome and attention deficit disorder with hyperactivity: are they genetically related? *J Am Acad Child Psychiatry* 1984; *23*:138–146.

Comings DE, Comings BG. A controlled study of Tourette syndrome. II. Conduct. *Am J Hum Genet* 1987a; *41*:742–760.

Comings DE, Comings BG. Hereditary agoraphobia and obsessive-compulsive behaviour in relatives of patients with Gilles de la Tourette's syndrome. *Br J Psychiatry* 1987b; *151*:195–199.

Comings DE, Comings BG. A controlled family history study of Tourette's syndrome, I: Attention-deficit hyperactivity disorder and learning disorders. *J Clin Psychiatry* 1990; *51*:275–280.

Debes NM, Hjalgrim H, Skov L. Predictive factors for familiality in a Danish clinical cohort of children with Tourette syndrome. *Eur J Med Genet* 2010a; *53*:171–178.

Debes NM, Lange T, Jessen TL et al. Performance on Wechsler intelligence scales in children with Tourette syndrome. *Eur J Paediatr Neurol* 2010b; *15*:146–154.

Draganski B, Martino D, Cavanna AE et al. Multispectral brain morphometry in Tourette syndrome persisting into adulthood. *Brain* 2010; *133*:3661–3675.

Eapen V. Genetic basis of autism: is there a way forward? *Curr Opin Psychiatry* 2011; *24*: 226–236.

Eapen V, Champion L, Zeitlin H. Tourette syndrome, epilepsy, and emotional disorder, a case of triple comorbidity. *Psychol Rep* 1997c; *81*:1239–1242.

Eapen V, Črnčec R. Tourette syndrome in children and adolescents: special considerations. *J Psychosom Res* 2009; *67*:525–532.

Eapen V, Fox-Hiley P, Banerjee S et al. Clinical features and associated psychopathology in a Tourette syndrome cohort. *Acta Neurol Scand* 2004; *109*:255–260.

Eapen V, Lees AJ, Lakke JP et al. Adult-onset tic disorders. *Mov Disord* 2002; *17*:735–740.

Eapen V, O'Neill J, Gurling HM et al. Sex of parent transmission effect in Tourette's syndrome: evidence for earlier age at onset in maternally transmitted cases suggests a genomic imprinting effect. *Neurology* 1997b; *48*:934–937.

Eapen V, Pauls DL, Robertson MM. Evidence for autosomal dominant transmission in Tourette's syndrome. United Kingdom cohort study. *Br J Psychiatry* 1993; *162*:593–596.

Eapen V, Robertson MM. All that tics may not be Tourette's. *Br J Psychiatry* 1994; *164*:708.

Eapen V, Robertson MM. Gilles de la Tourette Syndrome and attention deficit disorder - no evidence for a genetic relationship. *J Neuropsychiatr Neuropsychol Behav Neurol* 1996; 9:192–196.

Eapen V, Robertson MM, Alsobrook JP 2nd et al. Obsessive compulsive symptoms in Gilles de la Tourette syndrome and obsessive compulsive disorder: differences by diagnosis and family history. *Am J Med Genet* 1997a; 74:432–438.

Eapen V, Robertson MM, Zeitlin H et al. Gilles de la Tourette's syndrome in special education schools: a United Kingdom study. *J Neurol* 1997d; 244:378–382.

Eapen V, Robertson MM. Clinical correlates of Tourette's disorder across cultures: A comparative study between the United Arab Emirates and the United Kingdom. *Prim Care Companion J Clin Psychiatry* 2008; 10:103–107.

Earls F. Psychosocial factors in Tourette syndrome. *Adv Neurol* 1992; 58:55–59.

Elgen I, Sommerfelt K, Markestad T. Population based, controlled study of behavioural problems and psychiatric disorders in low birthweight children at 11 years of age. *Arch Dis Child Fetal Neonatal Ed* 2002; 87:F128–132.

Ercan-Sencicek AG, Stillmann AA, Ghosh AK et al. L-histidine decarboxylase and Tourette's syndrome N Engl J Med 2010; 362: 1901–1908.

Erenberg G, Cruse RP, Rothner AD. The natural history of Tourette syndrome: a follow-up study. *Ann Neurol* 1987; 22:383–385.

Fahim C, Yoon U, Das S et al. Somatosensory-motor bodily representation cortical thinning in Tourette: effects of tic severity, age and gender. *Cortex* 2010; 46:750–760.

Freeman RD. Tic disorders and ADHD: answers from a world-wide clinical dataset on Tourette syndrome. Eur *Child Adolesc Psychiatry* 2007; 16 Suppl 1:15–23.

Freeman RD, Fast DK, Burd L et al. An international perspective on Tourette syndrome: selected findings from 3,500 individuals in 22 countries. *Dev Med Child Neurol* 2000; 42:436–447.

Freudenberg F, Dieckmann M, Winter S et al. Selective breeding for deficient sensorimotor gating is accompanied by increased perseveration in rats. *Neuroscience* 2007; 148:612–622.

Garcia-Ribes A, Marti-Carrera I, Martinez-Gonzalez MJ et al. Factors related to the short term remission of tics in children with Tourette syndrome. *Rev Neurol* 2003; 37:901–903.

Garraux G, Goldfine A, Bohlhalter S et al. Increased midbrain gray matter in Tourette's syndrome. *Ann Neurol* 2006; 59:381–385.

Gershon ES, Goldin LR. Clinical methods in psychiatric genetics. I. Robustness of genetic marker investigative strategies. *Acta Psychiatr Scand* 1986; 74:113–118.

Gilles de la Tourette G. Étude sur une affection nerveuse caracterisée par l'incoordination motrice accompagnée d'écholalie et de coprolalie. *Archives de Neurologie [Paris]* 1885; 9:19–42 et 158–200.

Gottesman II, Gould TD. The endophenotype concept in psychiatry: etymology and strategic intentions. *Am J Psychiatry* 2003; 160:636–645.

Grados MA, Mathews CA. Latent class analysis of Gilles de la Tourette syndrome using comorbidities: clinical and genetic implications. *Biol Psychiatry* 2008; 64:219–225.

Haddad AD, Umoh G, Bhatia V et al. Adults with Tourette's syndrome with and without attention deficit hyperactivity disorder. *Acta Psychiatr Scand* 2009; 120:299–307.

Heinz A, Knable MB, Wolf SS et al. Tourette's syndrome: [I-123]beta-CIT SPECT correlates of vocal tic severity. *Neurology* 1998; 51: 1069–1074.

Hoekstra PJ, Steenhuis MP, Kallenberg CG et al. Association of small life events with self reports of tic severity in pediatric and adult tic disorder patients: a prospective longitudinal study. *J Clin Psychiatry* 2004a; 65:426–431.

Hoekstra PJ, Steenhuis MP, Troost PW et al. Relative contribution of attention-deficit hyperactivity disorder, obsessive-compulsive disorder, and tic severity to social and behavioral problems in tic disorders. *J Dev Behav Pediatr* 2004b; 25:272–279.

Horesh N, Zimmerman S, Steinberg T et al. Is onset of Tourette syndrome influenced by life events? *J Neural Transm* 2008; 115:787–793.

Hyde TM, Aaronson BA, Randolph C et al. Relationship of birth weight to the phenotypic expression of Gilles de la Tourette's syndrome in monozygotic twins. *Neurology* 1992; 42:652–658.

Hyde TM, Emsellem HA, Randolph C et al. Electroencephalographic abnormalities in monozygotic twins with Tourette's syndrome. *Br J Psychiatry* 1994; 164:811–817.

Hyde TM, Stacey ME, Coppola R et al. Cerebral morphometric abnormalities in Tourette's syndrome: a quantitative MRI study of monozygotic twins. *Neurology* 1995; 45:1176–1182.

Itard JEMG. Mémoire sur quelques fonctions involontaires des appareils de la locomotion, de la préhension et de la voix. *Archives Générales de Médecine* 1825; 8:385–407.

Jagger J, Prusoff BA, Cohen DJ et al. The epidemiology of Tourette's syndrome: a pilot study. *Schizophr Bull* 1982; 8:267–278.

Kalanithi PS, Zheng W, Kataoka Y et al. Altered parvalbumin-positive neuron distribution in basal ganglia of individuals with Tourette syndrome. *Proc Natl Acad Sci U S A* 2005; 102:13307–13312.

Kano Y, Ohta M, Nagai Y. Clinical characteristics of Tourette syndrome. *Psychiatry Clin Neurosci* 1998; 52:51–57.

Karlinsky H, Berg JM. Gilles de la Tourette's syndrome in Down's syndrome. *Br J Psychiatry* 1987; 151:707.

Karlinsky H, Sandor P, Berg JM et al. Gilles de la Tourette's syndrome in Down's syndrome—a case report. *Br J Psychiatry* 1986; 148:601–604.

Karp BI, Porter S, Toro C et al. Simple motor tics may be preceded by a premotor potential. *J Neurol Neurosurg Psychiatry* 1986; 61:103–106.

Kataoka Y, Kalanithi PS, Grantz H et al. Decreased number of parvalbumin and cholinergic interneurons in the striatum of individuals with Tourette syndrome. *J Comp Neurol* 2010; 518:277–291.

Keen-Kim D, Mathews CA, Reus VI et al. Overrepresentation of rare variants in a specific ethnic group may confuse interpretation of association analyses. *Hum Mol Genet* 2006; 15:3324–3328.

Kerbeshian J, Burd L. Comorbid Down's syndrome, Tourette syndrome and intellectual disability: registry prevalence and developmental course. *J Intellect Disabil Res* 2000; 44:60–67.

Khalifa N, von Knorring AL. Prevalence of tic disorders and Tourette syndrome in a Swedish school population. *Dev Med Child Neurol* 2003; 45:315–319.

Khalifa N, von Knorring AL. Tourette syndrome and other tic disorders in a total population of children: clinical assessment and background. *Acta Paediatr* 2005; 94:1608–1614.

Knell ER, Comings DE. Tourette's syndrome and attention-deficit hyperactivity disorder: evidence for a genetic relationship. *J Clin Psychiatry* 1993; 54:331–337.

Kurlan R, Eapen V, Stern J et al. Bilineal transmission in Tourette's syndrome families. *Neurology* 1994; 44:2336–2342.

Leckman JF. Phenomenology of tics and natural history of tic disorders. *Brain Dev* 2003; 25 Suppl 1:S24–28.

Leckman JF, Dolnansky ES, Hardin MT et al. Perinatal factors in the expression of Tourette's syndrome: an exploratory study. *J Am Acad Child Adolesc Psychiatry* 1990; 29:220–226.

Leckman JF, King RA, Gilbert DL et al. Streptococcal upper respiratory tract infections and exacerbations of tic and obsessive-compulsive symptoms: a prospective longitudinal study. *J Am Acad Child Adolesc Psychiatry* 2011; 50:108–118 e103.

Leckman JF, Pauls DL, Zhang H et al. Obsessive-compulsive symptom dimensions in affected sibling pairs diagnosed with Gilles de la Tourette syndrome. *Am J Med Genet B Neuropsychiatr Genet* 2003; 116B:60–68.

Leckman JF, Price RA, Walkup JT et al. Nongenetic factors in Gilles de la Tourette's syndrome. *Arch Gen Psychiatry* 1987; 44:100.

Leckman JF, Zhang H, Vitale A et al. Course of tic severity in Tourette syndrome: the first two decades. *Pediatrics* 1998; 102:14–19.

Lees AJ, Robertson M, Trimble MR et al. A clinical study of Gilles de la Tourette syndrome in the United Kingdom. *J Neurol Neurosurg Psychiatry* 1984; 47:1–8.

Leiser SC, Bowlby MR, Comery TA et al. A cog in cognition: how the alpha 7 nicotinic acetylcholine receptor is geared towards improving cognitive deficits. *Pharmacol Ther* 2009; 122:302–311.

Lewin AB, Murphy TK, Storch EA et al. A phenomenological investigation of women with Tourette or other chronic tic disorders. *Compr Psychiatry* 2012; 53:525–534.

Lieh-Mak F, Chung SY, Lee P et al. Tourette syndrome in the Chinese: a follow-up of 15 cases. In A Friedhoff & T Chase (Eds.), *Gilles de la Tourette syndrome* (pp. 281–283). New York: Raven, 1982.

Lin H, Katsovich L, Ghebremichael M et al. Psychosocial stress predicts future symptom severities in children and adolescents with Tourette syndrome and/or obsessive-compulsive disorder. *J Child Psychol Psychiatry* 2007; 48:157–166.

Lin H, Williams KA, Katsovich L et al. Streptococcal upper respiratory tract infections and psychosocial stress predict future tic and obsessive-compulsive symptom severity in children and adolescents with Tourette syndrome and obsessive-compulsive disorder. *Biol Psychiatry* 2010; 67:684–691.

Linet LS. Tourette syndrome, pimozide, and school phobia: the neuroleptic separation anxiety syndrome. *Am J Psychiatry* 1985; *142*:613–615.

Lipsitch M, Sousa AO. Historical intensity of natural selection for resistance to tuberculosis. *Genetics* 2002; *161*:1599–1607.

Liu J. Early health risk factors for violence: Conceptualization, review of the evidence, and implications. *Aggress Violent Behav* 2011; *16*:63–73.

Ludolph AG, Juengling FD, Libal G et al. Grey-matter abnormalities in boys with Tourette syndrome: magnetic resonance imaging study using optimised voxel-based morphometry. *Br J Psychiatry* 2006; *188*:484–485.

Makki MI, Govindan RM, Wilson BJ et al. Altered fronto-striato-thalamic connectivity in children with Tourette syndrome assessed with diffusion tensor MRI and probabilistic fiber tracking. *J Child Neurol* 2009; *24*:669–678.

Marsh R, Alexander GM, Packard MG et al. Habit learning in Tourette syndrome: a translational neuroscience approach to a developmental psychopathology. *Arch Gen Psychiatry* 2004; *61*:1259–1268.

Martino D, Dale RC, Gilbert DL et al. Immunopathogenic mechanisms in Tourette syndrome: A critical review. *Mov Disord* 2009a; *24*: 1267–1279.

Martino D, Defazio G, Church AJ et al. Antineuronal antibody status and phenotype analysis in Tourette's syndrome. *Mov Disord* 2007; *22*:1424–1429.

Mathews CA, Bimson B, Lowe TL et al. Association between maternal smoking and increased symptom severity in Tourette's syndrome. *Am J Psychiatry* 2006; *163*:1066–1073.

Mathews CA, Jang KL, Herrera LD et al. Tic symptom profiles in subjects with Tourette Syndrome from two genetically isolated populations. *Biol Psychiatry* 2007; *61*:292–300.

Mathews CA, Waller J, Glidden D et al. Self-injurious behaviour in Tourette syndrome: correlates with impulsivity and impulse control. *J Neurol Neurosurg Psychiatry* 2004; *75*:1149–1155.

McMahon WM van de Wetering BJ, Filloux F et al. Bilineal transmission and phenotypic variation of Tourette's disorder in a large pedigree. *J Am Acad Child Adolesc Psychiatry* 1996; *35*:672–680.

Mell LK, Davis RL, Owens D. Association between streptococcal infection and obsessive-compulsive disorder, Tourette's syndrome, and tic disorder. *Pediatrics* 2005; *116*:56–60.

Metcalfe A, Lail P, Ghali WA et al. The association between neighbourhoods and adverse birth outcomes: a systematic review and meta-analysis of multi-level studies. *Paediatr Perinat Epidemiol* 2011; *25*:236–245.

Min SK, Lee H. A clinical study of Gilles de la Tourette's syndrome in Korea. *Br J Psychiatry* 1986; *149*:644–647.

Moriarty J, Eapen V, Costa DC et al. HMPAO SPET does not distinguish obsessive-compulsive and tic syndromes in families multiply affected with Gilles de la Tourette's syndrome. *Psychol Med* 1997; *27*:737–740.

Motlagh MG, Katsovich L, Thompson N et al. Severe psychosocial stress and heavy cigarette smoking during pregnancy: an examination of the pre- and perinatal risk factors associated with ADHD and Tourette syndrome. *Eur Child Adolesc Psychiatry* 2010; *19*:755–764.

Muller-Vahl KR, Kaufmann J, Grosskreutz J et al. Prefrontal and anterior cingulate cortex abnormalities in Tourette Syndrome: evidence from voxel-based morphometry and magnetization transfer imaging. *BMC Neurosci* 2009; *10*:47.

Myers B, Puschel SM. Tardive or atypical Tourette's disorder in a population with Down syndrome? *Res Dev Disabil* 1995; *16*:1–9.

Neave LE, Robertson MM, Stern JS. Does the presence of putative aetiological factors in Tourette 's syndrome influence severity ? Paper presented at the Poster and Presentation at the Association of British Neurologists Annual Meeting, 2008.

Neuner I, Kellermann T, Stocker T et al. Amygdala hypersensitivity in response to emotional faces in Tourette's patients. *World J Biol Psychiatry* 2010; *11*:858–872.

Ni TL, Huang CC, Guo NW. Executive function deficit in preschool children born very low birth weight with normal early development. *Early Hum Dev* 2011; *87*:137–141.

Nomura Y, Segawa M. Gilles de la Tourette syndrome in Oriental children. *Brain Dev* 1979; *1*:103–111.

Nomura Y, Segawa M. Tourette syndrome in oriental children: clinical and pathophysiological considerations. *Adv Neurol* 1982; *35*:277–280.

Nomura Y, Kita M, Segawa M. Social adaptation of Tourette syndrome families in Japan. *Adv Neurol* 1992; *58*:323–332.

Obeso JA, Rothwell JC, Marsden CD. Simple tics in Gilles de la Tourette's syndrome are not prefaced by a normal premovement EEG potential. *J Neurol Neurosurg Psychiatry* 1981; *44*:735–738.

O'Roak BJ, Morgan TM, Fishman DO et al. Additional support for the association of SLITRK1 var321 and Tourette syndrome. *Mol Psychiatry* 2010; 15:447–450.

O'Rourke JA, Scharf JM, Platko J et al. The familial association of Tourette's disorder and ADHD: the impact of OCD symptoms. *Am J Med Genet B Neuropsychiatr Genet* 2011; 156:553–560.

Packer LE. Social and educational resources for patients with Tourette syndrome. *Neurol Clin* 1987; 15:457–473.

Pappert EJ, Goetz CG, Louis ED et al. Objective assessments of longitudinal outcome in Gilles de la Tourette's syndrome. *Neurology* 2003; 61:936–940.

Patel C, Cooper-Charles L, McMullan DJ et al. Translocation breakpoint at 7q31 associated with tics: further evidence for IMMP2L as a candidate gene for Tourette syndrome. *Eur J Hum Genet* 2011; 19:634–639.

Pauls DL, Hurst CR, Kruger SD et al. Evidence against a genetic relationship between Tourette syndrome and attention deficit disorder. *Am J Hum Genet* 1984; 36:68S.

Pauls DL, Leckman JF. The inheritance of Gilles de la Tourette's syndrome and associated behaviors. Evidence for autosomal dominant transmission. *N Engl J Med* 1986; 315:993–997.

Pauls DL, Leckman JF, Cohen DJ. Evidence against a genetic relationship between Tourette's syndrome and anxiety, depression, panic and phobic disorders. *Br J Psychiatry* 1994; 164:215–221.

Pauls DL, Raymond CL, Stevenson JM et al. A family study of Gilles de la Tourette syndrome. *Am J Hum Genet* 1991; 48:154–163.

Petek E, Windpassinger C, Vincent JB et al. Disruption of a novel gene (IMMP2L) by a breakpoint in 7q31 associated with Tourette syndrome. *Am J Hum Genet* 2001; 68:848–858.

Peterson BS, Leckman JF, Scahill L et al. Steroid hormones and CNS sexual dimorphisms modulate symptom expression in Tourette's syndrome. *Psychoneuroendocrinology* 1992; 17:553–563.

Peterson BS, Staib L, Scahill L et al. Regional brain and ventricular volumes in Tourette syndrome. *Arch Gen Psychiatry* 2001; 58:427–440.

Peterson BS, Thomas P, Kane MJ et al. Basal ganglia volumes in patients with Gilles de la Tourette syndrome. Arch Gen Psychiatry 2003; 60:415–424.

Pierre CB, Nolan EE, Gadow KD et al. Comparison of internalizing and externalizing symptoms in children with attention-deficit hyperactivity disorder with and without comorbid tic disorder. *J Dev Behav Pediatr* 1999; 20:170–176.

Pourfar M, Feigin A, Tang CC et al. Abnormal metabolic brain networks in Tourette syndrome. *Neurology* 2011; 76:944–952.

Pringsheim T, Sandor P, Lang A et al. Prenatal and perinatal morbidity in children with Tourette syndrome and attention-deficit hyperactivity disorder. *J Dev Behav Pediatr* 2009; 30: 115–121.

Randolph C, Hyde TM, Gold JM et al. Tourette's syndrome in monozygotic twins. Relationship of tic severity to neuropsychological function. *Arch Neurol* 1993; 50:725–728.

Rizzo R, Curatolo P, Gulisano M et al. Disentangling the effects of Tourette syndrome and attention deficit hyperactivity disorder on cognitive and behavioral phenotypes. *Brain Dev* 2007; 29:413–420.

Rizzo R, Gulisano M, Calì PV et al. ADHD and epilepsy in children with Tourette syndrome: a triple comorbidity? *Acta Paediatr* 2010; 99:1894–1896.

Robertson MM. Tourette syndrome, associated conditions and the complexities of treatment. *Brain* 2000; 123:425–462.

Robertson MM. The heterogeneous psychopathology of Tourette syndrome. In MA Bedard, Y Agid, S Chouinard, S Fahn, AD Korczyn & P Lesperance (Eds.), *Mental and behavioral dysfunction in movement disorders* (pp. 443–466). Totowa, NJ: Humana Press, 2003.

Robertson MM. Mood disorders and Gilles de la Tourette's syndrome: An update on prevalence, etiology, comorbidity, clinical associations, and implications. *J Psychosom Res* 2006; 61: 349–358.

Robertson MM. The prevalence and epidemiology of Gilles de la Tourette syndrome. Part 1: the epidemiological and prevalence studies. *J Psychosom Res* 2008a; 65:461–472.

Robertson MM. The prevalence and epidemiology of Gilles de la Tourette syndrome. Part 2: tentative explanations for differing prevalence figures in GTS, including the possible effects of psychopathology, aetiology, cultural differences, and differing phenotypes. *J Psychosom Res* 2008b; 65:473–486.

Robertson MM, Althoff RR, Hafez A et al. Principal components analysis of a large cohort with Tourette syndrome. *Br J Psychiatry* 2008; 193:31–36.

Robertson MM, Banerjee S, Hiley PJ et al. Personality disorder and psychopathology in Tourette's syndrome: a controlled study. *Br J Psychiatry* 1997; 171:283–286.

Robertson MM, Baron-Cohen S. *Tourette syndrome: The facts.* Oxford: Oxford University Press, 1998.

Robertson MM, Cavanna AE. The Gilles de la Tourette syndrome: a principal component factor analytic study of a large pedigree. *Psychiatr Genet* 2007; 17:143–152.

Robertson MM, Cavanna AE. *Tourette syndrome: The facts* (2nd ed.). Oxford: Oxford University Press, 2008d.

Robertson MM, Gourdie A. Familial Tourette's syndrome in a large British pedigree. Associated psychopathology, severity, and potential for linkage analysis. *Br J Psychiatry* 1990; 156: 515–521.

Robertson MM, Reinstein DZ. Convulsive tic disorder. Georges Gilles de la Tourette, Guinon and Grasset on the phenomenology and psychopathology of the Gilles de la Tourette syndrome. *Behav Neurol* 1991; 4:29–56.

Robertson MM, Shelley BP, Dalwai S et al. A patient with both Gilles de la Tourette's syndrome and chromosome 22q11 deletion syndrome: clue to the genetics of Gilles de la Tourette's syndrome? *J Psychosom Res* 2006b; 61:365–368.

Robertson MM, Trimble MR, Lees AJ. The psychopathology of the Gilles de la Tourette syndrome. A phenomenological analysis. *Br J Psychiatry* 1988; 152:383–390.

Robertson MM, Trimble MR, Lees AJ Self-injurious behaviour and the Gilles de la Tourette syndrome: a clinical study and review of the literature. *Psychol Med* 1989; 19:611–625.

Robertson MM, Verrill M, Mercer M et al. Tourette's syndrome in New Zealand. A postal survey. *Br J Psychiatry* 1994; 164:263–266.

Robertson MM, Williamson F, Eapen V. Depressive symptomatology in young people with Gilles de la Tourette Syndrome—a comparison of self-report scales. *J Affect Disord* 2006a; 91:265–268.

Roessner V, Overlack S, Baudewig J et al. No brain structure abnormalities in boys with Tourette's syndrome: a voxel-based morphometry study. *Mov Disord* 2009; 24:2398–2403.

Schneider SA, Robertson MM, Rizzo R et al. Fragile X syndrome associated with tic disorders. *Mov Disord* 2008; 23:1108–1112.

Shapiro AK, Shapiro E. An update on Tourette syndrome. *Am J Psychother* 1982; 36:379–390.

Shapiro AK, Shapiro E, Wayne HL et al. Tourette's syndrome: summary of data on 34 patients. *Psychosom Med* 1973; 35:419–435.

Shapiro AK, Shapiro ES, Young JG et al. *Gilles de la Tourette syndrome* (2nd ed.). New York: Raven Press, 1988.

Shelley BP, Robertson MM, Turk J. An individual with Gilles de la Tourette syndrome and Smith-Magenis microdeletion syndrome: is chromosome 17p11.2 a candidate region for Tourette syndrome putative susceptibility genes? *J Intellect Disabil Res* 2007; 51:620–624.

Silva RR, Munoz DM, Barickman J et al. Environmental factors and related fluctuation of symptoms in children and adolescents with Tourette's disorder. *J Child Psychol Psychiatry* 1995; 36:305–312.

Snijders AH, Robertson MM, Orth M. Beck Depression Inventory is a useful screening tool for major depressive disorder in Gilles de la Tourette syndrome. *J Neurol Neurosurg Psychiatry* 2006; 77:787–789.

Sowell ER, Kan E, Yoshii J et al. Thinning of sensorimotor cortices in children with Tourette syndrome. *Nat Neurosci* 2008; 11:637–639.

Spencer T, Biederman J, Harding M et al. Disentangling the overlap between Tourette's disorder and ADHD. *J Child Psychol Psychiatry* 1998; 39:1037–1044.

Spencer TJ, Biederman J, Faraone S et al. Impact of tic disorders on ADHD outcome across the life cycle: findings from a large group of adults with and without ADHD. *Am J Psychiatry* 2001; 158:611–617.

Staley D, Wand R, Shady G. Tourette disorder: a cross-cultural review. *Compr Psychiatry* 1997; 38:6–16.

Stephens RJ, Sandor P. Aggressive behaviour in children with Tourette syndrome and comorbid attention-deficit hyperactivity disorder and obsessive-compulsive disorder. *Can J Psychiatry* 1999; 44:1036–1042.

Stern JS, Robertson MM. Tics associated with autistic and pervasive developmental disorders. *Neurol Clin* 1997; 15:345–355.

Stewart SE, Illmann C, Geller DA et al. A controlled family study of attention-deficit/hyperactivity disorder and Tourette's disorder. *J Am Acad Child Adolesc Psychiatry* 2006; 45:1354–1362.

Storch EA, Murphy TK, Geffken GR et al. Further psychometric properties of the Tourette's Disorder Scale-Parent Rated version (TODS-PR). *Child Psychiatry Hum Dev* 2004; 35:107–120.

Sukhodolsky DG, Scahill L, Zhang H et al. Disruptive behavior in children with Tourette's syndrome: association with ADHD comorbidity, tic severity, and functional impairment. *J Am Acad Child Adolesc Psychiatry* 2003; 42:98–105.

Surwillo WW, Shafii M, Barrett CL. Gilles de la Tourette syndrome: a 20-month study of the effects of stressful life events and haloperidol on symptom frequency. *J Nerv Ment Dis* 1978; 166:812–816.

Sutherland Owens AN, Miguel EC, Swerdlow NR. Sensory gating scales and premonitory urges in Tourette syndrome. *Scientific World Journal* 2011; 11:736–741.

Swedo SE, Leonard HL, Garvey M et al. Pediatric autoimmune neuropsychiatric disorders associated with streptococcal infections: clinical description of the first 50 cases. *Am J Psychiatry* 1998; 155:264–271.

Termine C, Balottin U, Rossi G et al. Psychopathology in children and adolescents with Tourette's syndrome: a controlled study. *Brain Dev* 2006; 28:69–75.

Thomalla G, Siebner HR, Jonas M et al. Structural changes in the somatosensory system correlate with tic severity in Gilles de la Tourette syndrome. *Brain* 2009; 132:765–777.

Vettore MV, Gama SG, Lamarca Gde A et al. Housing conditions as a social determinant of low birthweight and preterm low birthweight. *Rev Saude Publica* 2010; 44:1021–1031.

Vicario CM, Martino D, Spata F et al. Time processing in children with Tourette's syndrome. *Brain Cogn* 2010; 73:28–34.

Wedenoja J, Loukola A, Tuulio-Henriksson A et al. Replication of linkage on chromosome 7q22 and association of the regional Reelin gene with working memory in schizophrenia families. *Mol Psychiatry* 2008; 13:673–684.

Wedenoja J, Tuulio-Henriksson A, Suvisaari J et al. Replication of association between working memory and Reelin, a potential modifier gene in schizophrenia. *Biol Psychiatry* 2010; 67:983–991.

Wells JC. The thrifty phenotype as an adaptive maternal effect. *Biol Rev Camb Philos Soc* 2007; 82:143–172.

Wolf SS, Jones DW, Knable MB et al. Tourette syndrome: prediction of phenotypic variation in monozygotic twins by caudate nucleus D2 receptor binding. *Science* 1996; 273:1225–1227.

Woods DW, Piacentini J, Himle MB et al. Premonitory Urge for Tics Scale (PUTS): initial psychometric results and examination of the premonitory urge phenomenon in youths with tic disorders. *J Dev Behav Pediatr* 2005; 26: 397–403.

Worbe Y, Gerardin E, Hartmann A et al. Distinct structural changes underpin clinical phenotypes in patients with Gilles de la Tourette syndrome. *Brain* 2010; 133:3649–3660.

World Health Organization. *The ICD-10 Classification of Mental and Behavioural Disorders: Diagnostic criteria for research.* Geneva: World Health Organization, 1992.

Yordanova J, Dumais-Huber C, Rothenberger A et al. Frontocortical activity in children with comorbidity of tic disorder and attention-deficit hyperactivity disorder. *Biol Psychiatry* 1997; 41:585–594.

Yordanova J, Heinrich H, Kolev V et al. Increased event-related theta activity as a psychophysiological marker of comorbidity in children with tics and attention-deficit/hyperactivity disorders. *Neuroimage* 2006; 32:940–955.

Zykov VP, Shcherbina AY, Novikova EB et al. Neuroimmune aspects of the pathogenesis of Tourette's syndrome and experience in the use of immunoglobulins in children. *Neurosci Behav Physiol* 2009; 39:635–638.

17

The Differential Diagnosis of Tic Disorders

ROGER KURLAN

Abstract

This chapter focuses on the differential diagnosis of tics and tic disorders. Tics need to be distinguished from other hyperkinetic movement disorders, such as chorea, myoclonus, and dystonia, as well as from movement disorders associated with psychiatric conditions (compulsions, sterotypies, mannerisms, habits). Tourette syndrome belongs to a family of primary tic disorders that include chronic motor or vocal tic disorder and transient tic disorder. However, tics may have different etiologies and can occur secondary to a number of conditions, including neurological disorders and medications, and as a psychogenic manifestation.

INTRODUCTION

This chapter will discuss the differential diagnosis of tic disorders at two levels. First will be a discussion about how to distinguish tics from other types of body movements and sounds. This will be followed by a discussion about the various etiological entities that can cause tics.

DISTINGUISHING TICS FROM OTHER TYPES OF MOVEMENTS AND NOISES

Other Neurological Movement Disorders

Tics encompass a complicated and heterogeneous clinical phenomenology, including motor and phonic types, simple and complex forms, and subtypes such as dystonic and tonic tics (Table 17.1). It is safe to say that virtually any movement or sound the human body is capable of making can be a manifestation of tics. This clinical complexity, on the one hand, may contribute to difficulties distinguishing tics from other movement disorders. On the other hand, it may assist with proper diagnosis. For example, myoclonus (lightning-like muscle jerks) or chorea (dance-like muscle jerks) can resemble the quick jerks of simple motor tics, but since simple motor tics are often accompanied by complex motor tics or vocal tics, they can be appropriately diagnosed by "the company they keep." Thus, the presence of vocal tics can allow the proper identification of body jerks as motor tics and vice versa. Thus, while diaphragmatic or respiratory muscle myoclonus or chorea can produce hiccough, sigh, or other noises reminiscent of simple vocal tics, a tic disorder can be diagnosed by the observation of other types (e.g., complex motor, dystonic) of tics. In addition, myoclonus and chorea tend not to be repetitive in the same location like tics. The presence of premonitory sensations (i.e., feelings of discomfort, pressure, or other uncomfortable sensations at the site of a tic or more generally in the head or body) (Leckman, Walker & Cohen, 1993) appears to be a feature of tics and not other neurological hyperkinetic movement disorders. Although voluntary suppressibility is a characteristic feature of tics, patients can sometimes suppress other types of hyperkinetic movement disorders temporarily.

Dystonic tics consist of slow, twisting movements resembling dystonia (twisting movements and postures) (Jankovic & Stone, 1991). Compared to dystonia, dystonic tics usually

Table 17.1 Other Movement Conditions Resembling Tics

Neurologic movement disorders: chorea, myoclonus, dystonia
Psychiatric-associated movement disorders: compulsions, stereotypies, mannerisms
Normal movements: habits

occur in brief bursts of movement, are not continuous, tend to produce abnormal postures that are not as sustained, and are often associated with premonitory sensations (Kwak, Dat Vuong & Jankovic, 2003). Dystonic tics are usually accompanied by other more typical motor tics or vocal tics, thus revealing their nature. It should be noted that tics and dystonia can occur together (Stone & Jankovic, 1991), sometimes in a familial pattern (Németh et al., 1999; Romstad et al., 2003).

Movement Disorders Linked to Psychiatric Conditions

Obsessive-compulsive disorder (OCD) is one of the most common psychiatric comorbidities of Tourette syndrome (TS). Compulsions and complex motor tics are sometimes difficult to distinguish, particularly when the two phenomena coexist. In contrast to tics, compulsions are carried out in response to an obsession (e.g., repeated hand washing to prevent contamination), to ward off future harm (e.g., repeated checking of stoves and other appliances to avoid danger), to decrease anxiety, or according to certain rules. This rule-based (ritualistic) quality is characteristic of compulsions, and clinicians should ask patients about the presence or absence of such rules. Typical rules relate to order, symmetry, number of repetitions, or time of day (e.g., morning or bedtime rituals). It is quite unusual for complex motor tics to occur in the absence of simple motor tics, thus helping to identify them. I have found that some individual actions, such as repetitive tapping or touching, may be difficult to classify as a tic or a compulsion and may have features of both. I refer to these as "compulsive tics" or "compultics" (Palumbo & Kurlan, 2007).

Probably the most common behavioral comorbidity of TS is attention-deficit/ hyperactivity disorder (ADHD). Some tics possess qualities of impulsiveness and sometimes aggressiveness and social inappropriateness often linked to ADHD. I call these "impulsive tics" or "impultics" (Palumbo & Kurlan, 2007). Examples include yelling out insults, punching self or others, or touching a hot stove. Reflecting the complex interrelationships between TS and its psychiatric comorbidities, there are actions that simultaneously have qualities of tics, compulsions, and impulsiveness (e.g., pushing someone after they have sneezed to prevent contamination), which can be considered "compulsive/impulsive tics" (Palumbo & Kurlan, 2007).

Motor and phonic tics should be distinguished from stereotypies, which occur in patients with congenital deafness and blindness, mental retardation, autism, Rett syndrome, encephalopathies, and psychosis. Stereotypies are coordinated, rhythmic, repetitive, and patterned movements, postures, or vocalizations that are carried out virtually the same way over and over again. Stereotypies can be quite complex, such as walking in circles, standing/sitting, and repeating words or phrases, and some can be self-harming (e.g., skin scratching or picking, eye poking, hand biting). Compared to tics, stereotypies are characteristically more stereotyped, with the same movement (e.g., hand flapping, body rocking, head nodding, head banging) or vocalization (e.g., yelling, moaning, hissing) occurring repeatedly for long periods of time. Patients with stereotypies usually have signs of severe auditory or visual sensory loss, global cognitive dysfunction, or psychosis. Stereotypies are not known to have premonitory sensations and may be more difficult to suppress than tics.

Mannerisms are peculiar or unusual characteristic ways of performing a normal activity. These include things like an odd gait, a peculiar speech, or a movement flourish. Mannerisms serve to attract attention to an individual and are usually associated with schizophrenia. Habits are repetitive, coordinated movements or sounds seen in normal individuals particularly during times of boredom, fatigue, self-consciousness, or anxiety. Common habits include foot tapping, abduction/adduction of thighs, finger drumming, thumb twiddling, popping finger joints, chewing fingernails, humming, pushing up glasses, and hair twirling. Some habits are developmental (e.g., thumb sucking) and some are socially inappropriate (e.g., nose picking, smoking). Like tics, habits are associated with stress and heightened anxiety and sometimes with fatigue. Habits are easier to suppress, at least temporarily, than tics.

CAUSES OF TICS

Primary Tic Disorders

Primary tic disorders are the most common causes of tics (Table 17.2). These are considered to be largely idiopathic, but with a strong genetic predisposition. Some evidence suggests a role for environmental factors in their etiology. TS is the main primary tic disorder and is the focus of this book. According to standard diagnostic criteria, patients with TS have childhood or adolescence onset of multiple motor and vocal tics with a duration of at least 1 year and no known cause (American Psychiatric Association, 2000). Traditionally, those with only motor tics are classified as having chronic motor tic disorder, and those with only vocal tics are classified as having chronic vocal tic disorder. Given that the production of vocal tics involves the contraction of laryngeal, pharyngeal, or respiratory muscles (i.e., motor activity), the separation of these latter conditions from TS does not have a strong neurobiological rationale (The Tourette Syndrome Classification Study Group, 1993).

Transient tic disorder is a type of primary tic disorder characterized by duration of less than 1 year. It has been suggested that tics might be a common occurrence during normal childhood development (termed "physiological tics"), reflecting normal basal ganglia-frontal lobe synaptogenesis (Kurlan, 1994). This is analogous to the mild chorea and dystonia that are often observed as infants and children grow. There is little evidence to support the common notion that transient tics in childhood are due to underlying emotional stress or anxiety. When childhood tics have a duration of less than 1 year at the time of initial evaluation, it is appropriate to defer the diagnosis until the transient or chronic nature can be established over time.

Secondary Tic Disorders

A variety of other conditions can cause tics. To achieve more homogeneity and clarity of diagnosis, I prefer to avoid using primary tic disorder diagnoses (e.g., TS) in these settings, instead indicating that the tics are secondary to another condition. Secondary tic disorders are often evident by the presence of other neurological dysfunction in addition to tics. Since they are much less common than primary tic disorders, diagnostic assessments for secondary causes of tics in the form of blood testing or neuroimaging are generally not necessary when confronted with a child who has tics in the absence of any other significant neurological deficits.

Just like other neurological movement disorders, tics can occur following generalized or more focal (usually the basal ganglia-frontal lobe pathways) brain insults. Probably most common are the brain developmental disorders, such as mental retardation, autism, Rett syndrome, and Asperger's syndrome (Comings & Comings, 1991; FitzGerald et al., 1990; Ringman & Jankovic, 2000). Many other genetic and chromosomal developmental disorders involving the brain have also been reported to be associated with tics (Jankovic & Mejia, 2006). In these brain developmental disorders, tics are often accompanied by stereotypies. Tics have been observed in patients with developmental stuttering (Abwender et al., 1998).

A few cases have been reported in which tics have been observed as a sequela of other brain disorders. Head trauma has been described as a cause of tics (Krauss & Jankovic, 1997; Majumdar & Appleton, 2002; Siemers & Pascuzzi, 1990; Singer, Sanchez-Ramos & Weiner, 1989). Stroke is another reported cause,

Table 17.2 The Causes of Tics

Physiological Tics

Primary Tic Disorders

    TS

    Chronic motor tic disorder

    Chronic vocal tic disorder

    Transient tic disorder

Secondary Tic Disorders

    Brain developmental disorders: mental retardation, autism, Asperger's syndrome, Rett syndrome, genetic and chromosomal abnormalities, developmental stuttering

    Brain insults: head trauma, stroke, infections

    Postinfectious: postencephalitis, Sydenham's chorea, PANDAS (?)

    Neurodegenerative diseases: Huntington's disease, neurodegeneration with brain iron accumulation

    Systemic illnesses: neuroacanthocytosis, Behçet's disease

    Peripheral trauma

    Medications: tardive tics, stimulants, antiepileptics, levodopa, antidepressants

    Toxins: carbon monoxide, mercury, wasp venom

    Psychogenic

---

including when localized to the basal ganglia (Gomis et al., 2008; Kwak & Jankovic, 2002; Ward, 1988) and following hemorrhage of a left frontal arteriovenous malformation (Yochelson & David, 2000). A few postencephalitic cases of tics have been published. A 6-year-old girl was reported who developed motor and vocal tics about 4 weeks after the onset of presumed herpes encephalitis with evident right temporal encephalomalacia by MRI (Northam & Singer, 1991). A 4-year-old boy developed motor and vocal tics about 2 months following acute varicella zoster encephalitis associated with MRI hyperintensities of the striatum and midbrain (Dale, Church & Heyman, 2003). Motor and phonic tics have been reported to be associated with other infections, including HIV encephalitis, *Mycoplasma pneumoniae*, and Lyme disease (Jankovic & Kwak, 2005).

It has been recognized that tics often occur as part of the movement disorder of Sydenham's chorea, the presumed autoimmune manifestation of acute rheumatic fever, particularly appearing after the chorea dissipates (de Teixeira et al., 2009). Based on this observation, a nonrheumatic form of poststreptococcal autoimmune encephalopathy has been hypothesized: pediatric autoimmune neuropsychiatric disorder associated with streptococcal infections (PANDAS) (Swedo et al., 1998) (see Chapter 9 for a detailed overview on this topic). Tics were originally proposed to be one of the key manifestations of PANDAS, although more recently this association has been downplayed because of a variety of inconsistencies and negative research studies (Kurlan et al., 2008).

Tics may accompany other neurological signs in certain neurological illnesses. Huntington's disease (HD) is an autosomal dominant neurodegenerative disease caused by expanded CAG repeats in the gene for huntingtin on chromosome 4. It is characterized by progressive dementia and chorea. Tics have been observed as potential manifestations of the HD movement disorder (Jankovic & Ashizawa, 1995). Neurodegeneration with brain iron accumulation (NBIA; formerly Hallervorden-Spatz disease) has been linked to mutations of the PANK-2 gene, which codes for pantothenate kinase, which is involved in the biosynthesis of coenzyme A, and typically presents in the second or third decade with progressive dementia, rigidity, spasticity, and dystonia. A few cases with tics have been described in association with NBIA (Carod-Artal et al., 2004; Nardocci et al., 1994). Some patients have been reported to experience tics secondary to neuroacanthocytosis (Saiki et al., 2004; Spitz, Jankovic & Killian, 1985). This autosomal recessive illness has variable clinical manifestations but tends to cause peripheral neuropathy, chorea, parkinsonism, and self-mutilatory lip and tongue biting. Tics have been described in the setting of the systemic illness Behçet's disease, a chronic relapsing and remitting vasculitic disorder that is characterized by oral and genital ulcers, skin lesions, and uveitis (Budman & Sarcevic, 2002). Beta-mannosidase deficiency is a rare inborn error of metabolism that typically leads to mental retardation, behavioral disturbances, hearing loss, and recurrent airway infections. One case with associated tics has been reported (Sedel et al., 2006). Two patients who developed tics after peripheral trauma have been described (Factor & Molho, 1997). The first experienced facial trauma followed by facial and sniffing tics, and the second suffered a neck injury followed by neck/head-turning tics.

Like other hyperkinetic movement disorders, tics can be the long-lasting and primary manifestation of tardive dyskinesia (tardive tics), which occurs following exposure to dopamine receptor antagonist drugs such as antipsychotics and antiemetics (Bharucha & Sethi, 1995). Several medications have been reported to temporarily induce tics, including psychostimulants (amphetamines, methylphenidate, pemoline, cocaine, heroin), antiepileptics (carbamazepine, phenytoin, phenobarbital, lamotrigine), levodopa, and antidepressants (Jankovic & Kwak, 2005). Since stimulants can induce tics, it had been recommended that these drugs should be avoided in children with ADHD who have tics or even a family history of tics. Randomized, blinded, and placebo-controlled trials have shown, however, that at least the stimulant methylphenidate does not exacerbate tics in children with TS and is effective in treating coexisting ADHD (Gadow et al., 2007; Tourette's Syndrome Study Group, 2002). Exposure to certain environmental toxins, including carbon monoxide, mercury, and wasp venom, has been reported as a rare cause of tics (Jankovic & Kwak, 2005).

Tics can be a manifestation of a psychogenic movement disorder, a type of conversion disorder in which intense, often subconscious psychodynamic conflicts are transformed into neurological symptoms. These have been referred to as pseudo-tics or psychogenic tics (Kurlan, Deeley & Como, 1992). Like pseudo-seizures, which often occur in patients with epilepsy, probably the most common group to experience psychogenic tics is patients with true tic disorders like TS. Patients embellish their TS symptoms by having pseudo-tics in addition to their actual tics. In the first description of psychogenic tics, patients were observed to have highly dramatic manifestations, such as falling to the floor or yelling very loudly (Kurlan, Deeley & Como, 1992). Other potentially helpful clinical features in establishing a psychogenic etiology include being incongruent with the typical appearance

---

Box 17.1. Key Points

- Tics need to be distinguished from other neurological movement disorders (chorea, myoclonus, dystonia).
- Tics also need to be distinguished from movement disorders associated with psychiatric conditions (compulsions, sterotypies, mannerisms, habits).
- TS is part of a family of primary tic disorders that include chronic motor or vocal tic disorder and transient tic disorder.
- Tics can occur secondary to a number of conditions, including neurological disorders, medications, and as a psychogenic manifestation.

of classical tics, accentuation with suggestion and reduction with distraction, absence of premonitory sensations, presence of other conversion symptoms or signs, associated histrionic or indifferent personality features, and evident psychodynamic problems or secondary gain (Jankovic et al., 2006).

REFERENCES

Abwender DA, Trinidad KS, Jones KR et al. Features resembling Tourette's syndrome in developmental stutterers. *Brain Lang* 1998; 62:455–464.

American Psychiatric Association. 2000. *Diagnostic and Statistical Manual of Mental Disorders* (4th ed., Text Revision). Washington, DC: American Psychiatric Association.

Bharucha K, Sethi KD. Tardive tourettism after exposure to neuroleptic therapy. *Mov Disord* 1995; *10*:791–793.

Budman C, Sarcevic A. An unusual case of motor and vocal tics with obsessive-compulsive symptoms in a young adult with Behçet's disease. *CNS Spectr* 2002; 7:878–881.

Carod-Artal FJ, Vargas AP, Marinho PB et al. Tourettism, hemiballism and juvenile parkinsonism: expanding the clinical spectrum of the neurodegeneration associated to pantothenate kinase deficiency (Hallervorden-Spatz syndrome). *Rev Neurol* 2004; 38:327–331.

Comings DE, Comings BG. Clinical and genetic relationships between autism-pervasive developmental disorder and Tourette syndrome: A study of 19 cases. *Am J Med Genet* 1991; 39:180–191.

Dale RC, Church AJ, Heyman I. Striatal encephalitis after varicella zoster infection complicated by tourettism. *Mov Disord* 2003; *18*:1554–1556.

de Teixeira AL, Cardoso F, Maia DP et al. Frequency and significance of vocalizations in Sydenham's chorea. *Parkinsonism Relat Disord* 2009; *15*:62–63.

Factor SA, Molho ES. Adult-onset tics associated with peripheral injury. *Mov Disord* 1997; 12:1052–1055.

FitzGerald PM, Jankovic J, Glaze DG et al. Extrapyramidal involvement in Rett's syndrome. *Neurology* 1990; 40:293.

Gadow KD, Sverd J, Nolan EE et al. Immediate-release methylphenidate for ADHD in children with comorbid chronic multiple tic disorder. *J Am Acad Child Adolesc Psychiatry* 2007; 46:840–848.

Gomis M, Puente V, Pont-Sunyer C et al. Adult-onset simple phonic tic after caudate stroke. *Mov Disord* 2008; 23:765–766.

Jankovic J, Ashizawa T. Tourettism associated with Huntington's disease. *Mov Disord* 1995; 10:103–105.

Jankovic J, Cloninger CR, Fahn S et al. Therapeutic approaches to psychogenic movement disorders. In M Hallet, S Fahn, J Jankovic, AE Lang, CR Cloninger, SC Yudofsky (Eds.), *Psychogenic movement disorders: Neurology and neuropsychiatry*. Philadelphia: Lippincott Williams & Wilkins, 2006.

Jankovic J, Kwak C. Tics in other neurological disorders. In R Kurlan (Ed.), *Handbook of Tourette's syndrome and related tic and behavioral disorders*. New York: Marcel Dekker 2005.

Jankovic J, Mejia NJ. Tics associated with other disorders. *Adv Neurol* 2006; 99:61–68. **A useful discussion of the causes of secondary tics.**

Jankovic J, Stone L. Dystonic tics in patients with Tourette's syndrome. *Mov Disord* 1991; 6:248–252.

Krauss JK, Jankovic J. Tics secondary to craniocerebral trauma. *Mov Disord* 1997; 12:776–782.

Kurlan, R. Hypothesis II: Tourette's syndrome is part of a clinical spectrum that includes normal brain development. *Arch Neurol* 1994; *51*:1145–1150. **Hypothesizes that tics can be a manifestation of basal ganglia synaptogenesis that occurs as part of normal brain development ("physiological tics"; chorea and dystonia are known to occur during normal childhood development) or as a manifestation of any condition that adversely interferes with this process.**

Kurlan R, Deeley C, Como PG. Psychogenic movement disorder (pseudo-tics) in a patient with Tourette's syndrome. *J Neuropsychiatry Clin Neurosci* 1992; 4:347–348. **The first article specifically discussing the phenomenon of pseudo- (psychogenic) tics. It points out that these may occur in patients with a true tic disorder, analogous to the fact that patients with epilepsy may experience pseudo-seizures.**

Kurlan R, Johnson D, Kaplan EL, and the Tourette Syndrome Study Group. Streptococcal infection and exacerbations of childhood tics and obsessive-compulsive symptoms: a prospective blinded cohort study. *Pediatrics* 2008; *121*:1188–1197.

Kwak C, Dat Vuong K, Jankovic J. Premonitory sensory phenomenon in Tourette's syndrome. *Mov Disord* 2003; *18*:1530–1531.

Kwak CH, Jankovic J. Tourettism and dystonia after subcortical stroke. *Mov Disord* 2002; *17*:821–825.

Leckman JF, Walker DE, Cohen DJ. Premonitory urges in Tourette's syndrome. *Am J Psychiatry* 1993; *150*:98–102.

Summarizes the prior literature about premonitory sensations (earlier called "sensory tics") and provides new information about the phenomenology of sensations occurrring in the setting of tics.

Majumdar A, Appleton RE. Delayed and severe but transient Tourette syndrome after head injury. *Pediatr Neurol* 2002; *27*:314–317.

Nardocci N, Rumi V, Combi ML et al. Complex tics, stereotypies, and compulsive behavior as clinical presentation of a juvenile progressive dystonia suggestive of Hallervorden-Spatz disease. *Mov Disord* 1994; *9*:369–371.

Németh AH, Mills KR, Elston JS et al. Do the same genes predispose to Gilles de la Tourette syndrome and dystonia? Report of a new family and review of the literature. *Mov Disord* 1999; *14*:826–831.

Northam RS, Singer HS. Postencephalitic acquired Tourette-like syndrome in a child. *Neurology* 1991; *41*:592.

Palumbo D, Kurlan R. Complex obsessive-compulsive and impulsive symptoms in patients with Tourette's syndrome. *Neuropsychiatric Dis Treat* 2007; *3*:687–693.

The first article to discuss the interplay between TS and commonly comorbid OCD and ADHD in causing a variety of complex behaviors that share overlapping features.

Ringman JM, Jankovic J. Occurrence of tics in Asperger's syndrome and autistic disorder. *J Child Neurol* 2000; *15*:394–400.

Romstad A, Dupont E, Krag-Olsen B et al. Dopa-responsive dystonia and Tourette syndrome in a large Danish family. *Arch Neurol* 2003; *60*:618–622.

Saiki S, Hirose G, Sakai K et al. Chorea-acanthocytosis associated with tourettism. *Mov Disord* 2004; *19*:833–836.

Sedel F, Friderici K, Nummy K et al. Atypical Gilles de la Tourette syndrome with beta-mannosidase deficiency. *Arch Neurol* 2006; *63*:129–131.

Siemers E, Pascuzzi R. Posttraumatic tic disorder. *Mov Disord* 1990; *5*:183.

Singer C, Sanchez-Ramos J, Weiner WJ. A case of post-traumatic tic disorder. *Mov Disord* 1989; *4*:342–344.

Spitz MC, Jankovic J, Killian JM. Familial tic disorder, parkinsonism, motor neuron disease, and acanthocytosis: a new syndrome. *Neurology* 1985; *35*:366.

Stone LA, Jankovic J. The coexistence of tics and dystonia. *Arch Neurol* 1991; *48*:862–865.

Swedo SE, Leonard HL, Garvey M et al. Pediatric autoimmune neuropsychiatric disorders associated with streptococcal infections: Clinical description of the first 50 cases. *Am J Psychiatry* 1998; *155*:264–271.

The Tourette Syndrome Classification Study Group. Definitions and classification of tic disorders. *Arch Neurol* 1993; *50*:1013–1016.

Tourette's Syndrome Study Group. Treatment of ADHD in children with tics: a randomized controlled trial. *Neurology* 2002; *58*:527–536.

Ward CD. Transient feelings of compulsion caused by hemispheric lesions: three cases. *J Neurol Neurosurg Psychiatry* 1988; *51*:266–268.

Yochelson MR, David RG. New-onset tic disorder following acute hemorrhage of an arteriovenous malformation. *J Child Neurol* 2000; *15*:769–771.

18

Comprehensive Assessment Strategies

ROBERT A. KING AND ANGELI LANDEROS-WEISENBERGER

Abstract

The objective of this chapter is to present the goals that a clinician should have beyond confirming a diagnosis of Tourette syndrome when assessing for the first time a patient with a tic disorder. Clinicians should assess the impact of the disorder on the patient and family, examine all the factors that exacerbate or mitigate symptoms, assess the burden of comorbidities, ensure the degree of understanding of the condition by the patient and family, and set up a collaborative relationship aiming at the correct identification of treatment objectives and priorities. The role of psychoeducational intervention will also be presented in general terms.

It is much more important to know what sort of patient has a disease, than what sort of disease the patient has.
—Attributed to Caleb Hillier Parry (1775–1822) [quoted in Blumer, 1955]

IN APPROACHING the assessment of a potential new or established case of tic disorder (see Chapter 17), the clinician has several goals that extend beyond confirming or clarifying the presence and severity of tics and the diagnosis of tic disorder (Cath et al., 2011; King et al., 2009; Leckman, 2012; Leckman et al., 1998). These include assessing the impact of the disorder on the patient and family; identifying the factors that exacerbate or mitigate the symptoms; determining the extent of comorbid conditions; clarifying the patient's and family's understanding of the disorder; and developing an alliance and shared perspective on the patient's problems in order to pursue the treatment goals and priorities that emerge from the assessment (King et al., 2009). These specific assessment tasks require understanding the patient's functioning in the domains of self-image, family relationships, peers, and school, as well as the patient's and family's overall adaptive strengths

and vulnerabilities. The patient's developmental stage and the duration, severity, and complexity of the condition all also shape the assessment process.

ASSESSING TICS AND THEIR IMPACT

As with all evaluations, the first task is identifying the manifest and latent concerns that bring the patient to the clinician. In long-established cases this may be clear, but with new cases it is important to establish a shared vocabulary for talking about the symptoms. Parents of younger children may have their own idiom or sensibilities about how the child's symptoms are discussed, preferring in the child's presence to talk about "habits," "twitches," "cramps," "tight feelings," or "sounds" rather than "tics." In some cases, parents may also be appropriately concerned about the suggestibility of tics, if discussing certain tics appears to provoke their occurrence. Even when children or parents cite "tics" or "[my] Tourette's syndrome" as the presenting problem, it is important to ask for specifics, since many non-tic behaviors can be mistakenly subsumed under those labels.

Having the patient or family complete a self-report tic inventory beforehand and reviewing it with them during the assessment is a useful means of organizing an overview of the location, frequency, intensity, and complexity of tics over time and their associated distress and impairment (see Fig. 18.1, Table 18.1, and Chapter 19). Children under the age of 8 years may genuinely be unaware of many of their tic symptoms or defensively deny their parents' accounts as perceived accusations or criticisms. In such cases, it helps set the child at ease by indicating that such symptoms are common in youngsters and familiar to the clinician. In other cases, children may be aware of premonitory urges, suppressed tics, or obsessive-compulsive symptoms that have not been apparent to the parents. Although the clinician will want to note what tics are actually observed in the interview, the absence of tics in the office does not invalidate the patient's or family's report, as many patients spontaneously suppress their tics in an unfamiliar setting.

Along with identifying current tic symptoms, the clinician will want to know about prior tics and their course. Beyond a catalogue of tic symptoms, what has their impact (if any) been on the patient in terms of distress, functional impairment, embarrassment, or social stigma? For some individuals, the internal bombardment of premonitory urges or the energy and vigilance required to suppress tics in public can be more burdensome or distracting than the movements or sounds themselves (Leckman et al., 1993; see also Chapter 1). For many adult patients with persistent tics, "Tourette syndrome (TS)" may have become a part of their "identity." This may build in part from the internal sensations associated with the disorder, but also from their anticipation of the likely response (e.g., surprise, curiosity, or critical glances) by people they encounter in their daily lives who are unfamiliar with TS.

Occasionally, parents may be much more upset than their child about symptoms that the child seems genuinely unaware of or unconcerned with. Indeed, some tics may be much more upsetting to one parent than the other or to the child. The nature of these parental apprehensions

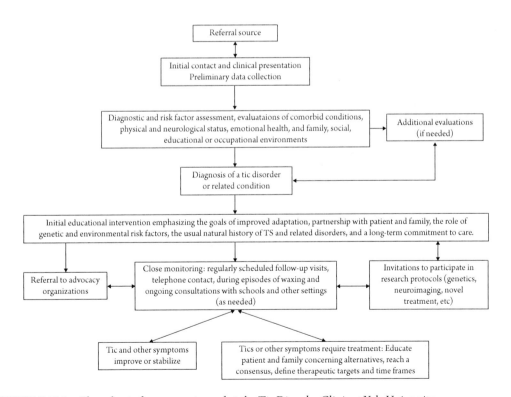

FIGURE 18.1   Flow chart of assessments used at the Tic Disorder Clinic at Yale University.

Table 18.1 Assessment Procedures and Rating Instruments Used in the Tourette Syndrome Clinic at Yale University

Topic	Measurement instrument in children	Measurement instrument in adults
Evaluation		
Demographics	Age, gender, ethnicity, grade in school, socioeconomic and marital status of parents	Age, gender, ethnicity, educational level, socioeconomic and marital status
Age at onset tics and/or of comorbid disorders	Age at onset, age at worst-ever symptoms	Age at onset, age at worst-ever symptoms
Tic disorder diagnosis, contextual issues influencing tic severity	Previous diagnosis yes/no, by whom, treatment	Previous diagnosis yes/no, by whom, treatment
Other diagnoses, especially ADHD, OCD, anxiety and mood disorders, autism spectrum disorder	Personal medical history / Previous medical records/ release of information from other practitioners	Personal medical history / Previous medical records/ release of information from other practitioners
Tic symptoms (past and present)	YGTSS	YGTSS
Sensory premonitory urges	PUTS	PUTS
Obsessive-compulsive symptoms (past/present)	CY-BOCS	Y-BOCS
ADHD	SNAP (self-report/parent/ teacher)	SNAP
Autism symptoms	ASSQ	
Family history	Family medical history, including disease in family members	Family medical history, including disease in family members
Monitoring Clinical Course		
Severity of tics	YGTSS (current and worst-ever items, age at worst ever)	YGTSS (current and worst-ever items, age at worst ever)
Severity of obsessive-compulsive symptoms	CY-BOCS severity (current and worst ever)	Y-BOCS severity (current and worst ever)
Severity of depression & anxiety	MFQ; SCARED; Hubbub Youth report	BDI/BAI
Level of psychosocial stress	PSS-P	PSS
Psychosocial functioning; quality of life	Ohio Scales for Youth; CGI; GTS-QOL	CGI; GTS-QOL

YGTSS, Yale Global Tic Severity Scale (Leckman et al., 1989); CY-BOCS, Children's Yale-Brown Obsessive Compulsive Scale (Scahill et al., 1997); Y-BOCS, Yale-Brown Obsessive Compulsive Scale (Goodman et al., 1989a, 1989b); SNAP, Swanson, Nolan and Pelham questionnaire (Bussing et al., 2008); PUTS, Premonitory Urge Tics Scale (Woods et al., 2005); CGI, Clinical Global Impression; MFQ, Mood and Feelings Questionnaire, youth form; PSS, Perceived Stress Scale (Cohen et al., 1983); PSS-P, Perceived Stress Scale-Parent rating (Cohen et al., 1983); SCARED, Screen for Child Anxiety and Related Emotional Disorders (Birmaher et al., 1997); BDI, Beck Depression Inventory II (Joe et al., 2008); BAI, Beck Anxiety Inventory (Steer et al., 1986). ASSQ, Autism Spectrum Screening Questionnaire (Ehlers et al., 1999); GTS-QOL, Gilles de la Tourette Syndrome Quality of Life Scale (Cavanna et al., 2008).

Questionnaires currently in use at the clinic are available upon request. See Chapter 19 for more detail on specific rating instruments.

is important to understand; hence, at some point in the assessment, parents of school-age children should be offered the opportunity to talk without the child present. Parents may be frightened of what the tics or a diagnosis of TS portends for the child's future and the possibility of future impairment or anticipated stigma or rejection. Inquiring about parental or other family history of tics, obsessive-compulsive disorder (OCD), trichotillomania, or anxiety is important, since a personal parental or family history of tic-related symptoms may color these parental concerns and heighten anxiety, empathy, or both. All of these issues help frame the psychoeducational aspects of the assessment when the discussion turns to the likely course of the disorder and potential impact for a particular child or adult (see Chapter 5).

What have the triggers, exacerbants, and alleviators of tics been, both over the months and during the course of the day? Stress, illness, exams, the beginning of the semester, or, later in life, interviews or presentations can all exacerbate tics; so can eagerly anticipated excitements, such as birthday parties, sports events, and vacations (King et al., 2009; see also Chapters 1, 9, and 14). Individuals with TS report experiencing higher levels of stress than their unaffected peers (Lin et al., 2007), and there is evidence that increased autonomic nervous system lability is a feature of TS, perhaps linked to anxiety-proneness (Chappell et al., 1994; see also Chapter 14). Individuals may spontaneously or with effort suppress tics in public—for example, at work or at school—and then habitually relax or let them emerge in a flurry at home or in private. Even without deliberate efforts at suppression, tics may be quiescent during coordinated or rhythmic motor activity (Sacks, 1995), particularly when it is associated with focused attention such as playing a musical instrument or athletic activities. Such observations are both theoretically intriguing in terms of the underlying pathophysiology of tics and, on a practical level, very important in terms of fostering areas of positive mastery and self-efficacy.

Impairment and distress due to tics can take several forms. The sense of having actions beyond one's full control can be deeply upsetting in its own right. The tics themselves, as well as premonitory urges and the need to resist them, can be very distracting even to children and adults with otherwise good concentration and attention. It is diagnostically important to differentiate between such individuals, whose attentional control is intact when their tics are quiescent, from other individuals with a long history of distractibility that often predates the onset of their tics. Beyond distraction and self-consciousness, do the tics interfere with or interrupt speaking, eating, writing, reciting in class, or sports activities? Does the tic cause pain or local irritation? Indeed, does the individual need to experience a certain level of pain for the tic to be "just right"?

Individuals with tics may be particularly "sticky" in acquiring bothersome or self-injurious habits such as repetitive nose, scab, or skin picking. A particularly vicious cycle can ensue when a tic, such as jaw stretching, cheek chewing, or self-hitting, causes pain or altered sensation that then becomes a nidus or trigger for further repetition of the tic, leading in turn to further pain/irritation. In those cases where severe tissue damage occurs—corneal abrasion, infection/bleeding, or orthopedic or dental damage—the need to break this cycle can become a challenging medical emergency.

Another area of assessment involves exploring what reactions the tics provoke from peers, family, or teachers and how the patient manages these responses (see Chapter 22). In newly diagnosed cases, parents may have scolded or exhorted the child to suppress tics they regarded as annoying or disruptive. In such cases, an important psychoeducational aim of the initial assessment is to "decriminalize" the tics by helping parents and teachers understand the largely involuntary (and only imperfectly suppressible) nature of most tics. Helping the child to become a "self-advocate" in explaining his or her tics to teachers or peers and coping with being teased or reproached is a central goal of treatment. Parents, school guidance personnel, or advocates from TS support organizations can be usefully enlisted in helping to educate teachers and peers about the patient's condition. A wealth of printed, video, and Web-based resources are available through the Tourette's Syndrome

Association (http://tsa-usa.org) and groups such as the New Jersey Center for Tourette's Syndrome (www.njcts.org) (see also Chapters 28 and 30). Some children, especially those with social anxiety or poor interpersonal skills, may be tormented by teasing and rejection in unsupportive school settings. On the other hand, other youngsters with good social skills often develop a protective and supportive nucleus of friends who provide a buffer against potential stigmatization, even in the face of prominent tics. The severity of youngsters' social difficulties with peers tends to be a function of the severity of attention-deficit/hyperactivity disorder (ADHD) comorbidity rather than tic severity *per se* (Bawden et al., 1998; see also Chapter 2).

One goal of the assessment is delineating the extent to which certain tics cannot be suppressed, and hence require greater tolerance and destigmatization; in contrast, other tics may be partially ameliorable by modifying antecedents likely to exacerbate them or by helping the affected individual develop "competing responses" as part of a comprehensive habit-reversal therapy approach (see Chapter 23). It may not initially be clear *a priori* which problematic tics are potentially modifiable. By exploring the antecedents and modifiers of particularly troublesome tic-related behaviors, such as aggressive or sexualized touching, hitting, or speech, the clinician can help the patient, family, and school staff to develop a stand that avoids unhelpful punitiveness, while finding ways to encourage the patient to exert whatever control is feasible.

BEYOND THE TICS: ASSESSING THE IMPACT OF COMORBID CONDITIONS

Although the history and assessment of the patient's tics are central to confirming the diagnosis of a tic disorder, tics and their immediate consequences may not be the patient's only or most impairing difficulty. Indeed, in clinical samples, only a minority of individuals have tics unaccompanied by the other comorbid conditions that commonly accompany TS: ADHD; obsessive-compulsive disorder (OCD);

vulnerability to anxiety, depression, or irritability; sleep problems; and learning difficulties, due to uneven cognitive profile, sensorimotor integration problems, or executive functioning impairments. The epidemiology, assessment, and treatment of each of these disorders are dealt with in separate chapters of this book (see in particular Chapters 2, 3, 4, and 25).

For many patients, impulsivity, irritability, distractibility, anxiety, or obsessions and compulsions may be more burdensome than their tics *per se*. Furthermore, the distress caused by these other difficulties often exacerbates the severity and impact of the tics. This can create a vicious cycle. In one clinical sample of youngsters with TS, over half reported one significant problem due to tics, and a third reported two or more problem areas. However, 70% of parents reported at least one area of non–tic-related impairment, most often impairment due to ADHD or OCD symptoms (Storch et al., 2007a; see also Chapters 2, 3, and 4, which review the most common co-occurring disorders). Individuals with tics alone may thus have a better functional prognosis than those with many comorbid symptoms, and the vicissitudes of these comorbid conditions often do not run the same time-limited course as tics (that is, commonly showing substantial spontaneous improvement by later adolescence) (see Chapter 5).

Although shared risk or pathophysiological factors presumably underlie the overlap of these conditions with tic disorders, they often do not respond therapeutically in parallel with tics but require distinctive behavioral, environmental, or pharmacological interventions of their own. Thus, clarifying the presence and clinical significance of various comorbidities and establishing treatment priorities between them is another central task of assessment.

Setting reasonable treatment goals is important as patients, families, and schools have finite resources of time and energy. In addition, polypharmacy in the form of pursuing multiple comorbidities with multiple simultaneous medications has its hazards, including cumulative metabolic interactions, sedation, and dysphoria. Medications intended to address one facet of the patient's difficulties may sometimes exacerbate problems in other areas; for example, selective serotonin reuptake inhibitors (SSRIs) targeting OCD symptoms can increase irritability, atypical neuroleptics targeting tics can increase weight and exacerbate self-consciousness, and high doses of stimulants occasionally exacerbate tics.

DEVELOPMENTAL, FAMILY, AND SCHOOL CONTEXTS

Individuals with tic disorders live in a developmental, family, social, and educational (or occupational) context, and the impact of their tic disorder cannot be understood in isolation from these broader contexts. Coexisting psychological difficulties, including family tensions and peer or school difficulties, are impairing not only in their own right, but can exacerbate tics and anxiety, leading to a vicious cycle. Because the diagnosis and management of tic disorders are unfamiliar to many families and their primary or mental health clinicians, it is important that the tic-specific features of the case, which may be perceived as exotic or esoteric, not distract from a balanced assessment and appreciation of the patient's and family's overall strengths and vulnerabilities.

Among children, the youngster's developmental stage provides one important context. Primary school children may be relatively unaware of their tics or any premonitory urges, as well as the reactions of their peers. By junior high school and early adolescence, youngsters may be most ill at ease and exquisitely sensitive to being perceived as "different." The embarrassment of tics is not the only threat to the youngster's acceptance and self-esteem; learning difficulties, impulsivity, and/or anxiety can heighten the young teen's sense of social marginalization. Unfortunately, this is often the age at which tics may be at their worst. Furthermore, the youngster's unhappiness and stress with peers can in turn increase tic severity. By mid-adolescence and high school, as attractiveness to the other sex, perceived stylishness, or athletic prowess becomes an important currency for popularity, tics or medication-associated weight gain may provoke teasing, bullying, ostracism, or shame. By the college years, even though tics have usually waned in severity and youngsters' intellectual, personal, and creative competencies become more socially salient, longstanding social anxiety, shame, or fear of rejection can still exact a toll.

Family life is the crucible in which the child's sense of self-worth and likeability is forged. Maintaining the child's sense of competency and self-esteem in the face of a chronic tic disorder and its comorbidities is a central therapeutic goal that must be reflected in the assessment process. It is often useful to begin an initial interview with inquiring about a youngster's hobbies and recreational interests. This conveys up front the clinician's interest in the youngster as a full person and not simply as a bearer of symptoms. It provides an opportunity to hear about positive aspirations and aspects of the self, as well as learning how they fit with the parents' interests and values. This approach also facilitates setting the child at ease and fostering an alliance, rather than immediately putting the youngster "on the spot" about symptoms that may be a source of self-consciousness or embarrassment. Additionally, it gives the clinician a chance to see what tics are apparent when attention is not specifically being focused on them, as it is when taking a tic inventory.

How the individual's tic disorder interacts with or exacerbates existing family tensions is an important dimension of assessment. A clinically significant chronic tic disorder places unusual burdens on family relationships. Especially when comorbid difficulties are present, families with a child affected by a chronic tic disorder have higher rates of parenting frustrations, marital difficulties, and family conflict, and poorer quality of parent–child interactions (Elstner et al., 2001). As with peer relationships (Bawden et al., 1998), interactions with parents and parents' perception of the quality of life may be more affected by the severity of the child's externalizing problems than by his or her tic severity *per se* (Cavanna et al., 2012; Elstner et al., 2001; Storch et al., 2007b).

School functioning is an essential arena for youngsters that serves as a test not only of intellectual ability and motivation, but also organizational and executive functioning, concentration, attitudes toward authority, ability to tolerate frustration or criticism, and social skills in relating to both teachers and classmates. Half of children with TS or chronic tic disorder report school-related difficulties such as concentrating on work, doing homework, writing in class, or taking exams. Assessing the child's academic and interpersonal "goodness of fit" with his or her school is a key area of inquiry, including classmates' and teachers' reactions to the child's tics. The clinician's assessment report is often an important vehicle for spelling out and mobilizing what accommodations or remedial resources are needed through the school to support the patient's learning and minimizing the educational and social impact of tics and any comorbid attentional, cognitive, organizational, anxiety, or behavior problems. The presence of a tic disorder may help qualify a child for special educational services with an "Other Health Impaired" disability. Serving as an advocate

for the child with the school and providing a broader context for understanding potential school problems is one of the clinician's most important functions.

For adults with TS, context is also critical. A comprehensive assessment should include the impact of the tics on the individual's interpersonal relationships, career trajectory, and life outside of the work environment.

PRIORITIZING PROBLEM AREAS TO BE ADDRESSED

The initial assessment should yield an overview of degree of impairment and distress caused by the patient's tics and comorbid difficulties. This in turn leads to a tentative prioritizing of symptoms and areas to be addressed in the treatment plan. Under ideal circumstances the clinician, the patient, and the accompanying family members can reach a consensus on what areas of symptoms (tic, ADHD, OCD, etc.) and problematic contexts

---

Box 18.1. Key Points

- In the assessment of a potential new or established case of tic disorder, the clinician has several goals that extend beyond confirming or clarifying the presence and severity of tics and the diagnosis of tic disorder. These include assessing the impact of the disorder on the patient and family; identifying the factors that exacerbate or mitigate the symptoms; determining the extent of comorbid conditions; clarifying the patient's and family's understanding of the disorder; and developing an alliance and shared perspective on the patient's problems in order to pursue the treatment goals and priorities that emerge from the assessment.

- To ensure the best outcomes, clinicians, teachers, parents, and peers should be educated regarding the key phenomenological features and natural course of TS and related disorders. This initial psychoeducational intervention should be part of what happens during the initial assessment.

- For children, although the family may focus on the upsetting and socially stigmatizing tics, the clinician needs to place the tics into the context of overall development so that the child's development is kept on track. This often involves refocusing the family's attention away from the tics and helping them find ways to build on the child's strengths and abilities.

- Social, emotional, and academic outcomes in adulthood do not always reflect tic outcomes given the chronic course, the negative impact on peer and family relationships, and the variable number of co-occurring conditions. Helping a child or an adult become a "self-advocate" rather than being ashamed of his or her tics is often a helpful approach (www.tsa-usa.org/aPeople/ForPeople_main.html). A comprehensive assessment of each of these domains will ensure that a consensus can be reached concerning treatment priorities.

should be addressed first. In the case of children, it is equally important that patients (and the individuals who are closest to them in the families) come away from an initial assessment with a perspective of what the presence of a tic disorder, if that is the diagnosis, means for the patient's development. Here, it is important to learn about how the patient thinks about the symptoms he or she is having. Some imaginative children may reveal their own personal, idiosyncratic theories about what is going on in their bodies or minds when tic urges or other tic-related phenomena present. For example, one boy imagined his efforts at symmetry and evening-up as a war between the "King of the Evens" (the good guys) and the "King of the Odds" (the bad guy, who got him to do things one more destabilizing time). He confided, however, that at times he was tempted to defect to the side of the Odds, because, after all, "one is an odd number, and if I could do something just once and quit, I wouldn't have a problem." Other children may have more intellectualized but less useful narratives concocted out of things they have heard about basal ganglia, dopamine, and so forth. Rather than the most sophisticated scientific understanding, the clinician's goal is for youngsters to come away from the assessment with a sense of themselves as cherished, competent individuals with strengths, talents, and virtues, no matter how besieged they may be by their tics and other difficulties. Thus, while explicating

what can be known of the patient's condition and what interventions may be helpful, the task is not to lose sight of the other aspects of the individual's development. To return to old Dr. Parry of Bath, the assessment should convey not just what diagnostic label applies to the patient, but who the patient (and family) are who bear the label, and with what resources, values, aspirations, and resiliencies.

REFERENCES

Bawden HN, Stokes A, Camfield CS et al. Peer relationship problems in children with Tourette's disorder or diabetes mellitus. *J Child Psychol Psychiatry* 1998; 39:663–668.

Birmaher B, Khetarpal S, Brent D et al. The Screen for Child Anxiety Related Emotional Disorders (SCARED): scale construction and psychometric characteristics. *J Am Acad Child Adolesc Psychiatry* 1997; 36:545–553.

Blumer G. Reminiscences of an old-time physician. *Yale J Med Biol* 1955; 28:15.

Bussing R, Fernandez M, Harwood M et al. Parent and teacher SNAP-IV ratings of attention deficit hyperactivity disorder symptoms: psychometric properties and normative ratings from a school district sample. *Assessment* 2008; 15:317–328.

Cath DC, Hedderly T, Ludolph AG et al. European clinical guidelines for Tourette syndrome and other tic disorders. Part I: assessment. *Eur Child Adolesc Psychiatry* 2011; 20:55–71.

The European clinical guidelines for TS and other tic disorders were recently compiled and published by the European Society for the Study of Tourette Syndrome and provide a useful step-by-step guide to assessment.

Cavanna AE, David K, Orth M, Robertson MM. Predictors during childhood of future health-related quality of life in adults with Gilles de la Tourette syndrome. *Eur J Paediatr Neurol* 2012 Feb 28. [Epub ahead of print]

Cavanna AE, Schrag A, Morley D et al. The Gilles de la Tourette – Quality of Life Scale (GTS-QOL). *Neurology* 2008; 71:1410–1416.

Chappell P, Riddle M, Anderson GA, et al. Enhanced stress responsivity of Tourette syndrome patients undergoing lumbar puncture. *Biological Psych* 1994; 36:35–43.

Cohen S, Kamarck T, Mermelstein R. A global measure of perceived stress. *J Health Soc Behav* 1983; 24:385–396.

Ehlers S, Gillberg C, Wing L. A screening questionnaire for Asperger syndrome and other high-functioning autism spectrum disorders in school age children. *J Autism Dev Disord* 1999; 29:129–141.

Elstner K, Selai CC, Trimble MR, Robertson MM. Quality of life (QOL) of patients with Gilles de la Tourette's syndrome. *Acta Psych Scand* 2001; 103:52.

Goodman WK, Price LH, Rasmussen SA et al. The Yale-Brown Obsessive Compulsive Scale. II. Validity. *Arch Gen Psychiatry* 1989b; 46:1012–1016.

Goodman WK, Price LH, Rasmussen SA et al. The Yale-Brown Obsessive Compulsive Scale. I. Development, use, and reliability. *Arch Gen Psychiatry* 1989b; 46:1006–1111.

Joe S, Woolley ME, Brown GK et al. Psychometric properties of the Beck Depression Inventory-II in low-income, African American suicide attempters. *J Pers Assess* 2008; 90:521–523.

King R, Schwab-Stone M, Peterson B et al. In VA Sadock, BJ Sadock, P Ruiz (eds.), *Kaplan and Sadock's comprehensive textbook of psychiatry*, Vol. 2. Wolters Kluwer/Lippincott Williams & Wilkins, 2009, pp. 3366–3399.

Leckman JF. Tic disorders. *BMJ* 2012; 344:d7659.

Leckman JF, King RA, Scahill L et al. Yale approach to assessment and treatment. In: JF Leckman, DJ Cohen (eds.), *Tourette's syndrome, tics, obsessions, compulsions—developmental psychopathology and clinical care*. New York: John Wiley and Sons, 1998, pp. 285–309.

Leckman JF, Riddle MA, Hardin MT et al. The Yale Global Tic Severity Scale: initial testing of a clinician-rated scale of tic severity. *J Am Acad Child Adolesc Psychiatry* 1989; 28:566–573.

Leckman JF, Walker DE, Cohen DJ. Premonitory urges in Tourette's syndrome. *Am J Psychiatry* 1993; 150:98–102.

Lin H, Katsovich L, Ghebremichael M et al. Psychosocial stress predicts future symptom severities in children and adolescents with Tourette syndrome and/or obsessive-compulsive disorder. *J Child Psychol Psychiatry* 2007; 48:157–166.

Sacks OW. *An anthropologist on Mars: seven paradoxical tales*. New York: Alfred A. Knopf, 1995.

Scahill L, Riddle MA, McSwiggin-Hardin M et al. Children's Yale-Brown Obsessive Compulsive Scale: reliability and validity. *J Am Acad Child Adolesc Psychiatry* 1997; 36:844–852.

Steer RA, Beck AT, Riskind GH, Brown G. Differentiation of depressive disorders from generalized anxiety by the Beck Depression Inventory. *J Clin Psychol*; 1986; 42:475–478.

Storch EA, Lack CW, Simons LE et al. A measure of functional impairment in youth with Tourette's syndrome. *J Pediatr Psychol* 2007a; 32:950–959.

Storch EA, Merlo LJ, Lack C et al. Quality of life in youth with Tourette's syndrome and chronic tic disorder. *J Clin Child Adolesc Psychol* 2007b; 36:217–227.

Woods DW, Piacentini J, Himle MB, Chang S. Premonitory Urge for Tics Scale (PUTS): initial psychometric results and examination of the premonitory urge phenomenon in youths with tic disorders. *J Dev Behav Pediatr* 2005; 26:397–403.

19

Clinical Rating Instruments in Tourette Syndrome

ANDREA E. CAVANNA AND JOHN C. PANSAON PIEDAD

Abstract

The complex motor and behavioral phenotype of Tourette syndrome presents a unique challenge to measurement and clinical observations. This chapter offers a systematic overview of the different clinician-, informant-, and self-report rating instruments for tics and associated phenomena that are available for use in clinical practice and/ or research settings. Each of the scales available to measure tics has strengths and limitations; among the latter, the difficulty of capturing all the different dimensions of tic symptoms, such as frequency, intensity, interference, and impairment, is one of the most common and is an object of future research. Moreover, the visible and audible nature of core Tourette syndrome symptoms allows direct observation of these symptoms using specific video protocols. A wide range of psychometrically validated clinician- and self-rated measures for obsessive-compulsive behavior, attention-deficit/hyperactivity disorder, and depressive and anxiety symptoms are also available for use in clinical practice and/or research settings. The use of behavioral measures with adequate psychometric indices is recommended. Clinicians and researchers ideally should combine information from professionals and patients (as well as informants if possible) to ensure that the information gathered is comprehensive and accurate.

INTRODUCTION

The clinical spectrum of Tourette syndrome (TS), described in detail in the first chapter of this book, encompasses motor and phonic tics, complex repetitive behaviors, such as copro-, echo-, and pali-phenomena, and comorbid behavioral disorders (Cavanna et al., 2009; Robertson, 2000). Both obsessive-compulsive behaviors (OCBs) and the combination of inattention, hyperactivity, and impulsivity (attention-deficit/ hyperactivity disorder [ADHD]) have been consistently reported across TS populations, as reviewed in Chapters 2 and 3. Similarly, the prevalence of affective and anxiety disorders, personality disorders, and impulse control disorders is higher compared to the general population (see Chapter 4). With such a broad range of clinical presentations, significant challenges arise for standardized assessments of the TS phenotype. A thorough neuropsychiatric examination with clinical history elicited from both patients and other informants is the current cornerstone of TS diagnostic protocols, although variability in practice and expertise can result in lack of rigorous standardization.

Rating scales perform the important task of assigning quantitative properties to clinically relevant phenomena in TS. This is particularly relevant to clinical research studies on behavioral, pharmacological, and surgical interventions, summarized in Chapters 23 to 26, which have the potential to inform optimal patient care. Use of standardized clinical rating scales in routine clinical practice also allows the monitoring of the natural course of tics and behavioral symptoms. For data to be accurate and of clinical utility, clinical rating scales need to have adequate psychometric properties, including validity and reliability. Validity represents how scales precisely capture the theoretical construct of what they aim to measure. Good reliability is an indication that the scale produces the same information when individuals are tested by the same raters at different times (test–retest), and when the same individual is assessed by different raters (interrater reliability). How scales capture information also differs, and this can affect their psychometric properties. Information can be provided by patients or by informants such as parents and teachers, through questionnaire constructs. Clinicians or appropriately trained observers may also obtain information from patients through their own versions of questionnaires and/or semistructured interview schedules. A more direct method of quantification is represented by video-based protocols where tics are observed and rated. Systematic reviews of the available instruments for the standardized measurement of the broad range of motor and nonmotor phenomena in TS are lacking. This chapter aims at filling this gap, focusing mainly on tic severity and behavioral scales that have proved useful in TS populations, as well as generic and disease-specific quality-of-life instruments (Table 19.1).

SELF- AND INFORMANT-RATED MEASURES

Tourette Syndrome Symptom List (TSSL)

The 41-item self- and parent-rated TSSL allows the daily subjective and informant assessment of tic and other behaviors throughout a week (Cohen et al., 1984). The TSSL is a revision of the original 29-item version (Cohen et al., 1980). The 35 questions about simple and complex motor and phonic tics are structured according to anatomical location and different noises, respectively. The severity of different tics and behaviors is rated on a scale of 0 to 5 for each day, with specific time periods indicated in the anchor points. These can be summed to give a weekly score. The number of symptoms for each subdomain is also counted over the week. A limitation of the TSSL is that only frequency dimensions of tics are captured; this does not include other relevant characteristics such as their intensity and the level of impairment they cause.

Nevertheless, it can be a useful adjunct measure capturing patient-rated tic symptoms in a diary fashion (e.g., Maciunas et al., 2007; Pringsheim & Marras, 2009; Sallee et al., 1997).

Tourette's Syndrome Questionnaire (TSQ)

The TSQ was initially developed for an epidemiological survey to record potential factors that mediate the prognosis of TS and its optimal treatment (Jagger et al., 1982). It is rated by the patient's parents or with their assistance. Thus, the TSQ is a useful tool for systematically eliciting relevant information such as sociodemographics, course of tic behaviors, and treatment, as well as prenatal, birth, developmental, and family histories. The TSQ could be appropriate in gathering data for patient registries in both clinical and research practice, such as in the screening stages, phenomenological studies, or treatment trials (Silva et al., 1995, 1996).

Ohio Tourette Survey Questionnaire

The 1987 Ohio Tourette Survey Questionnaire was developed as a postal questionnaire sent to patients and their families registered with the Ohio Tourette Syndrome Association (Bornstein et al., 1990). Patients were asked about TS symptoms, treatment history, and behavioral comorbidities. This instrument captures basic clinical data and can be useful as a template for patient datasets.

Motor Tic, Obsessions and Compulsions, Vocal Tic Evaluation Survey (MOVES)

The MOVES is a self-report assessment of motor and phonic tics, associated phenomena, obsessions, and compulsions (Gaffney et al., 1994). These scores can be combined to produce tic or obsessive-compulsive subscores. Individuals are asked to rate the presence of their symptoms from a list of 20 items in the previous 4 weeks, on a 4-point scale from "never" to "always." The MOVES is a relatively straightforward scale. Its acceptable validity was demonstrated with strong correlations to two clinician-rated tic scales and two OCB measures, with some sensitivity to

Table 19.1 Psychometric Instruments Relevant to Clinical Practice and Research in TS

Scales for different symptoms[a]	Respondent[b]	Administration time (minutes)[c]
Tics and associated symptoms		
Tourette Syndrome Symptom List (TSSL)	Patient, informant	–
Tourette's Syndrome Questionnaire (TSQ)	Child/adolescent, adults	–
Ohio Tourette Survey Questionnaire	Patient	–
Motor Tic, Obsessions and Compulsions, Vocal Tic Evaluation Survey (MOVES)	Child/adolescent, adult	1–5
Premonitory Urge for Tics Scale (PUTS)	Child (>10 years)/adolescent, adults	5
Parent Tic Questionnaire (PTQ)	Informant	–
Shapiro Tourette Syndrome Severity Scale (STSSS)	Clinician	5–10
Tourette Syndrome Global Scale (TSGS)	Clinician (child/adolescent, adult)	–
Global Tic Rating Scale (GTRS)	Informant, clinician	–
Tourette Syndrome-Clinical Global Impression (TS-CGI)	Clinician	–
Yale Global Tic Severity Scale (YGTSS)	Clinician (child/adolescent, adult)	15–20
Hopkins Motor and Vocal Tic Scale (HMVTS)	Clinician (child/adolescent, adult)	–
Tourette's Disorder Scale (TODS)	Informant (parent), clinician (child/adolescent)	5
University of São Paulo Sensory Phenomena Scale	Clinician (child/adolescent, adult)	–
Video-based ratings (various)	Clinician	Various
Automatic tic detection	Clinician	Various
Unified Tic Rating Scale (UTRS)	Clinician	–
Overall behavior		
Child Behavior Checklist (CBCL) and Youth Self-Report (YSR)	Informant (parent or teacher), child/adolescent	15–20
Obsessive-compulsive symptoms		
Leyton Obsessional Inventory (LOI)	Child/adolescent, adult	30–45
Obsessive Compulsive Inventory (OCI)	Child/adolescent, adult	5–10
Yale-Brown Obsessive Compulsive Scales (YBOCS, YBOCS-II, D-YBOCS; C-YBOCS)	Child/adolescent, adult, informant, clinician (child/adolescent, adult)	20–40 (clinician-administered YBOCS), 3–5 (patient/informant)

(Continued)

Table 19.1 (*Continued*)

Scales for different symptoms[a]	Respondent[b]	Administration time (minutes)[c]
Attention-deficit/hyperactivity symptoms		
Swanson, Nolan and Pelham Scale (SNAP-IV)	Informant (child/adolescent, adult)	5–10
ADHD Rating Scale IV (ADHD-RS-IV)	Informant (child/adolescent, adult)	8
ADHD Self-Report Scale (ASRS)	Adult	3
Conners' ADHD Rating Scales (CRS)	Child/adolescent, informant (parent or teacher), adult, clinician	10–20
Affective symptoms		
Beck Depression Inventory (BDI)	Adolescent, adult	5–10
Children's Depression Inventory (CDI)	Child/adolescent	10–15
Hamilton Depression Rating Scale (HDRS)	Adolescent, adult	10–20
Children's Depression Rating Scale (CDRS)	Child/adolescent	30–45 (when including adult informant interview)
Anxiety symptoms		
State-Trait Anxiety Inventory (STAI)	Children/adolescent, adult	10–20
Hamilton Anxiety Rating Scale (HARS)	Adolescent, adult	10–15
Hospital Anxiety and Depression Scale (HADS)	Patient	5
Revised Children's Anxiety and Depression Scale (RCADS)	Child/adolescent, parent	15–25
Quality of life		
Medical Outcomes Study 36-Item Short Form Health Survey (SF-36)	Patient	10–15
Gilles de la Tourette Syndrome-Quality of Life Scale (GTS-QOL)	Patient	10–15

[a]Scales in normal type have undergone comprehensive psychometric testing; scales in italic type have not (see references in text).
[b]For self- and clinician-report scales, the age target was derived from references of development study or systematic reviews of respective scales, where available (see references in text).
[c]Where available from references of development study or systematic reviews of respective scales.

clinically relevant changes (Gaffney et al., 1994). There are some issues with regard to its reliability, however, with some subscales showing below standard correlation coefficients (<.70): tic (.54), associated symptoms (.40), and total scores (.69) (Gaffney et al., 1994). Nevertheless, the MOVES is a useful adjunct to clinician ratings as a measure of patient perception of tic symptoms, for example during interventional or phenomenological studies (Haddad et al., 2009; Münchau et al., 2002; Orth et al., 2005).

Premonitory Urge for Tics Scale (PUTS)

The PUTS is a relatively brief scale designed to examine the phenomenon of premonitory sensations (also called premonitory urges or sensory tics) in tic disorders (Woods et al., 2005). It contains 10 descriptions of somatic sensations derived from phenomenological descriptions from the literature and clinical experience. The severity of urges is rated on a 4-point ordinal scale ranging from 1 (not at all true) to 4 (very much true). Although psychometric properties appear acceptable in older pediatric patients, initial testing revealed inadequate properties for patients younger than 10 years (Woods et al., 2005). A direct translation in Hebrew has recently become available in a study that provided independent testing of the PUTS, showing adequate properties in patients older than 10 years (Steinberg et al., 2010). Despite testing in pediatric populations only, adequate psychometric properties for older children may indicate utility in adults also. More recently, a study using the PUTS and a similar scale (USP-SPS, see below) demonstrated concurrent and discriminant validity (Sutherland Owens et al., 2011).

Child Tourette's Syndrome Impairment Scale (CTIM-P)

The CTIM-P is a 37-item parent-rated questionnaire that measures children's functional capabilities in school, home, and social activities over the previous month (Storch, Lack, Simons et al., 2007). Parents are asked to attribute how activities are affected by the child's tics or other behaviors (e.g., obsessionality, mood disturbances, hyperactivity) based on a 4-point scale, which produces tic-related and non–tic-related impairment scores. Initial psychometric testing of the CTIM-P demonstrated excellent properties.

Parent Tic Questionnaire (PTQ)

The PTQ is a recently developed measure of tics in children and adolescents (Chang et al., 2009). Parents are asked to assess the number of tics from a list of 14 common motor and phonic tics each over the previous week. Frequency and intensity are rated on a 4-point scale, and these are added for each tic to produce scores ranging from 0 (tic not present) to 8 (constant and intense tics). Psychometric testing against other tic and behavioral measures confirmed excellent validity.

CLINICIAN-RATED MEASURES

Shapiro Tourette Syndrome Severity Scale (STSSS)

The STSSS was developed to measure changes in tic symptoms during a clinical trial of pimozide (Shapiro & Shapiro, 1984; Shapiro et al., 1988). This clinician-rated scale addresses five factors: whether tics are noticeable, whether they elicit comments or curiosity, whether the patient is considered odd or bizarre, whether tics interfere with functioning, and whether they lead to incapacitation or to the patient being homebound or hospitalized. The item scores can be summed to produce total ratings, which are assigned a global severity rating on a 6-point scale from 0 (no tics) to 6 (very severe, total sum of ratings >8). The relative simplicity and brevity of the STSSS make it a convenient measure of tic symptoms, taking around 5 to 10 minutes to complete. However, the focus is clearly on social impairment, which somewhat limits the overall accurateness of this clinical assessment of tics. When compared with two measures of tic severity, the STSSS showed excellent reliability and validity (Walkup et al., 1992) and has been successfully applied in TS interventional studies (e.g., Müller-Vahl et al., 2002; Pringsheim & Marras, 2009; Pringsheim & Steeves, 2011).

Tourette Syndrome Global Scale (TSGS)

The TSGS is a clinician-rated measure of tics and social functioning in TS (Harcherik et al., 1984). The tic subscore measures simple and complex motor and phonic tics based on their frequency and resulting impairment. Frequency scores are rated on a scale of 0 to 5, with higher scores corresponding to higher tic frequencies. Impairment is measured on a scale of 1 to 5 based on how noticeable tics are and the resulting functional impairment. The social functioning subscore measures the level of functional impairment in behavioral conduct, motor restlessness, and school and learning or work and occupation problems (whichever is relevant). These are rated on a scale of 0 to 25 in increments of 5, with 0 indicating lack of issues in respective domains and 25 indicating severe functional impairment. The global measure of severity is calculated using both the tic and social functioning subscores. The advantage of the TSGS is its comprehensiveness in measuring different tic characteristics, as well as its multidimensionality by combining assessments of tics and their effects on social functionality. However, the formula for deriving global scores is relatively complicated and potentially produces social functioning subscores that are disproportionately weighted to tic symptoms (Kompoliti & Goetz, 1997). The TSGS has proven a useful instrument in interventional studies (e.g., Müller-Vahl et al., 2002; Pringsheim & Marras et al., 2009; Sallee et al., 1997). However, in a pharmacological trial of ondansetron, the TSGS detected a significant symptomatic change whereas a gold standard for measuring tic symptoms did not find differences compared to placebo ($p = .002$ vs. $.15$, respectively; Toren et al., 2005), suggesting potential concurrent validity issues.

Global Tic Rating Scale (GTRS)

The GTRS is a brief clinician measure of tic frequency (Gadow & Paolicelli, 1986). This checklist contains nine items, with the first five referring to the frequency of motor (three items) and phonic tics (two items) according to body region, which are summed to produce motor and phonic tic frequency subscores, respectively. The last four items refer to a tic severity dimension and are summed to produce a severity subscore. All items are rated on a scale from 0 (never) to 3 (very much). When compared with the Yale Global Tic Severity Scale (YGTSS; see below) and 2-minute tic count of the Unified Tic Rating Scale (UTRS; see below), the GTRS showed relatively small correlation coefficients (.01–.42), suggesting poor concurrent validity. Reliability appeared acceptable for motor and severity subscales with correlation coefficients of above .77, but less so with the vocal tic subscale (.58) (Nolan et al., 1994). It should be noted that, in this study, the GTRS was rated by teachers, who may not have the experience of skilled clinicians in adequately recognizing tics. The GTRS has been used in interventional trials for TS (Pringsheim & Steeves, 2011).

Tourette Syndrome-Clinical Global Impression (TS-CGI)

The CGI is a frequently used measure of disease severity. In preparation for a clinical trial in TS, three disease-specific versions of the CGI were developed (Leckman et al., 1988). These assess symptoms of TS, obsessive-compulsive disorder (OCD), and ADHD, based on DSM-III diagnostic criteria. The TS-CGI consists of seven items corresponding with descriptions of no identifiable symptoms (normal) to incapacitating tics or a high level of functional impairment associated with behavioral symptoms (extremely severe). The TS-CGI showed excellent reliability and validity indices when compared to the STSSS and YGTSS (Walkup et al., 1992) and has been used as an adjunctive clinician measure in interventional studies (e.g., Kwon et al., 2011; Pringsheim & Marras, 2009; Pringsheim & Steeves, 2011; Sallee et al., 1997).

Yale Global Tic Severity Scale (YGTSS)

The YGTSS is the most widely used measure of tic severity in TS (e.g., Porta et al., 2009; Pringsheim et al., 2009; Pringsheim & Marras, 2009; Pringsheim & Steeves, 2011) and other tic disorders (Leckman et al., 1989). It is based on a semistructured interview of symptoms over the past week, where the clinician is asked to record patients' motor and phonic tics. Subsequently, the tic symptoms are rated separately based on their number, frequency, intensity, complexity, and interference from 0 (no tic symptoms) to 5 (severe). The tic severity subscore consists of the motor and phonic tic severity scores. This is summed with the impairment subscore, which rates the severity of functional impairment from 0 to 50, to produce the total score (0–100). The YGTSS allows a multidimensional overview of tic characteristics, as well as the level of functional interference. The separation of motor and phonic tics is particularly useful, also for diagnostic purposes. Independent testing confirmed reliability and validity indices using the STSSS and TS-CGI (Walkup et al., 1992). A childhood and adolescent sample confirmed this scale's excellent psychometric properties, particularly its internal consistency and validity (Storch, Murphy, Geffken et al., 2005b). A factor analytic study also confirmed and validated the structure that was initially identified (Storch, Murphy, Fernandez et al., 2007). Cutoff scores for clinically relevant treatment response have been proposed: a reduction by 35% in total YGTSS scores or 6 or 7 points in the tic severity subscale (Storch, De Nadai, Lewin et al., 2011). A Spanish version (García-López et al., 2008) and a Polish adaptation (Stefanoff & Wolańczyk, 2005) of the YGTSS have been published. The YGTSS is an ideal instrument for busy routine clinical practice, as it takes only 15 minutes to complete.

The Hopkins Motor and Vocal Tic Scale (HMVTS)

The HMVTS is a parent- and clinician-rated scale that measures motor and phonic tics using a visual analog scale (VAS) (Walkup et al., 1992). Each tic is given a rating from 0 (not present) to 10 (most severe), with four intermediate ratings: "mild," "moderate," "moderately severe," and "severe." The severity of tics is rated across their frequency, intensity, and the level of interference and impairment they cause. An overall score is also assigned to each motor or phonic tic, ranging from 1 (no tic symptoms) to 5 (worst ever). The HMVTS is quite straightforward, and a particular strength is how comprehensively it assesses the various characteristics of tics. Initial psychometric testing demonstrated excellent reliability and validity indices when compared to the YGTSS, STSSS, and behavioral measures (Walkup et al., 1992). The HMVTS has been used in intervention studies to assess tic symptoms (Pringsheim & Steeves, 2011; Singer et al., 1995).

Tourette's Disorder Scale (TODS)

The TODS is an objective measure of the severity of tics plus a wide range of TS-related neuropsychiatric symptoms over a period of 1 month (Shytle et al., 2003). The 15-item scale contains questions about tics, inattention, hyperactivity, obsessions, compulsions, aggressions, and emotional symptoms. These were derived from a questionnaire in which parents were required to rate the occurrence and impact of 32 behavioral and emotional symptoms. Clinician- and parent-rated versions are available, both of which have been validated by further psychometric testing (Storch, Merlo, Lehmkuhl et al., 2007; Storch, Murphy, Geffken et al., 2004b).

University of São Paulo Sensory Phenomena Scale (USP-SPS)

Another scale specifically designed to capture sensory phenomena is the USP-SPS, which contains a checklist of past and current symptoms, including physical sensations, sensory-triggered experiences (e.g., tactical, auditory, visual), and inner "just right" perceptions (Rosario et al., 2009). Severity is rated on a 6-point scale indicating the frequency, distress, and interference of sensory phenomena, with a score of 15 representing the maximum severity of symptoms. Initial testing indicated adequate reliability and validity, and later studies demonstrated convergent validity with the PUTS (Sutherland Owens et al., 2011). Despite initial testing in adult patients only, utility in pediatric populations is suggested by an independent study showing concurrent and discriminant validity (Sutherland Owens et al., 2011).

Measures Based on Direct Observations of Tics

The visible and audible nature of tics permits quantification through video recording. Two standardized methods of video-based tic severity rating are widely used. In a clinical trial of pimozide for TS, Shapiro and Shapiro (1984) developed a video-based protocol for tic quantification (Shapiro et al., 1988). According to this protocol, motor and phonic tics are counted and rated in severity over three 2.5-minute test conditions: computation (adding a series of two numbers as quickly and accurately as possible), reading (three paragraphs of written text), and no stimulus (sitting in the office without the examiner).

During clinical trials of procholinergic agents (Tanner et al., 1982) and clonidine (Goetz et al., 1987a) for TS, Goetz and others (1987b) developed the Rush Video-Based Tic Rating Scale (RVBTRS), a more standardized tic rating protocol using video recording. Patients were filmed for 10 minutes, during which they were allowed to read, write, or draw as long as this did not obscure the camera's view. The recordings used a full frontal view of the patient and a head-and-shoulders view only. The conditions were with the examiner in the room and with the patient alone. Only the 5-minute recordings of the patients on their own are rated, based on the anatomical distribution of tics, with frequency derived from raw counts of discrete motor tics and vocalizations. The intensity of motor and phonic tics is rated on a 6-point scale of severity from 0 (absent tics) to 5 (extreme: complex behaviors or obscenities repeated more than four times). The RVBTRS was found to have adequate psychometric indices of stability, validity (in comparison to the YGTSS and TS-CGI), and reliability (Chappell et al., 1994). The same group modified the rating protocol for this scale in a talipexole clinical trial for TS (mRVBTRS) (Goetz et al., 1994, 1999). Keeping the original tic distribution, frequency, and intensity dimensions, the rating scales were reduced to a 0-to-4 arrangement by combining points 4 and 5. Cutoff points were also introduced to the tic distribution and frequency dimensions. Initial psychometric testing compared the five mRVB-TRS sections to the respective portions of the YGTSS. Moderate to large correlations were identified, with correlation coefficients of .49 to .90 (Goetz et al., 1999). Although other psychometric properties have not been adequately tested, interventional trials have successfully used the Rush protocol alongside clinician ratings (Feigin et al., 1996; Orth et al., 2005; Pringsheim & Steeves, 2011).

Himle and colleagues (2006) developed a different protocol within a pediatric sample in which the child was videotaped for 30 minutes while watching a television or computer monitor.

The authors suggested two recording methods. In the first method (event frequency), the total number of tics were counted and divided by the amount of time the patient was visible, to give an index of tics per minute. In the second method (partial-interval), the 30-minute recordings were divided into 10-second segments to be rated for the presence of tics. Both methods showed strong correlations and proved acceptable methods of tic quantification. However, small to moderate correlations were observed when the two scoring methods were applied for motor tics, whereas moderate to large correlations were observed with vocal tics when compared with respective YGTSS subscales. This may suggest validity issues (medium to large correlations are ideal for convergent validity), but it may be expected that differences arise because two different methods of measuring the same phenomenon are being compared (i.e., direct vs. indirect).

To maintain methodological rigor in research settings (particularly interventional studies), video recordings require randomization, blinded raters, and multiple testing (Goetz et al., 1987a, 1994; Leckman et al., 1991). For example, a modification to the Rush video protocols was introduced in a clinical trial for deep brain stimulation (DBS) (Maciunas et al., 2007). The 5-minute recordings were divided into ten 30-second segments, which were then presented to two blinded neurologists in a random order for rating. Other issues with video-based measurements are the duration and amount of video data to be collected. Due to the frequency of the fluctuations in tic expression, it is valid to question whether the captured data are an accurate clinical representation. In relation to this point, previous studies suggest that tic counts should be made based on a minimum of 5 minutes of recording (Chappell et al., 1994). However, a tic count modeling analysis on five of the ten 30-second segments from the Maciunas and colleagues (2007) study resulted in only a 10% increase in sample size necessary to maintain a specified statistical power (Albert et al., 2009).

As seen with the Shapiro and Rush protocols, there is variability in the environmental test conditions, with the patients sitting quietly and/

or performing a task, and with them alone and/ or with the examiner in the room. For example, another condition developed in a trial of psychobehavioral interventions for TS involved filming through a one-way mirror, with the patient aware that he or she is being recorded, but not when tic counts were to be performed (Azrin & Peterson, 1990). Given the clear demonstration that stress-inducing tasks can increase the expression of tics (Conelea et al., 2011), the task assigned to the patient during tic recording needs to be carefully chosen. However, since tics are highly responsive to stressful situations, it may be useful to try to collect tic data related to both stressful and nonstressful time periods. The authors of the Rush scales also noted during its development that tic counts rose by nearly fourfold when the examiner left the room (Goetz et al., 1987a). A comparison between tic quantification at home versus in the clinician's office, and with the patient alone versus with the observer, showed that tic frequencies were consistently higher with the patient alone and at home (Goetz et al., 2001). It has therefore been suggested that recordings be carried out at home to yield a more accurate quantitative clinical assessment; however, this issue is still debated, with conflicting data demonstrating a lack of difference in tic frequency according to the observer's presence or absence or a difference in settings (Himle et al., 2006; Piacentini et al., 2006). Video-based techniques have a few disadvantages: they require technical input and can be labor-intensive, and thus difficult to implement in research settings and more so in routine clinical practice without dedicated technicians.

More recently, an Italian group proposed an automatic tic detection mechanism (Bernabei et al., 2010). This apparatus involved a three-axial accelerometer worn by the patient on the trunk and measured tic-related events through an algorithm to fine-tune the kinematic signal. Scalar classifications of the intensity and frequency of tic events were rated on a 5-point scale based on the Goetz and colleagues (1994, 1999) classification, with the modification of intensity measured as g-force via accelerometer readings. During initial testing, study participants were concurrently videotaped and rated, with high correlation ($r = .91$) and concordance (98%) between clinician ratings and the automatic system. In terms of performance, the automated system showed mean 80% sensitivity, 77% specificity, and 80% accuracy. Furthermore, due to the positioning of the sensors, the automated system was limited to tics affecting the trunk region. The authors propose further research on different body locations and calibration to overcome individual tic phenotypes, but at the same modeling for homogenous tic types. Thus, this automatic system does show some promise and may be able to produce more accurate and *in situ* data, as well as overcoming limitations arising from clinician-based observations and from environmental influences of clinic rooms. There would still be a requirement for dedicated technicians to install and set the system and analyze the resulting data, with potential difficulties for applications of the technology in routine clinical practice.

The Diagnostic Confidence Index (DCI)

The difficulties with quantifying tics and their implications for clinical diagnosis led to the development of an index to measure the lifetime likelihood of having TS (Robertson et al., 1999). The clinician-rated items of the DCI for TS reflect the clinical features that are highly characteristic of this condition, based on the clinicians' experience and the published literature: copro-, echo-, and pali-phenomena; tic complexity and severity; temporal features of symptoms; sensory symptoms; tic suppressibility; duration of tics; corroborating informants; and lack of differential diagnoses. These factors are rated as "yes/ no" based on their probable or definite presence. Overall DCI scores range from 0 to 100, and the individual items are differentially weighted, with the highest weight for pathognomonic symptoms (particularly coprolalia), tic complexity, and waxing and waning course. The DCI is a useful tool during the assessment protocol within clinical or research settings because it allows the ascertainment of tic "traits" rather than tic "states" based on current severity or treatment regimens. The DCI is a relatively brief measure to rate, but it requires the expertise of a specialist on tic disorders. It has been used extensively in TS research (e.g., Haddad et al., 2009; Rickards & Robertson, 2003; Robertson et al., 2006).

Unified Tic Rating Scale (UTRS)

So-called "unified" measures, combining relevant dimensions or available scales within one measure, have been developed for different neuropsychiatric conditions, such as dystonia (Comella et al., 2003), Parkinson's disease (Fahn et al., 1987), and Huntington's disease (Huntington Study Group, 1996). Following a Tourette Syndrome Association-led motion toward developing a similar instrument for TS, the UTRS was developed by adopting and modifying existing scales, or developing new ones (Kurlan et al., 1988; Kurlan & McDermott, 2005). One of the aims of the UTRS is to minimize measurement errors and to ensure the comparability and consistent interpretation of clinical data on tic severity. The UTRS contains subscales rated by patients and/or informants and clinicians, which are summed to indicate overall tic severity. A 2-minute tic count is also incorporated to measure motor and vocal tics during conversation with the patient. The subscales contain items on the anatomical distribution of tics, types, frequency, intensity, and level of interference and suppression. Measures of ADHD and OCD symptoms and global functioning are also included. The multidimensionality of the UTRS and the inclusion of both subjective and objective data are its greatest advantages, and this instrument is likely to capture a broad range of clinically relevant data. The 2-minute tic count component was used in a phenomenological study in TS (Nolan et al., 1994), which demonstrated the versatility of the UTRS by focusing on relevant subscales. However, during field testing, the first edition of the UTRS showed poor psychometric properties and was cumbersome to complete, with ambiguity in item descriptions and anchor points (Kompoliti & Goetz, 1997). Revisions and piloting are currently under way, with a view toward improving the reliability, dimensionality, internal consistency, and validity (Kurlan & McDermott, 2005).

MEASURING BEHAVIORAL COMORBIDITIES

Although some of the aforementioned scales also include items that measure behavioral symptoms, such as the TS-CGI, specific scales are available that allow more in-depth assessments of the behavioral comorbidities of TS. A widely used scale addressing a broad range of behavioral problems in children and adolescents is the Child Behavior Checklist (CBCL), which assesses a child's overall emotional and behavioral function over the previous 6-month period (Achenbach, 1991a). Parents rate their child according to a 3-point scale. Achenbach (1991b) also developed a self-report version derived from the CBCL: the Youth Self-Report (YSR). Similar groups of questions form syndrome scales (withdrawn, somatic complaints, anxious/depressed, social problems, thought problems, attention problems, delinquent behavior, and aggressive behavior), which are further grouped into the internalizing and externalizing subscales. In its different age-appropriate versions, the CBCL is particularly useful for comprehensively assessing behavioral profiles and may be a valuable adjunct to more specific scales (e.g., Feigin et al., 1996; Pringsheim & Steeves, 2011; Termine et al., 2011). Of further use for diagnostic and severity measures are the factor structure-derived psychopathology scales embedded within the CBCL, which have been examined for their psychometric properties: OCBs (Nelson et al., 2001; Storch, Murphy, Bagner et al., 2006), ADHD symptoms (Biederman et al., 2001; Eiraldi et al., 2000), and affective and anxiety symptoms (Ferdinand, 2008).

Measuring OCBs

LEYTON OBSESSIONAL INVENTORY (LOI)

The LOI is a subjective measure of obsessions and compulsions using a card-sorting procedure (Cooper, 1970). This has been adapted into a questionnaire form (Kazarian et al., 1977) and has been routinely used in clinical studies on TS (e.g., Cavanna et al., 2007; Haddad et al., 2009; Rickards & Robertson, 2003; Robertson et al., 2006; Serra-Mestres et al., 2004). The original LOI version contains 69 questions about the presence ("yes/no") of OCB symptoms (46 items) and traits (23 items), with a subset of 39 items rated for interference caused by OCBs (4-point scale) and resistance (5-point scale) to OCBs. There are different wordings for male and female versions. Forty-four-item (Berg et al., 1986) and 20-item (Berg et al., 1988) versions are also available in the same format for children. A shortened 10-item version was recently developed, with some minor changes to the wording and the interference and resistance items (Bamber et al., 2002). Although the LOI is adequate in terms of psychometric indices (Grabill et al., 2008; Merlo et al., 2005), comprehensive, and flexible in its different versions, some drawbacks have been identified: high intercorrelation within the different LOI subscales, overrepresentation of cleanliness at the expense of other symptom domains, and overreliance of resistance items to the overall number of reported OCB symptoms (Taylor, 1995). Additionally, the LOI was inferior to the Yale-Brown Obsessive Compulsive Scales (YBOCS; see below) at detecting symptom changes in a clinical trial of clomipramine (Kim et al., 1990). This conclusion was also reached in a study comparing the child versions of these obsessionality scales (Stewart et al., 2005).

OBSESSIVE COMPULSIVE INVENTORY (OCI)

Another potentially useful self-report measure for OCBs in TS is the OCI (Foa et al., 1998). With this scale, subjects are asked to rate the presence of their symptoms from the previous month on a 5-point scale consisting of 42 items. The seven subscales correspond to specific OCB domains. Two global scores are available: the mean OCI distress score, which is the mean for the seven subscales, and the total score, which is the sum of individual items. A shorter 18-item version (OCI-R) was demonstrated to have retained the psychometric properties of its predecessor (Foa et al., 2002). The OCI-R has also

undergone further testing that has confirmed its adequate properties, with indications for both clinical and research purposes (Hajcak et al., 2004; Huppert et al., 2007). A German-language version has recently become available (Gönner et al., 2008). However, correlation between the new clinician-report YBOCS-II measure and the OCI-R was poorer compared to other clinician-rated measures (Storch, Rasmussen, Price et al., 2010). The authors also developed a version for children (OCI-CV; for ages 7–17 years), which demonstrated adequate psychometric properties and allows pediatric assessment using the adult conceptualization of the OCI-R (Foa et al., 2010). The OCI-CV contains 21 items, with modifications to questionnaire wording, and is rated on a simpler 3-point scale from 0 (never) to 2 (always).

YALE-BROWN OBSESSIVE COMPULSIVE SCALES (YBOCS)

The YBOCS is a group of scales that allow clinicians to measure OCBs based on the week prior to the assessment. Checklists of current and past symptoms are available and form the target symptom list for rating. The YBOCS contains 10 items, with an equal number of questions for obsessions and compulsions. These items explore the time spent on OCBs, associated functional interference and distress, efforts to resist OCBs, and degree of control over them. They are rated on a 5-point Likert-type scale ranging from 0 to 4, with higher scores indicating greater severity. The authors developed cutoff scores to indicate five levels of severity: subclinical, mild, moderate, severe, and extreme. Additional items, although not included in scoring, further explore OCB symptoms, including insight and avoidance. Versions for adults (Goodman et al., 1989a, 1989b) and children and adolescents (C-YBOCS) are available (Scahill et al., 1997). The YBOCS has undergone extensive independent testing (Frost et al., 1995; Kim et al., 1990; Mataix-Cols et al., 2004; Sulkowski et al., 2008; Woody et al., 1995). There are questions about its discriminant validity, particularly in relation to depression, but this may be a result of the high comorbidity of depressive symptoms with OCD (Robertson, 2006). However, there remain inconsistencies as to the factor structure of the YBOCS and some psychometric properties (Anholt et al., 2010; Deacon & Abramowitz, 2005; Garnaat & Norton, 2010; Storch, Shapira, Dimoulas et al., 2005), including sensitivity to clinically relevant symptomatic changes (Kim et al., 1994). Self-report versions of the YBOCS have been developed, which have proven useful alongside the interview version (Baer et al., 1993; Rosenfeld et al., 1992; Warren et al., 1993). The version developed by Baer and colleagues (1993) has been extensively tested (Federici et al., 2010; Steketee et al., 1996) and has been applied to interventional trials for OCD (e.g., Gabriëls et al., 2003). This version retains the core structure of the checklist and severity portions of the interview version, with plain-language examples to ensure comprehension. This may be a useful patient-rated adjunctive measure to the interview version by ensuring that information regarding OCBs comes from the same theoretical construct and conceptualization. Other self-report versions of the YBOCS symptom checklist have been independently developed, with different item components (Wu et al., 2007). These include the Dimensional YBOCS (D-YBOCS), which allows self- or informant-administered assessments of the presence and severity of specific OCB dimensions, such as aggressive, sexual, and religious obsessions and related compulsions (do Rosario-Campos et al., 2006). A clinician-rated part estimates global symptom ratings and overall impairment. Independent testing of the D-YBOCS confirmed the adequate psychometric properties identified by the developing authors (Pertusa et al., 2011).

The C-YBOCS has undergone similar extensive testing and has been found to be adequately reliable and valid in pediatric populations aged 4 to 18 years (Freeman et al., 2011; Gallant et al., 2008; Storch, Murphy, Geffken et al., 2004a). This instrument has been found to be particularly discriminative at the severe end of the OCB spectrum (Uher et al., 2008). However, a consistent C-YBOCS factor structure has yet to be elucidated (McKay et al., 2003; Storch, Murphy, Geffken et al., 2005a). Thus, a critical review of OCB rating methodology discourages the use

of the total YBOCS scores in routine clinical or research settings (Merlo et al., 2005). Child- and parent-rated versions of the C-YBOCS have been constructed, with adequate psychometric properties (Storch, Murphy, Adkins et al., 2006). A C-YBOCS version for pediatric patients with developmental disorders is also available (Scahill et al., 2006) and may be useful in TS populations.

A second edition of the adult YBOCS version (YBOCS-II) was recently developed and, like its predecessor, consists of a symptom checklist and a severity measure (Storch, Rasmussen, Price et al., 2010). The YBOCS-II reflects emerging phenomenological evidence regarding OCBs (e.g., the "resistance to obsessions" item has been replaced by "obsession-free interval") and has increased sensitivity to clinical change, particularly for more severe cases. The symptom checklist has also undergone further testing, showing adequate psychometric properties (Storch, Larson, Price et al., 2010). The YBOCS has often performed better than other OCB scales (Kim et al., 1990; Stewart et al., 2005) and has shown sensitivity to intervention-related symptomatic changes and adequately distinguishes between state and trait symptoms (Goodman & Price, 1992). Thus, the YBOCS is currently considered the gold standard for OCB assessment and is widely used (e.g., Maciunas et al., 2007; Porta et al., 2009; Pringsheim et al., 2009; Pringsheim & Steeves, 2011; Spencer et al., 2008). Dutch (Arrindell et al., 2002), French (Mollard et al., 1989), Hungarian (Harsányi et al., 2009), Japanese (Hamagaki et al., 1999; Nakajima et al., 1995), Spanish (Godoy et al., 2011; Pertusa et al., 2010; Ulloa et al., 2004; Vega-Dienstmaier et al., 2002), and Turkish (Tek et al., 1995; Yucelen et al., 2006) translations are available.

Measuring Inattention, Hyperactivity, and Impulsivity

SWANSON, NOLAN AND PELHAM SCALE (SNAP-IV)

The SNAP-IV is the newest edition of the Swanson, Nolan, and Pelham scale for measuring ADHD symptoms in clinical trials (Swanson,

1992; Swanson et al., 1983, 2001). The parent- and teacher-rated scales cover a wide range of the child's symptoms of inattention (items 1–9), hyperactivity and impulsivity (10–18), as well as oppositional-defiant disorder (ODD) symptoms (items 19–26). The presence of each symptom is rated on a 4-point scale from "not at all" to "very much." The three-factor structure seems robust and the psychometric properties of the SNAP-IV have been identified as adequate (Bussing et al., 2008). The brief administration and inclusion of ODD along with ADHD symptoms may be useful for research in this area.

ADHD RATING SCALE IV (ADHD-RS-IV)

The ADHD-RS-IV is an informant-rated scale that measures ADHD symptoms in children and adolescents (DuPaul et al., 1998). The 18 items of the ADHD-RS-IV correspond to DSM-IV diagnostic criteria for ADHD (inattentive and hyperactive/impulsive subtypes) and are rated on a scale from 0 (never or rarely) to 3 (very often) with reference to the week preceding the assessment. Further testing indicated adequate psychometric indices of reliability and validity (Zhang et al., 2005), as well as utility in adult patients (Kooij et al., 2005; Sandra Kooij et al., 2008). A Spanish translation is available (Rössler et al., 2006). The ADHD-RS-IV has been used in TS research, including interventional trials (Feigin et al., 1996; Kwon et al., 2011; Pringsheim & Steeves, 2011; Spencer et al., 2002, 2008).

ADHD SELF-REPORT SCALE (ASRS)

The World Health Organisation (WHO) developed the ASRS for patients to rate their symptoms of ADHD in the past 6 months (Kessler et al., 2005). Like the ADHD-RS-IV, the ASRS contains 18 items that address the DSM-IV diagnostic criteria for ADHD. These are measured on a 5-point scale rating how often symptoms are present, from "never" to "very often." The ASRS is comprehensive in capturing items that correspond to symptoms of inattention, hyperactivity, and impulsivity; is relatively simple to complete; and with the six-item screening

questions available for purposes of brevity is potentially useful in both clinical and research settings (Kessler et al., 2005, 2007). Initial testing showed excellent psychometric indices, which have been replicated by further testing (Adler et al., 2006; Reuter et al., 2006).

Conners' ADHD Rating Scales (CRS). The CRS is a widely used assessment tool that measures cognitive, behavioral, and emotional function and has been particularly useful for diagnosis and measurement of ADHD symptoms in children and adolescents as rated by parents or teachers (Conners, 1990, 1997). These symptoms are rated on a 4-point scale from 0 (not at all) to 3 (very much). The revised version was intended for patients aged 3 to 17 (Conners, 1997), while self-report versions are available for 12- to 17-year-olds and 8- to 18-year-olds. The version for adults is the Conners' Adult ADHD Rating Scale (CAARS), which is rated in the same format as for younger patients (Conners et al., 1999). In a review focusing on the psychometric properties of adult ADHD rating scales, the CAARS consistently demonstrated adequate validity and reliability indices (Taylor et al., 2011). Clinician- and self-administered versions are available, as are short and long versions for all Conners' scales. Their psychometric properties have been extensively investigated. A German translation is available (Rössler et al., 2006). The CRS has proven to be a useful measurement tool for ADHD rating in TS populations for both phenomenological studies (e.g., Pringsheim et al., 2009) and interventional studies (e.g., Kwon et al., 2011; Pringsheim & Steeves, 2011).

Measuring Depression

BECK DEPRESSION INVENTORY (BDI)

The Beck Depression Inventory (BDI) scales are a group of self-report measures that address the broad range of cognitive, affective, and somatic symptoms of depression. The BDI contains 21 items rated on a 4-point scale. The first edition (Beck et al., 1961) and its modified version (Beck & Steer, 1993) contained some item ambiguities and did not fully correspond to the DSM criteria for depressive disorders. The BDI-II (Beck et al., 1996) is intended for subjects aged 13 years or older and has the advantage of measuring not only depressive symptoms severity, but also direction of change for the "appetite" and "sleep" items. The psychometric properties of the BDI scales have been extensively researched (Brooks & Kutcher, 2001; Gray et al., 2009). The factor structure for the BDI-II is still under debate (e.g., Vanheule et al., 2008). According to a specific comparison of self-report scales, the BDI-II has been proposed as the assessment tool of choice for depression in TS (Snijders et al., 2006), and it has been used in TS research (e.g., Haddad et al., 2009; Rickards & Robertson, 2003; Servello et al., 2010).

HAMILTON DEPRESSION RATING SCALE (HDRS)

The HDRS is a clinician-administered assessment of depressive symptoms across 21 items (Hamilton, 1960). These are rated on 5-point scales and on 3-point scales when symptom quantification is difficult (i.e., just rating the presence of symptoms). Only the first 17 items are summed to generate the total score. The HDRS is generally considered as a gold standard for assessment of depressive symptoms (Brooks & Kutcher, 2001; Corruble & Hardy, 2005; Gray et al., 2009), although there are questions about its validity (Bagby et al., 2004). It has been pointed out that the use of the HDRS to measure depressive symptoms can generally tap into distress or vegetative symptoms such as appetite and concentration disturbances, which are potentially unrelated to depression itself (Palvuluri & Birmaher, 2004). This may be relevant to TS since symptoms of depression may cross-load onto TS or comorbidities such as OCD and ADHD (Robertson, 2006), and therefore this issue may be an intrinsic limitation to the measurement of affective symptoms. The TS literature appears to use self-rated scales disproportionately to clinician-based assessments of depression in adults. Therefore, the HDRS would be a useful objective assessment of depression in TS (Mantovani et al., 2006).

CHILDREN'S DEPRESSION INVENTORY (CDI)

The CDI was originally developed based on the BDI for children aged 7 years and older (Kovacs, 1982, 1985). It contains 27 items addressing the spectrum of depressive symptoms, rated on a 3-point scale and based on the 2 weeks preceding the assessment. Shortened versions exist (Kovacs, 1992), plus a revised and updated version (Kovacs, 2003). Although the CDI is widely used (Gray et al., 2009; Palvuluri & Birmaher, 2004), including in TS research (e.g., Spencer et al., 2002; Steinberg et al., 2010; Termine et al., 2011), and has been proposed as the assessment tool of choice for depression in children and adolescents with TS (Robertson et al., 2006), some problems have been raised with the discriminant validity of this scale, particularly in children (Brooks & Kutcher, 2001).

CHILDREN'S DEPRESSION RATING SCALES (CDRS)

The clinician-rated CDRS was developed to address the lack of psychometric data to support the use of the HDRS in young people (Brooks & Kutcher, 2001; Poznanski et al., 1979). A revised version of this instrument contains 17 items rated on a 7-point scale for 14 questions, and a 5-point scale for observations of children's speech, hypoactivity, and depressed affect (Poznanski et al., 1985). Information from adult informants is also sought. Psychometric data for 6- to 12-year-olds appear to be adequate, but are limited for adolescents (Brooks & Kutcher, 2001). Nonetheless, it has been used to measure depressive symptoms in childhood TS research (e.g., Allen et al., 2005; Spencer et al., 2008).

Measuring anxiety

STATE-TRAIT ANXIETY INVENTORY (STAI)

The STAI is a widely used self-report measure of anxiety (Spielberger et al., 1970, 1983). The 40-item scale is equally divided into two separate subscales, which correspond to state (current and temporary) and trait (chronic and pervasive) anxiety symptoms. Earlier (Spielberger et al., 1970) and later (Spielberger et al., 1983) versions of the STAI exist, differing on six items for both subscales to improve discriminant validity. Each item is rated on a 4-point Likert-type scale. A version for use with 9- to 12-year-old subjects (STAI-C) has also been developed (Spielberger et al., 1973). The psychometric properties of various versions of the STAI have been examined (Brooks & Kutcher, 2003). The differentiation between state and trait symptoms is an advantage of the STAI over other measures for anxiety, as evidenced in previous work in TS populations (e.g., Cavanna et al., 2007; Haddad et al., 2009; Rickards & Robertson, 2003; Servello et al., 2010).

HAMILTON ANXIETY RATING SCALE (HARS)

The HARS contains 14 self-report items that allow the standardized assessment of anxiety symptoms in both healthy and clinical populations by clinicians (Hamilton, 1959). Questions are rated on a 5-point scale from 0 (not present) to 4 (very severe). Not as widely used as the HDRS, the HARS has undergone in-depth psychometric testing, with adequate properties identified (Clark & Donovan, 1994; Matza et al., 2010). As with depression ratings, there are questions about the validity of rating anxiety in TS, a limitation that is likely to be shared across anxiety rating scales. The literature in TS shows extensive use of self-report anxiety measures. The HARS has been used in TS research (Mantovani et al., 2006) and would be a useful objective measure of anxiety alongside subjective ratings.

HOSPITAL ANXIETY AND DEPRESSION SCALE (HADS)

The HADS is a 14-item self-rated scale assessing anxiety and depressive symptoms (Zigmund & Snaith, 1983). Items are rated on a 4-point scale from 0 (not at all) to 3 (yes, definitely), with anhedonia and appetite change items reverse-scored and higher scores indicating greater severity. The total score can be split into anxiety and depression subscales, containing seven items

each. The HADS has been extensively investigated in nonpsychiatric populations, with adequate psychometric indices (Bjelland et al., 2002). The HADS can be a useful concurrent measure of depression and anxiety symptoms in TS (Robertson, 2006) and has proven useful in TS interventional studies (e.g., Münchau et al., 2002; Serra-Mestres et al., 2004).

REVISED CHILDREN'S ANXIETY AND DEPRESSION SCALE (RCADS)

The RCADS is the revised version of an anxiety-specific self-report measure developed for use in children (Spence, 1998). The RCADS consists of 47 items that address symptoms of specific anxiety syndromes (e.g., separation and generalized anxiety) and major depression, corresponding to DSM-IV diagnostic criteria (Chorpita et al., 2000). Psychometric tests have demonstrated adequate properties (Chorpita et al., 2005; de Ross et al., 2002). Items are rated on a 4-point scale, and a parent-administered version is also available (Ebusutani et al., 2010, 2011). The simultaneous assessment of anxiety and depressive symptoms within a single instrument is convenient for use in both research and clinical settings since anxiety and depression often co-occur.

MEASURING QUALITY OF LIFE

Quality of life (QoL) is of paramount importance in determining the impact TS has on individual experiences of everyday life (Eddy et al., 2011). Its measurement is particularly useful as it covers all aspects of disease burden and allows subjective perspectives to be captured (Devinsky, 1995). Therefore, studies need valid and reliable measures to capture QoL status in both cross-sectional and longitudinal studies, particularly when investigating potential therapeutic strategies.

Gilles de la Tourette Syndrome-Quality of Life Scale (GTS-QOL)

Health-related QoL (HR-QoL) scales allow assessment of the degree to which diagnosed disorders affect QoL, in a holistic sense.

Not surprisingly, over the past few decades, disease-specific HR-QoL scales have become available for a wide range of neuropsychiatric conditions, such as Parkinson's disease (Welsh et al., 2003) and epilepsy (Vickrey et al., 1993). The GTS-QOL was the first HR-QoL measure specifically developed for TS populations (Cavanna et al., 2008). The items included in this scale were derived from exploratory studies to capture clinically relevant issues through semistructured patient interviews, consultation with TS experts, and literature reviews. After the item-generation stage, an item pool of 102 questions was reduced to 40 questions by deleting duplicates and inappropriate items and grouping related questions. Further reductions to the questionnaire were endorsed by a principal component analysis to produce the final 27-item instrument. The GTS-QOL has a four-factor structure covering four domains: the "psychological" domain, with 11 items addressing affective and anxiety symptoms; the "physical and activities of daily living" domain, with 7 items addressing functional impairment due to motor dyscontrol; the "obsessive-compulsive" domain, with 5 items addressing OCBs; and the "cognitive" domain, with 4 items addressing memory and concentration. Each item is rated on a 5-point Likert-type scale from 0 (no problem) to 4 (extreme problem), and a 0-to-100 VAS is included to estimate overall satisfaction with life. Psychometric evaluations demonstrated that the GTS-QOL is a valid and reliable disease-specific instrument for the assessment of HR-QoL in TS (Cavanna et al., 2008). This scale has been used in two case series of DBS for TS (Martínez-Fernández et al., 2011; Porta et al., 2009) as an adjunct measure to capture the patients' perception of their overall HR-QoL.

Medical Outcomes Study 36-Item Short Form Health Survey (SF-36)

Generic HR-QoL measures are of clinical utility as they allow comparisons across different disease populations. The SF-36 has been widely used to examine perceived health status from a multidisciplinary perspective (Ware et al., 1993) and has proven particularly helpful in the development of disease-specific instruments (Cavanna et al., 2008; Vickrey et al., 1993; Welsh et al., 2003). The health domains examined by the SF-36 are physical functioning and related role limitations, psychological well-being and associated role limitations, social function, pain, vitality, and general health perceptions. The SF-36 has been psychometrically evaluated and can be a useful adjunct to the GTS-QOL in both research and clinical practice.

COMMENTARY

Limitations of Symptom Measurement in TS

There are significant difficulties with obtaining simple, accurate, and comprehensive measurements of TS symptoms, particularly due to the phenotypic variability in the expression of tics and behavioral problems. It is often not possible to encompass the multidimensionality of TS with generic available measures, and there is a need for the development or more diffuse use of other symptom/disorder-specific scales. For example, it is important that tic severity scales appropriately capture the wide characteristics of tic symptoms, such as number, frequency, intensity, complexity, and interference with normal behavior or speech. Conclusions from a study comparing the YGTSS and video-based tic frequency counts showed that there can be significant discrepancies between these methods, thus highlighting potential limitations for clinical applications (Himle et al., 2006). The cognitive and environmental effects on tic expression, such as voluntary suppression and suggestibility, can also affect accurate assessment and measurement of TS. This is a particularly important issue with video-based protocols (see above) but is also relevant with clinician-rated measures. The waxing and waning course that characterizes tics in TS introduces a further temporal dimension to tic symptoms and suggests the use of longer time periods for observation, although shorter timeframes are more likely to reduce recall biases.

The use of self-reports and informant reports of symptoms are always helpful because they capture subjective assessments of tics and behavioral symptoms, which might be missed or underestimated by the clinical assessment only. For example, highly relevant issues such as suicidality or disturbing thoughts may be uncomfortable to convey during clinician interviews or difficult to observe. These instruments are also useful in providing a quantitative overview of effects of symptoms on daily and family life. However, self-ratings and informant ratings may lack objectivity and therefore be less reliable, and the information yielded may be variable in quality. Informants would need specific instruction explaining what information is required to maintain the validity and the accuracy of the information collected. In a school-based study of tic symptoms, clinician- and teacher-rated measures showed poor correlation and different raters produced nonoverlapping assessments, thus confounding results (Nolan et al., 1994). Furthermore, the difficulty with self-report information may be a result of poor insight. Indeed, findings from phenomenological studies in TS (Pappert et al., 2003) and behavioral comorbidities such as OCD (Richter et al., 1994; Stewart et al., 2005) demonstrate the possible differences between self-report and clinician-report versions, highlighting the risk of misreporting symptoms. This is particularly relevant for the assessment of neurotic symptoms in TS, since most studies relied on self-report measures only. Whenever possible, it would be appropriate to obtain collateral information to supplement clinician and subjective ratings. Another issue related to the use of subjective measures is the impact of the level of insight displayed by specific patient populations, as this can change in different stages of a chronic disease (Brooks & Kutcher, 2001, 2003).

CONCLUSIONS AND RECOMMENDATIONS

The use of clinical rating scales for the comprehensive assessment of both core and peripheral symptoms of TS should be highly recommended. It is also important to consider the psychometric indices of these measures, since fewer tic measures have undergone comprehensive psychometric validation compared to instruments measuring behavioral comorbidities. We tentatively recommended a battery of standardized clinical rating scales for use in routine clinical practice and/or research (Table 19.2). There are, however, clear difficulties related to the variability in scale constructs and ways of obtaining clinical information. The YGTSS and YBOCS have been frequently used as standard measures for tic severity and OCB severity, respectively, during the development of newer instruments. However, this does not imply that these scales are the only ones with potential clinical and/or research utility. For example, during the development of the HMVTRS, comparisons of this scale with the STSSS, YGTSS, and TS-CGI showed that the newer instrument was an equally reliable and valid measure of overall tic severity (Walkup et al., 1992). Psychometric instruments can also be judged based on the ease and speed of administration, with the STSSS and TS-CGI perhaps being the quickest and most user-friendly. Different versions of an individual scale should be designed to allow assessments from different raters, such as the Conners' Scales for ADHD and YBCOS for OCBs. This permits comparability between data because it can be assumed the scale is derived from the same theoretical and clinical construct.

Since previous comprehensive reviews of rating instruments in TS (e.g., Kompoliti & Goetz, 1997; Kurlan & McDermott, 2005) were published, there have been significant developments, including revisions of original scales of particular relevance to TS (e.g., YBOCS-II, D-YBOCS) and development of new instruments (e.g., PUTS, CTIM-P, PTQ, TODS, USP-SPS, direct observation protocols, DCI). The PUTS and USP-SPS are welcome additions to the available assessment protocols, as these enable the standardized assessment of widely recognized sensory experiences playing an important role in tic expression and in the overall well-being of people who have such experiences.

A broad strategy for clinical measurement ensures that the phenomena related to TS are accurately captured. This may be time-consuming, an inherent limitation to TS psychometrics until a more comprehensive

Table 19.2 Recommendations for Use of Clinical Rating Instruments

Clinical variables	Recommended scale	Rationale
Tics—clinician observations	YGTSS	The most extensively validated tic rating instrument; allows comprehensive assessment of various tic dimensions
Tics—self-report[a]	TSSL	Allows comprehensive assessment of various tic symptoms and their frequency; allows informant corroboration
Tics—informant report	TODS (parent-report version)	Extensive psychometric testing carried out; brief construct; comprehensive assessment of motor and behavioral symptoms
Associated phenomena	PUTS	Extensive psychometric testing carried out; brief self-report construct
Diagnostic confidence	DCI	Measures TS "traits" as opposed to "states" and an index of diagnostic confidence
OCBs—clinician observations	YBOCS/C-YBOCS	Extensive psychometric testing carried out; comprehensive assessment of OCBs
OCBs—self-report	YBOCS/C-YBOCS	Extensive psychometric testing carried out; can be a useful adjunct to the YBOCS interview by measuring OCBs from the same theoretical constructs
ADHD—clinician observations	CRS	Extensive psychometric testing carried out; comprehensive assessment of ADHD symptoms
ADHD—self-report	CRS	Extensive psychometric testing carried out; can be a useful adjunct to the CRS interview by measuring ADHD symptoms from the same theoretical constructs
Depression—clinician observations	HDRS/CDRS	Extensive psychometric testing carried out
Depression—self-report	HADS/RCADS	Extensive psychometric testing carried out; allows concurrent measurement of depression and anxiety[b]
Anxiety—clinician observations	HARS	Extensive psychometric testing carried out
Anxiety—self-report	HADS/RCADS	Extensive psychometric testing carried out; allows concurrent measurement of depression and anxiety[c]
Quality of life	GTS-QOL	TS-specific QoL instrument

[a]No further psychometric evaluations have been carried out on self-report tic rating scales. If a brief tic self-report is required, the MOVES can be a useful alternative since it allows measurement of the frequency of tics, associated phenomena, and OCBs.

[b]If a specific depression scale is required, the BDI-II can be a useful alternative since it has undergone independent psychometric evaluation.

[c]If a specific anxiety scale is required, the STAI/STAI-C can be a useful alternative since it has undergone independent psychometric evaluation and has been shown to effectively differentiate between state and trait anxiety.

Box 19.1. Key Points

- The complex motor and behavioral phenotype of TS presents a unique challenge to measurement and clinical observations.
- Thorough neuropsychiatric assessments are the gold standard, although standardization and quantification of behavioral symptom severity is often difficult, posing a problem for interventional studies in particular.
- Different clinician-, informant- and self-report rating instruments are available for tics and associated phenomena, for use in clinical practice and/or research settings.
- Some scales fall short of measuring the different dimensions of tic symptoms, such as frequency, intensity, interference, and impairment.
- The visible and audible nature of core TS symptoms allows direct observation of these symptoms using specific video protocols.
- A wide range of psychometrically validated clinician- and self-rated measures for OCB, ADHD, depressive, and anxiety symptoms are also available for use in clinical practice and/or research settings.
- The use of behavioral measures with adequate psychometric indices is recommended.
- The potential differences between information gathered from clinicians and patients should always be taken into account.
- Clinicians and researchers should combine information from professionals and patients (as well as informants if possible) to ensure that the information gathered is comprehensive and accurate.

Box 19.2. Questions for Future Research

- **Factor structure of rating scales.** Factor analytic studies potentially allow "streamlining" of psychometric instruments, whereby one can observe which items capture the most variance. However, factor analytic studies of the existing rating instruments are characterized by heterogeneity of analytic methods and sample populations. Future research should be conducted to identify solid factor structures across clinical and nonclinical populations.
- **Unified Tic Rating Scale.** For ease of comprehensive assessment of the complex TS phenomena, a unified tic rating scale measuring tic and associated behavioral symptoms would be welcome for use in both research and clinical settings. Given their proven utility in clinical and research settings, currently available tic and behavioral measures can be incorporated into one comprehensive instrument that could be used as a whole or individual subscales as necessary. Thus, further testing of the UTRS, and modifications if necessary, could ensure that all dimensions of the TS spectrum are comprehensively addressed.
- **Automatic tic measurement device.** Initial testing of an automatic tic detection apparatus has shown some utility in measuring tic-related kinematic signals, although there are some limitations, particularly with regard to including detection of vocal and nontruncal tics. Developments are warranted to improve the measurement of vocal tics, sensor locations, tailoring to individual tic phenotypes, and modeling for homogenous tic types.

(Continued)

> • **Capturing tic phenotypes accurately.** There is controversy whether currently available indirect and direct measures can assess tic phenotypes accurately. Using self- and/or parent-rated measures as adjuncts to clinician-rated measures would help to overcome these limitations. However, more research is required to establish whether empirical differences exist between home and non-home environment tic phenotypes.

and accurate unified measure is developed. Depending on the type of study, flexible psychometric test batteries should be able to include assessments for both tic severity and behavioral comorbidities. Comorbid conditions are common in TS and are often more problematic for patients and their families than tics themselves (Leckman et al., 2006; Pringsheim et al., 2009). There seems to be a complex interplay between behavioral and tic symptoms (Robertson et al., 2006), and behavioral problems have been shown to significantly affect HR-QoL, particularly due to the presence of depression (Eddy et al., 2011; Müller-Vahl et al., 2010). This further highlights the importance of a holistic approach in assessing disease severity in TS, by also incorporating QoL measures.

REFERENCES

Achenbach TM. *Manual for the Child Behavior Checklist/4-18 and 1991 Profile.* Burlington, VT: University of Vermont Department of Psychiatry, 1991a.

Achenbach TM. *Manual for the Youth Self-Report and 1991 Profiles.* Burlington, VT: University of Vermont Department of Psychiatry, 1991b.

Adler LA, Spencer T, Faraone SV et al. Validity of pilot Adult ADHD Self Report Scale (ASRS) to rate adult ADHD symptoms. *Ann Clin Psychiatry* 2006; *18*:145–148.

Albert JM, Maddux BN, Riley DE, Maciunas RJ. Modelling video tic counts in a crossover trial of deep brain stimulation for Tourette syndrome. *Contemp Clin Trials* 2009; *30*:141–149.

Allen AJ, Kurlan RM, Gilbert DL et al. Atomoxetine treatment in children and adolescents with ADHD and comorbid tic disorders. *Neurology* 2005; *65*:1941–1949.

Anholt GE, van Oppen P, Cath DC et al. The Yale-Brown Obsessive-Compulsive scale: factor structure of a large sample. *Front Psychiatry* 2010; *1*:18.

Arrindell WA, de Vlaming IH, Eisenhardt BM et al. Cross-cultural validity of the Yale-Brown Obsessive Compulsive Scale. *J Behav Ther Exp Psychiatry* 2002; *33*:159–176.

Azrin NH, Peterson AL. Treatment of Tourette syndrome by habit reversal: A waiting-list control group comparison. *Behav Ther* 1990; *21*:305–318.

Baer L, Brown-Beasley MW, Sorce J, Henriques AI. Computer-assisted telephone administration of a structured interview for obsessive-compulsive disorder. *Am J Psychiatry* 1993; *150*:1737–1738.

Bagby RM, Ryder AG, Schuller DR, Marshall MB. The Hamilton Depression Rating Scale: has the gold standard become a lead weight? *Am J Psychiatry* 2004; *161*:2163–2177.

Bamber D, Tamplin A, Park RJ. Development of a short Leyton Obsessional Inventory for children and adolescents. *J Am Acad Child Adolesc Psychiatry* 2002; *41*:1246–1251.

Beck AT, Steer RA. *Manual for the Beck Depression Inventory.* San Antonio, TX: Psychological Corporation, 1993.

Beck AT, Steer RA, Brown GK. *Manual for the Beck Depression Inventory-II.* San Antonio, TX: Psychological Corporation, 1996.

Beck AT, Ward CH, Mendelson M et al. An inventory for measuring depression. *Arch Gen Psychiatry* 1961; *4*:561–571.

Berg CJ, Rapoport JL, Flament M. The Leyton Obsessional Inventory-Child Version. *J Am Acad Child Adolesc Psychiatry* 1986; *25*:84–91.

Berg CZ, Whitaker A, Davies M et al. The survey of the Leyton Obsessional Inventory-Child Version: norms from an epidemiological study. *J Am Acad Child Adolesc Psychiatry* 1988; *27*:759–763.

Bernabei M, Andreoni G, Mendez Garcia MO et al. Automatic tic detection of tic activity in the

Tourette syndrome. *Conf Proc IEEE Eng Med Biol Soc* 2010; 2010:422–425.

Biederman J, Monuteaux MC, Greene RW et al. Long-term stability of the Child Behavior Checklist in a clinical sample of youth with attention deficit hyperactivity disorder. *J Clin Child Psychol* 2001; 30:492–502.

Bjelland I, Dahl AA, Haug TT, Neckelmann D. The validity of the Hospital Anxiety and Depression Scale: an updated literature review. *J Psychosom Res* 2002; 52:69–77.

Bornstein RA, Stefl ME, Hammond L. A survey of Tourette syndrome patients and their families: the 1987 Ohio Tourette Survey. *J Neuropsychiatry Clin Neurosci* 1990; 2:275–281.

Brooks SJ, Kutcher S. Diagnosis and measurement of adolescent depression: a review of commonly utilised instruments. *J Child Adolesc Psychopharmacol* 2001; 11:341–376.
A useful review of rating instruments for depression.

Brooks SJ, Kutcher S. Diagnosis and measurement of anxiety disorder in adolescents: a review of commonly utilised instruments. *J Child Adolesc Psychopharmacol* 2003; 13:351–400.
A useful review of rating instruments for anxiety.

Bussing R, Fernandez M, Harwood M et al. Parent and teacher SNAP-IV ratings of attention deficit/hyperactivity disorder symptoms: psychometric properties and normative ratings from a school district sample. *Assessment* 2008; 15:317–328.

Cavanna AE, Robertson MM, Critchley HD. Schizotypal personality traits in Gilles de la Tourette syndrome. *Acta Neurol Scand* 2007; 116:385–391.

Cavanna AE, Schrag A, Morley D et al. The Gilles de la Tourette Syndrome-Quality of Life scale (GTS-QOL): development and validation. *Neurology* 2008; 71:1410–1416.
The report of the only disease-specific QoL measure in TS.

Cavanna AE, Servo S, Monaco F, Robertson MM. The behavioral spectrum of Gilles de la Tourette syndrome. *J Neuropsychiatry Clin Neurosci* 2009; 21:13–23.

Chang S, Himle MB, Tucker BP et al. Initial psychometric properties of a brief parent-report instrument for assessing tic severity in children with chronic tic disorders. *Child Fam Behav Ther* 2009; 31:181–191.

Chappell PB, McSwiggan-Hardin MT, Scahill L et al. Videotape tic counts in the assessment of

Tourette's syndrome: stability, reliability, and validity. *J Am Acad Child Adolesc Psychiatry* 1994; 33:386–393.

Chorpita BF, Moffitt CE, Gray J. Psychometric properties of the Revised Child Anxiety and Depression Scale in a clinical sample. *Behav Res Ther* 2005; 43:309–322.

Chorpita BF, Yim L, Moffitt C et al. Assessment of symptoms of DSM-IV anxiety and depression in children: a revised child anxiety and depression scale. *Behav Res Ther* 2000; 38:835–855.

Clark DB, Donovan JE. Reliability and validity of the Hamilton Anxiety Rating Scale in an adolescent sample. *J Am Acad Child Adolesc Psychiatry* 1994; 33:354–360.

Cohen DJ, Detlor J, Young JG, Shaywitz BA. Clonidine ameliorates Gilles de la Tourette syndrome. *Arch Gen Psychiatry* 1980; 37:1350–1357.

Cohen DJ, Leckman JF, Shaywitz BA. *The Tourette syndrome and other tics.* In: Shaffer DA, Ehrhardt AA, Greenhill LL (eds.), *The clinical guide to child psychiatry.* New York: Free Press, 1984, pp. 566–573.

Comella CL, Leurgans S, Wuu J et al. Rating scales for dystonia: a multicentre assessment. *Mov Disord* 2003; 18:303–312.

Conelea CA, Woods DW, Brandt BC. The impact of a stress induction task on tic frequencies in youth with Tourette syndrome. *Behav Res Ther* 2011; 49:492–497.

Conners K. *Manual For Conners' Rating Scales.* Toronto: Multi-Health Systems, 1990.

Conners K. *Conners' Rating Scales-Revised (CRS-R): technical manual.* New York: Multi-Health Systems, Inc., 1997.

Conners K, Erhardt E, Sparrow E. *Conners' Adult ADHD Rating Scales.* North Tonawanda, NY: Multi-Health Systems, Inc., 1999.

Cooper J. The Leyton obsessional inventory. *Psychol Med* 1970; 1:48–64.

Corruble E, Hardy P. Why the Hamilton Depression Rating Scale endures. *Am J Psychiatry* 2005; 162:2394.

Cullen B, Brown CH, Riddle MA et al. Factor analysis of the Yale-Brown Obsessive Compulsive Scale in a family study of obsessive-compulsive disorder. *Depress Anxiety* 2007; 24:130–138.

Deacon BJ, Abramowitz JS. The Yale-Brown Obsessive Compulsive Scale: factor analysis, construct validity, and suggestions for refinement. *J Anxiety Disord* 2005; 19:573–585.

de Ross RL, Gullone E, Chorpita BF. The Revised Child Anxiety and Depression Scale: a psychometric investigation with Australian youth. *Behav Change* 2002; *19*:90–101.

Devinsky O. Outcomes research in neurology: incorporating health-related quality of life. *Ann Neurol* 1995; *37*:141–142.

DuPaul GJ, Power TJ, Anastopoulos AD, Reid R. *ADHD Rating Scale-IV: checklists, norms, and clinical interpretation.* New York: Guilford, 1998.

Ebusutani C, Bernstein A, Nakamura BJ et al. A psychometric analysis of the Revised Child Anxiety and Depression Scale—a parent version in a clinical sample. *J Abnorm Child Psychol* 2010; *38*:249–260.

Ebusutani C, Chorpita BF, Higa-McMillan CK et al. A psychometric analysis of the Revised Child Anxiety and Depression Scale—a parent version in a school sample. *J Abnorm Child Psychol* 2011; *39*:173–185.

Eddy CM, Cavanna AE, Gulisano M et al. Clinical correlates of quality of life in Tourette syndrome. *Mov Disord* 2011; *26*:735–738.

Eiraldi RB, Power TJ, Karustis JL, Goldstein SG. Assessing ADDHD and comorbid disorders in children: the Child Behavior Checklist and the Devereux Scales for Mental Disorders. *J Clin Child Psychol* 2000; *29*:3–16.

Fahn S, Elton RL, UPDRS Development Committee. Unified Parkinson's Disease Rating Scale. In: Fahn S, Marsden CD, Calne DB, Goldstein M (eds.), *Recent developments in Parkinson's disease.* Florham Park, NJ: Macmillan, 1987, pp. 153–163.

Federici A, Summerfeldt LJ, Harrington JL et al. Consistency between self-report and clinician-administered versions of the Yale-Brown Obsessive-Compulsive Scale. *J Anxiety Disord* 2010; *24*:729–733.

Feigin A, Kurlan R, McDermott MO et al. A controlled trial of deprenyl in children with Tourette's syndrome and attention deficit hyperactivity disorder. *Neurology* 1996; *46*:965–968.

Ferdinand RF. Validity of the CBCL/YSR DSM-IV scales Anxiety and Affective Problems. *J Anxiety Disord* 2008; *22*:126–134.

Foa EB, Coles M, Huppert JD et al. Development and validation of a child version of the obsessive compulsive inventory. *Behav Ther* 2010; *41*:121–132.

Foa EB, Huppert JD, Leiberg S et al. The Obsessive-Compulsive Inventory: development and validation of a short version. *Psychol Assess* 2002; *14*:485–496.

Foa EB, Kozak MJ, Salkovskis PM et al. The validation of a new obsessive-compulsive disorder scale: the Obsessive-Compulsive Inventory. *Psychological Assess* 1998; *10*:206–214.

Frost RO, Steketee G, Krause MS, Trepanier KL. The relationship of the Yale-Brown Obsessive Compulsive Scale (YBOCS) to other measures of obsessive compulsive symptoms in a nonclinical population. *J Pers Assess* 1995; *65*:158–168.

Freeman J, Flessner CA, Garcia A. The Children's Yale-Brown Obsessive-Compulsive Scale: reliability and validity for use among 5- to 8-year-olds with obsessive-compulsive disorder. *J Abnorm Child Psychol* 2011; *39*:877–883.

Gabriëls L, Cosyns P, Nuttin B et al. Deep brain stimulation for treatment-refractory obsessive-compulsive disorder: psychopathological and neuropsychological outcome in three cases. *Acta Psychiatrica Scand* 2003; *107*:275–282.

Gadow KD, Paolicelli LM. *Global Tic Rating Scale.* Stony Brook, NY: State University of New York Department of Psychiatry, 1986.

Gaffney GR, Sieg K, Hellings J. The MOVES: a self-rating scale for Tourette's syndrome. *J Child Adolesc Psychopharmacol* 1994; *4*:269–280.

Gallant J, Storch EA, Merlo LJ et al. Convergent and discriminant validity of the Children's Yale-Brown Obsessive Compulsive Scale-Symptom Checklist. *J Anxiety Disord* 2008; *22*:1369–1376.

García-López R, Perea-Milla E, Romero-González J et al. [Spanish adaptation and diagnostic validity of the Yale Global Tics Severity Scale]. *Rev Neurol* 2008; *46*:261–266.

Garnaat SL, Norton PJ. Factor structure and measurement invariance of the Yale-Brown Obsessive Compulsive Scale across four racial/ethnic groups. *J Anxiety Disord* 2010; *24*:723–728.

Godoy A, Gavino A, Valderrama L et al. [Factor structure and reliability of the Spanish adaptation of the Children's Yale-Brown Obsessive-Compulsive Scale-Self Report (CY-BOCS-SR)]. *Psicothema* 2011; *23*:330–335.

Goetz CG, Leurgans S, Chmura TA. Home alone: methods to maximize tic expression for objective videotape assessments in Gilles de la Tourette syndrome. *Mov Disord* 2001; *16*:693–698.

Goetz CG, Pappert EJ, Louis ED et al. Advantages of a modified scoring method for the Rush Video-Based Tic Rating Scale. *Mov Disord* 1999; *14*:502–506.

Goetz CG, Stebbins GT, Thelen JA. Talipexole and adult Gilles de la Tourette's syndrome: double-blind, placebo-controlled clinical trial. *Mov Disord* 1994; 9:315–317.

Goetz CG, Tanner CM, Wilson RS et al. Clonidine and Gilles de la Tourette's syndrome: double-blind study using objective rating methods. *Ann Neurol* 1987a; 21:307–310.

Goetz CG, Tanner CM, Wilson RS, Shannon KM. A rating scale for Gilles de la Tourette's syndrome: description, reliability, and validity data. *Neurology* 1987b; 37:1542–1544.

Goodman WK, Price LH, Rasmussen SA et al. The Yale-Brown Obsessive Compulsive Scale. I. Development, use, and reliability. *Arch Gen Psychiatry* 1989; 46:1006–1011.

Goodman WK, Price LH, Rasmussen SA et al. The Yale-Brown Obsessive Compulsive Scale. II. Validity. *Arch Gen Psychiatry* 1989; 46:1012–1016.

Goodman WK, Price LH. Assessment of severity and change in obsessive compulsive disorder. *Psychiatr Clin North Am* 1992; 15:861–869.

Gönner S, Leonhart R, Ecker W. The Obsessive-Compulsive Inventory-Revised (OCI-R): validation of the German version in a sample of patients with OCD, anxiety disorders, and depressive disorders. *J Anxiety Disord* 2008; 22:734–749.

Grabill K, Merlo L, Duke D et al. Assessment of obsessive-compulsive disorders: a review. *J Anxiety Disord* 2008; 22:1–17.
A useful review of rating instruments for OCBs.

Gray LB, Dubin-Rhodin, Weller RA, Weller EB. Assessment of depression in children and adolescents. *Curr Psychiatry Rep* 2009; 11:106–113.
A useful review of rating instruments for pediatric depression.

Haddad ADM, Umoh G, Bhatia V, Robertson MM. Adults with Tourette's syndrome with and without attention deficit hyperactivity disorder. *Acta Psychiatr Scand* 2009; 120:299–307.

Hajcak G, Huppert JD, Simmons RF, Foa EB. Psychometric properties of the OCI-R in a college sample. *Behav Res Ther* 2004; 42:115–123.

Hamagaki, S, Takagi S, Urushihara Y et al. [Development and use of the Japanese version of the self-report Yale-Brown Obsessive-Compulsive Scale]. *Seishin Shinkeigaku Zasshi* 1999; 101:152–168.

Hamilton M. The assessment of anxiety states by rating. *Br J Med Psychol* 1959; 32:52–55.

Hamilton M. A rating scale for depression. *J Neurol Neurosurg Psychiatry* 1960; 23:56–62.

Harcherik DF, Leckman JF, Detlor J, Cohen DJ. A new instrument for clinical studies of Tourette's syndrome. *J Am Acad Child Adolesc Psychiatry* 1984; 23:153–160.

Harsányi A, Csiqó K, Demeter G et al. [Hungarian translation of the Dimensional Yale-Brown Obsessive-Compulsive Scale and our first experiences with the test]. *Psychiatr Hung* 2009; 24: 18–59.

Himle MB, Chang S, Woods DW et al. Establishing the feasibility of direct observation in the assessment of tics in children with chronic tic disorders. *J Appl Behav Anal* 2006; 39:429–440.

Huntington Study Group. Unified Huntington's Disease Rating Scale: reliability, and consistency. *Mov Disord* 1996; 11:136–142.

Huppert JD, Walther MR, Hajcak G et al. *J Anxiety Disord* 2007; 21:394–406.

Jagger J, Prusoff BA, Cohen DJ et al. The epidemiology of Tourette's syndrome: a pilot study. *Schizophr Bull* 1982; 8:267–278.

Kazarian SS, Evans DR, Lefave K. Modifications and factorial analysis of the Leyton Obsessional Inventory. *J Clin Psychol* 1977; 33:422–425.

Kessler RC, Adler L, Ames M et al. The World Health Organization Adult ADHD Self-Report Scale (ASRS): a short screening scale for use in the general population. *Psychol Med* 2005; 35:245–256.

Kessler RC, Adler LA, Gruber MJ et al. Validity of the World Health Organization Adult ADHD Self-Report Scale (ASRS) Screener in a representative sample of health plan members. *Int J Methods Psychiatr Res* 2007; 16:52–65.

Kim SW, Dysken MW, Kuskowski M. The Yale-Brown Obsessive-Compulsive Scale: a reliability and validity study. *Psychiatry Res* 1990; 34:99–106.

Kim SW, Dysken MW, Pheley AM, Hoover KM. The Yale-Brown Obsessive-Compulsive Scale: measures of internal consistency. *Psychiatry Res* 1994; 51:203–211.

Kompoliti K, Goetz CG. Tourette syndrome. Clinical rating and quantitative assessment of tics. *Neurol Clin* 1997; 15:239–254.

Kooij JJ, Buitelaar JK, van den Oord EJ et al. Internal and external validity of attention-deficit hyperactivity disorder in a population-based sample of adults. *Psychol Med* 2005; 35:817–827.

Kovacs M. *The Children's Depression Inventory: a self-rated depression scale for school-aged youngsters.* Pittsburgh, PA: University of Pittsburgh School of Medicine, 1982.

Kovacs M. The Children's Depression Inventory (CDI). *Psychopharmacol Bull* 1985; 21:995–998.

Kovacs M. *The Children's Depression Inventory*. North Tonawanda, NY: Mental Health Systems, 1992.

Kovacs M. *Manual for Children's Depression Inventory*. Toronto, ON: Multi-Health Systems, Inc., 2003.

Kurlan R, McDermott M, Como P. *Tourette Syndrome Unified Rating Scale*. New York: Tourette Syndrome Association, 1988.

The initial report of a comprehensive rating instrument, potentially capturing the complex aspects of the TS phenotype.

Kurlan R, McDermott MP. Rating tic severity. In: Kurlan R (ed.), *Handbook of Tourette's syndrome and related tic and behavioral disorders* (2nd ed.). New York: Marcel Dekker, 2005.

Kwon HJ, Lim WS, Lim MH et al. 1-Hz low frequency repetitive transcranial magnetic stimulation in children with Tourette's syndrome. *Neurosci Lett* 2011; 492:1–4.

Leckman JF, Bloch MH, Scahill L, King RA. Tourette syndrome: the self under siege. *J Child Neurol* 2006; 21:642–649.

Leckman JF, Hardin MT, Riddle MA et al. Clonidine treatment of Gilles de la Tourette's syndrome. *Arch Gen Psychiatry* 1991; 48:324–328.

Leckman JF, Riddle MA, Hardin MT et al. The Yale Global Tic Severity Scale: initial testing of a clinician-rated scale of tic severity. *J Am Acad Child Adolesc Psychiatry* 1989; 28:566–573.

Leckman JF, Towbin KE, Ort SI, Cohen DJ. Clinical assessment of tic disorder severity. In: Cohen DJ, Bruun RD, Leckman JF (eds.), *Tourette's syndrome and tic disorders: clinical understanding and treatment*. New York: John Wiley & Sons, 1988.

Leckman JF, Walker DE, Cohen DJ. Premonitory urges in Tourette's syndrome. *Am J Psychiatry* 1993; 150:98–102.

Maciunas RJ, Maddux BN, Riley DE et al. Prospective randomized double-blind trial of bilateral thalamic deep brain stimulation in adults with Tourette syndrome. *J Neurosurg* 2007; 107:1004–1014.

Mantovani A, Lisanby SH, Pieraccini F et al. Repetitive transcranial magnetic stimulation (rTMS) in the treatment of obsessive-compulsive disorder (OCD) and Tourette's syndrome (TS). *Int J Neuropsychopharmacol* 2006; 9:95–100.

Martínez-Fernández R, Zrinzo l, Aviles-Olmos I et al. Deep brain stimulation for Gilles de la Tourette syndrome: a case series targeting subregions of the globus pallidus internus. *Mov Disord* 2011; 26:1922–1930.

Mataix-Cols D, Fullana MA, Alonso P et al. Convergent and discriminant validity of the Yale-Brown Obsessive-Compulsive Scale Symptom Checklist. *Psychother Psychosom* 2004; 73:190–196.

Matza LS, Morlock R, Sexton C et al. Identifying HAM-A cutoffs for mild, moderate, and severe generalized anxiety disorder. *Int J Methods Psychiatr Res* 2010; 19:223–232.

McKay D, Piacentini J, Greisberg S et al. The Children's Yale-Brown Obsessive Compulsive Scale: item structure in an outpatient setting. *Psychol Assess* 2003; 15:578–581.

Merlo LJ, Storch EA, Murphy TK et al. Assessment of pediatric obsessive-compulsive disorder: a critical review of current methodology. *Child Psychiatry Hum Dev* 2005; 36:195–214.

A useful review of rating instruments for pediatric OCBs.

Mollard E, Cottraux, Bouvard M. [French version of the Yale-Brown Obsessive Compulsive Scale]. *Encephale* 1989; 15:335–341.

Müller-Vahl K, Dodel I, Müller N et al. Health-related quality of life in patients with Gilles de la Tourette's syndrome. *Mov Disord* 2010; 25:309–314.

Müller-Vahl KR, Schneider U, Koblenz A et al. Treatment of Tourette's syndrome with delta-9-tetrahydrocannabinol (THC): a randomized crossover trial. *Pharmacopsychiatry* 2002; 35:57–61.

Münchau A, Bloem BR, Thilo KV et al. Repetitive transcranial magnetic stimulation for Tourette syndrome. *Neurology* 2002; 59:1789–1791.

Nakajima T, Nakamura M, Taga C et al. Reliability and validity of the Japanese version of the Yale-Brown Obsessive Compulsive Scale. *Psychiatry Clin Neurosci* 1995; 49:121–126.

Nelson EC, Hanna GL, Hudziak JJ et al. Obsessive-compulsive scale of the Child Behavior Checklist: specificity, sensitivity, and predictive power. *Pediatrics* 2001; 108(1):E14.

Nolan EE, Gadow KD, Sverd J. Observations and ratings of tics in school settings. *J Abnorm Child Psychol* 1994; 22:579–593.

Orth M, Kirby R, Richardson MP et al. Subthreshold rTMS over pre-motor cortex has no effect on tics in patients with Gilles de la Tourette syndrome. *Clin Neurophysiol* 2005; 116:764–768.

Palvuluri M, Birmaher B. A practical guide to using ratings of depression and anxiety in child psychiatric practice. *Curr Psychiatry Rep* 2004; 6:108–116. **A useful review of rating instruments for pediatric depression and anxiety.**

Pappert EJ, Goetz CG, Louis ED et al. Objective assessments of longitudinal outcome in Gilles de la Tourette's syndrome. *Neurology* 2003; 61:936–940.

Pertusa A, Fernández de la Cruz L, Alonso P et al. Independent validation of the Dimensional Yale-Brown Obsessive-Compulsive Scale (DY-BOCS). *Eur Psychiatry* 2011 [E-pub ahead of print].

Pertusa A, Jaurrieta N, Real E et al. Spanish adaptation of the Dimensional Yale-Brown Obsessive-Compulsive Scale. *Compr Psychiatry* 2010; 51:641–648.

Piacentini J, Himle MB, Chang S et al. Reactivity of tic observation procedures to situation and setting. *J Abnorm Child Psychol* 2006; 34:649–658.

Porta M, Brambilla A, Cavanna AE et al. Thalamic deep brain stimulation for treatment-refractory Tourette syndrome: two-year outcome. *Neurology* 2009; 73:1375–1380.

Poznanski EO, Cook SC, Caroll BJ. A depression rating scale for children. *Pediatrics* 1979; 64:442–450.

Poznanski EO, Freeman LN, Mokros HB. Children's Depression Rating Scale-Revised. *Psychopharmacol Bull* 1985; 21:979–989.

Pringsheim T, Marras C. Pimozide for tics in Tourette's syndrome. *Cochrane Database Syst Rev* 2009;2:CD006996.

Pringsheim T, Lang A, Kurlan R et al. Understanding disability in Tourette syndrome. *Dev Med Child Neurol* 2009; 51:468–472.

Pringsheim T, Steeves T. Pharmacological treatment for attention deficit hyperactivity disorder (ADHD) in children with comorbid tic disorders. *Cochrane Database Syst Rev* 2011;4:CD007990.

Reiter M, Kirsch P, Hennig J. Inferring candidate genes for attention deficit hyperactivity disorder (ADHD) assessed by the World Health Organization Adult ADHD Self-Report Scale (ASRS). *J Neural Transm* 2006; 113:929–938.

Richter MA, Cox BJ, Direnfeld DM. A comparison of three assessment instruments for obsessive-compulsive symptoms. *J Behav Ther Exp Psychiatry* 1994; 25:143–147.

Rickards H, Robertson M. A controlled study of psychopathology and associated symptoms in Tourette syndrome. *World J Biol Psychiatry* 2003; 4:64068.

Robertson MM. Tourette syndrome, associated conditions and the complexities of treatment. *Brain* 2000; 123:425–462.

Robertson MM. Mood disorders and Gilles de la Tourette's syndrome: an update on prevalence, etiology, comorbidity, clinical associations, and implications, *J Psychosom Res* 2006; 61: 349–358.

Robertson MM, Banerjee S, Kurlan R et al. The Tourette syndrome diagnostic confidence index: development and clinical associations. *Neurology* 1999; 53:2108–2112.

Robertson MM, Williamson F, Eapen V. Depressive symptomatology in young people with Gilles de la Tourette syndrome—a comparison of self-report scales. *J Affect Disord* 2006; 91:265–268.

Rosario-Campos MC, Miguel EC, Quatrano S et al. The Dimensional Yale-Brown Obsessive-Compulsive Scale (DY-BOCS): an instrument for assessing obsessive-compulsive symptom dimensions. *Mol Psychiatry.* 2006; 11:495–504.

Rosario MC, Silva H, Borcato S et al. Validity of the University of São Paulo Sensory Phenomena Scale: initial psychometric properties. *CNS Spectr* 2009; 14:315–323.

Rosenfeld R, Dar R, Anderson D et al. A computer-administered version of the Yale-Brown Obsessive-Compulsive Scale. *Psychol Assess* 1992; 4:329–332.

Rössler M, Retz W, Thome J et al. Psychopathological rating scales for diagnostic use in adults with attention-deficit/hyperactivity disorder (ADHD). *Eur Arch Psychiatry Clin Neurosci* 2006; 256 (Suppl 1):1/3–1/11.

Sallee FR, Nesbitt L, Jackson C et al. Relative efficacy of haloperidol and pimozide in children and adolescents with Tourette's disorder. *Am J Psychiatry* 1997; 154:1057–1062.

Sandra Kooij JJ, Marije Boonstra A, Swinkels SH et al. Reliability, validity, and utility of instruments for self-report and informant report concerning symptoms of ADHD in adult patients. *J Atten Disord* 2008; 11:445–458.

Scahill L, McDougle CJ, Williams SK et al. Children's Yale-Brown Obsessive Compulsive Scale modified for pervasive developmental disorders. *J Am Acad Child Adolesc Psychiatry* 2006; 45:1114–1123.

Scahill L, Riddle MA, McSwiggin-Hardin M et al. Children's Yale-Brown Obsessive Compulsive

Scale: reliability and validity. *J Am Acad Child Adolesc Psychiatry* 1997; 36:844–852.

Serra-Mestres J, Ring HA, Costa DC et al. Dopamine transporter binding in Gilles de la Tourette syndrome: a [123I]FP-CIT/SPECT study. *Acta Pscyhiatr Scand* 2004; 109:140–146.

Servello D, Sassi M, Brambilla A et al. Long-term, post-deep brain stimulation management of a series of 36 patients affected with refractory Gilles de la Tourette syndrome. *Neuromodulation* 2010; 13:187–194.

Shapiro AK, Shapiro ES. Controlled study of pimozide vs. placebo in Tourette's syndrome. *J Am Acad Child Psychiatry* 1984; 23:161–173.

Shapiro AK, Shapiro ES, Young JG, Feinberg TE. Measurement in tic disorders. In: Shapiro AK, Shapiro ES, Young JG, Feinberg TE (eds.), *Gilles de la Tourette syndrome* (2nd ed.). New York, Raven Press, 1988, pp. 451–480.

Shytle RD, Silver AA, Sheehan KH et al. The Tourette's Disorder Scale (TODS): development, reliability, and validity. *Assessment* 2003; 10:273–287.

Silva RR, Muñoz DM, Daniel W et al. *J Child Psychol Psychiatry* 1995; 36:305–312.

Silva RR, Muñoz DM, Daniel W et al. Causes of haloperidol discontinuation with Tourette's disorder: management and alternatives. *J Clin Psychiatry* 1996; 57:129–135.

Singer HS, Brown J, Quaskey S et al. The treatment of attention-deficit hyperactivity disorder in Tourette's syndrome: a double-blind placebo-controlled study with clonidine and desipramine. *Pediatrics* 1995; 95:74–81.

Snijders AH, Robertson MM, Orth M. Beck Depression Inventory is a useful screening tool for major depressive disorder in Gilles de la Tourette syndrome. *J Neurol Neurosurg Psychiatry* 2006; 77:787–789.

Spence SH. A measure of anxiety symptoms among children. *Behav Res Ther* 1998; 36:545–566.

Spencer T, Biederman J, Coffey B et al. A double-blind comparison of desipramine and placebo in children and adolescents with chronic tic disorder and comorbid attention-deficit/hyperactivity disorder. *Arch Gen Psychiatry* 2002; 59:649–656.

Spencer TJ, Sallee FR, Gilbert DL et al. Atomoxetine treatment of ADHD in children with comorbid Tourette syndrome. *J Atten Disord* 2008; 11:470–481.

Spielberger CD, Edwards CD, Luschene RE et al. *Manual for the State-Trait Anxiety Inventory for Children*. Palo Alto, CA: Consulting Psychologists Press, 1973.

Spielberger CD, Gorsuch RL, Luschene RE. *Manual for the State-Trait Anxiety Inventory*. Palo Alto, CA: Consulting Psychologists Press, 1970.

Spielberger CD, Gorsuch RL, Luschene RE. *Manual for the State-Trait Anxiety Inventory (STAI Form Y)*. Palo Alto, CA: Consulting Psychologists Press, 1983.

Stefanoff P, Wolańczyk T. [Validity and reliability of Polish adaptation of Yale Global Tic Severity Scale (YGTSS) in a study of Warsaw schoolchildren aged 12–15]. *Przegl Epidemiol* 2005; 59:753–762.

Steinberg T, Baruch SS, Harush A et al. Tic disorders and the premonitory urge. *J Neural Transm* 2010; 117:277–284.

Steketee G, Frost R, Bogart K. The Yale-Brown Obsessive Compulsive Scale: interview versus self-report. *Behav Res Ther* 1996; 34:675–684.

Stewart SE, Ceranoglu TA, O'Hanley T, Geller DA. Performance of clinician versus self-report measures to identify obsessive-compulsive disorder in children and adolescents. *J Child Adolesc Psychopharmacol* 2005; 15:956–963.

Storch EA, De Nadai AS, Lewin AB et al. Defining treatment response in pediatric tic disorders: a signal detection analysis of the yale global tic severity scale. *J Child Adolesc Psychopharmacol* 2011; 21:621–627.

Storch EA, Lack CW, Simons LE et al. A measure of functional impairment in youth with Tourette's syndrome. *J Pediatr Psychol* 2007; 32: 950–959.

Storch EA, Larson MJ, Price LH et al. Psychometric analysis of the Yale-Brown Obsessive-Compulsive Scale Second Edition Symptom Checklist. *J Anxiety Disord* 2010; 24:650–656.

Storch EA, Merlo LJ, Lehmkuhl H et al. Further psychometric examination of the Tourette's Disorder Scales. *Child Psychiatry Hum Dev* 2007; 38:89–98.

Storch EA, Murphy TK, Adkins JW et al. The children's Yale-Brown obsessive-compulsive scale: psychometric properties of child- and parent-report formats. *J Anxiety Disord* 2006; 20:1055–1070.

Storch EA, Murphy TK, Bagner DM et al. Reliability and validity of the Child Behavior Checklist Obsessive-Compulsive Scale. *J Anxiety Disord* 2006; 20:473–485.

Storch EA, Murphy TK, Fernandez M et al. Factor-analytic study of the Yale Global Tic Severity Scale. *Psychiatry Res* 2007; *149*:231–237.

Storch EA, Murphy TK, Geffken GR et al. Psychometric evaluation of the Children's Yale-Brown Obsessive-Compulsive Scale. *Psychiatry Res* 2004a; *129*:91–98.

Storch EA, Murphy TK, Geffken GR et al. Further psychometric properties of the Tourette's Disorder Scale-Parent Rated version (TODS-PR). *Child Psychiatry Hum Dev* 2004b; 35:107–120.

Storch EA, Murphy TK, Geffken GR et al . *J Clin Child Adolesc Psychol* 2005a; 34:312–319.

Storch EA, Murphy TK, Geffken GR et al. Reliability and validity of the Yale Global Tic Severity Scale. *Psychol Assess* 2005b; *17*:486–491.

Storch EA, Rasmussen SA, Price LH et al. Development and psychometric evaluation of the Yale-Brown Obsessive-Compulsive Scale—Second Edition. *Psychol Assess* 2010; 22:223–232.

Storch EA, Shapira NA, Dimoulas E et al. Yale-Brown Obsessive Compulsive: the dimensional structure revisited. *Depress Anxiety* 2005; 22:28–35.

Sulkowski ML, Storch EA, Geffken GR et al. Concurrent validity of the Yale-Brown Obsessive-Compulsive Scale-Symptom checklist. *J Clin Psychol* 2008; 64:1338–1351.

Sutherland Owens AN, Miguel EC, Swerdlow NR. Sensory gating scales and premonitory urges in Tourette syndrome. *Scientific World J* 2011; 11:736–741.

Swanson JM. *School-Based Assessments and Interventions for ADD Students*. Irvine, CA: KC Publishing, 1992.

Swanson JM, Kraemer HC, Hinshaw SP et al. Clinical relevance of the primary findings of the MTA: success rates based on severity of ADHD and ODD symptoms at the end of treatment. *J Am Acad Child Adolesc Psychiatry* 2001; 40:168–179.

Swanson JM, Sandman CA, Deutsch C, Baren M. Methylphenidate hydrochloride given with or before breakfast: I. Behavioral, cognitive, and electrophysiologic effects. *Pediatrics* 1983; 72:49–55.

Tanner CM, Goetz CG, Klawans HL. Cholinergic mechanisms in Tourette syndrome. *Neurology* 1982; 32:1315–1317.

Taylor S. Assessment of obsessions and compulsions: reliability, validity and sensitivity to treatment effects. *Clin Psychol Rev* 1995; 15:261–296.

Taylor A, Deb S, Unwin G. Scales for the identification of adults with attention deficit hyperactivity disorder (ADHD): a systematic review. *Res Dev Disabil* 2011; *32*:924–938.
A useful review of rating instruments for adult ADHD.

Termine C, Selvini C, Balottin U et al. Self-, parent-, and teacher-reported behavioral symptoms in youngsters with Tourette syndrome: a case-control study. *Eur J Paediatr Neurol* 2011; 15:95–100.

Tek C, Uluğ B, Rezaki BG et al. Yale-Brown Obsessive Compulsive Scale and US National Institute of Mental Health Global Obsessive Compulsive Scale in Turkish: reliability and validity. *Acta Psychiatr Scand* 1995; *91*: 410–413.

Toren P, Weizman A, Ratner S et al. Ondasentron treatment in Tourette's disorder: a 3-week, randomized, double-blind, placebo-controlled study. *J Clin Psychiatry* 2005; 66:499–503.

Uher R, Heyman I, Turner CM, Shafran R. Self-, parent-report and interview measures of obsessive-compulsive disorder in children and adolescents. *J Anxiety Disord* 2008; *22*:979–990.

Ulloa RE, de la Peña Fm Higuera F, Palacios L et al. [Validity and reliability of the Spanish version of the Yale-Brown obsessive-compulsive rating scale for children and adolescents]. *Actas Esp Psiquiatr* 2004; *32*:216–221.

Vanheule S, Desmet M, Groenvynck H et al. The factor structure of the Beck Depression Inventory-II: an evaluation. *Assessment* 2008; 15:177–187.

Vega-Dienstmaier JM, Sal Y Rosas HJ, Mazzotti Suárez G et al. [Validation of a version in Spanish of the Yale-Brown Obsessive-Compulsive Scale]. *Actas Esp Psiquiatr* 2002; 30:30–35.

Vickrey BG, Perrine KR, Hays RD. *Quality of Life Scale in Epilepsy QOLIE-32 (Version 1.0) Scoring Manual*. Santa Monica, CA: RAND, 1993.

Walkup JT, Rosenberg LA, Brown J, Singer HS. The validity of instruments measuring tic severity in Tourette's syndrome. *J Am Acad Child Adolesc Psychiatry* 1992; 31:472–477.
An important review of clinical rating instruments for tics, comparing the STSSS, TS-CGI, and YGTSS, and reporting the development of the HMVTS.

Ware JE, Snow KK, Kosisnki M, Gandek B. *SF-36 Health Survey Manual and Interpretation Guide*. Boston: The Health Institute, 1993.

Warren R, Zgourides G, Monto M. Self-report versions of the Yale-Brown Obsessive-Compulsive Scale: an assessment of a sample of normals. *Psychol Rep* 1993; 73:574.

Welsh M, McDermott MP, Holloway RG et al. Development and testing of the Parkinson's disease quality of life scale. *Mov Disord* 2003; 18:637–645.

Woods DW, Piacentini J, Himle MB, Chang S. Premonitory Urge for Tics Scale (PUTS): initial psychometric results and examination of the premonitory urge phenomenon in youths with Tic disorders. *J Dev Behav Pediatr* 2005; 26:397–403. **The report of the first psychometric measure to assess TS sensory symptoms.**

Woody SR, Steketee G, Chambless DL. Reliability and validity of the Yale-Brown Obsessive Compulsive Scale. *Behav Res Ther* 1995; 33:597–605.

Wu KD, Watson D, Clark LA. A self-report version of the Yale-Brown Obsessive-Compulsive Scale Symptom Checklist: psychometric properties of factor-based scales in three samples. *J Anxiety Disord* 2007; 21:644–661.

Yucelen AG, Rodopman-Arman A, Topcuoglu V et al. Interrater reliability and clinical efficacy of Children's Yale-Brown Obsessive-Compulsive Scale in an outpatient setting. *Compr Psychiatry* 2006; 47:48–53.

Zigmund AS, Snaith RP. The Hospital Anxiety and Depression Scale. *Acta Psychiatr Scand* 1983; 67:361–370.

Zhang S, Faries DE, Vowles M, Michelson D. ADHD Rating Scale IV: psychometric properties from a multinational study as a clinician-administered instrument. *Int J Methods Psychiatr Res* 2005; 14:186–201.

Neuropsychological Assessment in Tourette Syndrome

TARA MURPHY AND CLARE M. EDDY

Abstract

Cognitive functioning is one of the most complex areas in Tourette syndrome (TS). The available evidence comes from a widely heterogeneous collection of studies, and the main objective of this chapter is to present a comprehensive and up-to-date summary of the existing literature on this topic. A thorough neuropsychological evaluation of TS patients can facilitate an individualized approach to meeting each patient's needs. Tailored neuropsychological testing for children with TS may be particularly useful. For example, in detecting specific learning disabilities. The impact of comorbid disorders is a very important aspect of cognitive assessment in TS. Although patients with comorbid attention-deficit/hyperactivity disorder are more likely display weaknesses in motor skills, cognitive flexibility, written expression, and attention, even individuals with pure TS may display problems with motor dexterity, sustained attention, emotion control, and social cognition. A group of TS patients might exhibit specific areas of neuropsychological strength. This area of research is in its dawning age but might contribute to promoting the individual's success and resiliency in life.

THE ASSESSMENT of neuropsychological function in Tourette syndrome (TS) is crucial in order to extend our understanding of both the cognitive changes involved in this condition and related alterations in brain structure and function. Furthermore, greater insight into the cognitive difficulties experienced by individuals with TS can inform the development of targeted therapeutic interventions. A review of the studies of cognitive function in TS and how this may apply to therapeutic and educational intervention is both pertinent and timely. In this chapter, we review evidence of the impact of TS on broader cognitive functions and more specific executive abilities. These skills can have a critical impact on both academic achievement (St Clair-Thompson & Gathercole, 2006) and everyday functioning (Hanks et al., 1999). Neuropsychological assessment will therefore prove particularly invaluable in young people with TS who experience complications related

to school-based learning or activities of daily living in association with their condition. In this chapter, we cover both child and adult neuropsychological assessment. However, it should not be assumed that findings at one developmental level will generalize across the lifespan, and assessment of the same cognitive domains may differ in children and adults.

Research to date indicates that individuals with TS may show problems with attention, memory, and language when compared with people without TS. Such challenges may affect performance in other cognitive or academic areas and may be associated with an increased rate of specific learning disabilities in people with TS. Executive functions (e.g., planning, organization, decision making, self-regulation) may also be vulnerable to impairment, although mixed performance across studies highlights a possible contribution of co-occurring conditions such as obsessive-compulsive disorder

(OCD) or attention-deficit/hyperactivity disorder (ADHD), detailed in Chapters 2 and 3. Aspects of cognition critical for social and emotional processes are only just beginning to be explored, but could offer greater understanding into the range of behavioral problems seen in people with TS.

While many studies have identified cognitive weaknesses associated with TS, recent investigations have uncovered intriguing evidence of possible strengths in certain aspects of neuropsychological functioning, including speeded processing of language or enhancement of cognitive control. The possibility of TS being associated with particular cognitive or behavioral strengths is also discussed in Chapter 29, which describes evidence of enhanced creative ability. Such findings emphasize the need for thorough neuropsychological assessment and encourage further study aimed at identifying ways in which these strengths may be drawn upon to compensate for areas of neuropsychological vulnerability.

INTELLECTUAL FUNCTION

Our review of neuropsychological function in individuals with TS will consider performance on tasks assessing a range of cognitive abilities. These include memory, learning, attention, linguistic ability, motor skills, and aspects of executive function. However, to achieve a good understanding of relative cognitive strengths and vulnerabilities, it is useful to consider where a level of global function might lie. We therefore first focus on the most usual evaluation of global function in cognition: the assessment of intellectual function. A measure of intellectual function in TS may guide assessment of other neuropsychological domains and, importantly, inform intervention.

There appears to be no obvious reason why people with TS should present with lower levels of general intellectual function. Rather, if there is reduced performance in intellectual function in specific indices, it is likely to be associated with factors such as the presence of a co-occurring condition. Schuerholz and colleagues (1996) administered the Wechsler

Intelligence Scale for Children (WISC-R) and the Woodcock-Johnson Psychoeducational Battery-Revised (WJ-R; Bracken & McCallum, 1993) to a group of 65 schoolchildren with TS. Twenty-one participants had TS alone (i.e., no comorbidities), 19 had TS+ADHD, and 25 exhibited attention difficulties that had not been evaluated in sufficient detail to reach a diagnosis of ADHD (TS ± ADHD). The TS-alone group had the highest Full-Scale IQ (FSIQ), with a mean of 117, followed by the TS±ADHD group (mean = 109). A control group (n = 27) also attained a FSIQ above the normal population (mean = 110), but below the pure-TS group. The TS+ADHD group attained a mean FSIQ closer to the general population mean (FSIQ = 103). There was a statistically significant difference between the pure-TS and TS+ADHD groups in terms of intellectual abilities. The authors did not offer an explanation for the stronger performance of the pure-TS group relative to the other groups, and similar results have not been replicated. Nonetheless, these data suggest that FSIQ in people with TS is unlikely to be lower than the general population average.

Controlling for ADHD is clearly important in the evaluation of general cognitive function in children with TS. Brand and colleagues (2002) reported that 23 children with TS alone scored significantly better than 17 children with TS+ADHD in terms of both verbal IQ (VIQ) and performance IQ (PIQ). Another study carried out by Huckeba and colleagues (2008) reported on 47 children with TS (including some with OCD or ADHD) and 18 controls. Mean scores for both groups fell within the average range. However, control participants attained significantly higher VIQ and PIQ than the TS group. This difference was largely attributable to performance on the Coding subtest of the WISC-R, a timed measure of visual-motor integration, which requires sustained attention. Interestingly, FSIQ and performance on the Test of Variables of Attention (TOVA; Greenberg, 1990), a measure of sustained attention and response inhibition, were positively correlated in the TS group. These findings suggest that IQ tasks requiring sustained attention/timed visual-motor abilities are most vulnerable to impairment in children with TS, and that therefore when the recorded FSIQ is lower, this may be due to attention problems. In relation to scholastic application, Brand and colleagues reported that TS participants with slower response time on the TOVA performed less well on a measure of math calculation (Kaufman Test of Educational Achievement [KTEA]; Kaufman & Kaufman, 1985). The authors noted that in children at risk for multiple diagnoses, standardized individual assessment of attention is preferable to reliance on diagnostic behavioral categories.

A recent study carried out by Debes and colleagues (2011) assessed 266 children with TS (including TS-alone, TS+ADHD, TS+OCD, and TS+ADHD+OCD groups) using the Wechsler Intelligence Scales–Third Edition. Controls exhibited significantly higher mean PIQ and FSIQ than patients with TS. The TS-alone group underperformed on the Block Design subtest (a measure of timed visual-spatial processing) and Coding (referred to as Digit Symbol in the paper) when compared with controls. The TS+ADHD group achieved lower scores on the Arithmetic subtest, a measure of active short-term memory/sustained attention. No effects of medication or tic severity (as assessed using the Yale Global Tic Severity Scale; Leckman et al., 1989) were noted, although the fluctuating nature of tics may complicate assessment of the latter factor. Of interest, Debes and colleagues (2011) found that for each year older the age of onset of tics had occurred, the child attained a PIQ one point higher. This outcome may be related to the severity of tics overall or the amount of subcortical involvement (Wang et al., 2011). Longitudinal assessment of the relationship between age of onset and PIQ alongside a measure of developmental neurophysiology could therefore prove informative.

In summary, studies investigating IQ in TS have raised the possibility of variation in relation to verbal and nonverbal abilities. Differences identified so far may relate to the chronicity or severity of tics, and/or the co-occurrence of other conditions. Whatever the case, it is important to consider how challenges with timed motor tasks may affect an individual with TS on a day-to-day basis. The addition of a measure of

adaptive behavior such as the Vineland Adaptive Behavior Scales (Sparrow et al., 2005) may also be beneficial in understanding an individual's general day-to-day function.

SPECIFIC LEARNING DIFFICULTIES

There is an overrepresentation of children with tics in special education placement (e.g., Kurlan et al., 2001), although the causes for this remain unclear. One obvious explanation for this is an increased need for educational support for children with tics, as is described comprehensively in Chapter 29. Specific learning disabilities (SpLDs) have traditionally been diagnosed based on a significant discrepancy between standardized scores of academic achievement and an individual's cognitive ability, although this is changing. More recent diagnostic approaches have emphasized the identification of selective cognitive deficits that are thought to underlie a particular behavioral SpLD. An example of this is the presence of phonological processing deficits and working memory impairments in children with developmental dyslexia (Morton & Frith, 1995). The prevalence of any single SpLD is difficult to estimate due to high levels of comorbidity but may be between 15% and 20% in the general child population (Brook and Boaz, 2005).

Different studies have offered different prevalence rates of SpLD in TS. Basing their estimates on discrepancy-based definitions, Burd and colleagues (1992) found that 51% of their sample met criteria for SpLD. Schuerholz and colleagues (1996) employed a similar definition (Maryland State Department of Education, 1986) and used cluster scores. In comparison to a prevalence of 9% in controls, they found no SpLD in the pure-TS group. Of participants with TS+ADHD, 31% were diagnosed with SpLD (mostly within the written language domain). Twenty-eight percent of participants with TS±ADHD met criteria for SpLD. The overall frequency of SpLD in participants with TS was 23%, in accordance with Abwender and colleagues (1996) but lower than estimates presented by Burd and colleagues (1991), perhaps because Burd and colleagues used achievement test composite scores in calculating discrepancy with IQ rather than single test scores. Across studies there are discrepancies not only in the prevalence but also in the type of SpLD. However, mathematics (particularly arithmetic skills) and written language appear to be the domains most vulnerable to impairment in individuals with TS.

Burd and colleagues (2005) presented more recent data from a registry database involving 5,500 individuals (the Tourette Syndrome International Consortium Database). In this clinical cohort, SpLD was diagnosed using the broad description of learning disorder not otherwise specified (LDNOS) criteria. Individuals with generalized learning disability were excluded and no standardized psychometric evaluation was carried out. From this large service-based cohort, the TS+LD subgroup consisted of 22.7% of the entire cohort, of whom 36% (about 8.1% of the whole cohort) had no comorbid disorders. Individuals with TS+LD were more likely to be male, have earlier tic onset (before age 8), exhibit coprophenomena, and have experienced perinatal complications (27%) in comparison to those with TS and no SpLD. Comorbid ADHD appeared to be a further risk factor for SpLD, highlighting the limitation associated with not controlling for this comorbidity.

In summary, it is difficult to draw conclusions from the literature due to inconsistencies across studies. However, it is likely that children with TS are at increased risk for SpLD, particularly when comorbid ADHD is present.

MEMORY

Memory encompasses different processes. Declarative memory relates to information that can be consciously recalled (e.g., remembering facts), while nondeclarative or procedural memory (e.g., how to ride a bicycle) is not easily available to consciousness (Squire & Zola, 1996). Given the complex neuropsychological profile of people with TS, consideration of many aspects of memory is critical for thorough assessment.

Studies have investigated declarative memory in relation to visual and verbal information. Evidence for deficits on measures of visual memory performance in TS was provided by Watkins and colleagues (2005), who reported spatial recognition memory deficits in a group of 20 adults with TS, of whom only 3 exhibited comorbid ADHD. Another study found evidence of poor performance on a design-recall task in 32 adolescents with TS (Sutherland et al., 1982). While aspects of visual memory appear vulnerable in people with TS, studies have provided equivocal evidence for deficits in verbal memory recall. Channon and colleagues (2003a) found little evidence of difficulties with story recall in children with TS who had no comorbidities and minor performance differences on a word list learning test between the TS group and controls. However, another study by Channon and colleagues (2003b) reported stronger evidence of impairment in adults with pure TS, who exhibited evidence of poor strategic encoding or retrieval when tested both immediately and after a delay.

It is probable that implicit memory processes, including procedural memory, nonassociative learning, and priming, could be affected in TS, given the likelihood of subcortical pathology (e.g., Baym et al., 2008; Peterson et al., 2003). Stebbins and colleagues (1995) investigated procedural memory in adults with TS without ADHD and reported deficits on a rotary pursuit task (participants were required to hold a stylus in their hand and maintain contact with a rotating spot). Marsh and colleagues (2005) used a similar task with 50 children and adults with TS and 55 controls. Learning on the task was intact in both age groups. These discrepant findings may be linked to the longer task used in Stebbins and colleagues' (1995) study that resulted in skill measurement at a different stage of learning, and thus associated with a different neural substrate (Marsh et al., 2005).

Stebbins and colleagues (1995) concluded that memory deficits were most apparent on measures of more effortful or strategic cognitive function in TS, which could explain the variation in findings across studies. However, deficits on some memory tasks could reflect problems with executive functioning or inhibitory processes, such as the intrusions reported on a list learning task in one study (Mahone et al., 2001).

In summary, there is inconsistent evidence of deficits in procedural (or "automatic") memory in TS, and this is likely to reflect the difference in measures used across studies. Visual and procedural aspects of memory appear worthy of further research, although studies should control for the possible influence of attention deficits.

LEARNING

The basal ganglia, which are thought to be dysfunctional in TS, appear to be important for learning implicit associations in addition to procedural skills. Keri and colleagues (2002) used a probabilistic classification task to assess implicit learning of associated probabilities in adults with TS. Participants were asked to decide whether combinations of geometric forms (cues) predicted good or bad weather, before being given feedback about the accuracy of their prediction. The geometric cues were probabilistically related to the weather outcomes, such that cue A would predict sunshine with high probability and cue B would predict rain with high probability. However, the relationship between the cue and weather outcome was not absolute (i.e., rain would occasionally follow cue A, and vice versa). Participants were therefore required to learn the likelihood of an association rather than a set cue–outcome rule. Previous studies have shown that people with amnesia (with medial temporal lobe damage) perform well on this kind of task (Knowlton, Squire & Gluck, 1994), whereas patients with degenerative conditions affecting the basal ganglia perform poorly (Knowlton et al., 1996). Keri and colleagues (2002) reported that children with TS performed significantly more poorly on this task than matched controls, especially those with more severe tics. In fact, there was a negative relationship between tic severity and performance.

Similar findings were reported by Marsh and colleagues (2004), who found deficits on "habit learning" weather prediction task in participants with TS. The presence of co-occurring conditions was not related to task performance, but rate of learning was better in participants with lower tic severity. These findings could have implications for behavioral interventions and perhaps decision-making processes in TS in that individuals with better control over tics/fewer tics/better executive function may benefit most from certain psychological interventions.

Findings from some studies suggest that performance on memory and learning tasks in TS may be related to neurochemical changes. Palminteri and colleagues (2009) examined the effects of dopaminergic drugs on a subliminal instrumental learning paradigm in TS. In this paradigm, participants had to learn the value of a risky choice from feedback about monetary outcomes (reward or punishment), which was masked and so could not be consciously perceived. Participants with TS taking dopamine antagonists showed poorer reward learning and good loss avoidance, but there was no significant difference between unmedicated patients and controls. These findings imply that neurochemical alterations in people with TS may have the potential to alter implicit learning processes.

In summary, it will be useful for future studies to further investigate both implicit and explicit learning in TS. Previous work has highlighted the importance of considering both the valence of cues and rewards, and controlling for medications when conducting studies of learning in TS.

ATTENTION

People with TS may experience reduced attentional resources due to tic suppression or comorbid ADHD. From an alternative perspective, individuals with TS could be less able to inhibit tics due to deficits with attention (Woods et al., 2008). In this section, two major types of attention control are discussed. The first is reflexively or exogenously driven attention, whereby stimulus-driven attention occurs via a bottom-up process due to a salient aspect of a stimulus (e.g., noticing a physical property of a stimulus). The second system involves selective or endogenously driven attention and is referred to as a top-down process (e.g., focusing on one detail while ignoring others). In this case the impulse to attend is goal-driven and controlled by the individuals themselves. Exogenous and endogenous attentional processes are proposed to involve different but associated brain mechanisms (Shomstein et al., 2010). Studies have used behavioral data and psychophysiological measurement to assess these attentional processes in people with TS.

Channon and colleagues (1992) reported behavioral deficits on endogenous attention tasks such as the Trail Making Test (TMT; Reitan, 1958), a serial addition task, and a vigilance test in adults with TS when compared to control participants with equivalent IQ. Another study (Bornstein & Yang, 2001) reported significant deficits on both the TMT and the Speech Sounds Perception Test (SSPT; Golden & Anderson, 1977; Halstead, 1947) when scores from children and adolescents with TS were compared to normative data. However, almost half of the sample exhibited ADHD in addition to TS. Conflicting findings were reported by Silverstein and colleagues (1995), who found no evidence that individuals with TS alone performed more poorly on the TMT than controls, whereas the co-occurrence of ADHD had a detrimental effect on performance. Other studies have failed to find evidence of attentional deficits in TS (Bornstein et al., 1991; Drake et al., 1992), even in individuals with comorbid ADHD (Brand et al., 2002). However, two studies did report attentional difficulties that appeared intrinsic to TS.

Shucard and colleagues (1997) assessed the performance of 22 boys with TS and 22 matched controls on a continuous performance task (CPT). The task consisted of 400 single-letter trials presented over a 12-minute period. Targets were designated as the letter "X" preceded by a specific letter. Children with TS showed significantly slower reaction times than controls. A relationship was found between complex vocal tics and reaction time, suggesting that longer reaction time may have resulted from tic suppression. A CPT was also used by Sherman and colleagues (1998), who assessed sustained attention in three groups of children: TS alone, TS+ADHD, and ADHD alone. Sustained attention was unaffected in the sample with pure TS. Deficits were noted in the ADHD and TS+ADHD groups, and of these, the TS+ADHD group performed better.

Some studies have looked at exogenous and endogenous attentional processes in groups with TS using event-related potentials (ERPs). Van Woerkom and colleagues (1994) used ERPs to assess a passive listening paradigm in a group of children with TS and matched controls. The groups attended to tones (exogenous attention task) and then had to press a button to identify deviant tones (discrimination paradigm involving endogenous attention). The TS group exhibited a significantly larger N1 and a significantly smaller P1 than control children during the discrimination paradigm, indicating reduced efficiency in orienting attention endogenously. Another ERP study (Johannes et al., 1997) found that despite similar performance to controls on simple attention tasks, adults with TS showed increased N2, demonstrating greater attentional effort. Adults with TS performed less accurately on a more complex feature conjunction task, and results indicated a speed-accuracy trade-off. Unfortunately, comorbidity was not controlled for in this study.

In summary, patients with TS are vulnerable to difficulties with focusing attention and can appear easily distracted. These attentional problems are likely to be more subtle in patients with TS alone, but the influence of tic suppression on performance has, as yet, not been well explored. It is important to supplement individual standardized testing with validated self-report measures from important others in the individual's life (i.e., parents, partners, teachers) to assess everyday function.

LINGUISTIC SKILLS

Available findings in relation to linguistic function may be considered preliminary, as a limited number of studies have investigated non–tic-related language and very few have applied specific linguistic measures. The focus of research carried out so far has been on vocal tic-related linguistic impairment (e.g., speech dysfluency) and has not addressed specific higher-order organizational levels of language, which again may be pertinent in relation to procedural language abilities.

Speech Dysfluency

A few studies have investigated speech dysfluency in association with TS. Abwender and colleagues (1998) found a history of tics in 11 of 22 participants (50%) with dysfluency. De Nil and colleagues (2005) also reported an increased prevalence of dysfluency (but not stuttering) in children with TS. The authors further noted that tics and dysfluency show several overlapping phenomenological features, such as a genetic link, higher frequency in males, childhood onset, waxing and waning developmental course with improvement with time, suppressibility, and exacerbation by stress. Assessment of stuttering in cases of TS may be complicated by the presence of palilalia (i.e., the repetition or echoing of one's own words).

Language

Language deficits in TS were reported by Brookshire and colleagues (1994), who compared 31 individuals with TS (aged 6–16 years) to 20 sibling controls and 10 individuals with arithmetic disabilities. Like the children with arithmetic disabilities, the TS group demonstrated poorer performance than controls on written arithmetic tasks. However, while the group with arithmetic disabilities demonstrated generalized nonverbal deficiencies, children with TS demonstrated more specific impairments on expressive language measures and measures of complex cognition compared with the sibling group. Unfortunately, no information about comorbid conditions was given for the TS sample.

Other studies have reported no evidence of language difficulties. For example, Channon and colleagues (2003b) reported intact performance on a stem completion task requiring analysis of established lexical representations and priming in TS. In another study, Schuerholz and colleagues (1996) analyzed lexical access using the Boston Naming Test (Kaplan & Goodglass, 1978) and the Rapid Automatized Naming Test (Denckla & Rudel, 1976) and rule-governed knowledge using a phoneme elision task (Vellutino & Scanlon, 1987). The TS-alone group performed better than either the TS+ADHD or TS±ADHD groups and no differently from controls.

Legg and colleagues (2005) assessed 10 adolescents with TS using a test battery sensitive to high-level language and discourse impairment (Test of Language Competence; Wiig & Secord, 1989). Participants with TS were compared to standardized data and a typically developing group. A relationship was observed between increased tic severity (rated as motor disturbance and tic severity) and poorer communicative competence (i.e., their language was verbose, dysfluent, tangential, or unrelated to the topic). Five participants exhibited communicative deficits involving disorganized output, concreteness of language, and poor language formulation abilities. Of note, all of these participants had co-occurring OCD or ADHD symptoms.

Concreteness of language could be linked to the difficulties found on a story task assessing pragmatic language skills in a group with TS (Eddy et al., 2010b). The authors documented impairment in understanding nonliteral sarcastic and metaphorical remarks in a sample of 18 adults with TS. Furthermore, deficits were present in participants with TS alone. The same individuals were able to correctly determine that literal remarks were contextually appropriate and that nonsense statements did not make sense. These rather specific difficulties interpreting nonliteral language could reflect changes in theory of mind (the understanding of mental states), as appreciation of the speaker's mental state is needed to understand a nonliteral remark. However, since many errors were linked to incorrect literal interpretations, the difficulties identified could also reflect a generally superficial style of language interpretation, perhaps as a result of reduced attentional resources.

At least one study has suggested that aspects of language function could be enhanced in children with TS. Walenski and colleagues (2007) tested the processing of idiosyncratic and rule-governed linguistic knowledge. While idiosyncratic knowledge (e.g., irregular past tense formation; *bring–brought*) is thought to be stored in a mental lexicon that depends on the temporal lobe-based declarative memory system, it is likely that rule-governed combination in grammar (e.g., in regular past tenses; *walk + -ed*) relies on the frontal/basal-ganglia-based procedural memory system (which may also subserve procedural motor skills). Walenski and colleagues found that children and adolescents with TS (n = 8: 1 TS+ADHD, 1 TS+OCD+ADHD) were significantly faster than control children in producing rule-governed past tenses (*slip–slipped*) but not irregular and other unpredictable past tenses (*bring–brought*). They were also faster than controls when naming pictures of physically manipulated items (e.g., *hammer*), but this was not the case for nonmanipulated items (e.g., *elephant*). The authors suggest that the processing of procedurally based knowledge, both in relation to grammar and manipulated objects, is speeded in TS. This finding is yet to be replicated.

In summary, there are difficulties drawing conclusions about the impact of TS on language processing, as few systematic studies have been conducted. However, previous studies suggest that comorbid ADHD may lead to an increased likelihood of expressive language problems. Further research should address more complex aspects of linguistic understanding such as interpretation of pragmatic communication in TS alone. It may also be helpful to assess the presence of speech dysfluency (particularly in children) and how this may affect other linguistic processes in people with TS.

VISUOMOTOR INTEGRATION AND VISUAL PERCEPTUAL SKILLS

Although studies on motor coordination in TS are few, findings tend to suggest that this domain may be vulnerable in children and adults with TS. One related drawback is that early studies often relied on the use of published normative data rather than matched control groups.

In the 1990s, Bornstein and colleagues (Bornstein, 1990, 1991; Yeates & Bornstein, 1994) evaluated over 160 people with TS on several tests of gross- and fine-motor skills. Individuals with TS performed well on tasks of simple motor speed that made few visual

perceptual demands, but exhibited impairment in skills dependent on visual perceptual processing (e.g., placing pegs into grooves of differing angles). This performance profile was apparent in both pure TS and TS+ADHD.

Bloch and colleagues (2006) assessed 32 children with TS (aged 8–14), using the Developmental Test of Visuomotor Integration (VMI; Beery, 1997) and the Purdue Pegboard test (Tiffin, 1968). Consistent with previous studies, performance in the TS group on the VMI task was noted to be impaired (Brookshire et al., 1994; Schultz et al., 1998) but was not predictive of tic severity or long-term outcome. Participants were reassessed an average of 7.5 years later. At follow-up assessment, poorer performance with the dominant hand on the Purdue Pegboard test predicted adulthood tic severity, and correlated with tic severity at the time of baseline childhood assessment. Deficits on the Purdue Pegboard test with both the dominant and nondominant hand also predicted lower global psychosocial functioning in adulthood. Bloch and colleagues suggested that performance on the Purdue Pegboard test may serve as a useful endophenotype, providing a crude measure of the degree of basal ganglia dysfunction present. However, some of the participants in this study were medicated with dopaminergic agents, which could have affected motor performance.

Similar measures (Purdue Pegboard test and Beery VMI-IV) were used in a later study by Sukhodolsky and colleagues (2010), who assessed the performance of 56 individuals with TS alone, 45 with TS+ADHD, 64 with ADHD alone, and 71 controls. The ADHD group was more impaired on measures of VMI than the other groups. Participants with pure TS exhibited no significant deficits on the VMI. However, boys (but not girls) with TS alone demonstrated significant difficulties with motor speed and manual dexterity in their dominant hand on the Purdue Pegboard test. Sukhodolsky and colleagues (2010) suggested that this finding could imply that tics have a different developmental course according to gender, which is in agreement with differences found in activation and thinning in the frontoparietal regions in males but not females (Fahim et al., 2010; Peterson et al., 2001).

A few studies have used the Rey Complex Figure Task (RCFT; Meyers & Meyers, 1995), a test in which participants first copy a complex line drawing and then reproduce the figure from memory. Evidence for deficits on the RCFT in TS populations is mixed. Lavoie and colleagues (2007) detected abnormalities on the RCFT in adults with TS compared to age-, gender-, and IQ-matched control participants. Moreover, lower RCFT scores were associated with tic severity. Harris and colleagues (1995) and Schuerholz and colleagues (1996) found evidence for deficits in children with TS+ADHD, but not in TS alone. Two studies that controlled for ADHD comorbidity found better RCFT performance in TS alone than TS+ADHD, suggesting that attention or impulsivity deficits may contribute to the visuomotor integration deficit previously reported in TS (Bloch et al., 2006). Schultz and colleagues (1998) showed that RCFT or VMI performance differences were not apparent between groups with TS alone and individuals with co-occurring ADHD. However, both groups with TS alone and TS+ADHD performed significantly worse than age-matched controls. The authors suggested that the VMI task was a better predictor of TS than the RCFT, which places a stronger emphasis on executive functions. Finally, Chang and colleagues (2007) showed that participants with OCD demonstrate difficulties on the RCFT, while deficits on this task were not evident in children with TS alone. If deficits are indeed evident on the RCFT, determining the cause of poor performance can be difficult, given that memory and attention are likely to contribute to performance in addition to visuomotor abilities. There is also the element of motor dexterity, which although critical for performance on the Purdue Pegboard test is not used as a scoring criterion in most of the RCFT scoring systems.

In summary, visuomotor performance appears to be poorer in TS if finer visual-perceptual discrimination is required, and when performance is timed. There is currently little evidence of deficits in visual-perceptual skills, although few studies have been conducted in this area. Earlier age of onset could be associated with poorer task performance. Studies indicate that slow motor dexterity could be linked with persistent tics into adulthood and poorer psychosocial outcome.

MOTOR SKILLS AND COORDINATION

Given that TS involves the motor system (Wang et al., 2011), it may be expected that aspects of motor coordination may differ in individuals with TS when compared with typically developing individuals.

Margolis and colleagues (2006) investigated interhemispheric interference and coordination in adults with TS. Participants with TS were impaired on the bimanual Purdue Pegboard test when compared to controls: right-hand performance was similar for the groups, but the expected left-hand advantage was not seen in the TS group. It is thought that the frontal cortex may contribute to the left-hand advantage during bimanual coordination by minimizing interference effects, so these findings could be indicative of frontal dysfunction in the TS group. The presence of TS was also associated with increased between-hemisphere interference on a verbal–manual interference task: the TS group were less able than controls to inhibit interference between right-hemisphere motor regions and left-hemisphere language systems. Margolis and colleagues therefore concluded that interhemispheric interference is greater in TS. The authors linked their findings to smaller dorsal anterior prefrontal cortex volumes and possible compensatory increases in the size of the corpus callosum in the TS group.

Another study (Avanzino et al., 2011) assessed bimanual coordination in children with TS. Young people with TS showed faster movement and longer touch time and made more errors than controls when performing sequential single-hand finger movements in comparison to healthy controls. The TS group did not show the loss of accuracy and increase in touch duration seen in controls when they performed the task bimanually. Perhaps of most interest was the finding that children with TS also showed less asymmetry than controls (in terms of movement accuracy) between right and left hands. Avanzino and colleagues suggested that their findings may be linked to altered structural and functional organization of interhemispheric connections in TS. These findings add to other reports of reduced asymmetry between hand movements (Georgiou et al., 1995). Such findings prompt the speculation that some of these differences in sensorimotor integration seen in TS could actually lead to enhanced performance of particular motor tasks.

Alterations in the timing of motor performance are also linked to the findings by Vicario and colleagues (2010). Time processing abilities were compared in young patients with pure TS and matched controls using a time reproduction task and another task involving the perceptual judgment of the length of time intervals. There was no difference between the groups for the perceptual judgment task. However, participants with TS showed better reproduction accuracy for intervals above 1 second, and were similar to controls for intervals below 1 second. Interestingly, tic severity was negatively correlated with reproduction accuracy for intervals over 1 second. Motor timing task performance was not related to performance on executive measures. Vicario and colleagues (2010) suggested that compensatory neural changes related to tic control (e.g., alterations in dorsolateral prefrontal cortex) could help explain their findings.

A recent study by Wang and colleagues (2011) showed a relationship between activation in sensorimotor loops (i.e., higher levels of activity in the motor portions of cortico-striato-thalamo-cortical circuits and reduced activity in the anterior cingulate and caudate) and self-reports of tics in participants with TS, which differed from participants who merely simulated tics. Such findings prompt further investigation of the sensorimotor components associated with tics, and whether these differ from those associated with voluntary movements in individuals without TS.

In summary, TS may be associated with enhanced abilities in terms of specific aspects of motor performance. Investigating interhemispheric interference effects or greater connectivity between motor and language systems in TS may have the potential to shed light on the neurocognitive mechanisms underlying more complex tics. For example, it may be interesting to consider how this increase in "mirroring" during bimanual actions may be linked to tics involving symmetry or "evening-up."

EXECUTIVE FUNCTION

Tests of executive function assess higher cognitive abilities, such as working memory (WM) and response inhibition. Evidence of dysexecutive behavior in everyday life in TS (Crawford et al., 2005) requires the investigation of specific executive abilities. Many executive tasks are thought to activate the dorsolateral prefrontal and anterior cingulate cortices, while the orbitofrontal cortex may make a more selective contribution to performance on tasks involving reward-related learning (Zgaljardic et al., 2006). Reviewing the pattern of performance in individuals with TS across tasks assessing different aspects of executive function could therefore offer insight into alterations within specific frontostriatal circuits in TS (Eddy et al., 2009).

Assessment of Everyday Executive Functioning in TS

Rasmussen and colleagues (2009) used parent and teacher ratings on the Behavioral Inventory of Executive Function (BRIEF; Gioia et al., 2000) to investigate neuropsychological profiles in a group of 38 children with TS alone, TS+OCD, or TS+ADHD. While no differences were found between TS+OCD and TS alone, TS+ADHD was associated with significantly poorer scores on the BRIEF parent rating scales for metacognition index and global executive composite. Teacher scores for the whole TS group indicated significantly more difficulties than parent report scores, which may suggest that executive function difficulties present more in the school-based rather than home-based context. These findings are in agreement with Mahone and colleagues (2001), who reported lower BRIEF scores in TS+ADHD versus TS alone, highlighting the importance of including multiple report sources whenever possible.

Working Memory

WM tasks require online manipulation of information in addition to encoding and recall processes. The N-back task has been used to assess WM in participants with TS. This task requires a participant to match a current stimulus with the same stimulus previously presented *n* times earlier in the sequence (Braver et al., 1997). Studies of participants with TS alone provide little evidence of verbal WM deficits in children (Crawford et al., 2005) or adults (Channon et al., 2006). Digit span performance can also be intact in adults with TS (Goudriaan et al., 2006). Another study (Eddy et al., 2010a) showed that a group of 16 adult patients (10 with TS alone) obtained similar manipulation span scores compared to controls on a digit reordering task. In relation to visual WM, Goudriaan and colleagues (2006) found no deficits on the Benton Visual Recognition Test (Sivan, 1992) in an adult TS group with a low prevalence of OCD and ADHD. However, Rasmussen and colleagues (2009) reported evidence of spatial WM deficits in a mixed group of children with TS, particularly in older children. Verte and colleagues (2005) reported that TS was a good predictor of visual WM on the Corsi Blocks Test (Corsi, 1972) in children with TS, although the effect disappeared when ADHD was controlled for. Comorbidity may also have contributed to a deficit on the Corsi Blocks Test in adults with TS who were not screened for this factor (Channon et al., 1992).

In summary, the evidence in favor of WM difficulties in TS is not particularly strong (Ozonoff & Strayer, 2001), and many reported deficits could reflect the effect of comorbid conditions. Visuospatial WM can appear more vulnerable than verbal WM in people with TS, although this finding remains equivocal.

Verbal Fluency

Verbal fluency tasks require attention, memory, and inhibition (e.g., of previously said words) and may therefore be considered to fall within the executive functioning category. Some findings are suggestive of verbal fluency impairments in children and adolescents (Bornstein, 1990; Sutherland et al., 1982) and in adults (Bornstein, 1991b) with TS, although many studies could have been influenced by the presence of comorbidities, with comorbid ADHD being particularly strongly implicated (Mahone et al., 2001; Schuerholz et al., 1998; Verte et al., 2005). Nonetheless, TS may still be a good predictor of poor verbal fluency performance in children (Schuerholz et al., 1998; Verte et al., 2005), and indeed a few studies have provided evidence of verbal fluency deficits even in TS alone (Schuerholz et al., 1996). For example, one recent study documented a deficit in phonological fluency in a subgroup of adult participants with TS alone (Eddy et al., 2011). Other studies reported no evidence of deficits in children or adolescents (Channon et al., 2003a) and adult TS samples (Stebbins et al., 1995). The likelihood of reliable deficits in verbal fluency in TS is further weakened by results from two studies that included measures of semantic fluency and reported no difficulties (Goudriaan et al., 2006; Watkins et al., 2005).

In summary, further work is needed to determine whether the mild deficits on verbal fluency tasks in TS could be linked to attention difficulties, inhibitory problems, or vocabulary limitations. Future studies should investigate the possibility that phonological fluency tasks are more vulnerable to impairment in TS than semantic fluency tasks.

Planning and Multitasking

A number of studies have reported that individuals with TS have no difficulty with tasks involving planning and problem solving, such as the Tower of London (Watkins et al., 2005) or Tower of Hanoi (Ozonoff & Jensen, 1999) tests. Intact performance has been demonstrated by both children (Verte et al., 2005) and adults (Goudriaan et al., 2006) with TS. Similarly, no deficits in multitasking were reported by two studies involving adults (Channon et al., 2003a, 2004). However, the presence of comorbid ADHD appears to make multitasking more vulnerable (Channon et al., 2003b).

In summary, although limited investigations have been carried out, planning and multitasking deficits look unlikely, at least in adults with TS. Having said this, further investigation of multitasking abilities in children may be merited, given that these tasks are likely to make considerable demands in terms of planning and attention shifting.

Shifting and Cognitive Flexibility

Switching or shifting deficits are fairly uncommon in TS on tasks involving object alternation (Change tal.,2007; Channon et al.,2006). Adults with TS alone have demonstrated intact shifting performance on a letter-and-digit-naming task (Channon et al., 2006). One study reported no set-shifting deficits in adults with TS, including individuals with comorbid ADHD (Brand et al., 2002), whereas another (Watkins et al., 2005) found evidence for poor extradimensional shifting in a group of adults with TS and a low prevalence of comorbid ADHD.

The Wisconsin Card Sorting Test (WCST; Berg, 1948) is often used to assess set shifting in TS, and many studies have reported intact performance on this task for children and adolescents with TS, even when comorbidities are present (Bornstein, 1991b; Bornstein & Yang, 2001; Channon et al., 2003b; Ozonoff & Jensen, 1999; Sutherland et al., 1982). Adults with TS alone also perform well (Channon et al., 2003b, 2004). Deficits on the WCST have been linked to dorsolateral prefrontal cortex damage (Milner, 1963), so intact performance may be suggestive of normal dorsolateral prefrontal functioning. Further research is needed in this area, given that some authors (Pennington & Ozonoff, 1996) suggest the WCST may not be sensitive enough to highlight subtle deficits.

In summary, cognitive flexibility may be relatively intact in TS, although problems may be more likely if comorbid OCD is present.

Inhibition

Attention has been drawn to the possibility of deficient inhibitory mechanisms in TS, as a tic is often preceded by an urge that the individual struggles to resist. On the other hand, there is growing evidence for possible strengths in cognitive control in TS. The assessment of inhibitory function is complicated by the definition of this construct and the likely existence of separable facets of this ability with different underlying neural substrates.

Many studies assessing inhibition in TS have used tasks that require inhibition of a motor response, such as a Go/No Go (GNG) task. This kind of task has revealed no deficits in pure TS (Ozonoff et al., 1994; Roessner et al., 2008) or in participants with comorbidities (Hershey et al., 2004). However, Eichele and colleagues (2010) found that young boys with TS showed slower correct responses than controls, and Müller and colleagues (2003) reported evidence of poor performance on a GNG in a group of 14 participants. These authors claimed that participants' commission errors reflected deficits in response inhibition, as the group performed well on attention measures. However, comorbid OCD could also have contributed to the reported deficits.

One study investigated underlying neural activity in TS during the GNG task. Serrien and colleagues (2005) found that despite no performance deficit, adults with TS exhibited greater activity than controls in the frontomesial network, which was also active during tic suppression. Serrien and colleagues (2005) suggested that these findings indicate decreased inhibitory control in TS, and related compensatory increases in brain activity. These findings are particularly important because compensatory mechanisms have the potential to confound study findings (Roessner et al., 2008).

Inhibitory impairment has been reported in children with TS playing Luria's hand game (Baron-Cohen et al., 1994) and during circle drawing and a change task, in association with comorbid OCD or ADHD (Verte et al., 2005). Goudriaan and colleagues (2006) tested 46 adults with TS (only 2 had comorbid ADHD) and found no deficit on the circle drawing task, but did report evidence of slower stop-signal reaction times in TS versus controls. A flanker task may also be used to assess inhibitory performance. The participant is required to respond to a central item surrounded by distracting symbols (e.g., arrows). Sometimes these distractors are "congruent" and all point to the same direction, but other times they are "incongruent," pointing in different directions. Responses to incongruent items are slower and less accurate due to interference. An adult study reported impaired performance compared to controls on incompatible trials of a flanker test in participants with pure TS (Crawford et al., 2005), although this deficit was not replicated by a later study (Channon et al., 2006). Georgiou and colleagues (1995) used a Simon task, in which adults with TS and controls were presented with an arrow located either to the left or right of center and pressed a button to indicate the direction of the arrow, which was either congruent with spatial location (e.g., a rightward-pointing arrow located to the right of center) or incongruent (e.g., a rightward-pointing arrow located to the left of center). The classic Simon effect, where participants are slower to respond on incongruent than congruent trials, was greater for the TS group than for controls. This finding could reflect greater effects of interference in TS, and less efficient inhibitory processes.

Individuals with TS can also have difficulty inhibiting verbal responses. For example, Baron-Cohen and colleagues (1994) reported deficits on a yes/no inhibition task in children with TS. However, children (Brand et al., 2002; Chang et al., 2007; Ozonoff & Jensen, 1999) and adults (Channon et al., 1992; Goudriaan et al., 2006; Sukhodolsky et al., 2010) with TS perform well on the Stroop task even when comorbidities are present. During this task the participant is asked to name the color of the ink of a list of color words (e.g., the word *blue* printed in red ink, the word *green* printed in yellow ink, etc.). It is assumed that to answer correctly, one must inhibit the automatic tendency to read the word. In one study, a simplified Stroop-style task using black and white boxes was used, which is similar to a traditional Stroop in that the automatic response must be inhibited (i.e., participants name the color or black boxes as being white, and vice versa). A significantly greater effect of interference according to time measures (but not errors) was seen in adults with TS, and this effect was apparent in participants with "pure"

TS (Eddy et al., 2010b). However, a more recent study (Eddy et al., 2011) didn't replicate this finding.

Reports of a deficit on the Hayling test (Burgess & Shallice, 1996) are more persuasive of inhibitory dysfunction in TS. During the Hayling test, participants are read sentences with a word missing at the end. Each sentence is designed to prompt a particular word. The inhibitory demand occurs in the second part of the test, when participants are told that they cannot say this obvious cued response (i.e., the first word they think of) but have to suppress this and think of an alternative answer. Channon et al. (1992, 2006) showed that both adults and children (Crawford et al., 2005) with TS alone tend to exhibit deficits on this test. Impairment on the Hayling test may implicate the involvement of the frontostriatal circuit involving the anterior cingulate cortex (Nathaniel James et al., 1997). As strategy use can influence performance on this task, one study used modified task instructions to help avoid strategy use and reported similar findings indicative of mild inhibitory impairment (Eddy et al., 2010a). However, more work is needed to determine whether participants' impairments may reflect deficits in verbal or conceptual processes (Crawford et al., 2005).

Further evidence of possible inhibitory dysfunction in TS was reported by Mahone and colleagues (2001), who found evidence of intrusions during list learning in children with TS and ADHD. Differences have also been reported in TS on tasks involving negative priming. The negative priming effect is the slower response made to a stimulus that has been shown before in a task but previously had to be ignored. Ozonoff and colleagues (1998) found evidence for reduced inhibition (a smaller negative priming effect) on a negative priming task in youths with TS and comorbidities. However, individuals without comorbidities performed similarly to controls. Such findings highlight the importance of controlling for ADHD when investigating inhibitory impairment in TS.

In summary, inhibitory performance is perhaps more vulnerable to impairment in TS than other executive functions, as possible deficits have been reported in response to motor and verbal stimuli. These deficits are more subtle in people with TS alone compared to those with co-occurring disorders.

A few studies have reported enhanced behavioral performance on certain tasks in carefully selected groups with TS. Mueller and colleagues (2006) used an oculomotor task involving switching between pro-saccade movements and anti-saccade movements. Nine adolescents with TS alone performed more accurately and fluently than controls on the high-demanding cognitive control (anti-saccade oculomotor) task. Mueller and colleagues suggested that the repeated demand to control involuntary tics could result in enhanced inhibitory control. Similar findings were reported by Jackson and colleagues (2007). The oculomotor tasks were modified and tested on seven adolescents with TS, who were carefully screened to exclude any possibility of comorbid conditions. Three of the seven participants were prescribed tic-controlling medication and showed a range of global tic scores on the day of testing. The modified task was less predictable and employed sequences in which the pro- or anti-saccades were presented in a randomized fashion without pre-cue information. Adolescents with TS exhibited greater levels of cognitive control on the eye-saccade task than controls. Finally, Roessner and colleagues (2008) used a GNG with a group of medication-naive adolescents with pure TS and matched controls. No differences were found between the groups in their ability to inhibit responses, and there was a trend for the TS group to respond more rapidly. The authors suggested that patients could be faster at the task because of compensatory mechanisms secondary to tic suppression. These findings could be related to the reduced motor interference reported in TS in studies discussed earlier in this chapter (under "Motor Skills and Coordination"). The findings of these latter studies are intriguing and may suggest areas of cognitive strength in neuropsychological function in certain groups with TS. However, it is unclear how the reported findings involving differences in the speed and accuracy of motor performance may be related to differences in cognitive inhibition processes. Furthermore, investigation is needed to

determine how such enhanced abilities could be reflected in everyday behavior.

Increased cognitive control due to practicing tic suppression could be associated with increased neural activation. In a recent event-related fMRI study (Baym et al., 2008), eighteen 7- to 13-year-old children with TS and 19 healthy controls performed three cognitive control tasks. Higher tic severity was correlated with slower task performance on the most demanding task conditions, and with enhanced activation of dopaminergic nuclei (substantia nigra/ventral tegmental area) and cortical, striatal, and thalamic regions during tasks. Higher tic severity was also associated with greater engagement of the subthalamic nucleus, and the clinical group engaged the left prefrontal cortex more strongly than controls. Unmedicated children with TS therefore exhibit increased activation in the direct pathway through the basal ganglia during demanding cognitive tasks, and increased compensatory activation in prefrontal cortex and the subthalamic nucleus.

Jackson and colleagues (2011) used a manual-switching task that created high levels of interhemispheric conflict with 14 children with TS alone and matched controls. Children with TS showed faster reaction times than controls during mixed switching trials. Furthermore, mixing costs (i.e., performance costs of mixing the two different tasks) and switch costs (i.e., performance costs between two sequentially presented tasks) were reduced in the TS group. Interestingly, there was a positive association between tic severity and reaction time switch costs. This could imply that adolescents with less severe tics had higher levels of cognitive control. Diffusion tensor imaging revealed that the TS group exhibited reduced fractional anisotropy in the corpus callosum and forceps minor, a pathway that connects the lateral and medial areas of the prefrontal cortex. Longitudinal studies are needed to establish whether the enhanced control identified on experimental tasks is due to neuroplastic changes in people with TS.

In translating these studies into clinical practice, the challenge will be to identify clinically relevant measures to determine which individuals with TS may benefit from behavioral therapies, such as habit reversal training (see Chapter 23), which capitalize and use this cognitive strength therapeutically.

EMOTION CONTROL

In this final section, we highlight study findings in an area that could be related to the cognitive alterations already posited to occur in TS. Changes in social and emotional processes could occur both directly through alterations in functioning within frontostriatal circuitry, or indirectly through difficulties with specific executive functions, such as inhibition, which contribute to emotion control and reasoning. We now discuss the evidence for emotion-related changes in TS, with a view to encouraging a broader perspective of the role of cognition in TS to encompass interactions between cognition, emotion, and behavior.

Emotion Regulation

Emotions influence tics, and individuals with TS report that negative emotions such as anxiety or sadness can exacerbate tics (Wood et al., 2003). In fact, emotion control difficulties such as rage or intermittent explosive disorder (IED) are fairly common in TS. Estimates indicate that 25% to 70% of patients with TS in clinical settings report episodic behavioral outbursts and anger control problems (Bruun & Budman, 1998; Budman et al., 2000; Freeman et al., 2000; Riddle et al., 1988; Santangelo et al., 1994; Stefl, 1984; Wand et al., 1993). These emotional outbursts are akin to IED and are precipitated by minimal stimuli that trigger a disproportionate emotional and behavioral reaction, often consisting of physical injury to self and others or damage to objects (Budman et al., 2003).

Episodes of emotion dyscontrol are most common at the more severe end of the TS spectrum. For example, Budman and colleagues (1998) reported that all 12 of their sample of children and adolescents with TS who presented with rage attacks met diagnostic criteria for OCD and ADHD. In a later study (Budman et al., 2008), 29 of 37 children demonstrated evidence of IED, with high rates of psychiatric comorbidity: 31

of 37 (84%) participants met criteria for OCD and 31 of 37 (84%) met criteria for ADHD. Another study reported a relationship between the presence of explosive outbursts and number of comorbid conditions, but not for tic severity (Budman et al., 2000). However, Cavanna and colleagues (2008) investigated anger outbursts in adults and children with TS alone (n = 19) and TS+ADHD (n = 16), and found that the TS-alone group scored significantly higher than the TS+ADHD group on the Anger Expression-Out and Anger Control-Out scales of the State-Trait Anger Expression Inventory-2 (Spielberger et al., 1999). These scales address the expression of anger toward other persons or objects in the environment and the control over such angry feelings, respectively. These findings imply that not all rage is associated with comorbid ADHD and that emotional control difficulties can be intrinsic to TS.

In summary, many people with TS report difficulties with controlling emotional reactions, and such problems may result from TS rather than comorbid conditions. Further work should investigate relationships between impulsive emotional behaviors in TS, inhibitory control, and decision-making processes.

Emotion-Related Reasoning and Social Cognition

Some individuals with TS exhibit changes in emotional processes and related social reasoning that can be associated with autistic spectrum disorders. Although the majority of individuals with TS do not exhibit such pertinent difficulties, a few studies have investigated emotion-related reasoning and social cognition in TS. Two studies reported no performance deficits. This included a study by Baron-Cohen and associates (1997) that included a small sample of individuals with TS as a control group for a study investigating theory of mind (ToM; reasoning about mental states) in autism and Asperger's syndrome. Another study (Channon et al., 2004) investigated the understanding of nonliteral language in adults with TS alone, but their performance indicated no difficulties in understanding the mental states of the story characters and interpreting remarks such as lies or sarcasm. However, another study conducted by Channon and colleagues (2003b) reported evidence of poor reasoning in adults with TS alone on a real-life–type problem-solving task involving difficult social situations. These difficulties were not related to executive deficits. Given the lack of difficulty demonstrated by people with TS on standard problem-solving tasks, it could be that more ecologically valid tasks involving social interaction are more sensitive to the form of difficulties individuals with TS present with.

Three studies carried out by Eddy and colleagues (Eddy et al., 2010a, 2010b, 2011) involving adults with TS have revealed evidence of difficulties on a range of tasks involving ToM. Participants with TS exhibited difficulties in understanding *faux pas* and nonliteral remarks such as sarcasm, and poorer performance than controls on four other tasks involving ToM, including a revised version of the Reading the Mind in the Eyes Task (Baron-Cohen et al., 2001), a task that involved making judgments about matching and conflicting emotional facial expressions and a task involving the understanding of humor in cartoons. Analysis excluding individuals with comorbid conditions revealed these difficulties were present in subgroups of participants with TS alone. Across these three studies, the clinical group exhibited limited evidence of executive dysfunction, and mild inhibitory deficits were uncorrelated with errors on the ToM tasks. However, given the possible insensitivity of some cognitive measures in TS, further research is needed to establish whether such changes are completely independent of subtle or selective difficulties with aspects of executive function.

The above findings indicate that TS can be associated with changes in reasoning on tasks involving emotion and social interaction. These changes may sometimes involve just thinking differently, or perhaps even too much, about emotions and other mental states. However, the performance of participants with TS on a economic decision-making task that involves reasoning about mental states may suggest that emotions can interact with reasoning processes in ways that lead to dysfunctional decision making (Eddy et al., 2011). This study employed a version of the Ultimatum Game, during which participants were asked whether they would accept an uneven split of £10, an amount offered to them by a proposer. They were told that if they did not accept the offer, both they and the proposer would receive nothing. An advantageous decision under these circumstances is to accept any offer, as rejection results in no personal gain. Indeed, the majority of neurologically intact individuals rejected few offers. Eddy and colleagues (2011) found that patients with TS rejected significantly more offers than matched healthy controls, including offers unanimously accepted by controls. Such behavior could reflect a difficulty in controlling negative emotional reactions resulting from feelings of unfairness, and may be related to the emotion dyscontrol seen in some individuals with TS. Future research should extend investigations of decision making in TS and aim to elucidate the relationship between cognitive control processes and the emotional symptomatology of TS.

In summary, it seems likely that TS is associated with changes in social cognition. However, while patients with TS exhibit differences in interpretation of social and emotional stimuli, they do not demonstrate an inability to appreciate people's mental states. One aim of future research should be to better characterize the complex interactions between emotion, cognition, and the dysfunctional social and behavioral problems seen in some people with TS.

CRITICAL COMMENTARY

A review of the data available on neuropsychological function in TS allows one to formulate a number of tentative conclusions. Firstly, the evidence of cognitive difficulties in TS is markedly inconsistent. This may partly reflect limitations in methodology and a lack of systematic assessment. Secondly, it would appear that difficulties are more commonly reported in child than adult samples, and this could be related in some way to the developmental trajectory of TS, changes in symptom severity over time, and possible compensatory mechanisms that develop in adolescence or adulthood. Longitudinal studies are clearly needed. Thirdly, based on the current evidence, it would appear that for individuals with TS alone, especially adults, cognitive difficulties are generally mild, and are likely to consist of subtle decrements in attention or inhibitory processes. A lack of substantial evidence for difficulties in executive functions makes the possibility of dysfunction in the dorsolateral prefrontal cortex rather unlikely. An explanation in terms of inconsistent anterior cingulate dysfunction is more convincing and would relate well with some recent imaging findings implicating structural changes in this neural region (Müller-Vahl et al., 2009) and functional activation during tics (Stern et al., 2000). Finally, a developing body of evidence suggests that subgroups of adolescents with TS alone may demonstrate certain strengths in aspects of cognitive control, with associated underlying neurobiological changes. The challenge for future studies will be to determine how these abilities may generalize in the everyday life of people with TS and could therefore be applied to enhance tic management.

There are difficulties in drawing clear conclusions from the TS literature, due to methodological limitations. The main limitation with studies carried out to date relates to sample selection. Most early studies did not control for or measure comorbidity, which leads to difficulties interpreting results and comparing findings across studies. Investigations that have controlled for comorbidity have often been limited by power. Task selection is a critical issue in assessing cognition in TS, as limitations may be associated with the use of particular assessment tools. Sometimes measures have not been sufficiently sensitive to detect subtle differences. In addition, the face and construct validities of some tasks (e.g., TMT and SSPT) are questionable, and it is difficult to specify the cause of impaired performance on measures that combine more than one cognitive domain (e.g., motor speed and cognitive flexibility; Arbuthnott et al., 2000; Shucard et al., 1997). Fundamental changes in learning or memory have the potential to affect performance across a wide variety of cognitive tasks, making it difficult to determine the basis of performance deficits. For example, in analyzing poor performance on

set-shifting tasks, it can be difficult to disentangle specific difficulties in withdrawing current attentional focus, re-engaging attentional focus, or remembering when a shift has been signaled. Furthermore, individuals with TS may perform more poorly on complex tasks because they involve several components. Task requirements, selection, and design should be carefully considered so that when deficits are identified, more precise judgments can be made about which cognitive processes are implicated. It is likely that a carefully considered, theoretically driven battery of tests will be more informative than individual tests in selected (and unrelated) cognitive domains. In test selection it is also helpful to be guided by the identified neurophysiology of TS, and to consider the inclusion of tasks linked to neural regions that previous studies suggest as being dysfunctional in TS.

In relation to the participants tested, there will be considerable variation within groups of individuals with TS in terms of tic symptoms, tic severity, medications, comorbid conditions, and accompanying emotional, social, and behavioral factors. Such differences may explain the variability in study findings. Comorbidity is a particularly important issue in TS. As illustrated by Peterson, Pine, Cohen, and Brook (2001), the relationships between the symptoms of TS and comorbid disorders are likely to be complex and may vary across the lifespan. Controlling for symptoms of co-occurring conditions may be difficult when many participants exhibit subthreshold symptoms of OCD or ADHD. The inclusion of measures assessing a range of clinical symptoms will therefore always be of use in drawing conclusions and recommendations for support and intervention. Another important consideration will be to control for IQ levels in studies that seek to measure specific cognitive domains in TS populations. Furthermore, tic severity characteristically waxes and wanes over time, which may be reflected in fluctuating cognitive performance. While many studies have tested children or adolescents, relatively few studies have included adult samples. Longitudinal studies are lacking and are critical to determine the relationship between age, disease chronicity, and neuropsychological performance.

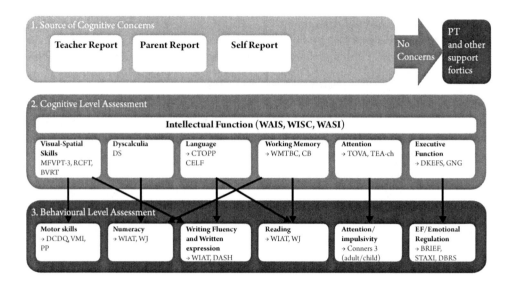

FIGURE 20.1 Proposed framework for assessing the cognitive needs of an individual with TS. BRIEF, Behavior Rating Inventory of Executive Function (Gioia et al., 2000); PT, Psychological Therapy (Comprehensive Behavioral Intervention for Tics, Exposure with Response Prevention); BVRT, Benton Visual Recognition Test (Siven et al., 1992); CELF-IV, Clinical Evaluation of Language Fundamentals (Semel, Wiig & Secord, 2005); CTOPP, Comprehensive Test of Phonological Processing (Wagner, Torgesen & Rashotte, 1999); Conners 3, Conners 3 (Conners, 2008); D S, Dyscalculia Screener (Butterworth, 2003); DASH, Detailed Assessment of Handwriting Speed (Barnett et al., 2007); DBRS, Disruptive Behavior Rating Scale (Barkley, 1997); DCDQ, Developmental Coordination Disorder Questionnaire (Wilson et al., 2000); DK-EFS, Delis Kaplan Executive Function System ((D-KEFS; Delis, Kaplan & Kramer, 2001); GNG, Go/No Go task; MFVPT-3, Motor Free Visual Perceptual Test (Colarusso & Hammill, 2003); PP, Purdue Pegboard (Tiffen, 1968); RCFT, Rey Complex Figure Test (Meyers & Meyers, 1995); TEA-ch, Test of Everyday Attention in Children (Manly et al., 1999); TOVA, Test of Variables of Attention (Greenberg, 1990); VMI-6th, Beery Developmental Test of Visual Motor Integration—Sixth Edition (Beery & Beery, 2010); WAIS, Wechsler Abbreviated Scale of Intelligence (Wechsler, 1999); WAIS, Wechsler Adult Intelligence Scale—Fourth Edition (Wechsler, 2008a); WIAT-III, Wechsler Individual Achievement Test—Third Edition (Wechsler, 2009); WISC, Wechsler Intelligence Scale for Children—Fourth Edition (Wechsler, 2005); WJIII, Woodcock Johnson Tests of Achievement (Woodcock, McGrew & Mather, 2007); WMTBC, Working Memory Test Battery for Children (Pickering & Gathercole, 2001).

The application of research study findings to clinical practice also presents many challenges. These include the problem that many of the tests used empirically are experimental in nature and do not necessarily offer strong ecological validity. Use of tests developed for adults to assess executive function in children is limited by poor sensitivity and specificity. It is likely that experimental studies of cognition in TS will be enhanced through the inclusion of scales assessing the impact of difficulties in everyday life (e.g., quality-of-life scales or adaptive behavior measures).

Since the findings related to cognitive function in populations with TS are diverse, they do not readily offer a clear set of guidelines for applied practice. Figure 20.1 offers suggestions in guiding the assessment, depending on the presenting cognitive or behavioral impairments identified. It can be assumed that there will be an overrepresentation of children and adults with ADHD in any TS population who will benefit from cognitive assessment. The screening aspect of the assessment is essential in any setting (school, clinic, or occupational). Reports, standardized information from schools and work, and previous history will provide the assessor with the information required to decide whether an assessment has the potential to be beneficial. Although cognitive difficulties would not be an exclusion criterion for behavioral or other therapy for tics, certain impairments, such as deficits with sustained attention, may present limitations (Woods et al., 2008). If reports do not indicate difficulty with day-to-day function, then there may be no real need to offer a cognitive assessment.

Once concerns have been identified, then behavioral difficulties can be formulated, usually through the use of questionnaires and standardized assessment in a range of domains. The role of the assessment is to identify the underlying cognitive difficulties that need to be addressed to support the child.

Including a measure of global intellectual function allows the assessor to interpret the results from specific cognitive testing within a baseline framework that reflects expectations for a given individual. It is then possible to identify the specific neuropsychological weaknesses that underlie specific learning difficulties, the most common of which relate to mathematical calculations and written expression for students within the educational setting. Potential underlying vulnerabilities are highlighted in Figure 20.1. For example, if a young person presents with written expression difficulties, a neuropsychologist will be able to identify if the vulnerabilities relate to motor challenges, language problems, attention difficulties, executive difficulties, and/or poor teaching relative to same-age peers. It is probable that multiple cognitive abilities underlie a complex behavior like written expression, but detailed assessment gives insight into the specific areas that will be most effective to advise educators in how to support the student (see Chapter 29 for more details). Certain measures may assess more than one neuropsychological domain.

One of many helpful tests is the RCFT, which measures a range of functions. The copy task assesses visual motor integration, in addition to motor planning. The subsequent recall trials assess retention of information, attention to detail, and motivation factors. The RCFT combined with a test of written expression such as the Detailed Assessment of Speed of Handwriting (Barnett et al., 2007) or the Wechsler Individual

Achievement Test (Wechsler, 2008b) encourages an understanding of how neuropsychological factors affect behavior.

In terms of gathering information from parents and teachers, the BRIEF covers a range of executive functions that will also add helpful information to the formulation (see Chapter 29 for additional strategies in how to address these difficulties through individual changes for the student and the school system) and is considered a clinically useful tool (Denckla, 2006). The behavioral profile associated with TS may lead to instances when such behaviors are mistakenly assumed to reflect specific cognitive difficulties in people with TS. For example, educators who lack understanding about tics may interpret fidgetiness for hyperkinetic behavior rather than tics, or poor school performance could be attributed to learning disability rather than problems sustaining attention while performing tics. Such possibilities make observation of the child in the classroom or clinic an important aspect of the assessment.

Figure 20.1 describes the process that an individual might undergo during a neuropsychological assessment. Concerns should be elicited from important sources in the individual's environment (teachers, family members, etc). This information is used to inform assessment at both the behavioral and cognitive levels. The arrows in Figure 20.1 demonstrate the cognitive areas likely to underlie the behavioral difficulties experienced by the individual. Figure 20.1 is not an exhaustive list of measures but identifies the most commonly used tests in published research or in specialist clinical practice. It is possible to use a reduced number of subtests within a battery, which can be used to screen and inform formulation. In certain cases where everyday function is compromised, use of an adaptive behavioral measure would also be contributory, especially in measuring the efficacy of a behavioral intervention. Some of the batteries of tests (e.g., Delis Kaplan Executive Function System) include a range of tests referred to previously in individual studies. It is beyond the scope of this chapter to give a detailed description of each test, but here we provide a framework for the clinician.

The framework for formulation is important. Once the general cognitive level is established for the individual, then educational attainments and specific cognitive impairments can be identified. From this information, the impact of these impairments on the individual's functioning at school or in the workplace can be monitored. It is important that relative cognitive strengths and other protective factors (e.g., well-developed social skills, supportive teachers or colleagues) are used as compensatory strategies to aid the individual with his or her difficulties.

Future Developments

Despite the limitations associated with studies investigating cognitive function in TS, the past 30 years of research in this area has yielded potentially fruitful avenues of further research. Controlled studies that adopt a more integrated approach addressing interactions between cognition, emotion, and behavior will be crucial to advance our understanding.

In general, more systematic studies are needed that compare the cognitive performance of matched groups of individuals with TS differing only in terms of age, comorbidity, or medication to examine the role of critical clinical and demographic variables. Measures of psychiatric symptoms (at least OCD, ADHD, depression, and anxiety) should be considered in all clinical work and empirical studies. The cognitive abilities being tested must be carefully defined, with a view to developing and employing tasks that allow more precise determination of identified deficits. For example, when assessing verbal memory, comparing performance on tests of recognition, recall, and cued-recall may help determine whether difficulties reflect poor encoding or retrieval of information. Tasks should also be presented across a variety of modalities (verbal, visual) to allow specification of any identified deficit, and both implicit and explicit skills should be considered where appropriate. Although some cognitive abilities may be largely inseparable experimentally, it is also advisable that tasks assessing attention and inhibition should always be included, as deficits in these abilities could lead to problems on a range of tasks.

Importantly, the application of empirical studies into translational research will be advantageous. As TS is a chronic neurodevelopmental disorder, longitudinal studies present the optimal research paradigm for understanding this condition. Such studies may encourage the development of predictive tools that will enable intervention to be focused where it is most needed. The benefits of cognitive screening will include the identification of those individuals who may benefit most from particular cognitive-behavioral treatments and educational interventions. For example, studies have indicated that response inhibition abilities may be predictive of the success of behavioral therapy for tic management (Deckersbach et al., 2006).

So far, research has largely neglected the possible interactions between cognition and the emotional and behavioral difficulties often seen in TS. Evidence of possible changes in social reasoning processes in TS could constitute one product of such interactions. The impact of mood and emotional experience on decision making is another area worthy of exploration. The development of an approach to research that can begin to appreciate the complexity of the interactions between processes within cognitive, social, and emotional domains on both a behavioral and neural level is critical.

The use of modern neurophysiological techniques will be invaluable in the exploration of cognition in TS. In a study using ERP, Johannes and colleagues (2001) found that although children and adults with TS showed normal behavioral performance on a dual-performance task, they demonstrated neural evidence of increased attention to irrelevant stimuli. Findings such as these raise the point that although the behavioral performance of participants with TS may not differ from controls, individuals with chronic tics may use a different approach or strategy when completing tasks. This could sometimes be related to reported compensatory changes. From an alternative angle, the top-down approach provided by the results of neuroimaging investigations may help to identify areas for which behavioral tasks can be developed. Development and availability of neurophysiological measurement such as magnetic reasoning imaging (especially diffusion tensor imaging) and electrophysiological measures such as ERPs will allow research to advance through a neurobiologically focused approach rather than relying on a complex behaviorally determined approach.

Another important issue raised by recent studies is the possibility of enhanced cognition, particularly related to inhibition, found in children and adults with TS. Structural alterations, increased activity, or improved transmission within frontostriatal circuitry may underlie skills in areas such as cognitive control or procedural language functions. One challenge for future research will therefore be to identify measures for which control populations do not perform at ceiling, in order to uncover potentially enhanced performance in individuals with TS.

Is there a neuropsychological endophenotype of TS? Much of the evidence reviewed in this chapter suggests that TS may well be associated

Table 20.1 Neuropsychological performance in Tourette syndrome alone and the likely impact of co-morbid obsessive compulsive disorder or attention deficit hyperactivity disorder

		Intellectual Function	Attention	Language	Executive Function
Pure TS	+	No evidence of global impairment		Processing and retrieval of verbal information from lexical store	**Cognitive Control**
	–	**Processing speed**	**Sustained and spatial attention** **Demanding attention measures (possible distraction through tic suppression)**	Higher level/ complex language skills	**Changes in Social Cognition (true nature/valence of impact needs further exploration)**
TS + OCD	+	Higher IQ			
	–		Visual memory	Higher level/ complex language skills	**Visual planning, organisation, visual retention and flexibility** **Cognitive flexibility, preoccupation with error / change**
TS + ADHD	–	**Lower IQ**	**Impulsivity and sustained attention**	**Written language** Slower motor output	Poorer verbal **fluency, inhibition, planning, and cognitive flexibility**

BOX 20.1. Key Points

- Although useful products of research may be the identification of broader neuropsychological traits associated with TS, it should of course be remembered that each individual with TS is unique from a neuropsychological perspective in terms of their strengths and weaknesses.
- Although performance on measures of intelligence in individuals with TS is similar to the general population, clinicians, parents and teachers and other professionals need to be vigilant to the special needs of children with TS.
- Individually tailored neuropsychological testing for children with TS may be particularly useful in detecting specific learning disabilities. Although cases with co-morbid ADHD are more likely display weaknesses in motor skills, cognitive flexibility, written expression and attention, even individuals with pure TS may display problems with motor dexterity, sustained attention, emotion control and social cognition.
- A select group of people with TS seem to display specific areas of neuropsychological strength, although this area of research is still in its infancy. It is important to note these areas of strength and where possible build on and utilise them in an effort to promote the individual's success and resiliency in life.

BOX 20.2. Questions for future research

- More integrated research is needed across a number of neuropsychological domains (see below). Ideally, future studies will include longitudinal designs that incorporate the latest imaging and electrophysiological techniques. The time is also ripe for meta-analytic studies that combine the existing data and test for the moderating effects of age, gender, IQ, tic severity, and the presence of co-occurring conditions such as ADHD, OCD, specific learning disabilities, and medication status. To detect whether there is a neuropsychological endophenotype for TS it will also be necessary to study unaffected family members. Considering each neuropsychological domain separately, some of the areas than need to be explored further are described below
- VISUOMOTOR INTEGRATION: Simple hand-eye co-ordination may not have been assessed. Procedural motor skills are linked to the basal ganglia, which may be dysfunctional in TS. Such abilities deserve further attention.
- VISUAL PERCEPTUAL SKILLS: Attention could influence performance. Studies should consider using different forms of assessment e.g. drawing, verbal descriptions etc. to better specify the level of any identified deficits.
- IQ: Problems with broader cognitive abilities such as attention could impact overall performance. Both VIQ and PIQ should be considered, and any areas of selective deficit highlighted. Further work is needed to determine the reason for deficits on WISC –III coding subtest.
- SPECIFIC LEARNING DISABILITIES: Screening for SpLD should be carried out for children and adults with TS. Incidence of SpLD in adults with TS has not yet been explored but difficulties are likely to persist into adulthood.

BOX 20.2. (*Continued*)

- MEMORY: Studies need to specify whether deficits reflect encoding or retrieval problems. Comparing recognition, recall, cued recall and input modalities could be useful. Studies should look specifically at procedural memory.
- LEARNING: Both implicit and explicit learning processes should be investigated. The valence of cues and rewards is important to consider.
- ATTENTION: Studies should investigate divided attention in addition to sustained attention. It may be useful to compare stimulus modalities. There is a need to determine if problems are due to tic suppression or attentional focus per se. What stage is the deficit e.g. disengaging, re-engaging?
- LINGUISTIC SKILLS: The possibility of enhanced language production/speed of articulation needs further exploration. The possible relationship between vocal tics and performance should be investigated. Longitudinal studies of written language skills are needed.
- MOTOR SKILLS AND CO-ORDINATION: Carefully designed studies are needed which determine the level of alterations in motor performance and the potential for changes in cognitive processes across development. Further work is needed to substantiate reports of enhanced performance on cognitive control tasks in TS and determine the therapeutic implications of such changes.
- WORKING MEMORY: Attention could make a key contribution to task performance. Studies should simultaneously test working memory for different modalities.
- VERBAL FLUENCY: It may be useful to directly compare semantic and phonological fluency. Studies should also consider design or ideational fluency.
- PLANNING/MULTI-TASKING: Further work is needed to assess multi-tasking performance in children. Both motor and cognitive aspects of planning should be considered.
- SHIFTING/COGNITIVE FLEXIBILITY: The relationships between inhibition, perseveration, set-shifting and repetitive behaviours are yet to be explored in TS.
- INHIBITION: Longitudinal studies would be useful. How is inhibition related to symptom improvement (throughout development and with behavioural therapy)? Is there any relationship between inhibition and pre-tic premonitory sensations?
- SOCIAL COGNITION: Studies should consider the impact of emotion on cognitive performance. Further work on social cognition and the role of emotion in decision making will improve our global understanding of TS.

with particular cognitive strengths and vulnerabilities. However, there are many complications associated with answering this question, including the spectrum of behavioral heterogeneity and frequency of comorbid conditions in TS. Table 20.1 aims to summarize the findings of studies that have assessed for particular cognitive strengths and weaknesses in samples with pure TS and the common comorbidities. Given the limitations associated with the available literature, here we present tentative conclusions based on more robust findings. Such difficulties prompt consideration of whether it is most appropriate to investigate the possible existence of multiple cognitive endophenotypes for subgroups of individuals with pure TS or TS plus associated conditions. However, such subgrouping may be of limited use, given that many individuals with TS will exhibit undiagnosed subthreshold symptoms of comorbid disorders. Perhaps a more informative way forward will be to develop more dimensional and less categorical approaches to the assessment of both the behavioral and cognitive features associated with TS.

The studies of neuropsychological functioning in TS carried out so far have highlighted the importance of research and assessment in this area. However, there is a great deal still to be achieved. As the literature stands, there is not a well-defined cognitive profile that can be considered to characterize individuals with TS. Future, better-designed studies will further elucidate the alterations in neuropsychological function associated with TS and their relevance for both the understanding and treatment of the cognitive, emotional, and behavioral aspects of this condition.

REFERENCES

Abwender DA, Como PG, Kurlan R et al. School problems in Tourette's syndrome. *Arch Neurol* 1996; 53:509–511.

Abwender DA, Trinidad KS, Jones KR et al. Features resembling Tourette's syndrome in developmental stutterers. *Brain Lang* 1998; 62:455–464.

Arbuthnott K, Frank J. Trail Making Test Part B as a measure of executive control: validation using a set-switching paradigm. *J Clin Exp Neuropsychol* 2000; 22:518–528.

Avanzino L, Martino D, Bove M et al. Movement lateralization and bimanual coordination in children with Tourette syndrome. *Mov Disord* 2011; 26:2114–2118.

Barkley RA. *Defiant children: A clinician's manual for assessment and parent training* (2nd ed.). New York: Guilford Press; 1997.

Barnett A, Henderson SE, Scheib B, Schulz J. *Detailed assessment of speed of handwriting.* Pearson Education Inc., Oxford, 2007.

Baron-Cohen S, Cross P, Crowson M, Robertson MM. Can children with Gilles de la Tourette syndrome edit their intentions? *Psychol Med* 1994; 24:29–40.

Baron-Cohen S, Jolliffe T, Mortimore C, Robertson MM. Another advanced test of theory of mind: Evidence from very high functioning adults with autism or Asperger's syndrome. *J Child Psychol Psychiatry* 1997; 387:813–822.

Baron-Cohen S, Wheelwright S, Hill J et al. The "Reading the Mind in the Eyes" test revised version: A study with normal adults, adults with Asperger's syndrome or high-functioning autism. *J Child Psychol Psychiatry* 2001; 42:241–251.

Baym CL, Corbett BA, Wright SB, Bunge SA. Neural correlates of tic severity and cognitive control in children with Tourette syndrome. *Brain* 2008; 131:165–179.

Beery KE. *The developmental test of visual motor integration.* Minneapolis, MN: NCS Pearson, Inc., 1997.

Beery KE, Beery NA. *The developmental test of visual motor integration, 6th edition.* NCS Pearson, Inc., Oxford 2010.

Berg EA. A simple objective technique for measuring flexibility in thinking. *J Gen Psychol* 1948; 39:15–22.

One of the few longitudinal studies in TS; identifies predictors of psychosocial outcome and tic persistence into early adulthood.
Bloch MH, Sukhodolsky DG, Leckman JF, Schulz RT. Fine-motor skill deficits in childhood predict adulthood tic severity and global psychosocial functioning in Tourette's syndrome. *J Child Psychol Psychiatry* 2006; 47:551–559.

Bornstein RA. Neuropsychological performance in children with Tourette's syndrome. *Psychiatry Res* 1990; 33:73–81.

Bornstein RA. Neuropsychological performance in adults with Tourette's syndrome. *Psychiatry Res* 1991a; 37:229–236.

Bornstein RA. Neuropsychological correlates of obsessive characteristics in Tourette Syndrome. *J Neuropsychiatry Clin Neurosci* 1991b; 3:157–162.

Bornstein RA, Baker GB, Baylewich T, Douglass AB. Tourette's syndrome and neuropsychological performance. *Acta Psychiatr Scand* 1991; 84:212–216.

Bornstein RA, Yang V. Neurological performance in medicated and unmedicated patients with Tourette's disorder. *Am J Psychiatry* 2001; 148:468–471.

Bracken BA, McCallum RS. *Woodcock-Johnson Psycho-Educational Battery - Revised.* Brandon, VT: Clinical Psychology Publishing Co., 1993.

Brand N, Geenen R, Oudenhoven M et al. Brief report: cognitive functioning in children with Tourette's syndrome with and without comorbid ADHD. *J Pediatr Psychol* 2002; 27:203–208.

Braver TS, Cohen JD, Nystrom LE et al. A parametric study of prefrontal cortex involvement in human working memory. *NeuroImage* 1997; 5:49–62.

Brook U, Boaz M. Attention deficit and learning disabilities (ADHD/LD) among high school pupils in Holon (Israel). *Patient Educ Couns* 2005; 58:164–167.

Brookshire B, Butler I, Ewing-Cobbs L, Fletcher J. Neuropsychological characteristics of children with Tourette syndrome: Evidence for a nonverbal learning disability? *J Clin Exp Neuropsychol* 1994; 16:289–302.

Bruun RD, Budman CL. Paroxetine treatment of episodic rages associated with Tourette's disorder. *J Clin Psychiatry* 1998; 59:581–584.

Budman C, Coffey BJ, Shechter R et al. Aripiprazole in children and adolescents with Tourette disorder with and without explosive outbursts. *J Child Adolesc Psychopharmacol* 2008; 18:509–515.

Budman CL, Bruun RD, Park KS, Olson ME. Rage attacks in children and adolescents with Tourette's disorder: A pilot study. *J Clin Psychiatry* 1998; 59:576–580.

Budman CL, Bruun RD, Park KS et al. Explosive outbursts with Tourette's disorder. *J Am Acad Child Adolesc Psychiatry* 2000; 39:1270–1276.

Budman CL, Rockmore L, Stokes J, Sossin M. Clinical phenomenology of episodic rage in children with Tourette syndrome. *J Psychosom Res* 2003; 55:59–65.

Burd L, Freeman RD, Klug MG, Kerbeshian J. Tourette syndrome and learning disabilities. *BMC Pediatr* 2005; 5:34.

Burd L, Kauffman DW, Kerbeshian J. Tourette syndrome and learning disabilities. *J Learn Disabil* 1992; 25:598–604.

Burgess PG, Shallice T. Response suppression, initiation and strategy use following frontal lobe lesions. *Neuropsychologia* 1996; 34:263–273.

Butterworth B. *Dyscalculia Screener*. Nelson Publishing Company Limited, London 2003.

Cavanna AE, Cavanna S, Monaco F. Anger symptoms and "delinquent" behavior in Tourette syndrome with and without attention deficit hyperactivity disorder. *Brain Dev* 2008; 30:308.

Chang SW, McCracken JT, Piacentini JC. Neurocognitive correlates of child obsessive compulsive disorder and Tourette syndrome. *J Clin Exp Neuropsychol* 2007; 29:724–733.

Channon S, Pratt P, Robertson MM. Executive function, memory, and learning in Tourette's syndrome. *Neuropsychology* 2003a; 17:247–254.

Channon S, Crawford S, Vakili K, Robertson MM. Real-life-type problem-solving in Tourette's syndrome. *Cogn Behav Neurol* 2003b; 16:3–15.

Channon S, Flynn D, Robertson MM. Attentional deficits in Gilles de la Tourette's Syndrome.

Neuropsychiatry Neuropsychol Behav Neurol 1992; 5:170–177.

Channon S, Gunning A, Frankl J, Robertson MM. Tourette's syndrome (TS): cognitive performance in adults with uncomplicated TS. *Neuropsychology* 2006; 20:58–65.

Channon S, Sinclair E, Waller D et al. Social cognition in Tourette's syndrome: intact theory of mind and impaired inhibitory functioning. *J Autism Dev Disord* 2004; 34:669–677.

Colarusso RP, Hammill DD. *Motor-Free Visual Perception Test, Third Edition (MVPT-3)*. Academic Therapy Publications, 2003.

Conners K. Conners (3rd ed.). Toronto, Ontario, Canada: Multi-Health Systems Inc., 2008.

Corsi PM. *Human memory and the medial temporal region of the brain*. Dissertation Abstracts International, 34 (02), 891B. (University Microfilms No. AAI05-77717), 1972.

Crawford S, Channon S, Robertson MM. Tourette's syndrome: performance on tests of behavioral inhibition, working memory and gambling. *J Child Psychol Psychiatry* 2005; 46:1327–1336.

Debes NM, Lange T, Jessen TL et al. Performance on Wechsler intelligence scales in children with Tourette syndrome. *Eur J Paediatr Neurol* 2011; 15:146–154.

Deckersbach T, Rauch S, Buhlmann U, Wilhelm S. Habit reversal versus supportive psychotherapy in Tourette's disorder: a randomized controlled trial and predictors of treatment response. *Behav Res Ther* 2006; 44:1079–1090.

Denckla M, Rudel R. Rapid autornized naming: dyslexia differentiated from other learning disabilities. *Neuropsychologia* 1976; 14:471–479.

Denckla MB. Attention-deficit hyperactivity disorder (ADHD) comorbidity: A case for "pure" Tourette syndrome? *J Child Neurol* 2006; 21:70.

De Nil LF, Sasisekaran J, Van Lieshout PH, Sandor P. Speech dysfluencies in individuals with Tourette syndrome. *J Psychosom Res* 2005; 58:97–102.

Drake MEJ, Hietter SA, Padamadan H et al. Auditory evoked potentials in Gilles de la Tourette syndrome. *Clin Electroencephalograph* 1992; 23:19–23.

Eddy CM, Mitchell IJ, Beck SR et al. Altered attribution of intention in Tourette syndrome. *J Neuropsychiatry Clin Neurosci* 2010a; 22:348–351.

Eddy CM, Mitchell IJ, Beck SR et al. Impaired comprehension of non-literal language in

Tourette syndrome. *Cogn Behav Neurol* 2010b; 23:178–184.

Eddy CM, Mitchell IJ, Beck SR et al. Social reasoning in Tourette syndrome. *Cogn Neuropsychiatry* 2011; 18:1–22.

Eddy CM, Rizzo R, Cavanna AE. Neuropsychological aspects of Tourette syndrome: A review. *J Psychosom Res* 2009; 67:503–513.

Eichele H, Eichele T, Hammar A et al. Go/NoGo performance in boys with Tourette syndrome. *Child Neuropsychol* 2010; 16:162–168.

Fahim C, Yoon U, Das S et al. Somatosensory-motor bodily representation cortical thinning in Tourette: effects of tic severity, age and gender. *Cortex* 2010; 46:750–760.

Freeman R, Fast D, Burd L et al. An international perspective on Tourette syndrome: selected findings from 3500 individuals in 22 countries. *Dev Med Child Neurol* 2000; 42:436–447.

Georgiou N, Bradshaw JL, Phillips JG et al. Advance information and movement sequencing in Gilles de la Tourette's syndrome. *J Neurol Neurosurg Psychiatry* 1995; 58:184–191.

Gioia GA, Isquith PK, Guy SC, Kenworthy L. *Behavior Rating Inventory of Executive Function.* Lutz, FL: Psychological Assessment Resources, Inc., 2000.

Golden CJ, Anderson SM. Short form of the Speech Sounds Perception Test. *Percept Mot Skills* 1977; 45:485–486.

Goudriaan AE, Oosterlaan J, de Beurs E, van den Brink W. Neurocognitive functions in pathological gambling: a comparison with alcohol dependence, Tourette syndrome and normal controls. *Addiction* 2006; 101:534–547.

Greenberg L. *Test of Variables of Attention 5.01.* St Paul, MN: Attention Technology Inc., 1990.

Halstead WC. *Brain and intelligence: A quantitative study of the frontal lobes.* Chicago: University of Chicago Press, 1947.

Hanks RA, Rapport LJ, Millis SR, Deshpande SA. Measures of executive function as predictors of functional ability and social integration in a rehabilitation sample. *Arch Phys Med Rehab* 1999; 80:1030–1037.

Harris EL, Schuerholz LJ, Singer HS et al. Executive function in children with Tourette syndrome and/or comorbid anxiety-deficit hyperactivity disorder. *J Int Neuropsychol Soc* 1995; 1:511–516.

Hershey T, Black KJ, Hartlein J et al. Dopaminergic modulation of response inhibition: an fMRI study. *Cogn Brain Res* 2004; 20:438–448.

Huckeba W, Chapieski L, Hiscock M, Glaze D. Arithmetic performance in children with Tourette syndrome: relative contribution of cognitive and attentional factors. *J Clin Exp Neuropsychol* 2008; 30:410–420.

Jackson GM, Mueller SC, Hambleton K, Hollis CP. Enhanced cognitive control in Tourette syndrome during task uncertainty. *Exp Brain Res* 2007; 182:357–364.

Jackson SR, Parkinson A, Jung J et al. Compensatory neural reorganization in Tourette syndrome. *Curr Biol* 2011; 21:580–585.

Evidence for enhanced control over motor output in TS and neural reorganization involving forceps minor pathways, which may underlie compensatory increases in self-regulation mechanisms.

Johannes S, Nager W, Wieringa BM et al. Electrophysiological measures and dual task performance in Tourette syndrome indicate deficient divided attention mechanisms. *Eur J Neurol* 2001; 8:253–260.

Johannes S, Weber A, Muller-Vahl KR et al. Event related potentials show changes attentional mechanisms in Gilles de la Tourette syndrome. *Eur J Neurol* 1997; 4:152–161.

Innovative application of ERP to show that individuals with TS exert increased effort to maintain attention performance at the same level as healthy controls.

Kaplan E, Goodglass H. *Boston Naming Test. Experimental Edition.* Philadelphia: Lea & Febiger, 1978.

Kaufman AS, Kaufman NL. *Kaufman Test of Educational Achievement.* Circle Pines, MN: American Guidance Service, 1985.

Keri S, Szlobodynik C, Benedek G et al. Probabilistic classification learning in Tourette syndrome. *Neuropsychologia* 2002; 40:1356–1362.

Knowlton BJ, Squire LR, Gluck MA. Probabilistic classification learning in amnesia. *Learn Mem* 1994; 1:106-120.

Knowlton BJ, Mangels JA, Squire LR. A neostriatal habit learning system in humans. *Science* 1996; 273:1399–1402.

Kurlan R, McDermott P, Deeley C et al. Prevalence of tics in schoolchildren and association with placement in special education. *Neurology* 2001; 57:1383–1388.

Lavoie ME, Thibault G, Stip E, O'Connor KP. Memory and executive functions in adults with Gilles de la Tourette syndrome and chronic tic disorder. *Cogn Neuropsychiatry* 2007; 12:165–181.

Leckman JF, Riddle MA, Hardin MT et al. The Yale Global Tic Severity Scale: Initial testing of a clinician-rated scale of tic severity. *J Am Acad Adolesc Psychiatry* 1989; 28:566–573.

Legg C, Penn C, Temlett J, Sonnenberg B. Language skills of adolescents with Tourette syndrome. *Clin Linguist Phon* 2005; 19:15–33.

Mahone EM, Kohn CW, Cutting L et al. Executive function in fluency and recall measures among children with Tourette's syndrome or ADHD. *J Int Neuropsychol Soc* 2001; 7:102–111.

Manly T, Robertson IH, Anderson V, Nimmo-Smith I. *TEA-Ch: The Test of Everyday Attention for Children Manual*. Bury St. Edmunds, UK: Thames Valley Test Company Limited, 1999.

Margolis A, Donkervoort M, Kinsbourne M, Peterson BS. Interhemispheric connectivity and executive functioning in adults with Tourette syndrome. *Neuropsychology* 2006; 20:66–76.

Investigation of motor performance on the Purdue Pegboard task revealed lack of left-hand advantage on the task (normally shown by controls), interpreted by the authors as evidence of alterations in interhemispheric connectivity and prefrontal dysfunction in TS.

Marsh R, Alexander GM, Packard MG et al. Habit learning in Tourette syndrome—a translational neuroscience approach to a developmental psychopathology. *Arch Gen Psychiatry* 2004; 61:1259–1268.

Marsh R, Alexander GM, Packard MG et al. Perceptual-motor skill learning in Gilles de la Tourette syndrome: Evidence for multiple procedural learning and memory systems. *Neuropsychologia* 2005; 43:1456–1465.

Maryland State Department of Education. *Learning Disabilities Guidelines*. Baltimore, 1986.

Meyers J, Meyers K. The Rey Complex Figure and Recognition trial under four different admin procedures. *Clin Neuropsychol* 1995; 9:65–67.

Milner B. Effects of different brain lesions on card sorting. *Arch Neurol* 1963; 9:90–100.

Morton J, Frith U. Causal modeling: Structural approaches to developmental psychopathology. In Cicchetti D, Cohen D (Eds.), *Developmental psychopathology*. New York: Wiley, 1995, pp. 357–390.

Mueller SC, Jackson GM, Dhalla R et al. Enhanced cognitive control in young people with Tourette's syndrome. *Curr Biol* 2006; 16:570–573.

Müller SV, Johannes S, Wieringa B et al. Disturbed monitoring and response inhibition in patients with Gilles de la Tourette syndrome and comorbid obsessive compulsive disorder. *Behav Neurol* 2003; 14:29–37.

Müller-Vahl KR, Kaufmann J, Gross Kreutz J et al. Prefrontal and anterior cingulate abnormalities in Tourette syndrome: Evidence from voxel-based morphometry and magnetization transfer imaging. *BMC Neurosci* 2009; 10:47.

Nathaniel-James DA, Fletcher P, Frith CD. The functional anatomy of verbal initiation and suppression using the Hayling Test. *Neuropsychologia* 1997; 35:559–566.

Ozonoff S, Jensen J. Brief report: specific executive function profiles in three neurodevelopmental disorders. *J Autism Dev Disord* 1999; 29:171–177.

Ozonoff S, Strayer DL, McMahon WM, Filloux F. Executive function abilities in autism and Tourette's syndrome: and information processing approach. *J Child Psychol Psychiatry* 1994; 35:1015–1032.

Ozonoff S, Strayer DL, McMahon WM, Filloux F. Inhibitory deficits in Tourette's syndrome: a function of comorbidity and symptom severity. *J Child Psychol Psychiatry* 1998; 39:1109–1118.

Ozonoff S, Strayer DL. Further evidence of intact working memory in autism. *J Autism Dev Disord* 2001; 31:257–263.

Palminteri S, Leberton M, Worbe Y et al. Pharmacological modulation of subliminal learning in Parkinson's and Tourette's syndromes. *Proc Natl Acad Sci USA* 2009; 106:19179–19184.

Offers insight into the potential influences of dopaminergic alterations in TS: blocking dopamine favored punishment-avoidance learning but impaired reward seeking.

Pennington BF, Ozonoff S. Executive functions and developmental psychopathology. *J Child Psychol Psychiatry* 1996; 37:51–87.

Peterson BS, Pine DS, Cohen P, Brook J. Prospective, longitudinal study of tic, obsessive-compulsive, and attention-deficit/hyperactivity disorders in an epidemiological sample. *J Am Acad Child Adolesc Psychiatry* 2001; 40:685–695.

Peterson BS, Staib L, Scahill L et al. Regional brain and ventricular volumes in Tourette syndrome. *Arch Gen Psychiatry* 2001; 58:427–440.

Peterson BS, Thomas P, Kane MJ et al. Basal ganglia volumes in patients with Gilles de la Tourette syndrome. *Arch Gen Psychiatry* 2003; 60:415–424.

Pickering SJ, Gathercole SE. *Working Memory Test Battery for Children*. London: Pearson Assessment, 2001.

Rasmussen C, Soleimani M, Carroll A, Hodlevsky O. Neuropsychological functioning in children with Tourette syndrome (TS). *J Can Acad Child Adolesc Psychiatry* 2009; *18*:307–315.

Reitan RM. Validity of the Trail Making test as an indicator of organic brain damage. *Percept Mot Skills* 1958; *8*:271–276.

Riddle M, Hardin M, Ort S et al. Behavioral symptoms in Tourette's syndrome. In: Cohen D, Bruun R, Leckman J (Ed.), *Tourette's syndrome and tic disorders: clinical understanding and treatment*. New York: Wiley, 1988, pp. 151–162.

Roessner V, Albrecht B, Dechent P et al. Normal response inhibition in boys with Tourette syndrome. *Behav Brain Funct* 2008; *4*:29.

Santangelo S, Pauls D, Goldstin J et al. Tourette's syndrome: what are the influences of gender and comorbid obsessive-compulsive disorder? *J Am Acad Child Adolesc Psychiatry* 1994; *33*:795–804.

Schuerholz LJ, Baumgardner TL, Singer HS et al. Neuropsychological status of children with Tourette's syndrome with and without attention deficit hyperactivity disorder. *Neurology* 1996; *46*:958–965.

One of few earlier studies to control for the effect of comorbid ADHD. Evidence that TS alone is less likely to be associated with learning difficulties but may be linked to specific deficits in executive functions.

Schuerholz LJ, Singer HS, Denckla MB. Gender study of neuropsychological and neuromotor function in children with Tourette syndrome with and without attention-deficit hyperactivity disorder. *J Child Neurol* 1998; *13*:277–282.

Schultz RT, Carter AS, Gladstone M et al. Visual-motor integration functioning in children with Tourette syndrome. *Neuropsychology* 1998; *12*:134–145.

Semel E, Wiig EH, Secord WA. *Clinical evaluation of language fundamentals* (4th ed). San Antonio, TX: The Psychological Corporation, 2005.

Serrien DJ, Orth M, Evans AH et al. Motor inhibition in patients with Gilles de la Tourette syndrome: functional activation patterns as revealed by EEG coherence. *Brain* 2005; *128*:116–125.

Sherman L, Sheppard M, Joschko M, Freeman RD. Sustained attention and impulsivity in children with Tourette Syndrome: comorbidity and confounds. *J Clin Exp Neuropsychol* 1998; *20*:644–657.

Shomstein S, Lee J, Behrmann M. Top-down and bottom-up attentional guidance: investigating the role of the dorsal and ventral parietal cortices. *Exp Brain Res* 2010; *206*:197–208.

Shucard DW, Benedict RHB, Tekokilic A, Lichter DG. Slowed reaction time during a continuous performance test in children with Tourette's syndrome. *Neuropsychology* 1997; *11*:147–155.

Silverstein SM, Como PG, Palumbo DR et al. Multiple sources of attentional dysfunction in adults with Tourette's syndrome: comparison with attention deficit–hyperactivity disorder. *Neuropsychology* 1995; *9*:157–164.

Sivan AB. *Benton Visual Retention Test* (5th ed.). San Antonio, TX: The Psychological Corporation, 1992.

Sparrow SS, Cicchetti DV, Balla DA. *Vineland Adaptive Behavior Scales*. PsychCorp, Pearson, London, 2005.

Spielberger CD. *State-Trait Anger Expression Inventory-2*. Odessa, FL: Psychological Assessment Resource Inc., 1999.

Squire LR, Zola SM. Structure and function of declarative and non-declarative memory systems. *Proc Natl Acad Sci USA* 1996; *93*:13515–13522.

St Clair-Thompson HL, Gathercole SE. Executive functions and achievements in school: Shifting, updating, inhibition and working memory. *Q J Exp Psychol* 2006; *59*:745–759.

Stebbins GT, Singh J, Weiner J et al. Selective impairments of memory functioning in unmedicated adults with Gilles de la Tourette syndrome. *Neuropsychology* 1995; *9*:329–337.

Stefl M. Mental health associated with Tourette syndrome. *Am J Public Health* 1984; *74*:1310–1313.

Stern E, Silbersweig DA, Chee KY et al. A functional neuroanatomy of tics in Tourette's syndrome. *Arch Gen Psychiatry* 2000; *57*:741–748.

Well-controlled study highlighting the potential influence of comorbid ADHD in TS on neuropsychological function, with an interesting discussion of possible underlying neurobiological mechanisms and compensatory changes.

Sukhodolsky DG, Landeros-Weisenberger A, Scahill L et al. Neuropsychological functioning in children with Tourette syndrome with and without attention-deficit/hyperactivity disorder. *J Am Acad Child Adolesc Psychiatry* 2010; *49*:1155–1164.

Sutherland RJ, Kolb B, Schoel WM et al. Neuropsychological assessment of children and adults with Tourette syndrome: a comparison with learning disabilities and schizophrenia. In: Friedhoff AJ,

Chase TN (Eds.), *Gilles de la Tourette syndrome*. New York: Raven Press, 1982, pp. 311–322.

Tiffin J. *The Purdue Pegboard: Examiner manual*. Chicago: Science Research and Associates, 1968.

van Woerkom TC, Roos RA, van Dijk JG. Altered attentional processing of background stimuli in Gilles de la Tourette syndrome: a study in auditory event-related potentials evoked in an oddball paradigm. *Acta Neurol Scand* 1994; 90:116–123.

Vellutino F, Scanlon D. Phonological coding, phonological awareness and reading ability: evidence from longitudinal and experimental studies. *Merrill Palmer Q*, 33, 321–363.

Verte S, Geurts HM, Roeyers H et al. Executive functioning in children with autism and Tourette's syndrome. *Dev Psychopathol* 2005; 17:415–445.

Vicario CM, Martino D, Spata F et al. Time processing in children with Tourette's syndrome. *Brain Cogn* 2010; 73:28–34.

Waber DP, Holmes JM. Assessing children's copy production of the Rey-Osterreith complex figure. *J Clin Exp Neuropsychol* 1985; 7:264–280.

Wagner R, Torgensen J, Rashotte C. *Comprehensive Test of Phonological Processing*. San Antonio, TX: The Psychological Corporation, 1999.

Walenski M, Mostofsky SH, Ullman MT. Speeded processing of grammar and tool knowledge in Tourette's syndrome. *Neuropsychologia* 2007; 45; 2447–2460.
One of the very few studies to investigate linguistic ability in TS; revealed intriguing evidence of faster processing of aspects of procedural language.

Wand R, Matazow G, Shady G et al. Tourette syndrome: associated symptoms and most disabling features. *Neurosci Biobehav Rev* 1993; 17:271–275.

Wang Z, Maia TV, Marsh R et al. The neural circuits that generate tics in Tourette's syndrome. *Am J Psychiatry* 2011; 168:1326–1337.

Watkins LH, Sahakian BJ, Robertson MM et al. Executive function in Tourette's syndrome and obsessive–compulsive disorder. *Psychol Med* 2005; 35571–35582.

Wechsler D. *Wechsler Intelligence Scale for Children—revised*. San Antonio, TX: The Psychological Corporation, 1971.

Wechsler D. *The Wechsler Abbreviated Scale of Intelligence*. San Antonio, TX: The Psychological Corporation, 1999.

Wechsler D. *The Wechsler Intelligence Scale for Children—Fourth Edition*. San Antonio, TX: The Psychological Corporation, 2003.

Wechsler D. *WISCIII DK*. Oversat af Henny Thomsen. Dansk Psykologisk Forlag, 2004.

Wechsler D. *The Wechsler Adult Intelligence Scale—Fourth Edition*. San Antonio, TX: Pearson, 2008a.

Wechsler D. *The Wechsler Individual Achievement Test—Third Edition*. San Antonio, TX: Pearson, 2008b.

Wiig EH, Secord W. *Test of Language Competence*. San Antonio, TX: Psychological Corporation, 1989.

Wilson BN, Kaplan BJ, Crawford SG et al. Reliability and validity of a parent questionnaire on childhood motor skills. *Am J Occup Ther* 2000; 54:484–493.

Wood BL, Klebba K, Gbadebo O et al. Pilot study of effect of emotional stimuli on tic severity in children with Tourette's syndrome. *Mov Disord* 2003; 18:1392–1395.

Woodcock R, McGrew N, Mather K. *Woodcock Johnson Tests of Achievement Third Edition*. Riverside Publishing, Rolling Meadows IL, 2007.

Woods D, Himle M, Miltenberger R et al. Durability, negative impact, and neuropsychological predictors of tic suppression in children with chronic tic disorder. *J Abnorm Child Psychol* 2008; 36:237–245.
This study is interesting in that it assesses the effects of tic suppression on cognition, which may have interesting implications for learning and psychological treatments.

Yeates KO, Bornstein RA. Attention deficit disorder and neuropsychological functioning in children with Tourette's syndrome. *Neuropsychology* 1994; 8:65–74.

Zgaljardic DJ, Borod JC, Foldi NS et al. An examination of executive dysfunction associated with frontostriatal circuitry in Parkinson's disease. *J Clin Exp Neuropsychol* 2006; 28:1127–1144.

21

Social and Adaptive Functioning in Tourette Syndrome

DENIS G. SUKHODOLSKY, VIRGINIA W. EICHER AND JAMES F. LECKMAN

Abstract

Many children, adolescents, and adults with Tourette syndrome have impairments across various domains of social and adaptive functioning, both as a result of the severity and particular features of tics and existing comorbidities. The relative contribution of tics and comorbid disorders to these impairments is under investigation. A thorough clinical assessment should also include standardized ratings of adaptive functioning. Psychosocial interventions for tics and associated behavioral disorders are constantly improving and show the potential to reduce symptom severity and associated functional impairment.

INTRODUCTION

Tourette syndrome (TS) is a neuropsychiatric disorder characterized by motor and vocal tics that affects approximately 0.6% of children in the general population (Centers for Disease Control and Prevention, 2009). As detailed in Chapter 1, tics are sudden, purposeless, and repetitive movements and vocalizations that vary in appearance, number, frequency, intensity, and complexity (Leckman, 2003). For example, blinking, nose twitching, and jerking of any part of the body are common motor tics, and throat clearing, coughing, and grunting are simple phonic tics. Tic severity may vary from mild and barely noticeable to disabling. Individuals with TS also experience premonitory urges, sensations of discomfort or pressure in the muscles involved in the tics, which are relieved by the performance of a tic (Banaschewski et al., 2003; Leckman et al., 1993). Another phenomenological feature of TS is that most tics can be suppressed for minutes or even hours, and there is increasing recognition that individuals with TS vary in their ability to suppress tics (Leckman et al., 2006). Tics usually appear around 6 years of age and, over the course of the disorder, multiply and worsen in number and complexity, with the period of worst severity between 10 and 12 years of age (Leckman et al., 1998). Afterward, as fully detailed in Chapter 5, tics follow a remitting course in many individuals, remain stable in some, or continue to worsen in a minority (Bloch et al., 2006).

TS often co-occurs with other disorders, most notably attention-deficit/hyperactivity disorder (ADHD), disruptive behavior, and anxiety disorders (see Chapters 2, 3, and 4). Clinically ascertained cases of TS may be associated with mood, anxiety, and disruptive behavior disorders. Up to 60% of clinically referred children with TS also have ADHD, while in community samples the rates of co-occurrence of TS and ADHD ranges from 8% to 58% (Sukhodolsky et al., 2009). Several controlled studies, including our own work, documented the negative impact of co-occurring ADHD on social and adaptive functioning in children with TS (Sukhodolsky et al., 2003, 2010).

The extent to which deficits in social and adaptive functioning in individuals with TS are associated with the tics, co-occurring conditions or their combination, or a nonspecific impact of a chronic illness is an area of active research. The questions of functional impairment and the relative contributions of tics and co-occurring conditions are also of critical importance in clinical evaluations and intervention planning. Furthermore, understanding the strengths, interests, abilities, and talents of individuals with TS has become a key principle of assessment and treatment planning for children with tics and their families toward the goal of not only reducing symptoms but optimizing adaptive functioning and personal well-being. We will first provide an overview of the field of social and adaptive functioning in child development and psychopathology. Then we will discuss empirical research on the role of tics and co-occurring disorders, focusing on our own research on co-occurring ADHD and disruptive behavior disorders in children with TS. We will conclude with an overview of clinical assessment and behavioral interventions that can be recommended for children with TS and their families.

SOCIAL AND ADAPTIVE FUNCTIONING IN TYPICAL CHILD DEVELOPMENT AND PSYCHOPATHOLOGY

The term "social functioning" usually reflects the level of a child's social interaction and information processing skills as well as the development and stability of peer relationships and friendships. Other closely related constructs include social skills, social performance, and social adjustment (Yeates et al., 2007). Social skills are commonly seen as the individual abilities or characteristics needed to behave competently in social settings. Social performance refers to children's actual behavior in social interactions and to whether their responses are effective both in achieving their own goals and in maintaining positive relationships. Social adjustment reflects the extent to which children attain socially desirable and developmentally appropriate goals. Social adjustment encompasses the quality of children's relationships as perceived by others

but also includes self-perceptions of loneliness, social support, or social self-esteem.

The broader construct of "adaptive functioning" comprises a variety of related concepts that reflect competences across multiple contexts such as school and family but also including socialization. For example, in the Vineland Adaptive Behavior Scales (VABS) (Sparrow et al., 1984, 2005), adaptive behavior is defined as the performance of activities required for personal and social sufficiency that is age-dependent and determined by social expectations. It is also emphasized that adaptive behavior is defined by typical performance, not ability. For example, if a child knows how to brush his or her teeth and has the ability to do it but seldom does, the adaptive behavior will be considered inadequate in this area. The term "functional impairment" is used to refer to deficits in specific or broad domains of adaptive functioning (Winters et al., 2005).

Several comprehensive reviews of social development and social skills deficits in children across ranges of developmental psychopathology are available (Beauchamp & Anderson, 2010). An individual's status in his or her peer group (e.g., popular, rejected), which is typically assessed using sociometric interviews, is a relatively stable characteristic that emerges early in childhood and may significantly affect psychosocial development. Peer rejection encompasses a broad range of behaviors aimed to exclude or hurt another person, ranging from not initiating social interaction to actively preventing a child from having access to social participation. More extreme forms of rejecting behavior include aggression, bullying, and harassment. The presence of a stable friendship with another child can moderate the negative effects of social exclusion. Children with friends are less likely to show the deleterious consequences of problems with peers in school than children who do not have close friends. For instance, Boivin and colleagues (1995) reported that having a close friend ameliorated the negative consequences of being victimized by bullies. Close friendships buffered children from problems in peer relationships during a transition into a new school, social isolation, and development of adjustment problems

(Lamarche et al., 2006; Laursen et al., 2007). Friends are essential confidants and sources of support in good times and bad, and provide benefits to mental health from childhood to old age. Furthermore, part of the protective effects of friendship may be rooted in self-efficacy, the individual's belief in his or her ability to form high-quality, lasting relationships with others (Poulin & Boivin, 2000).

While social impairment can be associated with any childhood psychiatric disorder, it is also a hallmark of autism spectrum disorders (Pelphrey et al., 2011) and one of the diagnostic features of social anxiety disorder (Beidel et al., 2010). Extensive literature is dedicated to social functioning in children with externalizing and internalizing psychopathology (Nijmeijer et al., 2008). Thus, children with externalizing disorders are more likely to be rejected by their non-aggressive peers, which leads to greater chances of affiliation with the delinquent peers and, in turn, greater levels of conduct problems via a process of socialization that has become known as deviancy training (Patterson et al., 1989). Children with internalizing disorders such as depression and anxiety are also more likely to be rejected by their peers or to avoid social interaction. Their withdrawal from social interactions in childhood also appears to be stable over time and across contexts (Reef et al., 2010).

SOCIAL AND ADAPTIVE FUNCTIONING IN TS

Lack of social acceptability, deficits in social self-esteem, and difficulty with establishing and maintaining friendships are commonly noted by children with TS and their parents during clinical evaluations. Involuntary movements and vocalizations, particularly the ones that are forceful and complex, can be perceived as strange or can be disruptive in social interactions. In our clinical experience, many children and families report high levels of support and understanding of tics in schools and communities, a positive trend that is likely due to increasing public awareness of TS. However, it is also common to hear about children being teased about their tics at school or parents and children

receiving upsetting comments about tics from passersby in public places. For example, in a recent survey of 211 children with chronic tics, 26% reported peer victimization (Zinner et al., 2012). Middle-school age seems to be the time when children can be particularly at risk of being teased or excluded by their peers because of noticeable tics. In the long run, this may contribute to the lack of opportunities to develop social skills and friendships. It is also possible that the lack of social skills makes children less capable of communicating with others about their tics, thus creating a vicious circle of peer problems. It has been observed that tic-related impairment is correlated with tic severity and tends to decease with age (Coffey et al., 2000, 2004). By adolescence, however, the issues of awareness of tics in social situations and social self-esteem become more prominent and may lead to avoidance of certain social situations.

For example, one of our patients with a loud vocal tic was persistently teased by another boy, who would mimic the tic (loud snort) when near the patient, making other children laugh and contribute offensive remarks. Justly upset by this situation, our patient, a 10-year-old boy, complained to the teacher and also to his parents, who in turn also communicated their concern to the school principal. Despite these steps, the teasing continued and the more socially skilled provocateur was able to successfully deny any wrongdoing. At one point our patient took the matter into his own hands and pushed the boy who had been teasing him. This incident happened to be witnessed by the teacher who did not hear the teasing, and our patient was suspended from school. Now the social functioning problem has also become a problem in a broader context of academic functioning. In this example, the act of pushing another child was preceded by a sequence of failed communications among multiple involved parties but fortunately led to the development of a comprehensive plan for addressing the bullying problem and increasing awareness about TS among the teachers and students at our patient's school.

One study examined social functioning in children with TS by using a peer-rated sociometric questionnaire (Pekarik et al., 1976) completed by the child's classmates. Twenty-one children with TS (mean age 11.4 years) who participated in this study were rated by their peers as more withdrawn and less likable by their classmates (Stokes et al., 1991). The level of tic severity was not correlated with the ratings of popularity, but the presence of co-occurring ADHD was associated with lower popularity scores. In a second study by the same researchers, 26 children with TS were compared to a matched group of children with diabetes mellitus on the same sociometric ratings of peer relationships as well as on children's self-report of social skills (Matson et al., 1983) and self-esteem across several areas of personal competences (Harter, 1985). Similar to the previous study, children with TS received more peer nominations for withdrawal, but self-reports of social skills and social self-esteem ratings were not different across the groups and within the norms of standardization samples.

Storch and colleagues (2007) examined the rates of peer victimization in 59 children with a chronic tic disorder compared to 52 children with type 1 diabetes and 52 healthy controls. Children completed self-reported measures of peer victimization (Schwartz et al., 2002) and loneliness (Asher & Wheeler, 1985), and parents completed the Child Behavior Checklist (CBCL). Using a cutoff score of 1 SD above the nonclinical mean of this sample (M = 9.8), 27% of children with tics were classified as reporting clinically significant peer victimization scores compared to 9% of children with type 1 diabetes and 9% of healthy controls. Using a cutoff score of 1 SD above the mean for the Asher and Wheeler's (1985) normative sample, clinically significant loneliness was reported by 26% of children with tics. Peer victimization was significantly and positively associated with phonic tics ($r = .28$, $p < .05$) but not motor tics ($r = .15$, $p > .05$).

TIC-RELATED FUNCTIONAL IMPAIRMENT

The extent to which functional impairment is related to tics versus co-occurring conditions such as ADHD or anxiety is an area of active research. One study used a parent-rating instrument that attempted to isolate tic-related impairment from impairment due to co-occurring disorders by asking the parents to differentiate between the two causes (Storch et al., 2007). Parents of 59 children, ages 8 to 17, with TS completed the 37-item Child Tourette Syndrome Impairment Scale, which asked them to rate how much tics caused difficulties in school, home, and social activities. The areas where parents reported the highest percentage of impairment due to tics were primarily related to school, such as writing during class (24.6%), doing homework (21.9%), concentrating on work (21.8%), and being prepared for class (18.5%), or to social activities, such as being teased by peers (17.5%) and having difficulty making friends (15.8%). The majority of the sample reported significant problems in one or more areas (52.1%), with 37.5% of the sample reporting significant problems in two or more areas. Across broad categories of impairment, 35.6% of children were reported as having at least one significant problem area in school, 23.7% were reported to have at least one significant problem area at home, and 25.4% were reported to have at least one problem area in social activities. Of those children with significant problems, 10.2% reported at least one problem area in each domain (school, home, and social activities). The levels of impairment were positively correlated with the Yale Global Tic Severity Scale (YGTSS) total tic severity score ($r = .51$) and CBCL social problems score ($r = .44$).

A recent study examined the association of tic severity with measures of functional impairment in a sample of 126 children, age 9 to 17 years, who participated in a study of Comprehensive Behavior Intervention for Tics (CBIT) (Specht et al., 2011). Tics were measured by the YGTSS conducted by experienced clinicians; adaptive functioning was evaluated by the clinician-rated Children's Global Assessment Scale (CGAS) and by the three competency scales and the total competency scale of the parent-rated CBCL. There was a negative correlation of a moderate magnitude between the YGTSS total tic score and global psychosocial functioning as measured by the CGAS ($r = -.46$) but not the CBCL total score ($r = -.13$). Then, the unique contributions of the YGTSS scores for the number, frequency, intensity, complexity, and interference of tics to functional impairment were evaluated by simultaneous linear regression. The YGTSS tic interference score independently predicted the CGAS scores and tic intensity predicted CBCL total impairment scores. In a study with a smaller sample of 38 children with TS, ages 8 to 16, there was a moderate but significant association between the CBCL total impairment score and the tic complexity domain of the YGTSS (Himle et al., 2007). Complexity refers to how long, involved, or purposeful a tic may appear (see Chapter 1 for more details). Complex tics may be more noticeable (e.g., jumping or hopping), interfere with surrounding activities (e.g., loud vocalizations in the classroom), or involve family members (e.g., touching or tapping). Some complex tics, such as coprolalia and copropraxia, may also be socially embarrassing (Kurlan et al., 1996).

Indeed, in our clinical work we are often asked about specific tics that cause particular concern or interference in one or more areas of functioning. These research findings and clinical experience highlight the importance of obtaining multi-informant evaluation of tics and associated impairment because different informants (child, parent, teachers) may be more aware of various dimensions and characteristics of tics.

Although most studies of functional impairment were conducted with clinic-referred or treatment-seeking samples of children with TS, community sample and survey studies also report significant impairment of social and adaptive functioning in children with TS. Thus, 25 children with TS who were identified as part of an extensive screening procedure, including all schoolchildren 7 through 15 years of age in a town in Sweden with a population of about 40,000, reported lower self-perceptions of social relations (Khalifa et al., 2010). In a study of 57 children with TS or chronic tic disorder who were identified in a community sample of 9- to 11-year-old children in Denmark, 19% were rated by parents on a Strengths and Difficulties Questionnaire (SDQ; Goodman, 2001) as having peer problems (Tabori Kraft et al., 2012).

A more fine-grained evaluation of functional impairment in a nonreferred sample was conducted by an Internet survey of 740 parents and 232 children (ages 10–17 years), members of the U.S. Tourette Syndrome Association. The majority of children and their parents reported that tics interfered with adaptive functioning across multiple domains. Thus, 43% of parents indicated that their children avoided social events or entertainment activities because of tics, 37% avoided public places, and 44% avoided group activities. Sixty percent of children reported that tics interfered with their schoolwork or made it hard to study (Conelea et al., 2011a). Similar survey methodology was employed in a study of 672 adults with self-reported chronic tic disorders (Conelea et al., 2011b). Approximately 40% of responders endorsed social difficulty such as avoiding social events, public places, or group activities. Responders who held a job within the past 12 months (N = 461) also reported that tics mildly interfered with their occupational functioning, although 7% reported quitting a job because of tics, 12.6% reported failure to pursue job advancement, and 12% reported avoiding job interviews.

Children with TS often experience difficulties at school, many of which may be tic-related, or related to associated disorders such as ADHD or anxiety (Kurlan et al., 2001; Packer, 2005; Sparrow et al., 1984, 2005). For example, Abwender and colleagues (1996) conducted a retrospective study of 138 children with TS ranging in age from 5 to 18 years and reported that 22% of children had a diagnosis of a specific learning disorder and an additional 33% had other school problems, such as grade retention and special education placement. In a community sample of children with TS, 80% of children had had school-related difficulties (Khalifa & Von Knorring, 2006). Even simple tics such as eye blinking may be time-consuming, so that the time spent performing a tic is time not spent doing schoolwork. More complex tics such as rewriting or rereading may also interfere with completing assignments on time. The waxing and waning nature of tics, as well as the partial suppressibility of tics, may give a false impression that tics are voluntary. Children may fidget in response to the urge, and the efforts to suppress tics may interfere with their ability to pay attention to academic tasks. Finally, children receiving medication for tics may experience side effects such as sedation or restlessness, which may interfere with their ability to learn. These and other scenarios of interference caused by tics often lead to accommodations such as extended time for tests, "friendly time-outs," and using tape-recorders and books on tape (Packer, 2005).

TS AND FAMILY FUNCTIONING

Adverse effects of TS on family functioning can include high caregiver stress (Cooper et al., 2003; Schoeder & Remer, 2007), reduced family cohesion and increased conflict (Carter et al., 2000), and impact on day-to-day functioning (Hubka et al., 1988; Pringsheim et al., 2009). For example, in a study of 26 children with TS who where compared to a matched sample of children with asthma, parents of children with TS reported greater strain in their daily activities, relationships, and well-being. Perceived caregiver burden was positively correlated with the presence of co-occurring behavioral problems (Wilkinson et al., 2008). In our study using the Family Environment Scale (Moos & Moos, 1986) in a relatively large sample of children with TS with and without co-occurring ADHD, we found that ADHD, but not the tics, was associated with reduced levels of family cohesion and increased levels of family conflict (Sukhodolsky et al., 2003). Similar results were reported in a study with parents of 45 children with chronic tics who completed the Impact on Family Scale (Woods et al., 2005). It is possible that the unique challenges of parenting children with co-occurring TS and ADHD can be partially explained by the difficulty parents have in distinguishing tics from impulsive behavior. Involuntary expression of tics on the one hand, contrasted with inappropriate behavior on the other hand, can make it difficult for parents to provide consistent discipline, leading to escalating family conflict and parenting stress (Scahill et al., 2006).

Consistent with studies of caregiver burden in children across neurodevelopmental disorders, parents of children with TS reported that social support lowered the perception of burden (Lee et al., 2007; Schoeder & Remer, 2007). This suggests the importance of interventions aimed at increasing social support toward the aim of reducing caregiver burden. One way to increase social support is to become involved with local and national TS associations (see Chapter 30). Parents of children with tics can be also encouraged to strengthen their ties with immediate and extended families. Indeed, we find that family support and education are critical components of comprehensive treatment for TS (see Chapters 22 and 28). Problem solving and assistance with daily activities are also likely to be useful interventions for alleviating parenting stress (Mendenhall & Mount, 2011; Silverstein et al., 2011), although this has not been formally studied in children with TS. There is also emerging evidence that tic exacerbations during the waxing and waning course of the disorder may be associated with psychosocial and family stress (see also Chapter 14; Lin et al., 2007), suggesting that treatment of TS should include stress management strategies.

QUALITY OF LIFE IN TS

There has been increasing recognition of the impact of TS on health-related quality of life, a term that reflects overall well-being and perceptions of the extent to which well-being is affected by the disorder. The first study of quality of life in TS included 103 adults who completed the Medical Outcomes Study 36-Item Short-Form Health Survey (SF-36) and Quality of Life Assessment Schedule, and were found to have significantly worse quality of life than a general population sample (Elstner, Selai, Trimble & Robertson, 2001). Storch and colleagues (2007) evaluated quality of life in children with TS (n = 56, age 8–17). Quality of life was defined as perceptions of the impact of disease and treatment on physical, emotional, social, and school functioning (Varni et al., 1999). Child self-reports and parent ratings of quality of life of children with TS were significantly lower than those of unaffected children. Other studies confirmed that the social dimension of the perceived quality of life is particularly vulnerable in TS (Eddy et al., 2011). Co-occurring ADHD and obsessive-compulsive disorder (OCD) were also found to be associated with lower quality of life in children with TS (Bernard et al., 2009).

Cavanna and colleagues have recently developed the Gilles de la Tourette Syndrome-Quality of Life Scale (GTS-QOL) (Cavanna et al., 2008), a 27-item questionnaire of overall well-being in individuals with TS (further details provided in Chapter 19). Using this scale in a large sample of 200 adults with TS, quality of life was considerably reduced and associated with greater levels of tics and depression (Müller-Vahl et al., 2010). In a recent longitudinal study of 46 children with TS who were re-evaluated at age 16 years or above with a mean follow-up period of 13 years, poorer quality of life in adulthood was predicted by greater tic severity in childhood (Cavanna et al., 2012). The results of this longitudinal study suggest a possibility that even when the association between tic severity and adaptive functioning does not reach statistical significance in cross-sectional studies with children, the impact of tics on functioning could accumulate over years and lead to functional impairment and reduced quality of life in adulthood.

IMPAIRMENT ASSOCIATED WITH ADHD AND DISRUPTIVE BEHAVIOR DISORDERS

Individuals with TS can also present with impairments in various domains of functioning. However, it may be difficult to determine whether the impairment is associated with tics or with the co-occurring condition. Several controlled studies documented the negative impact of co-occurring ADHD on psychopathology and functioning in children with TS. Spencer and colleagues compared 79 children with TS+ADHD and 18 children with TS without ADHD (Spencer et al., 1998). The rates of mood, disruptive, psychotic, and most anxiety disorders were similar in the TS+ADHD and ADHD-alone groups. Children with TS had a lower frequency of oppositional defiant disorder than the TS+ADHD group. The number of comorbid conditions and the Global Assessment

of Functioning Scale (GAF) scores did not differ significantly between children with mild (N = 43) and moderate to severe (N = 54) tic severity. By contrast, severe symptoms of ADHD in children with TS+ADHD were associated with a higher risk of mood disorders and lower GAF scores. Sukhodolsky and colleagues (2003) examined the association of disruptive behavior with social, family, and adaptive functioning in 42 children with TS alone and 52 children with TS+ADHD. Both TS groups were compared to age-matched children with ADHD alone and unaffected controls. Multiple domains of children's functioning were evaluated using parent and teacher ratings of disruptive behavior, and parent ratings of social and family functioning. Children with TS only did not differ from unaffected controls on the parent and teacher ratings of disruptive behavior. By contrast, children with TS+ADHD were significantly above unaffected controls and similar to children with ADHD alone on the measures of disruptive behavior. Children with TS, regardless of ADHD comorbidity, presented with age-appropriate levels of engagement in activities such as hobbies, clubs, and sports, as measured by the Activity Competence scale of the CBCL. However, children with TS+ADHD demonstrated significant impairment in all areas of social and adaptive functioning and were similar to the ADHD-alone contrast group. This pattern of scores on the CBCL Social Competence scale and the VABS is indicative of multiple deficits, such as having fewer friends, being rejected by peers, and failing to meet the demands of everyday life. Children with TS alone were also more impaired than unaffected controls on measures of social competency and daily living skills, but less so than those with TS+ADHD. These findings were generally consistent with other reports (Carter et al., 2000; Dykens et al., 1990; Hoekstra et al., 2004).

In contrast to findings of negative impact of ADHD on adaptive functioning in TS, tics contribute no or little impairment in children with ADHD (Spencer et al., 1999, 2001). Spencer and colleagues (1999) examined the course of tic disorders in 128 boys age 7 to 17 years. The distribution of tic disorders in this sample was 34% (43/128), including 18 cases of TS (14%). Boys with ADHD with and without tics were similar in terms of the average number of ADHD symptoms and ADHD age of onset. There were no differences between these two groups on the measures of cognitive, school, social, and family functioning. In all but three cases, the onset of ADHD preceded the onset of tics, and age-adjusted rates of remission were 20% for ADHD and 65% for tic disorders. Based on these data, it was concluded that tic disorders have a limited effect on the course and outcomes of ADHD. Similar conclusions were drawn from a study with 312 adults with ADHD, 36 of whom had tic disorders (Spencer et al., 2001).

Disruptive behavior may have additional negative impact on adaptive functioning in children with TS above that conferred by tics and co-occurring ADHD. Studies of clinically referred samples reveal that up to 80% of children and adolescents with TS also have co-occurring disruptive behavior problems (Coffey et al., 2000; Erenberg et al., 1986; Rosenberg et al., 1995). Survey studies of members of local chapters of the Tourette Syndrome Association also documented that anger-related problems were present in 36% to 67% of the respondents (Kadesjo & Gillberg, 2000; Stefl, 1984). The high rates of co-occurrence of disruptive behavior problems with TS in clinically referred samples is difficult to interpret in terms of etiology and may simply reflect the fact that patients with several disorders are more likely to seek medical attention (Pauls et al., 1994). The rates of disruptive behavior were somewhat lower in two community-ascertained samples of children with TS. In a sample of 13- and 14-year-old children (n =1,012), seven children had TS and three of them (43%) also had oppositional defiant disorder or conduct disorder (Hornsey et al., 2001). Other studies also demonstrated that children with tics had higher levels of disruptive behavior problems than children without tics (Gadow et al., 2002; Kurlan, 2002; Snider et al., 2002).

Due to their intensity and unpredictability in response to minimal provocation, anger outbursts in TS have been described as *rage attacks* or *rage storms*. The explosive and out-of-character nature of disruptive behavior in TS resembles characteristics of aggression noted in "episodic dyscontrol syndrome" (Gordon, 1999; Nunn, 1986), intermittent explosive disorder (Olvera, 2002), and "anger attacks" in depression (Fava et al., 1991). Using the modified DSM-IV criteria for intermittent explosive disorder, Budman and colleagues (1998) reported recurrent rage attacks resulting in destruction of property or personal injury in 12 consecutive children with TS referred to the movement disorders center of a general hospital. These episodes reportedly lasted from a few minutes to an hour, and were usually followed by remorse. The characteristics of rage attacks were further elaborated in a sample of 48 children age 7 to 17 (Budman et al., 2003). In this sample, over 90% of disruptive outbursts occurred at home and were triggered by being unable to get one's way or being told to give up what one was doing. In a study of children with TS with (n = 37) or without explosive anger (n = 31), the presence of anger was associated with higher rates of ADHD and OCD (Budman & Feirman, 2001).

In our 2003 study, we conducted hierarchical regression analyses using TS and ADHD diagnostic status and CBCL Aggression and Delinquency scores to predict the measures of functional outcome. A diagnosis of TS significantly predicted impairment only on the CBCL Social Competence scale. ADHD, on the other hand, significantly predicted all seven measures of functional outcome included in regression analyses. The CBCL Aggression and Delinquency scales, entered as one block, added a unique contribution to the CBCL Social Competence score, VABS Socialization score, and Family Environment Scale Conflict and Cohesion scores. Aggressive behavior was found to have the most detrimental effect on peer relationships in schoolchildren (Ladd & Burgess, 1999) and in children and adolescents with ADHD (Bagwell et al., 2001). Similarly, in this study, the diagnosis of ADHD was related to impairment across all measures of functional outcome, but the CBCL scores on the Aggression and Delinquency scales were associated with an additional increment in socialization impairment. Aggressive and delinquent behavior may also have a negative impact on family functioning, as evidenced by the measures of family conflict and cohesion. However, the direction of causality is unclear, as family dysfunction can contribute to child's disruptive behavior problems.

More than 50% of children with TS meet criteria for one or more anxiety disorders, and more severe tics can be associated with greater anxiety (Coffey et al., 2000). Anxiety itself can have deleterious effects on adaptive functioning, including social impairment and school problems (Manassis, 2012). In children with co-occurring anxiety and tic disorders, anxiety may require a separate treatment as well as moderate response to treatment of ADHD and behavioral problems (Gadow & Nolan, 2011). Anxiety disorders in children with TS and ADHD were found to be associated with more severe depression and disruptive behavior symptoms (Gadow et al., 2002). Using the data collected as part of a large Web-based Tourette Syndrome Impact Survey, Lewin and colleagues (2010) examined the moderating effects of anxiety and depression on the association of tics with functional impairment in 500 adults with self-reported TS. Participants completed the self-report version of the YGTSS, Sheehan Disability Scale (Leon et al., 1997), and Depression, Anxiety and Stress Scale (Lovibond & Lovibond, 1995). Hierarchical regression revealed that the strength of association of tics with functional impairment is indeed moderated by the levels of anxiety and depression. Specifically, in adults with higher levels of anxious or depressive symptoms, there is a stronger relationship between tic severity and functional impairment than among adults with fewer anxious and depressive symptoms. To our knowledge, the effects of anxiety on adaptive functioning in children with TS have not been directly evaluated. However, drawing on Lewin's findings in adults as well as on impairing features of anxiety in children without tics, it can be suggested that the clinical evaluation of children with tics should include careful assessment of possible co-occurring anxiety disorders.

COMMONLY USED MEASURES OF ADAPTIVE FUNCTIONING AND IMPAIRMENT

The YGTSS (Leckman et al., 1989) includes a one-item rating of tic-related impairment that is defined as the impact of tics *per se* on the individual's self-perception, relationships with family members, social relationships, and ability to perform in academic or occupational settings. This rating is assigned by an experienced clinician upon completion of the YGTSS interview to reflect the cumulative toll that the tic disorder has had on the individual. Operationally, ratings of impairment are based on a six-point scale (none, minimal, mild, moderate, marked, or severe impairment), with specific descriptions of anchors for each point. The interrater agreement of this one-item impairment rating was high in the YGTSS development sample (intraclass correlation coefficient = 0.80 for three raters and 20 subjects).

Tic-related impairment can be assessed using the Global Assessment of Functioning, both in children (C-GAS) (Shaffer et al., 1983) and in adults (Endicott et al., 1976), on a scale from 0 to 100, where 0 reflects the greatest levels of impairment, requiring complete dependence on others for care, and 100 reflects excellent functioning in all areas of personal development, school/work, and social activities.

A more detailed measure of tic-related impairment, the Child Tic Impairment Scale, has been developed by Storch and colleagues (2007). This is a 37-item parent-rated instrument that includes school, home, and social activities that may be impaired by the child's tics or co-occurring conditions such as obsessive-compulsive symptoms, depression, anxiety, oppositional/disruptive behavior, hyperactivity, or inattentiveness. Parents are instructed to rate how much their child's vocal and motor tics have caused difficulties for him or her over the past month on a 4-point rating system (not at all, just a little, pretty much, and very much). Items such as "Getting to school on time" and "Doing household chores" are first rated for tic-related impairment, and then for impairment due to a comorbid disorder known to the parents. A tic impairment score is derived by totaling all items in the tic dimension and a non-tic impairment score is derived by totaling all items in the non-tic dimension. Internal consistency of the scale for the tic-related and non–tic-related impairment was excellent, with Cronbach's alpha coefficients of .94 and .92, respectively.

The CBCL (Achenbach, 1991; Achenbach & Rescorla, 2001) is a standardized parent-report measure of problem behavior and adaptive functioning that has been most commonly used in research with children with TS. Adaptive functioning is measured by three competence scales (Activities, Social, and School) and a summary total competence score. The Activities competence scale reflects the number of sports, hobbies, and clubs the child participates in, as well as the parent's perception of how well the child performs in these activities compared to other children. The Social competence scale assesses the number of friends, time spent with friends, and the extent to which the child gets along with his or her peers. The School competence scale assesses the levels of performance in academic subjects, grade retention, and special services. The CBCL has been standardized on a large sample of typically developing children, and clinical samples of children with externalizing and internalizing disorders are available. The raw scores are converted to the T-scores with a mean of 50 and standard deviation of 10. On the competency scales higher scores correspond to greater levels of competency. Test–retest reliability coefficients for the competence scales range from .70 and .92.

The VABS (Sparrow et al., 1984, 2005) is a parent interview designed to measure adaptive behavior for ages birth through 90. This measure is standardized on a large national sample and extensive reliability and validity information is available. The Communication domain reflects receptive, expressive, and written communication skills. The Daily Living Skills domain samples personal living habits, domestic task performance, and behavior in the community. The Socialization domain assesses interaction with others, including friendships, play, and social appropriateness. In each domain, the interviewer begins with broad queries about the child's adaptive behavior. Additional questions are asked to identify skills that the child has acquired and performs on a regular basis (score of 2), skills that are performed sometimes (score of 1), or skills that are performed not at all (score of 0). Items are specific and arranged in increasing complexity. In general, however, the interviewer does not read the items from the page but asks the parent to respond indirectly. For example, rather than ask directly if the child can recite the alphabet, the interviewer engages in a discussion of letter recognition, word recognition, reading, and so forth. This semistructured approach permits the scoring of several clustered items. Finally, the scores on the first three domains are used to derive an adaptive behavior composite score, which is a global estimate of adaptive behavior. The VABS is considered a gold standard for the assessment of adaptive behavior, but only a few studies conducted with children with TS have used this measure (Carter et al., 2000; Dykens et al., 1990; Sukhodolsky et al., 2003).

The Behavioral Assessment System for Children (BASC) (Reynolds & Kamphaus, 2004) is a commonly used measure of psychopathology and adaptive functioning in children and adolescents. Although to our knowledge this scale has not been used in published studies of children with TS, it is among the most common measures used in psychological and psychoeducational assessments, and social and adaptive behavior of children with TS who undergo such assessments in the future are likely to be evaluated by the BASC. The parent-rating version of the BASC includes six adaptive scales: activities of daily living, adaptability, functional communication, leadership, social skills, and study skills. The scales are summed for an adaptive skills composite. Raw scores are converted to T-scores with a mean of 50 and standard deviation of 10, which are derived based on the large standardization sample. The internal consistency reliability coefficients for the adaptive scales range from .87 to .88.

BEHAVIORAL INTERVENTIONS

It is commonly suggested that children with tics may also benefit from informal (e.g., practicing with parents or siblings) or formal social skills training to prepare them to respond appropriately to teasing or rejection due to tics. Although social skills training has not been evaluated in children with tics, extensive literature on social skills training in children with behavioral and neurodevelopmental disorders suggests that this modality of psychosocial intervention may be helpful for addressing social skills deficits in children with TS. Procedures commonly involve techniques of instruction, modeling, rehearsal, corrective feedback, and reinforcement for appropriate performance aimed at improving specific social deficits and overall social adjustment (Spence, 2003). The theoretical background can be traced to behavioral and social-learning theories as well as to early behavioral approaches to psychotherapy (Wolpe, 1958). The broad goal of social skills training is to train specific behaviors relevant to improving deficits in social interaction. Deficits in social information processing skills such as consequential thinking and emotion regulation are also often addressed as part of social skills training. Social skills training is used in a variety of settings, such as residential facilities, hospitals, and schools. It can be administered individually, in groups, or with the participation of peer mediators. Applications vary broadly in terms of number, frequency, and duration of sessions, and sometimes treatment is conducted until the mastery criteria for performance of targeted social skills are reached. In addition to being used as a monomodal treatment, it is often used as part of multicomponent psychosocial treatments and preventive interventions. A recent review of meta-analyses of the effectiveness of social skills training with children and adolescents concluded that it is likely to be moderately effective for children with emotional and behavioral disorders (Cook et al., 2008). Application in children with developmental disorders and intellectual disabilities is also an area of active research (Reichow & Volkmar, 2010; Sukhodolsky & Butter, 2006).

Disruptive behavior, including anger, aggression, noncompliance, and explosive rage outbursts, is common in children and adolescents with TS and may be a source of greater impairment than tics (Sukhodolsky et al., 2003). We evaluated two forms of psychosocial interventions, parent management training (PMT) in school-age children and cognitive-behavioral therapy (CBT) for anger control in adolescents with TS. The PMT study included 24 children with TS and high levels of disruptive behavior who were randomized to 10 sessions of PMT or 10 weeks of treatment as usual (Scahill et al., 2006). Clinical ratings conducted by the independent evaluator as well as parent ratings of disruptive behavior showed a significant reduction of disruptive behavior in the PMT condition. In the study of CBT for anger control, 26 children and adolescents with TS were randomized to 10 sessions of CBT or 10 weeks of treatment as usual (Sukhodolsky et al., 2009). Participants in the CBT condition had a significant reduction of disruptive behavior on the clinical ratings by an independent evaluator as well as on parent ratings. In addition, there was a significant increase in the total competence score of the parent-rated CBCL in children who received CBT for anger control (Cohen's d effect size = .86). These results suggest that a reduction in disruptive behavior might have translated into an improvement in adaptive functioning, although this has to be replicated in larger studies.

There is also emerging evidence that behavior therapy for tics may be associated with improvement in social functioning (Woods et al., 2011). In a recently completed study of 126 children ages 9 to 17 years with chronic tic or Tourette disorder, comprehensive behavior intervention for tics was superior to psychological support control treatment for tic reduction (Piacentini et al., 2010). Children in the behavior therapy and control conditions did not differentially improve on psychosocial outcome measures at the end of active treatment. However, at the 6-month posttreatment assessment, a positive response to behavior therapy was associated with improved social functioning as measured by the self-report Social Adjustment Scale (Weissman et al., 1980). The authors noted that although children with ADHD, OCD, or other anxiety disorders were not excluded from the study, subjects were excluded if the co-occurring condition required more immediate treatment. Thus, few participants had elevated scores on these secondary symptom measures, and the baseline total competency scores on the CBCL were in the average range. Additional details on these management aspects are presented in Chapters 22 and 23.

CONCLUSIONS

Research studies show that approximately 50% of children with TS have impairments in social and adaptive functioning, and that co-occurring conditions such as ADHD, anxiety, and disruptive behavior may further exacerbate these functional deficits. Clinical evaluation of children with TS should include a detailed discussion of strengths and weaknesses in social and school functioning. More fine-grained analysis of adaptive behavior can be conducted by using standardized measures such as the VABS and CBCL. There is emerging evidence that behavioral therapy for tics and disruptive behavior in children with TS may be associated with improvements in social adjustment.

Clinical Implications

Focusing on personal strengths and building resilience has been at the center of our approach to caring for children with TS and their families. In addition to the evaluation of tics and possible co-occurring disorders, a comprehensive clinical evaluation of TS should involve a detailed discussion of social, family, and adaptive functioning. Whenever possible, the clinical interview should be complemented by standardized measures, some of which are listed in this chapter. Many families can benefit from a continuing discussion over the course of several visits about the relative contributions of tics versus ADHD, anxiety, or disruptive behavior disorders to the impairments in adaptive functioning.

Often pharmacological or behavioral interventions aimed at tics would lead to improvement in functioning. More focused interventions such as social skills training, family support, problem solving, or academic skills counseling can be helpful to address problems in social, family, and school functioning. There is emerging evidence that tics may be sensitive to environmental events, worsening during times of stress and fatigue and improving during engagement in activities that require mental focus or fine-motor skills. This can inform discussions with children and their families about the choice of hobbies and sports, scheduling of day-to-day

---

Box 21.1. Key Points

- Many children, adolescents, and adults with TS may have impairments across various domains of social and adaptive functioning. The degree of impairment may be associated with the overall severity of tics as well as particular characteristics of tics, such as high frequency or forcefulness.
- In addition to tics, impairment in adaptive functioning could be conferred by associated conditions such as ADHD, anxiety, and disruptive behavior disorders. The relative contribution of tics versus other co-occurring conditions to impairments in adaptive functioning is an active area of research.
- Careful clinical evaluation is required to understand profiles of strengths and weaknesses in adaptive functioning and to disentangle relative contributions of tics and co-occurring disorders to possible problems with peers, academic functioning, or family life. Whenever possible, clinical interviews should be supplemented by collecting standardized ratings of adaptive functioning.
- Recent advances in psychosocial interventions for tics and associated behavioral disorders suggest that these treatments are likely to improve the symptoms and associated functional impairment.

activities, and utilizing stress management strategies that may improve tics as well as optimize development across other important areas of functioning.

REFERENCES

Abwender DA, Como PG, Kurlan R et al. School problems in Tourette's syndrome. *Arch Neurol* 1996; 53:509–511.

Achenbach TM. *Manual for the Child Behavior Checklist/4-18 and 1991 Profile.* Burlington, VT: University of Vermont Press, 1991.

Achenbach TM, Rescorla LA. *Manual for the ASEBA School-Age Forms & Profiles.* Burlington, VT, University of Vermont, Research Center for Children, Youth, and Families, 2001.

Asher SR, Wheeler VA. Children's loneliness. A comparison of rejected and neglected peer status. *J Consult Clin Psychol* 1985; 53:500–505.

Banaschewski T, Woerner W, Rothenberger A. Premonitory sensory phenomena and suppressibility of tics in Tourette syndrome: developmental aspects in children and adolescents. *Dev Med Child Neurol* 2003; 45:700–703.

Beauchamp MH, Anderson V. SOCIAL: An integrative framework for the development of social skills. *Psychol Bull* 2010; 13:639–664.

Beidel DC, Rao PA, Scharfstein L et al. Social skills and social phobia: An investigation of DSM-IV subtypes. *Behav Res Ther* 2010; 48:992–1001.

Bernard BA, Stebbins GT, Siegel S et al. Determinants of quality of life in children with

Gilles de la Tourette syndrome. *Mov Disord* 2009; 24:1070–1073.

Bloch MH, Scahill L, Otka J et al. Adulthood outcome of tic and obsessive-compulsive symptom severity in children with Tourette syndrome. *Arch Pediatr Adolesc Med* 2006; 160:65–69.

Boivin M, Dodge KA, Coie JD. Individual–group behavioral similarity and peer status in experimental play groups of boys: The social misfit revisited. *J Pers Soc Psychol* 1995; 69:269–279.

Budman CL, Bruun RD, Park KS, Olson ME. Rage attacks in children and adolescents with Tourette's disorder: A pilot study. *J Clin Psychiatry* 1998; 59:576–580.

Budman CL, Feirman L. The relationship of Tourette's syndrome with its psychiatric comorbidities: Is there an overlap? *Psychiatr Ann* 2001; 31:541–548.

Budman CL, Rockmore L, Stokes J, Sossin M. Clinical phenomenology of episodic rage in children with Tourette syndrome. *J Psychosom Res* 2003; 55:59–65.

Carter AS, O'Donnell DA, Schultz RT et al. Social and emotional adjustment in children affected with Gilles de la Tourette's syndrome: Associations with ADHD and family functioning. *J Child Psychol Psychiatry* 2000; 41: 215–223.

Cavanna AE, David K, Orth M, Robertson MM. Predictors during childhood of future health-related quality of life in adults with Gilles de la Tourette syndrome. *Eur J Paediatr Neurol* 2012 [E-pub ahead of print].

This longitudinal study reported that greater severity of tics in children was associated with lower quality of life in adults with TS.

Cavanna AE, Schrag A, Morley D et al. The Gilles de la Tourette Syndrome-Quality of Life Scale (GTS-QOL): Development and validation. *Neurology* 2008; 71:1410–1416.

Centers for Disease Control and Prevention. Prevalence of diagnosed Tourette syndrome in persons aged 6–17 years—United States, 2007. *MMWR* 2009; 58:581–585.

Coffey BJ, Biederman J, Geller D et al. Distinguishing illness severity from tic severity in children and adolescents with Tourette's disorder. *J Am Acad Child Adolesc Psychiatry* 2000; 39:556–561.

Coffey BJ, Biederman J, Geller D et al. Reexamining tic persistence and tic-associated impairment in Tourette's disorder: findings from a naturalistic follow-up study. *J Nerv Ment Dis* 2004; 192:776–780.

Coffey BJ, Biederman J, Smoller JW et al. Anxiety disorders and tic severity in juveniles with Tourette's disorder. *J Am Acad Child Adolesc Psychiatry* 2000; 39:562–568.

Conelea CA, Woods DW, Zinner SH et al. Exploring the impact of chronic tic disorders on youth: Results from the Tourette Syndrome Impact Survey. *Child Psychiatry Hum Dev* 2011a; 42:219–242.

This survey study reports on a wide range of problems in adaptive functioning that may be associated with TS.

Conelea CA, Woods DW, Zinner SH et al. The impact of Tourette Syndrome in adults: Results from the Tourette Syndrome Impact Survey. *Commun Ment Health J* 2011b [E-pub ahead of print].

Cook CR, Gresham FM, Kern L et al. Social skills training for secondary students with emotional and/or behavioral disorders: A review and analysis of the meta-analytic literature. *J Emotional Behav Disord* 2008; 16:131–144.

Cooper C, Robertson MM, Livingston G. Psychological morbidity and caregiver burden in parents of children with Tourette's disorder and psychiatric comorbidity. *J Am Acad Child Adolesc Psychiatry* 2003; 42:1370–1375.

Dykens E, Leckman JF, Riddle M et al. Intellectual, academic, and adaptive functioning of Tourette syndrome children with and without attention deficit disorder. *J Abnorm Child Psychol* 1990; 18: 607–615.

Eddy CM, Rizzo R, Gulisano M et al. Quality of life in young people with Tourette syndrome: A controlled study. *J Neurol* 2011; 258:291–301.

Elstner K, Selai CE, Trimble MR, Robertson MM. Quality of life (QOL) of patients with Gilles de la Tourette's syndrome. *Acta Psychiat Scand* 2001; 103:52–59.

Endicott J, Spitzer RL, Fleiss JL, Cohen J. The global assessment scale. A procedure for measuring overall severity of psychiatric disturbance. *Arch Gen Psychiatry* 1976; 33:766–771.

Erenberg G, Cruse RP, Rothner AD. *Cleve Clin Q* 1986; 53:127–131.

Fava M, Rosenbaum JF, McCarthy M et al. Anger attacks in depressed outpatients and their response to fluoxetine. *Psychopharmacol Bull* 1991; 27:275–279.

Gadow KD, Nolan EE. Methylphenidate and comorbid anxiety disorder in children with both chronic multiple tic disorder and ADHD. *J Attent Disord* 2011; 15:246–256.

Gadow KD, Nolan EE, Sprafkin J, Schwartz J. Tics and psychiatric comorbidity in children and adolescents. *Dev Med Child Neurol* 2002; 44:330–338.

Goodman R. Psychometric properties of the strengths and difficulties questionnaire. *J Am Acad Child Adolesc Psychiatry* 2001; 40:1337–1345.

Gordon N. Episodic dyscontrol syndrome. *Dev Med Child Neurol* 1999; 41:786–788.

Harter S. *Manual for the Self-Perception Profile for Children*. Denver, CO: University of Denver Press, 1985.

Himle MB, Chang S, Woods DW et al. Evaluating the contributions of ADHD, OCD, and tic symptoms in predicting functional competence in children with tic disorders. *J Dev Phys Disabil* 2007; 19:503–512.

Hoekstra PJ, Steenhuis MP, Troost PW et al. Relative contribution of attention-deficit hyperactivity disorder, obsessive-compulsive disorder, and tic severity to social and behavioral problems in tic disorders. *J Dev Behav Pediatr* 2004; 25:272–279.

Hornsey H, Banerjee S, Zeitlin H, Robertson MM. The prevalence of Tourette syndrome in 13-14-year-olds in mainstream schools. *J Child Psychol Psychiatry* 2001; 42: 1035–1039.

Hubka GB, Fulton WA, Shady GA et al. Tourette syndrome: impact on Canadian family functioning. *Neurosci Biobehav Rev* 1988; 12:259–261.

Kadesjo B, Gillberg C. Tourette's disorder: epidemiology and comorbidity in primary school children. *J Am Acad Child Adolesc Psychiatry* 2000; 39:548–555.

Khalifa N, Dalan M, Rydell AM. Tourette syndrome in the general child population: Cognitive functioning and self- perception. *Nord J Psychiatry* 2010; 64:11–18.

Khalifa N, von Knorring AL. Psychopathology in a Swedish population of school children with tic disorders. *J Am Acad Child Adolesc Psychiatry* 2006; 45:1345–1353.

Kurlan R. Treatment of ADHD in children with tics: A randomized controlled trial. *Neurology* 2002; 58:527–536.

Kurlan R, Daragjati C, Como PG et al. Non-obscene complex socially inappropriate behavior in Tourette's syndrome. *J Neuropsychiatry Clin Neurosci* 1996; 8:311–317.

Kurlan R, McDermott MP, Deeley C et al. Prevalence of tics in schoolchildren and association with placement in special education. *Neurology* 2001; 57:1383–1388.

Lamarche V, Brendgen M, Boivin M et al. Do friendships and sibling relationships provide protection against peer victimization in a similar way? *Social Dev* 2006; 15:373–393.

Laursen B, Bukowski WM, Aunola K, Nurmi JE. Friendship moderates prospective associations between social isolation and adjustment problems in young children. *Child Dev* 2007; 78:1395–1404.

Leckman JF. Phenomenology of tics and natural history of tic disorders. *Brain Dev* 2003; 25 Suppl 1:S24–28.

Leckman JF, Bloch MH, Scahill L, King RA. Tourette syndrome: The self under siege. *J Child Neurol* 2006; 21:642–649.

Leckman JF, Riddle MA, Hardin MT et al. The Yale Global Tic Severity Scale: initial testing of a clinician-rated scale of tic severity. *J Am Acad Child Adolesc Psychiatry* 1989; 28:566–573.

Leckman JF, Walker DE, Cohen DJ. Premonitory urges in Tourette's syndrome. *Am J Psychiatry* 2003; 150:98–102.

Leckman JF, Zhang H, Vitale A et al. Course of tic severity in Tourette syndrome: the first two decades. *Pediatrics* 1998; 102:14–19.

Lee MY, Chen YC, Wang HS, Chen DR. Parenting stress and related factors in parents of children with Tourette syndrome. *J Nurs Res* 2007; 15:165–174.

Leon AC, Portera L, Olfson M et al. Assessing psychiatric impairment in primary care with the Sheehan Disability Scale. *Int J Psychiatry Med* 1997; 27:93–105.

Lewin AB, Storch EA, Conelea CA et al. The roles of anxiety and depression in connecting tic severity and functional impairment. *J Anxiety Disord* 2011; 25:164–168.

Lin H, Katsovich L, Ghebremichael M et al. Psychosocial stress predicts future symptom severities in children and adolescents with Tourette syndrome and/or obsessive-compulsive disorder. *J Child Psychol Psychiatry* 2007; 48:157–166.

This longitudinal study examined the effects of the severity of tics and associated symptoms of OCD and depression.

Lovibond SH, Lovibond PF. *Manual for the Depression Anxiety Stress Scales.* Sydney, Australia: Psychological Foundation of Australia, 1995.

Manassis K. Generalized anxiety disorder in the classroom. *Child Adolesc Psychiatr Clin North Am* 2012; 21:93–103.

Matson JL, Rotarori AF, Helsel WJ. Development of a rating scale to measure social skills in children: The Matson Evaluation of Social Skills with Youngsters (MESSY). *Behav Res Ther* 1983; 21:335–340.

Mendenhall AN, Mount K. Parents of children with mental illness: Exploring the caregiver experience and caregiver-focused interventions. *Families in Soc* 2011; 92:183–190.

Moos RH, Moos BM. *Family Environment Scale: Manual.* Palo Alto, CA: Consulting Psychologists Press, 1986.

Müller-Vahl K, Dodel I, Muller N et al. Health-related quality of life in patients with Gilles de la Tourette's syndrome. *Mov Disord* 2010; 25:309–314.

Nijmeijer JS, Minderaa RB, Buitelaar JK et al. Attention-deficit/hyperactivity disorder and social dysfunctioning. *Clin Psychol Rev* 2008; 28:692–708.

Nunn K. The episodic dyscontrol syndrome in childhood. *J Child Psychol Psychiatry* 1986; 27:439–446.

Olvera RL. Intermittent explosive disorder: epidemiology, diagnosis and management. *CNS Drugs* 2002; 16:517–526.

Packer LE. Tic-related school problems: Impact on functioning, accommodations, and interventions. *Behav Modif* 2005; 29:876–899.

Patterson GR, DeBarushe BD, Ramsey E. A developmental perspective on antisocial behavior. *Am Psychol* 1989; 44:329–335.

Pauls DL, Leckman JF, Cohen DJ. Evidence against a genetic relationship between Tourette's syndrome and anxiety, depression, panic and phobic disorders. *Br J Psychiatry* 1994; *164*:215–221.

Pekarik EG, Prinz RJ, Liebert DE. The pupil evaluation inventory. A sociometric technique for assessing children's social behavior. *J Abnorm Child Psychol* 1976; *4*:83–97.

Pelphrey KA, Shultz S, Hudac CM, Vanderwyk BC. Research review: Constraining heterogeneity: the social brain and its development in autism spectrum disorder. *J Child Psychol Psychiatry* 2011; *52*:631–644.

Piacentini J, Woods DW, Scahill L et al. Behavior therapy for children with Tourette disorder: a randomized controlled trial. *JAMA* 2010; *303*:1929–1937.

This large randomized controlled study confirmed that behavioral therapy is helpful for tics.

Poulin F, Boivin M. Reactive and proactive aggression: Evidence of a two-factor model. *Psychol Assess* 2000; *12*:115–122.

Pringsheim T, Lang A, Kurlan R et al. Understanding disability in Tourette syndrome. *Dev Med Child Neurol* 2009; *51*:468–472.

Reef J, van Meurs I, Verhulst FC, van der Ende J. Children's problems predict adults' DSM-IV disorders across 24 years. *J Am Acad Child Adolesc Psychiatry* 2010; *49*:1117–1124.

Reichow B, Volkmar FR. Social skills interventions for individuals with autism: evaluation for evidence-based practices within a best evidence synthesis framework. *J Autism Dev Disord* 2010; *40*:149–166.

Reynolds CR, Kamphaus RW. *BASC-2: Behavior Assessment System for Children*. Circle Pines, MN: AGS Publishing, 2004.

Rosenberg LA, Brown J, Singer HS. Behavioral problems and severity of tics. *J Clin Psychol* 1995; *51*:760–767.

Scahill L, Sukhodolsky DG, Bearss K et al. A randomized trial of parent management training in children with tic disorders and disruptive behavior. *J Child Neurol* 2006; *21*:650–656.

Schoeder CE, Remer R. Perceived social support and caregiver strain in caregivers of children with Tourette's disorder. *J Child Fam Studies* 2007; *16*:888–901.

Schwartz D, Farver JM, Chang L, Lee-Shin Y. Victimization in South Korean children's peer groups. *J Abnorm Child Psychol* 2002; *30*:113–125.

Shaffer D, Gould MS, Brasic J. A Children's Global Assessment Scale (CGAS). *Arch Gen Psychiatry* 1983; *40*:1228–1231.

Silverstein M, Feinberg E, Cabral H et al. Problem-solving education to prevent depression among low-income mothers of preterm infants: A randomized controlled pilot trial. *Arch Womens Ment Health* 2011; *14*:317–324.

Snider LA, Seilgman LD, Ketchen BR et al. Tics and problem behaviors in schoolchildren: prevalence, characterization, and associations. *Pediatrics* 2002; *110*:331–336.

Sparrow SS, Balla DA, Cicchetti DV. *Vineland Adaptive Behavior Scales*. Circle Pines, MN: American Guidance Service, 1984.

Sparrow SS, Balla DA, Cicchetti DV. *Vineland Adaptive Behavior Scales* (2nd ed.). Circle Pines, MN: American Guidance Service, 2005.

Specht MW, Woods DW, Piacentini J et al. Clinical characteristics of children and adolescents with a primary tic disorder. *J Dev Phys Disabil* 2011; *23*:15–31.

Spence SH. Social skills training with children and young people: Theory, evidence and practice. *Child Adolesc Ment Health* 2003; *8*:84–96.

Spencer T, Biederman J, Coffey B. The 4-year course of tic disorders in boys with attention-deficit/hyperactivity disorder. *Arch Gen Psychiatry* 1999; *56*:842–847.

Spencer T, Biederman J, Faraone S et al. Impact of tic disorders on ADHD outcome across the life cycle: findings from a large group of adults with and without ADHD. *Am J Psychiatry* 2001; *158*:611–617.

Spencer T, Biederman J, Harding M et al. Disentangling the overlap between Tourette's disorder and ADHD. *J Child Psychol Psychiatry* 1998; *39*:1037–1044.

Stefl ME. Mental health needs associated with Tourette syndrome. *Am J Public Health* 1984; *74*:1310–1313.

Stokes A, Bawden HN, Camfield PR et al. Peer problems in Tourette's disorder. *Pediatrics* 1991; *87*:936–942.

Storch EA, Lack CW, Simons LE et al. *J Pediatr Psychol* 2007; *32*:950–959.

This paper reports on the development of a measure of functional impairment that is specific to TS.

Storch EA, Merlo LJ, Lack C et al. Quality of life in youth with Tourette's syndrome and chronic tic disorder. *J Clin Child Adolesc Psychol* 2007; *36*:217–227.

Storch EA, Murphy TK, Chase RM et al. Peer victimization in youth with Tourette's syndrome and chronic tic disorder: Relations with tic severity and internalizing symptoms. *J Psychopathol Behav Assess* 2007; 29:211–219.
This is a large study with a sample of well-characterized children with TS with and without co-occurring ADHD that showed the negative impact of ADHD and disruptive behavior problems on adaptive functioning in children with TS.

Sukhodolsky DG, Butter E. Social skills training for children with intellectual disabilities. In Jacobson JW, Mulick JA (Eds.), *Handbook of mental retardation and developmental disabilities* (pp. 601–618). New York: Kluwer, 2006.

Sukhodolsky DG, Landeros-Weisenberger A, Scahill L et al. Neuropsychological functioning in children with Tourette syndrome with and without attention-deficit/hyperactivity disorder. *J Am Acad Child Adolesc Psychiatry* 2010; 49:1155–1164.

Sukhodolsky DG, Scahill L, Leckman JF. ADHD with Tourette syndrome. In Brown TE (Ed.), *ADHD comorbidities: Handbook for ADHD complications in children and adults* (pp. 293–303). Washington, DC: American Psychiatric Press, 2009.

Sukhodolsky DG, Scahill L, Zhang H et al. Disruptive behavior in children with Tourette's syndrome: Association with ADHD comorbidity, tic severity, and functional impairment. *J Am Acad Child Adolesc Psychiatry* 2003; 42:98–105.

Sukhodolsky DG, Vitulano LA, Carroll DH et al. Randomized trial of anger control training for adolescents with Tourette's syndrome and disruptive behavior. *J Am Acad Child Adolesc Psychiatry* 2009; 48:413–421.
This is a randomized controlled study of cognitive-behavioral therapy for anger, aggression, and noncompliance in adolescents with TS complicated by disruptive behavior.

Tabori Kraft J, Dalsgaard S, Obel C et al. Prevalence and clinical correlates of tic disorders in a community sample of school-age children. *Eur Child Adolesc Psychiatry* 2012; 21:5–13.

Varni JW, Seid M, Rode CA. The PedsQL™: Measurement model for the Pediatric Quality of Life Inventory. *Med Care* 1999; 37:126–139.

Weissman MM, Orvaschel H, Padian N. Children's symptom and social functioning self-report scales. Comparison of mothers' and children's reports. *J Nerv Ment Dis* 1980; 168:736–740.

Wilkinson BJ, Marshall RM, Curtwright B. Impact of Tourette's disorder on parent-reported stress. *J Child Fam Studies* 2008; 17:582–598.

Winters NC, Collett BR, Myers KM. Ten-year review of rating scales, VII: Scales assessing functional impairment. *J Am Acad Child Adolesc Psychiatry* 2005; 44:309–338.

Wolpe J. *Psychotherapy by reciprocal inhibition.* Stanford, CA: Stanford University Press, 1958.

Woods DW, Himle MB, Osmon DC. Use of the Impact on Family Scale in children with tic disorders: Descriptive data, validity, and tic severity impact. *Child Fam Behav Ther* 2005; 27:11–21.

Woods DW, Piacentini JC, Scahill L et al. Behavior therapy for tics in children: Acute and long-term effects on psychiatric and psychosocial functioning. *J Child Neurol* 2011; 26:858–865.
This paper shows that behavior therapy for tics can also lead to improvement in adaptive functioning.

Yeates KO, Bigler ED, Dennis M. Social outcomes in childhood brain disorder: a heuristic integration of social neuroscience and developmental psychology. *Psychol Bull* 2007; 133:535–556.

Zinner SH, Conelea CA, Glew GM et al. Peer victimization in youth with Tourette syndrome and other chronic tic disorders. *Child Psychiatry Hum Dev* 2012; 43:124–136.

SECTION 5

TREATMENT

22

Psychoeducational Interventions: What Every Parent and Family Member Needs to Know

ELI R. LEBOWITZ AND LAWRENCE SCAHILL

Abstract

It is important for patients and families to understand the complex manifestations of Tourette syndrome so they can cope efficiently with tics and related symptoms. This chapter examines all the different features (temporal fluctuation in severity, susceptibility to contextual factors, academic and social implications) contributing to the complexity of tics and discusses psychoeducational interventions for patients and families. The practical and emotional challenges faced by parents of children with tics are another important aspect of psychoeducation. Children with tics also face educational and social difficulties in school and are often targets of peer victimization. Psychoeducation for school staff as well as peers may alleviate these difficulties. Adults with tics face discrimination and social victimization in the workplace and tend to be underemployed. Psychoeducation for employers and colleagues about tics as well as about the legal obligations toward individuals with disabilities may mitigate such discrimination.

"What does this mean for his future? Will he still be able to go to college?"

"We try to act as if we don't notice the tics. We don't want to make her uncomfortable."

"His latest tic is jumping on his sistegr … he says he can't help it."

"How should we respond when she doesn't want to have friends over because of her brother's tics? She says it's embarrassing."

"I don't know how to explain this to my boss."

"I was fired because my coworkers were uncomfortable about my tics—what should I do?"

MOST TIC disorders have their onset in childhood (Freeman, 2000). A tic disorder will likely first be noticed between the ages of 4 and 8, although formal diagnosis may occur later. An important implication of this is that the treatment of tics must be considered in all the contexts relevant to childhood. Development, school performance, family relations, and parental attitudes and behaviors all need to be part of a successful treatment strategy for disorders that present most commonly in childhood.

For the clinician, psychoeducation of parents and other family members of children with tic disorders is a basic component in any successful treatment strategy. Adequately preparing parents to respond supportively to their child; supplying realistic information; allaying some of the inevitable parental anxiety without offering false promises; preparing parents to deal with the plethora of delicate interactions in the home, school, and other environments: all of these can make the difference between a well-balanced family rallied around a child with a difficulty and a family thrown into turmoil, confusion, or even hostility.

In this chapter we offer the most important information that parents will need to navigate their role as caretakers of children with tics.

Whether presented to parents in a series of discussions by a clinician or independently read by responsible parents seeking the necessary knowledge, we hope that the following sections will be useful in creating and maintaining an environment conducive to coping with and overcoming the challenge faced by the entire family. In the latter part of the chapter we review some of the educational and social challenges faced by children and adults with tics in school and the workplace and discuss the ways in which psychoeducation can be used to ameliorate those difficulties.

WHY DOES HE KEEP DOING THAT? INTRODUCTION TO TICS FOR "NON-TICCERS"

When parents of children with tics have a similar tendency themselves, or have experienced it in the past, they may gain an intuitive understanding of the phenomenology of tics. It is easier to understand why someone would repeatedly perform an action that causes so much distress if you have the same urges yourself. For those parents (and potentially clinicians) who do not share the tendency, the phenomenon can be considerably more puzzling. Below are some aspects pertinent to the experience of tics that may need clarification before caretakers can adopt a helpful attitude. For a more comprehensive review of the phenomenology of tics, see Chapter 1.

Control

One thorny issue that many parents grapple with is that of control. On the one hand their child may explain that she does the tics "because she can't help it," and this is evidenced by the clear frustration at needing to perform the repetitive, often embarrassing, and potentially painful behavior. On the other hand many parents see clear evidence pointing toward the conclusion that their child actually can exercise control over the tics. Most children, if asked to do so and accordingly motivated, can refrain from tics for some periods of time. These might range from seconds to minutes, or even longer. Clearly, control is not a simple yes/no question.

A helpful way to explain to parents the level of partial control typical of tics is to ask them to imagine that they needed to stop breathing. Almost anyone can hold the breath for a while. For some the maximum time will be measured in seconds, for others in minutes. Whoever the person is, though, as soon as breathing is withheld, the clock starts ticking, counting down the time until the urge to breathe becomes unbearably strong. A similar thing happens for children with tics. They can be controlled momentarily, sometimes even at some length, but the urge to perform the tic will eventually resurface or become unbearably strong.

Premonitory Urges

Children approximately 10 and older are often able to describe the inner feeling that drives them to perform the tic (Leckman et al., 1993; Woods et al., 2005). For most children this sensation will appear as a pressure that builds in the part of the body with which the tic is performed. This sensation has come to be called the *premonitory urge*. Although consciously experiencing a premonitory urge is not necessary for the performance of tics, being able to identify the feeling is useful in some of the interventions used to treat the disorders (see Chapter 23 on the behavioral treatment of tics). Some children will report having a premonitory urge that is not localized to the specific part of their body with which they would perform the tics.

For many children there exists the sensation that performing the tic "just one more time" or getting the tic to feel "just right" will allow them to stop the tics and give them respite. Unfortunately this is not the case, and the tic is soon followed by a renewal of the urge and accordingly a repetition of the behavior by the child.

Bouts and Bouts of Bouts

Tics are not a constant rhythmic phenomenon like the rise and fall of a person's relaxed breathing. Rather, they appear to be sporadic, intermittent, and irregular. A child may go for extended periods of time without having any tics and then have days on which the tics seem to be coming nonstop and rapid-fire. Analysis of the frequency of the seemingly unpredictable tics seems to point toward a hierarchical pattern of tic bursts (Peterson & Leckman, 1998). Over any specific unit of time, such as a minute, an hour, a day, etc., a child will likely exhibit times of increased tics (bouts) and other times of diminished tic frequency. If a somewhat longer unit of time is examined, those bouts of increased tics will accumulate into higher-order "bouts of bouts." It appears as though careful analysis of the time frequencies involved may indicate a fractal pattern of ever-increasing bout size based on the accumulation of lower-order bouts, but to an observer the tics will generally appear to wax and wane in severity without a clear or predictable pattern.

Some endogenous factors, such as a child's motivation to refrain from the tics (Verdellen et al., 2007), and some external variables, such as the presence of people in the child's environment, appear to interact with the intrinsic pattern of tic frequency in complex ways. Thus, for example, many children will make a concerted, and at times successful, effort to curb their tics while in school and then return home to a period of severe tics, which themselves will demonstrate a complex pattern of tic bouts.

Suggestibility of Tics

Another potentially confusing characteristic of tics is their typically high level of suggestibility (Robertson et al., 1999). For many people with tics, being reminded of them, hearing someone mention the tics, or being questioned about them can often bring about the need to perform them. This must be considered during any assessment of tics, as the questions posed can evoke tics that are otherwise not apparent. For many parents this suggestibility trait can also be a source of confusion, as it may appear as if a child is either "faking" the need to perform the tics ("He didn't think of them all day, but when I pointed it out to him he right away starting doing them again") or as if given the opportunity the child would simply forget about them completely. In actual fact this is clearly not the case. We have seen

many children with tics and have yet to be convinced that any child was faking a tic disorder simply for some secondary gains that might be earned in that way. The toll on the child of having the disorder far outweighs any potential benefits.

In fact, suggestibility in sensory phenomena is not limited to children or to tics. Even parents who have never experienced a tic can likely relate to other similar sensations. Thinking about an area of the body can cause many people to mentally "create" an itch in that area, and imagining biting into a lemon can easily cause many people to salivate. Whether the mechanism behind the suggestibility of tics is unique or shared with some other instances of suggestible sensory phenomena is unclear, but it is characteristic of many if not most children with tic disorders.

Stress and Fatigue

Another pattern recognized by many parents of children with tic disorders is the tendency for tics to be exacerbated at times of either stress or fatigue. In fact, psychosocial stress has been found to be a significant predictor of future severity of tic symptoms in children with Tourette syndrome (TS) (Lin et al., 2007). Although stress by definition can include both positive and negative experiences (an example of positive stress may be a nerve-wracking but much-anticipated date), it is the stress associated with negative events and situations that appears to be more likely to trigger bouts of tics (Findley et al., 2003).

The effects of stress and fatigue appear to interact with the natural tendency to a pattern of bouts of tics described above. For example, on a given day a child may exhibit considerably more tics in the evening when tired and in need of ,sleep and those tics will likely appear as bouts or bursts of tic behavior. On a larger time scale, a child may have many fewer tics over the summer vacation when away from the social and academic stresses of school, with tics re-emerging as the school year starts. For a comprehensive discussion of stress and tics see Chapter 14.

"Traveling" Tics

Tics can appear in most any part of the human body, head to toe. Some areas, such as the mouth and eyes, are "tic hot-spots" (Leckman et al., 1993) and are particularly vulnerable to urges, while others are much more rarely affected, but just about any muscle that can be contracted at will can become the locus of a tic.

For most children tics are not permanent and will seem to travel over time, "settling" in different parts of the body, at times temporarily disappearing completely only to resurface in another location. This tendency to shifting localization of tics has long been recognized as characteristic of tics (Borison et al., 1983). A child may at first exhibit eye-blinking behavior or the roll of a shoulder and sometime later have tics in a completely different part of the body, such as the need to tighten the abdominal muscles. Additionally, while many children will at first exhibit only motor tics, these may be followed, as an addition or a replacement, by vocal tics such as the need to inhale or exhale loudly, whistle, grunt, or say a certain word.

Blame and Guilt

A favorite topic for parents, but one shied away from by clinicians, is that of blame. Whether directed at the self in the form of feelings of guilt and responsibility or directed at the spouse as accusations, there are few feelings as unhelpful to a family contending with a child's disorder as those surrounding allocation of blame for the tics.

- I am to blame—I have tics and I "gave" them to him.
- It's your fault for picking on him!
- I wonder if I did something wrong.
- I should have treated them earlier.
- Should I have breastfed him? Kept him home longer with me?

Not only can this kind of rumination be destructive for the parent engaging in it, it can also have a negative impact on the child experiencing the tic disorder. Children with tics are often described to us as being particularly sensitive, empathic, and attuned to the feelings of others. Even a child who is not particularly sensitive will likely pick up on the fact that a problem of his or hers is causing significant emotional distress to a parent or straining the parents' relationship. Unfortunately, just as mothers or fathers may blame themselves for their child's problem, children's egocentric view of the world will usually lead them to consider themselves responsible for the current turmoil in the home.

Parental guilt is not only unhelpful, but it is also largely misplaced. Other chapters in this book examine the question of genetic variations and their potential role in the etiology of tic disorders (see Chapter 7 for an in-depth review), a field still a long way from maturity. But there are no data to support the idea that parenting style causes children to develop tics. In fact, there seems to be no factual evidence at all for the idea that parents can "give their children" tics through choices they make. Parents play an important role in supporting their children through dealing with the challenge of tics, they are responsible for supplying treatment as necessary, and they can potentially affect the course of the disorder by creating the kind of environment conducive to successful treatment, but they do not cause TS to appear.

TICS AND ASSOCIATED SYMPTOMS

Tic disorders represent a complex diagnostic conundrum. On the one hand, the diagnosis is for the most part straightforward. Patients with motor tics alone have a chronic tic disorder, as do those relatively rare patients who have only vocal tics. Those who have persistent motor and vocal tics have Tourette's disorder, as named in the DSM-IV. Ascertaining what behaviors are actually tics (as opposed to stereotypies, for example) can be tricky, but otherwise the diagnostic criteria are few and well defined (American Psychiatric Association, 2000). On the other hand, both research and clinical experience point to the conclusion that the reality is far less simple. The available data seem to indicate that although the diagnosis of a tic disorder is based entirely on the presence of tics, much of the time the syndrome will manifest with additional symptomatology (Kadesjo & Gillberg, 2000).

Some of the non-tic symptoms most frequently reported in cases of tic disorders are attentional difficulties, anger management problems such as explosive outbursts of rage, and obsessive-compulsive symptoms (Apter et al., 1993; Ivarsson et al., 2008; Walkup et al., 1995). Clearly delineating the boundaries between comorbid conditions (i.e., a child suffers from both tics and, say, attention-deficit/hyperactivity disorder [ADHD]) and secondary symptoms (i.e., the presence of the tic disorder is the cause of the attentional difficulty, although the latter is not part of the diagnosis) is a significant challenge for researchers, parents, and diagnosticians alike. For more information on symptoms associated with tic disorders, see Chapters 2 to 4 on the relationship to ADHD, obsessive-compulsive disorder (OCD), and other conditions, and Chapter 29 for a comprehensive review of educational needs associated with tics.

For example, in a study that looked at the course of illness among children diagnosed with both tics and ADHD, over the course of some years the tics were found to improve over time, while the ADHD continued to be a relevant diagnosis for longer term (Spencer et al., 1999). Yet in studies of the disruptive behaviors of children with tic disorders, most of the behavioral problems have been found to be associated directly with the presence of ADHD (Sukhodolsky et al., 2003). See Chapter 21 for a discussion of social functioning in the context of TS.

In the case of obsessive-compulsive behaviors, another category of symptoms often found to overlap with tic disorders, the questions can be even more complex. One issue often complicating the matter is that it's quite hard to decide whether a certain behavior is a tic (i.e., a movement that a person has an urge to complete against his or her will) or a compulsive ritual (i.e., another kind of behavior that a person feels compelled to complete) (Palumbo & Kurlan, 2007). Even Pierre Janet noted the overlap between compulsions and tics and hypothesized that they share a common etiology as behaviors that a person must perform until a sense of completeness is achieved (Pitman, 1987).

PARENTING THE CHILD WITH TICS

Creating and maintaining a balanced and supportive attitude toward tics can be major challenge for any parent. The emotional distress of discovering that one's child has any psychiatric disorder; the nightmarish way that TS is often portrayed in popular media; the difficulty of balancing one child's needs along with those of other children; the confusion around treatments and medications: all these and many other factors contribute to the distress experienced by parents of children diagnosed with tic disorders. We will attempt to answer some of the questions and provide a compass for navigating what can be a bewildering reality.

The Tic-Neutral Environment

The more emotion tics tend to arouse, the more likely they are recur (Conelea & Woods, 2008). At times it seems as though tics are deliberately targeted to evoke the most dramatic and emotionally charged response. For example, a person might feel the urge to say a disparaging word in the least appropriate setting. To read this behavior as being deliberate provocation on the part of the individual with a tic disorder, however, is tragically misguided. It is the very fear of the provocation that ensues that seems to make the urge to perform the tic appear and causes it to grow in strength.

Even when tics are not quite so clearly provocative, the need to perform them gains in strength when they arouse emotionally charged reactions (Carr et al., 1996; Scotti et al., 1994; Wood et al., 2003). It appears that the specific emotion actually matters less in this context than the level of drama that ensues. For instance, some parents may react to their child's tic with great sympathy, concern, or sadness. Yet the same parents whose eyes fill with tears as they watch their child perform a tic, or who immediately respond by tearfully hugging the child and voicing their pained devotion, are creating an environment in which tics are associated with much emotion. Similarly, parents who are deeply ashamed of the tics, blush furiously, furtively look around to see if anyone is observing, or mumble frantic apologies on their child's behalf are also associating the tics with a powerful emotion. Other examples are parents who are revolted by the sight of the tics and manifest disgust or repulsion, or parents who respond with frustrated and powerful anger at the child who "refuses" to stop what they perceive to be unacceptable behavior.

All these reactions share the element of emotion, although the specific emotional content is different in each, and all of them are likely to achieve exactly the opposite of what the parents hope for. Rather than serving to mitigate the tics or stop them entirely, they are actually considerably more likely to exacerbate them, producing a cycle in which the tics trigger emotion, which in turn leads to even more tics.

The solution to this problem is in striving for what can best be conceptualized as an emotionally neutral environment as to the tics. Parents can adopt a "matter-of-fact" attitude that conveys practical acknowledgement of the situation without charging it with emotion.

> The mother of a 14-year-old girl was intensely embarrassed by her daughter's vocal tic. The girl would have an uncontrollable need to mutter "fuck, fuck" whenever they were in a public place. The distraught mother would do her best to hush the girl but was generally unsuccessful, only causing both to feel frustrated and dismayed. She eventually hit on a trick that allowed her to maintain her neutrality when the tics occurred. Whenever the tics started, the mother would say to herself, "She's saying: flower, flower" until it seemed as if that is what she was hearing. After practicing this for some time she noticed the tics would actually recede much more quickly than before.

"Matter-of-factness" does not imply that parents should refrain from commenting on the tics altogether or act as though they do not notice them.

Reluctance to acknowledge the presence of the tics can actually create a very charged atmosphere, the very opposite of neutrality. By never being willing to address the topic of tics, a taboo is established that a child will easily perceive. The taboo will likely convey two unfortunate messages to the child. Firstly, a child will learn that the tics are so embarrassing or bad that his or her parents dare not even talk about them. No child will believe for long that parents who are attentive to other aspects of their life have actually failed to notice the tics. Any relief at not being seen will soon be replaced by confusion over the continued silence. We have seen children who have displayed multiple and very obvious motor or vocal tics for long periods of time whose parents had never asked the child about them or had any kind of discussion about them at all.

The second unhelpful message conveyed through parents' reluctance to talk about the tics with their child is that they are unable to offer any kind of help. A child whose parents make no comment on an ongoing problem he or she is obviously contending with can only conclude that the parents have no help to offer, or surely they would have approached the topic in order to do so. This can lead to unnecessary discouragement and loneliness in the place of care and support. Conversely, an empathic but pragmatic recognition of the child's tics without overbearing emotion attached to it can provide a child with hope and support. An example of how a parent might broach the subject of tics with a child is suggested below:

> I noticed you doing some movements (making some sounds) a while ago and it looked like you were having some trouble stopping it. Is that what was happening? You know, a lot of people actually feel like they really need to do something like that sometimes. It might feel like they need to move their hands or mouth a certain way or to breathe just so. I know it can get really uncomfortable and if it feels like it's bothering you, then we should probably talk about that. So many people have that, and there are some good ways of dealing

with feelings like that. Do you want to talk about what makes you do it?

When children are in treatment, it may be helpful to them if their parents remind them casually when they see the tics to practice the skills they have learned in therapy; clinicians can advise parents, based on the stage of treatment reached, on what techniques to mention. By doing this in a noncritical fashion, the child can feel supported rather than ashamed of the tics.

Helping parents to assume a matter-of-fact attitude toward tics can allow children to mirror the attitude in their own self-estimation. Rather than feeling as though they are the locus of a terrible and mysterious problem, they can view themselves as normal, healthy individuals with tics.

Keeping Sight of the Child

All too often clinicians fall into the unfortunate trap of losing sight of the person and seeing only the disorder. No diagnostic criteria or category, however fitting, can capture the human being, and no individual is the sum of his or her diagnoses. But however misguided it may be for clinicians or those engaged in research to think this way, it is even more unfortunate for parents to lose sight of their children and focus too strongly on the challenges they face. This kind of narrow focus will present children with a negative mirror in which to view themselves and the sad reflection of who they are.

By encouraging parents to maintain a positive and holistic view of the child that recognizes the tics as one element in a complex individual, a healthier stance is maintained. This can be accomplished in a number of ways.

Focus on Strengths

Even a child with very severe tics will have many other aspects to his or her personality as well, and letting the need to address the challenges become the sole point of contact leaves a child with little to feel proud of. This can be explained to parents in the following way:

Imagine that your child is in school and is not doing very well at mathematics. The teachers are concerned that he is falling behind, and you feel the need to bolster his performance so as to maintain his ability to progress throughout the year. Now imagine that to do that, you were to pull him out of every class in which he was doing well in order to devote that time to math practice. What would his school day be like? He would only have classes on the topics in which he was struggling. He would have no opportunities to show off, to demonstrate his competence, and to receive praise for being good at something. And if he ever did catch up with others, he'd find he'd probably fallen behind them in the very things he used to be best at.

In a similar way, making the daily life of a child with tics all about tics can remove all the opportunities to experience competence, mastery, and well-being. Just as neglecting tics completely is likely to be a mistake, overemphasizing them can be harmful as well. In addition, some research and experience point to the conclusion that children who are engaged in activities unrelated to the tics may experience fewer tics during that time (Kobets et al., *unpublished data*). This is likely to be particularly true for activities the child finds pleasurable and rewarding. Identifying, fostering, and encouraging areas of strength through which the child can feel successful and gain the admiration of others may be a powerful antidote to the potentially stigmatizing effect of the tics.

Parents should be encouraged to identify areas of social, physical, or academic competence and to actively support their child's engagement in these fields. Participating in Boy or Girl Scouts, engaging in team sports, socializing with peers, or engaging in a hobby can all be examples of such activities and can strengthen the message "You're a great child, who happens to have tics." Another context for pleasurable non–tic-related activities for the child can be time spent as a family or individually with parents. Driving a child to a doctor's office to seek treatment may well be a time for communication and support, but spending time with the child in arenas completely unrelated to the tics offers another kind of connection.

Maintaining Social Relationships

Occasionally a child may withdraw from peer interactions or fear taking part in them because of the embarrassment of being seen performing tics. In a study of 245 children and 177 adults with TS, over one third across all age groups reported social isolation associated with the tic disorder (Wand et al., 1993). In our experience, a specific child's social skills are generally a more significant predictor of peers' attitudes toward him or her than is the severity of tics, but it is easy to feel awkward or shy when tics focus the attention of others in aversive ways. This problem is at times exacerbated by the direct and uninhibited curiosity displayed by many children.

Helping children to preserve and maintain social ties and aiding them in developing strategies for handling uncomfortable situations can be a major contribution to their well-being. One potentially useful strategy is to assist parents in teaching children how to handle the puzzlement others express about the tics. This can be done in stages:

1. Reframing the interpretation of other's behavior. A child may say to himself or herself, "Those kids are looking at me. They think I'm weird!" Consequently the child is likely to avoid engaging with the other children and feel anxiety or hostility toward them. Teaching a child to say instead, "Those children don't know about tics. They are curious why I have them" can lead to considerably less negative emotion.

2. Self-representation. Most children are willing to accept unfamiliar phenomena at face value when these are introduced to them in a clear and nonjudgmental way. A child can practice saying to others, "I have tics. That means I sometimes need to move my hands like that. But I also like to play ball. Could I join your game?" or similar phrases. Many children will react positively, and as the novelty of the tics fades, the interest they arouse will soon be replaced by a focus on other shared interests.

3. Naturally, preexisting ties with friends and other acquaintances should also be maintained, and parents can take an active role in creating opportunities for the child to discover that despite the tics, nothing has changed in his or her ability to interact with others.

PARENT AND FAMILY INVOLVEMENT IN TICS

Ted was 14 years old and had been diagnosed with TS and OCD at age 9. Since that time he had experienced a variety of motor and vocal tics, including the need to sniff or lick things, to make a grunting sound, and to flex both his arms at once. He took medication that helped to moderate the tics and had been on a stable treatment regimen for over a year when his parents sought renewed counseling. Ted has recently developed two behaviors that were affecting the family in negative ways. The first was a renewed need to lick many objects and even people. Ted would take his mother, father, or sister's hand and lick it quickly. He did this repeatedly multiple times a day, much to the consternation of the others, particularly the sister. Ted would apologize when confronted but stated that he was not able to stop.

The second issue revolved around Ted's sensitivity to sounds and sensory experiences. He was extra careful to set down anything he was holding, just the right way. He needed to feel that the pressure created by things down was "just right"; otherwise, he was compelled to repeat the action. Recently Ted had begun insisting that others also set things down "just right." Mealtime had turned into a constant battle, with Ted pestering everyone to pick things up and put them down again correctly and the whole family becoming more and more frustrated and irritated with him.

Children who experience strong urges to do things "just so" are frequently liable to feel that others also need to comply with similar rules in order for them to feel comfortable (Lebowitz et al., 2011a, 2011b). The phenomenon can be described as a difficulty for the child in regulating unpleasant sensations and attempts to eliminate those sensations from the environment.

Misunderstanding of this pattern can often lead to one of two unhelpful parental and family patterns:

1. Compliance. Many parents naturally comply with a child's demands to accommodate the rules imposed by the aversive sensations that trouble the child with TS. This compliance can best be seen as a natural expression of the positive parental instinct to aid a child and protect him or her from distress. Additionally, some parents will feel the need to go along with the child's requests so as to avoid conflict or to maintain an efficient schedule in the home. When refusing to adhere to the child's demand leads to angry or disruptive outbursts, it may become more economical to acquiesce. To other parents it may appear as though any defiance of these kinds of demands exacerbates the tics or as though, because the child cannot control the behavior, it is unfair not to comply.

2. Confrontation. A second pattern encountered in some families of children who attempt to involve parents or siblings in their tics is one of aggressively and confrontationally resisting these attempts. Parents may interpret the demands as disrespectful, or the content of the behavior may seem inappropriate and cause embarrassment, leading to anger and repudiation. Children may be punished for their supposed "misbehavior" or identified as the "troublemaker" in the family who causes stress and irritation.

Our experience has shown that neither overly compliant nor harshly punitive attitudes on the part of parents are helpful in approaching these situations. Rather, the same practical "matter-of-fact" approach that is appropriate for other tics is most likely to work best in these cases as well. We recommend to clinicians working with parents of children who impose their tics on the family that they help the parents formulate responses to these behaviors or demands that convey two messages. The first part of the message entails recognition that the child's behavior stems from a real problem and is not an expression of voluntary disrespect or misconduct. The second, equally important, message is a clear statement about the degree to which

such demands will be met, and a rationale for the decision.

By recognizing that the child's behavior stems from a problem for which he or she is neither to blame nor responsible, much of the emotional turmoil surrounding the behavior can be mitigated. Additionally, by clarifying that the child is not being punished, the child can more easily see the changes made by the parents as reflecting his or her own best interests rather than a desire to chastise him or her. In this way, even if the child is initially opposed to the parents' decision, he or she is less likely to feel that they are directed against him or her rather than as a collaborative effort to overcome the problem. Here is an example of the way parents might make a supportive and determined explanation:

Ted, we love you so much and think you are wonderful! We understand how hard it is for you to feel that you need to perform the tics or behaviors, and we want you to know that we are not angry at you for them. We know if you could choose to "turn off" the feelings you absolutely would. We have thought a lot about this and consulted with some experts, and we know now that going along with your need for us to put things down "just right" isn't helping you. We know it makes it better just then, but afterwards the feelings always come back. We are sure you are strong enough to deal with this, and we have decided that from now on we will not agree to put things down again because of those feelings. We are not doing this to punish you, but because we believe this is best and we are confident you can cope with it. We love you very much.

PSYCHOEDUCATION AND COMORBIDITY

As discussed in detail in other chapters (see Chapters 2–4), children who have tic disorders also commonly meet the diagnostic criteria for at least one other psychiatric disorder as well. This is not unique to tic disorders—comorbidity has repeatedly been shown to be more the rule than the exception across the psychiatric spectrum—but it does magnify the burden for child and parents, an increase that often seems exponential in nature. In some cases the comorbidity might mean having to deal with additional hardship, but in many cases the presence of a comorbid condition seems to exacerbate the tics themselves as well.

Parents of children with comorbid tics and other disorders face unique challenges, for example the need to decide which problem to focus on at any given time. Many clinicians are expert in one area of psychopathology but insufficiently experienced in others to be able to adequately address them, creating a need to choose between target problems that become incompatible. Even when a clinician could be doing both this might be ineffective, detracting from the focus of treatment. Another challenge is in differentiating what symptoms or behaviors actually relate to the tic disorder and which do not. And more subtly, the ability to focus on a child's strengths and skills becomes increasingly harder as disorders and diagnoses "pile up."

Psychoeducation is an important tool in this regard. Providing parents with an understanding that comorbidity is in fact to be expected may help to alleviate some of the distress of feeling as though "my child got everything." Psychoeducation could also help parents understand which behaviors are tics and which are either normal behaviors or symptoms of a comorbid condition. For example, a child with a disruptive behavior disorder may use bad language, leading to confusion in parents over what constitutes coprolalia. Working out a treatment plan that addresses the various difficulties a child is facing and discussing priorities is an additional function that relies on providing parents with the necessary information to make informed decisions—for example, learning about the relative response rates of different disorders to the various available therapeutic techniques.

DEALING WITH SIBLINGS

In most cases parents of children with tics will also be the parents of additional children (who may or may not also suffer from a tic or other disorder), and the responsibilities and challenges they face are made correspondingly more complex. Parents need to address not only the issue of the tics themselves and how to cope with them but also the effect that the tic disorder can have on other siblings, the relationships between the siblings, and the importance of balancing the needs of multiple children when one has a particular problem (Conelea et al., 2011).

Siblings' Attitude Toward Tics

An advantage of the nonemotional, matter-of-fact attitude of parents toward the tics of a child is that it can model appropriate behavior for other children in the home as well. In most cases children will rapidly adapt to the unique attributes or eccentricities of a sibling if parents convey the sense that these are not an issue to focus attention on. It is often harder for adults and parents in particular to accept the tics of a child than for other children, and parents should be encouraged to foster this attitude of semi-indifference to the tics of a child on the part of his or her siblings.

When children voice genuine curiosity or concern regarding the tics of a sibling, parents can conduct an honest and age-appropriate conversation on the topic. Most children can easily grasp the concept of an urge to perform a certain behavior despite a desire to refrain from doing so, and many can offer similar examples from their own experience. Children who express additional fears about the topic, such as the fear that they will "catch the tics," can be offered factual information (i.e., tics are not contagious) and when relevant and appropriate can participate in a meeting with the therapist who is treating the sibling in order to raise their concerns. Much information for children can be found through the Tourette Syndrome Association (TSA) and its website, including videos and reading material.

Teasing

Teasing about the tics should always be actively discouraged by parents, and any hope that teasing will lead to increased motivation on the part of the child to stop the tics should be actively addressed by the clinician and removed. Parents should be advised to treat the teasing or mockery as they would other inappropriate behaviors on the part of one sibling toward another and should not make a special case of defending a "weaker child" because of a perceived disability.

PSYCHOEDUCATION IN SCHOOL

Children with TS and other tic disorders often face considerable confusion, misunderstanding, or prejudice on the part of adults and peer victimization by other children outside of the home (Zinner et al., 2011). Difficulties can stem both from the attentional and behavioral difficulties that sometimes make up part of the clinical picture (Sukhodolsky et al., 2003) and from attitudes of peers and adults toward children with tics. Although a child with exceptional social skills may well be popular and much liked despite even severe tics, the presence of tics is a risk factor for academic difficulties and for peer victimization by other children (Packer, 2005).

A number of studies have attempted to probe the typical attitudes of schoolchildren toward peers with tic disorders. In two such studies classmates of children with tics rated their whole class on a measure that assesses likeability, aggressiveness, and withdrawal (Bawden et al., 1998; Stokes et al., 1991). Both studies found that children with tics are perceived by peers as less likeable than others. Other studies have supported this conclusion, showing for example that children and adolescents who view a video of a peer with tics rate him or her less positively than the same child viewed without the tics (Boudjouk et al., 2000; Friedrich et al., 1996). Indeed, children with tic disorders have been shown to be disproportionately victimized by their peers, and the victimization appears to mediate the relationship between the severity of the tics and the experience of loneliness and isolation reported by the child (Storch et al., 2007).

Psychoeducation in the school can be directed at school staff such as teachers, principals, and mental health workers as well as at children (see also Chapter 29). Patients and their parents can also benefit from education specific to handling tics at school. In a 1998 paper on the relevance of tic disorders for school psychologists, the author called for more exposure to the topic during graduate training and emphasized the need to increase the ability of school psychologists to recognize tics in the classroom (Wodrich, 1998). A decade and a half later, these recommendations remain pertinent. Teachers should largely be encouraged to ignore the tics of a child during class, as focusing their attention on the tics will inevitably focus the attention of most of the other children in the classroom as well. Shining such a spotlight of attention on the tics will almost certainly cause embarrassment and is likely to lead to even more tics in the future. At times a child may need to be temporarily excused from class because of particularly disruptive or severe tics, and this should be achieved with as little fanfare as possible (Packer, 2005). When this eventuality is likely to take place, teachers should be adequately prepared so as to minimize the child's discomfort. In addition, when a child is having tics in school, it may be helpful to consider some of the institutional characteristics (Buckser, 2009) that may contribute to stress or exacerbate the tics and to seek ways to improve the overall experience for the child.

Equally important for teachers and school staff is education on how *not* to approach tics. Behavior modification plans, for example, that treat tics a negative behavior that requires extinction through a process of behavior modification can backfire, leading to negative results. The principle implicit in such a plan, but clear to teacher and child alike, is that the child should be able to control the tics, given adequate motivation and effort. This carries the potential for increased frustration on both sides, and ironically to increased tics resulting from the stress. Tics are not a ploy for attention in the classroom, nor are they are an attempt to undermine the authority of a teacher, and despite often being sporadic, irregular, or triggered by specific situations, teachers should be aware that they are not the "target" of the tics and need not seek to discipline the child for having them. As is the case with parental attitudes, assuming a punitive stance toward tics that cause disruption in the classroom can only serve to discourage the child, exacerbate the tics, and create an aversion to the class, teacher, or school in general.

Peers in the school may be educated about tic disorders by exposure to other children and adults with tics. In particular, highlighting successful or admired individuals who have a tic disorder may help to reframe the disorder and minimize stigmatization. Discussions about the experience of actually having tics and comparisons to other experiences more directly familiar to the children may help to counteract some of the effect of humorous or ridiculous ways that tic disorders are often portrayed in the media. Research into the effect of brief educational interventions such as viewing a video of a child explaining about his tics have had mixed results, but there is at least some support for the idea that these could minimize stigmatization or avoidance of the child (Friedrich et al., 1996), and more comprehensive interventions may have correspondingly greater impact. The TSA is often able to assist parents in organizing a psychoeducational intervention in a school, and representatives of that organization have been helpful in many cases by speaking with staff and peers when a child is experiencing social difficulties in class due to tics.

PSYCHOEDUCATION AND THE WORKPLACE

Researchers have paid relatively little attention to the effect of tics on the work life of adults with tic disorders. The extant literature points to the importance of further investigating this impact, as well to the need to ameliorate the current occupational conditions of individuals with tics. In one of the main contributions to this field, Shady and colleagues (1995) surveyed Canadian adults with TS about their work-life experiences. They found that adults with TS were disproportionately likely to be either unemployed or underemployed relative to their education, half reported that the disorder had affected their

choice of occupation, and over 20% reported having been dismissed or fired because of their disorder; an even greater percentage believed they had been denied promotion because of TS. These troubling results largely confirm the results of other reports about occupational difficulties related to tic disorders (Elstner et al., 2001; Stefle, 1983). Although individuals with TS are afforded some protections by law under the Americans with Disabilities Act, the results highlight the need for more education of employers and coworkers.

Psychoeducation for employers could include providing information about tics that might dispel some of the anxiety, and resulting discrimination, that can stem from the seeming strangeness of the tic behaviors; workshops that allow the employer to ask questions and meet other individuals with tics; information on the legal obligations and regulations relating to the treatment of people with disabilities; or providing guidelines for better decision making relating to the tics. For example, an employer might feel inclined to relocate a worker with tics to a location that would make the tics less visible, but could be coached not to make such decisions in a unilateral way without consulting the worker and inviting input about his or her point of view. Psychoeducation could also suggest better ways to handle interworker situations that stem from the tics, such as social shunning of a worker with TS or even more blatant forms of social aggression such as teasing, mocking, or imitation. By setting a clear example for other workers, the employer could potentially create a more protected and ultimately more productive work environment.

Psychoeducation could also directly target coworkers in addition to employers. Research has shown that brief psychoeducational interventions, such as watching a short video, has the potential to ameliorate negative views about people with tics and reduce the unfortunate tendency to avoid them (Woods et al., 1999, 2003). Providing coworkers with opportunities to become better acquainted with tics, ask pertinent questions, and address stereotypes associated with them in popular culture and media could all improve the likelihood of a positive work experience for individuals with tic disorders.

One issue pertinent to occupational difficulties for individuals with tics relates to the question of disclosure—that is, deciding if and when to discuss the disorder with colleagues and employers. Some individuals might prefer to raise the issue as early as possible, while others may choose never to discuss the matter at all. Preventive disclosure, or the strategy of providing information about a condition to others to minimize stigmatization, has been shown to be helpful in some other chronic conditions (Berlin et al., 2005). One study provided some support for the potential of preventive disclosure to reduce stigmatization in TS; however, this was a survey using a hypothetical vignette, and there are no reports on the actual effects of disclosure on work experience for people with tics.

DIRECTIONS FOR FUTURE RESEARCH

Tics are an easily misunderstood phenomenon that evokes strong emotional and cognitive reactions in patients, relatives, and others in the environment. Parents of children with tics face innumerable day-to-day dilemmas and decisions regarding their responses to the tics, and both children and adults are frequently confronted with negative reactions from others. Although there has been recognition of the need for psychoeducation, and psychoeducation has been incorporated in structured treatments for tics (see, for example, Woods, 2008), little is known about the actual relative contribution of education to treatment. Future research should attempt to identify the most important elements of psychoeducation for both individuals

---

Box 22.1. Key Points

- Gaining a better understanding of tics, their phenomenology, and complex manifestations can better prepare patients, parents, and others for the challenge of coping with tics and overcoming them.
- Tics represent a complicated behavior combining elements of controlled and uncontrollable behavior. They tend to wax and wane in frequency and severity and are often suggestible, in that they are exacerbated when attention is focused on them as well as when an individual is under fatigue or stress.
- Parents of children with tics face both practical and emotional challenges, including dealing with feelings of guilt or blame, and dilemmas such as when and how to respond to a child's tics.
- Overall, it is preferable not to respond in an emotional manner to tics, as charging the situation with emotion has the potential to exacerbate the tics.
- It is important to maintain sight of the individual and focus on strengths and interests, while supporting efforts to overcome the tics or better manage them.
- Parents often must contend with sibling-related issues such as teasing, jealousy, and misunderstanding. Modeling a "matter-of-fact" attitude that is neither hostile nor overly accommodating is a way of handling these difficulties.
- Children with tics face educational and social difficulties in school and are often targets of peer victimization. Psychoeducation for school staff as well as peers may alleviate these difficulties.
- Adults with tics face discrimination and social victimization in the workplace and tend to be underemployed. Psychoeducation for employers and colleagues about tics as well as about the legal obligations toward individuals with disabilities may help to mitigate such discrimination.

1. Can psychoeducation have an impact on tic severity and frequency, and would this effect be mediated by the effect of education on psychosocial stress?
2. Can more comprehensive psychoeducational programs with adult and child peers be effective in attenuating negative attitudes toward people with tics and tic disorders?
3. How important a component is psychoeducation in the treatment of tics, and would treatment with education be more effective than treatment without?
4. What is the role of parent guidance and training in the treatment of tic disorders in children?
5. In what ways should psychoeducation for adults differ from education in children?
6. What can be done to improve the way in which tics are portrayed in popular media?

in treatment and, in the case of children, their parents. Psychoeducation can encompass many different kinds of information, such as data on the prevalence of tics, their clinical course, or comorbidities, or it could include more practical information, such as preferable parental attitudes to adopt toward the tics. Another kind of psychoeducation teaches patients and relatives about the treatments available, including both behavioral and pharmacological interventions.

Another important question for future research relates to the attitudes of the general population toward tics and the people who exhibit them. Given the data reviewed above on discrimination and victimization of individuals with TS, and in particular given the relationship of tic severity to psychosocial stress, it is imperative to identify ways to educate the public and to battle discrimination. This kind of education too can take many forms, including public advocacy, dissemination of information, focused interventions in workplaces or schools, and attempts to influence media and discourage the negative portrayal of tics in movies and television. The evidence to date on the efficacy of any of these strategies is very scarce, and they would require concerted efforts on the part of clinicians, researchers, and families alike. Box 22.2 points to some specific questions that researchers could attempt to address in the course of furthering our understanding of psychoeducation for TS.

REFERENCES

American Psychiatric Association. Diagnostic and statistical manual of mental disorders: DSM-IV-TR, Washington, DC: American Psychiatric Association, 2000.

Apter A, Pauls DL, Bleich A et al. An epidemiologic study of Gilles de la Tourette's syndrome in Israel. *Arch Gen Psychiatry* 1993; 50:734–738.

Bawden HN, Stokes A, Camfield CS et al. Peer relationship problems in children with Tourette's disorder or diabetes mellitus. *J Child Psychol Psychiatry* 1998; 39:663–668.
Important study of the way children with tics are perceived by their classmates.

Berlin KS, Sass DA, Hobart Davies W et al. Cystic fibrosis disclosure may minimize risk of negative peer evaluations. *J Cyst Fibros* 2005; 4:169–174.

Borison RL, Ang L, Hamilton WJ et al. Treatment approaches in Gilles de la Tourette syndrome. *Brain Res Bull* 1983; 11:205–208.

Boudjouk PJ, Woods DW, Miltenberger RG, Long ES. Negative peer evaluation in adolescents: Effects of tic disorders and trichotillomania. *Child Family Behav Ther* 2000; 22:17–28.

Buckser A. *Institutions, agency, and illness in the making of Tourette syndrome. Human Organization* 2009; 68:293–306.

Carr JE, Taylor CC, Wallander RJ, Reiss ML. A functional-analytic approach to the diagnosis of a transient tic disorder. *J Behav Ther Exp Psychiatry* 1996; 27:291–297.

Conelea CA, Woods D, Zinner S et al. Exploring the impact of chronic tic disorders on youth: Results from the Tourette Syndrome Impact Survey. *Child Psychiatry Hum Dev* 2011; 42:219–242.
Comprehensive review of factors affecting tic expression, including emotional reaction to the tics.

Conelea CA, Woods DW. The influence of contextual factors on tic expression in Tourette's syndrome: A review. *J Psychosom Res* 2008; 65:487–496.

Elstner K, Selai CE, Trimble MR, Robertson MM. Quality of life (QOL) of patients with Gilles de la Tourette's syndrome. *Acta Psych Scand* 2001; 103:52–59.

Findley DB, Leckman JF, Katsovich L et al. Development of the Yale Children's Global Stress Index (YCGSI) and its application in children and adolescents with Tourette's syndrome and obsessive-compulsive disorder. *J Am Acad Child Adolesc Psychiatry* 2003; 42:450–457.

Freeman RD. An international perspective on Tourette syndrome: selected findings from 3,500 individuals in 22 countries. *Dev Med Child Neurol* 2000; 42:436–447.

Friedrich S, Morgan SB, Devine C. Children's attitudes and behavioral intentions toward a peer with Tourette syndrome. *J Pediatr Psychol* 1996; 21:307–319.

Ivarsson T, Melin K, Wallin L. Categorical and dimensional aspects of co-morbidity in obsessive-compulsive disorder (OCD). *Eur Child Adol Psychiatry* 2008; 17:20–31.

Kadesjo B, Gillberg C. Tourette's disorder: Epidemiology and comorbidity in primary schoolchildren. *J Am Acad Child Adolesc Psychiatry* 2000; 39:548–555.

Lebowitz ER, Omer H, Leckman JF. Coercive and disruptive behaviors in pediatric obsessive–compulsive disorder. *Depress Anxiety* 2011a; 28:899–905.

Lebowitz ER, Vitulano LA, Omer H. Coercive and disruptive behaviors in pediatric obsessive compulsive disorder: A qualitative analysis. *Psychiatry* 2011b; 74:362–371.

Leckman JF, Walker DE, Cohen DJ. Premonitory urges in Tourette's syndrome. *Am J Psychiatry* 1993;150:98–102.
One of the initial descriptive cross-sectional studies of premonitory urges.

Lin H, Katsovich L, Ghebremichael M et al. Psychosocial stress predicts future symptom severities in children and adolescents with Tourette syndrome and/or obsessive-compulsive

disorder. *J Child Psychol Psychiatry* 2007; 48:157–166.

Packer LE. Tic-related school problems: impact on functioning, accommodations, and interventions. *Behav Modif* 2005; 29:876–899.

Palumbo D, Kurlan R. Complex obsessive compulsive and impulsive symptoms in Tourette's syndrome. *Neuropsychiat Dis Treatment* 2007; 3:687–693.

Peterson BS, Leckman JF. The temporal dynamics of tics in Gilles de la Tourette syndrome. *Biol Psychiatry* 1998; 44:1337–1348.

Pitman RK. Pierre Janet on obsessive-compulsive disorder (1903). *Review and commentary. Arch Gen Psychiatry* 1987; 44:226–232.

Robertson MM, Banerjee S, Kurlan R et al. The Tourette syndrome diagnostic confidence index: development and clinical associations. *Neurology* 1999; 53:2108–2112.

Scotti JR, Schulman DE, Hojnacki RM. Functional analysis and unsuccessful treatment of Tourette's syndrome in a man with profound mental retardation. *Behav Ther* 1994; 25:721–738.

Shady G, Broder R. Tourette syndrome and employment: Descriptors, predictors, and problems. *Psych Rehab Journal* 1995; 19:35–42.
Important study of the occupational difficulties faced by individuals with TS.

Spencer T, Biederman J, Coffey B et al. The 4-year course of tic disorders in boys with attention-deficit/hyperactivity disorder. *Arch Gen Psychiatry* 1999; 56:842–847.

Stefle M. *The Ohio Tourette Study: An investigation of the special service needs of Tourette syndrome patients.* Cincinnati: Tourette Syndrome Association of Ohio, 1983.

Stokes A, Bawden HN, Camfield PR et al. Peer problems in Tourette's disorder. *Pediatrics* 1991; 87:936–942.

Storch EA, Murphy TK, Chase RM et al. Peer victimization in youth with Tourette's syndrome and chronic tic disorder: Relations with tic severity and internalizing symptoms. *J Psychopathol Behav Assess* 2007; 29:211–219.

Sukhodolsky DG, Scahill L, Zhang H et al. Disruptive behavior in children with Tourette's syndrome: association with ADHD comorbidity, tic severity, and functional impairment. *J Am Acad Child Adolesc Psychiatry* 2003; 42:98–105.

Verdellen CWJ, Hoogduin CAL, Keijsers GPJ. Tic suppression in the treatment of Tourette's syndrome with exposure therapy: The rebound phenomenon reconsidered. *Mov Disord* 2007; 22:1601–1606.

Walkup JT, Scahill LD, Riddle MA et al. Disruptive behavior, hyperactivity, and learning disabilities in children with Tourette's syndrome. *Adv Neurol* 1995; 65:259–272.

Wand RR, Matazow GS, Shady GA et al. Tourette syndrome: Associated symptoms and most disabling features. *Neurosci Biobehav Rev* 1993; 17:271–275.

Wodrich DL. Tourette's syndrome and tics: Relevance for school psychologists. *J School Psychol* 1998; 36:281–294.

Wood BL, Klebba K, Gbadebo O et al. Pilot study of effect of emotional stimuli on tic severity in children with Tourette's syndrome. *Mov Disord* 2003; 18:1392–1395.

Woods D, Koch M, Miltenberger R. The impact of tic severity on the effects of peer education about Tourette's syndrome. *J Dev Phys Disabil* 2003; 15:67–78.

Woods DW. *Managing Tourette syndrome: a behavioral intervention for children and adults: therapist guide.* Oxford, New York: Oxford University Press, 2008.

A detailed manual for treating TS, including psychoeducation in early sessions of treatment.

Woods DW, Fuqua R, Outman RC. Evaluating the social acceptability of persons with habit disorders: The effects of topography, frequency, and gender manipulation. *J Psychopathol Behav Assess* 1999; 21:1–18.

Woods DW, Piacentini J, Himle MB, Chang S. Premonitory Urge for Tics Scale (PUTS): initial psychometric results and examination of the premonitory urge phenomenon in youths with tic disorders. *J Dev Behav Pediatr* 2005; 26:397–403.

Zinner S, Conelea C, Glew G et al. Peer victimization in youth with Tourette syndrome and other chronic tic disorders. *Child Psychiatry Hum Dev* 2011; 43:124–136.

23

Cognitive-Behavioral Treatment for Tics

MATTHEW R. CAPRIOTTI AND DOUGLAS W. WOODS

Abstract

Cognitive-behavioral treatment (CBT) is efficacious in decreasing the severity of motor and vocal tics. This chapter reviews the different CBT approaches; among them, Habit Reversal Training (HRT) and related treatments such as Comprehensive Behavioral Intervention for Tics have the most empirical support. The efficacy of HRT-based interventions was shown to be similar to that provided by some pharmacological interventions in children, adolescents, and adults with various types of tics (e.g., motor, vocal, simple, complex). Attempts to enhance HRT-based treatments by adding cognitively oriented components (e.g., cognitive therapy, acceptance work), however, have not been successful to date. Premonitory urges are very important in the tic-management strategies taught in CBT for Tourette syndrome, and changing patients' response to them may be a key mechanism of change.

INTRODUCTION

Recently, greater attention has been directed toward the use of various nonpharmacological treatments for tic disorders. One of the primary treatments in this category is behavioral or cognitive-behavioral therapy (CBT). Although CBT is a blanket term used to describe a general approach to understanding and treating psychiatric dysfunction, it is important to understand that not all treatments falling under the CBT umbrella are the same. They differ in form and intended function. More importantly, they differ vastly in terms of evidence bases supporting their efficacy. Some CBT is ineffective, while other forms of CBT are quite effective in treating tics. The purpose of this chapter is to summarize an emerging behavioral model of tic disorders (Conelea et al., 2008a) and to review and describe the evidence for various forms of CBT for tic disorders. The greatest attention will be given to Habit Reversal Training (HRT) and a more recently enhanced version, Comprehensive Behavioral Intervention for Tics (CBIT), as these treatments have the greatest amount of empirical support.

BEHAVIORAL MODEL OF TICS

The use of a behavioral treatment for tics can be confusing to some readers who assume that the use of a treatment based on principles of learning (Pierce & Cheney, 2008) must imply that tics are learned (Jankovic, 2006). On the contrary, evidence is overwhelming that tics have a biological etiology (Mink & Pleasure, 2003), but research shows that the expression of tics is heavily and predictably influenced by their environmental (i.e., contextual) surroundings. Working within a framework established by operant and respondent principles, CBT constructively harnesses the power of the environment to bring about systematic tic reduction.

From a behavioral perspective, tics can be influenced by two broad classes of events, either of which can occur outside the person's body (external events such as social reactions, situations the person is in, etc.) or inside the body (internal events such as premonitory urges, anxiety, boredom, etc.). The first class of events, labeled "antecedents," is represented by those factors that occur immediately before a tic or bout of tics and make the tic happen more (or less) frequently or intensely. Examples of common external antecedent events include watching television, being around a certain person, or reading silently in a library or classroom (Conelea & Woods, 2008a; Silva et al., 1995). Internal antecedent events that influence tics often include stress, boredom, or fatigue (Bornstein et al., 1990; Conelea et al., 2011; Silva et al., 1995). Some antecedent events, such as emotional stress, appear to worsen tics for nearly all persons with Tourette syndrome (TS) (Bornstein et al., 1990; Eapen et al., 2004), and others, such as a state of relaxation, appear to reduce tics uniformly for virtually all patients (Silva et al., 1995). However, the effects of many antecedent events vary greatly from patient to patient. For instance, in one study, 45% of patients reported worsening of tics in social gatherings, while 42% reported ticcing less in these situations (Silva et al., 1995).

The second class of environmental events that can influence tics is represented by consequences. Consequences are factors that occur as the tic occurs or soon after it ends. Consequences can strengthen (or weaken) the tic (in terms of frequency, intensity, probability of occurring) and can include social reactions or even phenomenological changes in the person. For instance, research has consistently demonstrated that providing tic-contingent attention from a parent or other adult can increase the frequency of tics (Carr et al., 1996; Packer, 2005; Scotti et al., 1994; Watson & Sterling, 1998). In contrast, many laboratory studies have found that providing small monetary rewards for stopping tics can significantly reduce tic frequencies (Conelea & Woods, 2008b; Himle & Woods, 2005; Woods & Himle, 2004) and that these effects persist in the presence of stimuli that remind the person that he or she has been rewarded for stopping (Woods et al., 2009).

In addition to the various antecedent–tic and tic–consequence relationships that may influence tics, one particular type of functional relationship exists that plays a particularly important role in the behavioral model. As noted in earlier chapters, persons with tics often experience a premonitory urge. This urge is experienced as aversive and is often relieved temporarily as

the tic occurs or immediately upon its completion. In behavioral terms, it can be said that the removal of the urge following the tic serves as a reinforcer for the tic. In other words, the tic is strengthened because its immediate effect is to take away the unpleasant urge. This particular arrangement is quite powerful as it represents a situation in which the tic brings a bit of relief every time it occurs.

Despite our ability to discuss these environment–tic relationships (Bliss, 1980; Kane, 1994), it is important to understand that conscious awareness about the effects of these factors is not necessary for the environment to influence a person's tics. Patients are often unaware of the influences the environment has over their tics.

Based on this or similar behavioral models, various forms of CBT have been developed. Below, we will attempt describe some of these interventions. Roughly, these can broken down into two categories, "pre-habit reversal" approaches and "habit reversal-based" approaches.

PRE-HABIT REVERSAL APPROACHES TO TIC MANAGEMENT

In the 1950s and 1960s, researchers who focused on uncovering basic principles of operant and respondent conditioning began to translate their laboratory-based procedures into specific techniques geared at changing clinically important behavior, including tics. Some of these techniques included self-monitoring, massed negative practice (MNP), contingency management procedures, and relaxation training.

Self-Monitoring

Self-monitoring is done to increase a patient's awareness of his or her tics. Research on self-monitoring suggests that positive therapeutic effects can emerge either by making the patient aware of the target action so he or she can engage in counter-actions to stop the troubling behavior, or by making the aversive action salient, thus punishing the action (Nelson & Hayes, 1981; Peterson et al., 1999). As a treatment technique, self-monitoring usually involves asking the patient to engage in some overt monitoring activity whenever a tic occurs. For example, a patient may be asked to carry a note card around with him or her during the day and make a mark on the card each time a tic occurs. Existing evidence suggests that self-monitoring may be a useful adjunct to larger packages of CBT techniques (Ollendick, 1981; Varni et al., 1978), but little evidence exists to support its use as a standalone therapy (Woods et al., 1996).

Massed Negative Practice

MNP involves asking the patient to intentionally and repeatedly engage in the targeted tic for fixed durations of time during multiple periods throughout the day. This process was hypothesized to increase "reactive inhibition," which would prevent the actual tic from emerging (Tophoff, 1973). Although some early case studies suggested that MNP was an effective treatment for tics (e.g., Nicassio et al., 1972; Tophoff, 1973), a randomized controlled trial demonstrated that MNP had negligible impact on tics, and its effect was substantially lower than HRT, another form of CBT. Since that time, MNP has fallen out of favor as a treatment for tics and is not recommended in clinical practice (Cook & Blacher, 2007).

Contingency Management Procedures

Some early attempts at CBT focused directly on rewarding efforts to stop tics (e.g., Wagaman et al., 1995) or directly punishing tic occurrence (Alexander et al., 1973). Treatment procedures based solely on providing discrete reinforcers (i.e., small amounts of money or tokens that could later be exchanged for small rewards) for longer and longer periods of time without tics seem to yield some positive treatment effects in case studies (e.g., Doleys & Kurtz, 1974) and controlled single-case experiments (Wagaman et al., 1995). Contingency management procedures have never been evaluated in a randomized controlled trial, and thus their efficacy as a standalone treatment remains uncertain, but such procedures may be utilized as a part of

larger CBT packages for tics (e.g., Woods et al., 2008).

Often, the delivery of an electric shock contingent on an unwanted behavior is considered synonymous with CBT or behavior modification. However, very few studies report the use of electric shock or other aversive stimuli as a treatment for tics, no randomized trials on such a treatment have been conducted, and the limited evidence on these procedures suggests that they produce high dissatisfaction by the patient (e.g., Alexander et al., 1973). For these reasons and because the general trend in behavior therapy for the past 40 years has been to restrict dramatically the use of aversive treatment procedures, punishment procedures as treatments for tics are clinically unwarranted.

Relaxation

Another early form of CBT for tics was relaxation training. This form of therapy is based on the idea that tics are worsened by anxiety and stress. Through repeated exercises both in the clinic and at home, patients are taught to create a state of relaxation in themselves and to bring about this state when beginning to feel anxious (e.g., Turpin & Powell, 1984). Although case reports suggest that relaxation training may have some benefits, evidence from controlled trials suggests that relaxation training has marginal benefit and is probably not efficacious as a standalone treatment for tics (Bergin et al., 1998; Peterson & Azrin, 1992). Nevertheless, evidence does suggest that stress can disrupt efforts at tic control (Conelea et al., 2011), and thus relaxation training is often utilized as an adjunct to other CBT packages (e.g., Woods et al., 2008).

HABIT REVERSAL-BASED APPROACHES TO TIC MANAGEMENT

At the core of all second-phase CBT interventions is a behavior therapy technique known as habit reversal training. In 1973, Azrin and Nunn developed HRT for the treatment of motor tics and a host of other neuropsychiatric disorders in which repetitive movement was a core symptom (i.e., trichotillomania, stuttering; Woods & Miltenberger, 1995). From that point in time, variations of HRT, treatments that may be functionally similar to HRT (i.e., exposure), and attempted enhancements of HRT have emerged as a second phase of CBT for tics.

HRT is designed to teach the patient to manage his or her tics as they occur in real time. Using HRT, tics are treated one at a time according to how distressing/interfering the tic is for the patient (i.e., most distressing tics are treated first). Typically one or two therapy sessions are dedicated to doing HRT with each tic the patient wants to target. HRT is a multicomponent treatment package whose primary components are awareness training, competing response training, and social support.

Awareness training develops the patient's ability to detect his or her tics as they occur, as well as when the patient experiences premonitory urges signaling the onset of a tic. Many patients present to treatment with these skills well developed, but for some, especially younger children and those with attentional deficits, awareness training is a very important piece of the HRT intervention. To establish awareness, the patient and therapist first create a definition of the tic being targeted for treatment. These definitions are highly detailed and include all aspects of the tic, from the earliest feelings of the urge, to the beginning muscle movements of the tic, through completion of the tic. After spending time defining the tic, the therapist may simulate the tic for the patient in session and ask the patient to acknowledge (e.g., raise a finger) whenever the therapist simulates a tic. While the therapist is simulating tics, it is important that the therapist discuss non–therapy-related topics (e.g., the weather, movies, hobbies) with the patient. The purpose of this exercise is to have the patient recognize ticlike movements while not focusing solely on the awareness exercise. When the patient correctly acknowledges a tic, the therapist praises the patient but also reminds the patient when a tic occurs, but the patient does not acknowledge it. After the patient has shown that he or she can reliably detect 80% of the simulated tics, the process is repeated using the patient's actual tics as the to-be-detected response. In the final step of awareness training, the patient is instructed to raise a finger when he or she "feels a tic coming on" or experiences the urge.

After the patient has displayed mastery in detecting occurrence of tics and premonitory sensations, **competing response training** begins. Competing response training involves the selection and subsequent implementation of a physically incompatible behavior designed to prevent tics from occurring, or at least to make them more difficult. Competing responses should be incompatible with the tic they are designed to counteract, should be able to be performed in any physical position for a sustained period, and should be less noticeable/impairing than the related tic. For instance, a competing response for a lateral head jerking tic might be to gently tense one's neck muscles, to keep the chin level or slightly dropped, and to look straight ahead. Appropriate competing responses are devised for each tic the patient reports. The patient is instructed to perform the relevant competing response for about 1 minute or until the urge to tic diminishes (whichever is longer) whenever he or she tics or experiences the urge to perform a tic. After the therapist demonstrates the process, the patient practices the process in session, and the therapist provides appropriate praise and corrective feedback as necessary. Again, during this in-session practice, it is important for the patient and therapist to be engaged in discussion about the patient's life outside of the therapy context, as this may be helpful in transferring the therapeutic effects of HRT to the patient's day-to-day life.

The final major component of HRT is **social support**, which involves identifying a support person (e.g., parent, spouse, roommate) to promote use of HRT strategies (primarily use of the competing response) outside of therapy. Social support involves teaching the support person to praise the patient's efforts to use the competing response and to provide gentle prompts to use the competing responses when he or she is not attempting to do so. In children, social support may also involve the development of a concrete reward system for the use of competing responses and compliance with other aspects of HRT. Importantly, social support does *not* involve praising or admonishing the non-occurrence or occurrence of tics, but rather encouraging the use of skills learned in therapy.

Evidence for HRT

A large body of evidence now exists supporting the efficacy of HRT. One review (Himle et al., 2006) discussed 16 randomized controlled trials and smaller studies in which HRT consistently produced clinically significant decreases in tics. Cook and Blacher (2007) reviewed 20 published reports of HRT applied to the treatment of tic disorders (6 randomized controlled trials and 14 methodologically rigorous small-n analyses). Using varied outcome measures, 19 of the studies showed that HRT was an effective intervention for reducing tic symptoms (note: the authors of the study in which HRT failed reported that the treatment was not carried out as directed; Carr et al., 1996). More recently, a meta-analysis reviewing outcomes studies of HRT (Bate et al., 2011) found a large treatment effect size ($d = .8$), which is similar to that found for highly effective and widely used behavioral interventions for other disorders, such as exposure and response prevention for obsessive-compulsive disorder (OCD) (Abramowitz et al., 2005). Table 23.1 highlights some of the key controlled trials of HRT's efficacy in treating tic disorders.

Furthermore, evidence suggests that HRT's success is due to its specific behavioral techniques, as opposed to natural waxing and waning of tics or general treatment factors (e.g., an outlet to talk about tic-related frustrations, decreased feelings of abnormality upon learning more about tics, expectancy that one's tics will improve simply because one is in treatment; Deckersbach et al., 2006; Piacentini et al., 2010; Wilhelm et al., 2003). HRT has also proven more effective than relaxation training (Peterson & Azrin, 1992) and MNP (Azrin et al., 1980), further supporting the notion that HRT's success is due to its specific behavioral treatment features.

EXTENSIONS OF HRT

Soon after it was first presented, researchers sought to modify the HRT protocol in various ways. Here, we discuss three attempts to enhance HRT by using additional components.

HRT + Cognitive Therapy

Some clinical researchers have investigated the efficacy of a CBT treatment package that combines selected behavioral practices with cognitive components relevant to TS. This practice is in line with treatment development for other CBTs, which often combine analyses of patient cognitions and subsequent cognitive restructuring with in-session and out-of-session behavioral exercises. This variant of CBT, which we will refer to as Cognitive Behavioral Tension Reduction Therapy (CBTRT) to avoid confusion with the generic "CBT" label that its developers use, conceptualizes tics as serving a tension-reduction function (Bullen & Hemsley, 1983) and places a unique emphasis on directly addressing tension reduction to reduce tics (O'Connor, 2005). CBTRT includes the familiar HRT components of awareness training and competing response training, but also includes broad CBT components of self-monitoring (with emphasis on identifying tic-influencing antecedent settings and cues) and relaxation training. Additionally, CBTRT includes a cognitive restructuring component focused on changing patterns of thinking about tension and tics. The final face-to-face session in the CBTRT protocol addresses relapse prevention.

Studies suggest CBTRT is useful, but not superior to other existing treatments. Two studies have demonstrated that CBTRT significantly decreases tic symptoms in adults with TS (Lavoie et al., 2011; O'Connor et al., 2009), but neither of these studies included an active control condition. In the only study to use the Yale Global Tic Severity Scale (YGTSS), the "gold standard" measure of tic severity (Lavoie et al., 2011), CBTRT produced an average treatment effect of three points, a reduction of questionable clinical significance. Furthermore, a component analysis trial of

Table 23.1 The Most Relevant Controlled Trials Testing the Efficacy of HRT in Treating Tic Disorders

Authors (Year)	Participants	Treatments Evaluated	Primary Outcome Measure/Evaluator	Acute Results	Treatment Durability
Azrin et al., 1980	22 adolescents and adults	HRT, MNP	Patient self-monitoring	At 4-week follow-up, ~30% decrease for MNP, 92% decrease for HRT	HRT: 97% reduction from baseline at 18-month follow-up
Azrin & Peterson, 1990	10 children & adults	HRT, WL	Direct observation of tic frequency by independent observer, significant other, and self	Pretreatment to posttreatment symptom decreases: HRT: 93% mean reduction in self-reported tic frequency (95% for clinic observations). WL: no significant reduction.	Not clear due to use of repeated measures design with ongoing booster sessions
O'Connor et al., 1997	14 adults	HRT, HRT+CT	Patient diary of tic frequency	Pretreatment to posttreatment symptom decreases: HRT = 54%, HRT+CT= 57%	Reduction from baseline at 3-month follow-up: HRT, 77%; HRT+CT, 86%
Wilhelm et al. (2003)	32 adults	HRT, SP	YGTSS by treating clinician	Posttreatment mean symptom severity score: HRT: 19.8, SP: 26.9. Within-group effect size for HRT = 1.50; –.03 for SP	Tic severity not significantly changed from posttreatment to 10-month follow-up
Verdellen et al. (2004)	43 adults and children	HRT, ExRP	YGTSS and tic frequency registrations by blinded evaluator	Significant symptom reductions on both measures for HRT and ExRP. No significant differences between HRT and ExRP on outcome variables.	Not applicable due to immediate-crossover design

Study	Sample	Treatment	Measures	Outcomes	Follow-up
Dekersbach et al., 2006	30 adults	HRT, SP	YGTSS by treating clinician	Posttreatment mean symptom severity score: HRT: 18.3, SP: 26.8. Between-group effect size = 1.42	HRT group maintained gains at 6-month follow-up.
Piacentini et al., 2010	126 children and adolescents	CBIT, SP	YGTSS and CGI by blinded evaluator	Posttreatment CGI status: CBIT: 53% "much" or "very much" improved. SP: 18%. Pretreatment to posttreatment YGTSS decreases: CBIT: 7.6, SP: 3.5.	87% of CBIT responders maintained gains at 6 months, 50% for SP.
Wilhelm et al., 2012	122 adults	CBIT, SP	YGTSS and CGI by blinded evaluator	Percent "much" or "very much" improved (CGI) at posttreatment: CBIT: 38%, SP: 7%. Pretreatment to posttreatment YGTSS decreases: CBIT: 6.2, SP: 2.5.	80% of available CBIT responders maintained gains at 6 months, 25% for SP.

MNP, massed negative practice; WL, waitlist control; HRT+CT, Habit Reversal Training + Acceptance and Commitment Therapy; SP, supportive treatment; ExRP, exposure and response prevention; YGTSS, Yale Global Tic Severity Scale; CBIT, Cognitive-Behavioral Intervention for Tics; CGI, Clinician's Global Impression of Change

CBTRT found that removing the cognitive components of the intervention did not decrease its efficacy (O'Connor et al., 1997), suggesting that CBTRT works primarily because of its HRT-like features, as opposed to the adjunctive cognitive components.

HRT + Acceptance and Commitment Therapy

Recently, researchers (Franklin et al., 2011) have explored the possibility that adding acceptance-based cognitive components to HRT might enhance treatment outcomes. In this intervention, standard HRT was integrated with a tic-specific version of Acceptance and Commitment Therapy (ACT; Hayes et al., 2003). In general, ACT aims to improve patients' functioning by offering exercises to distance patients from distressing cognitions/urges and other distressing emotions. ACT has been shown to be an efficacious treatment, either as monotherapy or as an adjunct to other behavioral techniques, for a variety of psychiatric disorders and appears most promising in the treatment of anxiety disorders (for a review see Ruiz, 2010). As applied to TS, ACT focuses on teaching skills to behave flexibly in the presence of (1) aversive premonitory urges, (2) emotional disturbances resulting from tics (e.g., embarrassment upon ticcing in public or when meeting someone new), and/or (3) cognitive symptoms associated with comorbid psychiatric conditions such as OCD and attention-deficit/hyperactivity disorder (ADHD).

In the lone trial evaluating HRT + ACT (Franklin et al., 2011), 13 adolescents with TS were randomized to receive 10 weekly sessions of either HRT alone or HRT + ACT. Participants randomized to the HRT + ACT treatment condition received three sessions of HRT followed by seven sessions that focused on HRT and ACT (primarily ACT). After the 10-session acute treatment phase, participants received two booster sessions of the same therapy to which they had been randomized. Tics were assessed by a blinded evaluator's rating of clinical global severity and through the YGTSS. Adolescents and their parents each rated tic-related impairment using a validated paper-and-pencil measure of disorder-specific functional impairment. Participants in both treatment groups experienced similar clinically significant reductions in tic severity and tic-related impairment on all measures reported, thus suggesting that ACT procedures may not enhance the efficacy of standard HRT procedures.

COMPREHENSIVE BEHAVIORAL INTERVENTION FOR TICS

CBIT built upon the early HRT package by adding several new components based on research that had emerged since HRT was originally proposed.

The first technique added to the original HRT protocol was based on the understanding that contextual factors reliably influence tics in an individualized fashion. A process called function-based assessment results in individualized intervention strategies, designed to target the environmental or contextual factors that predictably worsen a patient's tics. During a functional assessment, the therapist talks with the patient (and parent, if the patient is a youth) to identify the contexts in which tics are exacerbated (e.g., at school, at restaurants, while watching television) and the consequences that follow the tics when they are exacerbated (e.g., verbal support from a family member, allowance of a break from an academic task). After the assessment of these antecedent and consequent events is complete, the therapist works with the patient and parent to determine therapeutic strategies to be implemented in the identified tic-triggering settings. These therapeutic strategies are designed to either minimize contact with tic-exacerbating situations or to teach the patient to cope with tic-exacerbating situations more effectively, so the effect of that situation on tics is reduced. Likewise, the functional interventions often require the patient and his or her family to minimize any inadvertent social reinforcement for tics. For instance, if a child indicates that his tics worsen while doing homework, and the parent reports that he or she gives the child a break from the homework when his tics are getting in the way, a function-based intervention might suggest that the child be given brief, regular breaks independent of tics and that the parent should not discuss the tics with the child during homework or break times.

CBIT also adds relaxation training and psychoeducation components to the core elements of HRT. Although evidence suggests that relaxation training as a monotherapy is ineffective for TS (Bergin et al., 1998), experimental evidence does suggest that tic suppression is more difficult when experiencing stress (Conelea et al., 2011). As a result, the CBIT protocol includes relaxation training as a stress-management tool, as opposed to a direct tic-management strategy. CBIT also includes psychoeducation about TS and its causes, as disorder-specific education has been found to have positive effects across multiple disorders (e.g., Kendall et al., 2008; Miklowitz et al., 2003).

Typical of outpatient psychological treatment for many disorders, CBIT is designed to be delivered in 1-hour-long, weekly sessions. To standardize CBIT for research studies, a detailed, manualized treatment protocol has been developed (Woods et al., 2008). In this protocol, tics are treated one at a time (most bothersome treated first). In addition, out-of-session homework assignments are an important part of the CBIT package. These assignments include regular implementation of competing response exercises and function-based interventions throughout daily activities, self-monitoring of tic frequency and tic-related impairment, and use of relaxation techniques in high-stress situations.

To evaluate the efficacy of CBIT, two multisite randomized controlled trials (one with pediatric patients, the other with adult patients) have been conducted. In each, a course of CBIT involving eight weekly sessions followed by three monthly booster sessions was compared to a control (PST) condition in which patients received a parallel course of supportive therapy and psychoeducation related to TS. In the pediatric trial (ages 9–17), CBIT produced significantly greater reductions in tic severity (as evaluated by an independent examiner who was blind to treatment condition) compared to PST. Following the acute treatment phase of the study, 52.5% of youngsters receiving CBIT were "very much improved" or "much improved," compared to 18.5% of those in the PST group. On average, patients receiving CBIT experienced a 7.6-point decrease on the total tic severity scale of the YGTSS (range, 0–50). These reductions were similar in magnitude to those seen with medications commonly used in the treatment of TS (e.g., olanzapine, risperidone; Piacentini et al., 2010). However, unlike these neuroleptic medications, which commonly produce adverse side effects, CBIT did not lead to adverse side effects, and attrition was uniformly low across both groups (8% for CBIT and 11% for PST). These findings speak to the tolerability of CBIT among pediatric patients and may help to dispel widespread concerns about potential negative side effects of behavior therapy for TS (Marcks et al., 2004).

Improvements produced by CBIT also proved to be highly durable, with 87% of those who responded to CBIT showing maintenance of treatment gains 6 months after treatment. Additionally, youngsters who responded to CBIT experienced long-term benefits beyond decreases in tics; these included decreases in disruptive behavior, anxiety, obsessive-compulsive symptoms, and family strain (Woods et al., 2011). These secondary benefits are intriguing given that CBIT is highly focused on addressing tics, as opposed to comorbid conditions or other behavioral or emotional issues.

The adult CBIT trial showed successes that paralleled the pediatric study (Wilhelm et al., 2012). This study also used masked assessors and a PST control condition. Following treatment, 38% (24/63) of the CBIT patients were rated as "very much improved" or "much improved" after treatment, compared to 6.8% (4/59) for PST. CBIT patients showed, on average, a 6.2-point reduction in YGTSS tic severity score, compared to an average 2.5-point reduction for the PST group. CBIT-associated treatment gains were durable: 80% of those assessed at 6-month follow-up showed continued benefit. Similar to the results of the pediatric trial, the efficacy of CBIT was not affected by potentially moderating patient factors (e.g., age, gender, education, symptom severity at baseline, comorbid psychopathology).

EXPOSURE AND RESPONSE PREVENTION

Although it is not based on HRT, another behavioral intervention, exposure and response prevention (ERP), has recently been adapted for the treatment of tics and other repetitive behaviors related to TS. ERP grew out of basic learning theory conceptualizations of OCD and has been widely used and validated as an effective behavioral intervention for OCD (Foa et al., 1998). In ERP for OCD, therapists guide patients to refrain from performing the ritualized compulsive behavior while performing the anxiety-provoking task at hand (i.e., they are *exposed* to the harm-related thoughts and settings and *prevented* from engaging in the compulsion as they normally would). Initially, patients experience increased anxiety, but these feelings later subside as the exposure session continues and tend to be less severe when the same exposure is conducted in subsequent sessions (Foa & Kozak, 1986). In the terms of behavior therapy, ERP facilitates both within-session and between-session habituation to the anxiety produced by intrusive cognitions, and by doing so, eliminates the motivation for performing the compulsive behavior.

As applied to tics, ERP focuses on exposure to premonitory urges. Exposure to the urge occurs by having the patient suppress the tics for long periods of time while the therapist "coaches" him or her through the process. Just as ERP allows patients with OCD to habituate to precompulsion obsessions and therefore no longer "need" to perform the compulsions, ERP provides patients with an experience that allows them to habituate to premonitory urges, thereby reducing motivation to tic. Unlike HRT/CBIT, ERP does not teach specific strategies for inhibiting tics, and ERP sessions consist almost exclusively of continuous practice of the exposure process described above, as opposed to the multitactic approach taken by HRT/CBIT.

In terms of clinical outcome, ERP is a promising but not yet well-established intervention for the treatment of tic disorders. In the only randomized controlled trial to date, ERP was compared to HRT in the treatment of 43 adults and youth with TS (Verdellen et al., 2004). ERP produced outcomes roughly equal to HRT. However, methodological limitations limit the extent to which its results can be clearly interpreted. In particular, the ERP treatment in this study involved over twice as much in-session time (12 2-hour sessions) as the HRT intervention (10 1-hour sessions). Also, HRT did not contain a social support component, which is one of the core elements of the treatment and has been shown to be a necessary component of the HRT package for it to be effective, at least in children (Woods et al., 1996).

POSSIBLE MECHANISMS OF CHANGE IN CBT FOR TS

Despite strong support for the efficacy of CBT, relatively little is known about the mechanisms underlying its effectiveness. Early explanations were varied and relatively atheoretical. For example, some assumed that tics were learned and could be eliminated by repeatedly pairing the tic with aversive stimulation (e.g., Tophoff, 1973). A second theory was that competing responses were simply functionally equivalent behaviors to the tic. In other words, it was thought that competing responses took away the urges in the same way that tics did, so the patient started doing the competing response instead of the tic because there were fewer negative social effects from doing the competing responses (Miltenberger et al., 1998). Finally, when introducing HRT, Azrin and Nunn (1973) proposed that tics were caused by an initial muscle injury or other physical ailment that resulted in tension, which was relieved by a repetitive behavior. It was thought that, over time, the person began to engage in the behavior habitually, even though the initial physical insult had healed (Azrin & Nunn, 1973; Yates, 1970). HRT was believed to be effective because it strengthened muscles that opposed tic motions. (Azrin & Nunn, 1973).

These early ideas about mechanisms of behavioral interventions for TS were earnest, well-founded attempts to make sense of the drastic treatment effects seen in early published reports (Azrin & Nunn, 1973; Azrin et al., 1980), but subsequent research raised questions as to the accuracy and completeness of these claims. For instance, studies have shown that when "dissimilar" competing responses are utilized (competing responses that do not utilize the muscles antagonistic to the tic and that are not physically incompatible with the tic), habit reversal can be effective for treating tics (Sharenow et al., 1989) and other repetitive behaviors (Woods et al., 1999). These findings run contrary to the notion that HRT works by strengthening tic-opposing musculature.

The theory about the counter-conditioning mechanism of behavior therapy (i.e., punishment/counter-conditioning) has not been tested, although evidence suggests that competing responses have to be done contingent on the tic or urge to tic to be effective (Miltenberger & Fuqua, 1985). Likewise, the theory that competing response exercises are functionally equivalent alternatives to ticcing is plausible, but there are holes in the empirical support. First, whereas tics provide immediate relief from aversive premonitory urges, using a competing response may initially *increase* the urge experience, with urge reduction occurring only after several minutes or longer (at least in the early stages of treatment; Woods et al., 2008). Thus, it does not follow that the instrumental consequences of engaging in a competing response are similar to those produced by performing a tic. A second piece of evidence arguing against the "replacement" behavior mechanism is that the literature on HRT does not report the continued use of competing responses over time. In fact, it appears that competing response use fades as tic frequency fades, indicating that the patient is not doing the competing response in exchange for the tic (Miltenberger et al., 1998).

More recently, noting that urges may initially increase when suppression occurs (Himle et al., 2007), researchers have begun to consider the possibility of a mechanism of change that explains why both ERP and HRT/CBIT

are effective. As mentioned earlier, it is thought that both forms of therapy operate by promoting habituation to the premonitory urge experience. The literature evaluating this idea in the context of treatment is sparse, but data consistent with this conceptualization do exist. For example, in a recent study, urges were tracked throughout the course of behavior therapy, and it was found that 11 2-hour sessions of ERP resulted in both between- and within-session habituation (Verdellen et al., 2008). No published reports have tested the possibility that similar habituation may occur throughout HRT and related therapies, but the specific clinical instructions given in HRT are to continue using the competing response for 1 minute or until the urge significantly diminishes, whichever takes longer. A habituation mechanism is also consistent with earlier findings that competing responses need not be physically incompatible with tics to be effective. This is consistent with such a mechanism because habituation should take place as long as the tic does not occur, regardless of what the patient does to keep it from occurring.

Although research to date is generally consistent with the idea that habituation to premonitory urges is a key mechanism of change in CBT for TS, other plausible explanations exist. For example, it is possible that practicing the competing response facilitates strengthening of generalized response inhibition capabilities. More colloquially, practicing use of a competing response may increase the individual's general ability to inhibit unwanted behaviors, including tics but also non-tic responses. Supporting this hypothesis, Lavoie and colleagues (2011) demonstrated that adults with TS performed better on tests of motor dexterity and demonstrated posttreatment normalization of previously abnormal EEG signals during response inhibition tasks following a course of CBT that included HRT. Likewise, children who responded to CBIT (discussed previously in this chapter) showed spontaneous, concomitant reduction in disruptive behavior from pretreatment to posttreatment assessment points (Woods et al., 2011). Future research could clarify the extent to which treatment for tics generalizes to clearly non-tic actions in those with TS.

LIMITATIONS OF CURRENT RESEARCH AND DIRECTIONS FOR FUTURE DEVELOPMENT

CBT for tic disorders has had a relatively long history. These nonpharmacological interventions have evolved tremendously from the early psychological but nonbehavioral "cures" for psychodynamic conflicts believed to form the basis of TS symptoms (Michael, 1957; Patrick, 1905) to efficacious forms of CBT that are based on careful research stemming from the behavioral sciences. In most contemporary forms, CBT for TS constitutes a safe and durable treatment tool as powerful as many pharmacological interventions. Research has shown that CBT for TS does not produce once-feared side effects, including exacerbation of tics for some individuals (Piacentini et al., 2010), postsuppression "rebound"-like exacerbation of tics (Himle & Woods, 2005; Leckman et al., 1986; Verdellen et al., 2007), or substitution of new tics for old (Nurnberger & Hingtgen, 1973; Woods et al., 2003).

Despite these successes, much work remains in terms of treatment development and dissemination/implementation. For advances in treatment development to occur, future research will have to follow two paths of inquiry. The first will require a series of studies on the existing form of CBT for tics. The second involves relying on translational science to enhance the power of existing CBT interventions, and to determine the most effective methods for making CBT for TS more available to patients.

Studies on Existing Forms of CBT for Tics

A number of questions remain about whether the current structure of CBT for tics is optimized for efficiency and effectiveness. For instance, the amount of in-session therapy time required to produce durable, clinically significant change in tics is unknown. Early studies of HRT showed large, durable gains following just 1 or 2 days of HRT therapy (e.g., Azrin & Nunn, 1973; Azrin & Peterson, 1988), but more recent randomized controlled trials that provide the most solid evidence for HRT/CBIT's efficacy delivered

therapy according to a more spaced schedule, with acute treatment lasting about 2 months. Interestingly, a meta-analytic review of HRT for the treatment of TS and other body-focused repetitive behaviors found that the amount of time spent in therapy sessions was not correlated with treatment outcomes (Bate et al., 2011), suggesting that efficacious treatment in relatively few sessions may be possible. Still, experiments involving direct comparison of the effects of the "massed" behavior therapy used in Azrin and colleagues' early work and the more "spaced" treatment schedule used in recent research are necessary to inform best practice in real-world practice settings.

Future research should also seek to evaluate the comparative efficacies of different behavioral and pharmacological interventions for TS. To date, controlled trials of CBT for TS have compared a single "active" treatment to either a waitlist (Himle et al., 2006) or a placebo-like control therapy (e.g., Deckersbach et al., 2006, Piacentini et al., 2010), but have rarely compared two efficacious behavioral interventions or compared a behavioral intervention to a pharmacological intervention. Given the lack of methodologically sound experiments directly comparing two or more efficacious treatments, practitioners, patients, and clinical researchers cannot truly answer the simple question "Which treatment works best?" Future research should generate evidence-based answers to this question by directly comparing multiple forms of efficacious behavioral and pharmacological interventions (e.g., CBIT, ERP, risperidone, and guanfacine). The Tourette Syndrome Association Behavioral Sciences Consortium could provide a network of clinical researchers well equipped to undertake this important, large-scale scientific endeavor.

Treatment Development Through Translational Science

To improve the efficacy of existing interventions, basic researchers must focus on understanding the underpinnings of tic suppression and the premonitory urge, while outcome researchers explain for whom CBT is and is not effective.

Both types of researchers will need to communicate with each other to move the research agenda forward. Basic researchers can follow-up on the outcome moderator data to determine why treatments fail at the neurobehavioral level and then provide insights to applied researchers, who can then use this information to modify interventions more effectively.

To understand the factors leading to effective tic suppression and the premonitory urge, serious attention also will need to be given to understanding the behavioral (separate but equal from neurological) factors that reliably control tic suppression, expression, and modification. Some of this work has already begun.

There exists a small but growing body of research on the basic processes involved in tic expression and suppression. To date, separate lines of investigation have progressed in areas of neuroscience and behavior analysis, but these lines have developed relatively independent of each other. These investigations have yielded coherent but incomplete accounts of the mechanisms involved in tic suppression and expression. For instance, research using functional magnetic resonance imaging has produced evidence suggesting that volitional suppression of tics is mediated by the prefrontal cortex and pathways between these regions and the basal ganglia, where abnormal neural signals are thought to give rise to tics (Peterson et al., 1998). Additionally, research has shown that premonitory urges to tic involve different neural circuitry than tic movement themselves and involve activation of the supplementary motor area, putamen, and amygdala (Wang et al., 2011). In parallel, behavioral research has indicated that premonitory urges may be enhanced through aversive consequences resulting from tics (Conelea et al., 2008a) and that suppression attempts are most successful when supported by external reinforcement for tic-free periods (Woods & Himle, 2004; Woods et al., 2009). Thus, two incomplete literatures have emerged. The neuroscience literature addresses processes involved in urge development and tic suppression but has not necessarily evaluated the neural mechanism under conditions in which urges may be most relevant or in which tics are most

effectively suppressed. On the other hand, the behavioral literature on urge development and tic suppression has investigated the effects of several important contextual variables (e.g., distraction, stress) but has done so without trying to explain how or why this is occurring at the level of the brain. Thus, researchers from either "camp" have yet to take the important step of translating their research to the others' level of analysis.

We believe such translational work can be achieved by examining the roadmaps followed by researchers who have developed consistent biobehavioral conceptualizations of other neuropsychiatric disorders (Hofmann, 2007; Risbrough & Stein, 2006). In these cases, early researchers produced empirically supported, behaviorally sound conceptualizations of the disorder and neuroscientists, in turn, used these conceptualizations to guide research elucidating neural mechanisms associated with the aberrant behavioral processes central to the disorder.

In TS, there are various areas in which such translational research may help the further development of CBT for TS by providing better understanding of the disorder.

Given the apparent clinical importance of habituation to premonitory urges, future research should explore contextual and biological factors that influence this process. Identification of habituation-enhancing factors can lead to procedural enhancements that improve the efficacy of CBT, and discovery of habituation-inhibiting factors can provide clues as to why certain variables may predict poor treatment outcome.

One barrier to understanding the urge-related habituation process involves problems with measuring the urge itself. Currently, subjective verbal rating of the premonitory urge serves as the primary mode of assessment, but development of behavioral and physiological measures of urge strength would likely facilitate more comprehensive, translational investigation. Once developed, these measures could be used to investigate habituation processes on both behavioral and biological levels. Insight into potential facilitators of the habituation process can be gained from research on ERP for other disorders, which suggests that within-session habituation is unnecessary for long-term habituation and clinical change in ERP (Craske et al., 2008). Data also suggest that ending sessions *before* within-session habituation (i.e., a decrease in anxiety in spider phobias) occurred produced *better* long-term fear reduction than ending exposure sessions once anxiety had decreased. If a similar finding was experimentally replicated in TS, the implementation of treatment sessions could be modified accordingly.

Finally, both humans and animal research shows that habituation proceeds more rapidly when multiple "conditioned excitors" (here, stimuli that increase the urge to tic) are present during exposure sessions. If experimental research supported that conducting ERP for TS in the presence of multiple urge-increasing cues resulted in faster and/or greater habituation effects, it would be advisable to first conduct a functional assessment to identify contextual antecedents that increase the urge for a specific patient, and then conduct exposure sessions or strongly encourage the use of HRT in these contexts.

Recently, research has demonstrated that systematic delivery of small monetary rewards can produce large decreases in tic frequency (e.g., Conelea & Woods, 2008b; Himle et al., 2007, Woods & Himle, 2004). Future imaging studies could hone in on the similarities and differences between neural processes involved in these two types of tic suppression by comparing patterns of brain activation during suppression with and without a supporting reinforcement contingency. This could help to further understand the brain–environment interactions that underlie the expression of TS symptoms.

Future research can also address gaps in the literature regarding behavioral and neural aspects of tic suppression maintained by various contextual factors. For instance, all laboratory investigations of reinforcement-maintained tic suppression to date have used a positive reinforcement paradigm in which monetary reinforcers are delivered after brief (e.g., 10-second) periods of suppression. However, in the real world, suppression might be more likely to be maintained by initial experiences with aversive consequences for tics, and subsequent maintenance of suppression by negative reinforcement contingencies. For example, a child might be teased for ticcing in front of schoolmates at recess, and then suppress tics at recess in the future to avoid being teased again. Indeed, several studies have shown that tics can be increased by providing social attention or breaks from academic tasks contingent on tic occurrence (e.g., Packer, 2005; Scotti et al., 1994; Watson & Sterling, 1998). More in-depth biobehavioral research comparing suppression maintained by social and nonsocial factors would further develop knowledge of the biological and behavioral processes involved in tic expression and suppression.

Other basic parameters of suppression situations, such as the magnitude and timing of reinforcement for abstaining from ticcing, also deserve further empirical evaluation. Although previous studies have found strong suppression using the positive reinforcement paradigm discussed above, a small but notable minority of individuals in these studies have not shown suppression under these conditions. Perhaps providing more frequent reinforcers (e.g., after every 5-second period of suppression instead of every 10 seconds) or more valuable reinforcers would have made suppression possible for these individuals. If monetary rewards arranged in tic suppression studies are viewed as "competing" with reinforcement that would be obtained from ticcing (i.e., reduction in the premonitory urge), it would be expected that momentary premonitory urge strength would be a determinant of whether a child ticced or suppressed at any given point in the tic suppression task. If a reliable real-time measure of urge could be developed (as discussed in this section), suppression could be enhanced by adjusting the magnitude of upcoming reinforcement based on the present urge strength. This might "up the ante" in terms of reinforcement for suppression when naturally occurring reinforcement for ticcing would not only create "better" tic suppression, but also facilitate exposure to high-intensity premonitory urges. As such, evidence suggesting that this is the case would not be merely an esoteric "proof-of-concept" laboratory demonstration, but rather a first step in developing a paradigm that could provide the foundation for enhanced behavior therapies for TS.

The other broad focus of future TS research involves the dissemination and implementation of existing CBT. Although future efforts are needed to understand why current CBT for TS works and how to further improve these interventions, the fact remains that effective non-pharmacological interventions do exist for TS but are not yet widely available (Conelea et al., 2011; Marcks et al., 2004). Likewise, it is not clear how and when CBT should be introduced in the continuum of care.

One important step in making effective CBT available to patients involves educating patients and their families about these treatments. The Tourette Syndrome Association (www.tsa-usa.org) is an excellent resource for patients and families seeking such information (see Chapter 30). Mass media has also helped to inform the public about the breakthroughs in behavioral therapy for TS, as indicated by the several published reports of the pediatric CBIT trial in popular news media (e.g., Harding, 2010; Holohan, 2011). As increasing numbers of patients learn that CBIT and some other CBTs are efficacious, patient demand for these services will likely increase. Even at present, many individuals with TS report that they are interested in receiving behavioral treatment but do not know where such treatments can be obtained, and/or find that no practitioners in their area offer CBT for TS (Conelea et al., 2011). This common patient experience is consistent with existing statistics about the number of treating professionals who provide CBT for TS. In a 2004 survey of psychiatrists, neurologists, general practitioners, and psychologists, only 35% had even heard of HRT and less than 5% actually knew how to implement the treatment.

These results indicate that efforts to disseminate the various forms of CBT for TS should be strengthened. To increase the number of professionals trained to implement CBT for tics, at least two possible avenues could be taken. First, effective training programs must be developed and implemented widely across multiple disciplines with requisite background training. However, it is unclear how effective instruction

programs should be structured. Is reading a printed manual sufficient for a therapist to become competent? Is a full training workshop necessary? Follow-up supervision? After an effective training program is established for psychologists, it should be modified to meet the needs of various disciplines, including school psychologists, board-certified behavior analysts, pediatric nurses and nurse practitioners, and occupational therapists. Of course, research will also be needed to evaluate the extent to which the efficacy of behavioral interventions is moderated when delivered by professionals from disciplines outside of clinical psychology, but the success of other behavioral therapies when applied by nonpsychologists (Wells et al., 2003) suggests that this type of dissemination is likely to succeed with appropriate adaptations.

The second pathway for increasing the availability of CBT for tics involves modifying the intervention so it is more easily adapted to practice settings in which tic referrals are most likely to occur. The first point of referral for most patients with tics is a pediatrician or general practitioner, followed by a neurologist or psychiatrist. However, the standard format of CBT (e.g., eight 60- to 90-minute sessions) does not fit well into the practice structure of such care providers. Attempts to simplify and streamline CBT procedures so they can be implemented by practitioners may improve accessibility.

In addition to increasing the number of practitioners able to provide effective CBT for TS, patient access to these treatments can also be improved by developing methods that maximize the number of patients a single provider can see within scheduling constraints. This could be accomplished by developing group delivery formats. In addition to increasing caseload capacity, such group adaptations might provide other benefits, such as promoting normalization of tic disorders and providing a supportive environment for patients to share their experiences with tics and related difficulties.

As far as increasing the local availability of CBT for tics in currently underserved regions, one of the more promising strategies is the use of telehealth. With recent breakthroughs in the accessibility and quality of videoconferencing technology, researcher and clinician interest in using telehealth methods to treat neurobehavioral conditions has dramatically increased (Postel et al., 2007). Research on the efficacy of telehealth-delivered CBT for TS is in its infancy, but a single study has suggested that HRT delivered via teleconferencing produced significant symptom changes in three children with TS (Himle et al., 2010). Of course, this preliminary study serves only as a first step in fully evaluating the efficacy of behavior therapy for TS via telehealth technology. Future research should involve well-designed, randomized controlled trials comparing the efficacy of CBT delivered via telehealth technology versus CBT delivered in the traditional face-to-face manner.

Ultimately, treatment outcome research should progress to focus on large-scale, practically oriented questions that provide clear answers to patients about effective courses of treatment. One such consideration involves answering the question, "For whom does CBT work, and for whom does it not?" Randomized controlled trials such as the CBIT trials have provided few answers to this question but have begun to inform thinking in regard to this matter. Although the separate child and adult CBIT papers found that certain factors such as the presence of various types of comorbid psychopathology, patient age, premonitory urge severity, baseline tic severity, and tic topography did *not* prove to moderate response to CBIT, our own clinical experience is that the presence of ADHD often makes treatment more difficult. In addition, one factor that approached statistical significance in predicting response to CBIT in children and adults was medication status. Pediatric and adult patients who were taking medications to reduce their tics while receiving the CBIT intervention were somewhat less likely to respond to treatment. Likewise, those who are not motivated to participate in the therapy process or who are not compliant with therapeutic instructions often receive less benefit. Future research is also needed to clarify the moderating effects of different classes of medication that may be prescribed for TS (e.g., atypical antipsychotics, alpha antagonists) on the response to CBT and on the fundamental behavioral processes that mediate the treatment response.

Research should also identify the optimal order of treatments given their presenting profile (e.g., answer questions such as "Is it better to try behavior therapy first and add medication later if necessary, or vice versa?"). Other questions might come after a patient has already failed to respond to one or more treatments (e.g., "If ERP didn't help my child, is it best to turn to another

---

Box 23.1. Key Points

- CBT is efficacious in decreasing the severity of motor and vocal tics.
- Of the different CBT approaches, HRT and related treatments such as CBIT have the most empirical support.
- HRT-based interventions produce symptom reduction similar to that provided by some pharmacological interventions.
- HRT has been proven efficacious in treating a wide variety of patients with TS, including:
  - Children, adolescents, and adults ages 8 to 65 years
  - Individuals with and without comorbid psychological conditions
  - Individuals currently taking medication for TS and those who are not
  - Individuals with various types of tics (e.g., motor, vocal, simple, complex)
- Attempts to enhance HRT-based treatments by adding cognitively oriented components (e.g., cognitive therapy, acceptance work) have not been successful to date.
- Premonitory urges play a key role in tic management strategies taught in CBT for TS, and changing patients' response to them may be a key mechanism of change.

form of CBT, medication, or both at the same time?"). We are aware of only one study that has systematically addressed questions of treatment sequencing. This study found that implementing ERP after a course of HRT produced further decreases in tic symptoms, but the opposite was not true: providing HRT after a course of ERP did not produce additional benefits (Verdellen et al., 2004). These questions are daunting topics for clinical outcomes researchers as they necessitate large, resource-intensive studies with very many participants. However, the information gained from them would be incredibly valuable to patients, and therefore these issues must be addressed.

Recently, researchers have used such adaptive trials (e.g., Tamura et al., 1994; for a review, see Murphy et al., 2007) in which patients are assigned to receive a given treatment first and are then assigned to subsequent treatments based on their response or lack of response to the first. In this sense, these trials parallel treatment in the real world. Patients try one therapy and continue it if it works for them. If they do not respond to the first treatment, patients shift treatment strategies following some predetermined but clinically justified order. These kinds of studies have provided very valuable information in recent studies of ADHD and other psychiatric disorders. As clinical scientists make progress in understanding the role of CBT in treating TS, as well as addressing the many other research questions discussed in this chapter, patients will benefit from enhanced access to varied, effective nonpharmacological treatment options for tic disorders.

Box 23.2. Questions for Future Research

1. What is the nature of the "dose–response" relationship for CBT for TS? What number of sessions and what session duration are best suited to produce good clinical outcomes in the most feasible way possible?
2. Through which mechanisms does CBT for TS operate? What key neurological and behavioral processes must CBT affect to bring about clinical change in tics? Do changes in premonitory urge severity and/or behavior in response to premonitory urges mediate the efficacy of CBT?
3. How can we use knowledge of change mechanisms to build more powerful interventions? What neurobiological and behavioral processes mediate response to CBT for TS? Based on this, what treatment strategies might serve as useful adjuncts to existing CBT interventions such as HRT? What role might novel intervention components (e.g., cognitive retraining, reinforced practice of tic suppression, building skills for premonitory urge tolerance) play in this endeavor?
4. How can we best predict who will respond to CBT? Currently, few factors are known to predict whether or not an individual will respond to CBT for TS. Can we identify demographic, clinical, and/or neuropsychological characteristics that can accurately predict who will and will not benefit from treatment?
5. Which sequencing of CBT and pharmacotherapy provides the best long-term outcomes for patients? Should first-time treatment seekers begin with CBT, pharmacotherapy, or both interventions simultaneously? How well does CBT work for patients receiving partial relief from pharmacological treatment?
6. How can CBT for TS be made more accessible? What is the best way to make CBT for TS available in a larger number of communities? Is it feasible to train an adequate number of clinicians using a typical model? Can telehealth technologies aid in this goal?

AUTHOR NOTE

The authors would like to thank Derek Spaeth for assistance in the preparation of this chapter.

REFERENCES

Abramowitz JS, Whiteside SP, Deacon BJ et al. The effectiveness of treatment for pediatric obsessive-compulsive disorder: A meta-analysis. *Behav Ther* 2005; 36:55–63.

Alexander AB, Chai H, Creer TL et al. The elimination of chronic cough by response suppression shaping. *J Behav Ther Exp Psychiatry* 1973; 4:75–80.

Azrin NH, Nunn RG. Habit-reversal: A method of eliminating nervous habits and tics. *Behav Res Ther* 1973; 11:619–628.
First published study of habit reversal for tic and other body-focused repetitive behaviors.

Azrin NH, Nunn RG, Frantz SE. Habit reversal vs. negative practice treatment of nervous tics. *Behav Ther* 1980; 11:169–178.

Azrin NH, Peterson AL. Habit reversal for the treatment of Tourette syndrome. *Behav Res Ther* 1988; 26:347–351.

Bate KS, Malouff JM, Thorsteinsson ET, Bhullar N. The efficacy of habit reversal therapy for tics, habit disorders, and stuttering: A meta-analytic review. *Clin Psychol Rev* 2011; 31:865–871.

Bergin A, Waranch HR, Brown J et al. Relaxation therapy in Tourette syndrome: A pilot study. *Pediatr Neurol* 1998; 18:126–142.

Bliss J. Sensory experiences of Gilles de la Tourette syndrome. *Arch Gen Psychiatry* 1980; 37:1343–1347.

Bornstein RA, Stefl ME, Hammond L. A survey of Tourette syndrome patients and their families: The 1987 Ohio Tourette Survey. *J Neuropsych Clin Neurosci* 1990; 2:275–281.

Bullen JG, Hemsley DR. Sensory experience as a trigger in Gilles de la Tourette's syndrome. *J Behav Ther Exp Psychiatry* 1983; 14:197–201.

Carr JE, Bailey JS, Carr CA, Coggin AM. The role of independent variable integrity in the behavioral management of Tourette syndrome. *Behavioral Interventions* 1996; 11:35–45.

Conelea CA, Brandt BC, Woods DW. The impact of a stress induction task on tic frequencies in youth with Tourette syndrome. *Behav Res Ther* 2011; 49:492–497.

Conelea CA, Woods DW. The influence of contextual factors on tic expression in Tourette syndrome: a review. *J Psychosom Res* 2008a; 65:487–496.

Conelea CA, Woods DW. Examining the impact of distraction on tic suppression in children and adolescents with Tourette syndrome. *Behav Res Ther* 2008b; 46:1193–1200.

Conelea CA, Woods DW, Zinner SH et al. Exploring the impact of chronic tic disorders on youth: results from the Tourette Syndrome Impact Survey. *Child Psychiatry Hum Dev* 2011; 42:219–242.

Cook CR, Blacher J Evidence-based psychosocial treatments for tic disorders. *Clin Psychol* 2007; 14:252–267.
Systematic review of the evidence base for various psychosocial treatments according to the American Psychological Association's classification system for empirically supported interventions.

Craske MG, Kircanski K, Zelikowsky M et al. Optimizing inhibitory learning during exposure therapy. *Behav Res Ther* 2008; 46:5–27.

Deckersbach T, Rauch S, Buhlmann U, Wilhelm S. Habit reversal versus supportive psychotherapy in Tourette's disorder: A randomized controlled trial and predictors of treatment response. *Behav Res Ther* 2006; 44:1079–1090.

Doleys DM, Kurtz PS. A behavioral treatment program for the Gilles de la Tourette syndrome. *Psychol Rep* 1974; 35:43–48.

Eapen V, Fox-Hiley P, Banerjee S, Robertson MM. Clinical features and associated psychopathology in a Tourette syndrome cohort. *Acta Neurol Scand* 2004; 109:255–260.

Foa EB, Franklin ME, Kozak MJ. Psychosocial treatments for obsessive-compulsive disorder: Literature review. In Swinson RP, Anthony MM, Richter MA (Eds.), *Obsessive compulsive disorder. Theory, research, and treatment.* New York: Guilford Press, 1998.

Foa EB, Kozak MJ. Emotional processing of fear: Exposure to corrective information. *Psychol Bull* 1986; 99:20–35.

Franklin ME, Best SH, Wilson MA et al. Habit reversal training and acceptance and commitment therapy for Tourette syndrome: A pilot project. *J Dev Phys Disabil* 2011; 23:49–60.

Harding A. (2010, May 18). Behavior therapy matches drugs for calming tics. Reuters. Retrieved October 20, 2011, from http://www.

reuters.com/article/2010/05/18/us-calming-tics-idUSTRE64H3P220100518.

Hayes SC, Strosahl KD, Wilson KG. *Acceptance and commitment therapy: An experiential approach to behavior change*. New York: The Guilford Press, 2003.

Himle MB, Olufs E, Himle J et al. Behavior therapy for tics via videoconference delivery: An initial pilot test in children. *Cogn Behav Pract* 2010; 17:329–337.

Himle MB, Woods DW. An experimental evaluation of tic suppression and the tic rebound effect. *Behav Res Ther* 2005; 43:1443–1451.

Himle MB, Woods DW, Conelea CA et al. Investigating the effects of tic suppression on premonitory urge ratings in children and adolescents with Tourette's syndrome. *Behav Res Ther* 2007; 45:2964–2976.

First study to empirically demonstrate that premonitory urge strength increases during tic suppression.

Himle MB, Woods DW, Piacentini JC et al. Brief review of habit reversal training for Tourette syndrome. *J Child Neurol* 2006; 21:719–725.

Hofmann SG. Enhancing exposure-based therapy from a translational research perspective. *Behav Res Ther* 2007; 45:1987–2001.

Holohan E (2011, April 21). Behavioral therapy may reduce Tourette tics, symptoms. *US News and World Report*. Retrieved October 20, 2011, from http://health.usnews.com/health-news/family-health/brain-and-behavior/articles/2011/04/21/behavioral-therapy-may-reduce-tourette-tics-symptoms.

Jankovic J. Tics and Tourette's syndrome. In Jankovic J, Tolosa E (Eds.), *The Parkinson's disease and movement disorders*. Philadelphia, PA: Lippincott Williams & Wilkins, 2006, pp. 356–375.

Kane MJ. Premonitory urges as `attentional tics' in Tourette's syndrome. *J Am Acad Child Adolesc Psychiatry* 1994; 33:805–808.

Kendall PC, Hudson JL, Gosch E et al. Cognitive-behavioral therapy for anxiety disordered youth: A randomized clinical trial evaluating child and family modalities. *J Consult Clin Psychol* 2008; 76:282–297.

Lavoie ME, Imbriglio TV, Stip E, O'Connor KP. Neurocognitive changes following cognitive-behavioral treatment in Tourette syndrome and chronic tic disorder. *Int J Cogn Ther* 2011; 4:34–50.

Leckman JF, Ort S, Cohen DJ et al. Rebound phenomena in Tourette's syndrome after abrupt withdrawal of clonidine: Behavioral, cardiovascular, and neurochemical effects. *Arch Gen Psychiatry* 1986; 43:1168–1176.

Marcks BA, Woods DW, Teng EJ, Twohig MP. What do those who know, know? Investigating providers' knowledge about Tourette syndrome and its treatment. *Cogn Behav Pract* 2004; 11:298–305.

Michael RP. Treatment of a case of compulsive swearing. *BMJ* 1957; 20:1506–1507.

Miklowitz DJ, George EL, Richards JA et al. A randomized study of family-focused psychoeducation and pharmacotherapy in the outpatient management of bipolar disorder. *Arch Gen Psychiatry* 2003; 60:904–912.

Miltenberger RG, Fuqua RW. A comparison of contingent vs. non-contingent competing response practice in the treatment of nervous habits. *J Behav Ther Exp Psychiatry* 1985; 16:195–200.

Miltenberger RG, Fuqua RW, Woods DW. Applying behavior analysis to clinical problems: Review and analysis of habit reversal. *J Appl Behav Anal* 1998; 31:447–469.

Mink JW, Pleasure DE. The basal ganglia and involuntary movements: Impaired inhibition of competing motor patterns. *Arch Neurol* 2003; 60:1365–1368.

Murphy SA, Collins LM, Rush AJ. Customizing treatment to the patient: Adaptive treatment strategies. *Drug Alcohol Depend* 2007; 88:S1–S3.

Nelson RO, Hayes SC. Theoretical explanations for reactivity in self-monitoring. *Behav Modif* 1981; 5:3–14.

Nicassio FJ, Liberman RP, Patterson RL et al. The treatment of tics by negative practice. *J Behav Ther Exp Psychiatry* 1972; 3:281–287.

Nurnberger JI, Hingtgen JN. Is symptom substitution an important issue in behavior therapy? *Biol Psychiatry* 1973; 3:221–236.

O'Connor KP. *Cognitive-behavioral management of tic disorders*. West Sussex, England: John Wiley and Sons Ltd, 2005.

O'Connor KP, Gareau D, Borgeat F. A comparison of behaviourial and a cognitive-behavioural approach to the management of chronic tic disorders. *Clin Psychol Psychother* 1997; 4:105–117.

O'Connor KP, Laverdure A, Taillon A et al. Cognitive behavioral management of Tourette's syndrome and chronic tic disorder in medicated and unmedicated samples. *Behav Res Ther* 2009; 47:1090–1095.

Ollendick TH. Self-monitoring and self-administered overcorrection: The modification of nervous tics in children. *Behav Modif* 1981; 5:75–84.

Packer LE. Tic-related school problems: Impact on functioning, accommodations, and interventions. *Behav Modif* 2005; 29:876–899.

Patrick HT. Convulsive tic. *JAMA* 1905; 44:437–442.

Peterson AL, Azrin NH. An evaluation of behavioral treatments for Tourette syndrome. *Behav Res Ther* 1992; 30:167–174.

Peterson BS, Skudlarski P, Anderson AW et al. A functional magnetic resonance imaging study of tic suppression in Tourette syndrome. *Arch Gen Psychiatry* 1998; 55:326–333.

Peterson LD, Young KR, West RP, Peterson MH. Effects of student self management on generalization of student performance to regular classrooms. *Educ Treat Children* 1999; 22:357–372.

Piacentini J, Woods DW, Scahill L et al. Behavior therapy for children with Tourette disorder: A randomized controlled trial. *JAMA* 2010; 303:1929–1937.
Largest trial of CBT for TS. Primary study evaluating efficacy of CBIT in children.

Pierce WD, Cheney CD. *Behavior analysis and learning.* New York: Taylor & Francis, 2008.

Postel GM, de Haan HA, de Jong CAJ. E-therapy for mental health problems: A systematic review. *Telemedicine J E Health* 2007; 14:707–714.

Risbrough VB, Stein MB. Role of corticotropin releasing factor in anxiety disorders: A translational research perspective. *Horm Behav* 2006; 50:550–561.

Ruiz FJ. A review of Acceptance and Commitment Therapy (ACT) empirical evidence: Correlational, experimental psychopathology, component and outcome studies. *Int J Psychol Ther* 2010; 10:125–162.

Scotti JR, Schulman DE, Honjacki RM. Functional analysis and unsuccessful treatment of Tourette's syndrome in a man with profound mental retardation. *Behav Ther* 1994; 25:721–738.

Sharenow EL, Fuqua RW, Miltenberger RG. The treatment of muscle tics with dissimilar competing response practice. *J Appl Behav Anal* 1989; 22:35–42.

Silva RR, Munoz DM, Barickman J, Friedhoff AJ. Environmental factors and related fluctuation of symptoms in children and adolescents with Tourette's disorder. *J Child Psychol Psychiatry* 1995; 36:305–312.

Tamura RN, Faries DE, Andersen JS, Heiligenstein JH. A case study of an adaptive clinical trial in the treatment of out-patients with depressive disorder. *J Am Stat Assoc* 1994; 89:768–776.

Tophoff M. Massed practice, relaxation, and assertion training in the treatment of Gilles de la Tourette syndrome. *J Behav Ther Exp Psychiatry* 1973; 4:71–73.

Turpin G, Powell GE. Effects of massed practice and cue-controlled relaxation on tic frequency in Gilles de la Tourette's syndrome. *Behav Res Ther* 1984; 22:165–178.

Varni JW, Boyd EF, Cataldo MF. Self-monitoring, external reinforcement, and timeout procedures in the control of high rate tic behaviors in a hyperactive child. *J Behav Ther Exp Psychiatry* 1978; 9:353–358.

Verdellen CWJ, Hoogduin CAL, Kato BS et al. Habituation of premonitory sensations during exposure and response prevention treatment in Tourette's syndrome. *Behav Modif* 2008; 32:215–227.
Most direct evidence for the hypothesized urge-reduction mechanism of CBT.

Verdellen CWJ, Hoogduin CAL, Keijsers GPJ. Tic suppression in the treatment of Tourette's syndrome with exposure therapy: The rebound phenomenon reconsidered. *Mov Disord* 2007; 22:1601–1606.

Verdellen CWJ, Keijsers GPJ, Cath DC, Hoogduin CAL. Exposure with response prevention versus habit reversal in Tourette's syndrome: A controlled study. *Behav Res Ther* 2004; 42:501–511.
Largest trial of ERP for TS to date.

Wagaman JR, Miltenberger RG, Williams DE. Treatment of a vocal tic by differential reinforcement. *J Behav Ther Exp Psychiatry* 1995; 26:35–39.

Wang Z, Maia TV, Marsh R et al. The neural circuits that generate tics in Tourette syndrome. *Am J Psychiatry* 2011; 168:1326–1337.

Watson TS, Sterling HE. Brief functional analysis and treatment of a vocal tic. *J Appl Behav Anal* 1998; 31:471–474.

Wells J, Barlow J, Stewart-Brown S. A systematic review of universal approaches to mental health promotion in schools. *Health Educ* 2003; 103:197–220.

Wilhelm S, Deckersbach T, Coffey BJ et al. Habit reversal versus supportive psychotherapy for Tourette's disorder: A randomized controlled trial. *Am J Psychiatry* 2003; *160*:1175–1177.

Wilhelm S, Peterson AL, Piacentini JC et al. Randomized trial of behavior therapy for adults with Tourette's disorder. *Arch Gen Psychiatry* 2012; *69*:795–803.

Woods DW, Himle MB. Creating tic suppression: Comparing the effects of verbal instruction to differential reinforcement. *J Appl Behav Anal* 2004; *37*:417–420.

Woods DW, Miltenberger RG. Habit reversal: A review of applications and variations. *J Behav Ther Exp Psychiatry* 1995; *26*:123–131.

Woods DW, Miltenberger RG, Lumley VA. Sequential application of major habit-reversal components to treat motor tics in children. *J Appl Behav Anal* 1996; *29*:483–493.

Woods DW, Murray LK, Fuqua RW et al. Comparing the effectiveness of similar and dissimilar competing responses in evaluating the habit reversal treatment for oral-digital habits in children. *J Behav Ther Exp Psychiatry* 1999; *30*:289–300.

Woods DW, Piacentini JC, Chang SW et al. *Managing Tourette syndrome: A behavioral intervention for children and adult (therapist guide).* New York: Oxford University Press, 2008.

Woods DW, Piacentini JC, Scahill L et al. Behavior therapy for tics in children: Acute and long-term effects on psychiatric and psychosocial functioning. *J Child Neurol* 2011; *26*:858–865.

Woods DW, Twohig MP, Flessner CA, Roloff TJ. Treatment of vocal tics in children with Tourette syndrome: Investigating the efficacy of habit reversal. *J Appl Behav Anal* 2003; *36*:109–112.

Woods DW, Walther MR, Bauer CC et al. The development of stimulus control over tics: A potential explanation for contextually-based variability in the symptoms of Tourette syndrome. *Behav Res Ther* 2009; *47*:41–47.

Yates AJ. *Behavior therapy.* New York: Wiley & Sons, 1970.

24

Pharmacological Treatment of Tics

VEIT ROESSNER AND ARIBERT ROTHENBERGER

Abstract

This chapter provides a literature review and a critical commentary of the available evidence on pharmacological treatment of tics in Tourette syndrome (TS). Because of the waxing and waning nature of tics, a meaningful appraisal of treatment efficacy in TS can be given in most cases only after a longer observation time. Environmental or situational factors have a modulating influence on tics, possibly biasing the appraisal of treatment efficacy. Many affected children, adolescents, and adults do not seek or require pharmacological treatment (tic severity: mild to moderate). Nonpharmacological and/or pharmacological interventions make sense for persons with subjective discomfort, social and/or emotional problems, functional interference, etc. The clinical experience is that pharmacotherapy induces faster and probably more prominent tic reduction than behavioral treatment options. The goal of pharmacological treatment is a reduction in tic symptoms. Antipsychotic drugs may produce the most reliable and fastest results, but they also pose the greatest risk of side effects. Risperidone can be considered a first-choice agent for treating tics; pimozide, tiapride, sulpiride, and aripiprazole are regarded as second-choice agents. Clonidine might be helpful mainly in case of TS plus attention-deficit/hyperactivity disorder. For high-quality evidence on pharmacological treatment in TS, future studies should include, for instance, longer observation periods, larger groups, a more standardized methodological approach, placebo controls, a double-blind design, etc.

PATHOPHYSIOLOGY-DRIVEN TREATMENT CONSIDERATIONS

Although the etiology and pathophysiology of tic disorders, including Tourette syndrome (TS), remain unclear (see Chapters 7–15), a dopaminergic hyperfunction is the most consentaneous view as the best target for pharmacological treatment in TS. This is supported not only by neuroscience studies but also by randomized controlled trials (RCTs), as well as the broad clinical experience over the past decades in treating TS with dopamine-blocking agents (Bloch et al., 2011).

So far, genetic studies have not detected clear and easily replicable deviations pointing to abnormalities in one or several neurochemical pathways of patients with TS (see Chapter 7). Nonetheless, clinical medication studies in combination with imaging studies and analyses of human material from cerebrospinal fluid, blood, urine, and postmortem brain tissue in rather small samples resulted mainly in hypotheses on dopaminergic deviances in TS (see Chapters 10 and 13). Studies showing an increased number of striatal and cortical dopamine receptors as well as differences in binding to dopamine transporters in the basal ganglia and release of dopamine following stimulant application leading to tic exacerbation in some patients have further strengthened the hypothesis of an imbalance in the dopaminergic system. Therefore, modulating the dopaminergic metabolism (particularly by blocking the postsynaptic D2 receptors) is the main action of drugs used in the pharmacological treatment of tics.

However, other neurochemical imbalances in TS, such as in the serotoninergic, noradrenergic, cholinergic, glutamatergic, opioid, and gamma-aminobutyric acid (GABA)-ergic metabolism, have also been reported (see Chapter 13). Taking into account that those systems function interactively, further studies should look in more detail at these interactions. Nondopaminergic agents, such as selective serotonin reuptake inhibitors (SSRIs) or noradrenergic drugs such as clonidine or atomoxetine, are used with great success in TS plus obsessive-compulsive disorder (OCD) or TS plus attention-deficit/hyperactivity disorder (ADHD) (see Chapter 25 for further details on the treatment of these comorbidities). Such an interaction between neurotransmitter systems is a crucial aspect to address in future research because, particularly due to knowledge gaps on the spectrum of comorbidity and pathophysiology of TS, at present it is difficult to hypothesize which novel pharmacological targets will prove most useful in the near future.

WHAT ARE THE PROBLEMS TO SOLVE WHILE INVESTIGATING THE PHARMACOLOGICAL TREATMENT OF TICS?

In view of this heterogeneous, and as yet incompletely defined, picture of possible pathophysiological deviations in TS with or without comorbid conditions, it is not surprising that there seems to be no imaginable neuropsychopharmacological option that has not been tested in treating tics. Nevertheless, compared to other neuropsychiatric disorders, high-quality evidence on pharmacological treatment of TS remains limited because a good proportion of available studies are far from being flawless in terms of design and methodology. This shortcoming is caused or aggravated by several issues, intrinsically related to TS, that are encountered while investigating treatment effectiveness in this condition.

The problem most specific to TS is the waxing and waning nature of the tics. These intra-individual fluctuations in intensity, frequency, location, complexity, and so forth of tics require longer observation periods to avoid making erroneous conclusions about causality. For example, a therapeutic intervention introduced at the climax of tic severity (date 1

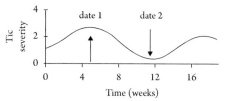

FIGURE 24.1   Evaluation of treatment efficacy in TS in light of its natural waxing and waning course. At date 1 a therapeutic intervention might be followed by tic reduction despite its potential to increase tics or its lack of effect on tics. This must be ascribed not to the causal mechanisms of the intervention but to the natural waxing and waning of the tics. Correspondingly, a therapeutic intervention at date 2 could be followed by an increase of TS symptomatology despite its potential to reduce tics. The therapeutic intervention might attenuate the natural waxing of the tics. Conclusion: Meaningful appraisal of treatment efficacy in TS can be made in most cases only after a longer time.

in Fig. 24.1) could be followed by tic reduction. This reduction might be due not to causal mechanisms related to the intervention, but to the natural waxing and waning of the tics. Likewise, a therapeutic intervention at a time point at which tic severity is only mild or moderate (date 2 in Fig. 24.1) could be followed by an increase of TS symptomatology despite its potential to reduce tics. An effective therapeutic intervention might, nonetheless, attenuate the natural waxing of tics. Therefore, in most cases a meaningful appraisal of treatment effectiveness in TS can be made only after longer observation periods (Roessner et al., 2011a). Hence, especially in TS, single-case or case-series observations of pharmacological treatment should be interpreted with extreme caution. This applies all the more as the well-known modulating influence of environmental or situational factors on tics (see Chapters 1, 8, and 14) could bias the intra-individual course of tics with or without pharmacological treatment (e.g., exacerbation during periods of stress, anxiety, excitement, anger, or fatigue; appearance during inquiries about specific movements; reduction during periods of concentration or active engagement). The same holds true for circumscribed situations of rating tic severity within a treatment study.

"NATURAL COURSE" OF TS

In addition to these shorter-term intrinsic, as well as externally triggered, fluctuations, the individual long-term course of tics over years varies within and between individuals. In general, after the period of worst-ever tic severity, occurring between the ages of 7 and 15 years, there is a gradual decline in tic severity (see Chapters 1 and 5). This also implies that adults who still have symptoms severe enough to come to clinical attention are unusual representatives of all subjects who have received a diagnosis of TS, and therefore studies on treatment effectiveness in TS should take this into account. Moreover, future tic severity can be predicted only approximately and not in a precise fashion, although some factors have been identified that correlate with a positive outcome regardless of baseline tic severity (e.g., intelligence, coping and social skills, meaningful daily activities, and good family and social support). Particularly, factors potentially interacting with age and neurotransmitters (e.g., age-related hormonal changes) await more detailed investigation and complicate the determination of whether an agent's primary mechanism of action is directly responsible for its efficacy (see some preliminary considerations on this in Chapter 14).

To date, the reliable measurement of TS severity is a matter of debate (see Chapter 20 for a review of rating instruments). This alone or in combination with the aforementioned aspects results in several problems of decision making related to the commencement, maintenance, or termination of pharmacological treatment, as well as to the design of a treatment study in TS. For example, some pharmacological interventions may be effective only in mild cases, whereas others may show an effect only in patients with more severe tics who have the potential to exhibit improvement across a wider scale. Undoubtedly, the variety of different approaches to assess treatment effectiveness in TS hinders us from making straightforward conclusions based on the available studies. Effectiveness could be defined in one study by the mean improvement in tic frequency or severity, or in terms of the percentage of patients whose symptoms were alleviated, whereas in another study treatment may be considered as effective if it led to a significant reduction of functional impairment. Because recently TS-specific quality-of-life assessment tools have been established, they might be another useful criterion to define treatment effectiveness.

Even more pronounced is the lack of any scientific data concerning the definition and investigation of treatment refractoriness in TS. Particularly, an assessment tool of refractoriness in TS would be of fundamental importance in the process of patient selection for other types of treatment, especially deep brain stimulation (see also considerations in Chapter 26).

Finally, the high rate of comorbid conditions, particularly in the more severely affected patients, could bias trial results on treatment effectiveness. This high rate of comorbid conditions in clinical trial populations is the result of a Berksonian bias (i.e., related to the higher mathematical chance for a patient with two or more coexisting disorders to be referred; referral rate for disorder A + referral rate for disorder B; Banaschewski et al., 2007) as well as of the referral bias. The latter mostly reflects the higher rate of referral due to higher impairment in case of two disorders (A + B) (Banaschewski, Neale et al., 2007). As an additional, pertinent example of the relevance of a bias due to comorbidity profile when assessing treatment effectiveness, a meta-analysis by Weisman and colleagues (2012) showed that alpha-2 agonists, including clonidine and guanfacine, were more effective in reducing tic symptoms in patients with TS+ADHD (medium to large effect size = .68), whereas in the absence of comorbid ADHD, the efficacy of these agents was small (effect size = .15) and nonsignificant. Therefore, these authors cautiously question whether this finding indicates a need to refine, or at least reconsider, existing treatment guidelines for TS and other chronic tic disorders, since some of them recognize alpha-2 agonists as the first-line pharmacological treatment for tics due to their more benign safety profile. All these problems not only hamper studies on treatment effectiveness of highest quality, but could also complicate the diagnosis of TS and the way to measure treatment response in individual patients.

DIAGNOSTIC ISSUES PRIOR TO PHARMACOLOGICAL TREATMENT

The above considerations notwithstanding, for the experienced clinician it is usually a simple task to diagnose TS, including in this diagnostic phase also the differentiation of tics from other movement disorders (see Chapters 1 and 17). However, in the context of planning treatment in a TS patient, it is crucial to detect coexisting conditions in order to understand their interplay and to disentangle the contribution of each to the patient's psychosocial impairment in everyday life. This is all the more important because the coexisting conditions often contribute to the patient's overall impairment more than the tics themselves (see Chapters 2–4).

Compared to more dimensionally diagnosed disorders such as ADHD, TS is a quite categorical (tics present/absent) diagnosis. In addition, diagnosing TS does not require functional impairment in the patient. Therefore, it is not surprising that many affected children, adolescents, and even adults with mild to moderate tic severity do not require or even seek pharmacological treatment. This view is supported by an often favorable prognosis that justifies a wait-and-see strategy after an appropriate psychoeducational intervention (see Chapter 22) and reassurance in case of a longer period of tic exacerbation.

Also, there is no evidence that the available pharmacological interventions have any impact on the longer-term prognosis of tics. Therefore, clear criteria are needed to define when the wait-and-see conservative approach should be abandoned and treatment should be initiated.

Such criteria were proposed for the first time in a consensus process within the European clinical guidelines for TS and other tic disorders (Roessner et al., 2011a). However, there are surprisingly few detailed statements in review articles that would explain the recommendations of the treatment algorithm presented in those guidelines (Fig. 24.2). One reason might be that, to our knowledge, in TS there is no study comparing the effectiveness of different treatment options, such as pharmacological versus behavioral treatment (see Chapter 23) or deep brain stimulation (see Chapter 26). Nevertheless, in the published literature there are some points that could be universally accepted:

- In TS, psychoeducation should be routinely offered to individuals and family members (see Chapter 22).
- The need for compliance by patients and parents and the lack of specially trained therapists and adequate insurance coverage limit the usefulness of habit reversal in clinical routine, although its effectiveness in the context of a multicenter study has recently been reported. The same is true for exposure with response prevention (see Chapter 23).
- In case of treatment refractoriness, combining or switching between different treatment options should be considered.

INDICATIONS FOR ACTIVELY TREATING TS

Nonpharmacological and/or pharmacological interventions should be considered for persons with clear impairment associated with tics, either at first referral or secondary to an exacerbation of symptoms. In particular the following circumstances, especially when persisting for some days, might require initiation of treatment, rather than persisting in the wait-and-see strategy.

Subjective Discomfort (e.g., pain or injury)

Pain in TS may arise from the actual performance of frequent or intense tics causing discomfort by sudden or repeated extreme exertion (e.g., in the head or neck). This kind of pain is usually musculoskeletal, although rare examples of neuropathic pain may occur. Tics can, in rare cases, cause injuries (Krauss & Jankovic, 1996).

A 13-year-old child was referred to a Pediatric Department with pain in his legs. The pain was relieved by rest and worsened during walking. Physical examination revealed spontaneous pain in the posterior region of both calves; the Lasegue sign was negative. At admission he had obsessive–compulsive behavior consisting of touching, polydipsia, intrusion of words and phrases, echolalia, poor impulse control, and a complex tic consisting of the need to sit down on his heels abruptly, then rapidly return to a standing position. He had been making this abnormal and marked repetitive movement for one month, many times a day. Obsessive–compulsive disorder and neuropsychiatric behavior had begun 2 years before admission to our hospital; no therapy was given. The child had no previous fractures. No family history of obsessive–compulsive disorder, TS or other neuropsychiatric illness was present. Routine laboratory tests, including antistreptolysin O titers, serum copper and ceruloplasmin, were negative. X-rays of the legs showed a fracture line in the upper third of both peroneal bones, more marked on left side. One month later the leg pain disappeared and the child presented with a simple motor tic (opening his mouth), which spontaneously disappeared some months after onset. Only analgesic treatment was administered. Finally, follow-up radiographs 3 months later showed complete healing of both fractures. (Fusco et al., 2006)

Striking or being struck by a moving body part involved in large-amplitude tics may also cause pain and is sometimes difficult to distinguish from deliberate self-injury. Additionally, some patients obtain relief from tics while experiencing pain, to such an extent that they will deliberately provoke pain to obtain benefit (Riley & Lang, 1989). A smaller number of patients complain of pain associated with the irresistible urge to tic or with aggravating premonitory urges during voluntary efforts to suppress their tics. Some patients report that tics worsen their headaches or migraines. Tic-suppressive medication may in those cases help to reduce the use of pain medication and should thus be considered.

Sustained Social Problems (e.g., social isolation or bullying)

Persistent complex motor tics and loud phonic tics can cause social problems. Tics may cause isolation, bullying, or social stigmatization; loud phonic tics may result in the child being put out of the classroom. In such cases a tic reduction, in addition to psychoeducation for the teacher, can be socially very helpful.

Tics do not lead to social impairments in all cases, however, so the issue of social problems needs to be assessed carefully. For example, parents of young children are often exceedingly worried about social problems, whereas adolescents sometimes overestimate the social consequences of their tics, and children in the early elementary grades are often tolerant of tics. When a primary school child becomes socially isolated by his or her peers, coexisting conditions are generally to be blamed more often than tics (Debes et al., 2010). In high school, bullying and social stigmatization due to tics become more common. After proper psychoeducation many children and adolescents will accept their tics and await their natural remission; sometimes, however, medication is indicated to avoid social stigmatization.

Social and Emotional Problems (e.g., reactive depressive symptoms)

In addition to the aforementioned sustained social problems that are a consequence of negative reactions to the social environment, some patients develop depressive and anxious symptoms, low self-esteem, and/or social withdrawal. In those cases, it is not fully clear the extent to which coexisting (sub)clinical symptomatology and self-triggered reactions cause the patient's social and emotional reactions to the tics.

Functional Interference (e.g., impairment of academic achievements)

Functional interference due to tics is relatively rare. However, bouts of tics can interfere with doing homework and falling asleep, and sleep may be disturbed, followed by hypoarousal during the day. Frequent phonic tics can impair fluency of speech and thus conversations. Moreover, children can expend mental energy in the classroom to suppress their tics, thus reducing their attention to schoolwork and interfering with their academic performance (Kurlan et al., 2001).

CRITERIA FOR SELECTING TREATMENT OPTIONS FOR TS

Compared to behavioral treatment options, pharmacotherapy seems to induce faster and probably more prominent tic reduction. Unfortunately, this observation is purely based on clinical experience and has never been tested in a clinical trial so far. Therefore, it is only possible to indirectly compare effect sizes reported in pharmacological and nonpharmacological studies. This is made even more difficult by the fact that there are few studies on pharmacological, let alone on psychotherapeutic, treatment options that meet rigorous quality criteria. The availability of behavioral therapists with expertise in habit reversal training or exposure with response prevention, as well as possible inadequate insurance coverage (see Chapter 23), also must be considered in treatment planning. For a general treatment algorithm, see Figure 24.2.

Latency and Extent of Treatment Effects

Pharmacological treatment works more quickly than behavioral treatment, so the urgency of reducing tic severity must be taken into consideration in each individual case. The clinician should inform patients and families that the realistic goal of pharmacological treatment in TS should not be to abolish tics, but rather to decrease their number in order to reduce the psychosocial impairment that they have generated. Unrealistic expectations as to the effectiveness of pharmacological treatment of TS will inevitably lead to frustration on the part of the child, the family, and the clinician. Also, the desire for complete tic remission can lead to an unfavorable benefit/risk ratio, causing more problems than the tics themselves. A common example is the "overmedication" of children to the point of excessive daytime sedation or unhealthy weight gain. Families should be informed that medication treatment typically results in only 25% to 50% reduction in tic symptoms.

Clinicians should also be aware of, and inform the family about, the biasing effects of the natural waxing and waning of tics in TS (Fig. 24.1). Hence, the use of formal tic severity rating scales can be recommended to more objectively assess responses to treatment over time. The most precise standardized instrument is the Yale Global Tic Severity Scale (YGTSS), a semistructured interview that records the number, frequency, intensity, complexity, and interference of motor and vocal tics separately (Leckman et al., 1989). In routine clinical practice the Tourette Syndrome Severity Scale (TSSS) can also be used; it is shorter and easier to apply (Shapiro et al., 1988; see Chapter 20 for more details).

Side Effects

The possibility of undesired side effects must be considered, but evidence is quite limited in TS. Most data on side effects of treatment with antipsychotic drugs have been collected in schizophrenic patients, and there is no evidence or at least expert consensus that identical problems could be seen to the same or even a similar extent in persons treated for TS. On average, compared to schizophrenia, the time of titration for antipsychotic agents is shorter and their mean dosage is lower in TS patients. Therefore, the core statements about the side effects of pharmacological treatment cannot be generalized from schizophrenia to TS, partly because there is good evidence that many side effects are dose-related. The incidence of tardive dyskinesia, a long-lasting side effect that does not fully remit even after stopping antipsychotic medication, might be lower in TS, but there are only preliminary data supporting such speculation deduced from clinical experience (Muller-Vahl & Krueger, 2011).

The actual evidence base, as well as clinical experience, indicates that antipsychotic drugs may produce the most reliable and fastest treatment effectiveness, but they also pose the greatest risk of side effects. While the typical

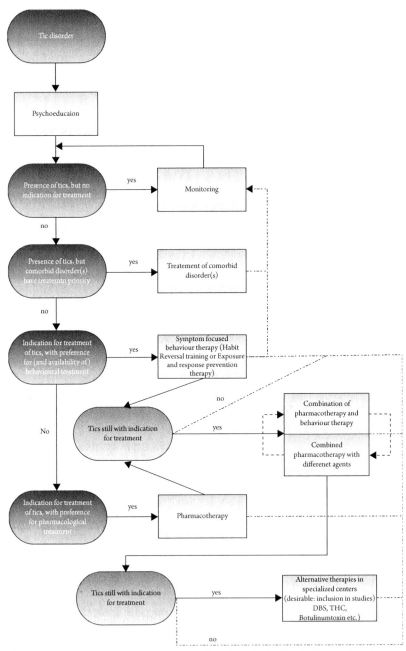

FIGURE 24.2 Decision tree for the treatment of tic disorders, including TS. DBS, deep brain stimulation; THC, tetrahydrocannabinol.

antipsychotic drugs (e.g., haloperidol, pimozide) seem to be somewhat more effective than the newer ones (e.g., risperidone, olanzapine, quetiapine, aripiprazole), they seem to be associated with more and more severe side effects. Also within the group of typical antipsychotic drugs there seem to be differences in the risk of side effects. For example, some studies suggest that pimozide (Sallee et al., 1997) and fluphenazine (Borison et al., 1983) may be as efficacious as haloperidol and produce fewer side effects. Whereas the most common side effects associated with typical antipsychotic drugs are relatively mild and include weight gain and drowsiness, some patients may experience detrimental effects on cognitive function and/or excessive sedation leading to difficulty in performing cognitive tasks. Additionally, the potential for them to lead to hyperprolactinemia (which is associated with amenorrhea, galactorrhea, and gynecomastia) and extrapyramidal symptoms, such as dystonia, parkinsonism, akathisia, and tardive dyskinesia, must be considered, particularly in view of the remitting "natural" course of tics in many cases. Hyperprolactinemia is reversible, but abnormal movements may persist after the cessation of treatment. Another serious but very rarely reported side effect in TS is the risk of neuroleptic malignant syndrome (Robertson & Stern, 2000).

Although the risk of extrapyramidal side effects may be lower with the atypical antipsychotic drugs, this complication can occur also with these drugs. The anticipated tolerability advantages of the atypical (second- and third-generation) antipsychotic drugs compared with the typical antipsychotics have not been clearly proven because patients treated with these newer drugs also experience side effects usually attributed to the typical antipsychotics, such as weight gain, hyperprolactinemia, sedation, sleep disturbance, and abnormal lipid metabolism. Additionally, newer antipsychotics like ziprasidone have a lower risk of weight gain but have generated concern because of the potential to alter cardiac conduction, especially QTc prolongation. As an alternative to antipsychotic drugs, benzamides seem comparably or only minimally less effective, and their use is much more rarely associated with extrapyramidal side effects. For example, tiapride is even recommended for the treatment of tardive dyskinesia because "clinical studies demonstrate its excellent efficacy in neuroleptic-induced tardive dyskinesia, […] tiapride is well tolerated, […] and adverse events are generally rare and mild" (Dose & Lange, 2000). "Typical" side effects of antipsychotic drugs, such as weight gain, hyperprolactinemia, and sedation, were seen during treatment of TS with benzamides, but in a less severe form and in fewer patients.

New analyses have questioned the effectiveness of alpha-2 agonists, including clonidine and guanfacine, in reducing tic symptoms (Weisman et al., 2012). Both agents have the advantage of a lower risk of side effects. The main side effects of clonidine are sedation and hypotension. Guanfacine is generally preferred over clonidine because it tends to cause less sedation and hypertension. Moreover, it acts longer than clonidine and therefore fewer daily doses are needed. Periodic blood pressure monitoring is advised during use, particularly because of possible rebound hypertension associated with abrupt discontinuation (Jankovic & Kurlan, 2011).

PHARMACOLOGICAL TREATMENT OPTIONS FOR TS

Although many drugs have been tested in single cases or case series of TS patients, there has not been much improvement in terms of evidence since the statement by Robertson and Stern (2000) that "the treatment of the Gilles de la Tourette syndrome has evolved from case reports, clinical experience and more recently blinded trials usually in small numbers of patients." This lack of high-quality studies is reflected by the fact that haloperidol is still the only drug that has been approved for TS widely in the world. Nevertheless, haloperidol is today usually not a drug of first choice in clinical practice because of its side effects. Additionally, the insufficient base of evidence results in a very heterogeneous and somewhat confusing situation of several available review publications presenting, at least in part, divergent recommendations on pharmacological treatment options for TS. In the past 2 years, six new general reviews have been published that included at least one section on pharmacological treatment of TS (Du et al., 2010; Eddy et al., 2011; Jankovic & Kurlan 2011; Kimber, 2010; Kurlan, 2010; Rickards, 2010) and three reviews have been dedicated to the pharmacological treatment of TS (Bestha et al., 2010; Parraga et al., 2010; Singer, 2010). The recommendations given by each of these groups reflect their individual clinical experience and tradition and therefore are highly diverse. For example, two U.S. TS experts (Jankovic & Kurlan, 2011) favor guanfacine and tetrabenazine, whereas the

German experts recommend the benzamide tiapride as first-line medication (Rothenberger et al., 2007). Both these recommendations are not based on best evidence from available RCTs. In addition to the agent selection, the selection of the outcomes differs between the reviews. For example, Singer (2010) gives very detailed and helpful, but mainly experience-driven, suggestions about dosing and dosage, whereas Eddy and colleagues (2011) give dosage information for only some of the included agents without explaining the selection criteria for this information. Jankovic and Kurlan (2011) did not report any information on dosage in their more general review on TS, although they recommended first- and second-line agents. Such a more subjective than systematic selection of recommended agents and associated outcome parameters in the existing reviews further emphasizes the need of well-designed RCTs in TS that could provide results of comparable methodological quality.

HIGH EVIDENCE BY COCHRANE REVIEWS

For their Cochrane review, Pringsheim and Marras (2009) identified six RCTs that used pimozide in TS (total 162 participants, age range 7–53 years). Pimozide was compared to placebo (one trial), haloperidol (one trial), placebo and haloperidol (two trials), and risperidone (two trials). The authors concluded that pimozide reduced tics more effectively than placebo. However, it was slightly less effective than haloperidol, while it showed fewer side effects. In terms of tic reduction or side effects, the two studies comparing pimozide and risperidone found no significant differences between the agents.

Pierce and Rickards (in press) screened the literature for all randomized, controlled, double-blind studies comparing atypical antipsychotics to placebo for the treatment of tics in TS. Because neither of the above-mentioned trials using risperidone included a control group receiving placebo, they did not include those studies in their Cochrane review. Parallel-group and crossover studies of children or adults, at any dose and for any duration, were included.

The authors identified only three randomized placebo-controlled trials, two comparing risperidone and one ziprasidone with placebo. In one trial risperidone was much more effective than placebo, although the 95% confidence intervals were large. The remaining two trials did not reveal a statistically significant superiority of treatment with risperidone or ziprasidone respectively compared to placebo. In particular, risperidone caused several extrapyramidal side effects and weight gain.

The third Cochrane review (Curtis et al., 2009) analyzed the effectiveness of delta-9-tetrahydrocannabinol (delta-9-THC) in the treatment of TS. A total of 28 different patients included in one double-blind, parallel-group trial and in one double-blind, crossover trial were studied. Although both trials reported a positive effect of delta-9-THC, the improvements in tic frequency and severity were small and apparent only on selected outcome measures.

In summary, all three Cochrane reviews on the pharmacological treatment of TS (Curtis et al., 2009; Pierce & Rickards, in press; Pringsheim & Marras, 2009) came to the conclusion that this very small and heterogeneous base of evidence not only for the effectiveness but also for the safety of potential drugs does not allow firm evidence-based recommendations to be made. The actual evidence based on RCTs not included in these Cochrane reviews is also alarmingly limited. An overview of all existing RCTs in TS (double-blind, placebo-controlled or comparator, parallel-group or crossover study) is presented in Table 24.1.

Therefore, broad clinical experience is still guiding both consensus findings of experts in terms of the pharmacological treatment of tics and the individual treatment decisions of clinicians.

SELECTED AGENTS

For a comprehensive review of the existing evidence on pharmacological treatment of TS, please see Roessner and colleagues (2011a). In the following section of the chapter, we present information about the agents that are most often

Table 24.1 Overview of All RCTs on TS that Represent Double-Blind, Placebo-Controlled or Comparator, Parallel-Group or Crossover Studies

MEDICATION	DESIGN	N; MEAN AGE (SD); RANGE; SEX[a]	DRUG DOSE[b]	REFERENCE
Alpha-Adrenergic Agonists				
Clonidine	Randomized, double-blind, parallel group, comparator: risperidone	Clonidine: 12; 12.1 (3.0); 7–17; 11 males, 1 female Risperidone: 9; 10.4 (2.7); 7–17; 8 males, 1 female	Clonidine: 0.005 mg/kg/d (highest) or 0.350 mg/d over 3–4 weeks (with a minimum target dose of 0.0025 mg/kg/d) Risperidone: 0.06 mg/kg/d (highest) with a minimum target dose of 0.03 mg/kg/d	Gaffney et al., 2002
	Randomized, double-blind, placebo-controlled parallel	Clonidine: 326; 10.5 (2.82); 6–18; 270 males, 56 females Placebo: 111; 9.89 (2.77); 6–18; 96 males, 15 females n = 6 dropouts	Clonidine: 1–2 mg/week Placebo	Du et al., 2008
Guanfacine	Randomized, double-blind, placebo-controlled, parallel group	34; 10.4 (2.01); 7–14; 31 males, 3 females Guanfacine: n = 17 Placebo: n = 17	Guanfacine: 1.5–3.0 mg/d Placebo	Scahill et al., 2001
	Randomized, double-blind, placebo-controlled parallel	Guanfacine: 12; 9.5 (2.0); 6–16; 12 males, 0 females Placebo: 12; 11.3 (2.4); 6–16; 8 males, 4 females	Guanfacine: initial dose: 0.5 mg/d; 1.0 mg/ b.i.d (highest) Placebo	Cummings et al., 2002

(Continued)

Table 24.1 (*Continued*)

MEDICATION	DESIGN	N; MEAN AGE (SD); RANGE; SEX[a]	DRUG DOSE[b]	REFERENCE
Typical Neuroleptics				
Haloperidol	Randomized, double-blind, placebo-controlled, parallel Comparator: pimozide	9; 18.7; 8–28; 7 males, 2 females	Haloperidol: initial dose: 2 mg/d; 12 mg/d (highest) Pimozide: initial dose: 2 mg/d; 12 mg/d (highest) Placebo	Ross & Moldofsky, 1978
	Randomized, double-blind, placebo-controlled parallel and crossover design Comparator: pimozide	57; 21.1 (11.0); 8–46; 44 males, 13 females Haloperidol: n = 18 Pimozide: n = 20 Placebo: n = 19	Haloperidol: 2–20 mg/d Pimozide: 2–48 mg/d Placebo	Shapiro et al., 1989
	Randomized, double-blind, placebo-controlled, double-crossover Comparator: pimozide	22; 10.2 (2.5); 7–16; 17 males, 5 females	Haloperidol: 3.5 mg/d (mean) Pimozide: 3.4 mg/d (mean) Placebo	Sallee et al., 1997
Pimozide	Randomized, double-blind, placebo-controlled, parallel Comparator: haloperidol	9; 18.7; 8–28; 7 males, 2 females	Pimozide: initial dose: 2 mg/d; 12 mg/d (highest) Haloperidol: initial dose: 2 mg/d; 12 mg/d (highest) Placebo	Ross & Moldofsky, 1978

Study design	Sample	Dosing	Reference
Randomized, double-blind, placebo-controlled parallel and crossover design Comparator: haloperidol	57; 21.1 (11.0); 8–46; 44 males, 13 females Pimozide: n = 20 Haloperidol: n = 18 Placebo: n = 19	Pimozide: 2–48 mg/d Haloperidol: 2–20 mg/d Placebo	Shapiro et al., 1989
Randomized, double-blind, placebo-controlled, double-crossover Comparator: haloperidol	22; 10.2 (2.5); 7–16; 17 males, 5 females	Pimozide: 3.4 mg/d (mean) Haloperidol: 3.5 mg/d (mean) Placebo	Sallee et al., 1997
Randomized, double-blind, parallel group Comparator: risperidone	Pimozide: 24; 23.5 (median); 11–45; 21 males, 3 females Risperidone; 26; 20.0 (median); 11–50; 23 males, 3 females n = 9 dropouts	Pimozide: 2.9 mg/d (mean); range 1–6 mg/d Risperidone: 3.8 mg/d (mean); range 0.5–6 mg/d	Bruggeman et al., 2001
Randomized, double-blind, crossover Comparator: risperidone	19; 11 (2.5); 7–17; 15 males, 4 females n = 6 dropouts	Pimozide: 1–4 mg/d; 2.4 mg/d (mean) Risperidone: 1–4 mg/d; 2.5 mg/d (mean) Placebo for 2 weeks before pimozide/risperidone	Gilbert et al., 2004
(Randomized ?), double-blind, crossover Comparator: olanzapine	4; 28.5; 19–40; 4 males, 0 females	Pimozide: 2 and 4 mg/d Olanzapine: 5 and 10 mg/d	Onofrj et al., 2000

(Continued)

Table 24.1 (*Continued*)

MEDICATION	DESIGN	N; MEAN AGE (SD); RANGE; SEX[a]	DRUG DOSE[b]	REFERENCE
Atypical Neuroleptics				
Olanzapine	(Randomized?), double-blind, crossover Comparator: pimozide	4; 28.5; 19–40; 4 males, 0 females	Olanzapine: 5 and 10 mg/d Pimozide: 2 and 4 mg/d	Onofrj et al., 2000
Risperidone	Randomized, double-blind, placebo-controlled, parallel group	34; 19.8 (17.01); 6–62; 30 males, 4 females Risperidone: n = 16 Placebo: n = 18	2.5 ± 0.85 mg/d (mean) Placebo	Scahill et al., 2003
	Randomized, double-blind, placebo-controlled, parallel group	Risperidone: 23; 31 (median); 17–49; 19 males, 4 females Placebo: 23; 33 (median); 14–45; 17 males, 6 females	Risperidone: 2.5 mg/d (mean); range 1–6 mg/d Placebo	Dion et al., 2002
	Randomized, double-blind, parallel group Comparator: clonidine	Risperidone: 9; 10.4 (2.7); 7–17; 8 males, 1 female Clonidine: 12; 12.1 (3.0); 7–17; 11 males, 1 female	Risperidone: 0.06 mg/kg/d (highest) (with a minimum target dose of 0.03 mg/kg/d) Clonidine: 0.005 mg/kg/d (highest) or 0.350 mg/d over 3–4 weeks (with a minimum target dose of 0.0025 mg/kg/d)	Gaffney et al., 2002
	Randomized, double-blind, parallel group Comparator: pimozide	Risperidone; 26; 20.0 (median); 11–50; 23 males, females Pimozide: 24; 23.5 (median); 11–45; 21 males, 3 females n = 9 dropouts	Risperidone: 3.8 mg/d (mean); 0.5–6 mg/d Pimozide: 2.9 mg/d (mean); range 1–6 mg/d	Bruggeman et al., 2001

	Study design	Sample	Dosage	Reference
	Randomized, double-blind, crossover; Comparator: risperidone	19; 11 (2.5); 7–17; 15 males, 4 females; n = 6 dropouts	Risperidone: 1–4 mg/d; 2.5 mg/d (mean); Pimozide: 1–4 mg/d; 2.4 mg/d (mean)	Gilbert et al., 2004
Ziprasidone	Randomized, double-blind, placebo-controlled, parallel group	Ziprasidone: 16; 11.3; 7–14; 14 males, 2 females; Placebo: 12; 11.8; 8–16; 8 males, 4 females; n = 4 dropouts	Ziprasidone: 28.2 ± 9.6 mg/d (mean); range 5–40 mg/d; Placebo	Sallee et al., 2000
Benzamides				
Sulpiride	Randomized, double-blind, placebo-controlled, crossover; Comparator: fluvoxamine	Sulpiride: 5; 29.6 (2.9); 3 males, 3 females; Fluvoxamine: 6; 28.3 (3.2); 5 males, 1 female	Sulpiride: 0.2 g–1 g/d; Fluvoxamine: 50–300 mg/d; Placebo	George et al., 1993
Tiapride	Randomized, double-blind, placebo-controlled, crossover	n = 17	Tiapride: 6 mg/kg/d; Placebo	Eggers et al., 1988

(*Continued*)

Table 24.1 (*Continued*)

MEDICATION	DESIGN	N; MEAN AGE (SD); RANGE; SEX[a]	DRUG DOSE[b]	REFERENCE
Baclofen	Randomized, double-blind, placebo-controlled, crossover	10; 11.7 (2.9); 8–14; 7 males, 3 females n = 1 dropout	Baclofen: 20 mg t.i.d Placebo	Singer et al., 2001
Botulinum toxin	Randomized, double-blind, placebo-controlled, crossover	20; 31.5; 15–55; 13 males, 5 females n = 2 dropouts	Treatment was with variable doses of botulinum toxin A (Botox; Allergan, Canada).	Marras et al., 2001
Fluvoxamine	Randomized, double-blind, placebo-controlled, crossover Comparator: sulpiride	Fluvoxamine: 6; 28.3 (3.2); 5 males, 1 female Sulpiride: 5; 29.6 (2.9); 3 males, 3 females n = 6 dropouts	Fluvoxamine: 50–300 mg/d Sulpiride: 0.2–1 g/d Placebo	George et al., 1993
Levetiracetam	Randomized, double-blind, placebo-controlled, crossover	22; 12.2 (2.3); 8–16; 21 males, 1 female n = 2 dropouts	Levetiracetam: initial dose: 10 mg/kg/d; 30 mg/kg/d (highest) Placebo	Smith-Hicks et al., 2007
Nicotine	Randomized, double-blind, placebo-controlled, (probably) crossover	23; 12.0 (2.8); 8–17; 19 males, 4 females n = 9 dropouts	Nicotine: 7 mg/d Placebo	Howson et al., 2004

Drug	Study design	Participants	Dose	Reference
Talipexole	Randomized, double-blind, placebo-controlled, crossover	13; 39.2; 19–63; 13 males, 0 females; n = 5 dropouts	Talipexole: initial dose: 0.3 mg/d; 2.4 mg/d (highest); Placebo	Goetz et al., 1994
Tetrahydro-cannabinol	Randomized, double-blind, placebo-controlled, crossover	12; 34 (13); 18–66; 11 males, 1 female	THC: 5–10 mg/d; Placebo	Muller-Vahl et al., 2002
	Randomized, double-blind, placebo-controlled parallel	24; 33 (11); 18–68; 19 males, 5 females; THC: n = 12; Placebo: n = 12; n = 7 dropouts	THC: 10 mg/d; Placebo	Muller-Vahl et al., 2003
Topiramate	Randomized, double-blind, placebo-controlled, parallel	29; 16.5 (9.89); 7–65; 26 males; 3 females; Topiramate: n = 15; Placebo: n = 14; n = 9 dropouts	Topiramate: 118 mg/d (mean); Placebo	Jankovic et al., 2010

[a] Not all data are available for each study. [b] Drug dose in mg/kg of body weight/day if available, otherwise in mg/day (mg/d); standard drug dose if available, otherwise mean drug dose if available, otherwise highest dose.

used and that have been intensively investigated and commonly mentioned. The order of the selected agents is arbitrary in both the text and in Tables 24.1 and 24.2, and does not reflect a recommendation or level of evidence. For a tentative attempt at recommendations, see the conclusions section of the chapter.

Noradrenergic Agents

In general, particularly U.S. experts favor the two alpha-2 adrenergic agonists clonidine and guanfacine as first-line treatment for mild to moderate tics (Singer, 2010). Such regional preferences seem to largely reflect differences in regional drug supply and experience (Jankovic & Kurlan, 2011; Muller-Vahl & Roessner, 2011). The tic-suppressing effects of both alpha-2 adrenergic agonists seem to be generally smaller, however, than those of antipsychotic agents (Robertson, 2000), although a small, single-blind, randomized trial showed similar effectiveness of clonidine and risperidone (Gaffney et al., 2002). The treatment effectiveness of clonidine and guanfacine is a good example of the large gaps of sufficiently qualitative evidence on the pharmacological treatment of TS (Weisman et al., 2012).

Although clonidine has been used for nearly three decades in the treatment of TS, there are only a few controlled studies supporting its use. At present, a transdermal clonidine patch is available that can be applied once weekly; however, it was found to cause local skin irritation and problems related to displacement (Du et al., 2008). Side effects of clonidine include sedation, irritability, dizziness, dry mouth, headache, orthostatic hypotension, dysphoria, and sleep disturbance. Although many authors report that these side effects are mild and usually self-limiting, this view is not fully supported, especially when moderate to severe tics require higher dosage. The initial dose of clonidine is 0.05 mg orally at bedtime. Because of its short half-life (about 6 hours), some suggest a more frequent dosage schedule for tics, and definitely for ADHD, than the usually recommended twice-a-day regimen. The maximum dose should not exceed 0.3 to 0.4 mg per day.

Guanfacine has also shown only modest effectiveness in reducing tics, with inconsistencies across studies of different quality and on heterogeneous clinical samples. The often-cited suggestion that guanfacine is better tolerated than clonidine requires caution because there has been no direct comparison study conducted between the two agents (Sandor, 2003). The main side effects of guanfacine are dizziness, drowsiness, confusion, fatigue, headache, hypotension, and mental depression. Constipation and dry mouth are common. Guanfacine, previously approved to treat hypertension in several European countries, has been withdrawn from the market in several of these countries. Guanfacine should be started at a dosage of 0.5 mg at bedtime and should be increased by 0.5 mg every 5 to 7 days, if necessary, to a maximum dose of 4 mg per day in a once-a-day or twice-a-day regimen.

For the selective noradrenergic reuptake inhibitor atomoxetine, the situation is quite similar to that for guanfacine. Atomoxetine was originally developed by Eli Lilly as a treatment for depression. Due to its unfavorable benefit/risk ratio in these trials, it was approved in late 2002 for ADHD. It was shown to be effective in randomized, placebo-controlled trials for ADHD in children, including patients with coexisting mild to moderate tics. As a result of its different mechanism of action, many patients who previously did not respond to stimulants have shown some response to atomoxetine (see Chapter 25). Common adverse effects of atomoxetine include nausea, emesis, diminished appetite, and insomnia. TS-specific doses have not been identified; hence, 0.5 to 1.2 mg per kg body weight could be seen as the optimal therapeutic range.

Antipsychotic Agents

During the past 40 years positive treatment effects in TS have regularly been reported for D2 dopamine receptor blockers (on average a marked decrease of tics in about 70% of cases; Shapiro & Shapiro, 1998). Although the blockade of striatal D2 dopamine receptors is thought to lead to reduction of tics, a high blockade of the receptors commonly correlates with the rate of unfavorable side effects, such as extrapyramidal symptoms or tardive dyskinesia (Bressan et al., 2004)—although it has been observed that the risk of tardive dyskinesia might be lower in TS (Muller-Vahl & Krueger, 2011).

TYPICAL ANTIPSYCHOTICS

The typical antipsychotics haloperidol and pimozide were the first ones shown to be effective in placebo-controlled treatment studies in TS. Although slight differences in effectiveness, as well as the rate and severity of side effects, were reported in available trials, no firm conclusions should be drawn. Several limitations and the small number of studies result in heterogeneity of findings. In a double-blind, 24-week, placebo-controlled, randomized double-crossover study of the most commonly used doses of haloperidol (mean dose 3.5 mg per day) and pimozide (mean dose 3.4 mg per day) conducted in 22 subjects aged 7 to 16 years, pimozide was significantly more effective than placebo in reducing tics, whereas haloperidol failed to have a significant effect, possibly due to the limited study power. Moreover, haloperidol exhibited a threefold higher frequency of serious side effects and significantly greater extrapyramidal symptoms than pimozide (Sallee et al., 1997).

The high frequency of side effects such as drowsiness, movement disorders (i.e., dystonia, akathisia, and pseudoparkinsonism, probably due to the strong dopaminergic blockade in the nigrostriatal pathways), anxiety, increased appetite, and hyperprolactinemia (with its complications such as gynecomastia, galactorrhea, irregular menses, and sexual dysfunction) limits the use of the typical antipsychotics at higher doses. In daily clinical practice, lower doses such as 1 to 4 mg per day for haloperidol and 2 to 8 mg per day for pimozide in divided doses are typically used today to treat TS. Doses above 5 mg per day for haloperidol and 10 mg per day for pimozide should be avoided.

ATYPICAL ANTIPSYCHOTICS

Like typical antipsychotics, atypical antipsychotics were found to be effective in the treatment of TS. We will review the most commonly used atypical antipsychotics in order of approval by the U.S. Food and Drug Administration (for non-TS indications).

Risperidone (FDA approval in 1993) is the atypical antipsychotic agent with the broadest base of evidence concerning the treatment of TS, which includes randomized, double-blind, placebo-controlled trials. Although similarly effective as haloperidol and pimozide in reducing tics, risperidone showed less frequent and less severe side effects. The most common side effects were mild to moderate sedation, fatigue, and somnolence, hypotension, metabolic adverse reactions (glucose and lipid metabolism), and hyperprolactinemia, which subsequently resolved with continued administration of the medication or with a dose reduction. Very rarely, clinically significant extrapyramidal symptoms have been observed. Weight gain as a consequence of increased appetite should be considered and, if necessary, suitable interventions started. The mean daily dose of about 2.5 mg (range 1–6 mg/day) should be given on a twice-a-day regimen.

For olanzapine (FDA approval in 1996), there are only some case reports and open-label studies suggesting effectiveness in the treatment of TS. Interestingly, in contrast to the other atypical antipsychotics, no European expert recommended olanzapine based on response to a survey questioning which medication expert clinicians would consider first, second, and third treatment choices (Roessner et al., 2011b). The side effects are very similar to those of risperidone, although olanzapine seems associated with a lower incidence of hyperprolactinemia and more severe weight gain. After starting with 2.5 mg orally every evening, a gradual escalation to 5 to 10 mg per day in divided doses, according to individual requirements, should be pursued. Maximum daily dose is 20 mg.

Evidence about TS treatment with quetiapine (FDA approval in 1997) is similarly very limited. Few reports document side effects with this drug during treatment of TS, but they seem to be less severe and frequent than those observed with other atypical antipsychotics. After initial dosing with 25 to 50 mg per day, quetiapine may be increased, as tolerated, to relatively high doses, up to 600 mg daily in two divided doses.

Only one randomized, double-blind, placebo-controlled study (Sallee et al., 2000) and one open-label study have shown effectiveness of ziprasidone (FDA approval in 2001) in reducing tics. The side effects were very mild and included sedation, weight gain, and hyperprolactinemia. Different dose recommendations are present in the literature; the usual range is 5 to 40 mg per day in divided doses.

Compared to olanzapine, quetiapine and ziprasidone, aripiprazole (FDA approval in 2002) has been studied much more extensively in TS and has shown a very promising benefit/risk ratio (Wenzel et al., 2012). A randomized, double-blind, placebo-controlled study is, however, still lacking. Even in "refractory" TS, aripiprazole has shown good effectiveness. It seems reasonably well tolerated; the most common adverse reactions include nausea, akathisia, weight gain, and sedation. As a starting dose 2 to 2.5 mg per day is often reported; the maximum dose is 30 mg per day.

BENZAMIDES

Two agents belonging to this family of drugs, tiapride and sulpiride, are used in the treatment of TS, although mainly in Europe (Roessner et al., 2011a). Despite its selective D2 dopamine receptor antagonism, these molecules have a low (sulpiride) or virtually absent (tiapride) antipsychotic effect compared to the typical antipsychotics, with fewer extrapyramidal and autonomic side effects than haloperidol. After early reports of success in treating TS with tiapride in the 1970s, only a few placebo-controlled studies with small sample sizes have been published. Nevertheless, due to its favorable benefit/risk ratio, tiapride still represents the recommended first-line treatment of tics in some European countries, such as Germany (Rothenberger et al., 2007). Its main side effects are drowsiness, moderate transient hyperprolactinemia, and weight gain (mean weight gain was 2–4 kg [Meisel et al., 2004] at a dose range of 100–900 mg per day). Tiapride has no impact on cognitive performance or neurophysiological recordings

such as EEG frequency analysis and sensory evoked potentials in children. The neurosecretory, hypothalamic-hypophyseal regulation of the sex hormones, thyroid stimulating hormone, growth hormone, or thyroid hormone, moreover, is not disturbed by tiapride. Likewise, positive effects of sulpiride on tics have been reported regularly since the 1970s (Robertson & Stern, 2000). In addition to its mild antipsychotic action, an antidepressant and anxiolytic effect has been observed with low doses of sulpiride; in addition, it seems to have positive effects on obsessive-compulsive symptoms co-occurring with tics as well as on OCD without tics. The most common side effects of sulpiride include sedation, drowsiness (in up to 25% of cases), and, less frequently, paradoxical depression; a few patients also complained of restlessness and sleep disturbances. Another important problem with sulpiride is the strong stimulation of prolactin secretion, causing galactorrhea/amenorrhea and a commonly observed increase of appetite leading to weight gain. Other side effects (hypotension, rarely long-QT syndrome, dry mouth, sweating, nausea, activation or sedation, insomnia, allergic rash, or pruritus) are rare. The titration of tiapride and sulpiride starts with a dose of 50 or 100 mg (2 mg per kg body weight) per day, and the dosage should not exceed 2 to 10 mg per kg body weight. Particularly at higher doses a division into three daily doses might be helpful.

Alternatives

Tetrabenazine for the treatment of TS has been discussed in previous reviews, especially by U.S. authors (Jankovic & Kurlan, 2011; Kurlan, 2010). This compound acts as a vesicular monoamine transporter type 2 inhibitor by depleting presynaptic dopamine and serotonin stores and by blocking postsynaptic dopamine receptors. Therefore, tetrabenazine might be an alternative to antipsychotic treatment due its divergent mechanism of action resulting in different efficacy and adverse reactions profiles compared to antipsychotics. However, even compared to the generally low level of evidence for other TS treatment options, very few clinical studies on hyperkinetic movement disorders are available with this drug, including small clinical samples of TS patients and two retrospective chart reviews. Possible side effects of tetrabenazine include drowsiness/fatigue, nausea, depression, parkinsonism, and akathisia, but all these side effects resolve with reduction of daily dosage. Weight gain seems to be less pronounced at doses of comparable anti-tic efficacy in respect to antipsychotics, and most patients who switched from an antipsychotic drug to tetrabenazine subsequently lost weight. The usual effective dose is 50 to 150 mg per day divided into three daily doses, with a maximum recommended dose of 200 mg per day.

The benzodiazepine clonazepam, which acts primarily on the GABAergic system, has a long history in the treatment of TS. It is included in many reviews *inter alia* due to its rapid onset of tic reduction. Only a few open-label and single-blind studies of clonazepam in TS have been carried out. In a single-blind comparison with clonidine in 20 children, clonazepam was superior in suppressing tics (Drtílková, 1996). As with all benzodiazepines, tolerance and side effects including sedation, short-term memory problems, ataxia, and paradoxical disinhibition often limit the use of clonazepam (Goetz, 1992). Clonazepam has been used at doses up to 6 mg per day to treat TS.

All of the aforementioned agents have systemic effects. Alternatively, botulinum toxin injections are used to treat persistent well-localized (noncomplex) motor and, sometimes, vocal tics by temporarily weakening the associated muscles. Since the 1990s, only case reports and case series of botulinum toxin treatment in TS have been published. The only exception is a randomized, double-blind, controlled clinical trial showing that the tic frequency and the premonitory urge were reduced by botulinum toxin injection (Marras et al., 2001). Yet patients subjectively perceived this treatment as overall not effective in improving their condition, perhaps because only a selected subset of tics can be addressed by local botulinum toxin injections. Side effects include temporary soreness, mild muscle weakness, and hypophonia when vocal tics are treated with vocal cord injections.

Additional treatment alternatives for TS in children have been used experimentally, for example dopamine agonists such as pergolide and ropinirole. Pergolide is a mixed D_1-D_2-D_3 dopamine receptor agonist. A study with 57 children showed that a low-dose treatment with pergolide (0.15–0.45 mg per day), compared to placebo, led to a significant improvement in tic severity (Gilbert et al., 2003). Likewise, in an open-label trial tic severity decreased in 75% of patients (24/32) during treatment with small doses of pergolide (0.1–0.3 mg per day). Side effects were relatively harmless and extrapyramidal side effects were absent (Lipinski et al., 1997). There are only a few studies on treatment effects of the dopamine agonist ropinirole. It does not interact with D1 receptors but has a high selectivity for D3 receptors and a weaker affinity for D2 receptors. The effectiveness of ropinirole at a dose of 0.25 to 0.5 mg twice a day was shown in a study with 15 patients (mean age 28.1 ± 6.1 years); of these, 10 reported a significant improvement in tic severity and frequency (Anca et al., 2004).

Antiandrogens such as finasteride and flutamide have also been tested in TS. Because of the preponderance of males affected by TS, androgens may possess a key role in its pathophysiology. During treatment with finasteride, patients displayed a reduction in total, motor, and phonic tics. Only 2 of 10 patients complained of a decline in libido and occasional difficulty in achieving erection (Muroni et al., 2011). A double-blind, placebo-controlled, crossover trial of flutamide (13 adults [10 men and 3 women]) showed a decrease in motor but not phonic tic severity, but the effects were relatively small in magnitude. Although subjects generally tolerated well a flutamide dose of 750 mg per day, this medication has caused in other conditions severe (sometimes fatal) liver dysfunction, in addition to a number of less severe but troublesome side effects such as diarrhea and gastric discomfort (Peterson et al., 1998).

CONCLUSIONS

There are unfortunately few studies on the pharmacological treatment of TS that fulfill high methodological standards. There are also very few studies directly comparing the effectiveness of different psychopharmacological agents, foremost with regard to longer-term effects or in cases refractory to previously tried medications. This has led to different recommendations in the literature, which depend heavily upon the authors' personal experiences and preferences. The question of the effectiveness of polypharmacy is another area in which evidence-based knowledge is virtually absent, even though it is not rare for clinicians to resort to polypharmacological treatment when dealing with treatment-refractory patients in their routine practice.

Based on the available, albeit insufficient, evidence base, as well as on experts' experience and preferences, risperidone can be recommended as a first choice for the treatment of tics. Side effects represent its biggest limitation, primarily weight gain and sedation. Pimozide has relatively good evidence, with a better adverse reaction profile than haloperidol. Tiapride and sulpiride can be recommended based on the broad clinical experience and favorable adverse reaction profile, although more controlled clinical studies are urgently required to prove this. Aripiprazole has great potential, especially in the treatment of refractory cases and probably less pronounced risk of severe weight gain. Finally, clonidine can be administered, especially when coexisting ADHD is present. All the other agents mentioned in Table 24.2 may be considered as alternatives, once the response to one or more of these medications has been unsatisfactory.

To overcome the dearth of high-quality evidence on pharmacological treatment in TS, all three available Cochrane reviews, as well as many experts on TS, urgently advocate for future trials with longer durations, larger groups, and a more standardized methodological approach to investigate the safety and efficacy of pharmacological treatment in TS. A double-blind design should also be chosen, although in the case of significant treatment effects there is the risk that participants can work out which condition they have been assigned to. Finally, the negative effects of excessively high dropout rates for different

causes should be considered with caution. In summary, treatment studies in TS require more effort than those for some other disorders.

As mentioned before and in other chapters, although TS is not a rare disease, only a minority of affected persons require pharmacological treatment. This creates obstacles to the development of new studies, given the lack of incentives (Fischer et al., 2005) and the limited interest on the part of the pharmaceutical industry. TS clinicians and researchers should be encouraged and, when possible, supported by TS patient associations (see Chapter 30) to develop, in the best-case scenario, worldwide consensus standards for all TS-specific methodological aspects of treatment studies (e.g., study duration, measurement of treatment and side effects, definition of refractoriness, etc.). Thereafter, lobbying for funding larger multicenter studies should be coordinated (e.g., in the United States and/or in Europe). Those studies should include the comparison of different agents and allow subgroup analyses of sufficiently homogenous groups in terms of age, comorbidity, etc.

In Box 24.2 we present outlooks for further studies on treatment agents, based on recent etiological and pathophysiological findings in TS. At first, the "old story" of TS as a "hyperdopaminergic illness" should be evaluated in more detail in view of recent work providing new evidence of the role of dopamine in TS, as well as its interactions with other neurotransmitters (e.g., glutamate, serotonin, and histamine). For example, in animal studies (see Chapter 15), systemic delivery of dopamine agonists and antagonists has identified differential stereotypical behavioral profiles depending on whether D1 receptors are stimulated through direct D1 specific agonists or upregulated through chronic exposure to specific D1 antagonists (Taylor et al., 2010). On the other hand, the idea underlying the use of dopamine agonists has been questioned in view of the news coming from the pharmaceutical company Boehringer Ingelheim, which arrested the clinical development of pramipexole, a D2/D3/D4 receptor agonist in pediatric TS, because there was no trend of improvement on pramipexole versus placebo in a 6-week, double-blind, randomized, placebo-controlled, flexible-dose

Table 24.2 Most Common and Important Medications for Treatment of TS and Other Chronic Tic Disorders

Medication	Indication	Start dosage (mg)	Therapeutic range (mg)	Frequent side effects	Physical examinations— at start and at control	Level of evidence
Alpha-Adrenergic Agonists						
Clonidine	ADHD/TS	0.05	0.1–0.3	Orthostatic hypotension, sedation, sleepiness	Blood pressure, ECG	A
Guanfacine	ADHD/TS	0.5–1.0	1.0–4.0	Orthostatic hypotension, sedation, sleepiness	Blood pressure, ECG	A
Typical Neuroleptics						
Haloperidol	TS	0.25–0.5	0.25–15.0	EPS, sedation, increased appetite	Blood count, ECG, weight, transaminases, neurological status, prolactin	A
Pimozide	TS	0.5–1.0	1.0–6.0	EPS, sedation, increased appetite	Blood count, ECG, weight, transaminases, neurological status, prolactin	A
Atypical Neuroleptics						
Aripiprazole	TS	2.50	2.5–30	Sedation, akathisia, EPS, headache, increased appetite (less than other neuroleptics), orthostatic hypotension	Blood count, blood pressure, weight, ECG, transaminases, blood sugar	C
Olanzapine	TS/OCB	2.5–5.0	2.5–20.0	Sedation, increased appetite, akathisia	Blood count, blood pressure, ECG, weight, electrolytes, transaminases, prolactin, blood lipids and sugar	B

(Continued)

Table 242 (*Continued*)

Medication	Indication	Start dosage (mg)	Therapeutic range (mg)	Frequent side effects	Physical examinations— at start and at control	Level of evidence
Quetiapine	TS	100–150	100–600	Sedation, increased appetite, agitation, orthostatic hypotension	Blood count, blood pressure, ECG, weight, electrolytes, transaminases, prolactin, blood lipids and sugar	C
Risperidone	TS/DBD	0.25	0.25–6.0	EPS, sedation, increased appetite, orthostatic hypotension	Blood count, blood pressure, ECG, weight, electrolytes, transaminases, prolactin, blood lipids and sugar	A
Ziprasidone	TS	5.0–10.0	5.0–30.0	EPS, sedation	Blood count, ECG, weight, transaminases, prolactin	A
Benzamides						
Sulpiride	TS/OCB	50–100 (2 mg/kg)	2–10 mg/kg	Problems with sleep, agitation, increased appetite	Blood count, ECG, weight, transaminases, prolactin, electrolytes	B
Tiapride	TS	50–100 (2 mg/kg)	2–10 mg/kg	Sedation, increased appetite	Blood count, ECG, weight, transaminases, prolactin, electrolytes	B

Listed in alphabetical order.
DBD, disruptive behavior disorder; OCB, obsessive-compulsive behavior; EPS, extrapyramidal symptoms. Evidence level: A (>2 RCTs), B (1 RCT), C (case studies, open trials).

study including a total of 63 patients aged 6 to 17 years with TS (43 on pramipexole, 20 on placebo; 58 of the 63 completed the trial) (http://trials.boehringer-ingelheim.com/res/trial/data/pdf/248.642_Statement.pdf). Secondly, two recent genetic studies (Ercan-Sencicek et al., 2010; Fernandez et al., 2012) reported evidence that diminished histaminergic neurotransmission might be associated with TS, at least in some patients. Accordingly, the authors suggested that raising brain histamine levels may decrease tics. To our knowledge, to date there is only one case report (Hartmann et al., 2011) of pharmacological treatment to modulate histaminergic neurotransmission in TS, describing a patient with comorbid narcolepsy without cataplexy, characterized by excessive daytime sleepiness and sleep disturbance; he received pitolisant, an inverse H3 receptor agonist that potentiates histaminergic neurotransmission. Previous trials of typical antipsychotics slightly decreased tics but induced fatigue and sedation, whereas stimulants exacerbated his tics

dramatically. Treatment with pitolisant alleviated the narcolepsy with a positive effect also on his tics. Therefore, the authors concluded that, apart from tics, pitolisant may be helpful in treating attention deficit in children with TS and in reversing antipsychotic-induced daytime sleepiness. There are several hints of a close interrelationship between histaminergic and dopaminergic neurotransmission, particularly in the striatum (Ferrada et al., 2008). Controlled clinical trials of agents modulating histaminergic neurotransmission in TS patients are under way.

A 9-year-old boy reported, over a period of approximately 2 years, a waxing and waning itching sensation, relieved by throat clearing and eye blinking. Additionally, he would stare at the ceiling lamp because this made his eyes feel better. Later on, facial grimacing, neck jerking, throat clearing, and high-pitched squeaking appeared, and he was referred to a TS

Box 24.2. Questions for Future Research

1. Does a specific drug really work in TS? Because of the limited evidence base and due to several difficulties in terms of the design of pharmacological trials in TS, more studies in larger and more homogeneous groups of affected persons with longer observation periods are urgently required.

2. How fast is the onset of effect of pharmacological versus behavioral treatment? What are the differences in their impact on the individual TS course? In daily clinical practice it seems likely that medication is associated with a faster onset of tic reduction but behavioral treatment might have a more "stable effect" (i.e., tic reduction remains after cessation of habit reversal).

3. What could be a definition of refractoriness of pharmacological treatment? Is there any evidence for polypharmacy? There is no evidence from clinical studies about polypharmacy, although it is often required in severe cases, particularly in the case of comorbid conditions such as ADHD, OCD, or depression or refractoriness to monotherapy.

4. Will medication reduce tics and/or premonitory urges? It is unclear if medication reduces tic severity and/or the premonitory urge. Maybe there are differences between the substances despite the same effect on tic amelioration.

5. How is stress modulated by anti-tic medication? Although there are several hints that stress has an impact on tic severity, there are no data about changes in stress by pharmacological treatment of tics.

6. What are the differences in efficacy and efficiency between pharmacological versus behavioral treatment (versus deep brain stimulation)? The evidence base (e.g., by comparing the effect sizes of single studies) concerning the efficacy and efficiency of pharmacological versus behavioral treatment or of their combination is very limited. Therefore, direct comparisons in one study (e.g., for ADHD) are urgently required.

7. Is it possible to develop individualized treatment plans based on genetic information? New and exciting genetic findings might open the possibility of starting the optimal individualized pharmacological treatment after genetic tests.

clinic. All symptoms could be controlled by volition, and there were no relevant problems during school hours. However, at home he reported a massive increase of symptom severity and subjective discomfort. Antihistaminic eyedrops and topical steroid nasal sprays had no positive effects. Prick testing to routine aeroallergens was negative. After TS was diagnosed, tiapride was initiated and after 8 weeks his tics had decreased dramatically.

Thirdly, and not only in the context of the poststreptococcal hypothesis (see Chapter 9), immunological abnormalities (Landau et al., 2012; Murphy et al., 2010) reported in TS patients (see Chapter 14) raise the question of whether antibiotic prophylaxis or immunomodulatory interventions can be helpful, at least in some susceptible TS patients (Hoekstra et al., 2004; Zykov et al., 2009). This question will remain unanswered until a clearer picture of the involvement of immunity in TS is provided by larger clinical studies that are under way (see www.emtics.eu).

Fourth, pharmacological modulation of GABAergic (inhibitory) and glutamatergic (excitatory) (Singer et al., 2010) neurotransmission in TS should be investigated in more detail. Finally, studies investigating the relationship of oxidative stress and TS are increasing, but therapeutic research is only just beginning (http://clinicaltrials.gov/show/NCT01172288).

REFERENCES

Anca MH, Giladi N, Korczyn AD. Ropinirole in Gilles de la Tourette syndrome. *Neurology* 2004; 62:1626–1627.

Banaschewski TB, Neale BM, Rothenberger A, Roessner V. Comorbidity of tic disorders & ADHD: conceptual and methodological considerations. *Eur Child Adolesc Psychiatry* 2007; 16 Suppl 1:5–14.

Bestha DP, Jeevarakshagan S, Madaan V. Management of tics and Tourette's disorder: an update. *Expert Opin Pharmacother* 2010; 11:1813–1822.

Bloch M, State M, Pittenger C. Recent advances in Tourette syndrome. *Curr Opin Neurol* 2011; 24:119–125.

An excellent review of the whole TS field.

Borison RL, Ang L, Hamilton WJ, et al. Treatment approaches in Gilles de la Tourette syndrome. *Brain Res Bull* 1983; 11:205–208.

Bressan RA, Jones HM, Pilowsky LS. Atypical antipsychotic drugs and tardive dyskinesia: relevance of D2 receptor affinity. *J Psychopharmacol* 2004; 18:124–127.

Bruggeman RC, van der Linden RC, Buitelaar JK, et al. Risperidone versus pimozide in Tourette's disorder: a comparative double-blind parallel-group study. *J Clin Psychiatry* 2001; 62:50–56.

Cummings DD, Singer HS, Krieger M, et al. Neuropsychiatric effects of guanfacine in children with mild tourette syndrome: a pilot study. *Clin Neuropharmacol* 2002; 25: 325–332.

Curtis A, Clarke CE, Rickards HE. Cannabinoids for Tourette's syndrome. *Cochrane Database Syst Rev* 2009:CD006565.

Debes N, Hjalgrim H, Skov L. The presence of attention-deficit hyperactivity disorder (ADHD) and obsessive-compulsive disorder worsen psychosocial and educational problems in Tourette syndrome. *J Child Neurol* 2010; 25:171–181.

Dion Y, Annable L, Sandor P, Chouinard G. Risperidone in the treatment of Tourette syndrome: a double-blind, placebo-controlled trial. *J Clin Psychopharmacol* 2002; 22:31–39.

Dose M, Lange HW. The benzamide tiapride: treatment of extrapyramidal motor and other clinical syndromes. *Pharmacopsychiatry* 2000; 33:19–27.

Drtílková I. Clonazepam, clonidine and tiapride in children with tic disorder. *Homeostasis* 1996; 37:216.

Du JC, Chiu TF, Lee KM, et al. Tourette syndrome in children: an updated review. *Pediatr Neonatol* 2010; 51:255–264.

Du YS, Li HF, Vance A, et al. Randomized double-blind multicentre placebo-controlled clinical trial of the clonidine adhesive patch for the treatment of tic disorders. *Aust N Z J Psychiatry* 2008; 42:807–813.

The only trial comparing directly two agents for treatment of TS with a large sample size (n = 437).

Eddy CM, Rickards HE, Cavanna AE. Treatment strategies for tics in Tourette syndrome. *Ther Adv Neurol Disord* 2011; 4:25–45.

Eggers C, Rothenberger A, Berghaus U. Clinical and neurobiological findings in children suffering from tic disease following treatment with tiapride. *Eur Arch Psychiatry Neurol Sci* 1998; 237:223–229.

Ercan-Sencicek AG, Stillman AA, Ghosh AK, et al. L-histidine decarboxylase and Tourette's syndrome. *N Engl J Med* 2010; 362: 1901–1908.

Fernandez TV, Sanders SJ, Yurkiewick IR, et al. Rare copy number variants in Tourette syndrome disrupt genes in histaminergic pathways and overlap with autism. *Biol Psychiatry* 2012; 71:392–402.

Ferrada C, Ferré S, Casadó V, et al. Interactions between histamine H3 and dopamine D2 receptors and the implications for striatal function. *Neuropharmacology* 2008; 55: 190–197.

Fischer A, Borensztein P, Roussel C. The European rare diseases therapeutic initiative. *PLoS Med* 2005; 2:e243.

Fusco C, Bertani G, Caricati G, Della Giustina E. Stress fracture of the peroneal bone secondary to a complex tic. *Brain Dev* 2006; 28:52–54.

Gaffney GR, Perry PJ, Lund BC, et al. Risperidone versus clonidine in the treatment of children and adolescents with Tourette's syndrome. *J Am Acad Child Adolesc Psychiatry* 2002; 41:330–336.

George MS, Trimble MR, Robertson MM. Fluvoxamine and sulpiride in comorbid obsessive-compulsive disorder and Gilles de la Tourette syndrome. *Hum Psychopharmacol* 1993; 8:327–334.

Gilbert DL, Batterson JR, Sethuraman G, Sallee FR. Tic reduction with risperidone versus pimozide in a randomized, double-blind, crossover trial. *J Am Acad Child Adolesc Psychiatry* 2004; 43:206–214.

Gilbert DL, Dure L, Sethuraman G, et al. Tic reduction with pergolide in a randomized controlled trial in children. *Neurology* 2003; 60: 606–611.

Goetz CG. Clonidine and clonazepam in Tourette syndrome. *Adv Neurol* 1992; 58:245–251.

Goetz CG, Stebbins GT, Thelen JA. Talipexole and adult Gilles de la Tourette's syndrome: double-blind, placebo-controlled clinical trial. *Mov Disord* 1994; 9:315–317.

Hartmann A, Worbe Y, Arnulf I. Increasing histamine neurotransmission in Gilles de la Tourette syndrome. *J Neurol* 2011; 259:375–376.

Hoekstra PJ, Minderaa RB, Kallenberg CG. Lack of effect of intravenous immunoglobulins on tics: a double-blind placebo-controlled study. *J Clin Psychiatry* 2004; 65:537–542.

Interesting paper because of the publication of negative findings concerning the possible therapeutic value of findings based on the pediatric autoimmune neuropsychiatric disorders associated with streptococcal infections (PANDAS) hypothesis.

Howson AL, Batth S, Ilivitsky V, et al. Clinical and attentional effects of acute nicotine treatment in Tourette's syndrome. *Eur Psychiatry* 2004; 19:102–112.

Jankovic J, Jimenez-Shahed J, Brown L. A randomized, double-blind, placebo-controlled study of topiramate in the treatment of Tourette syndrome. *J Neurol Neurosurg Psychiatry* 2010; 81:70–73.

Jankovic J, Kurlan R. Tourette syndrome: Evolving concepts. *Mov Disord* 2011; 26: 1149–1156.

Another interesting and important review of TS from a U.S. perspective; the selection of the presented findings on pharmacological treatment is subjective to a certain degree.

Kimber TE. An update on Tourette syndrome. *Curr Neurol Neurosci Rep* 2010; 10:286–291.

Krauss JK, Jankovic J. Severe motor tics causing cervical myelopathy in Tourette's syndrome. *Mov Disord* 1996; 11:563–566.

Kurlan R. Clinical practice. Tourette's Syndrome. *N Engl J Med* 2010; 363:2332–2338.

Kurlan R, McDermott MP, Deeley C, et al. Prevalence of tics in schoolchildren and association with placement in special education. *Neurology* 2001; 57:1383–1388.

Landau YE, Steinberg T, Richmand B, et al. Involvement of immunologic and biochemical mechanisms in the pathogenesis of Tourette's syndrome. *J Neural Transm* 2012; 119: 621–626.

Leckman JF, Riddle MA, Hardin MT, et al. The Yale Global Tic Severity Scale: initial testing of a clinician-rated scale of tic severity. *J Am Acad Child Adolesc Psychiatry* 1989; 28:566–573.

Lipinski JF, Sallee FR, Jackson C, Sethuraman G. Dopamine agonist treatment of Tourette disorder in children: results of an open-label trial of pergolide. *Mov Disord* 1997; 12:402–407.

Marras C, Andrews D, Sime E, Lang AE. Botulinum toxin for simple motor tics: a randomized, double-blind, controlled clinical trial. *Neurology* 2001; 56:605–610.

Meisel A, Winter C, Zschenderlein R, Arnold G. Tourette syndrome: efficient treatment with ziprasidone and normalization of body weight in a patient with excessive weight gain under tiapride. *Mov Disord* 2004; 19:991–992.

Muller-Vahl KR, Krueger D. Does Tourette syndrome prevent tardive dyskinesia? *Mov Disord* 2011; 26:2442–2443.

Muller-Vahl KR, Roessner V. Treatment of tics in patients with Tourette syndrome: Recommendations according to the European Society for the Study of Tourette Syndrome. *Mov Disord* 2011; 26:2447.

Muller-Vahl KR, Schneider U, Koblenz A, et al. Treatment of Tourette's syndrome with delta-9-tetrahydrocannabinol (THC): a randomized crossover trial. *Pharmacopsychiatry* 2002; 35:57–61.

The first trial on THC for treatment of TS. More studies are required.

Muller-Vahl KR, Schneider U, Prevedel H, et al. Delta-9-tetrahydrocannabinol (THC) is effective in the treatment of tics in Tourette syndrome: a 6-week randomized trial. *J Clin Psychiatry* 2003; 64:459–465.

Muroni A, Paba S, Puligheddu M, et al. A preliminary study of finasteride in Tourette syndrome. *Mov Disord* 2011; 26:2146–2147.

Murphy TK, Kurlan R, Leckman JF. The immunobiology of Tourette's disorder, pediatric autoimmune neuropsychiatric disorders associated with streptococcus, and related disorders: a way forward. *J Child Adolesc Psychopharmacol* 2010; 20:317–331.

Onofrj M, Paci C, D'Andreamatteo G, Toma L. Olanzapine in severe Gilles de la Tourette syndrome: a 52-week double-blind cross-over study vs. low-dose pimozide. *J Neurol* 2000; 247:443–446.

Parraga HC, Harris KM, Parraga KL, et al. An overview of the treatment of Tourette's disorder and tics. *J Child Adolesc Psychopharmacol* 2010; 20:249–262.

Peterson BS, Zhang H, Anderson GM, Leckman JF. A double-blind, placebo-controlled, crossover trial of an antiandrogen in the treatment of Tourette's syndrome. *J Clin Psychopharmacol* 1998; 18:324–331.

Pierce A, Rickards HE. Atypical antipsychotics for Tourette's syndrome. *Cochrane Database Syst Rev* (in press).

Pringsheim T, Marras C. Pimozide for tics in Tourette's syndrome. *Cochrane Database Syst Rev* 2009:CD006996.

Rickards H. Tourette's syndrome and other tic disorders. *Pract Neurol* 2010; 10:252–259.

Riley DE, Lang AE. Pain in Gilles de la Tourette syndrome and related tic disorders. *Can J Neurol Sci* 1989; 16:439–441.

Robertson MM. Tourette syndrome, associated conditions and the complexities of treatment. *Brain* 2000; 123:425–462.

Robertson MM, Stern JS. Gilles de la Tourette syndrome: symptomatic treatment based on evidence. *Eur Child Adolesc Psychiatry* 2000; 9 Suppl 1:160–75.

Roessner V, Plessen KJ, Rothenberger A, et al. European clinical guidelines for Tourette syndrome and other tic disorders. Part II: pharmacological treatment. *Eur Child Adolesc Psychiatry* 2011a; 20:173–196.

The first consensus-based international guidelines on pharmacologcial treatment of TS; it presents a comprehensive overview of all studies on pharmacological treatment of TS.

Roessner V, Rothenberger A, Rickards H, Hoekstra PJ. European clinical guidelines for Tourette syndrome and other tic disorders. *Eur Child Adolesc Psychiatry* 2011b; 20:153–154.

Ross MS, Moldofsky H. A comparison of pimozide and haloperidol in the treatment of Gilles de la Tourette's syndrome. *Am J Psychiatry* 1978; 135:585–587.

The first randomized, double-blind, placebo-controlled trial comparing directly two agents for treatment of TS.

Rothenberger A, Banaschewski T, Roessner V. *Tic-Störungen. Leitlinien zur Diagnostik und Therapie von psychischen Störungen im Säuglings-,* Kindes- und Jugendalter. P. u. P. Deutsche Gesellschaft für Kinder- u. Jugendpsychiatrie. Köln: Deutscher Ärzteverlag, 2007, pp. 319–325.

Sallee FR, Kurlan R, Goetz CG, et al. Ziprasidone treatment of children and adolescents with Tourette's syndrome: a pilot study. *J Am Acad Child Adolesc Psychiatry* 2000; 39:292–299.

Sallee FR, Nesbitt L, Jackson C, et al. Relative efficacy of haloperidol and pimozide in children and adolescents with Tourette's disorder. *Am J Psychiatry* 1997; 154:1057–1062.

Sandor P. Pharmacological management of tics in patients with TS. *J Psychosom Res* 2003; 55:41–48.

Scahill L, Chappell PB, Kim YS, et al. A placebo-controlled study of guanfacine in the treatment of children with tic disorders and attention deficit hyperactivity disorder. *Am J Psychiatry* 2001; 158:1067–1074.

Scahill L, Leckman JF, Schultz RT, et al. A placebo-controlled trial of risperidone in Tourette syndrome. *Neurology* 2003; 60:1130–1135.

Shapiro AK, Shapiro ES, Young JG, Feinberg TE. Measurement in tic disorders. In Shapiro AK, Shapiro ES, Young JG, Feinberg TE. *Gilles de la Tourette syndrome.* New York: Raven Press, 1988, pp. 127–193.

Shapiro E, Shapiro AK, Fulop G, et al. Controlled study of haloperidol, pimozide and placebo for the treatment of Gilles de la Tourette's syndrome. *Arch Gen Psychiatry* 1989; 46:722–730.

One of the rare trials comparing directly two agents for treatment of TS of larger sample size.

Shapiro E, Shapiro E. Treatment of tic disorders with haloperidol. In Cohen DJ, Bruun RD, Leckman JF (Eds.), *Tourette syndrome and tic disorders.* New York: John Wiley and Sons, 1998, pp. 267–280.

Singer HS. Treatment of tics and Tourette syndrome. *Curr Treat Options Neurol* 2010; 12:539–561.

Another interesting and important review of TS from a U.S. perspective; the selection of the presented findings on pharmacological treatment is subjective to a certain degree.

Singer HS, Morris C, Grados M. Glutamatergic modulatory therapy for Tourette syndrome. *Med Hypotheses* 2010; 74:862–867.

Interesting hypotheses for further research on pharmacological treatment of TS.

Singer HS, Wendlandt J, Krieger M, Giuliano J. Baclofen treatment in Tourette syndrome: a double-blind, placebo-controlled, crossover trial. *Neurology* 2001; 56:599–604.

Smith-Hicks CL, Bridges DD, Paynter NP, Singer HS. A double-blind randomized placebo control trial of levetiracetam in Tourette syndrome. *Mov Disord* 2007; 22:1764–1770.

Taylor JL, Rajbhandari AK, Berridge KC, Aldridge JW. Dopamine receptor modulation of repetitive grooming actions in the rat: potential relevance for Tourette syndrome. *Brain Res* 2010; 1322:92–101.

Weisman H, Qureshi IA, Leckman JF, et al. Meta-analysis: Alpha-2 agonists in the treatment of tic disorders: moderating effects of ADHD. *Neurosci Biobehav Rev* 2012; Oct 23. [Epub ahead of print].

An important meta-analysis revolutionizing the evaluation of clonidine in the pharmacological treatment of tics.

Wenzel C, Kleimann A, Bokemeyer S, Muller-Vahl KR. Aripiprazole for the treatment of Tourette syndrome: a case series of 100 patients. *J Clin Psychopharmacol* 2012; 32:548–550.

Zykov VP, Shcherbina AY, Novikova EB, Shvabrina TV. Neuroimmune aspects of the pathogenesis of Tourette's syndrome and experience in the use of immunoglobulins in children. *Neurosci Behav Physiol* 2009; 39:635–638.

25

Treatment of Psychiatric Comorbidities in Tourette Syndrome

FRANCESCO CARDONA AND RENATA RIZZO

Abstract

This chapter is a literature review and a critical commentary of the available evidence on pharmacological treatment of psychiatric comorbidities in Tourette syndrome (TS). Attention-deficit/hyperactivity disorder (ADHD) in TS may be initially approached with behavioral treatment, especially if the symptoms are mild or the parents refuse pharmacological treatments. The latter currently include different classes of drugs. Alpha-2 adrenoreceptor agonists (clonidine and guanfacine) showed efficacy in the treatment of both tics and ADHD symptoms and could be considered as first-line management, whereas psychostimulants and atomoxetine could represent a second choice. Although obsessive-compulsive disorder (OCD) and TS are closely related, no clinical trial to date has specifically evaluated the treatment of obsessive-compulsive symptoms in TS patients. The main source of information on OCD management in patients with chronic tics or TS comes from a few clinical trials testing medications for obsessive-compulsive symptoms that included also patients with tics. Monotherapy with serotonin reuptake inhibitors (SRI) or selective serotonin reuptake inhibitors (SSRI) yielded the highest efficacy in these studies, although nearly half of OCD patients do not respond completely, and only very few become asymptomatic. Several alternative strategies have been proposed for OCD nonresponders; among these, antipsychotic augmentation is discussed in greater detail. Finally, despite the high rate and the clinical relevance of other psychiatric comorbidities (non-OCD anxiety disorders, self-injurious and disruptive behaviors) in TS patients, only a few studies have been devoted to investigating a specific therapeutic approach in these patients.

INTRODUCTION

Tourette syndrome (TS) is a neurobiological, chronic, hereditary disease, characterized by the presence of motor and vocal tics. All the research data have suggested that TS is a discrete disorder with a wide range of increasingly complex and possible combinations of symptoms and comorbidities. In specialty clinics, up to 90% of TS patients will exhibit comorbidities.

Attention-deficit/hyperactivity disorder (ADHD) and obsessive-compulsive disorder (OCD) are the most frequent comorbid conditions, but elevated rates of sleep disorders, learning disabilities, anxiety disorders, mood disorders, self-injurious behaviors, and outbursts of extreme anger are also reported in TS patient series (Chapters 2, 3, and 4 are devoted to a detailed analysis of the complex spectrum of psychiatric comorbidities in TS).

The treatment of TS and its comorbidities is symptomatic, and multidisciplinary treatment is usually indicated. This includes an educational or supportive intervention, in some cases combined with pharmacological treatment. The choice of initial treatment is mainly based on the most disabling symptoms, on their severity, on the patient's sense of urgency for treatment, and on an evaluation of the risk of adverse effects.

The impact of the various symptoms on the patient's ability to function at school or work or in daily life is not directly related to the severity of symptoms because patients differ in their ability to tolerate a given degree of symptoms. Likewise, the people who come into contact with TS patients present different levels of tolerance for the patient's symptoms. However, the presence of comorbid symptoms seems to have a more significant influence on the patient's quality of life than the presence of tics alone, and therefore it can be associated with a stronger need for pharmacological intervention. This conclusion is supported by several studies that examined whether the pattern of pharmacological treatment was dependent on the presence of comorbidities. Ohta and colleagues (2003) examined 10 adults with TS alone and 14 adults with TS and comorbidity. Seventy percent of patients in the former group received medical treatment, 78.6% in the latter group. Freeman and colleagues (2000) examined the rates of medical treatment in four different groups with both children and adults with TS: TS alone, TS+ADHD, TS+OCD, and TS+ADHD+OCD. In these groups, 48%, 47%, 62%, and 64% of the participants received medications for tics, respectively. More recently, in a study on 314 TS children and adolescents (aged 5.3–20 years), Debes and colleagues (2009) found that only 36.4% of the patients with TS alone received medical treatment, compared with 77.6% in the group with TS+ADHD, 57.9% in the group with TS+OCD, and 88.2% in the group with TS+ADHD+OCD. Interestingly, in this population the pharmacological treatment was mainly started because of tics (38.4% of patients) and ADHD (36.8% of patients). Obviously, the presence of tics was the reason for starting medical treatment in the TS-alone group (63.6%), but also in the TS+OCD group (42.4%), while ADHD was the main reason in the groups in which this comorbidity was present (TS+ADHD and TS+ADHD+OCD: 63.5% and 41.7% respectively). Instead, OCD accounted for the institution of medical treatment in only a few cases (15.2% in the TS+OCD group and 11.7% in the TS+ADHD+OCD group).

Several factors complicate the treatment of psychiatric comorbidities in TS. Among these, the natural course of the disorder, characterized by the classical waxing and waning of symptoms, and the difficulty of reliably predicting the appearance of comorbidities (i.e., ADHD often precedes the occurrence of tics, while obsessive-compulsive symptoms usually develop later) represent challenges for evaluating the efficacy of treatments. Other difficulties in the treatment of comorbidities are the phenotypic variability of symptoms in each patient, hampering the establishment of a standardized therapeutic approach, and the need to treat the various concomitant symptoms with different drugs, even if there are still very few studies on combined therapies and on pharmacodynamic interactions among different drugs.

In this chapter we summarize the existing literature on the treatment of psychiatric comorbidities in TS and suggest a therapeutic approach for some of these comorbid conditions.

ADHD

The prevalence of coexisting ADHD in TS and details of the "nosological issue" of TS/ADHD co-occurrence are discussed in Chapter 2. The co-occurrence of TS and ADHD is in most cases associated with greater psychopathological, social, and academic impairment resulting from the negative impact of ADHD (Gorman, 2010; Rizzo et al., 2007). This co-occurrence often causes more clinical impairment and may be more responsive to treatment than tics themselves (Bloch, 2008). For these reasons, treatment of tics and coexisting conditions should be prioritized according to the impairment caused by each problem in order to treat the target symptoms.

In the past 11 years 13 guidelines on diagnosis and/or management of ADHD from 10 medical associations have been published (Seixas et al., 2011); all guidelines agree that the diagnosis of ADHD is based on a full clinical interview, which includes a mental state examination, assessments of impairment, development, comorbidity, and family history as well as a physical examination. All guidelines for children recommend a family interview, and all agree that the clinical interview remains the gold standard for the assessment of ADHD, whereas the use of rating scales has become standardized and has improved the reliability, breadth, and efficiency of assessments. The importance of the exclusion of physical and

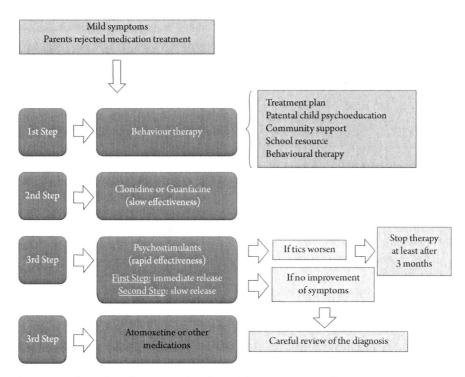

FIGURE 25.1 Evidence-based summary flowchart of the management of coexisting ADHD in TS.

psychiatric comorbidity is also highlighted in all guidelines (Seixas et al., 2011). The U.S. Tourette Syndrome Association Medical Advisory Board Association Guidelines for the Pharmacotherapy of TS published a set of recommendations regarding the treatment of ADHD in patients with comorbid tics. These state that, given the added disability attributable to ADHD in children and adolescents with TS, aggressive treatment of ADHD in these cases is warranted (Scahill et al., 2006). Clinical guidelines for pharmacological treatment of TS and other tic disorders produced by the European Society for the Study of Tourette Syndrome also affirm that primary treatment of ADHD may reduce stress, improve attentional resources, and sometimes reduce tics by enhancing the individual's ability to suppress tics (Roessner et al., 2011). Figure 25.1 summarizes our proposed approach to the management of coexisting ADHD in TS.

Nonpharmacological Treatments

Therapeutic options for ADHD represent a multitude of pharmacological, cognitive-behavioral,

psychoeducational, and psychosocial interventions, allowing creation of an individualized treatment regimen that caters to a patient's needs in terms of the suppression of symptoms, coping, and overall psychological well-being. The idea behind a multimodal treatment approach is that once attentional challenges and motor restlessness are dealt with pharmacologically, training in underdeveloped social skills and improvements in self-structuring capabilities will help patients to catch up with their peers (Geissler & Lesch, 2011). Considering the potential benefits associated with both forms of treatment as well as their combination, discussions between clinicians, patients, and families are pivotal. Psychological interventions, educational changes, and medications should be guided by a treatment plan drawn up for the individual. This plan should include psychoeducation about TS and ADHD for the parents, the child, and the child's school, linkage with community supports, and additional school resources, as appropriate. Psychoeducation is distinguished from psychosocial interventions such as behavioral therapy and is the main topic of Chapter 22.

The efficacy of behavioral therapy in ADHD was studied in the Multimodal Treatment of Attention Deficit Hyperactivity Disorder (MTA) study (MTA Cooperative Group, 1999). Children with ADHD were randomized into four groups: medication management alone, medication and behavioral management, behavioral management alone, and standard community treatment. Children in all four groups showed reduced symptoms of ADHD at 14 months relative to baseline. The two groups that received algorithmic medication management showed a superior outcome with regard to ADHD symptoms compared to those who received intensive behavioral treatment alone or community treatment. Those who received behavioral treatment alone did not improve more significantly than those who received community treatment. One fourth of the subjects randomized to receive behavioral treatment alone required treatment with medication during trials because of the lack of effectiveness of the behavioral treatment. It seems to have been established that a pharmacological intervention for ADHD associated with behavioral treatment is more effective than behavioral treatment alone (AACAP, 2007). In our opinion, behavioral therapy should be recommended as an initial treatment for patients with TS/tic disorder and ADHD, especially if symptoms are mild or the parents reject pharmacological treatment. An advantage of behavioral treatments may be their better long-term effects, lasting beyond the duration of the treatment, and the fact that they appear to cause less severe adverse reactions. In a recent review, Jankovic and Kurlan (2011) recommended behavioral therapy as the first line of intervention in patients with TS and comorbid ADHD, as did Roessner and colleagues (2011) in the European clinical guidelines for TS.

Pharmacological Treatments

Currently, three classes of drugs are used in the treatment of ADHD: alpha-agonists (clonidine and guanfacine), psychostimulants (amphetamine enantiomers [Adderall], methylphenidate enantiomers [Ritalin], or slow-release preparations [Concerta]), and a selective norepinephrine reuptake inhibitor [atomoxetine (Strattera)].

ALPHA-2-ADRENOCEPTOR AGONISTS

Clonidine was the first drug in this class to be used off-label. Although clonidine has been used for nearly three decades in the treatment of TS, there are few controlled studies evaluating its effects on ADHD (Robertson, 2000). A recent contribution in this respect was provided by the meta-analysis performed by Bloch and colleagues (2009). A single-blind placebo-controlled trial (Leckman et al., 1985) demonstrated a significant improvement in behavioral problems and motor and phonic tics in 6 of the 13 patients treated for 60 weeks. A randomized controlled study on 47 TS patients (age 7–48 years) treated for 12 weeks demonstrated that clonidine was more effective than placebo on parent-rated measures of impulsivity and hyperactivity and on clinician-rated measures of tics (Leckman et al., 1991), while Goetz and colleagues (1987), in their double-blind study on 30 children and adults with TS, concluded that clonidine did not significantly reduce either impulsivity/hyperactivity or tics. Singer (1995) conducted a 6-week double-blind, placebo-controlled study on 34 children (7–13 years) randomly assigned to clonidine 0.05 mg four times per day versus placebo and desipramine 25 mg four times per day versus placebo. The outcome of ADHD symptoms was measured with the Child Behavior Checklist (CBCL), continuous performance tests, and neuropsychological tests for the executive functions. Clonidine did not alter ADHD or tic severity significantly but improved the "nervous/overactive" subscale score of the CBCL. Gaffney and colleagues (2002) conducted a double-blind placebo-controlled trial in 21 TS patients (age 7–17 years), randomly assigned to 8 weeks of treatment with clonidine or risperidone. Fifty percent of the clonidine-treated group versus 29% of the risperidone group were considered ADHD symptom-responders on the Du Paul Attention Deficit Hyperactivity Scale (ADHDRS). Hedderick and colleagues (2009) compared the efficacy of clonidine and levetiracetam in a double-blind crossover 6-week study on 10 TS patients (age 8–27 years). No significant changes were reported in the ADHDRS score for clonidine or levetiracetam. In this study, a small but statistically significant improvement in total tic score was found with clonidine, whereas no improvement occurred with levetiracetam. The Tourette Syndrome Study Group (2002) conducted the largest, well-designed, randomized, double-blind trial using orally administered clonidine and methylphenidate. One hundred thirty-six children with TS+ADHD were treated for 16 weeks and randomly assigned to clonidine alone (n = 34), methylphenidate alone (n = 37), clonidine and methylphenidate (n = 33), and placebo (n = 32). Clonidine alone and clonidine plus methylphenidate significantly improved hyperactivity/impulsive symptoms of ADHD on the ADHD Conners Abbreviated Symptoms Questionnaire for Teachers (ASQ). Yale Global Tic Severity Scale (YGTSS) scores showed a statistically significant improvement with clonidine alone and clonidine plus methylphenidate. The proportion of subjects reporting a worsening of tics was no higher in the active arm compared to the placebo arm.

Two recent double-blind placebo-controlled Chinese studies (Du et al., 2008; Zhong, 2007) using clonidine patches evaluated only the improvement on YGTSS scores, without other behavioral measures, and showed significant tic amelioration with clonidine transdermal patches (Table 25.1).

Guanfacine was reported as effective in the combined hyperactive/inattentive ADHD subgroup, showing less efficacy in the inattentive subtype (Heal et al., 2011). Chappell and colleagues (1995) conducted an open-label study of guanfacine in 10 children with TS+ADHD, aged 8 to 16 years. The duration of follow-up was 4 to 20 weeks. Ratings of tic severity and ADHD symptoms were obtained using the YGTSS, the Tic Symptom Self Report (TSSR), and the Conners Parent Rating Scale. In addition, blind Continuous Performance Tests (CPTs) were performed at baseline and at two follow-up intervals in eight subjects. Guanfacine was associated with significant decreases in both commission errors ($p < .02$) and omission errors ($p < .01$) on the CPT. In addition, guanfacine caused a significant decrease in the severity of motor ($p < .02$) and phonic ($p < .02$) tics, as measured by the TSSR and the YGTSS,

respectively. Boon-Yasidhi and colleagues (2005) evaluated the efficacy and safety of guanfacine in children with ADHD and tic disorders in an 8-week open-label study. They studied 25 medication-free subjects, aged 7 to 16 years. Outcome measures included the Hyperactivity Index of the Conners Parent Rating Scale, the teacher-rated ADHD Rating Scale, and the YGTSS. Guanfacine was associated with mean improvement of 27% on the Hyperactivity Index (N = 25; $t = 4.61$; $p < .001$), 32% on the total score of the teacher-rated ADHD Scale (N = 19; $t = 5.27$; $p < .001$), and 39% on the total tic severity scale (N = 19; $t = 4.17$; $p < .001$). Scahill and colleagues (2001) conducted a randomized, double-blind, placebo-controlled clinical trial in 34 children aged 7 to 15 years who met DSM-IV criteria for ADHD and chronic tic disorder. They were treated with guanfacine (1.5–3 mg/day) or placebo for 8 weeks. Guanfacine significantly reduced symptoms of ADHD and tics as measured by the ASQ. Only Cummings and colleagues (2002), in a double-blind placebo-controlled study evaluating the efficacy of guanfacine on tic severity, cognitive functioning, and parent rating of behavior before and after treatment, found that guanfacine, prescribed at a moderate dose and for a short course of treatment, did not provide significant neuropsychiatric benefits in this group of children with mild TS. Guanfacine is empirically considered better than clonidine but is not available in many European countries.

Frequently reported adverse events with clonidine and guanfacine include somnolence, fatigue, sedation (often dissipated with continued treatment [Bloch et al., 2009]), upper abdominal pain, dry mouth, nausea, dizziness, and depression. Reductions in blood pressure and heart rate were also found. Most changes were not clinically relevant, but serious episodes of orthostatic hypotension and syncope have been reported in about 2% of subjects in long-term trials (Biederman et al., 2008). Also, rebound hypertension can occur with abrupt discontinuation. Kollins and colleagues (2011) conducted a phase 3, double-blind, placebo-controlled trial in 198 children and adolescents with ADHD to assess the efficacy and safety of clonidine combined with stimulants. Somnolence, headache, fatigue, upper abdominal

Table 25.1 Characteristics of Included Studies

Drug	Author(Year)	Study Design	Sample Size	Outcome	
				ADHD	TIC
Clonidine	Leckman (1985)	SB	6/13	+++	+++
	Goetz (1987)	DB	30	–	–
	Leckman (1991)	RC	47	+	+
	Singer (1995)	DB	34	++	–
	Gaffney (2002)	DB	21	++	++
	Zhong (2007)	DB (patch)	—	No measures of behavior	+
	Du (2008)	DB (patch)	437	No measures of behavior	+
	Hedderick (2009)	DB	10	–	++
Guanfacine	Chapell (1995)	OL	10	+++	+++
	Scahill (2001)	DB	34	+++	+++
	Cummings (2002)	DB	24	–	–
	Boon-Yasidhi (2005)	OL	25	+++	+++
Clonidine/ Methylphenidate	TS Study Group (2002)	RDB	34/136 (clonidine) 33/136 (methylphenidate + clonidine)	+++	+++
Methylphenidate	Sverd (1989)	SB	4	+++	–
	Gadow (1995)	DB	34	+++	++
	Gadow (1999)	PS	34	+++	–
	Gadow (2007)	DB	71	+++	++
Dextroamphetamine/ Methylphenidate	Castellanos (1997)	PC/DB	20	+++	—
Atomoxetine	Allen (2005)	DB	76/148	+++	+++

SB, single-blind placebo-controlled study; DB, double-blind controlled study; RC, randomized controlled study; OL, open-label; RDB, randomized double-blind; PS, prospective study; PC, placebo-controlled.

+++ improvement, ++ mild improvement, + More effective than placebo, – no improvement, — increase in tic severity pain, nasal congestion, and mean systolic and diastolic blood pressure decreases were most frequently reported in patients treated with clonidine plus stimulants compared with those who received placebo plus stimulants.

More recently, Weisman and colleagues (2012), in their meta-analysis of six randomized, placebo-controlled trials, demonstrated a modest but significant benefit of alpha-2-agonists in the treatment of children with chronic tics. Alpha-2-agonists had a medium to large effect in reducing tic symptoms in clinical trials in which participants also had ADHD. In the absence of ADHD, however, the efficacy of these agents was small and nonsignificant. Presuming that pharmacotherapy is chosen as a treatment option in patients with TS and coexisting ADHD, we therefore suggest alpha-2-agonists (either clonidine or guanfacine in monotherapy) as first-line management, given the combined benefit relating to both ADHD and tic symptoms (Fig. 25.1).

PSYCHOSTIMULANTS

Amphetamine and methylphenidate are commonly referred to as psychostimulants. Psychostimulant medications are currently the first line of treatment for children with ADHD (Pliskza et al., 2007; Taylor et al., 2004). Psychostimulants have demonstrated superior short-term efficacy compared to both nonpsychostimulant medications and psychosocial treatment for ADHD (MTA Cooperative Group, 1999; Van der Oord et al., 2008).

Because stimulants cause dopamine release, there has been a theoretical concern that these drugs could exacerbate tics. There has also been a concern that tic disorders could be primarily provoked in this way, and there have been reports of children with isolated ADHD being treated with stimulants and subsequently developing tics or TS. For some time the use of psychostimulants in the treatment of ADHD in children with comorbid tics has been controversial because they were thought to worsen tics (Borcherding et al., 1990; Denckla et al., 1976; Lowe et al., 1982). Controlled clinical trials have not indicated a deterioration of tics in patients treated with stimulants (Castellanos et al., 1997; Gadow et al., 1999; Nolan & Gadow, 1997; Tourette Syndrome

Study Group, 2002). It has become apparent that clinical data do not substantiate the concern. The emergence of tics after ADHD treatment is instituted probably reflects the underlying natural chronology of TS, and the observed worsening of the tics in some patients after the initiation of stimulant therapy may represent natural fluctuations in tic severity that can obscure drug effects.

Methylphenidate

In the past decade several studies of short-term treatment of individuals with TS or tic disorder and ADHD have been published. Sverd and colleagues (1989) reported the effects of methylphenidate in a single-blind trial in individuals with TS+ADHD compared to placebo; clinical ratings showed improvement in ADHD and no effects on tics. Gadow and colleagues (1995), in a double-blind placebo-controlled study, examined 34 children with a tic disorder (age 6.1–11.9 years) who received three doses of methylphenidate (0.1, 0.3, and 0.5 mg/kg) for 2 weeks. Each boy was observed for 20 hours in the school setting. Results showed that methylphenidate effectively suppressed hyperactive/disruptive behaviors in the classroom and physical aggression in the lunchroom and on the playground. Methylphenidate also reduced the occurrence of vocal tics. None of the motor tic measures revealed drug effects. On the minimal effective dose, only one boy experienced motor tic exacerbation (the study sample included 11 children who were described in preliminary reports: Gadow et al., 1992; Sverd, 1989). The data from this trial were subsequently analyzed in a separate report (Nolan, 1997). Gadow and colleagues (1999) analyzed the long-term effect of methylphenidate therapy in 34 prepubertal children evaluated at 6-month intervals for 2 years as part of a prospective observational study. Treatment effects were assessed using videotaped sessions in a simulated classroom and ADHD measures. Treatment gains that were experimentally demonstrated in the previous 8-week controlled drug trial were still present after a 2-year follow-up and were documented in the simulated classroom setting. There was no evidence that motor or vocal tics changed in frequency or severity during maintenance therapy compared with diagnostic or initial double-blind, placebo-controlled evaluations. Castellanos and colleagues (1997), in a 9-week, placebo-controlled, double-blind crossover study, compared methylphenidate's and dextroamphetamine's effects on tic severity in boys with ADHD and TS. Methylphenidate significantly decreased hyperactivity at all doses, as measured by day program teachers, although there was no significant interaction between drug and dose, indicating that additional improvements in hyperactivity were not observed with higher doses. Higher doses of methylphenidate (45 mg b.i.d) and dextroamphetamine (22.5 mg b.i.d.) resulted in a significant, albeit reversible, increase in tic severity. In the TS Study Group work (2002), a statistically significant treatment effect on the ASQ from baseline to 16 weeks compared to placebo was observed with methylphenidate alone and with clonidine plus methylphenidate. In this study the authors also found that although more subjects reported tics as a dose-limiting side effect for methylphenidate therapy, the reported frequency of tic worsening was about the same across all treatments: 20% in the methylphenidate-alone group, 26% in the clonidine-alone group, and 22% in the placebo group. Gadow and colleagues (2007) conducted a double-blind long-term observation study (1989–2004) to examine the safety and efficacy of immediate-release methylphenidate for the treatment of ADHD in 71 children (ages 6–12 years) with TS (96%) or chronic motor tic disorder (4%). The study sample included two cohorts of children. The initial group (cohort 1) was recruited primarily to assess the short-term effects of immediate-release methylphenidate (n = 39; Gadow et al., 1995), followed by a naturalistic observation study through age (Gadow et al., 1999). During the follow-up study, a second sample was recruited (n = 32, cohort 2). The two cohorts received placebo and three doses of methylphenidate (0.1, 0.3, and 0.5 mg/kg) twice daily for 2 weeks each (Table 25.1). Treatment effects were assessed with an extensive battery of parent-, teacher-, child-, and physician-completed rating scales and laboratory tasks. Immediate-release methylphenidate effectively suppressed ADHD, oppositional defiant disorder, and peer aggression behaviors. There was no evidence that immediate-release methylphenidate altered the overall severity of tic disorder or OCD. Teacher ratings indicated a decrease in tic frequency and severity.

In conclusion, methylphenidate appears to be a safe and effective short-term treatment for ADHD in the majority of children with chronic tic disorder.

Dextroamphetamine

Castellanos and colleagues (1997) conducted a crossover trial of 3 weeks to compare methylphenidate and dextroamphetamine to placebo on tic severity in boys with ADHD and TS or chronic tic disorder. Weekly dextroamphetamine doses were 7.5, 15, and 22.5 mg b.i.d. A significant decrease in hyperactivity was seen on ADHD measures. However, when the data from subjects who received high doses were combined, the overall effect of methylphenidate and dextroamphetamine were significant. Dextroamphetamine had a significantly greater effect than placebo upon tic severity, while the effect of methylphenidate on tic severity was indistinguishable from that of placebo. Long-term open follow-up of this study supported an advantage for methylphenidate: in contrast with five subjects taking dextroamphetamine at discharge, only one had an excellent long-term course. It is notable that summer and other briefer drug holidays produced consistent improvements in tic severity even in subjects whose tics were mild while taking stimulants.

Stimulants are generally considered to be safe medications, with few contraindications to their use. Side effects occur early in treatment and tend to be mild and short-lived (Graham & Coghill, 2008). The most common side effects are decreased appetite, abdominal pain or headache, delayed sleep onset, jitteriness, or social withdrawal. Most of these symptoms can be successfully managed by adjusting the dosage or schedule of medication.

The use of stimulant medications in patients with ADHD and chronic tic disorder remains a subject of debate. However, long-term treatment with methylphenidate is not associated with increases in tic severity (Gadow, 1999), and controlled clinical trials have not indicated a deterioration of tics in persons treated with stimulants (Bloch et al., 2009; Tourette Syndrome Study Group, 2002). The package insert warning that stimulant medications are contraindicated in children with preexisting tic disorders was based primarily on uncontrolled case reports and animal experiments using high doses of stimulants. Stimulant medications were reported to cause elevations of blood pressure. A small increase of mean heart rate was observed during treatment with stimulants (Vetter et al., 2008). Prolongation of the QT interval above 500 msec, sudden death, and increased heart rate have all been reported with methylphenidate and dextroamphetamine (Nissen, 2006). Significant QT prolongation is known to result in a risk of potentially fatal arrhythmias such as torsades de pointes (Noda et al. 2004). Pretreatment checking and monitoring of pulse, blood pressure, and ECG are recommended when stimulant medication is used in children with tics or TS and ADHD. If there may truly be a cardiac risk (e.g., congenital QT syndrome), the clinician should inform the patient and the family; a discussion of these aspects between the family, the neuropsychiatrist, and the cardiologist should help to refine the acceptability of the risk for the patient (Graham et al., 2011; Gulisano et al., 2011). The impact of stimulants on growth is a common concern; current data indicate that the initial reduction in both height and weight observed in some children (Faraone et al., 2008) appears to attenuate over time (Swanson et al., 2007).

In our opinion, stimulants should be the second choice of drugs, given the quicker onset of action of any of these agents, which may be particularly beneficial in children who need immediate improvement. Clinicians should begin with a low dose of medication and titrate upward. In addition, a short-acting preparation should be used in the first instance and subsequently once-a-day formulations, as there may be individual cases in which stimulants appear to exacerbate tics. If short-term dose reversal clearly indicates tic exacerbation, switching to another stimulant or a new drug class may be useful (Gadow, 2007). However, because tics are naturally waxing and waning, the "cause-and-effect"

interpretation of drug effects and clinical implications could be difficult (see also Chapter 24). Therefore, a long-term observation of at least 3 months is sometimes required before a clinical decision can be made, and in this case stimulants may be combined with an antipsychotic agent for tics. Finally, clinicians should avoid starting patients on two medications simultaneously (Roessner et al., 2011; Fig. 25.1).

SELECTIVE NOREPINEPHRINE REUPTAKE INHIBITORS: ATOMOXETINE

Atomoxetine is a relatively new, nonstimulant drug used to treat ADHD (Perwien et al., 2006). It acts as a presynaptic blocker of norepinephrine reuptake (Swanson et al., 2006). Unlike other medications used in ADHD, such as amphetamine and methylphenidate, atomoxetine has no appreciable affinity for dopamine receptors or the dopamine transporter. Although the nondopaminergic action of atomoxetine appears at first sight to contradict the dopamine hypothesis, it actually increases dopamine concentration specifically in the prefrontal cortex, because the norepinephrine transporter (NET) plays an important role in clearance of dopamine in this region. This regional specificity on dopamine function, plus a lower affinity for the serotonin (5-HT) transporter than methylphenidate, may account for differences in clinical effects (Swanson et al., 2006; Wickens et al., 2011). Compared to stimulants, atomoxetine has a relatively slow onset of action (day to weeks compared to minutes to hours; Biederman & Faraone, 2005).

Atomoxetine was shown to be a well-tolerated and efficacious treatment for ADHD in a double-blind, placebo-controlled study (Kelsey et al., 2004; Michelson et al., 2002; Spencer et al., 2002; Weiss et al., 2005).

The efficacy of atomoxetine in treating children with ADHD and comorbid TS or chronic tic disorder was examined in an 18-week parallel-group study of 148 children (age 7–17 years) that aimed to test the hypothesis that atomoxetine does not significantly worsen tic severity compared to placebo (Allen et al., 2005). In this large, industry-sponsored, multicenter study, patients were randomly assigned to double-blind treatment with placebo (n = 72) or atomoxetine (0.5–1.5 mg per day, n = 76). The primary efficacy measure for this study was the YGTSS total score, and secondary assessment measures included the ADHDRS-IV-Parent, CGI-Overall-S (a single-item rating of the clinician's assessment of both neurological and psychiatric symptom severity), and the CGI-ADHD/Psych-S (a subscale rating of the clinician's global assessment of the severity of ADHD and other psychiatric symptoms). On YGTSS total score, atomoxetine showed improvement at the endpoint compared to placebo, although this did not reach statistical significance. Atomoxetine led to greater improvement compared to the placebo group in the ADHDRS Parent total score (–10.9 vs. –4.9; $p < .001$) and in both the inattentive (–5.7 vs. –2.7; $p < .001$) and hyperactive/impulsive subscale scores (–5.2 vs. –2.1; $p < .001$); on the CGI-ADHD/Psych-S, both treatment groups showed improvement from baseline, but the difference in atomoxetine improvement relative to placebo was significant (–0.8 vs. 0.3; $p < .001$) (Table 25.1). Concerns were raised, however, that children with severe ADHD or tics might not have been enrolled in the study (Gilbert, 2006), which had a fairly high dropout rate in both the active (34%) and placebo (26%) arms. A *post hoc* subgroup analysis of the study by Allen and colleagues (2005) focusing specifically on those patients with TS comorbid with ADHD (79.1% of the original population; atomoxetine n = 61, placebo n = 56) showed that atomoxetine was effective in treating the symptoms of ADHD in these patients (ADHD-RS total score: 10.4 vs. 4.4 for placebo; $p = 0.027$). In addition, there was a significantly greater response to atomoxetine on the YGTSS (–5.1 vs. –2.0; $p = .027$) and the CGI-Tic/Neuro-S (–0.7 vs 0.0; $p = .003$) (Spencer et al., 2008).

Atomoxetine was reported to cause elevations of blood pressure. Controlled-trial data during atomoxetine administration showed elevations in blood pressure above the 95th percentile in 6.8% of patients (systolic) and 2.8% (diastolic), in comparison to 3% and 0.5%, respectively, of patients treated with placebo (Wernicke et al., 2003). Moreover, a small increase of heart rate

average was observed during the use of stimulant and nonstimulant medications (Vetter et al., 2008), with a small proportion of patients developing mean rate increases who were treated with atomoxetine (Wernicke et al., 2003). For these reasons, pretreatment checking and monitoring of pulse, blood pressure, and ECG are recommended also for nonstimulant medications in all children with tics or TS and ADHD. Spencer and colleagues (2005, 2007) evaluated, in a two-part study, atomoxetine's effect on growth during short- and long-term (i.e., up to 5 years) treatment and found a small effect for short-term treatment but no effect for long-term treatment. However, considering that there are few studies to allow firm conclusions to be drawn, physicians should monitor height, weight, and appetite at least once every 6 months in children and adolescents receiving this agent (Taylor et al., 2004). In a meta-analysis of adverse event data from the atomoxetine clinical trials database, Bangs and colleagues (2008) identified a statistically significant risk increase of suicidal thoughts among atomoxetine-treated patients compared with those taking placebo. Suicide-related events are rarely associated with stimulant treatment (Graham et al., 2011). Nonetheless, a detailed psychiatric history, with special attention to emotional and behavioral changes, is in any case recommended before prescribing these medications, and active monitoring to detect any emotional and behavioral changes should be pursued during treatment (Graham et al., 2011).

We therefore suggest that the third-line treatment should be atomoxetine, as it does not appear to worsen tics, although occasional case reports suggesting this exist and should not be neglected.

In their meta-analysis on the treatment of ADHD in children with comorbid tic disorder that included nine studies, Bloch and colleagues (2009) demonstrated that methylphenidate, alpha-2-agonists, atomoxetine, and desipramine have shown efficacy in treating ADHD symptoms. They also support the following conclusion from the Medical Advisory Board of Tourette USA (Scahill et al., 2006): "after a review of the alternatives and the family's preference, treatment may start with an alpha-2 agonist (guanfacine or clonidine) or stimulant medication. Combined treatment with an alpha-2 agonist and stimulant medications may produce better outcomes than either treatment alone." Pringsheim and Steeves (2011) conducted a Cochrane review on pharmacological treatment of ADHD in children with comorbid tic disorder that included eight randomized controlled studies. Three of these trials assessed multiple agents, including methylphenidate, clonidine, desipramine, dextroamphetamine, guanfacine, atomoxetine, and selegiline. Participants were children between 5 and 17 years of age with a diagnosis of ADHD and TS or chronic motor or vocal tic disorder based on DSM-III-R or DSM-IV-TR. All trials included both ADHD and tic outcomes. All studies used YGTSS as one measure of tic severity. The findings of this review suggested that there are a number of effective treatment options available to treat children with tic disorders and comorbid ADHD, including methylphenidate, alpha-2-agonists, desipramine, and atomoxetine. Pringsheim and Steeves (2011) concluded that, given the methodological difficulties inherent in comparing effect size across studies with divergent inclusion criteria, efficacy measures, and designs, the review did not provide evidence-based recommendations for choosing between treatment options.

Beyond the comparison of efficacy of the available ADHD and TS medications, there is now a greater focus on safety concerns, and pharmaceutical manufacturers are required to provide patients with detailed medication guides. Further research is needed to provide guidelines regarding the challenges of combination therapy. The safety of ADHD medications is not fully known. The risk/benefit ratio of treatment is seen as favorable in most cases, but with a caveat that there are several areas of uncertainty about the nature of these risks. We recommend that clinicians be vigilant for side effects throughout treatment. Clinicians should also review over time the need for pharmacological treatment in each patient. Often the value of washout becomes clear in patients treated as children or adolescents before their brains have matured, while using street drugs, or in the midst of a hormonal storm. Yet many of these patients are never taken off their medications to see whether they are still necessary once psychological and neurophysiological maturity is completed (Hoffman et al., 2011).

FUTURE TREATMENT APPROACHES

Drug candidates in the late stages of development for ADHD treatment tend to be marked by the application of formulation technologies to existing drugs. Pharmaceutical companies have applied a range of formulation technologies (bead formulations, slow-release matrices, and transdermal patches) to methylphenidate or amphetamine to produce novel, once-daily medications. In the search for alternative pharmacological approaches, drug candidates have been evaluated with a wide diversity of mechanisms, many of which act as modulators of catecholaminergic function in the central nervous system, or acting on various novel molecular targets have been evaluated to determine their efficacy and safety as potential ADHD medications.

Genetic and neurobiological studies of ADHD support the strong role of dysfunctional catecholamine neurotransmission in the presentation of the disorder (Pliszka, 2005). The majority of the research into the neurobiology of ADHD has targeted the dopaminergic system as the main neurotransmitter responsible for the disorder. Thus, one of the first genes shown to be associated with ADHD was the dopamine receptor D4 (DRD4; Li et al., 2006). Less emphasis has been placed on serotonin (5-HT), although studies have shown that 5-HT has a modulating effect on the dopaminergic system (Hawi et al., 2002). It has been established that 5-HT is involved in behavioral disinhibition, including aggression and impulsivity (Quist et al., 2003). Eltoprazine hydrochloride, a serotonergic agent under development, was recently investigated in a clinical trial in adult ADHD patients; in the limited research conducted in this population, it appeared to show efficacy and tolerability (Wigal & Duong, 2011).

Several nonselective monoamine reuptake inhibitors have been explored in ADHD, although for four of them (DOV102677, GSK372475,

(R)-Sibutramine, and SPD473) development has been interrupted, mostly for lack of efficacy, suggesting that this type of pharmacological approach is not appropriate for the treatment of ADHD (Heal et al., 2011). Development of nicotinic receptor agonists (pozanicicline, sofinicline, lobeline) also received great attention; however, the available data suggest that nicotinic alpha-4/beta-2 receptor agonists are unlikely to provide a significant advance in pharmacotherapy (Heal et al., 2011; Wilens et al., 2006). Histamine H3 antagonists and AMPA receptor modulators are in clinical evaluation for ADHD. As highlighted also in Chapters 7 and 13, histaminergic neurotransmission may also be involved in the pathobiology of TS. Preliminary clinical data indicate that none of these compounds has comparable efficacy to the stimulants or provides adequate safety (Heal et al., 2011).

OCD

The literature indicates that OCD and TS are closely related, although the percentage of patients with TS who also show OCD varies from 11% to 80% (Cavanna et al., 2009). The reason for these discrepancies in the rate of comorbidity between OCD and TS is difficult to ascertain: one of the causes could stem from the fact that there is no agreement regarding categorization of a series of repetitive behaviors, which are frequently present in TS patients and are also referred to as "impulsions" or "tic-like compulsions." Controversy exists over whether they are manifestations of OCD or rather represent complex tics (Worbe et al., 2010; see also Chapters 3 and 17).

To our knowledge, no clinical trial has specifically evaluated the treatment of obsessive-compulsive symptoms in TS patients. Therefore, the main source of information about the treatment of OCD in patients with chronic tics or TS is drawn from the small number of clinical trials on efficacy of anti-obsessional drugs that have also included patients with tics and compared their clinical effects in OCD subjects with and without tics. The paucity of similar studies has been due to the fact that earlier double-blind, randomized clinical trials of treatment with selective serotonin reuptake inhibitors (SSRIs) for OCD have used numerous exclusion criteria for study entry. Most studies have excluded subjects with comorbid TS or ADHD. In addition, all studies have excluded subjects with comorbid primary mood and psychotic disorders, most have excluded patients with eating and pervasive developmental disorders, and some have even excluded patients with non-OCD anxiety disorders (for a comprehensive list, see Geller et al., 2003a). However, comorbid psychopathology is the rule and not the exception in patients with OCD, mainly in youth, even in nonspecialized settings. Therefore, the common use of exclusionary criteria in all randomized controlled trials of anti-obsessional medications over the past two decades raises questions as to how well the results of these studies may generalize to naturalistic clinical samples of children and adolescents with OCD (Geller et al., 2003a).

The results of the clinical trials that have compared the efficacy of serotonin reuptake inhibitor (SRI) treatment in OCD patients with and without tics are particularly useful for the management of TS subjects with prominent OCD symptoms. In fact, the main entry criterion in these studies was the diagnosis of OCD as defined in the DSM-IV-R. At the same time, all guidelines and reviews on the treatment of TS agree on the need for a careful assessment of patients in order to identify target symptoms that are interfering with the patient's quality of life, and thereby to plan a therapeutic strategy.

OCD Treatment

OCD was considered until the mid-1960s to be resistant to treatment with both psychodynamic psychotherapy and medication. Nonetheless, due to lack of alternatives, psychodynamic psychotherapy continued to be administered to patients with OCD despite limited clinical benefit. At present, it is widely recognized that, for OCD, psychodynamic approaches have limited evidence to justify their use. With regard to psychodynamic therapy and psychoanalysis, one of the most current expert guidelines notes that "there is doubt as to whether it has a place in mental health services for OCD" at all (NICE, 2006).

In the following years, several behavioral interventions were developed to alleviate OCD-related distress, with varying degrees of success. Systematic desensitization and aversion therapy were used in OCD with limited or no success. The first real breakthrough came in the mid-1960s, when Meyer (1966) described two patients successfully treated with a behavioral therapy program that included prolonged exposure to distressing objects and situations, combined with strict prevention of rituals— exposure and ritual prevention (EX/RP). Since then, the efficacy of EX/RP and its durability in reducing OCD symptom severity have been established, as demonstrated by results from numerous studies. Cognitive therapy is another behavioral approach designed to help patients to identify obsessional thoughts and change their interpretations, in order to decrease anxiety levels and decrease compulsive behaviors.

DRUG TREATMENT

Parallel to the development of effective cognitive-behavioral therapy (CBT) for OCD, there was a development of medication treatment for the disorder. The first case report indicating that the tricyclic antidepressant clomipramine might have some benefit in patients with OCD was published more than 40 years ago (Fernandez-Cordoba et al., 1967). Since then, clomipramine has been studied thoroughly, and it was the first drug approved by the FDA for the treatment of OCD. Clomipramine acts by inhibiting the reuptake of norepinephrine and serotonin, but serotonin inhibition is more pronounced. The selectivity of clomipramine for serotonin led to the hypothesis that a serotonin deficit is responsible for obsessive-compulsive symptoms. This hypothesis also gave impetus to the study of SSRIs in OCD, in the hope that those agents would be more efficacious and better tolerated than clomipramine.

Monotherapy with SRIs In the past decade, several meta-analyses of short-term treatment studies of adult OCD patients have been published. Early meta-analyses suggested that both SSRIs and clomipramine were more effective

than placebo. It is remarkable that, when the data for clomipramine were compared with the SSRIs, the former generally had greater effect sizes. However, head-to-head studies have found similar efficacy for clomipramine and SSRIs. This may partly be explained by the fact that clomipramine studies were typically conducted earlier, patients were treatment-naive, and placebo response was low. In contrast, the SSRI studies may have included patients who had previously failed to respond to other agents, and placebo responses were higher (Decloedt & Stein, 2010).

A recent Cochrane review analyzed efficacy and tolerability in OCD, comparing the different molecules (Soomro et al., 2008). The SSRIs of interest were fluoxetine, fluvoxamine, sertraline, paroxetine, and citalopram. Seventeen studies were included in the review, involving 3,097 participants. Based on all 17 studies, SSRIs as a group were more effective than placebo in reducing the symptoms of OCD, measured using the Yale-Brown Obsessive Compulsive Scale (Y-BOCS), between 6 and 13 weeks after treatment. The weighted mean differences for individual SSRIs were similar and not statistically significant. Based on 13 studies (2,697 participants), SSRIs were more effective than placebo in achieving clinical response after treatment. The pooled relative risk was shown to be similar between individual SSRI drugs.

Similarly, a systematic review of long-term medication studies in OCD showed that agents that are effective in short-term treatment are typically effective also during long-term treatment (Fineberg & Gale, 2005). For example, studies of clomipramine, escitalopram, fluoxetine, and sertraline showed that treatment effect was maintained beyond 12 weeks. Relapse prevention trials also showed significant advantages for patients remaining on medication. Thus, evidence does not support superior efficacy of clomipramine over SSRIs, or of one SSRI over the others, with different tolerability and drug interaction profiles.

The efficacy of many of these agents has been shown also in pediatric OCD. Clinically significant reductions in OCD symptoms have been documented in children and adolescents using the SRI clomipramine and the SSRIs sertraline, fluoxetine, paroxetine, and fluvoxamine. Up to now, at least 21 studies reporting on medication experience in OCD and including over 1,300 pediatric subjects have been published. All showed that serotonergic medications are effective in the short- and medium-term treatment of OCD (Mancuso et al., 2010).

The suggested duration of an adequate trial of a serotonin reuptake inhibitor in OCD is no less than 10 to 12 weeks, with at least 4 weeks at the maximally tolerated dose. However, there is some disagreement regarding what constitutes an adequate dose. Some but not all fixed-dose trials of SSRIs indicate that higher doses are significantly superior to lower doses in treating OCD. In a meta-analysis examining differences in efficacy and tolerability between different doses of SSRIs, Bloch and colleagues (2010) observed that higher doses of SSRIs are associated with greater efficacy on OCD symptoms, although with a worse side-effect profile. However, caution is warranted because it not clear that the conclusions of this meta-analysis can be generalized to all patients with pediatric-onset OCD and comorbid tics.

MANAGEMENT OF TREATMENT-RESISTANT OCD

Despite the clinical improvement provided by the pharmacological treatment of OCD with clomipramine or SSRIs, nearly half of all patients do not respond completely. Furthermore, even among responders, few become asymptomatic. The profiles of nonresponders are difficult to cluster due to ambiguities in diagnostic criteria, the possibility of subtypes, and high rates of comorbidity. Moreover, the findings of current studies of the so-called nonresponsive cases currently cannot be generalized because of the lack of an operational definition for nonresponders.

These findings have given rise to studies aimed at identifying factors responsible for poor or no response to SRI or SSRI treatment and a search for alternative strategies. Taking into consideration the previous methodological issues, various strategies have been proposed: (1) increasing doses; (2) switching to another drug; (3) augmentation strategies; and (4) novel treatments.

A small number of uncontrolled case reports suggested that OCD patients who had tolerated maximal doses of an SSRI without adverse effects could benefit from further increasing the dose beyond formulary limits. However, their symptom scores remained higher than those of a less treatment-resistant group of patients receiving standard doses over a similar time period, suggesting enduring treatment resistance (Pampaloni et al., 2010).

The results of a series of clinical trials showed that SSRIs have equivalent efficacy in the treatment of OCD. In particular, a meta-analysis of studies on treatment of pediatric OCD patients showed that the SSRIs were statistically indistinguishable from each other with respect to overall effect (Geller et al., 2003a). However, a large degree of intersubject variability in response to individual SSRIs is actually observed in clinical practice. Hence, a decision to use a specific one may depend more on adverse-event profiles and individual pharmacokinetic properties than on efficacy. Accordingly, other possibilities in the pharmacotherapy of resistant OCD are sequential trials of different SSRIs. However, the likelihood of experiencing a response to one SSRI diminishes with each consecutively failed trial. Obviously, if the patient does not tolerate one specific SSRI, it is advisable to try a different one, selected on the basis of the expected side-effect profile (Goodman et al., 2006). No randomized trials have been carried out on this topic in OCD patients, either adults or children.

Evidence of the potential involvement of the dopamine system in OCD gave impetus to the study of whether antipsychotics could augment SSRIs in the treatment of the disorder. In 2006, Bloch and colleagues conducted a systematic review of previous studies on antipsychotic augmentation in treatment-refractory OCD. Only randomized clinical trials that were conducted in a double-blind manner were included in the analysis. The author identified and selected nine studies. All of the selected studies included only adult OCD patients, with a total of 278 OCD patients (143 receiving antipsychotic augmentation and 135 receiving placebo augmentation).

The analyses gave the following results. Treatment response was significantly more likely in the antipsychotic augmentation group than in the placebo augmentation group (treatment response rates of 32% and 11%, respectively). Haloperidol and risperidone augmentation demonstrated significant efficacy compared to placebo, whereas quetiapine and olanzapine augmentation failed to demonstrate efficacy. There was no evidence suggesting a treatment effect of antipsychotic augmentation in OCD patients who received less than 12 weeks of maximal SRI treatment; this might have been due to the high rate of treatment response (25.6%) to continued SRI monotherapy among these subjects, compared to 4.3% in those receiving maximal SRI monotherapy for 12 weeks or longer. There was no difference in the number of dropouts in the antipsychotic augmentation versus placebo augmentation arms of included randomized controlled clinical trials. A more recent meta-analysis of double-blind, randomized, placebo-controlled trials on the efficacy of antipsychotic augmentation therapy in treatment-resistant OCD (Dolt el al., 2011) substantially confirmed these results.

Based on the reported efficacy of aripiprazole alone or added to SSRIs or clomipramine in treatment-resistant OCD, a 16-week, double-blind, randomized, placebo-controlled trial was performed to explore the efficacy of aripiprazole (15 mg/day) add-on pharmacotherapy on clinical symptoms and cognitive functioning in a sample of 30 adults with treatment-resistant OCD receiving SSRIs (Muscatello et al., 2011). Results indicated that aripiprazole added to stable SSRI treatment substantially improved obsessive-compulsive symptoms (OCS) as measured by changes on the Y-BOCS total scores and subscores. Regarding cognitive functioning, improvement was observed in some areas, such as attentional resistance to interference and executive functioning. In another single-blind, randomized study comparing the efficacy of aripiprazole and risperidone as augmenting agents in adults with treatment-resistant OCD, half of all patients exhibited a treatment response to aripiprazole augmentation. However, a significantly higher response rate was found with risperidone than aripiprazole (Selvi et al., 2011).

Beside antipsychotics, other drugs have been tested in augmentation strategies in OCD patients, including agents that modulate the serotonin system (e.g., tryptophan, lithium, and buspirone). A Cochrane review of the pharmacotherapy of treatment-resistant anxiety disorder concluded that more than twice as many patients with treatment-resistant OCD respond to pharmacotherapy augmentation with various drugs than to placebo; however, a substantial proportion of the efficacy evidence was for augmentation with antipsychotic agents (Ipser et al., 2006). Two recent clinical trials investigated the effects on adults with resistant OCD of augmentation with topiramate, with mixed results (Berlin et al., 2011; Mowla et al., 2010). Information regarding augmentation of SRIs with stimulants is limited and has provided mixed results. While some suggest that dextroamphetamine may be effective in reducing symptoms (Koran et al., 2009), case studies point to stimulant treatment leading to worsening of symptoms.

Novel therapeutic approaches are derived from clinical, translational, and basic research. The focus on association at common polymorphisms in several serotonin transmitter system genes has shifted to include interest in glutamatergic mechanisms and the glutamate transporter gene SLC1A1 (Arnold et al., 2006). For example, approaches manipulating glutamatergic, gamma-amino-butyric acid (GABA)-ergic, and peptide neurotransmitter pathways are under way and will likely be informed by genome-wide association studies. Numerous glutamatergic modulating agents are being tested in the treatment of OCD, but at the moment none of these meets minimal evidence-based standards that permit recommendation for their routine use.

Riluzole is believed to reduce glutamate release in the brain via multiple presynaptic mechanisms. The results of several trials with riluzole have been remarkably consistent, with roughly half of the patients treated thus far experiencing significant treatment response. Memantine, a noncompetitive N-methyl-d-aspartic acid (NMDA) receptor antagonist, has exhibited positive effects in treatment-resistant OCD. In a single-blinded case-control study augmenting intensive residential treatment with memantine, responders showed clinically significant improvement; however, only 36% of patients were found to be responders (Stewart et al., 2010), raising the possibility of a subtype of OCD for which this approach is beneficial. Amantadine is structurally and functionally related to memantine and has recently been shown to inhibit marble burying in mice. Consistent with glutamatergic interventions, glycine, an NMDA glutamate receptor agonist, has proved to be efficacious in the treatment of OCD in several studies. N-acetyl-cysteine (NAC) augmentation of SRI treatment resulted in decreased symptoms in a single OCD case or in open-label studies. Such findings require replication before they can be generalized, and a double-blind, placebo-controlled study is under way at the National Institute of Mental Health. d-Cycloserine, a partial agonist of NMDA, has been found to enhance extinction effects in combination with exposure-based behavioral therapy (Wilhelm et al., 2008). A meta-analysis of d-cycloserine augmentation of CBT in adults suggests efficacy (Norberg et al., 2008), and a pilot randomized controlled trial in children also showed promising results (Storch et al., 2010). Overall, Bhattacharyya and Chakraborty (2007) concluded that glutamatergic dysfunction is a relevant novel target for anti-OCS drugs.

Opiate drugs for treatment-refractory OCD have recently been explored. One study found evidence to support the convergent effects of the serotoninergic and opiate systems in brain areas (Rojas-Corrales et al., 2007). In adults, morphine was shown to be effective and well tolerated in a treatment-refractory OCD population, but given its potential for abuse, such approaches are unlikely to be useful in children (Koran et al., 2005).

Based on the discovery of the role of orbitofrontal cortex in OCD from functional imaging studies, repetitive transcranial magnetic stimulation is being explored as a noninvasive and safe treatment approach. Although repetitive transcranial magnetic stimulation treatment of OCD has not been studied extensively, nor focused on a specific brain region, one study found that magnetic stimulation of the left orbitofrontal cortex showed short-term improvement

of OCS in adults, with symptom reduction lasting up to 10 weeks (Ruffini et al., 2009).

SSRI MONOTHERAPY IN OCD PATIENTS WITH AND WITHOUT TICS

In a retrospective study in adults, McDougle and colleagues (1993) studied 33 OCD patients with tics treated for 8 weeks with fluvoxamine, and compared them with 33 age- and sex-matched OCD patients without tics who received the same treatment. Criteria for treatment response of OCS to fluvoxamine included (1) 35% or greater improvement in the Y-BOCS score from the beginning of treatment trial and a final Y-BOCS score of less than 16; (2) a final Clinical Global Impression (CGI) rating of "much" or "very much improved"; and (3) the consensus of two of the primary investigators. In both groups, fluvoxamine treatment was associated with a statistically significant improvement in scores on the Y-BOCS (17% decrease in OCD+tics patients, 32% decrease in OCD-alone patients). There were statistically significant differences between OCD patients with and without tics also on the final CGI rating. In addition, on the basis of the treatment response criteria, 21% of OCD patients with comorbid chronic tic disorders responded to fluvoxamine, compared with 52% of OCD patients without tics.

Recently Husted and colleagues (2007) replicated the McDougle and colleagues' work, carrying out an 8-week prospective open-label trial of fluoxetine in adults with OCD, investigating whether SSRI monotherapy was an effective treatment of OCD in patients with tics and, if so, whether it was equally efficacious in OCD patients with tics as in OCD patients without tics. This open-label fluoxetine treatment was part of a randomized, placebo-controlled trial of fluoxetine plus placebo versus fluoxetine plus olanzapine for subjects who were either partial responders or nonresponders to 8 weeks of treatment with fluoxetine (Shapira et al., 2004). Of the 74 subjects overall, 15 subjects withdrew from the 8-week study, 44 were partial or nonresponders to fluoxetine, and 15 were full responders to fluoxetine. The results demonstrated a significant response over time in both OCD subjects with tics (29% decrease in Y-BOCS score) and those without tics (34% decrease) when treated with fluoxetine over the 8-week period. The two study groups did not differ statistically from each other in terms of mean decrease in Y-BOCS scores. In terms of a clinically meaningful improvement, the treatment responses of the two study groups did not differ statistically from each other. In contrast, when evaluating the number of subjects with at least a 25% decrease in Y-BOCS scores, there were 70.5% subjects without tics versus only 38.5% in the study subjects with tics. Interestingly, although study subjects were taking no psychotropic other than fluoxetine, there was a significant decrease in YGTSS scores from baseline to week 8 for OCD subjects with tics.

In pediatric OCD, Geller and colleagues (2003b) found that coexisting ADHD or chronic tic disorder was associated with a lower response rate to SSRIs compared with OCD alone. The data were derived *post hoc* from a previously reported 32-week, multicenter, double-phase study of the safety, efficacy, and long-term maintenance of efficacy of paroxetine in 335 children and adolescents with OCD. The first phase was a 16-week, open-label, flexible-dose study. Patients achieving a therapeutic response, defined as 25% or more improvement in baseline CY-BOCS total score and a Clinical Global Impression–Improvement Scale (CGI-I) score of 1 (very much improved) or 2 (much improved) at week 16, were eligible to participate in the second phase. This was a 16-week, double-blind, placebo-controlled withdrawal phase in which patients were randomly assigned (1:1) to continue paroxetine or to placebo substitution. Three hundred thirty-five children and adolescents with OCD as their predominant psychiatric diagnosis were included in the first phase (open-label), and 193 (paroxetine = 95, placebo = 98) entered the second phase (double-blind). At study entry, most patients (193/335, 58%) had at least one comorbid psychiatric illness, and the most common comorbid disorders were generalized anxiety disorder (20%), ADHD (19%), specific phobia (16%), tic disorder (15%), separation anxiety disorder (10%), dysthymia (8%), oppositional defiant disorder (8%), and major

depressive disorder (6%). The mean CY-BOCS total score was reduced from 26.3 at baseline to 13.0 at the endpoint of the first phase. Almost 71% of patients met the responsiveness criteria. Response rates in OCD subjects with comorbid ADHD (56%), tic disorder (53%), and oppositional defiant disorder (39%) were all associated with a significantly lower likelihood of response compared to the total patient group (71%). At the end of the second phase, the overall relapse rate was approximately 10% greater in the placebo group than in the paroxetine group (43.9% vs. 34.7%, respectively). This difference increased with the number of comorbid disorders present: 20% greater relapse in placebo subjects for any (one or more) and 30% greater relapse in placebo subjects for multiple (two or more) comorbid diagnoses. For the placebo group but not the paroxetine group, any (one or more) and multiple (two or more) comorbid disorders were associated with a significantly higher rate of relapse compared with subjects without comorbid illnesses.

More recently, March and colleagues (2007) examined the potential effect of tic comorbidity on the treatment of children and adolescents with OCD. Using data from the Pediatric OCD Treatment Study (POTS, 2004), the authors found an interaction between tic comorbidities and the difference between the effects of sertraline and placebo on OCD symptom severity. A sample of 112 subjects ages 7 to 17, including a primary DSM-IV diagnosis of OCD, entered the multisite study. Seventeen of the 112 patients (15.2%) exhibited either TS or a chronic motor tic disorder. Combined treatment, CBT and sertraline, proved significantly superior to placebo; combined treatment was significantly superior to CBT and to sertraline; and CBT was significantly superior to sertraline. These analyses replicated the previously published intent-to-treat outcomes, which were ordered as follows: combined treatment > CBT > sertraline > placebo (POTS, 2004). The posttreatment CY-BOCS score mean (SD) was slightly lower for patients with (15.5) than for those without (17.0) a tic disorder; the main effect of tic disorder was not statistically significant, whereas the tic disorder/treatment interaction term was statistically significant. Only the comparison between sertraline and placebo showed a statistically significant shift in presence of comorbid tic disorder: specifically, sertraline did not differ from placebo in the presence of comorbid tic disorder but was superior to placebo in the absence of comorbid tic disorder. Hence, the tic disorder/treatment interaction appeared to arise from a reduction in magnitude of the impact of sertraline on OCD symptoms when tics were also present.

AUGMENTATION STRATEGIES IN OCD PATIENTS WITH AND WITHOUT TICS

The first study on augmentation strategy in OCD patients with and without a comorbid chronic tic disorder refractory to adequate SSRI monotherapy was that by McDougle and colleagues (1994). Sixty-two patients with a primary diagnosis of OCD received fluvoxamine for 8 weeks: 34 of them were refractory to fluvoxamine and were randomized in a double-blind fashion to 4 weeks of treatment with either haloperidol or placebo, as add-on to fluvoxamine. Haloperidol augmentation was significantly better than placebo in reducing the severity of OCS measured by the Y-BOCS; 11 of 17 patients responded to haloperidol, but none responded to placebo; also, all 8 patients with comorbid chronic tic disorders responded to double-blind haloperidol add-on augmentation, showing also a significant reduction in tic frequency as measured by the YGTSS. On the other hand, haloperidol augmentation was of little benefit in treating OCD patients without tics.

In the above-mentioned systematic review of studies on antipsychotic augmentation in treatment-refractory OCD, Bloch and colleagues (2006) identified five of nine selected trials that included OCD subjects with a comorbid tic disorder. Apart from the above-mentioned study by McDougle and colleagues (1994) that reported a significantly increased rate of response to antipsychotic augmentation in OCD patients with comorbid tics, none of the four subsequent studies confirmed this, likely due to their small sample sizes. Nonetheless, OCD patients with comorbid tic disorders overall seemed to experience a better response than OCD patients without comorbid tics.

NON-OCD ANXIETY DISORDERS

Although the majority of studies on TS comorbidity have focused on OCD, the literature suggests that other anxiety disorders may also complicate the clinical course of TS. In fact, elevated rates of trait anxiety, phobias, generalized anxiety disorder, and separation anxiety have been described in people with TS (Coffey et al., 1992; Cohen & Leckman, 1994; Comings & Comings, 1987b; Robertson et al., 1993; see for details Chapter 4).

Whereas comorbidity with OCD has long been recognized as being associated with a more severe TS phenotype (Bornstein, 1991; Comings & Comings, 1987c; Leonard et al., 1992), we have limited knowledge of the role of non-OCD anxiety disorders in TS patients. Since non-OCD anxiety disorders encompass a wide range of conditions that can also be associated with morbidity and dysfunction, it is important to clarify the impact of these comorbid conditions on the clinical picture of TS. In a study of anxiety disorders and tic severity in children and adolescents (Coffey et al., 2000) separation anxiety was found to be most predictive of tic severity. Furthermore, anxiety was found to be overrepresented in patients with severe TS.

If it is true that non-OCD anxiety disorders influence tic severity, there are important clinical implications, since anxiety disorders require a different treatment strategy than that used for tics. Thus, clarification of this issue could facilitate the development of more appropriate intervention strategies for affected patients. Evidence that severe tics could be anxiety-mediated is supported in the typical exacerbation of tics that occurs in children with TS before they return to school, and in the tic-ameliorative effects of the high-potency benzodiazepine anxiolytic clonazepam (Borison et al., 1982; Goetz, 1992). The alpha-adrenergic agonist clonidine and tricyclic antidepressants such as desipramine may also ameliorate tics through their putative anxiolytic effect (Bruun, 1982b; Leckman et al., 1991; Singer et al., 1995). Considering the documented anxiogenic effects of neuroleptics in TS patients (Bruun, 1982a; Linet, 1985), it is possible to speculate that increased doses of neuroleptics during periods of tic exacerbation may render the patient more susceptible to anxiety, and thus more likely to experience increased tics. On the other hand, in clinical practice, a better control of tics following an increase of the dose of neuroleptics often leads to a reduction of anxious symptoms.

It is worth noting that patients with anxiety comorbidity exhibit greater OCS severity than patients with OCD alone, particularly in the domain of compulsions. This suggests a possible synergistic effect whereby OCD symptoms are exacerbated or exaggerated by the presence of comorbid symptoms. One possible explanation for this relationship is that comorbid symptoms (e.g., mood instability, inattention, behavioral outbursts, interpersonal problems) promote increased stress, which the patient may attempt to manage by increasing engagement into compulsive rituals.

So, when planning the treatment strategy for patients with comorbidities, the most impairing disorder in each child should be taken into special consideration. Moreover, the treatment strategy should be determined by distinguishing between children who experience anxiety secondary to their tics and those with a primary anxiety disorder that might be worsening their tic symptoms. In every case, research on the course of anxiety disorders indicates the importance of intervening early to address symptoms of anxiety, whether primary or secondary to TS.

Traditional approaches to anxiety disorders in childhood were predominantly psychological. Few controlled studies assessing the efficacy of such treatment modalities are available (Target & Fonagy, 1994), but studies of cognitive-behavioral strategies in adolescent anxiety disorders are encouraging (Kendall et al., 1997). The results of a Cochrane review of CBT for pediatric anxiety disorders (James et al., 2005), as well as behavioral therapy and CBT for OCD in children and adolescents (O'Kearney et al., 2006), also emphasize a role for this treatment modality. Interestingly, the patients with only anxiety disorder comorbidity did not significantly differ from those with "pure" OCD with regard to treatment response, suggesting that CBT for OCD is not negatively

influenced by the presence of other anxiety symptoms (Storch et al., 2010).

The perception of pediatric anxiety disorders as the initial manifestation of the same disorders found in adults (Kessler et al., 2007) is consistent with expert consensus that SSRIs should be regarded as first-line agents in treating anxiety disorders in both children/adolescents and adults. Sertraline, fluoxetine, and fluvoxamine have all been approved by the FDA for the treatment of pediatric OCD. SSRIs have also been compared favorably to other medications in treating pediatric anxiety disorders: these drugs typically cause fewer side effects and a longer treatment effect than tricyclic antidepressants, and they do not present the risk of dependency associated with benzodiazepines. Nevertheless, the need for systematic comparison of the risk/benefit profiles of the different medication classes in treating pediatric anxiety disorders is highlighted by concerns that the benefits of certain SSRIs in treating depression do not outweigh the risks associated with their use among patients under 18 years of age (MHRA, 2003).

DISRUPTIVE BEHAVIORS

Many people with TS, or at least many clinically referred patients, report disruptive behavioral symptoms characterized by sudden and unpredictable anger, irritability, temper outbursts, self-injurious behavior (SIB), and aggression. In many patients these symptoms are intertwined with each other and with OCD and ADHD symptoms, and this contributes to the typical phenotypic variability of TS. However, because these symptoms have not been systematically evaluated, their etiology and true prevalence within the TS population is unknown. These symptoms are often a leading cause of dysfunction and disability and result in increased family distress, maladaptive educational and/or occupational functioning, interpersonal conflicts, and increased rates of psychiatric hospitalization. However, there are relatively few studies investigating the treatment of these highly disruptive symptoms in TS. In fact, many reports are open-label trials in relatively small group of patients or single case reports; hence, most of the therapeutic advice for clinicians derives from studies of treatment of the same symptoms in other neuropsychiatric conditions. Moreover, it is not known if the treatment of these symptoms in TS patients implies the same problems already seen for ADHD or OCD.

SIB

Despite its prevalence, SIB is probably one of the least studied among the comorbidities of TS. Gilles de la Tourette noted SIB in three of the nine patients in his initial description of the disorder. More recent studies report that 25% to 50% of clinically referred individuals with TS exhibit SIB, although estimates vary depending on the definition of self-injury (Robertson et al., 1989). Generally speaking, SIB is a feature of some genetic disorders, such as Lesch-Nyhan syndrome, and a wide variety of psychiatric disorders, including mental retardation, schizophrenia, borderline personality disorder, pervasive developmental disorders, and stereotypic movement disorder. Depending on the criteria and methods used, estimates of the prevalence of SIB range from 400 to 1,400 per 100,000 population (Favazza, 1998). Thus, SIB seems to be a heterogeneous disorder and, like other behaviorally defined disorders, it is reasonable to assume that SIB can be the consequence of a variety of etiologies, which in turn involve a variety of environment–brain–behavior relationships (Schroeder et al., 2001). Consequently, a number of biological and behavioral models have emerged in the past two decades. Neurobiological models of SIB have identified roles for opiatergic (Sandman, 1988; Sandman et al., 1990, 1991), dopaminergic (Breese et al., 1989), and serotonergic (Cook & Leventhal, 1996) systems in the pathophysiology of SIB.

From a clinical point of view, a systematic delineation of self-injury from other types of self-harming behavior is necessary for the establishment of reliable research on the prevalence, explanation, and management of these behaviors. In the majority of studies, SIB is defined as any socially unaccepted behavior involving deliberate and direct injury to one's own body surface without suicidal intent. Many researchers and clinicians have attempted to categorize self-injury using different dimensions, but there is currently no consistent classification system. The most widely used schema divides SIB into four major categories: stereotypic, major, compulsive, and impulsive. However, the available studies on SIB in TS divide SIB simply into moderate and severe categories. Moderate SIB includes behaviors that result in moderate tissue damage, such as skin picking or scratching that leads to profuse bleeding, scarring, or infections requiring antibiotic treatment. Severe SIB includes extreme self-injurious or mutilating behaviors that lead to permanent, potentially impairing sequelae, such as self-cutting, deliberate eye enucleation, or castration. However, the majority of studies examining SIB in TS have not differentiated severe from mild to moderate types of SIB, which may account for the high prevalence estimates and the variability across studies. Recently, Cheung and colleagues (2007) proposed a new category, "malignant TS," for those cases in which TS and its comorbid behavioral symptoms can result in potentially life-threatening outcomes due to the result of severe tics, extreme rage attacks, depression with suicidal ideation, and disabling SIB. This categorization is based on the consequences of different behaviors (tics, OCD, SIB, rage attacks) rather than on clinical symptoms or pathophysiological mechanisms and is therefore relatively unhelpful for treatment purposes.

Retrospective cohort studies have suggested that SIB in TS is correlated with severity of tic symptoms and high levels of obsessionality and hostility as measured by a number of subjective rating scales (Robertson et al., 1989). The largest study to date, a retrospective assessment of 3,500 individuals with TS from all over the world, found that SIB was present in 14% of cases (range 4–43%). Individuals who had TS plus at least one other psychiatric comorbidity had a fourfold increase in SIB, and there was a positive linear relationship between the number of psychiatric comorbidities and the presence of SIB (Freeman et al., 2000). SIB in other neuropsychiatric disorders appears to be related to problems in impulse control. Impulse dysregulation is seen in a number of neuropsychiatric disorders that affect children with TS, including ADHD, depression, and bipolar disorder. However, despite evidence for impulse dysregulation in ADHD and mood disorders, previous studies in TS have indicated that SIB is not correlated with the presence of either of these syndromes alone. The major source of data on SIB in TS is the study by Mathews and colleagues (2004), who retrospectively examined the relationship between SIB and other behavioral features in nearly 300 subjects with TS participating in three genetic studies. Unexpectedly, they found little overlap in the predictors for SIB and those for severe SIB. For SIB, the most important predictor variables appeared to be related to OCS. Contrary to the study hypothesis, impulse/affect dysregulation was not significantly correlated with SIB. For severe SIB, the opposite was true: the most important predictor variables were related not to OCS, but to tic severity and to the strongest clinical indicators of lack of impulse control (rages and risk-taking behaviors). These findings suggested that SIB and severe SIB may be different phenomena and could have some implication on the treatment of SIB of TS patients. If it is true that mild SIB in TS is primarily compulsive, for example, the optimal treatment for behaviors such as persistent skin picking may be the treatments traditionally reserved for OCD, including the use of SSRIs, perhaps in conjunction with atypical antipsychotics, and CBT directed specifically at reducing the behavior. Serotonergic agents have proved to be effective in reducing SIB in mental retardation and in autism, as have the atypical neuroleptics. These medications have also been found to be helpful in disorders thought to be related to TS, OCD, and SIB, such as trichotillomania and skin picking (Schroeder et al, 2001).

Severe SIB presents a more difficult problem, and can be approached in two ways. Nonrepetitive forms of severe SIB, such as those commonly seen in patients with mood disorders or personality disorders, appear to be related to problems with impulse or affective dysregulation, and may be most effectively treated as such with mood stabilizers. It has been shown that in adults with severe, long-lasting SIB and aggression, agents such as divalproex and gabapentin have been effective in reducing SIB. For severe repetitive SIB such as repeated eye poking or very severe skin picking, on the other hand, the opiate blocker naltrexone may be the treatment of choice; indeed, severe repetitive SIB is hypothesized by some to be caused by abnormalities in sensation at the body site, perhaps due to dysregulation in the opiate (endorphin/encephalin) system. Symons and colleagues (2004) comprehensively reviewed studies on naltrexone hydrochloride for the treatment of self-injury among individuals with mental retardation and related developmental disorders. Overall, 80% of individuals with predominantly severe or profound mental retardation showed reductions in self-injury during short-term treatment with naltrexone. Forty-seven percent of the total pooled sample showed clinically significant reductions of 50% or greater during naltrexone treatment relative to baseline. Outcomes (i.e., changes in SIB as a function of naltrexone treatment) were not significantly related to age, autism status, or SIB topography. Although there have been reports suggesting that specific SIB topographies—head banging, hand biting—may be more responsive to treatment with naltrexone than others—body hitting, skin picking (Herman et al., 1987)—the data reviewed here neither refute nor support this notion. Finally, positive long-term effects of naltrexone treatment for self-injury of 1 year or longer have been reported (Casner et al., 1996; Crews et al., 1993; Sandman et al., 2000).

AGGRESSIVE BEHAVIOR AND EXPLOSIVE OUTBURSTS (RAGE ATTACKS)

The distinction between aggressive symptoms and explosive outbursts and their therapeutic management have been poorly explored. Aggressive symptoms, typically of an impulsive nature, have been reported to occur in 25% to 70% of clinically referred youths with TS (Budman et al., 2003; Comings & Comings, 1987a; Wand et al., 1993). Explosive outbursts, also called rage attacks, are seen in up to 50% of TS patients (Budman et al., 2000). Although they may be part of impulsivity/ADHD, oppositional defiant disorder, or OCD (frustration over unmet needs), they often represent one of the most disabling manifestations. Moreover, antisocial and oppositional behaviors are frequently encountered in TS, although psychosocial, familial, and economic settings may be more relevant in understanding these pathological relational behaviors. Overlap with OCD, ADHD, and impulse control disorder probably plays a significant role in these behaviors (Stephens & Sandor, 1999).

Children with this type of disruptive behavior are a difficult-to-treat population, as they are noncompliant almost by definition. The frequent co-occurrence of a number of biological, functional, and psychosocial risk factors for the development of conduct disorder suggests a need for multimodal interventions (Burke et al.,

---

Box 25.1. Key Points

- Behavioral treatment should be recommended as initial treatment for patients with TS or another tic disorder and ADHD, especially if symptoms are mild or parents refuse pharmacological treatment.
- Currently, the following classes of drugs are used in the treatment of ADHD:
  - Alpha-2 adrenoreceptor agonists: Clonidine and guanfacine have been proven to be efficacious in the treatment of children with tics or TS and ADHD and could be considered as the first-line management.
  - Psychostimulants should be the second choice of drugs in the treatment of tics or TS and ADHD. The use of stimulant medications in patients with tics or TS and ADHD in controlled trials have not indicated a deterioration of tics.
  - The efficacy of atomoxetine in the treatment of children with tics or TS and ADHD has been shown.
- Although OCD and TS are closely related, no clinical trials have specifically evaluated the treatment of OCD symptoms in TS patients.
- The main source of information about the treatment of OCD in patients with chronic tics or TS is drawn from the small number of clinical trials on the efficacy of anti-OCD drugs that have also included patients with tics and compared their clinical effects in OCD subjects with and without tics.
- Monotherapy with SRIs or SSRIs has been proven to be efficacious in the treatment of OCD patients, adults and children, in the short as well the long term.
- No individual drug in these classes demonstrated a superior efficacy to the others.
- However, nearly half of OCD patients do not respond completely to SRI/SSRI monotherapy, and even among the responders few become asymptomatic.
- Various strategies have been proposed for OCD nonresponders: increasing doses, switching to another drug, augmentation strategies, and novel treatments.
- OCD patients with comorbid chronic tics or TS show a lower response rate than those without tics, both in terms of percentage of responders as well as in terms of symptom reduction.
- An increased rate of response to antipsychotic augmentation in OCD patients with comorbid tics compared to those without was reported in only one old study.
- Despite the high rate and the clinical relevance of other psychiatric comorbidities (non-OCD anxiety disorders, SIB, disruptive behaviors) in TS patients, only a few studies have been devoted to investigating a specific therapeutic approach in these patients.
- Indeed, there are not any special strategies for their treatment in TS patients. The effects of combined therapies need to be scrutinized.

2002). Familial intervention should be tried first when facing difficult impulse control problems, also in TS patients.

Pharmacological interventions may be tried, but efficacy and safety data, mainly in children, are scant. Studies that dealt with the treatment of these disruptive symptoms in TS are few, are often open-label, and do not clearly distinguish between aggressive behavior and rage attacks. The potential efficacy of atypical antipsychotics on impulsive aggression symptoms in children with TS has been explored through a retrospective review of treatment response (Sandor & Stephens, 2000). Case notes of 28 patients with TS (aged 5–18 years; mean age 11.1 years) who presented with aggressive behavior at baseline (i.e., before the start of treatment with risperidone) were analyzed; an assessment of tic and aggression severity was made 2 weeks to 4 months later (mean 2 months). Twenty-two of the 28 showed decreased aggression scores at the end of the treatment period; overall, the decreases in aggressive behavior and tic severity ratings by the end of treatment were significant, suggesting that risperidone could be an effective monotherapy for impulsive aggression in these youths.

More recently, Stephens and colleagues (2004) treated 10 youngsters (aged 7–13 years) with TS and impulsive aggression with the atypical agent olanzapine in a single-blind, 2-week, placebo run-in, 8-week treatment trial. Olanzapine produced clinically and statistically significant reductions of aggression and tic severity from baseline to trial completion, as measured by the Achenbach Child Behavior Checklist and YGTSS. Weight gain during the treatment period was the most common adverse effect. Another study exploring the efficacy of olanzapine on tics and aggressive behaviors was conducted by McCracken and colleagues (2008) as a single-site, 6-week, open-label, flexible-dose trial. These authors enrolled 12 patients with TS (age range 7–14; mean age 11.3), 9 of whom met the criteria for at least one disruptive behavior disorder (ADHD, oppositional defiant disorder, or conduct disorder). Statistically significant pretreatment to posttreatment decreases were noted for all motor tic category variables and for some of the vocal tic categories. Analyses also identified statistically significant within-subject decreases for hyperactivity, aggression, and other disruptive behaviors, as measured by the parent version of the SNAP-IV Rating Scale (Swanson,

---

Box 25.2. Questions for Future Research

- Is a multimodal approach (behavioral plus pharmacological) to the treax`tment of coexisting ADHD in TS truly more beneficial thaCn unimodal approaches?
- How can we predict a negative outcome on tics when treating coexisting ADHD with stimulants?
- What is the real impact of atomoxetine treatment on tics, and what is its overall safety profile when used in the long term?
- How should "drug holidays" be used when treating coexisting ADHD in TS?
- Which of the newer agents under investigation is most likely to become a mainstay of treatment of coexisting ADHD in TS?
- What is the efficacy of currently available treatment approaches for childhood-onset OCD on coexisting OCD in TS?
- Can antipsychotic augmentation be exploited for the treatment of coexisting OCD in TS? Which antipsychotic agents are most likely to help in this context?
- What is the best management approach for SIB in TS?
- Should antipsychotics be used in all TS patients manifesting "rage attacks," and which antipsychotic agent provides the best risk/benefit ratio?

Nolan and Pelham Questionnaire revision). Moreover, when the researchers analyzed the number of aggression episodes, as defined by the Overt Aggression Scale, statistically significant between-subject decreases were found.

Finally, Budman and colleagues (2008), assessed the efficacy of aripiprazole in a retrospective chart review of 37 patients (age range 8–18 years) with TS with and without intermittent explosive disorder. At the end of treatment (12 weeks, at the mean daily dose of 11.7 mg), a reduction in tic severity was noted in all 29 patients who completed the study. Twenty-four of the 25 subjects with explosive outbursts showed at the endpoint a reduction in rage, measured by the Clinical Global Impression-Rage Scale.

CONCLUSIONS

There appears to be a dissimilar state of the art for each of the most relevant psychiatric comorbid disorders associated with TS. The amount of literature data on the treatment of ADHD in children with TS has allowed us to propose a flowchart with suggestions on how to manage these disabling symptoms. Even in the absence of controlled studies, the treatment of aggressive behavior and explosive outbursts with antipsychotics seems to be well established. Moreover, the usefulness of augmentation with antipsychotics in TS patients with OCD symptoms poorly responsive to monotherapy is supported by some studies. Finally, regarding SIB and non-OCD anxiety disorders, the paucity of data does not allow us to conclude unequivocally in favor of one or more specific therapeutic strategies. More generally, this review highlights the compelling need to improve our knowledge in these fields.

REFERENCES

AACAP Official Action. Practice Parameter for the Assessment and Treatment of Children and Adolescent With Attention-Deficit/Hyperactivity Disorder. *J Am Acad Child Adolesc Psychiatry* 2007; 46:824–921.

Allen AJ, Kurlan RM, Gilbert DL et al. Atomoxetine treatment in children and adolescents with ADHD and comorbid tic disorders. *Neurology* 2005; 65:1941–1949.

Arnold PD, Sicard T, Burroughs E et al. Glutamate transporter gene SLC1A1 associated with obsessive-compulsive disorder. *Arch Gen Psychiatry* 2006; 63:769–776.

Bangs ME, Tauscher-Wisniewski S, Polzer J et al. Meta-analysis of suicide-related behavior events in patients treated with atomoxetine. *J Am Acad Child Adolesc Psychiatry* 2008; 47:209–218.

Berlin HA, Koran LM, Jenike MA et al. Double-blind, placebo-controlled trial of topiramate augmentation in treatment-resistant obsessive-compulsive disorder. *J Clin Psychiatry* 2011; 72:716–721.

Bhattacharyya S, Chakraborty K. Glutamatergic dysfunction—newer targets for anti-obsessional drugs. *Recent Pat CNS Drug Discov* 2007; 2:47–55.

Biederman J, Faraone SV. Attention-deficit hyperactivity disorder. *Lancet* 2005; 366:237–248.

Biederman J, Melmed RD, Patel A et al. Long-term, open-label extension study of guanfacine extended release in children and adolescents with ADHD. *CNS Spectr* 2008; 13:1047–1055.

Bloch MH. Emerging treatments for Tourette's disorder. *Curr Psychiatry Rep* 2008; 10:323–330.

Bloch MH, Landeros-Weisenberger A, Kelmendi B et al. A systematic review: antipsychotic augmentation with treatment refractory obsessive-compulsive disorder. *Mol Psychiatry* 2006; 11:622–632.

An interesting review on antipsychotic augmentation in the treatment of patients with refractory OCD.

Bloch MH, McGuire J, Landeros-Weisenberger A etal. Meta-analysis of the dose-response relationship of SSRI in obsessive-compulsive disorder. *Mol Psychiatry* 2010; 15:850–855.

Bloch MH, Panza KE, Landeros-Weisenberger A, Leckman JF. Meta-analysis: treatment of attention-deficit/hyperactivity disorder in children with comorbid tic disorders. *J Am Acad Child Adolesc Psychiatry* 2009; 48:884–893.

This article analyzed nine double-blind, randomized, placebo-controlled trials examining the efficacy of six medications for ADHD and comorbid tic disorders. Methylphenidate, alphaa-2-agonists, desipramine, and atomoxetine yielded the greatest improvement in ADHD and tic symptoms.

Boon-Yasidhi V, Kim YS, Scahill L. An open-label, prospective study of guanfacine in children with ADHD and tic disorders. *J Med Assoc Thai* 2005; 88 Suppl 8:S156–162.

Borcherding BG, Keysor CS, Rapoport JL et al. Motor/vocal tics and compulsive behaviors on stimulant drugs: is there a common vulnerability? *Psychiatry Res* 1990; 33:83–94.

Borison RL, Ang L, Chang S et al. New pharmacological approaches in the treatment of Tourette syndrome. *Adv Neurol* 1982; 35:377–382.

Bornstein RA. Neuropsychological correlates of obsessive characteristics in Tourette syndrome. *J Neuropsychiatry Clin Neurosci* 1991; 3:157–162.

Breese GR, Criswell HE, Duncan GE, Mueller RA. Dopamine deficiency in self-injurious behavior. *Psychopharmacol Bull* 1989; 25:353–357.

Bruun RD. Dysphoric phenomena associated with haloperidol treatment of Tourette syndrome. *Adv Neurol* 1982a; 35:433–436.

Bruun RD. Clonidine treatment of Tourette syndrome. *Adv Neurol* 1982b; 35:403–405.

Budman C, Coffey BJ, Shechter R et al. Aripiprazole in children and adolescents with Tourette disorder with and without explosive outbursts. *J Child Adolesc Psychopharmacol* 2008; 18:509–515.

Budman CL, Bruun RD, Park KS et al. Explosive outbursts in children with Tourette's disorder. *J Am Acad Child Adolesc Psychiatry* 2000; 39:1270–1276.

Budman CL, Rockmore L, Stokes J, Sossin M. Clinical phenomenology of episodic rage in children with Tourette syndrome. *J Psychosom Res* 2003; 55:59–65.

The first study on treatment of rage attacks in TS patients.

Burke JD, Loeber R, Birmaher B. Oppositional defiant disorder and conduct disorder: a review of the past 10 years, part II. *J Am Acad Child Adolesc Psychiatry* 2002; 41:1275–1293.

Casner JA, Weinheimer B, Gualtieri CT. Naltrexone and self-injurious behavior: a retrospective population study. *J Clin Psychopharmacol* 1996; 16:389–394.

Castellanos FX, Giedd JN, Elia J et al. Controlled stimulant treatment of ADHD and comorbid Tourette's syndrome: effects of stimulant and dose. *J Am Acad Child Adolesc Psychiatry* 1997; 36:589–596.

Cavanna AE, Servo S, Monaco F, Robertson MM. The behavioral spectrum of Gilles de la Tourette syndrome. *J Neuropsychiatry Clin Neurosci* 2009; 21:13–23.

Chappell PB, Riddle MA, Scahill L et al. Guanfacine treatment of comorbid attention-deficit hyperactivity disorder and Tourette's syndrome: preliminary clinical experience. *J Am Acad Child Adolesc Psychiatry* 1995; 34:1140–1146.

Cheung MY, Shahed J, Jankovic J. Malignant Tourette syndrome. *Mov Disord* 2007; 22:1743–1750.

Coffey B, Frazier J, Chen S. Comorbidity, Tourette syndrome, and anxiety disorders. *Adv Neurol* 1992; 58:95–104.

Coffey BJ, Biederman J, Smoller JW et al. Anxiety disorders and tic severity in juveniles with Tourette's disorder. *J Am Acad Child Adolesc Psychiatry* 2000; 39:562–568.

Cohen DJ, Leckman JF. Developmental psychopathology and neurobiology of Tourette's syndrome. *J Am Acad Child Adolesc Psychiatry* 1994; 33:2–15.

Comings DE, Comings BG. A controlled study of Tourette syndrome. II. Conduct. *Am J Hum Genet* 1987a; 41:742–760.

Comings DE, Comings BG. A controlled study of Tourette syndrome. III. Phobias and panic attacks. *Am J Hum Genet* 1987b; 41:761–781.

Comings DE, Comings BG. A controlled study of Tourette syndrome. IV. Obsessions, compulsions, and schizoid behaviors. *Am J Hum Genet* 1987c; 41:782–803.

Cook EH, Leventhal BL. The serotonin system in autism. *Curr Opin Pediatr* 1996; 8:348–354.

Crews WD Jr, Bonaventura S, Rowe FB, Bonsie D. Cessation of long-term naltrexone therapy and self-injury: a case study. *Res Dev Disabil* 1993; 14:331–340.

Cummings DD, Singer HS, Krieger M et al. Neuropsychiatric effects of guanfacine in children with mild Tourette syndrome: a pilot study. *Clin Neuropharmacol* 2002; 25:325–332.

Debes NM, Hjalgrim H, Skov L. The presence of comorbidity in Tourette syndrome increases the need for pharmacological treatment. *J Child Neurol* 2009; 24:1504–1512.

Decloedt EH, Stein DJ. Current trends in drug treatment of obsessive-compulsive disorder. *Neuropsychiatr Dis Treat* 2010; 6:233–242.

Denckla MB, Bemporad JR, MacKay MC. Tics following methylphenidate administration. A report of 20 cases. *JAMA* 1976; 235:1349–1351.

Du YS, Li HF, Vance A et al. Randomized double-blind multicentre placebo-controlled clinical trial of the clonidine adhesive patch for the treatment of tic disorders. *Aust N Z J Psychiatry* 2008; 42:807–813.

Faraone SV, Biederman J, Morley CP, Spencer TJ. Effect of stimulants on height and weight: a review of the literature. *J Am Acad Child Adolesc Psychiatry* 2008; 47:994–1009.

Favazza AR. The coming of age of self-mutilation. *J Nerv Ment Dis* 1998; *186*:259–268.

Fernandez-Cordoba E, Lopez-Ibor Alino J. Monochlorimipramine in mental patients resisting other forms of treatment. *Actas Luso Esp Neurol Psiquiatr* 1967; *26*:119–147.

Fineberg NA, Gale TM. Evidence-based pharmacotherapy of obsessive-compulsive disorder. *Int J Neuropsychopharmacol* 2005; 8:107–129.

Freeman RD, Fast DK, Burd L et al. An international perspective on Tourette syndrome: selected findings from 3,500 individuals in 22 countries. *Dev Med Child Neurol* 2000; *42*:436–447.

Gadow KD, Nolan E, Sprafkin J, Sverd J. School observations of children with attention-deficit hyperactivity disorder and comorbid tic disorder: effects of methylphenidate treatment. *J Dev Behav Pediatr* 1995; *16*:167–176.

Gadow KD, Nolan EE, Sverd J. Methylphenidate in hyperactive boys with comorbid tic disorder: II. Short-term behavioral effects in school settings. *J Am Acad Child Adolesc Psychiatry* 1992; *31*:462–471.

Gadow KD, Sverd J, Nolan EE et al. Immediate-release methylphenidate for ADHD in children with comorbid chronic multiple tic disorder. *J Am Acad Child Adolesc Psychiatry* 2007; *46*:840–848.

Gadow KD, Sverd J, Sprafkin J et al. Efficacy of methylphenidate for attention-deficit hyperactivity disorder in children with tic disorder. *Arch Gen Psychiatry* 1995; *52*:444–455.

Gadow KD, Sverd J, Sprafkin J et al. Long-term methylphenidate therapy in children with comorbid attention-deficit hyperactivity disorder and chronic multiple tic disorder. *Arch Gen Psychiatry* 1999; *56*:330–336.

Gaffney GR, Perry PJ, Lund BC et al. Risperidone versus clonidine in the treatment of children and adolescents with Tourette's syndrome. *J Am Acad Child Adolesc Psychiatry* 2002; *41*:330–336.

Geissler J, Lesch KP. A lifetime of attention-deficit/hyperactivity disorder: diagnostic challenges, treatment and neurobiological mechanisms. *Expert Rev Neurother* 2011; *11*:1467–1484.

Geller DA, Biederman J, Stewart SE et al. Which SSRI? A meta-analysis of pharmacotherapy trials in pediatric obsessive-compulsive disorder. *Am J Psychiatry* 2003a; *160*:1919–1928.

Geller DA, Biederman J, Stewart SE et al. Impact of comorbidity on treatment response to paroxetine in pediatric obsessive-compulsive disorder: is the use of exclusion criteria empirically supported in randomized clinical trials? *J Child Adolesc Psychopharmacol* 2003b; *13* Suppl 1:S19–29.

Gilbert DL, Ridel KR, Sallee FR et al. Comparison of the inhibitory and excitatory effects of ADHD medications methylphenidate and atomoxetine on motor cortex. *Neuropsychopharmacology* 2006; *31*:442–449.

Goetz CG. Clonidine and clonazepam in Tourette syndrome. *Adv Neurol* 1992; *58*:245–251.

Goetz CG, Tanner CM, Wilson RS et al. Clonidine and Gilles de la Tourette's syndrome: double-blind study using objective rating methods. *Ann Neurol* 1987; *21*:307–310.

Goodman WK, Storch EA, Geffken GR, Murphy TK. Obsessive-compulsive disorder in Tourette syndrome. *J Child Neurol* 2006; *21*:704–714.

Gorman DA, Thompson N, Plessen KJ et al. Psychosocial outcome and psychiatric comorbidity in older adolescents with Tourette syndrome: controlled study. *Br J Psychiatry* 2010; *197*:36–44.

Graham J, Banaschewski T, Buitelaar J et al. European guidelines on managing adverse effects of medication for ADHD. *Eur Child Adolesc Psychiatry* 2011; *20*:17–37.

Graham J, Coghill D. Adverse effects of pharmacotherapies for attention-deficit hyperactivity disorder: epidemiology, prevention and management. *CNS Drugs* 2008; *22*:213–237.

Gulisano M, Calì PV, Cavanna AE et al. Cardiovascular safety of aripiprazole and pimozide in young patients with Tourette syndrome. *Neurol Sci* 2011; *32*:1213–1217.

Ipser JC, Carey P, Dhansay Y et al. Pharmacotherapy augmentation strategies in treatment-resistant anxiety disorders. *Cochrane Database Syst Rev* 2006; (4):CD005473.

Hawi Z, Dring M, Kirley A et al. Serotonergic system and attention deficit hyperactivity disorder (ADHD): a potential susceptibility locus at the 5-HT(1B) receptor gene in 273 nuclear families from a multi-centre sample. *Mol Psychiatry* 2002; 7:718–725.

Heal DJ, Smith SL, Findling RL. ADHD: Current and Future Therapeutics. *Curr Top Behav Neurosci* 2012; 9:361–390.

Hedderick EF, Morris CM, Singer HS. Double-blind, crossover study of clonidine and levetiracetam in Tourette syndrome. *Pediatr Neurol* 2009; *40*:420–425.

Herman BH, Hammock MK, Arthur-Smith A et al. Naltrexone decreases self-injurious behavior. *Ann Neurol* 1987; *22*:550–552.

Hoffman DA, Schiller M, Greenblatt JM, Iosifescu DV. Polypharmacy or medication washout: an old tool revisited. *Neuropsychiatr Dis Treatment* 2011; 7:639–648.

Husted DS, Shapira NA, Murphy TK et al. Effect of comorbid tics on a clinically meaningful response to 8-week open-label trial of fluoxetine in obsessive compulsive disorder. *J Psychiatr Res* 2007; 41:332–337.

James A, Soler A, Weatherall R. Cognitive behavioural therapy for anxiety disorders in children and adolescents. *Cochrane Database Syst Rev* 2005; (4):CD004690.

Jankovic J, Kurlan R. Tourette syndrome: evolving concepts. *Mov Disord* 2011; 26:1149–1156.

Kelsey DK, Sumner CR, Casat CD et al. Once-daily atomoxetine treatment for children with attention-deficit/hyperactivity disorder, including an assessment of evening and morning behavior: a double-blind, placebo-controlled trial. *Pediatrics* 2004; 114:e1–8.

Kendall PC, Flannery-Schroeder E, Panichelli- Mindel SM et al. Therapy for youths with anxiety disorders: a second randomized clinical trial. *J Consult Clin Psychol* 1997; 65:366–380.

Kessler RC, Angermeyer M, Anthony JC et al. Lifetime prevalence and age-of-onset distributions of mental disorders in the World Health Organization's World Mental Health Survey Initiative. *World Psychiatry* 2007; 6:168–176.

Kollins SH, Jain R, Brams M et al. Clonidine extended-release tablets as add-on therapy to psychostimulants in children and adolescents with ADHD. *Pediatrics* 2011; 127:e1406–1413.

Koran LM, Aboujaoude E, Bullock KD et al. Double-blind treatment with oral morphine in treatment-resistant obsessive-compulsive disorder. *J Clin Psychiatry* 2005; 66:353–359.

Koran LM, Aboujaoude E, Gamel NN. Double-blind study of dextroamphetamine versus caffeine augmentation for treatment-resistant obsessive-compulsive disorder. *J Clin Psychiatry* 2009; 70:1530–1535.

Leckman JF, Detlor J, Harcherik DF et al. Short- and long-term treatment of Tourette's syndrome with clonidine: a clinical perspective. *Neurology* 1985; 35:343–351.

Leckman JF, Hardin MT, Riddle MA et al. Clonidine treatment of Gilles de la Tourette's syndrome. *Arch Gen Psychiatry* 1991; 48:324–328.

Leonard HL, Swedo SE, Rapoport JL et al. Tourette syndrome and obsessive-compulsive disorder. *Adv Neurol* 1992; 58:83–93.

Li J, Zhang X, Wang Y et al. The serotonin 5-HT1D receptor gene and attention-deficit hyperactivity disorder in Chinese Han subjects. *Am J Med Genet B Neuropsychiatr Genet* 2006; 141B:874–876.

Linet LS. Tourette syndrome, pimozide, and school phobia: the neuroleptic separation anxiety syndrome. *Am J Psychiatry* 1985; 142:613–615.

Lowe TL, Cohen DJ, Detlor J et al. Stimulant medications precipitate Tourette's syndrome. *JAMA* 1982; 247:1729–1731.

Mancuso E, Faro A, Joshi G, Geller DA. Treatment of pediatric obsessive-compulsive disorder: a review. *J Child Adolesc Psychopharmacol* 2010; 20:299–308.
A recent and comprehensive review on the treatment of pediatric OCD.

March JS, Franklin ME, Leonard H et al. Tics moderate treatment outcome with sertraline but not cognitive-behavior therapy in pediatric obsessive-compulsive disorder. *Biol Psychiatry* 2007; 61:344–347.
This study investigated the effects of comorbid tics upon treatment outcome of pediatric OCD patients.

Mathews CA, Waller J, Glidden D et al. Self-injurious behaviour in Tourette syndrome: correlates with impulsivity and impulse control. *J Neurol Neurosurg Psychiatry* 2004; 75:1149–1155.
This is the broadest study on SIB in TS patients.

McCracken JT, Suddath R, Chang S et al. Effectiveness and tolerability of open-label olanzapine in children and adolescents with Tourette syndrome. *J Child Adolesc Psychopharmacol* 2008; 18:501–508.

McDougle CJ, Goodman WK, Leckman JF et al. The efficacy of fluvoxamine in obsessive-compulsive disorder: effects of comorbid chronic tic disorder. *J Clin Psychopharmacol* 1993; 13:354–358.
The first study on the impact of comorbid tics upon the treatment of OCD.

McDougle CJ, Goodman WK, Leckman JF et al. Haloperidol addition in fluvoxamine-refractory obsessive-compulsive disorder. A double-blind, placebo-controlled study in patients with and without tics. *Arch Gen Psychiatry* 1994; 51:302–308.

Medicines & Healthcare Products Regulatory Authority. Selective serotonin reuptake inhibitors (SSRIs): overview of regulatory status and CSM advice relating to major depressive disorder (MDD) in children and adolescents including a summary of available safety and efficacy data. Available at http://www.mhra.gov.uk/Safetyinformation/

Safetywarningsalertsandrecalls/
Safetywarningsandmessagesformedicines/
CON019494 (last accessed 18 April 2007).

Meyer V. Modification of expectations in cases with obsessional rituals. *Behav Res Ther* 1966; 4:273–280.

Michelson D, Allen AJ, Busner J et al. Once-daily atomoxetine treatment for children and adolescents with attention deficit hyperactivity disorder: a randomized, placebo-controlled study. *Am J Psychiatry* 2002; 159:1896–1901.

Mowla A, Khajeian AM, Sahraian A et al. Topiramate augmentation in resistant OCD: A double-blind placebo-controlled clinical trial. *CNS Spectr.* 2010 Nov 1 [E-pub ahead of print].

MTA Cooperative Group. Multimodal Treatment Study of Children with ADHD. A 14-month randomized clinical trial of treatment strategies for attention-deficit/hyperactivity disorder. *Arch Gen Psychiatry* 1999; 56:1073–1086.

Muscatello MR, Bruno A, Pandolfo G et al. Effect of aripiprazole augmentation of serotonin reuptake inhibitors or clomipramine in treatment-resistant obsessive-compulsive disorder: a double-blind, placebo-controlled study. *J Psychopharmacol* 2011; 31:174–179.

National Institute for Health and Clinical Excellence (NICE). Obsessive-compulsive disorder: core interventions in the treatment of obsessive-compulsive disorder and body dysmorphic disorder. The British Psychological Society & The Royal College of Psychiatrists. 2006. Available at: www.nice.org.uk.

Nissen SE. ADHD drugs and cardiovascular risk. *N Engl J Med* 2006; 354:1445–1448.

Noda T, Shimizu W, Satomi K et al. Classification and mechanism of torsades de pointes initiation in patients with congenital long QT syndrome. *Eur Heart J* 2004; 25:2149–2154.

Nolan EE, Gadow KD. Children with ADHD and tic disorder and their classmates: behavioral normalization with methylphenidate. *J Am Acad Child Adolesc Psychiatry* 1997; 36:597–604.

Norberg MM, Krystal JH, Tolin DF. A meta-analysis of D-cycloserine and the facilitation of fear extinction and exposure therapy. *Biol Psychiatry* 2008; 63:1118–1126.

Ohta M, Kano Y. Clinical characteristics of adult patients with tics and/or Tourette's syndrome. *Brain Dev* 2003; 25 Suppl 1:S32–36.

O'Kearney RT, Anstey KJ, von Sanden C. Behavioural and cognitive behavioural therapy for obsessive compulsive disorder in children and adolescents. *Cochrane Database Syst Rev* 2006;(4):CD004856.

Pampaloni I, Sivakumaran T, Hawley CJ et al. High-dose selective serotonin reuptake inhibitors in OCD: a systematic retrospective case notes survey. *J Psychopharmacol* 2010; 24:1439–1445.

Pediatric OCD Treatment Study (POTS) Team. Cognitive-behavior therapy, sertraline, and their combination for children and adolescents with obsessive-compulsive disorder: the Pediatric OCD Treatment Study (POTS) randomized controlled trial. *JAMA* 2004; 292:1969–1976.

Perwien AR, Kratochvil CJ, Faries DE et al. Atomoxetine treatment in children and adolescents with attention-deficit hyperactivity disorder: what are the long-term health-related quality-of-life outcomes? *J Child Adolesc Psychopharmacol* 2006; 16:713–724.

Pliszka S; AACAP Work Group on Quality Issues. Practice parameter for the assessment and treatment of children and adolescents with attention-deficit/hyperactivity disorder. *J Am Acad Child Adolesc Psychiatry* 2007; 46:894–921.

Pliszka SR. The neuropsychopharmacology of attention-deficit/hyperactivity disorder. *Biol Psychiatry* 2005; 57:1385–1390.

Pringsheim T, Steeves T. Pharmacological treatment for attention deficit hyperactivity disorder (ADHD) in children with comorbid tic disorders. *Cochrane Database Syst Rev* 2011; (4):CD007990.

Quist JF, Barr CL, Schachar R et al. The serotonin 5-HT1B receptor gene and attention deficit hyperactivity disorder. *Mol Psychiatry* 2003; 8:98–102.

Rizzo R, Curatolo P, Gulisano M et al. Disentangling the effects of Tourette syndrome and attention deficit hyperactivity disorder on cognitive and behavioral phenotypes. *Brain Dev* 2007; 29:413–420.

Robertson MM. Tourette syndrome, associated conditions and the complexities of treatment. *Brain* 2000; 123:425–462.

Robertson MM, Channon S, Baker J, Flynn D. The psychopathology of Gilles de la Tourette's syndrome. A controlled study. *Br J Psychiatry* 1993; 162:114–117.

Robertson MM, Trimble MR, Lees AJ. Self-injurious behaviour and the Gilles de la Tourette syndrome: a clinical study and review of the literature. *Psychol Med* 1989; 19:611–625.

Roessner V, Plessen KJ, Rothenberger A et al. European clinical guidelines for Tourette syndrome and other tic disorders. Part II: pharmacological treatment. *Eur Child Adolesc Psychiatry* 2011; 20:173–196.
Interesting and comprehensive guidelines in the treatment of TS and chronic tic disorder.

Rojas-Corrales MO, Gibert-Rahola J, Mico JA. Role of atypical opiates in OCD. Experimental approach through the study of 5-HT(2A/C) receptor-mediated behavior. *Psychopharmacology* 2007; 190:221–231.

Ruffini C, Locatelli M, Lucca A et al. Augmentation effect of repetitive transcranial magnetic stimulation over the orbitofrontal cortex in drug-resistant obsessive-compulsive disorder patients: a controlled investigation. *Prim Care Companion J Clin Psychiatry* 2009; 11:226–230.

Sandman CA. Beta-endorphin dysregulation in autistic and self-injurious behavior: a neurodevelopmental hypothesis. *Synapse* 1988; 2:193–199.

Sandman CA, Barron JL, Chicz-DeMet A, DeMet EM. Plasma B-endorphin levels in patients with self-injurious behavior and stereotypy. *Am J Ment Retard* 1990; 95:84–92.

Sandman CA, Barron JL, Chicz-DeMet A, DeMet EM. Brief report: plasma beta-endorphin and cortisol levels in autistic patients. *J Autism Dev Disord* 1991; 21:83–87.

Sandman CA, Hetrick W, Taylor DV et al. Long-term effects of naltrexone on self-injurious behavior. Am J Ment Retard 2000; 105:103–117.

Sandor P, Stephens RJ. Risperidone treatment of aggressive behavior in children with Tourette syndrome. *J Psychopharmacol* 2000; 20:710–712.

Scahill L, Chappell PB, Kim YS et al. A placebo-controlled study of guanfacine in the treatment of children with tic disorders and attention deficit hyperactivity disorder. *Am J Psychiatry* 2001; 158:1067–1074.

Scahill L, Erenberg G, Berlin CM Jr et al. Contemporary assessment and pharmacotherapy of Tourette syndrome. *NeuroRx* 2006; 3:192–206.

Schroeder SR, Oster-Granite ML, Berkson G et al. Self-injurious behavior: gene-brain-behavior relationships. *Ment Retard Dev Disabil Res Rev* 2001; 7:3–12.

Seixas M, Weiss M, Müller U. Systematic review of national and international guidelines on attention-deficit hyperactivity disorder. *J Psychopharmacol* 2012; 26:753–765.

Selvi Y, Atli A, Aydin A et al. The comparison of aripiprazole and risperidone augmentation in selective serotonin reuptake inhibitor-refractory obsessive-compulsive disorder: a single-blind, randomised study. *Hum Psychopharmacol* 2011; 26:51–57.

Shapira NA, Ward HE, Mandoki M et al. A double-blind, placebo-controlled trial of olanzapine addition in fluoxetine-refractory obsessive-compulsive disorder. *Biol Psychiatry* 2004; 55:553–555.

Singer HS, Brown J, Quaskey S et al. The treatment of attention-deficit hyperactivity disorder in Tourette's syndrome: a double-blind placebo-controlled study with clonidine and desipramine. *Pediatrics* 1995; 95:74–81.

Soomro GM, Altman D, Rajagopal S, Oakley-Browne M. Selective serotonin re-uptake inhibitors (SSRIs) versus placebo for obsessive compulsive disorder (OCD). *Cochrane Database Syst Rev* 2008; (1):CD001765.

Spencer TJ, Biederman J, Wilens TE, Faraone SV. Novel treatments for attention-deficit/hyperactivity disorder in children. *J Clin Psychiatry* 2002; 63 Suppl 12:16–22.

Spencer TJ, Kratochvil CJ, Sangal RB et al. Effects of atomoxetine on growth in children with attention-deficit/hyperactivity disorder following up to five years of treatment. *J Child Adolesc Psychopharmacol* 2007; 17:689–700.

Spencer TJ, Newcorn JH, Kratochvil CJ et al. Effects of atomoxetine on growth after 2-year treatment among pediatric patients with attention-deficit/ hyperactivity disorder. *Pediatrics* 2005; 116:e74–80.

Spencer TJ, Sallee FR, Gilbert DL et al. Atomoxetine treatment of ADHD in children with comorbid Tourette syndrome. *J Atten Disord* 2008; 11:470–481.

Stephens RJ, Bassel C, Sandor P. Olanzapine in the treatment of aggression and tics in children with Tourette's syndrome-a pilot study. *J Child Adolesc Psychopharmacol* 2004; 14:255–266.

Stephens RJ, Sandor P. Aggressive behaviour in children with Tourette syndrome and comorbid attention-deficit hyperactivity disorder and obsessive-compulsive disorder. *Can J Psychiatry* 1999; 44:1036–1042.

Stewart SE, Jenike EA, Hezel DM et al. A single-blinded case-control study of memantine in severe obsessive-compulsive disorder. *J Psychopharmacol* 2010; 30:34–39.

Storch EA, Lewin AB, Farrell L et al. Does cognitive-behavioral therapy response among adults with obsessive-compulsive disorder differ as a function of certain comorbidities? *J Anxiety Disord* 2010; *24*:547–552.

Storch EA, Murphy TK, Goodman WK et al. A preliminary study of D-cycloserine augmentation of cognitive-behavioral therapy in pediatric obsessive-compulsive disorder. *Biol Psychiatry* 2010; *68*:1073–1076.

Sverd J, Gadow KD, Paolicelli LM. Methylphenidate treatment of attention-deficit hyperactivity disorder in boys with Tourette's syndrome. *J Am Acad Child Adolesc Psychiatry* 1989; *28*:574–579.

Swanson CJ, Perry KW, Koch-Krueger S et al. Effect of the attention deficit/hyperactivity disorder drug atomoxetine on extracellular concentrations of norepinephrine and dopamine in several brain regions of the rat. *Neuropharmacology* 2006; *50*:755–760.

Swanson JM, Elliott GR, Greenhill LL et al. Effects of stimulant medication on growth rates across 3 years in the MTA follow-up. *J Am Acad Child Adolesc Psychiatry* 2007; *46*:1015–1027.

Symons FJ, Thompson A, Rodriguez MC. Self-injurious behavior and the efficacy of naltrexone treatment: a quantitative synthesis. *Ment Retard Dev Disabil Res Rev* 2004; *10*:193–200.

Target M, Fonagy P. Efficacy of psychoanalysis for children with emotional disorders. *J Am Acad Child Adolesc Psychiatry* 1994; *33*:361–371.

Taylor E, Döpfner M, Sergeant J et al. European clinical guidelines for hyperkinetic disorder—first upgrade. *Eur Child Adolesc Psychiatry* 2004; *13* Suppl 1:I7–30.

Tourette's Syndrome Study Group. Treatment of ADHD in children with tics: a randomized controlled trial. *Neurology* 2002; *58*: 527–536.

Van der Oord S, Prins PJ, Oosterlaan J, Emmelkamp PM. Efficacy of methylphenidate, psychosocial treatments and their combination in school-aged children with ADHD: a meta-analysis. *Clin Psychol Rev* 2008; *28*:783–800.

Vetter VL, Elia J, Erickson C et al. Cardiovascular monitoring of children and adolescents with heart disease receiving medications for attention deficit/hyperactivity disorder [corrected]: a scientific statement from the American Heart Association Council on Cardiovascular Disease in the Young Congenital Cardiac Defects Committee and the Council on Cardiovascular Nursing. *Circulation* 2008; *117*:2407–2423.

Wand RR, Matazow GS, Shady GA et al. Tourette syndrome: associated symptoms and most disabling features. *Neurosci Biobehav Rev* 1993; *17*:271–275.

Weisman H, Qureshi IA, Leckman JF et al. Systematic review: Pharmacological treatment of tic disorders – Efficacy of antipsychotic and alpha-2-adrenergic agonist agents. *Neurosci Biobehav Rev* 2012; Oct 23. [Epub ahead of print].

Weiss M, Tannock R, Kratochvil C et al. A randomized, placebo-controlled study of once-daily atomoxetine in the school setting in children with ADHD. *J Am Acad Child Adolesc Psychiatry* 2005; *44*:647–655.

Wernicke JF, Faries D, Girod D et al. Cardiovascular effects of atomoxetine in children, adolescents, and adults. *Drug Saf* 2003; *26*:729–740.

Wickens JR, Hyland BI, Tripp G. Animal models to guide clinical drug development in ADHD: lost in translation? *Br J Pharmacol* 2011; *164*:1107–1128.

Wigal SB, Duong S. Pharmacokinetic evaluation of eltoprazine. *Expert Opin Drug Metab Toxicol* 2011; *7*:775–781.

Wilens TE, Verlinden MH, Adler LA et al. ABT-089, a neuronal nicotinic receptor partial agonist, for the treatment of attention-deficit/hyperactivity disorder in adults: results of a pilot study. *Biol Psychiatry* 2006; *59*:1065–1070.

Wilhelm S, Buhlmann U, Tolin DF et al. Augmentation of behavior therapy with D-cycloserine for obsessive-compulsive disorder. *Am J Psychiatry* 2008; *165*:335–341.

Worbe Y, Mallet L, Golmard JL et al. Repetitive behaviours in patients with Gilles de la Tourette syndrome: tics, compulsions, or both? *PLoS One* 2010; *5*:e12959.

Zhong YQ, Zhou WZ, Hu WG. Randomized double-blind controlled study on treatment of tic disorders in children with transcutaneous patch of clonidine. *Zhonghua Er Ke Za Zhi* 2007; *45*:785–787.

26

Surgical Treatment of Tourette Syndrome

MAURO PORTA, MARCO SASSI AND DOMENICO SERVELLO

Abstract

This chapter presents an overview of the literature on the surgical approach to the treatment of Tourette syndrome (TS) and summarizes current recommendations for the use of this treatment. Attention is given to pending issues related to this invasive treatment, which will need to be addressed in future research. Some technical notes based on the authors' longstanding experience using this treatment are given at the end of the chapter. Deep brain stimulation (DBS) for TS must still be considered an investigational procedure: it is not curative and in some cases does not improve tics. Drugs in TS are prescribed according to the patient's symptoms, and although the same tailored approach is conceivable in choosing the best target for DBS, evidence is still insufficient to provide a sound clinical guidance for target selection. The ongoing technological advances in the surgical procedure (e.g., the introduction of the O-arm and other imaging modalities) may improve its safety and applicability in routine clinical practice. A robust treatment algorithm, based on evidence from randomized controlled trials and multidisciplinary experiences from tertiary referral centers, is lacking and is definitely needed.

INTRODUCTION

The onset of tics in Tourette syndrome (TS) usually occurs between the ages of 6 and 8 years. The severity of tics then follows a waxing and waning course, reaching a climax at around 10 to 12 years of age (Leckman, 2003), as summarized in greater detail in Chapter 1. Subsequently, as reviewed in Chapter 5, most patients improve significantly during adolescence and early adulthood (Bloch et al., 2006; Leckman et al., 1998; Peterson et al., 2001). In adulthood, only a subgroup of patients with persisting tics require treatment, which often consists of conservative behavioral and/or pharmacological interventions (for a wide discussion of these aspects, see Chapters 23, 24, and 27). There are, however, a few adults whose tics are severe or disabling despite medication use (Cavanna et al., 2008). In some cases, tics are self-injurious and, in extreme circumstances, life-threatening. These are generally patients with one or more coexisting disorders, such as attention-deficit/hyperactivity disorder (ADHD), obsessive-compulsive disorder (OCD) or obsessive-compulsive behavior, poor impulse control, learning difficulties, limited interpersonal skills, self-injurious behavior (SIB), anxiety, depression, and various forms of personality disorder (see Chapters 2, 3, 4, and 25). Once less-invasive established and experimental interventions have been tried and failed, some of these cases should be considered for more experimental interventions, including deep brain stimulation (DBS) surgery (Sassi et al., 2011).

Although our understanding of the core pathomechanisms of TS is steadily advancing (see Chapters 10–15), there is no definitive agreement on when, in whom, or indeed which surgical anatomical target should be used in this condition. Both North American (Jankovic & Kurlan, 2011; Mink et al., 2006) and European (Muller-Vahl et al., 2011) authors agree that DBS surgery in TS should be restricted to adult patients who are very severely affected and refractory to conservative and less-invasive experimental treatments. DBS for TS remains experimental and there is a clear need for more extensive investigation, including long-term follow-up, before patients and clinicians can be sufficiently well informed concerning the immediate and long-term risks and benefits of this type of intervention (Ackermans et al., 2012).

LESIONAL SURGERY IN TOURETTE SYNDROME: A SHORT HISTORICAL PREAMBLE

The history of functional neurosurgery in TS began, as for all the main indications for this treatment approach, in the form of lesional or ablative procedures. In general terms, these procedures are now not easily justifiable from an ethical perspective, given their irreversible nature. There are two excellent reviews of the lesional approach to functional neurosurgery in TS (Rauch et al., 1995; Temel & Visser-Vandewalle, 2004). The first reports date back to 1955. Prior to 2003, there were at least 24 reports describing the results of lesional surgery undertaken in more than 60 individuals with severe TS. The target sites were diverse and included the frontal lobe (e.g., in prefrontal lobotomy and bimedial frontal leucotomy) as well as the limbic system (e.g., in limbic leucotomy and anterior cingulotomy). The first

thalamotomy was undertaken in 1970 by Hassler and Dieckmann (1970), who targeted the centromedian/parafascicular (CM/Pf) complex plus the nucleus ventralis oralis internus (Voi) of the thalamus; they reported a clear improvement of tic severity. Their seminal work has been critically reappraised by Rickards and colleagues (2008).

Subsequently, a number of other regions were targeted, including intrathalamic lesions at the level of the zona incerta and ventrolateral/lamella medialis thalamus; cerebellar dentatotomies also were performed (Temel & Visser-Vandewalle, 2004). Figure 26.1 presents a schematic drawing of targeted areas for TS (see also Ackermans et al., 2008a, 2008b). Imprecise target localization, often in the absence of a robust rationale, unclear diagnostic criteria in patient selection, major adverse side effects ranging from dystonia to tetraplegia, and the young age of some of these patients represent the major limits of these early surgical procedures.

FUNCTIONAL NEUROSURGERY OF TS TODAY: DBS

Neuroscientists have long attempted to use electrical signals to modulate brain function.

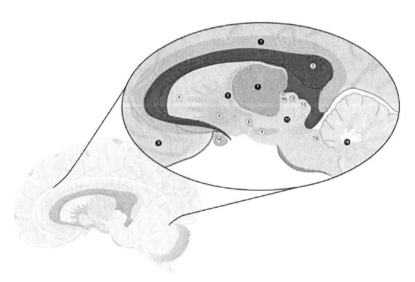

FIGURE 26.1   Anatomical targets for DBS in TS (Ackermans et al., 2008b): (1) cingulate cortex, (2) corpus callosum, (3) frontal lobe, (4) caudate-putamen, (5) zona incerta, (6) globus pallidus, (7) thalamus, (8) subthalamic nucleus, (9) substantia nigra, (10) posterior commissure, (11) Forel H fields, (12) superior colliculus, (13) inferior colliculus, (14) optic chiasm, (15) superior cerebellar peduncle, and (16) dentate nucleus.

In 1874, Bartholow reported his early experience of cortical stimulation (Harris & Almerigi, 2009). Deeper structures of the brain started to be investigated with stimulation procedures using stereotactic approaches by Spiegel and colleagues in 1947. In the 1970s and 1980s, scattered reports of DBS for tremor and other movement disorders began to be published. In 1987, Benabid and colleagues published a report of stimulation of the ventral intermediate thalamic nucleus in a patient with Parkinson's disease. DBS began to be applied more frequently to treat common hyperkinetic movement disorders, including essential tremor (Benabid et al., 1991) and dystonia (Krauss et al., 1999; Loher et al., 2000).

Table 26.1 summarizes the available scientific reports concerning TS patients treated with DBS. Unfortunately, the vast majority of these articles describe single cases. To date, at least seven major brain areas have been targeted, although thalamic stimulation has been used in more than 50% of all the patients reported so far. All the targets used belong to the ventral striatal-thalamo-cortical circuitry, which is thought to be dysfunctional in TS (see Chapters 10, 12, and 13). Another important general consideration is that the specific anatomical coordinates for any given neuroanatomical location targeted in different clinical centers may differ slightly.

TARGETS FOR DBS IN TS: THERAPEUTIC EFFECT AND ADVERSE EVENTS

CM/Pf–Substantia Periventricularis– Nucleus Voi Crosspoint of the Thalamus

In 1999, DBS was introduced in treatment-refractory, severely affected TS patients by Visser-Vandewalle and colleagues. They introduced bilateral stimulation of the medial part of the CM/Pf or the Voi nuclei of the thalamus. They chose this anatomical location on the basis of the favorable results obtained by Hassler and Dieckmann (1973) with thalamotomy. The initial patient showed 90% improvement in tics at 1 year of follow-up. Subsequently, three additional cases were described by the same group

using the same target (Visser-Vandewalle et al., 2003), and improvement was reported for each of these cases; their follow-up durations ranged between 8 months and 5 years, and adverse effects included stimulation-induced erectile dysfunction and reduced energy levels in two of the three cases (Visser-Vandewalle et al., 2003). Bajwa and colleagues (2007) reported another case of a 48-year-old man with severe TS manifesting with dangerous self-injurious motor tics characterized by violent and continuous head jerks that had produced a permanent left-sided weakness secondary to spinal cord injury. Bilateral implantation of electrodes at the level of the CM, substantia periventricularis, and Voi resulted in substantial tic improvement at more than 24 months of follow-up. A subsequent case report showed efficacy of the same target in a 40-year-old woman with TS whose severe tics had caused unilateral blindness, and following incomplete improvement obtained after placement of deep brain stimulators in the anterior limb of the internal capsule (Shields et al., 2008). Similar efficacy was confirmed in a Chinese patient with self-injurious tics (Lee et al., 2011).

Subsequent work from our group described a larger case series of bilateral DBS in the same brain region (Servello et al., 2008, 2009). Eighteen patients received bilateral DBS using a thalamic target located 2 mm anteriorly to the one reported by Visser-Vandewalle and colleagues (2003) (Fig. 26.2); their follow-up duration ranged between 3 and 18 months, with observed decreases in the severity of tics, premonitory urges, obsessive-compulsive symptoms, OCD, SIB, and anxiety. Fifteen of these 18 patients were re-evaluated at a 24-month follow-up and marked improvement was confirmed in terms of tic severity, obsessive-compulsive symptoms, anxiety and depressive symptoms, and subjective perception of social functioning and quality of life (Porta et al., 2009a). Importantly, there was no detrimental effect of thalamic stimulation upon cognitive measures. An even longer follow-up (6 and 10 years) has been reported on two patients, in whom tic improvement was maintained (Ackermans et al., 2010). One of these two individuals, however, exhibited an

Table 26.1 Summary of Case Series or Controlled Studies of DBS in TS

Authors	No. of patients	Targets	Stimulation parameters	Follow-up (months)	Tic severity improvement	Comments
Vanderwalle et al. (1999)/ Visser-Vanderwalle (2003)	3	CM/Pf, Voi	Bipolar all contacts 100 Hz, 210 μs, 2.4 V right, 2.2 V left; Right double monopolar 65 Hz, 210 μs, 3 V; left one monopolar 100 Hz, 210 μs; Right one monopolar 2.8 V, 130 Hz, 210 μs; left one monopolar 2.4 V, 100 Hz, 210 μs	60; 12; 8	90% 72% 83%	Feeling of decreased energy. Increased libido and decreased libido in 1 patient each.
Diederich et al. (2005)	1	Posteroventral GPi	One monopolar 2 V, 185 Hz, 60 μs	14	75%	Small symptomatic bleeding right globus pallidus. Bradykinesia left hand.
Houeto et al. (2005)/ Houeto et al. (2005); Welter et al. (2008)	2 1	CM/Pf and anteromedial GPi	CMPf: double monopolar 1.5–1.7 V Gpi: single or double monopolar 1.5–3.5 V	60,27 20	82%, "stable reduction", 74%	Prospective randomized double-blind sham. Pallidal better than thalamic stimulation, both better than sham.
Flaherty et al. (2005)/ Shields et al. (2008)	1 Same patient	Anterior capsule CM/Pf, Voi	Bipolar 4.1 V, 185 Hz, 210 μs 7 V, 90 μs, 185 Hz	18 3	25% 32%	Electrode breakage. DBS in another target.
Gallagher et al. (2006)	1	Posteroventral GPi	Not available	Several months	Disappearance of tics	Infection and explantation
Ackermans et al. (2006, 2007)	1 1	CM/Pf, Voi Posteroventral GPi	Double monopolar 6.4 V, 130 Hz, 120 μs Triple monopolar 3.1 V, 170 Hz, 210 μs	12 12	Tics from 20 to 3/min Tics from 28 to 2/min	Decreased libido Vertical gaze palsy Both: decreased energy

Kuhn et al. (2007)	1	NAC	Tetra monopolar 7 V, 90 μs, 130 Hz	30	41%	Y-BOCS improved >50%.
Shahed et al. (2007)	1	Posteroventral GPi	6	Monopolar 5 V, 156 Hz, 90 μs	84%	Y-BOCS improved 69%, fewer obsessions.
Bajwa et al. (2007)	1	CM/Pf, Voi	Bipolar 2 V, 130 Hz, 90 μs	24	66%	Y-BOCS improved 75%.
Maciunas et al. (2007)	5	CM/Pf, Voi	Bipolar 2 V, 130 Hz, 90 μs	3	66%	Three patients improved. Quality-of-life scale was used.
Vilela Filho et al. (2007)	2	GPe	Variable polarity 3.5–3.6 V, 90–210 μs, 130–185 Hz	23	Mean 43%	Ongoing study of external pallidal DBS
Servello et al. (2008)	18	CM/Pf, Voi	Not available	3	81%	Progressive improvement
				18	65%	
Dehning et al. (2008)	1	Posteroventral GPi	Bipolar, 2.5–4 V, 90–120 μs, 130 Hz	12	88%	
Zabek et al. (2008)	1	Right NAC	Monopolar 4.2 V, 145 Hz, 210 μs	28	80%	Unilateral SIB disappeared.
Porta et al. (2009)	15	CM/Pf, Voi	Not available	24	52%	Y-BOCS improved 60%.
Neuner et al. (2009)	1	NAC	Double monopolar 6 V, 145 Hz, 90 μs	36	44%	Incidental finding: loss of desire to smoke
Vernaleken et al. (2009)	1	Thalamus Dorsomedial nucleus	Double monopolar 4.4 V, 130 Hz, 180 μs	6	36%	Previously ineffective GPi stimulation
Martinez-Torres et al. (2009)	1	STN	Monopolar 3 and 3.2 V, 130 Hz, 60 μs	12	76%	Concomitant Parkinson's disease and TS
Servello et al. (2009)	36	CM/Pf, Voi	Variable polarity	24	47.7%	Largest patient series reported to date

(Continued)

Table 26.1 (*Continued*)

Authors	No. of patients	Targets	Stimulation parameters	Follow-up (months)	Tic severity improvement	Comments
Dueck et al. (2009)	1	Posteroventral GPi	Monopolar, 4 V, 130 Hz, 120 μs	12	No improvement	Comorbidity: learning disability
Burdik et al. (2010)	1	ALIC/NAC	Bipolar, 6.5 V, 135 Hz, 90 μs	30	Fewer tics by 17% Unchanged severe OCD	First negative report
Takanobu et al. (2010)	3	CM/Pf, Voi	Bipolar 2.3–2.6 V, 80–130 Hz, 180–210 μs	12	52–71%	Blurred vision
Lee et al. (2011)	1	CM/Pf, Voi	Double monopolar 3.5–5 V 150–200 Hz, 150–180 μs	18	81%	No adverse effect reported
Martinez-Fernandez et al. (2011)	5	Posteroventral or anteromedial GPi	Monopolar 2.5 V, 170 Hz, 150 μs, Double monopolar. Bipolar	3–24	29%	Capsular effects, infection
Ackermans et al. (2011)	6	Voi–CM–substantia periventricu-laris	Monopolar and bipolar 1–7.3 V	12	49%	Oculomotor dysfunction, decreased energy, parenchymal hemorrhage, infection

Studies are listed in chronological order.

CM/Pf, centromedian/parafascicularis thalamic nuclei; GPi, globus pallidus internus; Voi, ventralis oralis internus nucleus of thalamus; DBS, deep brain stimulation; NAC, nucleus accumbens; Y-BOCS, Yale-Brown Obsessive-Compulsive Rating Scale; GPe, globus pallidus externus; TS, Tourette syndrome; STN, subthalamic nucleus; ALIC, anterior limb of the internal capsule increase in anger and aggression with problems of psychosocial adaptation.

The first controlled trial assessing the efficacy of this thalamic target was conducted by Maciunas and colleagues (2007). These authors assessed tic severity and quality of life for 4 weeks in five adult subjects with severe TS, with each week spent in one of four states of unilateral and bilateral stimulation. The primary outcome measure was the modified Rush Video-Based Rating Scale (MRVBRS) score, on which a significant reduction was shown in the bilateral on state; there was also improvement on the Yale Global Tic Severity Scale (YGTSS) and quality-of-life indices. Importantly, the therapeutic benefit persisted after 3 months of open stimulator programming. The long-term benefit, however, was accounted for mainly by a marked response in three of the five patients, whereas the other two did not exhibit a significant benefit.

The effect of CM–substantia periventricularis–Voi stimulation was more recently assessed in another small-scale, prospective, randomized, double-blind crossover trial, with evaluation at 1-year follow-up (Ackermans et al., 2011). The anatomical coordinates of the target were 2 mm posterior to those used by Servello and colleagues (2008). Initially, eight patients were enrolled in the randomized study, and six completed a 12-month follow-up. In one of the two groups (on/off group), the stimulator was switched on after surgery for 3 months, and this was followed by an off period of 3 months; in the other, the stimulator was switched "off" in the first 3 months and then switched on for the following 3 months (off/on group). However, only two patients completed the full 3 months off and 3 months on, whereas the other four asked for rescheduling after a few weeks in the on or off condition. YGTSS scores were significantly lower (37%) when the stimulator was on than when it was off; compared to the preoperative period, the subjects on average showed a 49% improvement after 1 year. However, no changes were observed on the Conners Adult ADHD Rating Scale, the Yale-Brown Obsessive Compulsive Scale, and the Beck Anxiety and Depression Inventories. In addition, on neurocognitive testing the patients showed poorer performance on the Stroop Color Word Card test, a measure of selective attention and response inhibition. Other adverse events included

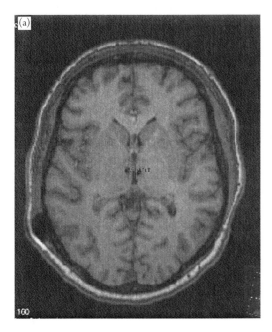 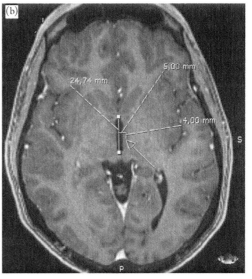

FIGURE 26.2 MRI of the CM/Pf complex target.

subtle oculomotor dysfunction, varying from blurred vision to fixation problems and vertical gaze palsy in one participant who intraoperatively had a small parenchymal hemorrhage at the tip of one electrode. Most of these patients, moreover, reported a substantial, albeit generally tolerated, restriction in daily activities due to reduced energy levels.

Globus Pallidus Internus (Ventroposterolateral Motor Part)

The first report of successful treatment of tics with bilateral globus pallidus internus (GPi) stimulation was published in abstract form in 2002, and described the case of a 27-year-old man with refractory TS (van der Linden et al., 2002). Soon after, Diederich and colleagues (2005) reported on a 14-month follow-up study of a patient with refractory TS who exhibited a 73% reduction in tic frequency in the postoperative phase of a bilateral GPi DBS, with permanent, albeit tolerated, left-sided bradykinesia. Success was also shown in one case reported by Ackermans and colleagues (2006). Another noteworthy case is that of a 26-year-old man who experienced a marked improvement of his motor and phonic tics following bilateral GPi DBS (Gallagher et al., 2006): however, after that the left stimulator lead was removed due to infection, and motor tics reappeared in the right side of his face and in his right arm. Dehning and colleagues (2008) reported successful bilateral GPi DBS in a female TS patient. Shahed and colleagues (2007) described the results of the same procedure in a 16-year-old boy with severe, drug-refractory TS. In this case the MRVBRS score improved to a moderate degree; however, there was also a more considerable improvement in comorbid symptoms and quality of life, as well as improvement in cognitive measures of verbal reasoning, psychomotor speed, mental flexibility, and visual perception. Another case of bilateral GPi DBS in a 16-year-old boy with longstanding, severe, and treatment-refractory TS associated with learning disabilities did not result in a similar degree of improvement (Dueck et al., 2009). A case series of four TS patients treated with ventroposterolateral GPi stimulation showed good response in two of them, whose predominant symptoms were SIB and vocal tics (Dehning et al., 2011). Interestingly, these two patients responded also to electroconvulsive therapy, which was ineffective in the two patients who were nonresponders to DBS.

Globus Pallidus Internus (Anteromedial Limbic Part)

The limbic part of GPi was stimulated for the first time in a TS patient in the context of a prospective, double-blind, randomized "N of 1" study of a 36-year-old woman with a severe form of TS manifesting also with coprolalia and dangerous SIB (Houeto et al., 2005). She was treated with bilateral stimulation of the CM/Pf complex of the thalamus, anteromedial GPi, or both. The severity and frequency of her tics were ameliorated by about 70% with disappearance of SIB on each of the three different stimulation approaches. No potentiation or interference between the two targets was observed when both sets of electrodes were switched on. The same group subsequently enlarged the series to three patients (Welter et al., 2008). In this study, thalamic and/or pallidal stimulation produced a marked improvement in tic severity in comparison with preoperative and sham evaluations, with better improvement obtained with anteromedial GPi stimulation (80%, 90%, and 67% reduction in motor and phonic tic subscore of the YGTSS) compared to CM/Pf thalamic stimulation (64%, 30%, and 40% reduction). Once again no additional improvement on combined thalamic and pallidal stimulation was observed. Interestingly, persisting adverse effects on pallidal stimulation included nausea, vertigo, and anxiety, whereas CM/Pf stimulation led to a decrease in libido, consistent with some of the preliminary findings from the Dutch-Flemish group (Visser-Vandewalle et al., 2003). Another important finding of this work is the long-term benefit observed with both stimulation targets (Fig. 26.3).

Another noteworthy experience of GPi DBS in TS comes from the National Hospital for

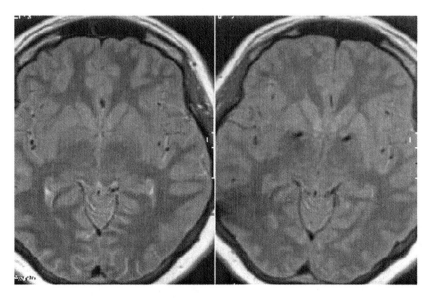

FIGURE 26.3   MRI of the anteromedial GPi target.

Neurology & Neurosurgery, Queen Square, London (Martinez-Fernandez et al., 2011). In their small series of four cases treated with bilateral GPi DBS, in two the ventroposterolateral part was the target selected, whereas the anteromedial part was the target in the other two. All patients improved, but to a variable degree. The more convincing effect was seen in patients with electrodes sited in the anteromedial part, with mean reduction in the MRVBRS score of 54% in the former and 37% in the ventroposterolateral site. Although no clinical data was reported in 2012 Saleh et al. (Saleh et al., 2012) described simultaneous dual pallidal stimulation for TS by targeting the medial/limbic and the posteroventral/motor pallidal sections. Clinical data for this approach is pending.

Nucleus Accumbens/Anterior Limb of Internal Capsule

The anterior limb of the internal capsule has been previously used as a target for DBS of drug-refractory OCD (Flaherty et al., 2005). This area is mostly occupied by pallidostriatal fibers and by fibers traveling between the orbitofrontal cortex and the anterodorsal thalamus. Flaherty and colleagues (2005) reported on the results of a single case of severe TS and OCD.

This patient showed a 25% reduction of tic severity 18 months after the surgery. Adverse effects included apathy and hypomania (Fig. 26.4).

The nucleus accumbens (NAC) is presumed to have a modulatory role on limbic cortico-basal ganglia networks, and its activity is strongly influenced by dopaminergic neurotransmission. DBS of the NAC showed some efficacy in treating obsessive-compulsive symptoms (Sturm et al., 2003). The first report of efficacy of NAC DBS in TS was published in 2007 (Kuhn et al., 2007). This patient exhibited a 41% improvement in the YGTSS severity score at a follow-up assessment conducted 30 months after the surgery. A second case of intractable TS was treated with unilateral DBS where the right NAC was the target (Zabek et al., 2008). This patient, who had severe, drug-refractory tic disorder and associated compulsions and SIB, was treated with unilateral right-sided NAC stimulation. At the 28-month follow-up visit, a good response was observed on tics, compulsions, and SIB. However, subsequent single case reports have been inconsistent in showing sustained benefit of this target (Burdick et al., 2010; Neuner et al., 2009, 2010). For example, in one case report of bilateral DBS of the anterior inferior internal capsule, there was incomplete improvement of tics, and the patient subsequently underwent CM/Pf stimulation with better results

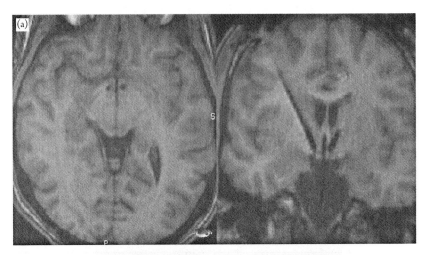

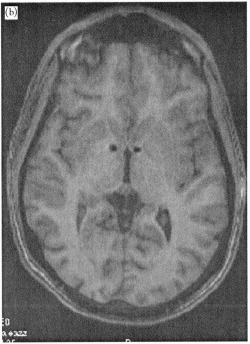

FIGURE 26.4   MRI of the NAC (**A**) and NAC/anterior limb of the internal capsule (**B**) targets.

(Shields et al., 2008). Additional observations on larger, better-characterized series of TS patients are needed to justify controlled studies on this specific target. Along this line, Servello and colleagues (2010) reported on ten patients with complicated TS who underwent DBS targeting the NAC. Three of these ten patients had already gained improvement over tic frequency and severity after a first DBS procedure that targeted the CM/Pf or GPi. The decision to target the NAC was made on the basis of persistent behavioral comorbidities (obsessive-compulsive features, anxiety, and depression). A moderate degree of improvement was observed with NAC stimulation.

Subthalamic Nucleus

An interesting serendipitous observation came from Martinez-Torres and colleagues (2009), who described a 38-year-old man with an 8-year history of Parkinson's disease secondary to an exon deletion in the parkin gene, who also had a history of typical childhood-onset tics that had improved around puberty and worsened later in adulthood before the diagnosis of Parkinson's disease. A bilateral subthalamic nucleus (STN) stimulation to treat severe Parkinson's disease led also to improvement of his tics; this improvement was observed even before stimulation was started, likely due to a microlesion effect. Tic frequency diminished by 89% at 6 months and 97% at 1 year, based on videotape count. Switching off the stimulation led to an immediate increase in tic frequency. Interestingly, stimulation of the anterior portion of the STN reduced stereotypies in a primate model (Baup et al., 2008). Stimulation of the STN might allow modulation of both limbic and sensorimotor territories. Given its small size and characteristic electrophysiology, the STN may be a promising target for the treatment for TS as well as related behavioral disorders.

Other Neuroanatomical Targets

Additional targets reported to show efficacy only in small case series are the dorsomedial thalamic nucleus (Vernaleken et al., 2009) and the globus pallidus externus (Vilela Filho et al., 2008, 2010). The latter experience comprises seven patients but has been published to date only in abstract form. The choice of the globus pallidus externus as a target derives from the observation of stereotyped tic-like movements following microstimulation of this structure in nonhuman primates with a gamma-aminobutyric acid (GABA) antagonist, bicucullin (François et al., 2004; Grabli et al., 2004). Given the high number of single case observations of DBS in TS, a relevant publication bias is highly likely, particularly with respect to targets for which only isolated case reports are currently available.

In summary, at present no clear recommendation can be given as to which target is the optimal one, given that data from large active comparative trials are lacking. Based on the grade of evidence present and the general experience, CM/Pf-Voi and GPi seem the most reasonable targets (Muller-Vahl et al., 2011). DBS does not work for everyone with severe TS, and a complete cessation of tics is the exception rather than the rule. More research is needed to demonstrate whether

specific targets can provide amelioration of specific symptoms, in the view of an individually tailored approach. In a few TS patients with severe comorbid OCD, the addition of the NAC/anterior internal capsule target to the CM/Pf-Voi target has been proposed as a form of "rescue procedure" (Servello et al., 2010).

ADVERSE EVENTS ASSOCIATED WITH DBS

In general, serious adverse events of DBS in TS are, overall, not specific to this condition. Complications can be divided into those related to the surgery, the hardware, and the stimulation. The most serious potential surgery-related complication is intracerebral hemorrhage (Servello et al., 2011), potentially caused by the repeated passages of the test electrode during microelectrode recording and macrostimulation to confirm correct electrode positioning (Hariz et al., 2002). One case treated with bilateral GPi DBS led to unilateral bradykinesia which was permanent, but well tolerated (Diederich et al., 2005). As noted above, Ackermans and colleagues (2007, 2011) reported a small hemorrhage caudal to the tip of a thalamic electrode that caused transient vertical gaze palsy. An additional case of bilateral subcortical hematomas was also reported in a patient who subsequently was noted to have low levels of coagulation factor XIIIa (Idris et al., 2010).

Infections leading to removal of the stimulator have also been reported as an emerging surgery- and hardware-related adverse event (Gallagher et al., 2006; Servello et al., 2011). Servello and colleagues (2011) retrospectively reviewed their experience of 531 procedures on 272 patients treated for various movement disorders. This total included 39 individuals with severe TS. Remarkably, among these TS cases they found a significant number of infectious complications at the stimulator site. It is intriguing to speculate whether this finding may be somehow related to the overactive immune response in these patients (see Chapter 14).

Stimulation-related adverse events of DBS in TS have been mostly associated with CM/Pf-Voi stimulation. The most commonly reported side effect is a combination of sedation, fatigue, reduced energy, apathy, and lethargy, reported by both patients and caregivers; this has been observed following thalamic (Ackermans et al., 2011; Visser-Vandewalle et al., 2003), GPi (Diederich et al., 2005; Foltynie et al., 2009), and anterior capsule (Flaherty et al., 2005) procedures. Visual abnormalities have also been reported with relative frequency. All patients in the randomized trial by Ackermans and colleagues (2011) reported visual disturbances, varying from blurred vision to fixation problems. However, thus far no objective abnormalities have been detected by optometrists or neuro-ophthalmologists; also, vestibular tests confirmed normal vestibular and oculomotor function in these patients, suggesting that these might have been due to visual processing problems. Servello and colleagues (2008) also reported subjective vertigo, blurring of vision, and upward ocular deviation after thalamic DBS, although these side effects were transient in their series. Other adverse events reported anecdotally have been changes (predominantly a decrease) in sexual function (libido, potency, ejaculation), vertigo, anxiety, nausea, weight loss, psychosis, depression or hypomania, social avoidance, and short dystonic jerks when GPi stimulators were switched on (Muller-Vahl et al., 2011).

PATIENT SELECTION

The selection of TS patients for DBS is difficult and remains controversial. Given the paucity of sufficiently powered randomized controlled trials proving the efficacy of this therapeutic approach in adult patients with severe TS, national and international consensus-based guidelines are needed. The issues of target selection and number of stimulated electrodes have been summarized above. At present, the clinical judgment concerning the eligibility of patients to undergo DBS is guided by different sets of recommendations from expert clinicians (Cavanna et al., 2011; Mink et al., 2006; Muller-Vahl et al., 2011; Steeves et al., 2012). Table 26.2 summarizes these recommendations. Some of the key issues that need to be considered include the following points.

Patients must have received a diagnosis of TS or chronic tic disorder by a clinician with experience in the diagnosis and treatment of tic disorders. The confidence in the diagnosis is an undisputable condition to define a patient's eligibility for DBS. Relying on diagnostic checklists or the diagnostic confidence index for TS (see Chapter 20 for further details on this instrument) might further help to fulfill this condition. In general, until DBS becomes more widely used in these conditions, it is advisable that the diagnosis of every patient for whom DBS is considered should be confirmed in a tertiary referral center for TS and related disorders. Ideally, patients should be assessed by an expert multidisciplinary team that includes neurologists, psychiatrists, psychologists, and experienced functional neurosurgeons.

Tics should be the patient's main symptom. They should be sufficiently severe and impair significantly the patient's quality of life. In chronic tic disorders the efficacy of DBS has been tested primarily in respect to the alleviation of tics rather than other manifestations, such as psychiatric comorbid symptoms. Whereas it seems pure common sense that tics should be severe enough to justify an invasive procedure like DBS, the threshold of severity for DBS eligibility is highly disputed. The U.S. Tourette Syndrome Association's series of recommendations for DBS (Mink et al., 2006) suggested a cutoff at more than 35 of the maximal 50 points of the YGTSS severity subscore (see Chapter 20 for further detail on the properties of this scale as well as other severity and quality-of-life rating scales for tics). As discussed also in the European Society for the Study of Tourette Syndrome (ESSTS)'s recommendations (Muller-Vahl et al., 2011), this score requires a mean tic score of 4 for one of the two types of tics (motor or phonic) and of 3 for the other type. Although this threshold seems reasonable, it has never been formally tested in routine clinical practice. Moreover, the severity of tics should be persistent, and not simply related to a restricted period of time. If tics remain severe and disabling for at least 1 year in adults, the chances of subsequent improvement in the following period of time are generally low.

However, patients may score lower on the YGTSS but nevertheless be markedly impaired

Table 26.2 Selected Recommendations for DBS in TS

	TSA USA-MDS (Mink et al., 2006)	Dutch Flemish study group (Ackermans et al., 2006)	Italian study group (Porta et al., 2009b)	ESSTS (Muller-Vahl et al., 2011)
Patient age	25 or over, with rare exceptions	25 or over	18 or over with rare exceptions	18 or over
Symptom severity	YGTSS >35/50 for 12 months (videotaped and family interview assessment)	YGTSS >20/50 and Overall impairment >5/50 (videotaped assessment)	YGTSS ≥35/50 with motor tic subscore ≥15, tics causing distress, SIB	YGTSS ≥35/50, tics should be severe for ≥1 year and lasting ≥5 years before DBS
Comorbidities	Baseline assessment of comorbidities and stable treatment for 6 months	Tics should be the primary clinical problem (e.g, not OCD or SIB as primary problem)	Extensive assessment recommended	Tics should be the primary problem.
Treatment refractoriness criteria	Failure to respond to (or severe side effects from) alpha-adrenergic agonists, typical and atypical antipsychotics, benzodiazepine, behavioral therapy	None/partial response to 3 medications (for 12 weeks), including typical and atypical antipsychotics and "experimental" drugs, and to 12 sessions of behavioral therapy	Lack of response to or intolerable adverse effects from typical and atypical antipsychotics and "experimental" treatments	Treatment with 3 different drugs, including both a typical and an atypical antipsychotic in adequate dosage over an adequate period of time proving not effective or leading to unacceptable adverse events; behavioral treatment for 12 sessions without effect
Other patient specifications	Willingness to engage in ongoing treatment, good compliance, consider psychosocial difficulties	Ability to make a "complete decision" to participate, emphasis on ethics and right to withdraw	Assessment of treatment compliance, symptom-related difficulties in social life	Tics cause social impairment in quality of life (relationships, home environment, school/work). Compliance and stable psychosocial environment.

(Continued)

Table 26.2 (*Continued*)

	TSA USA-MDS (Mink et al., 2006)	Dutch Flemish study group (Ackermans et al., 2006)	Italian study group (Porta et al., 2009b)	ESSTS (Muller-Vahl et al., 2011)
Patient exclusion criteria	Tics attributable to other disorder, severe/contraindicated medical or psychiatric conditions	Tics attributable to other disorders, severe/contraindicated medical or psychiatric conditions or mental deficiency	Cognitive dysfunction, substance abuse, tics due to medication or other tic disorder, previous brain surgery or abnormal imaging findings	No tics, obsessive-compulsive behavior, or SIB that could cause electrodes or stimulator damage. No major depression and/or suicidal thoughts at time of operation. No other conditions increasing risks in anesthesia, operative procedure, DBS.
Postoperative assessment (noteworthy points)	Determine site (CT preferred); blinded (stimulator on/off) assessment at 6–12 months including neuropsychological assessment	Blinded assessment	Comparison between planning and postoperative MRI, evaluation of tics and comorbidity	Supportive psychotherapy should be recommended after surgery.

TSA USA, Tourette Syndrome Association USA; ESSTS, European Society for the Study of Tourette Syndrome; YGTSS, Yale Global Tic Severity Scale severity subscore; SIB, self-injurious behaviors; DBS, deep brain stimulation; OCD, obsessive-compulsive disorder; ADHD, attention-deficit/hyperactivity disorder.

in their relationships, home environment, and academic or professional achievements, thus requiring efficacious treatment. The suitability of the disease-specific quality of life for TS, recently proposed by Cavanna and colleagues (2008), has never been adequately confronted with the problem of eligibility for DBS. Another possible scenario is that of patients with severe tics "by history," despite the documentation of lower severity ratings using the YGTSS or other scales when assessed in the clinic. This may occur as a consequence of the fluctuating course of tics (see Chapter 1 for more detail on this phenomenological aspect). In some cases, patients and reliable relatives, partners, or friends may provide strong evidence in favor of severe and disabling tics. Sometimes videotaped documentation of the high severity of tics in contexts other than the hospital might be of help to judge with higher sensitivity the degree of impairment caused by tics in the individual patient. On the other hand, if tics are repeatedly less severe during clinic visits, this might indicate that they are suppressible, and this would therefore justify the use of noninvasive procedures, such as behavioral therapy programs (habit reversal training or exposure-response prevention; see Chapter 23 for more details), before considering the patient for surgery. Specific types of tics or complex stereotyped tic-like behavior such as SIB, albeit infrequent, may be very dangerous for the patient and justify resorting to invasive treatments (Cavanna et al., 2011; Cheung et al., 2007). More work is certainly needed to standardize the assessment and eligibility criteria for DBS in respect to severity and functional impairment in patients with chronic tic disorders.

Patients should have a tic disorder that persists into adulthood. DBS is considered only for adult patients (older than 18); some authors recommend a minimum age of 25 years. This age threshold is not simply related to the risk of the procedure in youngsters, but even more to the possibility, which is typical of the natural history of the disorder, that tics will improve spontaneously with age. Over the past decade, almost 20% of the TS patients who underwent DBS were younger than 25, highlighting the heterogeneity

of approach in respect to the age factor across specialized clinical centers. Longitudinal, prospective studies analyzing possible predictive factors for persistence and severity of tics in adulthood might provide more robust evidence that could be useful to define eligibility for DBS even in younger patients. Chapter 5 provides an overview of the available evidence on natural history.

Tics should be resistant to less-invasive standard and experimental therapies. This is probably the most complex issue in respect to patient selection for DBS. Similar to what has been pointed out for severity, there are no universally accepted definitions of refractoriness to treatment for patients with tics. Future standardization of this definition is highly desirable in the context of eligibility for surgery. Muller-Vahl and colleagues (2011) proposed an assumption of "treatment resistance" if treatment with three different medications, including both a first- and a second-generation antipsychotic, at an adequate dosage over an adequate period of time, does not lead to significant tic reduction, or, alternatively, leads to unacceptable adverse effects (Table 26.2). In addition, a good adherence to the medication regimen should be present in the definition of "treatment resistance"; this may be related to the psychosocial environment in which the patient lives. An additional problem is the fact that, in many countries, only a very limited number of medications (in Europe, often only haloperidol) are licensed for tics and TS, so the trial of different medications may not always be feasible in routine clinical practice. The ESSTS recommendations (Muller-Vahl et al., 2011) also state that, if available, behavioral treatment should have been performed for at least 12 sessions without significant benefit. The limited availability of this treatment approach poses a similar problem to that of drug licensing in the practical application of a definition of "treatment resistance." In other words, if a patient is assessed in a center that has the facility to provide DBS, but where behavioral treatment is not available and clinicians are limited in their capability of prescribing drugs due to licensing restrictions, he or she might be offered surgery even if theoretically responsive to less-invasive treatments. The risk of this paradoxical situation seems real in many countries and should be taken seriously.

Patients and their families need to know that, thus far, DBS is not curative and in some cases does not even diminish tics, and that the procedure and the placement of the stimulators and the electrodes can cause serious adverse events. They also need to be aware that the most beneficial neuroanatomical target remains open to question, and that the long-term benefits and risks (greater than 5–10 years after the surgery) have not been assessed in more than a handful of individuals. Likewise, patients need to be aware that postsurgical programming is needed to optimize the stimulator settings. This can take a substantial period of time (weeks to months; see below).

DETAILS CONCERNING THE SURGICAL PROCEDURE

Surgical Planning

In our experience, a preoperative brain 1.5 Tesla magnetic resonance imaging (MRI) is routinely performed in all patients. T1 contrast-enhanced sequences with 1 mm in thickness are obtained when the preferred target is CM/Pf-Voi, whereas T1- and T2-weighted sequences with 1.5-mm slices are used when targeting nucleus accumbens or the anterior limb of the internal capsule. On the day of surgery, a brain computed tomography (CT) scan is performed after positioning of the stereotactic frame. MRI and CT images are transferred to a neuronavigation device; the images are fused together and target coordinates are calculated using the AC-PC (anterior commissure and posterior commissure) plane as an anatomical reference.

Anesthesia

Scanty data are available on the anesthetic and surgical procedures for DBS in TS (Ackermans et al., 2008a). Visser-Vandewalle and colleagues (1999) pointed out that general anesthesia could preclude intraoperative interrogation of the patient and monitoring of symptoms; if local anesthesia and sedation are used, patients can undergo clinical evaluation, which is also useful for the monitoring of adverse events during stimulation (Visser-Vandewalle, 2007). Our current experience is mainly with general anesthesia using propofol, curare, and clonidine, along with remifentanil.

Electrode Implantation, Intraoperative Neurophysiology, and Internal Pulse Generator Positioning

At the beginning of the surgical procedure, the patient is positioned on the operating table, the frame is secured, and the intraoperative CT scanner is positioned at the head of the patient. A sterile drape covers the CT to separate the operating field from the rest of the room. This strategy was introduced after experience with the mobile fluoroscopic system (C-arm) utilized for intraoperative control (Fig. 26.5). The Medtronic O-arm permits the surgeon to obtain x-ray images of the descending electrodes and an intraoperative CT scan after definitive electrode positioning (Fig. 26.6).

When thalamic nuclei are targeted, we obtain intraoperative microrecording by means of a computer-guided robot for simultaneous multi-track recording. One microelectrode is inserted in the central track corresponding to the planned trajectory and the other two are inserted in the anterior and the posterior tracks, respectively. Microelectrode recordings are obtained starting from a site positioned 10 mm cranially to the planned target and ending 1 mm caudally to the planned target. Microelectrodes are advanced in 0.5-mm steps. The electrical activity in each position is recorded for about 30 to 60 seconds. Signals are band-pass filtered (250 Hz to 5 kHz), visualized, and stored in a personal computer for further offline analysis. Central microelectrode signals are considered for the analysis. Segments containing artifacts are excluded. Along the track approaching the target there are three distinct firing patterns: "irregular firing" 6 to 4 mm above the target, "oscillatory bursting" 3 to 1 mm above the target, and a relatively "silent area" at the target. The zona incerta has

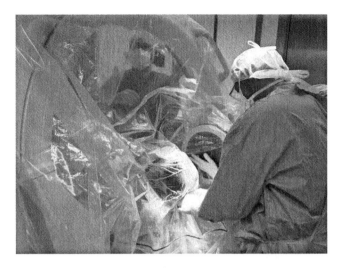

FIGURE 26.5   Mobile fluoroscopic system (C-arm) used for intraoperative control.

a silent pattern of neuronal activity (Hutchison et al., 1998). The area of decreased activity could be related to the approaching zona incerta below the targeted nuclei.

After electrode implantation, an intraoperative brain CT scan is obtained and then

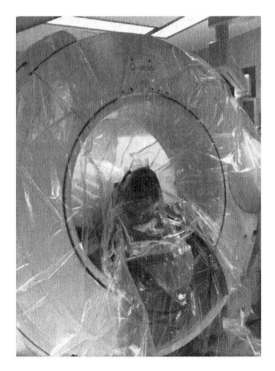

FIGURE 26.6   Medtronic O-arm used to obtain x-ray imaging of the descending electrodes.

transferred to the neuronavigation device, where it is fused with the preoperative CT scan to evaluate the correct electrode position. After confirming the correct electrode positioning, the internal pulse generator (IPG) is inserted. The IPG is placed in a submuscular pouch in the subclavian region (in earlier cases the abdominal wall was used). Interaction with the stimulator becomes feasible through an external device that communicates with the implanted stimulator by means of a wireless connection. Thus, it is possible to vary the stimulation parameters (frequency, amplitude, pulse width), to change the separate electrical contacts into anode, cathode, or neutral, and to obtain the history of the stimulation and the battery life.

Programming

Before programming the IPG, the accurate positioning of the leads must be verified. Two days after surgery a brain MRI (T1-weighted) with a 1-mm slice thickness is performed, and an experienced functional neurosurgeon and a neuroradiologist evaluate the electrode position. Currently standardized and homogenous guidelines for IPG programming are not available. Mink and colleagues (2006) recommend a defined procedure including on/off evaluation, which in our experience has provided unpredictable results in the short term; only long-term periods in on or off stimulation states are likely to have a substantial impact on symptoms. In our department, programming starts from setting the deepest contacts in monopolar fashion, and subsequently extending to bipolarity if results are not satisfying after a few days. In only a few patients does the regulation of contacts produce immediate/rapid results on motor and vocal tics. It takes at least 3 to 4 weeks to observe significant results.

The initial pulse duration and the frequency settings in our series are, respectively, 60 to 90 microseconds and 130 Hz. In some patients, more satisfactory results may be obtained by increasing the pulse width rather than modifying the intensity. Amplitude varies between 2 and 5 V, with pulse width ranging between 90 and 140 microseconds and frequency between 60 and 180 Hz (Servello et al., 2009). DBS programming in TS still seems to be a matter of trial and error, guided by the best clinical effects and the fewest adverse events.

Postoperative Monitoring

The clinical assessment of patients after DBS surgery is performed during both the on and the off stimulation states. According to Mink and colleagues (2006), efficacy and safety assessments are performed several weeks after surgery to allow time for stimulator settings to be optimized and stabilized.

Patients are evaluated at discharge and subsequently after 1, 3, 6, and 12 months, or on demand if any problem appears. The postoperative clinical assessment includes evaluation of tics and comorbidities using the same protocol employed in the preoperative assessment, which includes also the MRVRS. Another useful tool is the 10-point Visual Analogue Scale (VAS), as proposed by de Boer and colleagues (2004), which grades the subjective extent of impairment in social functioning after the DBS.

REFERENCES

Ackermans L, Duits A, Temel Y et al. Long-term outcome of thalamic deep brain stimulation in two patients with Tourette syndrome. *J Neurol Neurosurg Psychiatry* 2010; *81*:1068–1072.

Ackermans L, Duits A, Van der Linden C et al. Double-blind clinical trial of thalamic stimulation in patients with Tourette syndrome. *Brain* 2011; *134*:832–844.

Ackermans L, Kuhn J, Neuner I et al. Surgery for Tourette syndrome. *World Neurosurg* 2012; Jun 18 [E-pub ahead of print].

Ackermans L, Temel Y, Bauer NJC, Visser-Vandewalle V. Vertical gaze palsy after thalamic stimulation for Tourette syndrome: case report. *Neurosurgery* 2007; *61*:E1100.

Ackermans L, Temel Y, Cath D et al. Deep brain stimulation in Tourette's syndrome: two targets? *Mov Disord* 2006; *21*:709–713.

Ackermans L, Temel Y, Visser-Vandewalle V. Deep brain stimulation in Tourette's syndrome. *Neurotherapeutics* 2008a; 5:339–334.

Ackermans L, Temel Y, Visser-Vandewalle. Deep brain stimulation in Tourette's Syndrome. In: Tarsy D, Vitek JL, Starr PA, Okun MS (Eds.), *Deep brain stimulation in neurological and psychiatric disorders*. Totowa, NJ: Humana Press, 2008b, pp. 321–332.

These authors report the results of the largest double-blind randomized crossover study of DBS in TS to date. The stimulation of CM–substantia periventricularis–Voi remarkably ameliorated tics, but adverse side effects were observed.

Bajwa RJ, de Lotbinière AJ, King RA et al. Deep brain stimulation in Tourette's syndrome. *Mov Disord* 2007; *22*:1346–1350.

Baker EF. Gilles de la Tourette syndrome treated by bimedial frontal leucotomy. *Can Med Assoc J* 1962; *86*:746–747.

Baup N, Grabli D, Karachi C et al. High-frequency stimulation of the anterior subthalamic nucleus reduces stereotyped behaviors in primates. *J Neurosci* 2008; *28*:8785–8788.

Benabid AL, Pollak P, Gervason C et al. Longterm suppression of tremor by chronic stimulation of the ventral intermediate thalamic nucleus. *Lancet* 1991; *337*:403–406.

Benabid AL, Pollak P, Louveau A et al. Combined (thalamotomy and stimulation) stereotactic surgery of the VIM thalamic nucleus for bilateral Parkinson disease. *Appl Neurophysiol* 1987; *50*: 344–346.

The first major paper reporting DBS treatment in a patient with Parkinson's disease.

Bloch MH, Peterson BS, Schahill L et al. Adulthood outcome of tic and obsessive-compulsive symptom severity in children with Tourette syndrome. *Arch Pediatr Adolesc Med* 2006; *160*:65–69.

Burdick A, Foote KD, Goodman W et al. Lack of benefit of accumbens/capsular deep brain stimulation in a patient with both tics and obsessive-compulsive disorder. *Neurocase* 2010; 1–10.

Cavanna AE, Eddy CM, Mitchell R et al. An approach to deep brain stimulation for severe treatment-refractory Tourette syndrome: the UK perspective. *Br J Neurosurg* 2011; *25*:38–44.

Cavanna AE, Schrag A, Morley D et al. The Gilles de la Tourette Syndrome-Quality of Life scale (GTS-QOL): development and validation. *Neurology* 2008;*71*:1410–1416.

Despite the production of several clinical guidelines, in North America and Europe, for DBS in TS patients, a number of unresolved issues persist. Eligibility criteria and brain targets are discussed in this paper.

Cheung MY, Shahed J, Jankovic J. Malignant Tourette syndrome. *Mov Disord* 2007; *22*:1743–1750.

Coubes P, Roubertie A, Vayssiere N et al. Treatment of DYT1-generalised dystonia by stimulation of the internal globus pallidus. *Lancet* 2000; *355*:2220–2221.

de Boer AG, van Lanschot JJ, Stalmeier PF et al. Is a single-item visual analogue scale as valid, reliable and responsive as multi-item scales in measuring quality of life? *Qual Life Res* 2004; *13*:311–320.

Dehning S, Feddersen B, Cerovecki A et al. Globus pallidus internus-deep brain stimulation in Tourette's syndrome: can clinical symptoms predict response? *Mov Disord* 2011; *26*: 2440–2441.

Dehning S, Mehrkens JH, Muller N, Botzel K. Therapy-refractory Tourette syndrome: beneficial outcome with globus pallidus internus deep brain stimulation. *Mov Disord* 2008; 23:1300–1302.

Diederich NJ, Kalteis K, Stamenkovic M et al. Efficient internal pallidal stimulation in Gilles de la Tourette syndrome: a case report. *Mov Disord* 2005; 20:1496–1499.

Dueck A, Wolters A, Wunsch K et al. Deep brain stimulation of globus pallidus internus in a 16-year-old boy with severe Tourette syndrome and mental retardation. *Neuropediatrics* 2009; 40:239–242.

Flaherty AW, Williams ZM, Amirnovin R et al. Deep brain stimulation of the anterior internal capsule for the treatment of Tourette syndrome: technical case report. *Neurosurgery* 2005; 57(4 Suppl):E403.

Foltynie T, Martinez-Torres I, Zrinzo L et al. Improvement in vocal and motor tics following DBS of motor Gpi for Tourette syndrome, not accompanied by subjective improvement in quality of life: A case report. *Mov Disord* 2009; 24:S497–S498.

François C, Grabli D, McCairn K et al. Behavioural disorders induced by external globus pallidus dysfunction in primates II. Anatomical study. *Brain* 2004; 127:2055–2070.

Gallagher CL, Garell PC, Montgomery EB. Hemi tics and deep brain stimulation. *Neurology* 2006; 66:E12.

Grabli D, McCairn K, Hirsch EC et al. Behavioural disorders induced by external globus pallidus dysfunction in primates: I. Behavioural study. *Brain* 2004; 127:2039–2054.

Hariz MI. Complications of deep brain stimulation surgery. *Mov Disord* 2002; 17(Suppl 3):S162–166.

Harris LJ, Almerigi JB. Probing the human brain with stimulating electrodes: the story of Roberts Bartholow's (1874) experiment on Mary Rafferty. *Brain Cogn* 2009; 70:92–115.

Hassler R, Dieckmann G. Stereotaxic treatment of tics and inarticulate cries or coprolalia considered as motor obsessional phenomena in Gilles de la Tourette's disease. *Rev Neurol* 1970; 123:89–100.

A seminal paper. The lesional target described by Hassler and Dieckmann was the first to be used in DBS for TS.

Hassler R, Dieckmann G. Relief of obsessive-compulsive disorders, phobias and tics by stereotactic coagulations of the rostral intralaminar and medial thalamic nuclei. In: Laitinen LV, Livingston K (Eds.), *Surgical approaches in psychiatry. Proceedings of the Third International Congress of Psychosurgery.* Cambridge, UK: Garden City Press, 1973, pp. 206–212.

Houeto JL, Karachi C, Mallet L et al. Tourette's syndrome and deep brain stimulation. *J Neurol Neurosurg Psychiatry* 2005; 76:992–995.

Clear discussion of the rationale of choosing different targets for DBS in TS.

Hutchison WD, Allan RJ, Opitz H et al. Neurophysiological identification of the subthalamic nucleus in surgery for Parkinson's disease. *Ann Neurol* 1998; 44:622–628.

Idris Z, Ghani AR, Mar W et al. Intracerebral haematomas after deep brain stimulation surgery in a patient with Tourette syndrome and low factor XIIIA activity. *J Clin Neurosci* 2010; 17:1343–1344.

Jankovic J, Kurlan R. Tourette syndrome: Evolving concepts. *Mov Disord* 2011; 26:1149–1156.

Kuhn J, Lenartz D, Mai JK et al. Deep brain stimulation of the nucleus accumbens and the internal capsule in therapeutically refractory Tourette syndrome. *J Neurol* 2007; 254: 963–965.

The authors report their experience in DBS for TS targeting limbic nuclei (NA-ALIC).

Leckman JF. Phenomenology of tics and natural history of tic disorders. *Brain Dev* 2003; 25(Suppl1):S24–S28.

Leckman JF, Zhang H, Vitale A et al. Course of tic severity in Tourette syndrome: the first two decades. *Pediatrics* 1998; 102:14–19.

Lee MWY, Au-Yeung MM, Hung KN, Wong CK. Deep brain stimulation in a Chinese Tourette's syndrome patient. *Hong Kong Med J* 2011; 17:147–150.

Maciunas RJ, Maddux BN, Riley DE et al. Prospective randomized double-blind trial of bilateral thalamic deep brain stimulation in adults with Tourette syndrome. *J Neurosurg* 2007; 107:1004–1014.

The first paper reporting data from a prospective, randomized, double-blind controlled trial of DBS in TS.

Martinez-Fernandez R, Zrinzo L, Aviles-Olmos I et al. Deep brain stimulation for Gilles de la Tourette syndrome: a case series targeting subregions of the globus pallidus internus. *Mov Disord* 2011; 26:1922–1930.

Martinez-Torres I, Hariz MI, Zrinzo L et al. Improvement of tics after subthalamic nucleus deep brain stimulation. *Neurology* 2009; 72:1787–1789.

Mink JW, Walkup J, Frey KA et al. Patient selection and assessment recommendations for deep brain stimulation in Tourette syndrome. *Mov Disord* 2006; 21:1831–1838.

Muller-Vahl KR, Cath DC, Cavanna AE et al. European clinical guidelines for Tourette syndrome and other tic disorders. Part IV: deep brain stimulation. *Eur Child Adolesc Psychiatry* 2011; 20:209–217.

This paper presents a series of recommendations from an ad hoc working group within the European Society for the Study of Tourette Syndrome.

Neuner I, Halfter S, Wollenweber F et al. Nucleus accumbens deep brain stimulation did not prevent suicide attempt in Tourette syndrome. *Biol Psychiatry* 2010; 68:e19–e20.

Neuner I, Podoll K, Lenartz D et al. Deep brain stimulation in the nucleus accumbens for intractable Tourette's syndrome: follow-up report of 36 months. *Biol Psychiatry* 2009; 65:e5–e6.

Peterson BS, Pine DS, Cohen P, Brook JS. Prospective, longitudinal study of tic, obsessive-compulsive, and attention-deficit/hyperactivity disorders in an epidemiological sample. *J Am Acad Child Adolesc Psychiatry* 2001; 40:685–695.

Porta M, Brambilla A, Cavanna AE et al. Thalamic deep brain stimulation for treatment-refractory Tourette syndrome: two-year outcome. *Neurology* 2009a; 73:1375–1380.

Porta M, Sassi M, Ali F et al. Neurosurgical treatment for Gilles de la Tourette syndrome: the Italian perspective. *J Psychosom Res* 2009b; 67:585–590.

Rauch SL, Baer L, Cosgrove GR, Jenike MA. Neurosurgical treatment of Tourette's syndrome: a critical review. *Compr Psychiatry* 1995; 36:141–156.

Rickards H, Wood C, Cavanna AE. Hassler and Dieckmann's seminal paper on stereotactic thalamotomy for Gilles de la Tourette syndrome: translation and critical reappraisal. *Mov Disord* 2008; 23:1966–1972.

Sassi M, Porta M, Servello D. Deep brain stimulation therapy for treatment-refractory Tourette's syndrome: A review. *Acta Neurochir (Wien)* 2011;153:639–645.

Servello D, Porta M, Sassi M et al. Deep brain stimulation in 18 patients with severe Gilles de la Tourette syndrome refractory to treatment: the surgery and stimulation. *J Neurol Neurosurg Psychiatry* 2008; 79:136–142.

This paper presents the results obtained from a series of 18 patients with severe and refractory TS. DBS was used to stimulate mostly thalamic nuclei.

Servello D, Sassi M, Brambilla A et al. De novo and rescue DBS leads for refractory Tourette syndrome patients with severe comorbid OCD: a multiple case report. *J Neurol* 2009; 256:1533–1539.

The importance of this paper lies in the presentation of the concept of "rescue" DBS, paving the way for a clinically based tailored approach to target selection in DBS for TS.

Servello D, Sassi M, Brambilla A et al. Long-term, post-deep brain stimulation management of a series of 36 patients affected with refractory Gilles de la Tourette syndrome. *Neuromodulation* 2010; 13:187–194.

Servello D, Sassi M, Gaeta M et al. Tourette syndrome (TS) bears a higher rate of inflammatory complications at the implanted hardware in deep brain stimulation (DBS). *Acta Neurochir (Wien)* 2011; 153:629–632.

Discussion of complications related to DBS in TS.

Shahed J, Poysky J, Kenney C et al. GPi deep brain stimulation for Tourette syndrome improves tics and psychiatric comorbidities. *Neurology* 2007; 68:159–160.

Shields DC, Cheng ML, Flaherty AW et al. Microelectrode-guided deep brain stimulation for Tourette syndrome: within-subject comparison of different stimulation sites. *Stereotact Funct Neurosurg* 2008; 86:87–91.

Spiegel EA, Wycis HT, Marks M, Lee AJ. Stereotaxic apparatus for operations on the human brain. *Science* 1947; 106:349–350.

Steeves T, McKinlay BD, Gorman D et al. Canadian guidelines for the evidence-based treatment of tic disorders: behavioural therapy, deep brain stimulation, and transcranial magnetic stimulation. *Can J Psychiatry* 2012; 57:144–151.

Sturm V, Lenartz D, Koulousakis A et al. The nucleus accumbens: a target for deep brain stimulation in obsessive-compulsive and anxiety disorders. *J Chem Neuroanat* 2003; 26:293–299.

Discussion of the role of nucleus accumbens and its stimulation to reduce obsessive-compulsive symptoms and anxiety in patients with refractory TS.

Temel Y, Visser-Vandewalle V. Surgery in Tourette syndrome. *Mov Disord* 2004; 19:3–14.

van der Linden C, Colle H, Vandewalle V et al. Successful treatment of tics with bilateral internal pallidum (GPi) stimulation in a 27-year-old male patient with Gilles de la Tourette's syndrome. *Mov Disord* 2002; 17:S341.

Vernaleken I, Kuhn J, Lenartz D et al. Bithalamical deep brain stimulation in Tourette syndrome is associated with reduction in dopaminergic transmission. *Biol Psychiatry* 2009; 66:e15–17.

Vilela Filho O, Ragazzo P, Silva D et al. Bilateral GPe-DBS for Tourette's syndrome [abstract]. *Neurotarget* 2008; 3:65.

Vilela Filho O, Ragazzo P, Souza J et al. Bilateral GPe-DBS for Tourette syndrome: a double-blind prospective controlled study of seven patients [abstract]. In: *Abstract book of the ASSFN (American Society for Stereotactic and Functional Neurosurgery), 2010 biennial meeting: Bridging the Future of Neurosurgery*, New York. **The first case series of DBS for intractable TS is reported in this article.**

Visser-Vandewalle V, Temel Y, Boon P et al. Chronic bilateral thalamic stimulation: a new therapeutic approach in intractable Tourette syndrome. Report of three cases. *J Neurosurg* 2003; 99:1094–1100.

Visser-Vandewalle V, van der Linden C, Groenewegen HJ, Caemaert J. Stereotactic treatment of Gilles de la Tourette syndrome by high-frequency stimulation of thalamus. *Lancet* 1999; 353:724.

Visser-Vandewalle V. DBS in Tourette syndrome: rationale, current status and future prospects. *Acta Neurochir Suppl* 2007; 97:215–222.

Welter ML, Mallet L, Houeto JL et al. Internal pallidal and thalamic stimulation in patients with Tourette syndrome. *Arch Neurol* 2008; 65:952–957.

Zabek M, Sobstyl M, Koziara H, Dzierzecki S. Deep brain stimulation of the right nucleus accumbens in a patient with Tourette syndrome. Case report. *Neurol Neurochir Pol* 2008; 42:554–559

27

Alternative Treatments in Tourette Syndrome

BEATA ZOLOVSKA AND BARBARA J. COFFEY

Abstract

Complementary and alternative medicine (CAM) approaches are among the most popular and widely used treatments for Tourette syndrome (TS). This chapter is a systematic and critical review of the scattered evidence available on this topic. The five major groups of CAM practices are mind–body medicine, biologically based therapies, manipulative and body-based therapies, energy medicine, and whole medical systems. Research on CAM approaches is limited but rapidly expanding and improving in its quality. The CAM approaches most frequently reported to be used by patients with TS are dietary modification, allergy treatment, prayer, vitamins, massage, nutritional and dietary supplements, chiropractic manipulation, meditation, yoga, acupuncture, hypnosis, homeopathy, and biofeedback. Research evidence suggests that a number of CAM approaches are potentially useful in TS, yet there are methodological limitations in all studies. The approaches that appear to have the most promise based on the evidence to date are hypnosis, biofeedback, omega-3 fatty acids, cannabinoids, and traditional Chinese medicine (Ningdong granule).

Integrative Medicine is the practice of medicine that reaffirms the importance of the relationship between practitioner and patient, focuses on the whole person, is informed by evidence, and makes use of all appropriate therapeutic approaches, healthcare professionals and disciplines to achieve optimal health and healing.
—The Consortium of Academic Health Centers for Integrative Medicine

INTRODUCTION

In recent years, a growing scientific evidence base has accrued around the complexities of the Tourette syndrome (TS) phenotype. In addition to multiple tics, clinically referred individuals with TS may experience many other non-tic symptoms, such as obsessions, compulsions, inattention, impulsivity, and mood and anxiety symptoms. Tic and psychiatric symptoms may range from mild to severe and impairing. Despite the spectrum of symptom type and severity, there are only two formally approved treatments for TS: haloperidol and pimozide, typical neuroleptics. At best these medications result in only partial relief of tic symptoms, and unfortunately they are often associated with significant adverse effects, such as fatigue, weight gain, and extrapyramidal symptoms (Faridi & Suchowersky, 2003).

As a result, many individuals with TS discontinue treatment because of the intolerable adverse effects of these agents (Silva, 1996); one study reported that only 20% to 30% of TS patients taking haloperidol or pimozide continue with treatment (Chappell, 1995). The newer, atypical neuroleptics, while efficacious, have a different adverse-effect profile than conventional agents. Of these, risperidone has been the most extensively studied in the treatment of tics. Risperidone's efficacy is supported by results from at least two randomized, placebo-controlled trials, but adverse metabolic effects are also often reported. Despite efficacy, tic reduction with neuroleptics is limited to about 30% to 62%

of treated TS patients (Bruggeman et al., 2001). A full review of pharmacotherapy for treatment of tics in TS can be found in Chapter 24, and for treatment of psychiatric comorbid symptoms in Chapter 25.

Most recently, behavioral treatment has been found to be efficacious in the treatment of tics in youth with TS (Piacentini et al., 2010), but it is often difficult for patients to access trained behavioral therapists. A full review of cognitive-behavioral treatment of tics can be found in Chapter 23.

Taken together, given the limited efficacy, tolerability, or availability of these established interventions, a range of other treatments of TS has been explored in recent years, including complementary and alternative treatments, deep brain stimulation, transcranial magnetic stimulation, botulinum toxin, and novel medication approaches. Of these interventions, complementary and alternative medicine (CAM) treatments have been among the most popular and widely used. Patients with TS turn to CAM because of incomplete resolution of symptoms and significant adverse effects associated with conventional treatment. Although there is little scientific evidence base for the efficacy of these approaches, CAM treatments have been frequently used in patients with TS.

OVERVIEW OF CAM

Because of the widespread use of CAM practices, in 1992 the National Institutes of Health (NIH) established the Office of Alternative Medicine, which later became the NIH National Center for Complementary and Alternative Medicine (NCCAM). NCCAM has spearheaded educational efforts and funding of research on CAM. Defining and categorizing CAM treatments pose a challenge, as the field is broad, diverse, complex, and constantly changing. NCCAM defines CAM as a "diverse group of medical and health care systems, practices, and products that are not part of conventional Western medicine" (http://nccam.nih.gov). The boundaries between conventional and alternative approaches are fluid, and alternative therapies can become integrated into conventional

medicine as the research evidence base accrues to support the use of particular treatments. For example, guided imagery, a CAM intervention, has been proven to be effective in the treatment of pain in controlled studies, and as a result is now part of many pain-management protocols. In addition, what is considered conventional in the United States can be considered alternative in another country or culture, and what is conventional in another country might be alternative in the United States.

The NCCAM defines five major groups of CAM practices:

1. Mind-body medicine
2. Biologically based therapies
3. Manipulative and body-based therapies
4. Energy medicine
5. Whole medical systems

CAM approaches can be either integrated with or used in place of conventional medicine. Complementary medicine is used *in conjunction with* conventional medicine—for example, using a relaxation technique in addition to medication. Alternative medicine is used *in place of* conventional medicine—for example, using an herbal treatment instead of a medication. The term "CAM" is increasingly being replaced by "holistic," "integrative," or "integrative holistic" medicine.

Integrative holistic medicine is guided by a number of principles that focus on wellness and prevention; belief in the body's inherent drive toward healing; the importance of the relationship between the patient and the practitioner; use of all appropriate therapies, both conventional and alternative; use of least-invasive and toxic approaches first; focus on the whole person; and practitioners teaching by example and striving for balance in their own life (www.imconsortium.org).

Many large academic institutions have centers for CAM practice and research, and many hospitals have CAM programs. The Consortium of Academic Health Centers for Integrative Medicine currently has 50 members consisting of academic medical centers and affiliated institutions (www.imconsortium.org).

CAM USE: EPIDEMIOLOGY AND RESEARCH

The use of CAM has grown in recent decades in the United States and abroad. The estimates of prevalence of use of CAM vary dramatically, depending on how CAM is defined. The World Health Organization estimates that 80% of the world's population regularly uses some form of CAM. In the United States, more than one third of adults have used CAM (Eisenberg, 1993). The number of visits to CAM providers increased by 47.3% from 1990 to 1997, and in that same year there were more visits to CAM providers than to primary care physicians. Americans spent $21.2 billion on CAM services in 1997 (Eisenberg, 1998).

Notably, children and adolescents also increasingly use CAM. The pediatric utilization literature identified a huge range of rates of use: from 2% to 89% of youth, depending on the study (Braganza, 2003; Yussman, 2004). More than 50% of children with chronic, recurrent, and incurable conditions such as cerebral palsy, inflammatory bowel disease, or cancer use CAM (Armishaw, 1999; McCann, 2006).

Research on CAM is growing and the evidence base is expanding. The NCCAM increased its fiscal-year appropriations from $50 million in 1998 to $123 million in 2006 (http://nccam.nih.gov). Total funding by all Institutes and Centers of the NIH for research and training on CAM exceeded $225 million in 2006. Between 2002 and 2007, NCCAM funded 543 clinical research studies. Unfortunately, research on children and problems that primarily affect children is not a priority of NCCAM, and only 39 (7%) of the 543 studies included children.

The quality and amount of scientific studies of CAM are reported to be improving; in one review, the quality of CAM randomized controlled trials was judged as good as that of conventional randomized controlled trials (Klassen, 2005). Another study judged the quality of systematic reviews of CAM as better than that of conventional medicine systematic reviews (Lawson, 2005).

CAM POLICY ISSUES

The U.S. Food and Drug Administration (FDA) passed the Dietary Supplements Health and Education Act of 1994 (DSHEA) amending prior FDA statutes to include dietary supplement-specific provisions. Under DSHEA, a dietary supplement is a product (other than tobacco) intended to supplement the diet that bears or contains one or more of the following ingredients: a vitamin, mineral, herb or other botanical, or an amino acid. The classification of dietary supplements is separate from food and drug categories and lies outside the jurisdiction of the safety and regulatory rules that cover food and drugs (DSHEA, 1994). Because of these provisions, unlike pharmaceuticals, dietary supplements, which are often used as CAM interventions, can be marketed without studies documenting either safety or efficacy.

CAM USE IN TS

Despite the availability of established and FDA-approved medications for TS, CAM treatments are of interest to many individuals with TS. CAM treatments that have been frequently associated with TS can be grouped into the following categories; these are based on the NCCAM categories of CAM practices, published research on CAM in TS, and the results of two studies on the prevalence of CAM use in TS (Kompoliti et al., 2009; Mantel et al., 2004):

1. Mind-body
   - Relaxation
   - Biofeedback
   - Hypnosis
   - Meditation
   - Yoga
2. Biologically based therapies
   - Dietary modifications
   - Nutritional supplements
   - Herbal treatments
   - Tetrahydrocannabinol (THC)
   - Allergy treatment
   - Environmental modifications
3. Manipulative and body-based therapies
   - Massage
   - Spinal manipulation
   - Chiropractic
4. Energy medicine
   - Prayer (not strictly an energy medicine approach, but related)

5. Whole systems
- Chinese medicine
- Ayurveda
- Homeopathy

The focus of this section will be on evidence for these CAM approaches published in peer-reviewed manuscripts and book chapters; an evidence summary table is included at the end (Table 27.1). Bear in mind that the studies reported in this chapter are generally limited by small sample size and in many cases by methodological problems.

As an overview, two studies examined the prevalence of CAM use for treatment of TS. One study was a survey with a focus on nutritional supplements mailed to 1,250 potential responders; 115 returned the questionnaire. Of those, 87.8% reported using one or more nutritional supplements to control tic symptoms. In addition, 42.6% used dietary modification, 24.3% allergy treatment, 5.7% homeopathy, 13% environmental modification, 6% biofeedback, and 2% acupuncture (Mantel et al., 2004).

A second study, also a survey on CAM approaches, of 100 consecutive TS patients at Rush University Medical Center reported that 64% used at least one CAM modality (Kompoliti et al., 2009). Study participants averaged 21.5 ± 13.5 years of age; 76% were male and 87% were Caucasian. CAM treatments reported were prayer (28), vitamins (21), massage (19), dietary supplements (15), chiropractic manipulation (12), meditation (10), diet alteration (9), yoga (9), acupuncture (8), hypnosis (7), homeopathy (6), and EEG biofeedback (6). With regard to rationale for use, 35% of the participants reported using CAM modalities for additional benefits to their prescribed treatment, 28% for hope for cure, 25% for the belief that CAM is harmless, 23% for the belief that CAM is safer than traditional treatments, 23% for personal empowerment, 22% for the desire for a natural therapy, and 17% for a desire to achieve inner peace and harmony. Overall, 56% of the CAM users reported some improvement, and 47% paid out of pocket for the treatments. Interestingly, in this Rush University study, 80% of individuals reported that they initiated CAM use without informing their doctor.

As noted in other studies of CAM utilization, many individuals do not reveal their use of CAM treatments to their doctors. As some CAM treatments have the potential for interactions with medications and allopathic medicine treatments, a lack of communication between CAM consumers and their doctors poses a potential risk and highlights a limitation in communication.

CAM IN TS PSYCHIATRIC COMORBID DISORDERS

Clinically referred patients with TS often have comorbid psychiatric disorders or symptoms, such as attention-deficit/hyperactivity disorder (ADHD), obsessive-compulsive disorder (OCD), and mood and non-OCD anxiety disorders (Coffey et al., 2000; Robertson et al., 1988). A recent review of CAM in children with ADHD found predominant evidentiary support for zinc, iron, *Pinus marinus*, and Ningdong herbal formula and mixed evidence for omega-3 and L-acetyl carnitine (Sarris et al., 2011). In addition, a recent meta-analysis on the use of omega-3 in children with ADHD found that omega-3 supplementation, particularly with higher doses of eicosapentaenoic acid, was modestly effective in the treatment of ADHD (Bloch et al., 2011). A recent review of CAM in OCD and OCD spectrum disorders found evidentiary support from methodologically weak studies for mindfulness meditation, electro-acupuncture, and kundalini yoga, and evidence from better-designed studies for glycine, milk thistle, borage, movement decoupling, and N-acetylcysteine (Sarris et al., 2012). A review of research on CAM use in disorders frequently comorbid with TS, while much needed, is beyond the scope of this chapter.

CAM IN TS: RESEARCH AND EVIDENCE BASE

The evidence base for CAM treatments in TS remains limited and is generally of poor methodological quality. Nevertheless, the high level of interest and use of CAM treatments in TS appears to be unimpeded by the lack of high-quality research evidence for efficacy and

Table 27.1 Summary Table of CAM Treatment Modalities

Treatment Modality	Author, Date	Design and Measure	Sample Size	Outcome	Key Points
Mind/Body					
Relaxation	1. Turpin et al., 1984 2. Michlutka et al., 1984 3. Bergin et al., 1998	1. Case series 2. Case reports 3. Unblinded RCT	1. N = 4 2. N = 1 3. N = 23 Overall N = 28 (children)	Trend toward improvement, not significant	No convincing evidence of efficacy
Hypnosis	Raz et al., 2007; Lazarus et al., 2010; Additional case reports	Several case reports and case series; no standardized measures used	Largest study with N = 33 (children)	Positive	Potentially useful, but methodological limitations
Biofeedback	1. Tansey et al., 1986 2. Nagai et al., 2009	1. Case report 2. Case series using standardized measures	1. N = 2 2. N = 15 Overall N = 17 (adults)	Positive	Potentially useful, but methodological limitations
Yoga Meditation	No studies No studies				No studies No studies
Biological					
Dietary modification	Müller-Vahl et al., 2008	Questionnaire	1,887 mailed, 224 received	Significant correlation	Potentially useful, but no studies
Omega-3 fatty acids	Gabbay et al., 2012	RCT	N = 33children (children)	Negative; significant on tic-related impairment measure	Potentially useful for reduction of impairment

(*Continued*)

Table 27.1 (Continued)

Treatment Modality	Author, Date	Design and Measure	Sample Size	Outcome	Key Points
Magnesium	Grimaldi et al., 2002	Hypothesis and report of anecdotal self-reports	N/A	N/A	No studies
Cannabinoids	Müller-Vahl et al. 2002, 2003; Also other case reports	RCT, standardized measures used	N = 12 N = 24 Overall N = 36	Positive	Potentially useful, but small sample size
Allergy treatment	No studies				No evidence
Environmental modification	No studies				No evidence
Body Manipulation					
Massage	No studies				No evidence
Chiropractic	Elster, 2003	Case report	N = 1	Positive	Potentially useful, but methodological limitations
Energy medicine	No studies				No evidence
Whole Medical Systems					
Traditional Chinese medicine	Li, 2009 Zhao et al., 2010	Double-blind, placebo controlled RCT, standard measures used	N = 90 N = 64 Overall N = 154	Positive	Likely useful. Evidence from Chinese studies is positive; no U.S. or European studies.
Ayurveda	No studies				No evidence
Homeopathy	No studies				No evidence

safety of these approaches. Unfortunately, at this time, none of the commonly used CAM therapies has been subjected to large, controlled randomized trials in patients with TS. The available evidence is summarized in Table 27.1.

This section will focus on NCCAM's five general groups of CAM practices as they apply to TS.

Mind-Body Treatments for TS

RELAXATION

Relaxation techniques incorporate a variety of systematically applied relaxation exercises such as controlling and slowing down the breath, scanning the body for areas of tension, directing attention to specific areas of the body to relax various muscles, and using a variety of techniques to lower physical and emotional tension. Progressive muscle relaxation involves first tensing the muscles and then relaxing them, while cue-controlled relaxation involves relaxing muscles without initially tensing them. One case report, one case series and one randomized controlled trial were identified in the literature on relaxation for TS.

Turpin and Powell (1984) used cue-controlled relaxation and reported a reduction in tic symptoms in one of three patients with TS.

Michultka, Blanchard, and Rosenblum (1989) reported on a 19-year-old individual with TS receiving haloperidol 3 mg daily who was treated with relaxation and desensitization training. The first phase of treatment consisted of six sessions of progressive muscle relaxation. The emphasis was on application of techniques outside of the training session with use of anti-stress imagery, muscle discrimination (body scanning throughout the day for tension), and cue-controlled relaxation procedures. The second phase included six sessions of systematic desensitization training with imaginary exposures to anxiety-provoking situations combined with relaxation exercises. The authors reported a 40% to 50% reduction in distress and frequency and intensity of tics, both by patient and parent reports.

Bergin and colleagues (1998) reported on a 3-month, randomized, nonblinded trial of relaxation therapy in 23 patients with TS. Only 16 patients, mean age 11.8 years, completed the study, which included either weekly, hour-long relaxation training sessions, or for the control group, minimal therapy awareness and quiet time training. At 6 weeks, the relaxation group showed a trend toward improvement in tic severity, but there was no difference between the groups at 3 months.

HYPNOSIS

Hypnosis is a state characterized by heightened suggestibility, relaxation, and imagination. It is usually produced by a procedure called hypnotic induction, which comprises a series of preliminary instructions and suggestions linking external states and internal states. Hypnotic suggestions may be delivered by a hypnotist or administered as self-suggestions. Hypnosis is related to relaxation training and other self-regulatory techniques, and several case reports and a case series on the use of hypnosis in TS have been published (Raz et al., 2007).

Raz and colleagues (2007) described hypnosis as a "lens" for understanding TS, noting the importance of the partially controllable phenomenology of tics. They reported on several cases that illustrate the effectiveness of hypnosis in TS and the critical role of patient motivation. Among the examples Raz and colleagues give is that of a 25-year-old man with TS treated with hypnosis for severe tics. Hypnotic treatment was initially combined with haloperidol, but eventually the haloperidol was discontinued. Hypnotic suggestions were that "habits" might be necessary only during morning classes, and later suggestions that they could be omitted entirely at school. Within a few weeks, the habits were manifested only at home (occasionally) and at public places in the presence of his parents. Results indicated that the patient became tic-free while under hypnosis, and hypnotic suggestions were effective at reducing tic frequency.

Another of Raz's clinical illustrations reported a case series of self-hypnosis (relaxation and mental imagery) with four children with TS ranging in age from 6 to 10 years. Three children were taking haloperidol. Three patients learned self-hypnosis at the first visit and demonstrated reduction in tic frequency immediately after the self-hypnosis training. The improvement was sustained over time. A third illustration was that of a 16-year-old boy with TS treated with nine hypnosis sessions with full resolution of symptoms. Raz and colleagues concluded that hypnotic suggestion, a minimal-risk procedure, causes specific changes at the neural level and supports the concept that volitional control can be gained over involuntary processes.

More recently, Lazarus and Klein (2010) reported on a case series of 33 children with TS between the ages of 6 and 19 years who received self-hypnosis training aided by the viewing of a videotape of a boy undergoing self-hypnosis training. The self-hypnosis training involved teaching a number of procedures, for example imagining placing a STOP sign before a tic, thinking about a tic and then throwing it into a trash can, transferring the tic urge to a different part of the body, or depersonalization of tics with imagining the color or shape of the tic. Clinical response was defined as subjective verbal report of decrease in tic activity following the intervention; no standardized measures were used. Over the 2.5-month treatment interval evaluated, 79% of the participants achieved enough improvement in tic control to report personal satisfaction with the technique. Of the 33 patients, 12 experienced a dramatic response in tic control after two visits, 13 after three visits, and 1 after four visits.

BIOFEEDBACK

Biofeedback is a process that involves learning to control brain waves, muscle tone, skin conductance, heart rate, and pain perception through use of instruments that provide information on the activity of these parameters. Biofeedback relies on the connection between thoughts and emotions and body physiology. The procedure involves the presentation of a covert physiological response, such as heart rate, galvanic skin response (GSR), or brain wave (EEG) pattern, to the participant through an online visual or auditory feedback, allowing the individual to learn to actively modify his or her physiological state. The evidence for use of biofeedback in TS is limited.

Tansey (1986) reported on two cases of EEG biofeedback: one was a 32-year-old man with a 17-year history of a simple motor tic, and the other was a 14-year-old boy with a 6-year history of TS, characterized by symptoms of coprolalia, jaw movements, jerky forward head movements, and attention-deficit problems. The treatment consisted of weekly, 30-minute sessions using single-channel EEG aimed at training the participants to emit 14 ± 0.5-Hz neural discharge rhythm over the central rolandic cortex. The subjects received the instructions: "Now, let yourself become hollow and heavy. Just let yourself be a heavy, hollow rock; quiet, hollow, and heavy—and let the beeps (feedback tones reflective of neural discharge production in the targeted range) come out." The subjects received verbal praise every few minutes for "beep" production. In both cases, the EEG training resulted in improvement in tics. In the patient with the simple motor tic, the tic was completely eliminated, and remission was sustained on follow-up 3 years later. Tic symptoms resolved completely in the TS patient, and he remained free of tics and attention-deficit problems at the 6-month follow-up.

Another study, which examined the effect of biofeedback using GSR in 15 adults with TS, reported positive results. GSR reflects the activity of sympathetic nerves innervating the skin's sweat glands and is a measure of peripheral autonomic arousal associated with emotional and physical reactivity. Peripheral manipulation of GSR may influence central neural activity, and biofeedback training has been used to reduce seizure frequency in patients with drug-resistant epilepsy (Nagai, 2004). GSR biofeedback was used to induce either sympathetic arousal or relaxation. The study examined how changes in sympathetic arousal, induced using GSR biofeedback, affected tic frequency. The authors reported significantly fewer tics in subjects during relaxation feedback compared to arousal biofeedback (Nagai, 2009).

YOGA AND MEDITATION

In the Kompoliti (2009) survey of the use of various CAM approaches in 100 adults with TS, yoga was reported by 9 individuals and meditation by 10. No studies of either mediation or yoga for TS were identified.

Biological Treatments for TS

DIETARY MODIFICATION

One questionnaire study investigated the influence of 32 different foods and drinks on tics in patients with TS (Müller-Vahl et al., 2008). Of 887 mailed questionnaires, 224 were returned and used for analyses. A significant positive correlation was found for caffeine- and theine-containing drinks such as Coca-Cola, coffee, and black tea, as well as for preservatives and refined sugar and sweeteners. The authors speculated that since 34% and 47% of responders, respectively, reported that coffee and Coca-Cola exacerbated tics, caffeine may stimulate an already overactive dopaminergic system in TS and thus increase tics.

OMEGA-3 FATTY ACIDS

In a recently published study, Gabbay and colleagues (2012) randomized 33 children and adolescents with TS, ages 6 to 18 years, in a double-blind trial to omega-3 fatty acids or placebo for 20 weeks. The omega-3 fatty acids consisted of combined eicosapentaenoic acid (EPA) and docosahexaenoic acid (DHA), with an EPA:DHA ratio of 2:1 (i.e., total 250 mg or 500 mg of EPA+DHA per capsule), and the placebo was olive oil. Results indicated that at endpoint, subjects treated with omega-3 fatty acids did not have significantly higher response rates or lower mean scores on the Yale Global Tic Severity Scale (YGTSS)-Total Tic scale than those in the placebo group (53% vs. 38%; 15.6 ± 1.6 vs. 17.1 ± 1.6, $p > .1$). However, significantly more subjects taking omega-3 fatty acids were considered responders on the YGTSS-Tic-Related Impairment measure (59% vs. 25%, $p < .05$) and on the YGTSS-Global Severity measure (53% vs. 31%, $p = .05$). Mean YGTSS-Global Severity scores were significantly lower in the omega-3 fatty acid group than the placebo group (31.7 ± 2.9 vs. 40.9 ± 3.0, $p =.04$). Obsessive-compulsive, anxiety, and depressive symptoms were not significantly affected by omega-3 fatty acid use. Longitudinal analysis did not yield group differences on any of the measures. The authors concluded that omega-3 fatty acids did not reduce total tic scores but may be beneficial in reducing tic-related impairment for some children and adolescents with TS. Study limitations included the small sample size and possible therapeutic effects of olive oil.

MAGNESIUM SUPPLEMENTATION

Grimaldi (2002) proposed a central role of magnesium deficiency in TS. Grimaldi noted that there are many similarities between the symptomatology and biochemistry of TS and magnesium deficiency. In addition, 11q23 is the chromosomal site for renal magnesium loss, as well as a proposed site for TS. Grimaldi described many (>90) separate, self-reported anecdotal accounts of improvement in TS and comorbid symptomatology with magnesium-containing supplements. These reports claim that TS-associated symptoms recur with supplement discontinuation and improve with reintroduction of the supplements. In addition, Grimaldi noted anecdotal reports of symptom reduction with elimination of airborne and food allergens. Grimaldi called for systematic research on the use of supplements for TS and proposed a sample supplementation regimen.

A randomized, placebo-controlled, double-blind phase 4 study of the effectiveness and safety of magnesium and vitamin B6 for TS is under way in Spain (Garcia-Lopez et al., 2009).

CANNABINOIDS

Cannabis contains over 60 cannabinoid compounds, of which THC is the most psychoactive. The cannabinoid receptor CB1 is found throughout the brain, with the highest concentration in the basal ganglia, hippocampus, and cerebellum (Romero, 2002). The endocannabinoid system regulates synaptic transmission. Smoking is the usual mode of delivery of THC, yet in clinical practice this mode of delivery is not feasible due to the risk associated with smoke inhalation; instead, oral preparations such as nabilone and dronabinol have been used. However, oral preparations are problematic due to significant first-pass liver metabolism and uptake of cannabinoids into fatty tissue. The use of cannabinoids is associated with a number of risks, including dose-related impairments in short-term memory, attention, vigilance, and perception.

Two controlled studies of THC in adults with TS have been reported. In a single-dose, randomized, double-blind, placebo-controlled crossover study in 12 adult TS patients, THC significantly reduced tics on the self-reported Tourette Syndrome Symptom List compared to placebo. No serious adverse effects occurred, and no impairment on neuropsychological performance was observed (Müller-Vahl, 2002). In another 6-week, randomized, double-blind placebo-controlled trial in 24 TS patients, THC was administered in gelatin capsules of either 2.5 mg or 5 mg. Patients were treated over a period of 6 weeks with six visits and dose titration. Dose range was 5 to 10 mg, depending on weight and age. Tics were evaluated with a variety of measures, including both self-reports and investigator measures, and results indicated there was either a significant difference, or a trend toward significant difference, between drug and placebo groups on multiple tic outcome measures. No adverse effects were reported (Müller-Vahl, 2003).

A 2009 Cochrane review by Curtis and Rickards on the use of cannabinoids for TS concluded that there is not enough evidence to support their use in treatment of tics and obsessive-compulsive behavior in individuals with TS.

OTHER BIOLOGICAL TREATMENTS

While the use of allergy treatment and environmental modifications is prevalent among those with TS (Mantel, 2004), no relevant studies were identified in the literature. A discussion of the potential role of autoimmunity in TS is beyond the scope of this chapter and can be found in Chapter 14.

Manipulative and Body-Based Therapies

In the survey of the use of various CAM approaches in 100 adults with TS reported by Kompoliti (2009), massage was reported by 19 individuals and chiropractic manipulation by 12.

Chiropractic manipulation aims to address various traumatic and chronic injuries through manual manipulation of the spine, joints, and soft tissues. One case report described use of upper cervical chiropractic care in a 9-year-old boy with TS, ADHD, depression, asthma, insomnia, and headaches, and with history of traumatic birth with forceps delivery and subsequent cervical subluxation (Elster, 2003). Elster reported that after 6 weeks of treatment, all tic symptoms resolved and remained absent at 5-month follow-up. In addition, the patient was able to discontinue multiple medications.

While massage is used by patients with TS (Kompoliti, 2009), there are no published studies on massage for the treatment of TS.

Energy Medicine

Energy medicine is based on the belief that body energy can be manipulated; there is thought to be an energy body and the ability of healers to manipulate that energy for healing purposes. Some energy medicine approaches include biofield energy healing, therapeutic touch, and Reiki. While prayer is not a true energy medicine but rather a spiritual practice, it has some commonalities with energy medicine.

In the Kompoliti (2009) survey of the use of various CAM approaches in 100 adults with TS, prayer was reported by 19 individuals. No studies on the use of energy medicine or prayer for TS could be identified in the literature.

Whole Medical Systems

Whole medical systems such as Ayurveda, traditional Chinese medicine, homeopathy, and other traditional health systems offer an integrated perspective on health and disease that often have little in common with Western medicine. Many cultures developed their own medical systems that correspond to the beliefs of the people and offer unique explanatory models of disease, as well as diagnostic and treatment approaches.

While homeopathy use was reported by about 6% of individuals with TS (Kompoliti, 2009; Mantel, 2004), no studies of homeopathy for TS were identified in the literature.

TRADITIONAL CHINESE MEDICINE

Chinese medicine refers to a broad range of practices sharing common theoretical concepts developed in China and dating back at least 2,000 years. Chinese medicine treatments include herbs, acupuncture, massage, exercise (*qigong*), and dietary therapies. These approaches are commonly used in Asia but are considered alternative in the United States. Chinese medicine focuses on functional entities that regulate digestion, breathing, aging, and other functions. Health is perceived as harmony among the elements, and disease is related to disharmony. Some of the key concepts include *yin-yang*, *chi*, five elements theory, energy body, acupuncture, and pulse diagnosis.

In Chinese medicine, TS is classified in the categories of convulsions, muscular twitch, and cramps. The pathogenesis of TS in Chinese medicine relies on the concepts of *Xin* (contains the spirit and masters the mind and speech) and *Gan* (functions to disperse, masters tendons and speech) and is seen as a *Xin-Gan* insufficiency. The therapeutic approach aims to nourish *Xin* and smooth *Gan*.

A study in the Chinese language (Wu, 1996) reported on the use of acupuncture in 156 patients with TS, with improvement in 92.3% of those studied.

A study by Li and colleagues (2009) reported on the use of the traditional Chinese medicine herbal preparation Ningdong granule in combination with haloperidol. Ninety children with TS were randomized; 60 children in the treatment group received Ningdong granule plus haloperidol, while the 30 control-group children received haloperidol alone. Haloperidol was started at 0.5 mg per day and increased by 0.25 mg per day as needed, up to 2 to 6 mg per day. The Ningdong granule dose was 3 to 6 mg, and the composition of the granule was reported as gastrodia tuber, asiabell root, lilyturf root, white peony root, dragon's bone, oyster shell, earthworm, and licorice root. Study duration was 6 months. Symptoms were assessed with the YGTSS. Significant improvement was reported in 95% of the treatment group versus 73% of the control group ($p < .05$). At 6-month follow-up, the improvement rate in the treatment group was 86.7%, compared to 30% in the control group ($p < .01$). The treatment group was reported to have lower rates of adverse effects and a lower recurrence rate of tics.

Zhao and colleagues (2010) reported on an 8-week, randomized, placebo-controlled, double-blind clinical study of Ningdong granule in pediatric subjects (age 7–18 years) with TS. The eight main ingredients of the Ningdong granule were *Rhizoma Gastrodiae*, *Codonopsis pilosula*, dwarf lilyturf tuber, White Peony Alba, Keel, oyster shell, *Pheretima asaitica*, and liquorice. The proportions of these eight components in the Ningdong granule were 2:3:2:4:5:5:2:2, respectively. In this study, TS was reported to belong to the traditional Chinese medicine categories of "chronic infantile convulsion" and "hyperspasmia," and the putative primary pathogenesis was considered to be *yin* insufficiency of the heart and liver. Ningdong granule aims to relieve convulsions and spasms by nourishing heart and liver *yin*. Thirty-three subjects received 1 g/kg per day Ningdong granule and 31 subjects received a placebo. After 8 weeks of treatment tic reduction on the YGTSS (Chinese version) was seen in 41.4% of the Ningdong granule group and 10.7% of the placebo group ($p < .001$).

AYURVEDA

Ayurveda originated in India several thousand years ago as a comprehensive medical system and a lifestyle guide. The goal of Ayurveda is a balance of the body, mind, and spirit to create health and prevent illness. Ayurvedic treatments aim to cure disease by cleansing the body of substances that are considered toxic. Ayurveda recommendations typically include lifestyle changes, herbs, special diets, yoga, meditation, and massage.

The Ayurvedic treatment recommended for TS is *shirodhara*, which involves warmed,

Box 27.1. Key Points

- CAM approaches are among the most popular and widely used treatments in TS.
- CAM is defined as a "diverse group of medical and health care systems, practices, and products that are not part of conventional Western medicine."
- The five major groups of CAM practices are mind-body medicine, biologically based therapies, manipulative and body-based therapies, energy medicine, and whole medical systems.
- Research on CAM approaches is limited but rapidly expanding.
- While NIH funding of CAM research has increased in recent years, only 7% of the studies included children.
- The quality and quantity of scientific research on CAM is reported to be improving, and one review reported that the quality of CAM randomized controlled trials was as good as studies of conventional controlled trials.
- The CAM approaches most frequently reported to be used by patients with TS are dietary modification, allergy treatment, prayer, vitamins, massage, nutritional and dietary supplements, chiropractic manipulation, meditation, yoga, acupuncture, hypnosis, homeopathy, and biofeedback.
- Research evidence suggests that a number of CAM approaches are potentially useful in TS, yet there are methodological limitations in all studies. The approaches that appear to have most promise based on the evidence to date are hypnosis, biofeedback, omega-3 fatty acids, cannabinoids, and traditional Chinese medicine (Ningdong granule).

Box 27.2. Questions for Future Research

1. What is the prevalence of use of CAM approaches in TS?
2. What is the prevalence of CAM use in children, adolescents, and adults with TS, and which CAM approaches are most commonly used?
3. Which CAM approaches are efficacious in reducing tic symptoms in TS?
4. What are the safety concerns with the use of CAM approaches in TS?
5. Which CAM approaches are appropriate for the treatment of symptoms of the psychiatric comorbid disorders that frequently co-occur in TS, such as ADHD or OCD?
6. Additional research of good methodological quality and with large enough sample sizes is needed on the approaches for which there is already some research evidence, such as cannabinoids, omega-3 fatty acid, traditional Chinese medicine (Ningdong granule), hypnosis, and biofeedback. High-quality research is also needed for CAM approaches that are used by the TS population yet lack any evidence base, such as yoga, meditation, chiropractic, magnesium supplementation, dietary modification, allergy treatment, environmental modification, massage, and homeopathy.

medicated oil, milk, or water streamed onto the forehead of a patient lying on his or her back on a massage table. It is commonly used to treat mental health problems and stress (Tirodkar, 2010). No studies could be identified in English language on the use of Ayurveda for TS.

CLINICAL COMMENTARY

In summary, despite increasing popularity and widespread use, the evidence base on CAM approaches to the treatment of TS remains extremely limited. The field of CAM is broad, and a wide variety of interventions are used by individuals with TS. Controlled studies are limited in number, sample sizes are small, and standardized measurements are infrequently used. Several alternative treatments, such as omega-3 fatty acids and THC, showed positive results in small studies or case series. Given the burgeoning use of these approaches in TS patients, increased awareness among medical providers and clinicians of CAM practices might facilitate communication between patients and clinicians. Whether CAM approaches will result in improved treatment outcomes awaits further investigation.

ACKNOWLEDGMENTS

We would like to thank Resham Gellatly and Sarah Matson for their assistance in the preparation of this chapter.

REFERENCES

Armishaw J, Grant CC. Use of complementary treatment by those hospitalized with acute illness. *Arch Dis Child* 1999; 81:133–137.

Bergin A, Waranch HR, Brown J et al. Relaxation therapy in Tourette syndrome: A pilot study. *Pediat Neurol* 1998; 18:136–142.

Bloch M, Qawasmi A. Omega-3 fatty acid supplementation for the treatment of children with attention-deficit/hyperactivity disorder symptomatology: systematic review and meta-analysis. *J Am Acad Child Adolesc Psychiatry* 2011; 50:991–1000.

Braganza S, Ozuah PO, Sharif I. The use of complementary therapies in inner-city asthmatic children. *J Asthma* 2003; 40:823–827.

Bruggeman R, van der Linden C, Buitelaar JK. Risperidone versus pimozide in Tourette's disorder: A comparative double-blind parallel-group study. *J Clin Psychiatry* 2001; 62:50–56.

Chappell PB, Leckman JF, Riddle MA. The pharmacological treatment of tic disorders. *Child Adolesc Psychiat Clin North Am* 1995; 4:197–216.

Coffey BJ, Biederman J, Spencer T et al. Informativeness of structured diagnostic interviews in the identification of Tourette's disorder in referred youth. *J Nerv Ment Dis* 2000; 188:583–588.

Consortium of Academic Health Centers for Integrative Medicine website. www.imconsortium.org. Accessed January 29, 2012.

Curtis A, Clarke CE, Rickards H. Cannabinoids for Tourette's syndrome. *Cochrane Database Systematic Reviews* 2009; 4:CD006565.

Dietary Supplement Health and Education Act of 1994. Public law No. 103–417, 1994. www.fda.gov/opacom/laws/dshea.html. Accessed January 29, 2012.

Eisenberg DM, Davis RB, Ettner SL et al. Trends in alternative medicine use in the United States, 1990–1997: Results of a follow-up national survey. *JAMA* 1998; 280:1569.
Key study of the prevalence of CAM use in the United States.

Eisenberg DM, Kessler RC, Foster C et al. Unconventional medicine in the United States: prevalence, costs, and patterns of use. *N Engl J Med* 1993; 4:246–252.

Elster EL. Upper cervical chiropractic care for a nine-year-old male with Tourette syndrome, attention deficit hyperactivity disorder, depression, asthma, insomnia, and headaches: a case report. *J Vertebral Subluxation Res* 2003, 1–11.

Faridi K, Suchowersky O. Gilles de la Tourette's syndrome. *Can J Neurol Sci* 2003; 30:64–71.

Gabbay V, Babb J, Klein R et al. A double-blind, placebo-controlled trial of omega-3 fatty acids in Tourette's disorder. *Pediatrics* 2012; 129:e1493–e1500.

Garcia-Lopez R, Perea-Milla E, Garcia CR et al. New therapeutic approach to Tourette syndrome in children based on a randomized placebo-controlled double-blind phase IV study of the effectiveness and safety of magnesium and vitamin B6. *Trials-Electronic Resource* 10:16, 2009.

Grimaldi BL. The central role of magnesium deficiency in Tourette's syndrome: causal relationships between magnesium deficiency, altered biochemical pathways and symptoms relating to Tourette's syndrome and several reported comorbid conditions. *Med Hypotheses* 2002; 58:47–60.

Klassen TP, Pham B, Lawson M L, Moher D. For randomized controlled trials, the quality of reports of complementary and alternative medicine was as good as reports of conventional medicine. *J Clin Epidemiol* 2005; 58:763–768.

Kompoliti K, Fan W, Leurgans S. Complementary and alternative medicine use in Gilles de la Tourette syndrome. *Mov Disord* 2009; 24:2015–2019.

A survey of prevalence of use of various CAM approaches.

Lawson ML, Pham B, Klassen TP, Moher D. Systematic reviews involving complementary and alternative medicine interventions had higher quality of reporting than conventional medicine reviews. *J Clin Epidemiol* 2005; 58:777–784.

Lazarus JE, Klein SK. Nonpharmacological treatment of tics in Tourette syndrome adding videotape training to self-hypnosis. *J Dev Behav Pediat* 2010; 31:498–504.

Li A, Cong S, Lu H et al. Clinical observation on treatment of Tourette syndrome by integrative medicine. *Chinese J Integrative Med* 2009; 15:267–271.

Mantel BJ, Meyers A, Tran QY et al. Nutritional supplements and complementary/alternative medicine in Tourette syndrome. *J Child Adolesc Psychopharmacol* 2004; 14:582–589.

Study of the prevalence of use of various CAM approaches in TS.

McCann LJ, Newell SJ. Survey of pediatric complementary and alternative medicine use in health and chronic illness. *Arch Dis Child* 2006; 91:173–174.

Michultka DM, Blanchard EB, Rosenblum EL. Stress management and Gilles de la Tourette's syndrome. *Appl Psychophysiol Biofeedback* 1989; 14:115–123, 1989.

Müller-Vahl KR, Buddensiek N, Geomelas M, Emrich HM. The influence of different food and drink on tics in Tourette syndrome. *Acta Paediat* 2008; 97:442–446.

Müller-Vahl KR, Prevedel H, Theloe K et al. Treatment of Tourette syndrome with delta-9-tetrahydrocannabinol (THC): no influence on neuropsychological performance. *Neuropsychopharmacology* 2003; 28:384–388.

Müller-Vahl KR, Schneider U, Koblenz A et al. Treatment of Tourette syndrome with delta-9-tetrahydrocannabinol (THC): a randomized crossover trial. *Pharmacopsychiatry* 2002; 35: 57–61.

Müller-Vahl KR, Schneider U, Prevedel H et al. Delta 9-tetrahydrocannabinol (THC) is effective in the treatment of tics in Tourette syndrome: a 6-week randomized trial. *J Clin Psychiatry* 2003; 64:459–465.

Nagai Y, Cavanna A, Critchley H. Influence of sympathetic autonomic arousal on tics: implications for a therapeutic behavioral intervention for Tourette syndrome. *J Psychosom Res* 2009; 67:599–605.

Nagai Y, Goldstein LH, Fenwick PBC, Trimble MR. Clinical efficacy of biofeedback treatment on reducing seizures in adult epilepsy: a preliminary randomized controlled study. *Epilepsy Behav* 2004; 22:243–51.

National Center for Complementary and Alternative Medicine website. http://nccam.nih.gov. Accessed January 29, 2012.

National Institutes of Health. National Center for Complementary and Alternative Medicine website. http://nccam.nih.gov. Accessed January 29, 2012.

Piacentini J, Woods DW, Scahill L et al. Behavior therapy for children with Tourette disorder: A randomized controlled trial. *JAMA* 2010; 303:1929–1937.

Raz A, Keller S, Norman K, Senechal D. Elucidating Tourette's syndrome: perspectives from hypnosis, attention and self-regulation. *Am J Clin Hypn* 2007; 49:289–309.

Robertson MM, Trimble MR, Lees AJ. The psychopathology of Gilles de la Tourette syndrome. A phenomenological analysis. *Br J Psychiatry* 1998; 152:383–390.

Romero J, Lastres-Becker I, de Miguel R et al. The endogenous cannabinoid system and the basal ganglia: biochemical, pharmacological, and therapeutic aspects. *Pharmacol Ther* 2002; 95:137–152.

Sarris J, Camfield D, Berk M. Complementary medicine, self-help, and lifestyle interventions for obsessive compulsive disorder (OCD) and the OCD spectrum: A systematic review. *J Affect Disord* 2012; 138:213–221.

Sarris J, Kean J, Schweitzer I, Lake J. Complementary medicines (herbal and nutritional products) in the treatment of attention deficit hyperactivity disorder (ADHD): A systematic review of the evidence. *Complement Ther Med* 2011; 19: 216–227.

Silva RR, Munoz DM, Daniel W et al. Causes of haloperidol discontinuation in patients with Tourette's disorder: management and alternatives. *J Clin Psychiatry* 1996; 57: 129–135.

Tansey MA. A simple and a complex tic (Gilles de la Tourette's syndrome): Their response to EEG sensory motor rhythm biofeedback training. *Int J Psychophysiol* 1986; 4:91–97.

Tirodkar M. Tourette syndrome in Indian ayurvedic medical practice. *J Dev Behav Pediat* 2010; 31:173–174.

Turpin G, Powell G. Effects of massed practice and cue-controlled relaxation on tic frequency in Gilles de la Tourette's syndrome. *Behav Res Ther* 1984; 22:165–178.

Wu L, Li H, Kang L. 156 cases of Gilles de la Tourette's syndrome treated by acupuncture. *J Tradit Chin Med* 1996; 16:211–213.

Yussman S, Ryan SA, Auinger P, Weitzman M. Visits to complementary and alternative providers by children and adolescents in the United States. *Ambul Pediatr* 2004; 4:429–439.

Zhao L, Li AY, Lv H et al. Traditional Chinese medicine Ningdong granule: the beneficial effects in Tourette's disorder. *J Int Med Res* 2010; 38:169–175.

SECTION 6

RESOURCES AND SUPPORT

28

Information and Social Support for Patients and Families

KIRSTEN R. MÜLLER-VAHL

Abstract

This chapter summarizes the current experience on information and psychoeducation, predominantly from a European perspective. Due to the wide spectrum of symptoms associated with Tourette syndrome (TS), patients with tics may seek doctors from different specialties, including not only neurologists and psychiatrists but also general practitioners, ear/nose/throat physicians, ophthalmologists, pediatricians, allergists, speech and language therapists, dermatologists, and even dentists. The delay to diagnosis has among its possible causes the insufficient knowledge and awareness of this condition among professionals. Psychoeducation should always be the first step in the treatment of patients with TS, informing decisions on the best management approach to take in the short, medium, and long term. With respect to treatment, a shared decision-making model is recommended where the physician provides tailored, unbiased, and up-to-date information about the benefits and disadvantages of alternative treatment choices, while the patient makes the decision about whether treatment will be initiated. Knowledge on potential restrictions and limitations regarding daily functioning represent an important aspect of the psychoeducational intervention. The economic burden of adult patients with TS is high, with indirect costs having a greater impact than direct costs; this represents an underinvestigated aspect of this condition.

INTRODUCTION

For the vast majority of patients and parents, it is a relief and not a burden to receive the diagnosis of Tourette syndrome (TS). However, the diagnosis process should always be accompanied by detailed information about different aspects of the condition. Although the type and amount of information that should be given vary on an individual basis, some basic education should be provided to all patients. As described in Chapter 22, psychoeducation should be the first step in the treatment of patients with TS (Roessner et al., 2011), since it improves patients' knowledge and results in better coping with the condition.

Recent studies have clearly demonstrated that quality of life is significantly impaired in many patients with TS, especially those with comorbid attention-deficit/hyperactivity disorder (ADHD), obsessive-compulsive disorder (OCD), and depression (Eddy et al., 2011a, 2011b; Müller-Vahl et al., 2010; Pringsheim et al., 2009). In contrast, the vast majority of young children with transient or mild tics are either not disturbed by or even completely unaware of their tics. Thus, the question of whether, and if so, which kind of social support is needed strongly depends on widely different aspects, including the patient's age, tic severity, comorbidities, quality of life, school situation, occupation, marital status, and social life.

THE RIGHT NOT TO BE INFORMED

Tics are common and occur in up to 15% of all primary-school children (Robertson, 2008; see also Chapter 6). Because in most of these children the tics are transient or mild, their parents will never seek medical advice and the children will never be diagnosed with tics. In families where both child and parents are completely unaware of the tics, medical doctors should refrain from concentrating their attention on this symptom. When tics are very mild, they cause no social impairment at all, and they are noticed only by the attending physician or by an expert consultant, it is appropriate to pursue a "watch-and-wait" strategy. Alerting the child and parents to the tics may raise a previously nonexisting problem. In daily clinical practice, it happens quite often that parents turn to a doctor because of their child's tics, but at the same time the whole family—including the parent—completely overlooks the fact that the parent also has mild tics. In other cases, the parent is perfectly aware that he or she had tics in childhood but is erroneously convinced that in the meantime his or her tics have disappeared. In such a situation, the medical doctor should not confront the parent with his or her tics unless he or she refers to them spontaneously without being asked. This procedure is well-founded, since the parent obviously is totally unaffected by his or her tics without any impairment to health and quality of life. To inform a person who is feeling healthy about otherwise unnoticed tics might be disturbing.

THE DIAGNOSIS OF TS: A RELIEF AND NOT A BURDEN

If a patient or parents are aware of the tics, then further information has to be given. For example, many parents not only are worried about the child's tics, but also feel guilty and responsible for them. Furthermore, parents often hear statements such as "the child's tics are caused by poor parenting," "the tics are provoked by extensive TV watching," "the tics are caused by playing too much on the computer," or "the tics are related to a traumatic experience." Thus, the correct diagnosis of a tic disorder relieves the parents' guilt and, moreover, may prevent the child from receiving ineffective and inappropriate treatment. In this context, it can be helpful for parents to know that TS is not a "modern disease," but was first described in 1885 (Gilles de la Tourette, 1885).

Most adult patients, whose tic onset dates back many years, feel relief when receiving the correct diagnosis of TS. For most of these patients—who have been aware of their tics for a long time—the main problem is not the tics themselves, but the fact that no irrefutable medical diagnosis has been made so far. This situation may result not only in uncertainty and anxiety about the future, but also in depression. In contrast, for the parents of a young child, the correct diagnosis of a tic disorder often produces both relief (because the disorder is now precisely named) and shock (because they have to accept that their child has a chronic disorder, which is sometimes difficult to treat). Especially for children who have not only tics but also comorbidities like ADHD and OCD, it can be hard for the parents to accept that their child is diagnosed with more than one disorder and possibly requires different treatment strategies. In such cases, it can be very helpful for the patients and their parents not only to learn about disabilities and restrictions that may be associated with the disease, but also to learn that a few "positive" aspects as well may be closely linked to TS. People with TS, for example, may have positive personality characteristics and talents such as punctuality, correctness, conscientiousness, a sense of justice, quick comprehension, good intelligence, creativity, musicality, and athletic abilities. For that reason, some people with TS even hesitate when asked whether they wish the disorder would disappear completely.

DID MOZART HAVE TS?

In this context, it might be very helpful to tell the patient that there are several prominent and successful people known all over the world, both currently and in the past, who also probably had tics. There is an ongoing debate whether the musician and composer Wolfgang Amadeus Mozart (1756–1791) had TS (Ashoori & Jankovic, 2007; Aterman, 1994; Monaco et al., 2009). This question cannot be answered conclusively because the available documents provide insufficient information, but there is no doubt that in his time Mozart's behavior was often bizarre and unusual. His passion for using obscene words, gestures, and writing (expression of coprophenomena?) is well documented

(Simkin, 1992). Between 1771 and 1781 Mozart wrote the so-called series of Bäsle letters to his cousin Maria Anna Thekla Mozart, which contain a large variety of inappropriate and obscene words. Some of these obscenities are repeated several times; some repetitions are incomplete and with no context. Furthermore, Mozart's temperament has been described as childlike or immature and his profanity is well documented (Monaco et al., 2009). In contrast, reports about inappropriate or involuntary movements that in retrospect could be interpreted as motor tics are limited. All in all, some of Mozart's bizarre, inappropriate, and obscene behavior is in fact consistent with the diagnosis of TS, although reports about motor tics are scarce, and several other explanations for his behavior have been suggested (Ashoori & Jankovic, 2007).

Without doubt, Mozart's musical brilliance does not rule out the diagnosis of TS, since today there are many talented musicians known who have this condition, such as the jazz pianist and composer Michael Wolf, the classical pianist Nick van Bloss, the composer Tobias Picker, the drummer Matt Giordano, the musician Jonas Altberg (Basshunter), and the singer Nick Tatham (Müller-Vahl, 2010). In addition, the versatile scholar and writer Samuel Johnson, the writer and politician André Malraux, and the author Quim Monzo had TS. Furthermore, a large number of very successful athletes have made public their diagnosis of TS, including baseball, soccer, and basketball players as well as skeleton, motocross, and stock car racers (Müller-Vahl, 2010).

All these examples illustrate vividly that an individual with TS can still be a successful athlete, musician, politician, author, or scholar. Both patients and parents should know that the vast majority of people with this condition can take up any profession they like and can be very successful in their chosen career.

DELAY IN DIAGNOSIS

The diagnosis of TS is often delayed, mainly due to insufficient knowledge of the condition among professionals (Mol Debes et al. 2008). The erroneous belief that TS is a rare and severe disorder always associated with coprolalia is unfortunately still tenacious—even among medical doctors. Regretfully, until today many medical doctors worldwide have not been taught about TS at all during their university education. The consequence of this omission is documented in several scientific studies. In a Danish study in 2008, Mol Debes and colleagues (2008) investigated 314 children with TS and found a median delay from the onset of tics until diagnosis of 2.8 years, and a delay from the onset of the presenting symptoms until diagnosis of 5.3 years. Families had consulted an average of two or three professionals before the diagnosis was made. Of interest, in 88.2% of cases, the child's parents were the first to notice symptoms, followed by kindergarten teachers in 4.5%, nursery staff in 1.9%, other family members in 1.3%, schoolteachers in 1%, and others in the remaining 3.2% (Mol Debes et al., 2008). Because tics are not necessarily the presenting symptoms of TS, Mol Debes and colleagues (2008) suggested that physicians should be aware that children presenting with ADHD and/or obsessive-compulsive symptoms could develop tics later in life. Finally, they emphasized that a delay in diagnosis results in delayed initiation of the necessary support (Mol Debes et al., 2008).

In 2005, Khalifa and von Knorring (2005) examined 4,479 children aged 7 to 15 years in Sweden. Twenty-five of these children (0.6%) met the diagnostic criteria for TS. Altogether, 96% of these children had already been in contact with medical services prior to the study, but only in two thirds of cases had the correct diagnosis of TS been made. In 2000, Freeman and colleagues analyzed data from a worldwide multicenter study comprising 3,500 individuals diagnosed with TS (Freeman et al., 2000). They found a mean age of tic onset of 6 to 7 years. While in 92.7% of all patients tics started before the age of 11 years, the correct diagnosis was made in only 56% before that age; 16% of all patients were not even diagnosed before adulthood, even though only 1% of all patients had onset of their tics after the age of 15. While Freeman and colleagues (2000) and Khalifa and von Knorring (2005) found a median delay of diagnosis from the onset of tics of 4 and 6.4 years, respectively, in a German study conducted between 1995 and 2007, which included 763 patients with TS, a mean delay of 11.9 years was found (Müller-Vahl, 2010). However, this was a long-running study that started in 1995; also, in Germany the first self-help group for TS was founded until 1992; around that time there was only one child and adolescent psychiatry center that specialized in tic disorders; and the first tertiary referral center caring for adult patients with tic disorders was established only in 1994. Assuming that the health care systems for patients with tic disorders today are comparable in Sweden, Denmark, and Germany, it can be hypothesized that—at least in these countries—the delay between tic onset and diagnosis has shortened tremendously (from more than 10 years to less than 6 years). It can be speculated that different factors contributed to this improvement: (1) the expansion of specialist TS outpatient departments, (2) the unstinting work of national and local self-help groups, and (3) the increasing media coverage of TS.

COMMUNICATION OF THE DIAGNOSIS

In a Spanish study, Rivera-Navarro and colleagues (2009) investigated the way in which a diagnosis of TS is communicated to patients, and the impact of the diagnosis on patients and their relatives. Although this study was performed quite recently, patients and their relatives still found that it was difficult to receive the diagnosis of TS. While patients still had a general lack of knowledge accountable for this delay, relatives stated that the symptoms were often hidden due to a sense of guilt within the family. Parents reported that the communication of the diagnosis was inadequate due to poor understanding and interpretation of the clinical terminology (Rivera-Navarro et al., 2009).

WHICH SPECIALTY?

Not only is the clinical spectrum of TS very wide, including a variety of comorbid disorders, but even the motor and vocal tics can be highly diverse (for details, see the first four chapters).

Therefore, patients with TS and their parents may initially present to doctors from different medical specialties, including general practitioners (77.7%), ear/nose/throat specialists (9.9%), ophthalmologists (11.1%), psychiatrists (11.8%), psychologists (46.5%), pediatricians (30.9%), or others (such as allergy specialists, speech and language therapists, etc., 31.2%; Mol Debes et al. 2008). In exceptional cases, the presenting feature may consist of lesions caused by the dysfunctional behavioral pattern. A patient described by Jankovic and Sekula (1998) manifested initially with skin lesions and presented first to a consultant dermatologist; indeed, tics, obsessive-compulsive symptoms, and self-injurious behavior can all cause skin damage due to biting, scratching, skin picking, and burning. In rare cases, patients may initially present to a dentist because motor tics can result in teeth grinding leading to dental lesions, or even self-extraction of a tooth (Leksell & Edvardson, 2005). In children, however, motor and vocal tics are most often misdiagnosed as asthma, bronchitis, allergy, nervousness, and epilepsy, or attributed to psychological causes (Müller-Vahl, 2010).

Today, many parents thoroughly acquaint themselves with TS via the Internet before bringing their child to the doctor. It is the rule rather than the exception that parents, and not professionals, first suspect the correct diagnosis of a tic disorder (Mol Debes et al., 2008).

IMPACT ON QUALITY OF LIFE

Although even younger children can be severely impaired by their tics, in several cases parents can be more impaired than their child (Pringsheim et al., 2009). When considering medical treatment, this aspect has to be taken into account. Quite often, the unimpaired child receives medical treatment to reduce tics, when instead the parents should more appropriately receive psychoeducation and social support to better cope with the condition. Several studies have provided evidence that psychosocial health in children with TS alone (i.e., without comorbidities) is comparable to that of "healthy" children, while quality of life is significantly impaired in the majority of those children with TS "plus" (i.e., with coexisting ADHD, OCD, depression, or other comorbidities) (Cutler et al., 2009; Eddy et al., 2011a, 2011b; Mol Debes et al., 2010; Pringsheim et al., 2009; Storch et al., 2007). Social adjustment of children with TS is most heavily influenced by comorbid ADHD (Bawden et al., 1998; Stokes et al., 1991; see also Chapter 22). However, it has also been demonstrated that functional impairment is positively correlated with tic severity and perceptions of discrimination (Conelea et al., 2011; Cutler et al., 2009). Accordingly, many children with TS avoid leisure activities due to the experience of discrimination secondary to their tics (Mol Debes et al., 2010). Thus, comorbidities such as ADHD and OCD have a considerably greater impact on quality of life in children with TS than tics. This aspect has to be considered when medical treatment will be administered. In most children with TS "plus," treatment of ADHD and OCD is paramount, as detailed in Chapter 25.

In adults with TS, tics have a greater influence on physical, social, occupational/academic, and psychological functioning than in children (Altman et al., 2009; Conelea et al., 2011; Elstner et al., 2001; Müller-Vahl et al., 2010). Adults often report social or public avoidance and experiences of discrimination resulting from their tics (Conelea et al., 2011). Moreover, vocal tics can have a greater negative impact than motor tics (Altman et al., 2009). However, also in adults symptoms of depression and OCD have a considerably greater impact on quality of life than tic severity (Conelea et al., 2011; Müller-Vahl et al., 2010). The negative influence of different symptoms of TS on psychosocial well-being is documented in a very limited way by the fact that the financial burden of adult patients with TS is high, with a greater impact of indirect compared to direct costs (Dodel et al., 2010).

INFORMATION ON CLINICAL AND PATHOLOGICAL ISSUES

Patients and parents should both know that the diagnosis of TS is a clinical diagnosis, made on the basis of knowledge obtained by medical history and a psychiatric and neurological examination including direct observation of tics, but generally without further benefit coming from laboratory tests, including electroencephalography or neuroimaging. One of the first and most important pieces of information that should be shared with patients is that TS is a neuropsychiatric and not a psychogenic disorder. Most parents feel relieved when they learn that tics are not caused by the psychosocial environment, traumatic experiences, poor parenting, extensive TV watching, excessive computer use, unhealthy eating, bad habits, or psychological conflicts. Professionals should remember that parents often feel guilty about their child's tics.

When TS is diagnosed, especially parents of young children must be informed that, in the vast majority of patients, a favorable course of the disease may be expected; a "malignant" course with severe tics, significant coprolalia, and a variety of comorbidities will occur in only a minority of patients. Even though TV documentaries about TS in most cases are informative and educational, often the patients portrayed in these programs suffer from very severe, or even extreme, tics. This incorrect and exaggerated characterization of the disease often causes concern and uncertainty, especially among parents of young children; it also strengthens among both laypeople and professionals the belief that TS is always associated with severe tics and coprolalia.

In particular, the parents of young children with tics are interested in the future course of the disease. Unfortunately, there are still no reliable and generally accepted prognostic factors for long-term clinical outcome (for further details, see Chapter 5). In most patients a reliable prognosis on the course can be made around the age of 14 to 16 years, after the climax of tic severity has passed (Müller-Vahl, 2010).

Parents and patients should also know that TS is a chronic disorder, and that tics (1) fluctuate spontaneously, with a typical waxing and waning course, (2) are influenced by environmental factors (most commonly they increase under stress and decrease at rest or with high concentration), (3) are age-dependent, with a climax of severity at the age of 10 to 12 years (Bloch et al., 2006), and (4) decrease in adolescence and adulthood in the majority of patients, but disappear completely in only a few adult patients (see Chapters 1 and 5).

Most patients and parents of children with tics are unaware of the fact that tics are often associated with comorbid disorders such as ADHD, OCD, depression, anxiety disorder, self-injurious behavior, sleep disorders, addiction, and learning disorders. It is the physician's responsibility to disentangle and classify all the different symptoms within the TS spectrum. In doing this, however, the terminology used by patients or parents should not be automatically adopted. For example, patients may use the term "tic," but in fact the presenting symptom is not a tic but a compulsion or hyperactivity—or vice versa, the patient may talk about "compulsions" but in fact exhibit complex motor tics. The same is true in most cases when parents report that their child is "inattentive." "Inattention" in children with TS can be caused by ADHD but can also be related to tics, tic suppression, OCD, depression, or even sedation due to medical treatment.

DECISION ON TREATMENT

TS can be regarded as an exemplary disease where a shared decision-making model is recommended. The physician should provide tailored, unbiased, and up-to-date information about the disease, as well as the benefits and disadvantages of alternative treatment choices, while engaging the patient in decision making and taking into account his or her preferences, values, and lifestyle (Rivera-Navarro et al., 2009). Involving the patient in this process will not only improve the patient–physician partnership but will also increase patient satisfaction, treatment compliance, clinician satisfaction, and outcomes (Rivera-Navarro et al., 2009).

Patients and parents should be informed that available therapy for TS aims simply to reduce tics (generally, by about 50%), but complete remission cannot be obtained with the available treatment options. Different treatment strategies should be explained, including behavioral therapy, medication, and—in adults with severe, treatment-resistant disease—surgical

therapy. Patients should know that there is no clear evidence that available treatments influence the underlying cause or the course of the disease, although more research is needed on this. According to current views, tics respond to treatment regardless of the point in time when it is initiated. Unfortunately, there are still no known predictive factors for treatment outcome.

With respect to treatment, professionals should bear in mind that two thirds of all patients try "alternative" treatments to reduce TS symptoms (Kompoliti et al., 2009). Most interestingly, 80% of these patients do not inform their attending physician about this "co-treatment." Since nearly half of the patients are willing to pay a lot of money for "alternative treatment" (Kompoliti et al., 2009), professionals should feel obliged to inform their patients about not only effective but also ineffective treatments. Although many patients and parents are convinced that special diets improve tics, there is only weak evidence that caffeine (coffee and tea) might increase tics in predisposed people (Müller-Vahl et al., 2008).

TS AND SCHOOL PROBLEMS

As discussed in more detail in Chapter 29, many symptoms associated with TS can cause social disability and disadvantages at school. Difficulties at school in children with TS can be caused either by social problems (including exclusion, discrimination, teasing, less popularity, confrontation with criticism and prejudice) or directly by different symptoms associated with TS, including tics, OCD, ADHD, and learning difficulties (Mol Debes et al., 2010). Children with TS often have poorer peer relationship than their classmates. However, in most cases peer relationship problems are related to ADHD and OCD, not to tic severity (Bawden et al., 1998; Mol Debes et al., 2010; Stokes et al., 1991). Unfortunately, teasing occurs quite often in a school-related setting. Some children with TS are afraid of being teased by their peers, even when this never really occurred. However, both teasing and fear of teasing may lead to withdrawal from social life and can even result in depression.

Teachers must realize (and accept) that tics (and even coprolalia) are involuntary and not meaningful and are not performed deliberately. Only if this is clearly understood can teachers help to prevent the child with TS from being teased and reprimanded. Depending on the individual situation, it can be reasonable and helpful to inform not only teachers but also classmates and their parents to prevent teasing of children with TS in the school environment.

Coprolalia, as well as other less common coprophenomena such as copropraxia and coprographia, can cause significant social problems. For teachers and parents, sometimes it is difficult to distinguish coprolalia from "normal" swearing, which is not uncommon among youngsters at the age of 10 to 15 years. This differentiation, however, is important because coprolalia is an involuntary complex vocal tic and therefore should be tolerated, whereas "normal" swearing is a deliberate behavior that may have to be punished. The following specific characteristics of coprolalia may help to differentiate it from swearing. Coprolalia typically manifests rather as a heckle than a spoken word, and most often appears in modified loudness and articulation. In addition, coprolalia has no context of meaning compared with swearing, although it can be triggered by environmental factors (see also Chapter 1).

Teachers should also realize that the severity of tics fluctuates spontaneously over time and space, and tics are influenced by different factors—for example, stress, the presence of specific people, or even daytime. Furthermore, they should know that, with increasing age, children become able to suppress their tics, but only for short periods of time. Teachers should not ask a child with TS to suppress his or her tics, because tic suppression can be exhausting, unpleasant, and attention-demanding and can result in a subsequent rebound bout of tics. Pestering a child to suppress his or her tics may cause stress, resulting in tic deterioration. These factors can lead to a varying degree of tic severity at school compared to home, so teachers may underestimate the extent of the problems at home (Mol Debes et al., 2010).

DISABILITY COMPENSATION FOR CHILDREN WITH TS

In most countries, rights of disabled persons, including education, employment, and the living environment, are regulated by legislation. In Germany, and probably in many other countries worldwide, students are eligible for disability compensation according to the Disabled Persons Act. However, at school individual compensations have to be defined by teachers and parents.

In severely affected children, individual case support can be a very effective way to enable them to keep attending school. A social worker may assist the child at school for single lessons, for the full school day, or even at home (to help with homework or supervise leisure activities). The costs, in general, are covered by youth welfare services.

Sometimes simple tricks or special arrangements can be very helpful for children with TS. For example, it can be a great relief for a child with tics to be allowed to leave the classroom from time to time "to tic." Being allowed to chew chewing gum may reduce vocal tics during class. For some children with TS, it helps to type on a laptop instead of writing exercises in longhand. Not only repetitive motor tics but also compulsions can make handwriting very difficult. Furthermore, poor or illegible handwriting is not uncommon in children with TS (Müller-Vahl, 2010). Children may need additional time on tests to compensate for the time lost as a result of tics or compulsions. They should be given the chance to choose between taking an oral and a written examination, depending on their current tics. While a verbal examination might be fairer for a child with severe motor tics, a written examination might be more suitable for a child with frequent and loud vocal tics. In general, for many children with tics it is a great relief to take their written examination in a separate room, where they will not feel compelled to suppress their tics and will be able to better concentrate on the exam.

Not only tics but also OCD can cause impairment at school. Due to OCD, children may be incapable of arriving at school on time (e.g., because of washing or dressing rituals at home or because of "just-right" phenomena on the way to school). In addition, compulsions can affect handwriting, for example when the child has to write words "just right," or has to draw specific patterns in the exercise book, or has to start over and over again at the beginning due to a slight mistake.

Both "learning difficulties" as well as "inattentiveness" in children with TS can be caused by specific learning disabilities and ADHD, respectively, but also by tics, the attempt to suppress them, OCD, depression, sleeping problems, autism, and sedation due to medical treatment. Thus, a thorough examination is indicated when teachers report these symptoms in a child with TS.

Supervising homework can be very exhausting and time-consuming for parents of a child with TS. Several symptoms, including ADHD, tics, and OCD, can cause time delays and may complicate homework completion. For parents it can be a great relief, when this task is taken over by a third party, ideally a social worker in the context of individual case support.

Usually children with TS should attend a regular school, but teachers should be informed in advance about the child's tics. Parents and teachers should refrain from sending a child with TS to a special school only because of the tics. Bright pupils with tics should attend a grammar school independent of TS. Both parents and teachers should be informed that tics most typically reach a climax of severity exactly at the age when secondary school has to be chosen, but they will decrease with increasing age.

SOCIAL PROBLEMS, SEVERE DISABILITY, AND TS

Compared to the general population, patients with TS have significantly lower levels of self-esteem and self-confidence, and higher social anxiety (Carter et al., 1994; Robertson et al., 2002). Studies investigating personality disorders in patients with TS demonstrated that there are—in addition to the well-known comorbidities—a wide variety of personality traits associated with TS, predominantly schizotypal traits, borderline personality disorder, and avoidant personality traits (Cavanna et al., 2007; Robertson et al., 1997; Schneider et al., 2011).

When assessing the degree of disability in people with TS, tics, comorbidities, and psychopathologies, as well as their impact on quality of life, have to be considered. In general, patients with TS are entitled to apply for recognition as a disabled person. The pension office will determine the individual degree of disability, which may vary from 0% to 100%. In patients with "only" mild tics, motor tics are predominantly located in the cranial district and, therefore, will be recognized by other people even during short conversations. While mild vocal tics such as sniffing and clearing one's throat may be not heard in everyday life, they may be striking and annoying when attending classical concerts, opera, lectures, or movies. Thus, even mild tics can cause relevant social impairment and may strengthen the person's tendency to withdraw from social life, also due to comorbid avoidant personality traits and anxiety spectrum disorders. In Germany, for example, the status of "severe disability" in TS patients may lead to improved employment protection, extra paid days of leave, or reduced taxes. Depending on the individual situation, job seeking, however, can be made either easier or more difficult: if asked, the job seeker must acknowledge his or her status as a disabled person.

RESTRICTIONS DUE TO TS

Parents need to be informed whether they will have to impose specific restrictions on their child with TS. However, neither restrictions on food nor on sporting activities, hobbies, or exposure to media are reasonable and necessary. In general, children with TS—in the absence of additional problems or disabilities caused by other conditions—should attend a regular school. Choices related to career and occupation should mainly be determined by the child's personal tendencies and interests. Otherwise, professional life will not give pleasure, resulting in unease, stress, and, finally, worsening of tics. People with tics have to decide whether or not they will inform their colleagues and social acquaintances. If the tics are obvious, as a general rule it is best to inform acquaintances to prevent prejudice and rumors and unbearable sustained efforts to suppress tics.

Only patients who have loud vocal tics, noticeable or socially disruptive tics, marked coprolalia, or significant comorbidities should take into account the presence of TS when making decisions about their future professional life. However, even in these severely affected patients, these choices should not be made at the age when tics are at their worst (10–12 years), since in most cases tics will spontaneously decrease later on. Therefore, there is no adequate basis for making such far-reaching decisions at this period of life.

DRIVING AND TS

Only some patients with TS need to advise their driving school teacher and the driving test supervisor about their disease before starting driver's training. This does not apply to patients who have very mild tics that will not be likely noticeable during the driving test under stress. In general, people with TS can drive a car without any restrictions. Fitness to drive in people with TS should be assessed in a completely different way than patients who have other involuntary movement disorders, because tics occur intermittently and can be suppressed. Only a very few very severely affected patients are not qualified for a driver's license. This includes not only patients with extreme eye-blinking or eye-rolling tics and severe motor tics of the head, arms, trunk, and legs, but also patients with specific complex motor tics or compulsions such as the urge to bang on the car window, to manipulate the car's controls, or to touch objects inside the car again and again until they feel "just right." Within the context of a driver's license assessment, comorbidities such as severe depression as well as the adverse effects of medical treatment must also taken into account.

All in all, the risks of car accidents among persons with TS seem to be no different from those in healthy people. The fact that there are even people with TS who work as professional race drivers underscores the fact that, in general, people with TS are qualified for a driving license.

MILITARY SERVICE AND TS

In countries that still have compulsory military service, people with TS should be released from military service. The main reason for this recommendation is the high probability that they will be teased because of their tics. In addition, tics may occur while using a firearm. Comorbidities such as OCD and depression may further reduce fitness for military service. In general, people with TS should be considered unfit for military service.

ECHOPHENOMENA AND TS SELF-HELP GROUPS

As discussed in Chapter 30, in many countries there are very active national self-help and patient advocacy groups providing information and organizing meetings for patients, parents, and professionals. When attending such a meeting, patients with TS are often concerned that they might echo tics seen or heard in other people. Although echophenomena are quite common in patients with tics, and there is evidence that many of these patients are unaware of their echopraxia (Jonas et al., 2010), in only a minority of patients will new and persistent tics occur as a result of echoing. Thus, for the majority of patients the advantages of attending a self-help group will outweigh the disadvantages.

WHO GIVES SOCIAL SUPPORT TO PATIENTS WITH TS? THE EUROPEAN PERSPECTIVE

Since health care systems differ considerably between different countries, there are substantial differences in the pathways of care for patients with TS. In most European countries, patients with tics are seen primarily by a general practitioner or a pediatrician and will subsequently be referred to either a psychiatrist or neurologist. Today, in several European countries and in North America, specialized TS outpatient clinics are being offered, most commonly associated with university clinics, either at the department of child and adolescent psychiatry, adult psychiatry, or neurology. At these centers patients are primarily seen by medical doctors and/or psychologists. Only in some clinics are they assisted by social workers. While in some centers all the services (including diagnosis, information, treatment, and general social counseling) are performed by medical doctors alone, other centers have social workers who function as intermediaries among government agencies, the clinic, and families; for example, they may communicate with youth care and other social and therapeutic services, establish contact with authorities such as the youth welfare office, and give practical advice on various matters (e.g., questions related to educational counseling, problems at school, or how to fill out forms).

Box 28.1. Key Points

- Receiving the correct diagnosis of a tic disorder is a relief and not a burden for most patients and parents. Parents no longer need to blame themselves for the tics, and patients can avoid receiving ineffective and inappropriate therapies.
- Due to the wide spectrum of TS symptoms, patients may consult different specialists, including not only neurologists and psychiatrists but also general practitioners, ear/nose/throat physicians, ophthalmologists, pediatricians, allergists, speech and language therapists, dermatologists, and even dentists.
- Lack of knowledge among professionals is the main reason why the diagnosis of TS is often delayed for several years.
- A delay in diagnosis results in delayed initiation of the necessary support for children and their families.
- So that they do not miss the diagnosis of a tic disorder, physicians should remember that children presenting with ADHD and/or OCD can develop tics later in life.
- Psychoeducation should always be the first step in the treatment of patients with TS. It improves patients' knowledge and results in better coping with the disease.
- In the majority of younger children, the parents are much more impaired by the child's tics than the child. Therefore, it has to be decided whether the child should receive medical treatment to reduce the tics or the parents should receive psychoeducation and social support to better cope with the disease.
- With respect to treatment, a shared decision-making model is recommended where the physician provides tailored, unbiased, and up-to-date information about the benefits and disadvantages of alternative treatment choices, while the patient makes the decision whether treatment will be initiated.
- Comorbidities such as ADHD and OCD have a considerably greater impact on quality of life in children with TS than tics.
- The economic burden of adult patients with TS is high; indirect costs have a greater impact than direct costs.
- People with TS—apart from a few severely affected patients—are able to drive a car without any restrictions.
- Specific restrictions (such as diets, sports, hobbies, or exposure to media) should not be imposed on children with TS.
- In general, patients with TS are entitled to apply for recognition as a disabled person.
- There are several renowned and successful musicians, athletes, and writers who have TS.

Adult patients, in contrast, may be supported by social workers in terms of professional training, employment, retirement, driver's license, and insurance. In most European countries, there are no dedicated social support programs available for children or adults with TS. However, in some countries this gap is at least partly filled by special offers from the national TS self-help groups. For example, TS support groups publish informational brochures and material for educators, organize informational events, and offer further training for teachers, workshops for families (e.g., on quality of life, social skills, partnership), and TS camps for youngsters.

CONCLUSIONS

It is important for people with TS to receive the correct diagnosis as early as possible. This is a prerequisite not only for appropriate and best therapy, but also for the necessary psychosocial support from social authorities. Only with an early diagnosis it is possible to manage different social problems and to facilitate understanding in the social environment. However, there is still a delay of several years between tic onset and diagnosis. In addition, patients and their relatives still often complain of a general lack of knowledge among professionals. Psychoeducation as a meaningful supplement to treatment should be the first step in treatment and should be offered to all patients and families with TS.

REFERENCES

Altman G, Staley JD, Wener P. Children with Tourette disorder: a follow-up study in adulthood. *J Nerv Mental Dis* 2009; 197:305–310.

Ashoori A, Jankovic J. Mozart's movements and behaviour: a case of Tourette's syndrome? *J Neurol Neurosurg Psychiatry* 2007; 78:1171–1175.

Aterman K. Did Mozart have Tourette's syndrome? Some comments on Mozart's language. *Perspect Biol Med* 1994; 37:247–258.

Bawden HN, Stokes A, Camfield CS et al. Peer relationship problems in children with Tourette's disorder or diabetes mellitus. *J Child Psychol Psychiatry* 1998; 39:663–668.

Bloch MH, Peterson BS, Scahill L et al. Adulthood outcome of tic and obsessive-compulsive symptom severity in children with Tourette syndrome. *Arch Pediatr Adolesc Med* 2006; 160:65–69.

Carter AS, Pauls DL, Leckman JF, Cohen DJ. A prospective longitudinal study of Gilles de la Tourette's syndrome. *J Am Acad Child Adolesc Psychiatry* 1994; 33:377–385.

Cavanna AE, Robertson MM, Critchley HD. Schizotypal personality traits in Gilles de la Tourette syndrome. *Acta Neurol Scand* 2007; 116 385–391.

Conelea CA, Woods DW, Zinner SH et al. Exploring the impact of chronic tic disorders on youth: results from the Tourette Syndrome Impact Survey. *Child Psychiatry Hum Dev* 2011; 42:219–242.

A study on a large, "virtual" community sample of children with chronic tic disorders using an Internet-based survey completed by families,

exploring the functional impact of tics among youth.

Conelea CA, Woods DW, Zinner SH et al. The impact of Tourette syndrome in adults: results from the Tourette Syndrome Impact Survey. *Community Ment Health J* 2012 [E-pub ahead of print].

A valuable survey from a large sample of adults with chronic tic disorders, highlighting the type and extent of social impairment secondary to tics in adulthood.

Cutler D, Murphy T, Gilmour J, Heyman I. The quality of life of young people with Tourette syndrome. *Child Care Health Dev* 2009; 35:496–504.

Dodel I, Reese JP, Muller N et al. Cost of illness in patients with Gilles de la Tourette's syndrome. *J Neurol* 2010; 257:1055–1061.

The first study specifically dedicated to economic issues related to TS.

Eddy CM, Cavanna AE, Gulisano M et al. Clinical correlates of quality of life in Tourette syndrome. *Mov Disord* 2011a; 26:735–738.

Eddy CM, Rizzo R, Gulisano M et al. Quality of life in young people with Tourette syndrome: a controlled study. *J Neurol* 2011b; 258:291–301.

Elstner K, Selai CE, Trimble MR, Robertson MM. Quality of life (QOL) of patients with Gilles de la Tourette's syndrome. *Acta Psych Scand* 2001; 103:52–59.

Freeman RD, Fast DK, Burd L et al. An international perspective on Tourette syndrome: selected findings from 3,500 individuals in 22 countries. *Dev Med Child Neurol* 2000; 42:436–447.

Gilles de la Tourette G. Etude sur une affection nerveuse caracterisée par de l'incoordination motrice accompagnée d'echolalie et de coprolalie. *Arch Neurol* 1885; 9:19–42.

Jankovic J Sekula S. Dermatological manifestations of Tourette syndrome and obsessive-compulsive disorder. *Arch Dermatol* 1998; 134:113–114.

Jonas M, Thomalla G, Biermann-Ruben K et al. Imitation in patients with Gilles de la Tourette syndrome—a behavioral study. *Mov Disord* 2010; 25:991–999.

Khalifa N, von Knorring AL. Tourette syndrome and other tic disorders in a total population of children: clinical assessment and background. *Acta Paediatr* 2005; 94:1608–1614.

Kompoliti K, Fan W, Leurgans S. Complementary and alternative medicine use in Gilles de la Tourette syndrome. *Mov Disord* 2009; 24:2015–2019.

Leksell E, Edvardson S. A case of Tourette syndrome presenting with oral self-injurious behaviour. *Int J Paediatr Dent* 2005; 15:370–374.

Mol Debes N, Hjalgrim H, Skov L. Limited knowledge of Tourette syndrome causes delay in diagnosis. *Neuropediatrics* 2008; 39:101–105.

One of the very few systematic studies addressing the issue of latency between onset and diagnosis in TS.

Mol Debes N, Hjalgrim H, Skov L. The presence of attention-deficit hyperactivity disorder (ADHD) and obsessive-compulsive disorder worsen psychosocial and educational problems in Tourette syndrome. *J Child Neurol* 2010; 25:171–181.

Looks at the psychosocial and educational consequences of ADHD comorbidity in children with TS.

Monaco F, Servo S, Cavanna AE. Famous people with Gilles de la Tourette syndrome? *J Psychosom Res* 2009; 67:485–490.

Müller-Vahl K. *Tourette-Syndrom und andere Tic-Erkrankungen im Kindes- und Erwachsenenalter. 1.* Aufl. Berlin: Medizinisch Wissenschaftliche Verlagsgesellschaft, 2010.

Müller-Vahl KR, Buddensiek N, Geomelas M, Emrich HM. The influence of different food and drink on tics in Tourette syndrome. *Acta Paediatr* 2008; 97:442–446.

Müller-Vahl KR, Dodel I, Muller et al. Health-related quality of life in patients with Gilles de la Tourette's syndrome. *Mov Disord* 2010; 25: 309–314.

Pringsheim T, Lang A, Kurlan R et al. Understanding disability in Tourette syndrome. *Dev Med Child Neurol* 2009; 51:468–472.

A valuable study assessing physical and psychosocial health in different groups of TS patients, with a special look at the impact of comorbidities.

Rivera-Navarro J, Cubo E, Almazan J. The diagnosis of Tourette's Syndrome: communication and impact. *Clin Child Psychol Psychiatry* 2009; 14:13–23.

An original study exploring communication issues and skills related to sharing the diagnosis of TS with patients and families.

Robertson MM. The prevalence and epidemiology of Gilles de la Tourette syndrome. Part 1: the epidemiological and prevalence studies. *J Psychosom Res* 2008; 65:461–472.

Robertson MM, Banerjee S, Eapen V, Fox-Hiley P. Obsessive compulsive behaviour and depressive symptoms in young people with Tourette syndrome. A controlled study. *Eur Child Adolesc Psychiatry* 2002; *11*: 261–265.

Robertson MM, Banerjee S, Hiley PJ, Tannock C. Personality disorder and psychopathology in Tourette's syndrome: a controlled study. *Br J Psychiatry* 1997; *171*:283–286.

Roessner V, Plessen KJ, Rothenberger A et al. European clinical guidelines for Tourette syndrome and other tic disorders. Part II: pharmacological treatment. *Eur Child Adolesc Psychiatry* 2011; *20*:173–196.

Schneider M, Trillini M, Bokemeyer S, Müller-Vahl K. *Persönlichkeitsakzentuierungen bei Patienten mit Gilles de la Tourette-Syndrom.* P-019-005, DGPPN-Kongress 2011.

Simkin B. Mozart's scatological disorder. *BMJ* 1992; *305*:1563–1567.

Stokes A, Bawden HN, Camfield PR et al. Peer problems in Tourette's disorder. *Pediatrics* 1991; *87*:936–942.

Storch EA, Merlo LJ, Lack C et al. Quality of life in youth with Tourette's syndrome and chronic tic disorder. *J Clin Child Adolesc Psychol* 2007; *36*:217–227.

29

Information and Support for Educators

SHERYL K. PRUITT AND LESLIE E. PACKER

Abstract

Students with tics or Tourette syndrome face numerous academic, behavioral, and social challenges. Most of the impairment appears due to associated disorders. Comprehensive psychoeducational and functional behavioral assessments enable the school team to develop appropriate accommodations and interventions. Providing a supportive environment, nurturing the child's strengths and talents, and providing resources and support for the parents in service of the child can help the student overcome any challenges and have a successful school year. This chapter examines the various issues that teachers and educators should be familiar with when facing the social and academic challenges of Tourette syndrome patients.

M, a bright teenager with Tourette syndrome (TS) and obsessive-compulsive disorder (OCD), was frustrated by eye tics when reading but tormented by the number 4. She could not calculate math problems if the digit 4 was part of the problem. She compulsively counted how many letters were in words to see if they were multiples of 4 and compulsively checked to determine if the number of words in a sentence was a multiple of 4. As her grades slipped precipitously, her tics and anxiety worsened, and her parents requested school accommodations for her symptoms. District personnel were shocked to learn of the severity of M's problems and promised to provide the accommodations but did not follow through, even when M's parents contacted them again. Two months later, never having been given the accommodations and now failing her courses, M attempted suicide.

PREVIOUS CHAPTERS have described the cardinal features of TS and its associated disorders. This chapter describes their impact on academic, behavioral, and social functioning and gives information about school-based accommodations and intervention strategies.

TS AND LEARNING DIFFICULTIES

As discussed in Chapter 20, although some studies suggest possible differences in IQ scores between students with TS and their non-TS peers, most studies report that IQ scores of students with uncomplicated TS (TS only) follow the normal curve model. But lack of impact on IQ scores does not mean lack of significant impact on school functioning. Studies investigating the educational placement of students with TS consistently report higher-than-expected rates of students with TS in special education settings (Comings & Comings, 1987; Cubo et al., 2011; Kurlan et al., 2001). The overrepresentation of students with TS in special education may not be due to tics, however, as much as to the presence of learning disabilities and interference from associated disorders (Packer, 2005).

The rate of learning disability (LD) in TS has been a somewhat contentious issue. Although early studies reported higher-than-expected rates of LD in the presence of TS, these studies often lacked adequate controls. Failure to extend time as an accommodation for tic interference and failure to control for associated disorders may have contributed to overestimates of the rate of LD in students who have TS only. For students who have TS in combination with associated disorders, the most common LDs are in written expression and math calculations. Chapters 4 and 20 provide additional information on LD in TS.

Whereas TS only does not increase referrals to special education, the addition of attention-deficit/hyperactivity disorder (ADHD) strongly predicts referral to special education, even after controlling for the presence of LD. Children diagnosed with TS+ADHD and children with ADHD only do not differ from each other in rate of placement in special education. Significantly, tic symptom severity does not correlate with placement in special education, but ADHD symptom severity does (Spencer et al., 2001). OCD, which is also commonly comorbid with TS, does not appear to be a significant factor in removal from regular education placement by itself (OCD only) but does contribute to learning difficulties and occurs in higher-than-expected rates in special education settings for students with severe behavior-emotional problems (Cubo et al., 2011). Other associated disorders that increase the likelihood of removal from regular education include executive dysfunction (EDF), autism spectrum disorder (ASD), and bipolar disorder.

IMPACT OF TICS ON SCHOOL FUNCTIONING

Even if TS only is not a significant risk factor for removal from regular education placement, tics can significantly interfere with learning and performance. In a recruited sample of parents and guardians of students with TS and associated disorders, Packer (2005) found that approximately three fourths of the children reportedly experienced some degree of tic-related interference in academic functioning; approximately half of the sample described the impact as moderate to severe. Simple motor tics involving the eyes, head and/or neck region, and upper extremities were reported as interfering with reading and handwritten work, while vocal tics reportedly interfered with reading aloud and participating in class discussions. These reports are consistent with other parent surveys on the impact of TS (Hagin et al., 1980, in Silver & Hagin, 1990; Hagin & Kugler, 1988).

Tics also interfere indirectly with learning or performance, such as when an urge to tic builds up. Some students may be acutely aware of these internal sensations (premonitory urges), while others are unaware. Awareness of premonitory urges emerges developmentally between the ages of 8 and 10 (Leckman et al., 2006). Awareness of an inner itch or tingle that precedes a tic or bout of tics distracts the student from paying attention, while attempts to suppress tics for fear of peers noticing may distract the student and decrease the accuracy of his or her work (Conelea & Woods, 2008b). Efforts to suppress tics may also lead to a build-up in frustration, fatigue, and irritability over the course of the school day.

Impact from tic interference will vary, in part, with the waxing and waning cycles of tics. Even when tics remit, however, most students continue to experience impaired academic functioning. Persisting academic impairment may be due to the impact of associated disorders that do not also remit (Packer, 2005).

STRESS AND TICS

Stressors do not cause tics, but they may exacerbate them (Silva et al., 1995). Stressors that may affect a student in school include time pressure (especially on tests), overarousal due to holidays or special events, fatigue, anxiety, infection, being overheated, feeling conspicuous or being observed, allergy seasons, and some social situations. In contrast, tics often decrease when the student is non-anxiously engrossed in an activity or a skilled task, using a special gift or talent, reading for pleasure, talking with friends, or during a novel task. For some students, allowing them to read for pleasure or work on an interesting puzzle or on the computer may provide short-term relief from severe or frequent tics.

School personnel need to be aware, however, that some factors may have different effects on different students or even on the same student at different times. As one example, relaxation is often associated with a decrease in tics, but as the student first starts to relax, more tics may come out. See Table 1.2 in Chapter 1 of this volume and Conelea and Woods (2008a) for more information on environmental factors that may affect tic frequency and severity.

OTHER TS-RELATED IMPAIRMENT

In addition to direct and indirect interference from tics, TS has also been linked to other potential sources of impairment in school functioning. As discussed in Chapter 20, however, the research has produced somewhat equivocal results as to whether some sources of impairment are attributable to TS *per se* or if they are better explained by the presence of associated disorders. As one example, although a number of earlier studies suggested visual-motor integration (VMI) deficits in TS, other studies suggest the VMI deficits are better explained by the presence of comorbid ADHD and OCD. In contrast, deficits in mental and written math (Brookshire et al., 1994; Burd et al., 1992) have been reported in individuals with TS only and may be due to attentional difficulties that are hypothesized to be intrinsic to TS (Chang et al., 2007; Huckeba et al., 2008; Schuerholz et al., 1996). Other deficits that have been linked directly to TS include deficits in habit acquisition (Marsh et al., 2004); inhibiting verbal responses or blurting, homework issues (Dornbush & Pruitt, 2009; Packer & Pruitt, 2010), and speech dysfluencies (De Nil et al., 2005).

Although questions as to whether specific deficits are directly or only indirectly linked to TS are fascinating, on a practical level educators simply need to know that a significant subset of students with TS will have the problems identified above. Each of these challenges may require accommodations, not only so that the student can learn and perform but so that tics are not exacerbated by the stress of these other challenges.

COMMON SENSE ACCOMMODATIONS FOR TICS IN SCHOOL SETTINGS

Most students with TS require accommodations for their tics. Respondents in one small survey reported that their children received an average of more than four accommodations for tic-related interference (Packer, 2005). Although there has been no adequately controlled research on the effectiveness of in-school accommodations, parental and student reports consistently identify a number of accommodations as being useful.

Extended time is one of the most crucial accommodations. Because stress, especially time pressure, often increases tics, school personnel need to extend the amount of time provided for classwork, quizzes, and tests, and allow extra time to record assignments and pack up materials. *Testing in a separate location* with a proctor with whom the student feels comfortable allows the student to concentrate on the test without having to worry that others are noticing or being distracted by the student's tics. *Preferential seating* also helps, but it is important to allow the student to determine where to sit. Students may prefer to avoid the front row or high-traffic areas and to sit off to the side or close to the door so they can discreetly leave if their tics become overwhelming. *Allowing students to leave the room* at their discretion and without having to call attention to themselves is also a helpful accommodation. School personnel need to collaborate with students to identify locations where they can go to either release tics in a private setting or restore themselves to a calmer state. For a student with prominent vocal tics, the school team may need to *excuse the student from tasks or settings* where the tics will be very noticeable or distracting (such as reading aloud, the school library, or study hall). When tics or the effort to suppress tics distracts the student from paying attention or taking notes, teachers will need to *provide the student with a hard copy of any lecture notes or board work*.

Other important accommodations for tics include reducing the amount to be read or written at any one time if tics are interfering directly or indirectly, reducing handwriting demands, reducing copying from the board, and using assistive technology such as books on tape, keyboarding, or voice dictation software. School personnel are encouraged to ask the student and the parents what accommodations are needed. In cases of severe, prominent, or socially problematic tics, peer education may be one of the most important accommodations, as discussed later in this chapter.

Two of the most helpful strategies teachers can use are to *refrain from commenting on or responding visibly to a student's tics* and to *model acceptance and support.* Ignoring the tics publicly does not mean that the teacher cannot privately discuss the student's tics with him or her to determine necessary supports or to empathize with the student. During any tic-oriented discussions, the student's vocal tics temporarily increase (Woods et al., 2001), but in our experience, any temporary exacerbation is offset by the benefit of empowering the student in determining what supports or accommodations are needed.

Having a supportive teacher is one of the most significant protective factors in minimizing the potential negative impact of tics. Other protective factors of note include having supportive parents who encourage autonomy, having friends, an internal locus of control, and involvement in non-athletic activities (Cohen et al., 2008). Environments that nurture any enhanced creativity (discussed later in this chapter) are also protective.

Communicating with the student's parents on an ongoing and regular basis is often an important piece of any plan for a student with TS. Tics will change over the course of the school year, and parents often see more tics at home than the teacher will see in the classroom. Through ongoing communication, parents can alert teachers to the student's current stressors and tics so that the school can implement accommodations. Parents can also inform the teacher about medication side effects or changes the student may be experiencing that may interfere with functioning. In a mutually supportive relationship, educators support the parent in service of the student by ensuring that parents have sufficient information to assist their child with homework and by providing parents with helpful community resources and online resources for information and TS support. Chapter 30 provides some resources educators may wish to share with parents.

IMPACT OF ASSOCIATED DISORDERS ON SCHOOL FUNCTIONING

Most students with TS have features of one or more associated disorders; some of the commonly associated disorders are discussed in Chapters 2, 3, and 4. Educators need to be aware that the student with TS may have symptoms of one or (usually more) of the following challenges in addition to TS: ADHD, OCD, depression or bipolar disorder, non-OCD anxiety disorders, EDF, memory impairment, slow processing speed, behavioral disinhibition, anger issues, hypersensitivity to sensory stimuli, emotional dysregulation, deficits in VMI, impaired fine-motor control, and/or impaired graphomotor skills. Some students with TS will also have comorbid ASD, which, as discussed in Chapter 4, predicts significant academic and social challenges.

Because the associated disorders are usually a greater source of impairment in academic functioning than the tics of TS (Du et al., 2010; Packer, 1997, 2005), educators also need to be aware of the impact of the associated disorders. Because most students with TS have comorbid disorders, a referral for a comprehensive assessment and a psychiatric evaluation to clarify the student's diagnoses is often necessary. For many students, referral to the school's occupational therapist and speech and language pathologist will be important in addressing academic, behavioral, and social skills issues. For students with ASD, the school's autism consultant will need to identify additional necessary accommodations and interventions.

In the remainder of this chapter, students with TS who have associated disorders or features of associated disorders are denoted as having "TS+." Although the most common TS+ pattern may be TS+ADHD+OCD (Packer, 1997), in the following material "TS+" can indicate any pattern of associated disorders.

Handwriting

Handwriting is often impaired for students with TS+ (Packer, 1997; Packer & Gentile, 1994), but the nature of the deficit varies as a function of comorbid conditions. Tics can interfere with the production of neat handwriting, but comorbid OCD may also interfere if there are writing rituals such as erasures and rewriting. Similarly, while students with severe OCD tend to have very small handwriting, students with ADHD tend to have large and sloppy handwriting. The classroom teacher may need the assistance of the school's occupational therapist to assess the student's graphomotor skills and the advice of both the occupational therapist and assistive technology specialist to suggest necessary accommodations or devices to compensate for the student's handwriting problems. Handwriting is one of the biggest sources of frustration for students with TS. Accommodating production problems and difficulty copying from the board can make the difference between a successful school year and an unsuccessful one.

Homework

Most students with TS+ also have significant homework issues. Sleep problems may interfere with completion of work, and for students with comorbid OCD, perfectionistic rituals may interfere with completion. For students with comorbid ADHD of the inattentive subtype (ADHD-I), sluggish cognitive tempo or slow processing speed may impede their ability to complete homework, while students with comorbid EDF may fail to complete their homework because they failed to record all of their assignments and pack up all necessary materials. For some students, homework time may be after any medication they take for school wears off. Homework is a frequent source of "storms" or "meltdowns" in the home. School personnel need to screen for homework issues that may require accommodations (see Packer and Pruitt, 2010, for a homework problems screening tool teachers can use). Homework

needs to be on the student's independent level and parents need to let the school know if the child cannot complete assignments independently or if the parent is actually doing the homework for the child to prevent a "storm."

Executive Dysfunction, Memory Impairment, and Processing Speed Deficits

Some of the most influential aspects of TS+ are "hidden" disabilities such as EDF, memory impairment, and processing speed deficits. EDF may impair the student's organizational skills, social functioning, and academic tasks such as written expression and long-term projects (Dornbush & Pruitt, 2009). Although students with TS only generally do not have deficits in planning or problem solving (see Chapter 20), and not all students with TS+ have comorbid EDF, school personnel need to be especially alert to it in students who are disorganized, fail to complete and turn in homework, and/or have poor social skills. Students with EDF may require accommodations and direct instruction in skills such as recording assignments completely, packing up necessary materials, breaking big tasks into smaller tasks with intermediate deadlines, study skills, and generating prioritized to-do lists. Students with EDF-related homework problems may benefit from appropriate organizational skills interventions (Evans et al., 2005; Langberg et al., 2008a, 2008b, 2010). Screening for organizational problems can help identify students who will require accommodations (see Packer and Pruitt, 2010, for a screening tool teachers can use). It is especially helpful for schools to use the Behavior Rating Inventory of Executive Function (BRIEF; Gioia et al., 2000) to evaluate students with suspected EDF or students who are having significant academic issues. The BRIEF helps teachers, parents, and students appreciate the impact of EDF on functioning, highlights specific areas of weakness that require accommodations and remediation, and changes the conversation from "lazy student" to "neurologically impaired student." Drs. Murphy and Eddy review some of the research on EDF in Chapter 20.

Memory deficits also impair academic functioning. In Chapter 20, Drs. Murphy and Eddy review some of the research on memory functions and TS. From an applied perspective, school personnel need to be especially aware of, and screen for, *working memory* deficits. Working memory deficits impair the student's ability to retain information while skills are being applied or to comply with multistep directions. Such deficits are common in ADHD (Kofler et al., 2010, 2011; Martinussen et al., 2005) and depression (Klimkeit et al., 2011).

Other types of memory impairment include *procedural memory* and *strategic memory* deficits. These deficits reduce the student's ability to automate certain skills or sequences and reduce their use of strategies to recall important information. For a subset of students with TS, handwriting is a skill that never becomes fully automatic. While their peers are simply recording the content of a lecture, such students have to actively think about how to form the letters they are writing. Deficits in *prospective memory* affect the ability to remember what needs to be done in the future, while deficits in *metamemory* impair the ability to understand and appreciate one's memory strengths and weaknesses. Students with memory impairments require accommodations as well as instruction in strategies for enhancing memory.

Speed of processing affects the efficiency of working memory and the student's ability to process orally presented material in a timely fashion. As a consequence, the student often misses important information or does not have adequate time to consolidate it with previously acquired information. Slow speed of processing is associated with inattentive behavior and has been reported in students with TS (Khalifa et al., 2010), OCD, ADHD-I (Weiler et al., 2000), anxious/depressed symptoms (Lundy et al., 2010), and bipolar disorder (Doyle et al., 2005). Teachers can accommodate slow processing speed by simply pausing more in their speech to give the student time to catch up, by giving one instruction at a time for multistep instructions, and by extending time on tests.

Although an in-depth discussion of the impact of the associated disorders and their management in school settings is beyond the scope of this chapter, Table 29.1 provides a highly simplified overview of just a few of the types of impact educators may observe in the school setting, along with a few suggested accommodations for each problem. Note that ADHD is omitted from the table as a separate diagnosis in favor of treating impulsivity and attentional problems as challenges that are also features of other disorders. ASD and some other challenges mentioned in this chapter are also omitted although they, too, need to be addressed. Because there is almost no controlled research on the efficacy of particular accommodations, the tips in Table 29.1 are based on our experience as well as parental reports in published surveys on school experiences.

As can be seen in Table 29.1, students with TS+, regardless of whether they meet full diagnostic criteria for any associated disorders, are likely to experience numerous sources of interference in the school setting. Resources with additional information on impact and accommodations can be found elsewhere (Adams, 2011; Dornbush & Pruitt, 2009; Killu & Crundwell, 2008; Packer, 2009; Packer & Pruitt, 2010).

REFERRING STUDENTS FOR ASSESSMENT

As suggested by the preceding material, students with TS+ may have a complex and confusing array of symptoms and challenges. For many students, referral to the school's occupational therapist and speech and language pathologist will be important in addressing academic, behavioral, and social skills issues. For other students, an autism consultant may need to assist the team in identifying additional necessary accommodations and interventions. For students with TS+ who are not performing commensurate with their potential, a referral for a comprehensive assessment that includes a neuropsychological assessment is often crucial to developing an appropriate set of accommodations and interventions. A referral to a psychiatrist may also be needed to clarify the student's diagnoses and to help the school team understand the student's behavior.

Table 29.1 Associated Disorders or Challenges, Potential Impact, and Accommodations or Strategies for Educators in TS

Disorder or challenge	Potential impact	Accommodations or strategies
Attention or focus deficits	Student misses information and directions. Student takes longer to complete work. Student misses social cues, resulting in inappropriate responses to peers.	Provide hard copy of all information. Allow extra time for classwork and tests. Provide direct instruction and practice in areas where student misses social cues.
OCD and non-OCD anxiety disorders	Disorder interferes with processing and memory. Student avoids certain tasks or settings. Student gets "stuck" and cannot move on with work until it is "just right." Student has difficulty making transitions.	Do not assign more work than can be completed in available time. Reduce environmental triggers. Reduce work if symptoms interfere with timely completion. Pre-warn about transitions.
Mood disorders	Mood disorders carry an increased risk of suicide and severely impulsive and self-injurious behaviors. Mood disorders present as severe irritability in some students. Mood disorders vary in impact by type of mood episode.	Refer for psychiatric evaluation if mood or behavioral changes last more than 2 weeks or if there are safety concerns. Allow student to go to a "safe person or place." More than one accommodation plan is needed as mood status changes.
Homework problems	Homework problems create conflict at home and school and result in lower grades. Medication may have less impact later in the day. Student may fail to record assignments and pack necessary materials. Student will require parental supervision and assistance with homework. Homework problems lead to feelings of failure and hopelessness.	Screen for homework problems. Do not penalize for lateness. Modify and reduce homework. Make sure assignments are recorded accurately and needed materials are packed. Ensure parents have adequate information and support so they can assist their child. Ensure that student achieves homework success.
Visual-motor integration, graphomotor, fine-motor deficits	Student produces sloppy handwriting. Student has difficulty copying from the board. Student has reduced endurance for written tasks. Student avoids lengthy writing tasks.	Reduce handwriting demands. Give copy of notes from the board. Refer to occupational therapist. Refer for assistive technology.

(Continued)

Table 29.1 (*Continued*)

Disorder or challenge	Potential impact	Accommodations or strategies
Executive dysfunction	Executive dysfunction impairs organization. Student has difficulty planning and completing work. Student struggles with prioritization. Student lacks adequate study skills.	Color-code books and materials by subject. Assist with planning reports and projects. "Chunk" big projects and monitor progress. Use syllabus and provide partial notes. Teach and rehearse study skills.
Impulsive or disinhibited behavior	Impulsive or disinhibited behavior increases safety risks. Student loses temper inappropriately. Student interrupts others. Student makes careless errors in work.	Increase adult supervision. Teach coping skills. Teach strategy of covering mouth. Provide cues such as editing strips.
Memory impairments	Student cannot hold information in mind long enough to act on it and to store it. Memory impairments reduce the student's ability to retrieve information, impair the automaticity of sequences, and decrease memory for strategies.	Reduce amount of material presented at one time and use electronics to externalize memory. Use cognitive strategies to assist with retrieval. Teach mnemonics for sequences. Have student collect strategies to use.
Sensory defensiveness	Student overreacts to sensory stimuli, which may lead to "storms." Student avoids strong sensory experiences. This may lead to reduced social interactions.	Refer to occupational therapy. Allow the student to avoid sensory overload. Strategies may include letting the students leave class early to avoid noises in hall, and encouraging the student to eat lunch with a friend in a quiet setting.
Sleep disorders	Student has difficulty waking up, resulting in attendance issues. Student falls asleep while doing homework. Sleep disorders impair the student's focus and memory, possibly leading to aggressive behavior.	Recommend a sleep hygiene program and do not penalize for lateness. Reduce and modify homework. Modify classwork and provide notes. Refer for functional behavioral assessment.
Difficulties with written expression and long-term projects	Student has great difficulty starting, planning, and completing work. Student feels overwhelmed by long-term projects and avoids work. Student cannot organize and sequence ideas. Student cannot edit while writing. Student can edit only one thing at a time.	"Chunk" big assignments into smaller tasks with intermediate deadlines. Enter deadlines in planner and monitor progress toward intermediate goals. Provide visual or graphic organizer. Allow separate time for editing. Use a cognitive or visual cue strip to edit.

When referring a student for assessment, the following types of information will help the assessment team determine what specific assessments may be needed:

1. A teacher narrative describing the student's academic, behavior, and social-emotional functioning with a statement of teacher concerns. We find teacher narratives particularly helpful over and above any teacher-completed scale or checklist on attention and behavior.

2. Handwritten work samples that illustrate what the student typically produces when asked to write more than a sentence by hand. Work samples that involve written expression and copying from the board are particularly helpful. Such work samples may also usefully include a sample of math calculations if there are handwriting issues.

3. Report cards from previous year(s) and current year if significant deterioration in performance has been noted.

4. A narrative or statement from the parent as to the parent's concerns about the child's school functioning. Having parents complete the BRIEF and screening tools in Packer and Pruitt (2010) about their child's sleep, homework, and organization can provide valuable information to assessors.

5. A statement from the student (if possible) outlining his or her concerns about school functioning. Students with suspected EDF can also be asked to complete the student survey tools in Packer and Pruitt (2010) about their study and homework habits.

6. A description of the student's strengths or special talents. Capitalizing on the student's strengths and talents is an important element in developing school-based plans.

Although not every student requires a neuropsychological assessment, for those who do, a helpful report will include both a full description of the deficits and sources of interference the student faces in school as well as a description of necessary and appropriate accommodations and interventions for each area of deficit. For students who are being treated pharmacologically for symptoms of TS+, the report also needs to clarify how the current medications may be affecting the student's performance.

"NAUGHTY OR NEUROLOGY?" BEHAVIOR PROBLEMS IN SCHOOL

Students with TS+ are often misunderstood as engaging in intentional misbehavior because school personnel may not recognize the behaviors as neurological symptoms. Educators often ask us, "Is this a behavior or a symptom?" as if something is one or the other. To be clear, when using the term "behavior," there is no implication that it is wholly voluntary. Similarly, labeling something a "symptom" does not imply that it cannot be modified by self-regulation, treatment, interventions, or altering the environment and antecedents to its occurrence. And although parents may be reluctant to allow the school to target a medical symptom, it is incumbent on schools to appropriately address self- or other-injurious symptoms or symptoms that may result in expulsion or removal to a more restrictive placement. Other symptoms may need to be addressed because they seriously impair the development of normal social and peer relationships. To address them safely and effectively, however, schools generally need to obtain professional guidance.

WHY SCHOOL-BASED BEHAVIOR PLANS OFTEN FAIL—OR BACKFIRE

Attempting to modify tics or symptoms of TS+ is fraught with pitfalls. The school will need to conduct a functional behavioral assessment and secure the assistance of professionals with expertise in these disorders, in behavioral analysis, and in modifying behavior. Often, the first step is educating personnel that (1) the symptom is not willful or voluntary, (2) the root cause of the problem is not motivational, and (3) the student cannot behave appropriately just by "trying harder." The confusion is understandable: symptoms often look purposeful and may be highly variable, leading some educators to wonder if a student's noncompliance on a particular day indicates lack of motivation. After all, he could behave appropriately yesterday, right?

If the solution were really to motivate the student to "just try harder," then a simple incentive plan whereby the student earns immediate and student-selected rewards for appropriate or desirable behavior might suffice. In actual practice, consequence-based plans often fail because the cause of the problem is not lack of motivation. Not only do some plans fail, but inappropriately applied positive-based interventions may lead to demoralization, frustration, and worsening symptoms. Just as medications may have adverse effects, so, too, can behavioral interventions (Packer, 2005). Thankfully, one tool, if administered properly, can often help school personnel avoid some pitfalls.

THE ALL-IMPORTANT FUNCTIONAL BEHAVIORAL ASSESSMENT

In our experience, the single most common explanation for inappropriate school-based interventions is failure to conduct comprehensive assessments. Functional behavioral assessments pinpoint the antecedents for the problematic symptom and identify other factors that need to be addressed. At the very least, the school team needs to:

1. Collect objective and quantifiable baseline data on the to-be-targeted behavior in an A-B-C (Antecedent, Behavior, Consequences) format across settings, tasks, and times of day
2. Assess the student for other factors that may contribute to the behavioral problem, including handwriting issues, working memory or processing speed deficits, sleep problems, deficits in social skills, deficits in executive functions, homework hassles, and sensory defensiveness
3. Interview all teachers to determine under what conditions the behavior occurs in their class and under what conditions it does not occur
4. Interview the parents to determine whether the behavior also occurs in the home or community, and if so, under what conditions it does occur and under what conditions it does not occur
5. Interview the student (if possible) to determine his or her awareness and understanding of

the behavior's impact on himself or herself and others. Determine the student's willingness to address it, and what supports are needed to help regulate or modify the behavior.

School personnel are also encouraged to ask the student's prescribing physician whether the observed behavioral concerns might be an adverse effect of medications. Some medications may have adverse behavioral effects such as activation or increased impulsivity, school phobia, or agitation and restlessness.

Conducting a functional behavioral assessment is especially important if the student exhibits school avoidance or school refusal. There may be a variety of factors that need to be addressed. A functional behavioral assessment is also crucial if the student has "meltdowns" or "storms" in school.

"MELTDOWNS" OR "STORMS"

Some students experience what are variously called "meltdowns" (Greene, 1998), "storms" (Dornbush & Pruitt, 1995), or "rage attacks" (Budman et al., 1998). These incidents are not temper tantrums or attempts to manipulate the teacher: they indicate a temporary loss of control that can be due to a variety of factors or combination of factors. During such incidents, the student may yell, curse, or say and do things he or she would not normally say or do. Afterwards, the student may be genuinely remorseful or have no recollection of what he or she said during the incident. Some of the relevant research on rage attacks is described in Chapters 4, 20, and 25.

Loss of control is easier to prevent than to deal with once it has occurred. A comprehensive assessment is crucial so that school personnel can eliminate or reduce triggers, provide stress-reducing accommodations, and implement remedial training in any deficient academic or social skills that contribute to the problem. As part of such remediation, students may require direct instruction in how to handle frustration in acceptable ways.

In some cases, teachers may detect warning signs of an impending meltdown (some students suddenly get louder or may seem more frustrated and unable to tolerate anything). School personnel may help avert a storm by encouraging the student to take a break out of the classroom, to take a walk, or to engage in some physical activity. If the student is accompanied by a paraprofessional during any such walk, the aide needs to avoid touching the student or initiating conversation with the student.

If a storm has not been avoided, then after the storm, the teacher should allow the student to go to some place to calm down or to engage in a quiet and calming activity. Some students may need to sleep. School personnel should not attempt to analyze the meltdown with the student right after the incident; this may lead to a rekindling of the problem. There is plenty of time to discuss it later.

DISCIPLINE MEANS TRAINING, NOT PUNISHMENT

As concerned as we are about ineffective and potentially harmful positive-based interventions, we are more concerned about punitive or aversive consequences applied to symptoms. As examples, we have seen students directed to, taken to, or even forcibly dragged to time-out rooms because they were "stuck" and could not cooperate with their teachers; we have seen students suspended for lashing out at teachers who did not appreciate the "fight-or-flight" nature of panic attacks or OCD; and we have seen students suspended for having a "storm" in situations where the school had not provided necessary accommodations and supports. When staff is adequately trained to recognize and accommodate symptoms of the student's disability, many situations do not escalate or become problematic.

Punishment is basically an attempt to motivate the student not to do something again. However, if the problem is due to a skills deficit such as inability to make a transition, attempting to boost motivation by punishing the student will not result in the desired outcome and will often backfire. It is easier, and more effective, to change the environment and what we do *before* behavior occurs than to try to deal with undesirable behavior after it occurs.

EMPATHY AS AN INTERVENTION

"I've come to the frightening conclusion that I am the decisive element in the classroom. It's my personal approach that creates the climate. It's my daily mood that makes the weather. As a teacher, I possess a tremendous power to make a child's life miserable or joyous. I can be a tool of torture or an instrument of inspiration. I can humiliate or humor, hurt or heal. In all situations, it is my response that decides whether a crisis will be escalated or de-escalated and a child humanized or dehumanized." (Dr. Haim Ginott, 1975)

Based on our experiences working with students and in school settings, the most important single intervention is to arrange for professional staff development that increases teachers' awareness of symptom interference and accommodations. Including experiential activities and quotes from students will enhance the effectiveness of training and promote empathy for the student. Although we have made significant progress in some countries and areas, there are still too many areas where TS is neither recognized nor understood. Thus, Wei (2011), describing the situation in Taiwan, writes:

> *"Only recently has the disorder gained national attention, in part because a middle school student with Tourette syndrome was accused of cheating because he repeatedly shook his head and made disruptive noises while taking the National High School Entrance Examination; the student was unfairly given a score of 'zero.' Still, the public has little understanding of the disorder."*

Academic failure, such as that experienced by "M," whom we described at the beginning of this chapter, or the student who was failed because his teachers did not understand TS, can increase the risk of suicide by a factor of five, even after controlling for self-esteem, locus of control, and depressive symptoms (Richardson et al., 2005).

We can do better and we must do better.

SOCIAL ISSUES IN STUDENTS WITH TS+

"The school is not quite deserted," said the Ghost. "A solitary child, neglected by his friends, is left there still." (Charles Dickens, 1843)

Tics, TS, and Peer Problems

Tics have been associated with significantly increased rates of peer harassment, bullying, and rejection (Conelea et al., 2011; Packer, 2005; Storch et al., 2007; Wei, 2011). Students with TS are more likely to withdraw from their peers, who may view students with tics as being less socially acceptable. As a consequence, students with TS report poorer perceived quality of life (Eddy et al., 2011). Even what school personnel may consider "mild" cases of tics may have significant social and emotional consequences (Bernard et al., 2009) that persist even when tics remit or wane (Packer, 2005).

For students experiencing peer harassment or rejection due to their tics, a peer awareness program may help. In conducting peer education programs, it is helpful to include what Pruitt calls a "Bully Blaster" comment, something like, "I am so glad that you are all fifth graders because you are too mature to tease students with tics like some first graders do." The few available studies on peer education report that such programs may lead to improvement in peers' stated *attitudes* toward students with tics (Holtz & Tessman, 2007; Woods et al., 2003), but the improved intentions may not translate into improved peer relationships without additional supports (Woods & Marcks, 2005). In some cases, using a "Circle of Friends" technique (a community-based inclusion program) may be of benefit, although there is no research on this approach as applied to students with TS (Dykens et al., 1999). Pairing the student with a supportive peer for academic activities may also promote greater social acceptance.

Before conducting a peer education program in which a student is identified, school personnel need to secure parental and student consent. Some students feel empowered by having an opportunity to explain TS to their peers, while others will not want to be identified or to participate. There is some research on adults that suggests that self-disclosure may be helpful (Marcks et al., 2007), and while there is no guarantee that students will not be teased if they self-disclose, our experience has been that students' tics decrease once they are no longer under self-imposed stress to hide their tics or keep them a secret.

Impact of Associated Disorders on Peer Relationships

Just as associated disorders contribute significantly to academic problems, they also contribute significantly to peer and social problems. ADHD is a significant contributor to peer problems. Children with ADHD are categorized as victims, bullies, and bully/victims more often than their non-ADHD peers (Wiener & Mak, 2009); up to 80% are rejected by their peers or have no dyadic friendships (Erhardt & Hinshaw, 1994; Hoza, 2007). Students with the combined subtype of ADHD appear interfering, noncompliant, and aggressive and are actively rejected by their peers, while those with AHDH-I appear shy, anxious, and withdrawn and are neglected by their peers.

OCD, with its obsessions, often bizarre compulsions, and resulting inflexibility, may lead to victimization and peer problems (Piacentini et al., 2003; Storch et al., 2006). The student who *has to* have everything "just right" or gets "stuck," the student who is overly sensitive to mistakes and criticism, and the student who feels morally obligated to point out others' failings is less popular with peers.

Mood disorders such as dysthymia, depression, and bipolar disorder also have a significant impact on peer and social relationships. Students experiencing a loss of enjoyment or energy may withdraw from their peers, while students who are in the throes of a manic episode may be irritable, grandiose, paranoid, or aggressive. Even when not in an obvious mood episode, a subset of students with bipolar disorder have difficulty reading facial emotions accurately and will miss important nonverbal cues in their interactions with peers (Schenkel et al., 2007).

As with academic impairment, EDF is one of the most socially influential disorders. It may be helpful to think about the child with EDF as being socially "clueless" (Pruitt, 1995, in Dornbush & Pruitt, 2009), where the "clues" are missing pieces of information or skills that need to be directly taught or provided. Deficits in problem solving, setting realistic goals, time management, prioritizing, organizing, sequencing, flexibility, initiating, executing, self-monitoring, using feedback appropriately, and inhibiting may all impair the child or teen's ability to be socially successful.

Students who have working memory deficits will be impaired socially due to difficulty following social directions, forgetting what they want to say while speaking, difficulty holding on to complex social situations, and difficulty keeping important information in mind long enough to record it for the future. Imagine the challenges a teenager with working memory deficits faces if he receives an oral invitation and cannot record it immediately. If he is told, "We're going to meet at Northcrest Mall, at 7 p.m., in front of the movie theater on the south side of the mall, and then go for pizza with Dan, Darin, Jory, and Julianna," the odds are he will not be in the right place at the right time.

Processing deficits or delays also may impair the ability of the student with TS+ to socialize. The normal give-and-take of conversations requires rapid processing and rapid ability to generate responses as well as the ability to sift through complex social information such as multiple directions.

As suggested by the preceding discussion, there are numerous possible sources of negative social impact for students with TS+, and the more diagnoses or comorbid conditions they have, the greater their challenges and the greater the need for the school's support.

Remediating Social Skills Deficits

A social skills deficit not only impairs current interactions but also increases the risk of substance abuse, depression, atypical friendships, delinquency, school failure, and school dropout (Barkley, 2006). Impaired social skills may also limit the student's future ability to obtain a job, make and keep friends, and form a lasting relationship with a spouse. It is not just students with ASD who need social skills curricula; students with TS+ who do not have ASD may require direct instruction in social skills, especially if they have EDF. Although a description of such a curriculum is beyond the scope of this chapter, information and resources for a social skills curriculum are detailed in Dornbush and Pruitt (2009).

In the remainder of this section, we describe some simple school-based coaching interventions that school personnel can employ. Just as a sports coach tells an athlete what to do at the point of performance, so, too, can school personnel provide point-of-performance direct instruction in how to be socially successful. As students gain skills or can participate in analyzing their own behavior and interactions, the approach shifts to an interactive and cooperative problem-solving technique, also described below. Discussion of these techniques can be found in Packer and Pruitt (2010).

Instant Replay is a technique used to review and correct a past social blunder right before the student is in the same type of situation again. In a calm voice, the teacher privately tells the student the impact of his or her previous behavior on peers and provides concrete directions as to what to do this time instead. The student then immediately tries to implement the coach's directions and comes back to evaluate its success. If the student forgets to report back, the teacher initiates the follow-up. As an example:

Justin and his best friend Loren were chatting amiably over lunch until Loren asked Justin if she could have one of his cookies and Justin refused. The teacher, observing Loren's hurt and angry expression, walked over and told Justin she needed his help. Outside of the cafeteria, the teacher neutrally told Justin that Loren had felt hurt by his response, and reminded him how Loren had shared her desserts with him in the past. The teacher suggested Justin go back and offer Loren his remaining cookie with a cheery, "Friends share!" Justin followed the suggestion and reported back that Loren was smiling and happy with him.

Coached behaviors will not automatically generalize, and rehearsal and repetition across settings is required—for example, Justin may need to be coached how to share crayons during tasks, how to share equipment on the playground, etc. Instant Replay can also be used to spontaneously reinforce appropriate social skills by pointing out what the student just did, how it positively affected his or her peers, and how the peers reacted positively to the student's behavior.

Cooperative Problem Solving (P.L.A.N.) can be used for students who have the potential to think about their own problems and generate possible solutions. For many students, recognizing a problem or defining it is a major hurdle. An adult may need to initiate the process by identifying the problem for the student and asking the student to consider how to solve it. The mnemonic "P.L.A.N." (Pruitt & Pruitt, 2001, in Packer & Pruitt, 2010) can remind the student of the steps: **P**roblem defined, **L**ist options, **A**ct on one, **N**ow evaluate. As one example:

When Michael dropped his papers in front of his peers, he felt embarrassed. His friend David offered to help pick them up, but Michael yelled, "Get away — I can do it myself!" David walked away, and instead of sitting with Michael at lunch, he joined others. Michael was confused and did not understand why David was ignoring him. He asked his teacher what happened. The teacher explained that David had felt hurt by what Michael had said, and she asked Michael what he might do to repair the relationship. Michael generated a few ideas: he could give David time to cool off, he could try apologizing, or he could try apologizing and offering to let David play with a new toy that he knew David wanted to try. Michael decided to implement the third option, and he came back to the teacher afterwards to let her know

that his "P.L.A.N." had worked well and the boys had played together at recess.

In the P.L.A.N. approach, it is important to encourage the student to generate the possible solutions; the teacher should refrain from offering suggestions unless the student cannot come up with any ideas and requests a suggestion. That said, school personnel may help the student by asking questions that point out possible problems with the plan.

One technique to help students avoid embarrassment is to use a "Graceful Exit" system (Pruitt, 1995, in Dornbush & Pruitt, 1995). Students are given their own pass to keep with them. The pass is used when they feel that staying in the classroom might lead to negative peer reactions—for instance, if they are having a bout of tics or an anxiety attack, are "stuck," or are about to have a meltdown. The pass allows the student to go to an agreed-upon location to calm down, to take a brief walk, or to go discharge tics without having to first ask the teacher for permission to leave the room. The plan may also include the teacher using previously agreed-upon cues to alert the student to leave. Graceful exits are not always as graceful as one would hope. Even if the student appears to grumble or mutter while leaving the room in response to the teacher's signal, the teacher should consider it a success and reinforce the student for leaving. Learning to extricate themselves from situations before they embarrass themselves is an important life skill that students will need to help them keep jobs and maintain family relationships. When students do not know how or when to remove themselves, direct instruction is crucial.

Reparations is one of the most effective tools for teaching students how to take responsibility for the impact of their behavior on others and how to clean up after they have made a social blunder or hurt others' feelings. In the P.L.A.N. example above, Michael not only apologized to David, but he went further to try to help reestablish their friendship by inviting him to play with his new toy. Using P.L.A.N. with a reparation approach, Michael restored the damaged relationship and learned that sometimes strained relationships can be repaired.

THE "UP" SIDE OF TS: ENHANCED CREATIVITY

Having described some of the challenges students with TS or TS+ may encounter in school, we would be remiss if we did not explore some of the advantages TS or TS+ may confer.

Anecdotally, clinicians have often noted the extraordinary creativity exhibited by some individuals with TS and TS+ (c.f., Sacks, 1992). Recent research by Zanaboni and Porta provides preliminary confirmation that children and adolescents with TS and TS+ are more likely than their peers to demonstrate heightened creativity. Using samples of children in both Italy and the United States, and employing measures of divergent thinking, Zanaboni and Porta found that children with TS score significantly higher than control children on measures of flexibility and fluidity (Zanaboni, 2011). Enhanced fluidity and flexibility enable the student to rapidly process numerous alternative ideas and to quickly generate a large number of valid responses.

Combined with the flexibility to quickly adjust to new information or circumstances, a subset of students with TS will be extraordinarily creative thinkers and problem-solvers. School personnel can capitalize on these strengths and assist students in using their problem-solving skills to address challenges they may face academically and socially. That said, we would remind teachers that many students with TS are not able to adjust quickly to new circumstances due to comorbid disorders such as OCD. They may still be extraordinarily creative, but unable to adjust quickly.

Although Zanaboni and Porta's findings are exciting and articulate nicely with reports of differences in neural network connections that may be associated with divergent thinking (Church et al., 2009), not all available research has supported claims of increased creativity. Using different measures, Wei (2011) found no evidence of enhanced creativity and in fact some evidence of decreased creativity on a measure of picture elaboration. Wei's findings may be confounded,

---

Box 29.1. Key Points

- Students with tics or TS face numerous academic, behavioral, and social challenges, some of which are summarized in Table 29.2.

Table 29.2 Summary Table of Key Points

	Impact of TS+	Strategies
Academic	Focus and memory issues	Provide staff development.
	LD in written expression and math calculations	Screen for learning disabilities
		Chunk tasks and monitor progress
	Handwriting issues	Decrease handwriting demands
	Decreased productivity	Provide copies of lecture notes
	Inability to complete work in a timely fashion	Screen for assistive technology
		Extend time
	Organizational deficits	Use testing accommodations
	Homework issues	Teach executive function skills
		Reduce and modify homework

(Continued)

Box 29.1. (*Continued*)

	Impact of TS+	Strategies
Behavioral Symptoms	Dysregulated behavior Irritable or aggressive "Storms" or "rage attacks"	Conduct functional behavioral assessment Use "Graceful Exit" system Teach reparations
Social Relations	Peer rejection or bullying Cannot keep up with social pace Social skills deficits Lonely, depressed	Educate peers Coach and use "Instant Replay" Teach problem-solving (P.L.A.N.) Provide social skills curriculum Community peer support

- Most of the impairment appears due to associated disorders rather than tics. Comprehensive psychoeducational and functional behavioral assessments enable the school team to develop appropriate accommodations and interventions.
- Providing a supportive environment, nurturing the child's strengths and talents, and providing resources and support for the parents in service of the child can help the student overcome challenges and have a successful school year.

Box 29.2. Questions for Future Research

- Research evaluating the efficacy of accommodations and interventions is sorely needed; this is an area ripe for investigation. Some important questions to address include the following.
- What are the elements of an effective peer education program on TS for elementary school students? Studies including behavioral measures of peer acceptance are needed because stated intentions do not always translate into actual changes in behavior.
- To what extent does the use of assistive technology increase productivity in students with tics or TS?
- What is the impact of allowing extended time for students with OCD-related writing rituals? Does it foster greater work completion, does it unintentionally reinforce unwanted compulsive behavior, or both?
- Does direct instruction in executive function skills such as planning and "chunking" a big project improve academic productivity and timely completion of tasks?
- Does providing students with hard copies of all board work and lecture notes improve test performance in high school students with handwriting impairment due to TS?

however, by the potential impact of grapho-motor deficits that do not appear to have been assessed nor controlled for. Because so many children and adolescents with TS have significant graphomotor problems and are reluctant to write by hand, paper-and-pencil measures may significantly underestimate their creativity. An anecdote from our experience may illustrate why schools may need to provide accommodations in their screening for gifted and talented programs:

An intellectually gifted student with TS+ scored poorly on a creative uses test used to determine admission to his school's gifted program. The standard administration of the task had required him to write down the uses he could generate for the object but after listing two uses, his hand cramped and he simply stopped writing. When he was denied admission to the gifted program, his surprised parents requested that the school reassess him and provide accommodations that would allow him to respond orally. When retested with appropriate accommodations, he quickly generated a long list of uses. He was admitted to the district's gifted program, where he quickly rewarded their decision by earning first place in a regional competition to create an eco-friendly power generation system.

REFERENCES

Adams GB. *Students with OCD: a handbook for school personnel*. Campton Hills: Pherson Creek Press, 2011.

Barkley RA. *Attention deficit hyperactivity disorder: a handbook for diagnosis and treatment* (3rd ed.). New York: Guilford Press, 2006.

Bernard BA, Stebbins GT, Siegel S et al. Determinants of quality of life in children with Gilles de la Tourette syndrome. *Mov Disord* 2009; 24:1070–1073.

Brookshire BL, Butler IJ, Ewing-Cobbs L, Fletcher JM. Neuropsychological characteristics of children with Tourette syndrome: evidence for a nonverbal learning disability? *J Clin Exp Neuropsychol* 1994; 16:289–302.

Budman CL, Bruun RD, Park KS, Olson ME. Rage attacks in children and adolescents with Tourette's disorder: a pilot study. *J Clin Psychiatry* 1998; 59:576–580.

Burd L, Kauffman DW, Kerbeshian J. Tourette syndrome and learning disabilities. *J Learn Disabil* 1992; 25:598–604.

Burd L, Freeman RD, Klug MG, Kerbeshian J. Tourette syndrome and learning disabilities. *BMC Pediatrics* 2005; 5:34.

Controlled comparison of learning disabilities in TS with or without ADHD derived from an international database.

Chang SW, McCracken JT, Piacentini JC. Neurocognitive correlates of child obsessive compulsive disorder and Tourette syndrome. *J Clin Exp Neuropsychol* 2007; 29: 724–733.

Church JA, Fair DA, Dosenbach NU et al. Control networks in paediatric Tourette syndrome show immature and anomalous patterns of functional connectivity. *Brain* 2009; 132:225–238.

Cohen E, Sade M, Benarroch F et al. Locus of control, perceived parenting style, and symptoms of anxiety and depression in children with Tourette's syndrome. *Eur Child Adolesc Psychiatry* 2008; 17:299–305.

Comings DE, Comings BG. A controlled study of Tourette syndrome. I. Attention-deficit disorder, learning disorders, and school problems. *Am J Hum Genet* 1987; 41:701–741.

The first of a series of reports by the investigators on school-related difficulties and comorbidity in students with TS.

Conelea CA, Woods DW. The influence of contextual factors on tic expression in Tourette's syndrome: a review. *J Psychosom Res* 2008a; 65:487–496.

An extensive review of research on environmental factors that affect tic frequency and severity.

Conelea CA, Woods DW. Examining the impact of distraction on tic suppression in children and adolescents with Tourette syndrome. *Behav Res Ther* 2008b; 46:1193–1200.

Conelea CA, Woods DW, Zinner SH et al. Exploring the impact of chronic tic disorders on youth: results from the Tourette Syndrome Impact Survey. *Child Psychiatry Hum Dev* 2011; 42:219–242.

Cubo E, Trejo Gabriel Y Galn JM, Villaverde VA et al. Prevalence of tics in schoolchildren in central Spain: a population-based study. *Pediatr Neurol* 2011; 45:100–108.

De Nil LF, Sasisekaran J, Van Lieshout PH, Sandor P. Speech disfluencies in individuals with Tourette syndrome. *J Psychosom Res* 2005; 58:97–102.

Dickens C. *A Christmas Carol.* London: Chapman and Hall, 1843.

Dornbush MP, Pruitt SK. *Teaching the Tiger: A handbook for individuals involved in the education of students with attention deficit disorders, Tourette syndrome or obsessive-compulsive disorder.* Duarte: Hope Press, 1995.

Dornbush MP, Pruitt SK. *Tigers, too: executive functions/speed of processing/memory—Impact on academic, behavioral, and social functioning of students with ADHD, Tourette syndrome, and OCD: Modifications and interventions.* Marietta: Parkaire Press, 2009.

Doyle AE, Wilens TE, Kwon A et al. Neuropsychological functioning in youth with bipolar disorder. *Biol Psychiatry* 2005; 58:540–548.

Du JC, Chiu TF, Lee KM et al. Tourette syndrome in children: an updated review. *Pediatr Neonatol* 2010; 51:255–264.

Dykens EM, Sparrow SS, Cohen DJ et al. Peer acceptance and adaptive functioning. In Leckman JF, Cohen DJ (Eds.), *Tourette's syndrome—tics, obsessions, compulsions: Developmental psychopathology and clinical care* (pp. 104–117). Hoboken, NJ: John Wiley & Sons Inc., 1999.

Eddy CM, Rizzo R, Gulisano M et al. Quality of life in young people with Tourette syndrome: a controlled study. *J Neurol* 2011; 258:291–301.

Erhardt D, Hinshaw SP. Initial sociometric impressions of attention-deficit hyperactivity disorder and comparison boys: Predictions from social behaviors and from nonbehavioral variables. *J Consult Clin Psychol* 1994; 62:833–842.

Evans SW, Langberg J, Raggi V et al. Development of a school-based treatment program for middle school youth with ADHD. *J Atten Disord* 2005; 9:343–353.

Ginott HG. *Teacher and child: a book for parents and teachers.* New York: Macmillan, 1975.

Gioia GA, Isquith PK, Guy SC, Kenworthy L. *Behavior Rating Inventory of Executive Function* Lutz, FL: Psychological Assessment Resources, Inc., 2000.

Greene RW. *The explosive child: a new approach for understanding and parenting easily frustrated, chronically inflexible children.* New York: Harper Collins, 1998.

Hagin RA, Beecher R, Pagano G, Kreeger H. *Final report to the Gatepost Foundation*, 1980.

Hagin RA, Kugler J. School problems associated with Tourette's syndrome. In Cohen DJ, Bruun RD, Leckman JF (Eds.), *Tourette's syndrome and tic disorders: Clinical understanding and treatment* (pp. 223–236). Oxford: John Wiley & Sons, 1988.

Holtz KD, Tessman GK. Evaluation of a peer-focused intervention to increase knowledge and foster positive attitudes toward children with Tourette syndrome. *J Dev Phys Disabil* 2007; 19:531–542.

Hoza B. Peer functioning in children with ADHD. *Ambul Pediatr* 2007; 7:101–106.

Huckeba W, Chapiesk IL, Hiscock M, Glaze D. Arithmetic performance in children with Tourette syndrome: relative contribution of cognitive and attentional factors. *J Clin Exp Neuropsychol* 2008; 30:410–420.

Khalifa N, Dalan M, Rydell A. Tourette syndrome in the general child population: Cognitive functioning and self-perception. *Nord J Psychiatry* 2010; 64:11–18.

Killu K, Crundwell RMA. Understanding and developing academic and behavioral interventions for students with bipolar disorder. *Intervention in School and Clinic* 2008; 43: 244–251.

Klimkeit EI, Tonge B, Bradshaw JL et al. Neuropsychological deficits in adolescent unipolar depression. *Arch Clin Neuropsychol* 2011; 26:662–676.

Kofler MJ, Rapport MD, Bolden J et al. ADHD and working memory: the impact of central executive deficits and exceeding storage/rehearsal capacity on observed inattentive behavior. *J Abnorm Child Psychol* 2010; 38:149–161.

Kofler MJ, Rapport MD, Bolden J et al. Working memory deficits and social problems in children with ADHD. *J Abnorm Child Psychol* 2011; 39 805–817.

Kurlan R, McDermott MP, Deeley C et al. Prevalence of tics in schoolchildren and association with placement in special education. *Neurology* 2001; 57:1383–1388. **School-based study that compared the rates of tics and TS in regular education and special education settings.**

Langberg J, Epstein J, Altaye M et al. The transition to middle school is associated with changes in the developmental trajectory of ADHD symptomatology in young adolescents with ADHD. *J Clin Child Adolesc Psychol* 2008; 37: 651–663.

Langberg J, Epstein J, Graham A. Organizational-skills interventions in the treatment of ADHD. *Expert Rev Neurother* 2008; 8:1549–1561.

Langberg JM, Arnold LE, Flowers AM et al. Parent-reported homework problems in the MTA study: evidence for sustained improvement with behavioral treatment. *J Clin Child Adolesc Psychol* 2010; 39:220–233.
A seminal report indicating that homework issues related to executive dysfunction can be remediated.

Leckman JF, Bloch MH, Scahill L, King RA. Tourette syndrome: the self under siege. *J Child Neurol* 2006; 21:642–649.

Lundy SM, Silva GE, Kaemingk KL et al. Cognitive functioning and academic performance in elementary school children with anxious/depressed and withdrawn symptoms. *Open Pediatr Med J* 2010; 14:1–9.

Marcks B, Berlin K, Woods D, Davies W. Impact of Tourette syndrome: a preliminary investigation of the effects of disclosure on peer perceptions and social functioning. *Psychiatry* 2007; 70:59–67.

Marsh R, Alexander GM, Packard MG et al. Habit learning in Tourette syndrome: a translational neuroscience approach to a developmental psychopathology. *Arch Gen Psychiatry* 2004; 61:1259–1268.

Martinussen R, Hayden J, Hoog-Johnson S, Tannock R. A meta-analysis of working memory impairments in children with attention-deficit/hyperactivity disorder. *J Am Acad Child Adolesc Psychiatry* 2005; 44:377–384.

Packer LE. Social and educational resources for patients with Tourette syndrome. *Neurol Clin* 1997; 15:457–473.

Packer LE. *Educating children with Tourette syndrome: Understanding and educating children with a neurobiological disorder. I: Psychoeducational implications of Tourette syndrome and its associated disorders.* New York State Education Dept., Albany, NY, 1995.

Packer LE. Tic-related school problems: impact on functioning, accommodations, and interventions. *Behav Modif* 2005; 2:876–899.

Packer LE. *Find a way or make a way: checklists of helpful accommodations for students with attention-deficit hyperactivity disorder, executive dysfunction, mood disorders, Tourette's syndrome, obsessive-compulsive disorder, and other neurological challenges.* Marietta: Parkaire Press, 2009.

Packer LE, Gentile M. Tourette's syndrome: A maze of pathologies for unsuspecting OTs. *ADVANCE for Occupational Therapists* 1994; 10:16.

Packer LE, Pruitt SK. *Challenging kids, challenged teachers: teaching students with Tourette's, bipolar disorder, executive dysfunction, OCD, ADHD, and more.* Bethesda, MD: Woodbine House, 2010.

Piacentini J, Bergman RL, Keller M, McCracken J. Functional impairment in children and adolescents with obsessive-compulsive disorder. *J Child Adolesc Psychopharmacol* 2003; 13 Suppl 1:S61–S69.

Richardson AS, Bergen HA, Martin G et al. Perceived academic performance as an indicator of risk of attempted suicide in young adolescents. *Arch Suicide Res* 2005; 9:163–176.

Sacks O. Tourette's syndrome and creativity. *BMJ* 1992; 305:1515–1516.

Schenkel LS, Pavuluri MN, Herbener ES et al. Facial emotion processing in acutely ill and euthymic patients with pediatric bipolar disorder. *J Am Acad Child Adolesc Psychiatry* 2007; 46:1070–1079.

Schuerholz LJ, Baumgardner TL, Singer HS et al. Neuropsychological status of children with Tourette's syndrome with and without attention deficit hyperactivity disorder. *Neurology* 1996; 46:958–965.

Silva RR, Munoz DM, Barickman J, Friedhoff AJ. Environmental factors and related fluctuation of symptoms in children and adolescents with Tourette's disorder. *J Child Psychol Psychiatry* 1995; 36:305–312.

Silver AA, Hagin RA. *Disorders of learning in childhood.* New York: John Wiley & Sons, Inc, 1990.

Spencer T, Biederman J, Coffey B et al. Tourette disorder and ADHD. *Adv Neurol* 2001; 85: 57–77.

Storch EA, Ledley DR, Lewin AB et al. Peer victimization in children with obsessive-compulsive disorder: relations with symptoms of psychopathology. *J Clin Child Adolesc Psychol* 2006; 35:446–455.

Storch EA, Murphy TK, Chase RM et al. Peer victimization in youth with Tourette's syndrome and chronic tic disorder: relations with tic severity and internalizing symptoms. *J Psychopathol Behav Assess* 2007; 29:211–219.

Wei MH. Social adjustment, academic performance, and creativity of Taiwanese children with
Tourette's syndrome. *Psychol Rep* 2011;
108:1–8.

Weiler MD, Bernstein JH, Bellinger DC, Waber DP.
Processing speed in children with
attention deficit/hyperactivity disorder,
inattentive type. *Child Neuropsychol* 2000;
6:218–234.

Wiener J, Mak M. Peer victimization in children
with attention-deficit/hyperactivity disorder.
Psychology in the Schools 2009; *46*:116–131.

Woods DW, Koch M, Miltenberger RG. The impact
of tic severity on the effects of peer education

about Tourette's syndrome. *J Dev Phys Disabil*
2003; *15*:67–78.

Woods DW, Marcks BA. Controlled evaluation
of an educational intervention used to modify
peer attitudes and behavior toward persons
with Tourette's syndrome. *Behav Modif* 2005;
29:900–912.

Woods DW, Watson TS, Wolfe E et al.
Analyzing the influence of tic-related talk
on vocal and motor tics in children with
Tourette's syndrome. *J Appl Behav Anal* 2001;
34:353–356.

Zanaboni C. Does Tourette syndrome have a link to
creativity? *In the Loop* 2011; *9*:13–15.

30

Tourette Syndrome Support Organizations Around the World

LOUISE ROPER, PETER J. HOLLENBECK AND HUGH E. RICKARDS

Abstract

This chapter presents and discusses the results of a survey that collected extensive information on patient advocacy and support groups for Tourette syndrome (TS) worldwide. TS associations and support groups are in different stages of development in different countries, probably as a result of different self-help/advocacy cultural approaches. Funding derives from different sources, including the government. Only a few organizations are involved in political and scientific agenda setting (e.g., in directing and funding research, providing guidelines, and lobbying governments). Current austerity measures due to the worldwide financial crisis are likely to affect the future activities of patient support groups, which may need to adapt their operational strategies.

INTRODUCTION

Patient advocacy and support is a modern phenomenon. It has gained ground in developed countries in the past 30 years, supported by a variety of social factors, including the dominance of consumerist and self-help models, challenges to "medical narratives," and the rise of IT-based social networking. Groups have often been started by highly motivated individuals with personal experience of an illness, either themselves or through their family. Most groups have grown and gone through the often-painful process of professionalization. The aim of this chapter is to describe the current state of Tourette syndrome (TS) support groups throughout the world and to document the history of their development. To this aim, we conducted a survey to gather relevant information from TS support groups around the globe.

SURVEY

We attempted to contact the lead members of all the TS associations throughout Europe, in North America, and in a number of other Western countries. For a complete list of countries contacted, see Figure 30.1 and Appendix 1. Having established a primary contact within each association, we sent a list of questions, covering features such as the number of members, funding, services, involvement with government and public policy, and participation in research and its evaluation (see Appendix 2). Having received the answers from the groups, we collated the information. If a country had more than one association, we analyzed the information from each separately.

We received full information on Tourette syndrome associations (TSA) from 12 (41%) of the 29 countries addressed in the survey (Fig. 30.2). Of these 29 countries, only 4 did not have a TSA, while 2 countries (Germany and Australia) had more than 1 association.

In all of the associations we interviewed, membership entitled patients, as well as their friends, family, and caregivers, to access the help and services the group provides. Almost all organizations had a website and a phone and e-mail helpline, with the only exceptions being

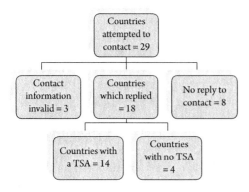

FIGURE 30.1   Summary of the TSAs contacted around the world as part of the survey. Details on the participation rate to the survey are provided.

TSAs from the Czech Republic and Denmark. Many of the associations produced their own newsletters for their members and were also involved, to varying degrees, in educating the public about TS. A number of the TSAs in Europe receive the bulk of their funding from their governments. Like most organizations in this line of work, all the groups we consulted relied on volunteers to form the majority of their staff. Some of the groups had regular, active roles in influencing public policy, but few groups carried out or formally evaluated research. TSAs from two countries (Belgium and Australia) require all their staff to be either personally affected by TS or have a close family member who is affected.

DETAILS FROM INDIVIDUAL COUNTRIES

Australia

The Tourette Syndrome Association of Victoria (TSAV) was established in 1990. The organization is run by nine volunteers, including one medical doctor (the group's medical adviser), a president, and a treasurer. There is no board of trustees. All of the volunteers either have TS themselves or have a family member with the condition. TSAV serves the Australian state of Victoria, covering about one third of New South Wales, in the southeastern corner of the continent. With a membership of 87, TSAV provides a phone line and offers an e-mail helpline and a website (www.tsavic.org.au). TSAV endeavors to enhance the profile of TS by holding an annual "Awareness Week," as well as via its website and by attending public meetings.

TSAV is a small organization, with no full-time, salaried staff; patients and staff combined number less than 100. Due to its small size, it cannot take on their own research, formally evaluate the research of others, or influence policymaking. However, it has established strong links with much larger associations, particularly in the United Kingdom and North America. This allows them to share the information and experiences of much larger organizations.

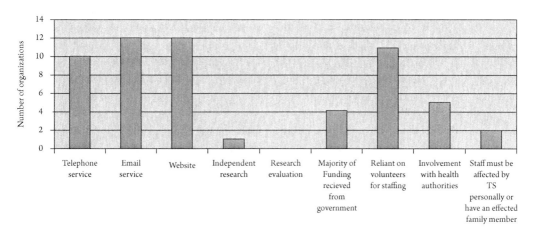

FIGURE 30.2   General features on the services provided and the organization of the TSAs around the world.

TSAV relies on government grants to finance most of its work. Some money is also collected in membership fees and from small private donations.

Belgium

The Tourette Association Belgium (TAB) was established at the end of 1994. Although there are just six staff members, all volunteers, there are over 1,600 members. This is quite a considerable number in light of the fact that TAB covers only the Flemish part of Belgium. TAB has one trustee, a permanent telephone manager, and an editor for its regular news magazine. A board of four doctors gives medical advice to TAB.

TAB receives no money from the government and raises its annual income of 8,000 Euros from its members, from both membership fees and gifts.

TAB allocates most of its resources to raising awareness of TS. It regularly gets involved in TV documentaries and even has its own visual media, through which it recently produced a DVD entitled *I'm a Regular Kid*. TAB also encourages student interest in TS by helping students to write papers on the subject.

TAB campaigns reach both professionals and the wider community by means of posters and leaflets that are published and distributed to doctors' offices, schools, and community areas. TAB runs regular symposia for professionals, to which doctors and teachers are invited. TAB uses this as a way to influence the diagnosis and management of TS patients. TAB also aims to influence politicians and is currently lobbying for facilities and support for TS children in schools.

For the members and their families, TAB provides a phone line, which is constantly staffed, and an e-mail helpline that is answered every day. The group has a Facebook page. Informal "adventure weekends" are currently held for TAB members.

To work for the association, a person must either have TS himself or herself or have a first-degree relative with the condition. At present, all members of staff are parents of children with by TS.

TAB maintains strong links with other TSAs around the world. It regularly exchanges newsletters with Canadian and American groups and has a close bond with the association in the Netherlands, to whose meetings they often send delegates.

Canada

The Tourette Syndrome Foundation of Canada/ La Fondation Canadienne du syndrome de la Tourette (TSFC; www.tourette.ca) was founded in 1976 by two fathers of patients with TS who had faced a dearth of information and support. This national voluntary organization's mission is to "improve the quality of life for those with or affected by Tourette syndrome through programs of education, advocacy, self-help and the promotion of research." The national office, located in Mississauga, Ontario, is operated by an executive director and a small staff. TSFC has a dedicated board of directors comprising individuals from across the country and a volunteer professional advisory board comprising researchers and clinicians. The TSFC has always collaborated broadly with other patient and family foundations and was a charter member of the Neurological Health Charities Canada (NHCC; www.mybrainmatters.ca).

From the modest newsletter of the mid-1970s to the comprehensive website it manages today, TSFC has been providing information and services to Canadian families affected by TS for 35 years. The national organization and its local affiliates organize and connect families to support groups, sponsor workshops and discussion forums, provide in-service presentations, and put on an annual national conference. The national office provides a toll-free line for information and referral, and its website provides families, educators, and clinicians with news, information, access to publications and seminars, connections to support groups, and information for advocacy. TSFC has also supported a variety of research programs over the years, particularly in TS genetics.

The national office also acts as a liaison to local affiliates across Canada. These are functionally categorized into provincial and regional chapters, and the less formally organized resource units and contact representatives (http://www.tourette.ca/connect-chaptersaffiliates.php). These legally affiliated local groups carry out the TSFC's mission in a less structured but more immediate manner. They provide first contact and support for families and newly diagnosed patients, publish local newsletters, and sponsor special programs and events.

Czech Republic

The Tourette Association in Czech Republic (ATOS) was established in 2001. The group consists of doctors, a psychologist, and volunteers. ATOS provides services for the whole of the Czech Republic, as well as for part of the Slovak Republic, via its website (www.atos-os.cz) and e-mail help service, but at present does not have a phone line. These services are staffed by the doctors and the psychologist working in the team, as well as by additional volunteers. The main objective of ATOS is to raise awareness of TS, and it achieves this by frequently participating in television documentaries, radio programs, and any other media opportunities as they arise. ATOS receives most of its financial aid from private companies or, in the case of specific projects, from grants.

ATOS does not conduct or evaluate research, either in a formal or informal capacity. However, it is involved in developing public policy and in designing diagnostic and treatment guidelines for professionals in the Czech Republic.

Denmark

Dansk Tourette Forening (DTF), the TSA in Denmark, helps approximately 730 TS patients around the country, with an overall membership of about 1,300. For its members DTF offers support via three websites (main one: www.tourette.dk), an e-mail queries service, and, informally, a phone service. DTF endeavors to raise awareness of TS by participating in conferences, running workshops, and publishing a newsletter twice a year.

The group was founded in 1984 by a group of patients and parents and is now a small but well-established organization. Their 10 staff members are all volunteers, and two doctors are associated with their work. The board has seven members. Like a number of European TSAs, DTF receives over half its annual income from the country's government, amounting to 27,000 Euros per annum.

DTF does not initiate its own research, nor does it evaluate the scientific findings of others. It has a few contacts with other European countries.

Germany

Tourette Gesellschaft Deutschland (TGD e.V), the older of the two principal TSAs in Germany, was founded in 1993. Today the society has approximately 800 members. The group is run by a board of three volunteers. In addition, it employs two part-time office staff and two technicians, who are responsible for the website (www.tourette-gesellschaft.de). TGD e.V has a board of scientific advisors made up of TS specialists. TGD e.V provides a list of recommended specialists. A number of TGD e.V's workers have TS themselves.

TGD e.V acts in the capacity of an umbrella organization, supporting 17 smaller, independent, regional self-help groups, set up across the 16 German states. They describe themselves as providing "help for self-help." Fundraising is a large part of this support; money comes from subsidies from health insurance companies and donations. However, a generous amount also comes from their members' fees. For its members, TGD e.V provides a website, phone line, and an e-mail service, manned by the staff.

TGD e.V is committed to educating the public and professionals alike about TS. Their staffers frequently attend conferences, run training courses for teachers, and participate in media and fundraising events. However, the group's interaction with government, and hence their involvement with public policy, is limited and carried out on a purely case-by-case basis, despite their endeavors to increase this in recent years.

TGD e.V is active in funding research carried out by other centers, but the group does not conduct its own research studies, nor is it involved in officially evaluating any such work. To stay up to date with the European TS community, TGD e.V often web-links and exchanges information with associations in Switzerland and Poland and self-help groups in Austria. Further afield, it is seeking to establish relationships with that in Australia.

Interessenverband TS (IVTS e.V) is the younger TSA in Germany, founded in 2007. This group serves wide catchment area, comprising the territories of Germany, Austria, and parts of Switzerland, as required. However, despite its large geographical catchment area, IVTS e.V is a much smaller group than TGD e.V, with 50 TS patients and just over 100 family members. It has only one paid member of staff, who works 5 hours per week, and 10 volunteers. Additionally, eight doctors are associated with the group.

IVTS e.V has a website (www.iv-ts.de), telephone helpline, and e-mail service. However, due to the small number of staff, the group is not involved in determining public policy, conducting professional training, or performing or evaluating research. Thus, its main role in the TS community is to provide support to patients at the point of need and to raise awareness of the condition. It enhances its public image by participating in television documentaries and articles. IVTS e.V receives the majority of its annual income from health insurance funds as well, approximately 25,000 Euros in 2010. Currently, IVTS e.V has little European collaboration.

Italy

The Italian association (Associazione Italiana Sindrome di Tourette, AIST), established in 1991, provides support services to TS patients across all of Italy (www.tourette.it). Some of the staff members have TS. The group has an income of 10,000 to 20,000 Euros per year and maintains contacts with other TSAs around Europe.

The Netherlands

Netherlands Stichting Gilles de la Tourette Syndrome (NSGTS) was founded in 1981 by parents and patients, with the help of TS specialists. Currently, the group has an associate board, headed by a chairman. This group directs 30 members of staff. Besides these volunteers, NSGTS has an advisory board of doctors, including neurologists, child and adult psychiatrists, and behavioral therapists.

The group has approximately 1,000 members. These consist of "donors" (members, contributors to the organization's activities, and financial donors) and their family members (numbering approximately 600). The donors contribute around 35% of NSGTS's annual income of approximately 80,000 Euros. The government provides the remainder.

The services offered by NSGTS include a website (www.tourette.nl), with a question-and-answer discussion forum. It also provides phone and e-mail helplines, as well as educational media such as films and a newsletter. Furthermore, NSGTS has established smaller regional groups. The group also uses the media to increase the general population's understanding of TS, via articles in the press as well as events and lectures.

Norway

Norsk Tourette Forening (NTF) is one of the larger European TSAs, with 1,000 affected members and a further 300 family members. The group was founded 1984. NTF has 1 full-time staff member, 2 part-time members, and a board of 11 members. Three doctors volunteer to give medical advice. NTF does not keep a record of whether its staff members are affected by TS, but several of them are.

The majority of NTF's funding comes from the government. It also applies for grants each year from the local councils of the regions in which it operates. NTF uses this money to maintain a website (www.tourette-foreningen.no), phone line, and e-mail service. The group is also heavily involved in the education of schoolteachers and has written a leaflet of management guidelines to be used in schools. Upon request, NTF will liaise with family doctors about an individual's diagnosis.

Scotland

Tourette Scotland (http://www.tourettescotland.org) was set up in 1994. The association has 809 members and 514 caregiver contacts. The association employs two full-time and three part-time office staff. There are 35 volunteer support staff and 11 volunteer trustees. STSA is in contact with 115 hospitals and 326 health centers or general practices, and has a register of 129 consultants, with whom they correspond on matters regarding research and training. The medical advisory group is led by a consultant neurologist and neurological therapist nurse.

STSA is a constituted charitable organization with a board of 12 trustees and advisors. STSA covers all of Scotland, including the islands, running outreach support groups staffed by 15 "organisational support leaders" whose duties include house visits and review meetings. There are also local support groups in at least six regions across the country. STSA offers a regular training service to school staff, involving parents and adults with TS as co-trainers. As part of its education program, presentations are given regularly to a number of professional bodies, including health care professionals, employees of the criminal justice system, lobbyist societies, and conferences.

STSA runs both a helpline and an e-mail contact service, in addition to a counseling unit and regular respite adventure weekends. Over 75% of the group's volunteers have TS, as do a number of the committee members and paid staff. The group obtains all its money from a fundraising program. It often receives private sector grants and runs events such as backpacking or sponsored walks.

STSA aids medical, educational, and legal practitioners with projects and studies by providing statistics and qualitative information where possible from their data collection program. It also conducts its own, limited, studies. The Association endeavors to affect public policy via its involvement with a number of political parties across Scotland. Currently, the charity is involved in developing diagnostic criteria for TS by liaising with general practitioners and other health care professionals and campaigns

to broaden acceptance of treatment approaches within Scottish health services.

Switzerland

Tourette Romandie (TR) has only 88 members, including patients, family, and caregivers, suggesting that this organization is by far the smallest of those described here. This is surprising because the organization serves a considerable area: all of the French-speaking part of Switzerland (1.8 million inhabitants and 13,000 square kilometers).

TR has only four members of staff and one additional doctor. It was founded in 2004. The organization has a budget of 9,000 francs per year. Each member pays 20 francs per year as a subscription, and the rest of the group's income comes from private donations. TR has a website (www.tourette-romandie.ch), a phone line, and an e-mail service. The group also writes to schools via their health services and works with pediatricians. The group organizes conferences on medical subjects, and although it does not fund or carry out research, it prints out information leaflets for the general public. Two members of staff have TS and the other two are parents of TS patients.

United Kingdom

Tourette Action UK (TA UK), formerly known as Tourette Syndrome Association (UK), was founded in 1981. It has flourished as an organization and now has six members of staff, four of them full time, as well as a board of trustees. While there is only one official doctor on the team, many other doctors are involved informally. Also working as part of the team, TA UK has a chief executive, an events manager, a services manager, and groups and accounts managers.

TA UK covers all of the UK, including newly established groups in Northern Ireland and Wales. Scotland, however, has its own TSA, described above. TA UK does not routinely collect data on membership numbers, but in the past year TA UK collected just under 1,000 subscription fees. In the same time period, about

45,000 people contacted TA UK, either via the telephone helpline, by downloading information from the website (www.tourettesaction. org.uk), or by e-mail. TA UK provides support for TS patients and their families, friends, and caregivers. The helpline is staffed by non-health care professionals. TA UK also provides an e-mail contact, which in most cases is answered within 24 hours.

TA UK has three longstanding patrons. It receives no statutory funding and so relies entirely upon fundraising, grants, and donations. In the past year its annual income was £324,000, approximately £200,000 of which came from donations and a further £100,000 from grants. The source of these grants may be charitable organizations; however, often the families involved in TA UK will take it upon themselves to hold a fundraising or sponsored event, generating further income.

TA UK gives education and advice to school staff and educational services as well as to general practitioners and children and adolescent mental health teams. However, TA UK has no official training programs. Two members' conferences are held each year. The themes presented in these vary, from a summary of the latest research to a discussion of the efficacy of complementary therapies. TA UK runs a research network, the Tourette Action Research Network, which includes researchers, psychiatrists, doctors, and other health care professionals in the field. TA UK holds an annual Research Network conference, the aim of which is to share progress in research and new ideas. TA UK applies for grants to fund projects run by other specialist centers and act as a co-applicant for grants applied for by other centers. However, while taking a primary role in supporting the research of others, TA UK does not carry out research of its own.

TA UK analyzes and simplifies research papers for posting to the website in a format that the members can understand. This both allows the members to gain access to research that they otherwise would not and ensures that TA UK staff and members are kept abreast of any developments and changes in practice. However, TA UK has no official arm for evaluating evidence by academic standards.

An important part of the group's work involves interacting with members of Parliament to raise awareness of TS. In all such endeavors, TA UK recognizes the importance of remaining in touch with TS patients. Although TA UK does not have a specific quota to fill in terms of the number of employees with TS, a number of the staff are either directly affected by TS or have family members who are: three of the trustees have TS and three others have children with TS.

United States

The National Tourette Syndrome Association (TSA-US) is an American organization founded in 1972 by a small group of parents in New York. Its mission, then as now, is to "identify the cause, find the cure and control the effects of Tourette syndrome." Its paid membership, which stood around 6,000 in 2011, comprises individuals, families, and medical professionals. The organization is run by a professional staff located in New York and a volunteer board of directors. The latter comprises individuals from many walks of life whose lives have been touched by TS. Many of the original board members were parents of TS children; today a number are themselves successful adults with TS.

TSA-US assembled its first medical advisory board in 1974, and this group of clinicians and clinical scientists began by representing TSA-US at medical meetings. It has since evolved to provide national and international leadership in TS education, clinical best practices, and clinical research. TSA-US's commitment to advancing TS research was formalized in 1984 with the formation of its research fund, which has since distributed several million dollars in research grants to TS investigators in the United States and throughout the world. Scientific guidance is provided by a scientific advisory board, established in the late 1970s. This panel of basic and clinical researchers provides the organization with scientific and policy advice, helps the group organize collaborative research consortia, and performs peer review of the applications made by investigators annually for research funds. The strategic use of the group's research funds, its encouragement of young researchers, and its stimulation of the formation of multisite research collaborations have resulted in many researchers turning the pilot studies funded by TSA-US into major government-funded research efforts. Over the past 30 years TSA-US and its medical and scientific advisory boards have organized numerous scientific and medical conferences, including five international scientific symposia on TS, two young investigators forums, and many ad hoc meetings on specific topics such as clinical trials, neuroimmunology, and deep brain stimulation.

Through its national office and website (www.tsa-usa.org), TSA-US provides a variety of resources for TS patients and their families, doctors, and teachers. A quarterly newsletter contains articles about and by TSA-US members, Q&A columns by leading clinicians, layman's research updates, and other information. The TSA-US website provides a wealth of information, including basic medical facts, research news, access to seminars and advice from leading clinicians and researchers, problem solving for school and workplace issues, and social support for all ages. A key event for TSA-US members is the national conference, held each spring since 1978 near Washington DC. This event brings together members, newly diagnosed patients and families, successful TS adults, scientists, and doctors for several days of presentations, Q&A sessions, networking, and visits to members of the U.S. House of Representatives and Senate.

TSA-US carries out education and advocacy efforts across the United States. It sponsors education programs for medical and education professionals and public awareness campaigns to educate the public and counter harmful stereotypes about TS. It has been involved with the production of several popular documentary films about life with TS, including the Emmy Award-winning HBO film *I Have Tourette's But Tourette's Doesn't Have Me*. It also organizes visits by TSA-US members to Capitol Hill, where they meet with their representatives in Congress to discuss policy and legislation affecting those with TS. A notable success was TSA-US's role in getting TS included under the Individuals with Disabilities Education Act, the result of which was the provision of educational accommodations and support for TS schoolchildren. A significant part of the public information effort is carried out by Youth Ambassadors, people under 18 with TS who participate in TSA-US training workshops and go on to educate and advocate in their schools, communities, and state and national legislatures.

While the national organization was formed with the missions of research and advocacy, local chapters have evolved in response to the need for local help. The 33 currently incorporated chapters and approximately 125 local support groups of TSA-US are the first line of contact for many newly diagnosed patients and their families. With the knowledge and experience that chapter members have in their own region, they can serve to connect people with doctors and help solve problems in schools. Local chapters sponsor or coordinate support groups and organize local events, youth camps, and many other

---

Box 30.1. Key Points

Here is a summary of the TSA characteristics we found in our survey:

- Most TSAs have a telephone line, an e-mail account, and an active website.
- All organizations rely heavily on volunteers to provide the majority of their staff.
- Most European associations (excluding the UK) receive significant government funding.
- The size of the associations ranges from less than 100 members (Australia) to over 6,000 (United States).
- At present there is little collaboration between the European associations.

To decrease the stigma caused by the condition

- Community-based fundraisers
- School initiatives
- Leaflets, distributed around public forums such as doctors' waiting rooms

To inform public and professionals

- Training days for teachers run by parent volunteers
- Get professionals on board by contacting the doctors of the group's members
- Small-scale conferences for interested professionals
- Political lobbying

To facilitate research execution and dissemination

- Patient advisory boards to research groups
- Provision of data to research projects
- Layman's explanations of current research published in regular newsletters

activities. They also serve as the main source of information for the physician referral list that is vetted and maintained by the national TSA-US organization. Although most chapter activities are organized by volunteers, some chapters have paid staff.

CONCLUSION

We believe this to be the first attempt at a survey of TSAs throughout the world. It shows organizations in different stages of development. Most organizations start "around the kitchen table" with concerned parents and patients. Initially they tend to provide written and telephone information. Funding appears to come from a variety of sources, including governments. Most of the organizations become "professionalized" as their size grows. Only a few organizations are involved in political and scientific agenda setting (directing and funding research, providing guidelines, lobbying government). We can only guess at the reasons for the differences in the developmental stages of organizations in

different countries. In general, more affluent countries tend to have more developed patient support groups, and in some countries, such as the United States, there is a stronger self-help/ advocacy culture.

In the future, the existing groups worldwide will probably continue to develop. However, worldwide austerity measures may lead to organizations becoming less reliant on government funding. Emerging nations (including those in Eastern Europe, Russia, India, China, and parts of Africa) may develop TS patient support groups as standards of living and expectations about health rise. As well as providing support for people with TS, support groups should be providing a voice so that people with TS can shape the narrative of their condition.

ACKNOWLEDGMENTS

Many thanks go to all the association leaders and staff, without whom this survey would not have been possible. Special thanks go to Renata Rizzo and Wim Buisman for their help and contributions.

Appendix 1. Countries Contacted and Contact Information

Country	Contact e-mail address
Australia	Tourette.syndrome@msaustralia.org.au
	president@tourette.org.au
Austria	Personal contact
Belgium	info@tourette.be
Bulgaria	No organization
Canada	tsfc@tourette.ca
Czech Republic	atos@email.cz
Denmark	Personal contact
Estonia	No organization
Egypt	Personal contact
France	Personal contact
Germany	Personal contact
Greece	No organization
Hungary	No organization
Iceland	tourette@tourette.is
Ireland	support@tsireland.ie
Israel	Personal contact
Italy	sindrometourette@tiscali.it
Japan	tsaj@tourette.jp
The Netherlands	info@tourette.nl
Norway	post@tourette.foreningen.no
Poland	msobor@gmx.net
Scotland	info@tourettescotland.org
Switzerland	info@tourette-romandie.ch
South Africa	moosamy@medicine.wits.ac.za
Turkey	Personal contact
United Kingdom	admin@tourettes-action.org.uk
United States	Visit www.tsa-usa.org
We Move Worldwide education and awareness for movement disorders	http://www.wemove.org/aso/default.asp?dis=13

Attempts were made to contact other 3 countries (Croatia, Finland, Sweden), but no valid contact details were available.

1. How many members do you have? This includes:
   - patients with Tourette Syndrome
   - carers
   - family members
   - staff (how many salaried staff do you have? How many are full time and how many part time? How many volunteer staff do you have?)
   - Doctors
   - Who are your main patrons?
2. How old is the organization?

Who set the organization up?

3. Please can you describe the infrastructure of your organization?

i.e.: Do you have a board of directors or trustees?

Do you have a chief executive?

Who is in charge of the organization and who organizes the staff?

Do you have any doctors working for or affiliated to the organization?

4. Which geographical area do you serve?

5. What was your income for the last year and how do you do most of your fundraising?

Does most of your money come from patrons, the government, grants or individuals doing their own fundraising?

6. Are you involved in raising awareness and understanding about Tourette syndrome?

If so, how do you achieve this?

7. What support services do you offer?

Do you have a website? A phone helpline? An email service? Who staffs these services (i.e.: volunteers, health care professionals, and other paid staff)?

8. Do you fund research?

9. Do you do your own research?

If so, do you publish your research in academic journals?

10. Is the organization involved in evaluating other people's research?

If so, do you ever publish your analysis in academic journals?

11. Do you interact with local or national government or get involved in public policy?

12. Are you involved in creating guidelines for health care professionals regarding diagnosis or treatment?

13. Do any of the staff or volunteers in your organization have Tourette syndrome? Is this something that is of high importance in your organization?

14. Do you have contacts in other European countries?

If so, how do you work together with them and how is this useful to your organization?

Disclosure

Pedro G. de Alvarenga has nothing to disclose.

Kevin J. Black is a site investigator for a multisite study in Parkinson's disease sponsored by Acadia Pharmaceuticals, and has research projects funded by the Tourette Syndrome Association and by the NIH.

Michael H. Bloch acknowledges support from NIMH: Research Support; Trichotillomania Learning Center: Research Support; APIRE/Eli Lilly Psychiatric Research Fellowship: Research Support; AACAP/Eli Lilly: Research Support; NARSAD: Research Support; and the Associates Yale Child Study Center: Program Support.

Kathryn Bradbury has nothing to disclose.

Matthew R. Capriotti has nothing to disclose.

Francesco Cardona has nothing to disclose

Danielle C. Cath is supported by a grant from the Foundation Nuts- Ohra (grant nr. 1003-69), by a grant from the VCVGZ (grant nr. MF25059), and by a Marie Curie intial training network grant (2012: Eurotrain, PI: dr. Paschou). She gives lectures for Pfizer and Lundbeck pharmaceutical companies.

Andrea E. Cavanna serves on the Medical Advisory Board of the USA-Tourette Syndrome Association.

Barbara J. Coffey reports affiliations with the American Academy of Child and Adolescent Psychiatry: Honoraria; Boehringer Ingelheim: Research Support; Bristol Myers Squibb: Research Support; Catalyst: Research Support; Eli Lilly: Research Support / Advisory Board; Genco Sciences, Advisory Board; Jazz Pharmaceuticals: Advisory Board; Eli Lilly: Research Support / Advisory Board; NIMH: Research Support; NINDS: Research Support; Novartis: Advisory Board; Otsuka: Research Support; Pfizer: Research Support; Shire: Research Support; and Tourette Syndrome Association: Research Support, Former Medical Advisory Board, Speakers Bureau

Soren Dalsgaard acknowledges support from the Danish Council for Independent Research and the Foundation for Psychiatric Research in the Region of Southern Denmark.

Valsamma Eapen reports funds from the Australian Government

Clare M. Eddy has nothing to disclose.

Virginia W. Eicher has nothing to disclose.

Thomas V. Fernandez reports National Institutes of Health USA: Research Support (NIMH); Psychiatry Research Scholars Program: Research Support.

Ygor A. Ferrao has nothing to disclose.

Deanna J. Greene has nothing to disclose.

Pieter J. Hoekstra has nothing to disclose

Peter Hollenbeck's research is supported by NS 027073.

Ana G. Hounie reports funding from the Brazilian governmental agencies FAPESP, CNPq and CAPES/PRODOC

Yukio Imamura has nothing to disclose

Masaki Isoda has nothing to disclose

Yuko Kataoka-Sasaki has nothing to disclose

Robert A. King reports program support from the Associates Yale Child Study Center.

Roger Kurlan receives research support from Otsuka and is on the speakers bureau for Teva and UCB.

Angeli Landeros-Weisenberger has nothing to disclose.

Eli R. Lebowitz reports program support from the Associates Yale Child Study Center.

James F. Leckman reports National Institutes of Health USA: Research Support (NICHD), Program Support (NIMH); Grifols, S.A.: Research Support; Associates Yale Child Study Center: Program Support; AÇEV (Mother-Child Education Foundation): Program Support; and Tourette Syndrome Association: Research Support, Speaker Bureau.

Jessica B. Lenningtonhas nothing to disclose.

Andrea G. Ludolph reports support from Shire Pharmaceuticals, Janssen-Cilag, Medice Pharma, Lilly, Novartis, and has carried out clinical trials in cooperation with the Janssen-Cilag, Otsuka, Shire, and Boehringer Ingelheim companies.

Davide Martino has nothing to disclose.

Maria A. De Mathis reports funding from the Brazilian governmental agencies FAPESP and CNPq

Kevin W. McCairn has nothing disclose

Euripedes C. Miguel has nothing to disclose.

Kirsten R. Müller-Vahl 's research is supported by Lundbeck, Otsuka, FP7-EMTICS-278367, PF7-PEOPLE-2012-ITN-TS-EUROTRSAIN-316978, COST Action BM0905.

Tanya K. Murphy has received research support in the past 3 years from National Institutes of Health, F. Hoffmann-La Roche Ltd, Otsuka, International OCD Foundation, Tourette Syndrome Association, Shire, All Children's Hospital Research Foundation, Centers for Disease Control, Shire, and Transcept Pharmaceuticals, Inc. Dr. Murphy is on the Medical Advisory Board for Tourette Syndrome Association and Scientific Advisory Board for the International OCD Foundation. She receives textbook honorarium from Lawrence Erlbaum, and research support from the Maurice and Thelma Rothman Endowed Chair.

Tara Murphy has nothing to disclose.

Michael Orth's research is supported by the CHDI Foundation, Inc.

Leslie E. Packer has nothing to disclose.

John C. Pansaon Piedad has nothing to disclose

Mauro Porta has nothing to disclose

Sheryl K. Pruitt has nothing to disclose.

Hugh E. Rickards has nothing to disclose.

Renata Rizzo has nothing to disclose

Mary Robertson has received grants from the Tourette's Action-UK (Grant to support Dr A E Cavanna at University College London, working on Factor Analytic studies and the Tourette Syndrome phenotype[s] - 2007) and jointly with Professors H Critchley and E Joyce and Dr Y Nagai (from the USA

Tourette Syndrome Association, to study biofeedback in patients with Tourette syndrome). She has also received honoraria from Janssen-Cilag, and has received Royalties for co-authored books from Wiley - Blackwell, David Fulton/Granada/Taylor Francis, Oxford University Press and also Jessica Kingsley Publishers. She is a Patron of Tourette's Action (UK), sits on the Medical Advisory Board of the Italian Tourette Syndrome Association and The Tourette Syndrome Foundation of Canada (all honorary). She is Honorary Life President of ESSTS (European Society for the Study of Tourette Syndrome).

Veit Roessner has nothing to disclose

Louise Roper has nothing to disclose

Maria C. do Rosario reports funding from the Brazilian governmental agencies FAPESP and CNPq and has received honoraria from Shire and Novartis

Aribert Rothenberger has nothing to disclose

Marco Sassi has nothing to disclose.

Lawrence Scahill has served as a consultant for BioMarin, Pfizer, Roche, and Bracket, and received research support from Shire, Pfizer, and Roche. This work was supported by National Institute of Mental Health grants R01 MH069874 to Dr. Scahill and R01 MH070802 to Dr. John Piacentini (with subcontract to Dr. Scahill). Dr Scahill also received support from the Yale University Clinical and Translational Sciences Award (UL1 RR024139 from the National Center for Research Resources, NIH) and a grant from the Tourette Syndrome Association.

Bradley L. Schlaggar has nothing to disclose

Domenico Servello has nothing to disclose

Harvey S. Singer's study, "Developing new treatments for Tourette syndrome: Therapeutic trials with modulators of glutamatergic neurotransmission" is supported by a grant from the NIH R34-MH085844. He serves on the editorial board for the Neurologist.

Mathew W. State has nothing to disclose

Denis G. Sukhodolsky's research has been supported by the NIMH (K01 MH079130; R03 MH94583) and research award from the Tourette Syndrome Association

Flora M. Vaccarino has nothing to disclose.

Douglas W. Woods is on the medical advisory board for the Tourette Syndrome Association. He receives royalties from Guilford Press, Oxford University Press, and Springer Press.

Beata Zolovska has nothing to disclose

Index